Hale & Hartmann's

Textbook of Human Lactation

First Edition

Hale & Hartmann's

Textbook of Human Lactation

Editors

— Thomas W. Hale, RPh, PhD
Professor
Department of Pediatrics
Texas Tech University Health Sciences Center
School of Medicine
Amarillo, Texas, USA

— Peter Hartmann, BRurSc, PhD
Professor
School of Biomedical, Biomolecular, and Chemical Sciences
Faculty of Life and Physical Sciences
The University of Western Australia
Crawley, WA
Australia

SPRINGER PUBLISHING COMPANY
NEW YORK

Springer Publishing Company, LLC
11 West 42nd Street
New York, NY 10036
www.springerpub.com

ISBN: 9780826160096
e-book ISBN: 9780826160119

17 18 19 20 / 5 4 3 2 1

The author and the publisher of this Work have made every effort to use sources believed to be reliable to provide information that is accurate and compatible with the standards generally accepted at the time of publication. Because medical science is continually advancing, our knowledge base continues to expand. Therefore, as new information becomes available, changes in procedures become necessary. We recommend that the reader always consult current research and specific institutional policies before performing any clinical procedure. The author and publisher shall not be liable for any special, consequential, or exemplary damages resulting, in whole or in part, from the readers' use of, or reliance on, the information contained in this book. The publisher has no responsibility for the persistence or accuracy of URLs for external or third-party Internet websites referred to in this publication and does not guarantee that any content on such websites is, or will remain, accurate or appropriate.

Library of Congress Cataloging-in-Publication Data
CIP data is available from the Library of Congress.

Printed in the United States of America.

To our wives

Quetha and Robyn

Without whose patience we could not have accomplished this task.

CONTRIBUTING AUTHORS

Dawit Aregawi, MD
Cholesterol Center
Jewish Hospital
Cincinnati, OH

Clare A. Berry, BSc (Hons)
School of Biomedical, Biomolecular, and Chemical Sciences
The University of Western Australia
Crawley, Western Australia

Pamela D. Berens, MD
Associate Professor
Department of Obstetrics and Gynecology
University of Texas Medical School
Houston, TX

E. Stephen Buescher, MD
Eastern Virginia Medical School
Department of Pediatrics
Norfolk, VA

Mark Cregan, PhD
School of Biomedical, Biomolecular, and Chemical Sciences
The University of Western Australia
Crawley, Western Australia

Charles Czank, BSc (Biomed Sc) (Hons)
School of Biomedical, Biomolecular, and Chemical Sciences
The University of Western Australia
Crawley, Western Australia

Kathryn G. Dewey, PhD
Professor of Nutrition
Department of Nutrition
University of California
Davis, CA

Lawrence M. Gartner, MD, FAAP
Professor
Department of Pediatrics
University of Chicago
Chicago, IL

Donna Geddes, PhD
Research Fellow
School of Biomedical, Biomolecular, and Chemical Sciences
The University of Western Australia
Crawley, Western Australia

Lee T. Gettler, BA
Department of Anthropology
Notre Dame University
Notre Dame, IN

Charles J. Glueck, MD
Director
Cholesterol Center
Jewish Hospital
Cincinnati, OH

L. Peter Hackett, MRSC
Research Scientist
Clinical Pharmacology and Toxicology Laboratory
Path West Laboratory Medicine
Nedlands, Western Australia

Thomas W. Hale, RPh, PhD
Professor
Assistant Dean of Research
Department of Pediatrics
Texas Tech University Health Sciences Center
School of Medicine
Amarillo, Texas

Lars A. Hanson, MD, PhD
Professor Emeritus
Clinical Immunology
Goteborg University
Sweden

Peter E. Hartmann, BRurSc, PhD
School of Biomedical, Biomolecular, and Chemical Sciences
The University of Western Australia
Crawley, Western Australia

Jennifer J. Henderson, RN, RM, PostGrad Dip Adv Nursing, MPH, PhD
School of Biomedical, Biomolecular, and Chemical Sciences
The University of Western Australia
Crawley, Western Australia

Daniel S. Hirsch, MD, FAAP
Daniel S. Hirsch, MD, FAAP
Assistant Professor of Pediatrics
Robert Wood Johnson University Hospital
University of Medicine & Dentistry of New Jersey
New Brunswick, NJ

Judy Hopkinson, PhD, IBCLC
Associate Professor of Pediatrics
USDA/ARS Children's Nutrition Research Center
Baylor College of Medicine
Houston, TX.

Sheila Humphrey, BSc, RN, IBCLC
Lactation Consultant
Fairview Lakes Regional Hospital
Marine on St. Croix, Minnesota

Kenneth F. Ilett, BPharm, PhD
Emeritus Professor of Pharmacology
Pharmacology and Anaesthesiology Unit
School of Medicine and Pharmacology
University of Western Australia
Crawley, Western Australia, and
Consultant Pharmacologist
Clinical Pharmacology & Toxicology Laboratory
Path West Laboratory Medicine
Nedlands, Western Australia

Robert P. Kauffman, MD
Associate Professor
Director, Reproductive Medicine and Infertility
Department of Obstetrics & Gynecology
Texas Tech University Health Sciences Center
School of Medicine
Amarillo, Texas

Jacqueline C. Kent, PhD
School of Biomedical, Biomolecular, and Chemical Sciences
The University of Western Australia
Crawley, Western Australia

Judith H. Kristensen, BPharm
Senior Pharmacist
Department of Pharmacy
King Edward Memorial Hospital for Women
Women and Newborn Health Service
Subiaco, Western Australia

Miriam Labbok, MD, MPH, FACPM, FABM, IBCLC
Professor of the Practice of Maternal and Child Health
Director, Center for Infant and Young Child Feeding and Care
Department of Maternal and Child Health
School of Public Health
University of North Carolina at Chapel Hill
Chapel Hill, NC

Ching Tat Lai, MSc, PhD
School of Biomedical, Biomolecular, and Chemical Sciences
The University of Western Australia
Crawley, Western Australia

Thomas Martin, MSc, PhD
School of Biomedical, Biomolecular and Chemical Sciences
The University of Western Australia
Crawley, Western Australia

Ghia McAfee, BPharm, MSc, PhD
Fort Worth, Texas

James J. McKenna, PhD
Professor
Department of Anthropology
Director, Mother-Baby Behavioral Sleep Lab
University of Notre Dame
Notre Dame, IN

Julie A. Mennella, PhD
Director of Education Outreach
Monell Chemical Senses Center
Philadelphia, PA

Leon Mitoulas, BSc (Hons), PhD
Breastfeeding Research Scientist
Medela, AG
Baar, Switzerland

Jane A. Morton MD, FABM
Director of Breastfeeding Medicine
Pediatrics-Neonatal
Stanford University
Palo Alto, CA

Kristin M.E. Piper, BSc (Hons)
School of Biomedical, Biomolecular, and Chemical Sciences
The University of Western Australia
Crawley, Western Australia

Danielle Prime, BSc (Hons)
School of Biomedical, Biomolecular, and Chemical Sciences
The University of Western Australia
Crawley, Western Australia

Jonathan Rampono, MB ChB, FRANZCP
Consultant Psychiatrist and Head of Department,
Department of Psychological Medicine
King Edward Memorial Hospital for Women
Women and Newborn Health Service
Subiaco, Western Australia

Kathleen Rasmussen, ScD, RD
Professor
Division of Nutritional Sciences
Cornell University
Ithaca, NY

Marzieh Salehi, MD
Cholesterol Center
Jewish Hospital
Cincinnati, OH

Luann Sieve, BS
Cholesterol Center
Jewish Hospital
Cincinnati, OH

Elizabeth C. Thomas, BSc (Hons)
School of Biomedical, Biomolecular, and Chemical Sciences
The University of Western Australia
Crawley, Western Australia

Nancy E. Wight, MD, IBCLC, FABM, FAAP
Neonatologist
Rady Children's Hospital San Diego
and Sharp Mary Birch Hospital for Women
Medical Director
Sharp Health Care Lactation Services
San Diego, CA

Ping Wang, PhD
Cholesterol Center
Jewish Hospital
Cincinnati, OH

PREFACE

Human lactation not only provides nourishment that is tailored to the developmental needs of the baby, but also has an equally, if not more important role of providing innate immunological protection to the baby against pathogenic microorganisms. Furthermore, breastfeeding itself brings the mother and baby into a close contact, and the act of breastfeeding has been found to have subtle positive influences on physiological responses in both the mother and her baby. An understanding of the unique importance of human lactation has led to the successful promotion of breastfeeding in developed countries as a public health strategy. However, such initiatives require an evidence-based understanding of the physiology and biochemistry of human lactation to facilitate the appropriate clinical care of mothers and their breastfeeding babies.

In the past decade, there has been an exponential increase in our understanding of human lactation. While we have grown to understand many of the wonders of human milk and the reasoning for its existence, there is still much to learn about this wonderful process. While breastmilk is not the only single food that can sustain human life, in the last decade, we've learned that infants who breastfeed have far fewer infectious diseases, fewer visits to the doctor, higher intelligence, and enhanced neurobehavioral development, better eyesight, and even fewer deaths. With hundreds of new publications arriving annually, no one has yet tried to collect a major part of the wisdom in this field into one book. Thus, this first edition of the *Textbook of Human Lactation* was designed to provide the higher science of this field.

While there are numerous books that cover the various experienced-based clinical aspects of human lactation, our purpose in compiling this textbook was to present the current state of knowledge in the field of human lactation, direct from researchers who work in this field. An authoritative text of this magnitude requires the profound effort of many authors who labored under minimal guidance and who were willing to meet deadlines and conform to our editorial requirements. For this, we are most grateful.

The reader will find this volume full of new and interesting research findings about human milk, lactation, and breastfeeding behavior. We are mindful of areas of omission, but hope you agree with us that the first edition of *Textbook of Human Lactation* at least attempts to provide a comprehensive review of the state of the science of human lactation.

Thomas Hale
Peter Hartmann

CONTENTS

Contributing Authors vii
Preface xi

INTRODUCTION

1 Mammary Gland: Past, Present, and Future 3
Peter E. Hartmann

Section I
ANATOMY AND BIOCHEMISTRY

2 Gross Anatomy of the Lactating Breast 19
Donna T. Geddes

3 The Histology and Cytology of the Human Mammary Gland and Breastmilk 35
Clare A. Berry, Elizabeth C. Thomas, Kristin M.E. Piper, and Mark D. Cregan

4 Human Milk Composition - Fat 49
Charles Czank, Leon R. Mitoulas, Peter E. Hartmann

5 Human Milk Composition - Carbohydrates 69
Charles Czank, Leon R. Mitoulas, and Peter E. Hartmann

6 Human Milk Composition - Nitrogen and Energy Content 75
Charles Czank, Leon R. Mitoulas, and Peter E. Hartmann

7 Hormonal Control of the Lactation Cycle 89
Charles Czank, Jennifer J. Henderson, Jacqueline C. Kent, Ching Tat Lai, and Peter E. Hartmann

8 Molecular Aspects of Mammary Gland Development 113
Thomas Martin and Charles Czank

9 Oxytocin: Milk Ejection and Maternal-Infant Well-being 141
Danielle K Prime, Donna T. Geddes, and Peter E. Hartmann

Section II
IMMUNOBIOLOGY

10 The Role of Breastfeeding in the Defense of the Infant 159
Lars A. Hanson

11 Human Milk and Infectious Diseases 193
E. Stephen Buescher

Section III
MANAGEMENT - INFANT

12 Human Milk, Breastfeeding, and the Preterm Infant 215
Nancy E. Wight and Jane A. Morton

13 Hyperbilirubinemia and Breastfeeding 255
Lawrence M. Gartner

14 Mother-Infant Cosleeping with Breastfeeding in the Western Industrialized Context 271
James J. McKenna and Lee T. Gettler

Section IV
MANAGEMENT - MOTHER

15 Breastfeeding, Birth Spacing, and Family Planning 305
Miriam Labbok

16 Reproductive Bioenergetics, Infertility, and Ovulation Induction in the Lactating Female 319
Robert P. Kauffman

17 Polycystic Ovary Syndrome: Pathophysiology, Endocrinopathy, Treatment, and Lactation 343
Charles J. Glueck, Marzieh Salehi, Dawit Aregawi, Luann Sieve, and Ping Wang

18 Management of Lactation in the Puerperium 355
Pamela Berens

Section V
MATERNAL AND INFANT NUTRITION

19 Nutrition in Lactation 371
Judy Hopkinson

20 Maternal Obesity and the Outcome of Breastfeeding 387
Kathleen M. Rasmussen

21 Chemical Senses and the Development of Flavor Preferences in Humans 403
Julie A. Mennella

22 Nutrition, Growth, and Complementary Feeding . of the Breastfed Infant 415
Kathryn G. Dewey

23 Vitamin D and the Breastfed Infant 425
Daniel S. Hirsch

Section VI
MEDICATIONS

24 The Transfer of Medications into Human Milk 465
Thomas W. Hale, Judith H. Kristensen, and Kenneth F. Illett

25 Medications that Alter Milk Production 479
Thomas W. Hale

26 Analgesics and Anti-Inflammatory Drugs 491
Kenneth F. Ilett and Judith H. Kristensen

27 Anesthetic and Analgesic Medications: Implications for Breastfeeding 501
Thomas W. Hale

28 Antibiotic, Antifungal, Antiviral, and Antiretroviral Drugs 513
Judith H. Kristensen and Kenneth F. Illett

29 Anthelmintics and Antiprotozoals; Scabicides and Pediculicides; Antimalarials and Antimycobacterials 523
Kenneth F. Ilett and Judith H. Kristensen

30 Antidepressants and Antipsychotics 535
Jonathan Rampono, Judith H. Kristensen, and *Kenneth F. Ilett*

31 Antihypertensives, Diuretics, and Anticoagulants 557
Judith H. Kristensen and Kenneth F. Ilett

32 Antihistamines, Anticholinergics, and Endocrine Drugs 565
Kenneth F. Ilett and Judith H. Kristensen

33 Drugs of Abuse and Breastfeeding 575
Chia McAfee

34 Study Design and Data Analysis for Assessing Drug Transfer into Milk 611
Kenneth F. Ilett and L. Peter Hackett

35 Herbal Therapeutics During Lactation 629
Sheila Humphrey

INDEX 655

INTRODUCTION

Chapter 1

Mammary Gland: Past, Present, and Future

Peter E. Hartmann

"The longer you look back the further you look forward." (Winston Churchill, 1948)

SUMMARY

The evolution of the mammary gland holds a place of privilege in mammals because it is the site of an activity vital to the survival of these species, including humans. Milk (and breastmilk in particular) contains an enormous array of innate immune protection factors. Lactation probably evolved initially to protect the young against infection and subsequently took on a nutritional role. However, infant formula is focused on nutrition rather than protection. Therefore, it is not surprising that the mortality rate of formula-fed infants in the USA today is at least 21% higher than breastfed babies. Furthermore, it is not widely known that breastfeeding also has significant health benefits for the mother, including intellectual development, decreased incidence of some cancers, and improved bone structure.

The proportion of Australian mothers who choose to breastfeed their babies has increased from about 48% in 1972 due to experience-based support from the Australian Breastfeeding Association and, subsequently, from health professionals. Now, more than 90% of mothers choose to breastfeed their babies. Whereas, WHO recommends that mothers should be encouraged to exclusively breastfeed their babies for the first six months, many Australian mothers experience difficulties in sustaining lactation and about 40-50% cease breastfeeding by six months post-partum.

This lack of success is perhaps not surprising when the evidence-based care of the lactating breast is compared to that of other metabolically equivalent organs in the body. The lactating breast requires 30% of resting energy compared to only 23% by the brain, but the medical evidence-based support for human lactation is almost non-existent. For example, there is no medical speciality dedicated to the normal function of the lactating breast.

Now that health education programs have been effective and almost all mothers choose to breastfeed, there is an obligation for health authorities to support research directed towards the development of evidence-based diagnosis and treatment protocols for human lactation to ensure that the mothers who commence breastfeeding receive appropriate support to enable them to have a sustained and successful breastfeeding experience. To this end, the lactating breast must be accorded the same scientific and medical status as other equivalent organs in the human body.

MAMMALS

The Swedish monk, Carl Linnaeus, developed the current systematic scientific system for naming, ranking, and classifying plants and animals and became known as the 'Father of Taxonomy.' He introduced the term Mammalia (meaning 'of the breast') into zoological taxonomy in Systema Naturae in 1758 (Schiebinger, 1993). Oddly enough, at the time his work was very controversial as it was considered that the basic premise of his classification system was obscene. Fortunately, this concern was not directed to the fact that he had focused on the breast as an anatomical symbol for the grouping of animals, including humans, into the class 'Mammalia.' The criticism was provoked because he had classified plants on the basis of differences in their flowers, that is, differences in the plants' reproductive organs. At the time, this was considered by the Encyclopaedia Britannica to be "*disgusting strokes of obscenity in a system of botany*" (Fara, 2003). Fortunately, prejudices come and go and now the classification of plants in relation to their floral parts does not evoke prudish comment. On the other hand, the human mammary gland undergoes accelerated growth at puberty and its prominence in adulthood has unfortunately resulted in the non-lactating breast replacing the flower fantasies of the 18th century, particularly in Western cultures, to the detriment of its essential role in the nurturing of human infants. Linnaeus recognized the uniqueness of the mammary gland. This feature, together with several other common characteristics (hair, three ear bones, and four chambered heart), united whales, dolphins, and porpoises (previously grouped as fish) with terrestrial quadrupeds.

During this period, the wet-nursing of babies by affluent people was common. Haden (1827) stated:

"*Wet nurses are unfortunately a necessary evil. Without them the children of the better classes would suffer very materially.*"

Cadogan (1748) observed:

"*The mother who has only a few rags to cover her child loosely, and little more than her own breast to feed it, sees it healthy and strong and very soon able to shift for itself, while the puny insect, the heir and hope of a rich family, lies languishing under a load of finery that overpowers his limbs, abhorring and rejecting the dainties he is cramm'd with, 'till he dies a victim to the mistaken care and tenderness of his fond mother.*"

Evidence suggests that Linnaeus supported breastfeeding and opposed wet nursing and that he chose the term mammalia ('of the breast') to emphasize that these animals fed their own young (Schiebinger, 1993). Nevertheless, wet nursing remained popular for another 150 years when the arrival of the 'pocket wet nurse' (the baby feeding bottle) not only replaced the wet nurse, but also extended the option of abandoning maternal breastfeeding of infants to the middle and lower socio-economic classes in Western countries. Now, pictures of baby feeding bottles are used widely as baby symbols.

EVOLUTION OF THE MAMMARY GLAND AND ITS SECRETION

Mammals are the only animals that secrete a complex fluid from an elaborate skin gland to both provide innate protection and nourishment for their young. Since body stores can contribute precursors for milk secretion, lactation has enabled mammals to reproduce successfully in habitats where food is either scarce or only available in a form suitable for adults (Pond, 1984). There are more than 4,000 species of mammal with striking similarities in the structure and function of their mammary glands, as well as in their unique milk components, such as the caseins, α-lactalbumin, lactoferrin, lactose, and milk fat, but nevertheless exhibiting profound variations in the arrangement and number of mammary glands, milk composition (**Table 1**), and suckling strategies (Akers, 2002). This has resulted in a number of theories

Table 1. The Macro-Nutrient Content of Milk from Domestic, Laboratory, and Aquatic Mammals Compared to Human Milk

Milk Composition (g/L)			
Mammal	Lactose	Protein	Fat
Women	70	8	41
Horse	62	19	13
Pig	55	56	83
Cow	48	32	37
Goat	41	29	38
Sheep	48	55	74
Dog (she-wolf)	38	75	95
Rabbit	22	103	151
Harp Seal	1	87	422

being advanced on the evolutionary origin of both the mammary gland and its secretion (Oftedal, 2002a; 2002b). Based on the observation that sea horses hatched and reared their young in a brood pouch, Darwin, in 1859, proposed that cutaneous glands evolved in a pouch to undertake the specialized function of providing nourishment for the young. This explanation was refuted with the subsequent discovery of the egg-laying platypus that produced milk from a brood patch, but did not possess a pouch. This would not have been of concern to Darwin because Short (1985) reported that:

'It is said that he (Darwin) *always carried in his coat pocket a piece of paper on which he recorded only those facts that were contrary to his views, realizing that therein lay a source of new inspiration.'*

Oftedal (2002a) reviewed the hypotheses that have been put forward to explain the development of specialized skin secretions in the egg-laying reptilian lineage that separated from other taxa more than 310 million years ago and evolved into mammals. This lineage, the synapsid, had a glandular rather than scaled integument and gradually evolved mammalian features. Oftedal noted that the various hypotheses of the origin of the mammary gland were not mutually exclusive and some built on and extended prior approaches. Various proposals suggested that the mammary gland evolved from either sweat glands, sebaceous glands, apocrine glands, or a combination of all three glands. However, Oftedal concluded that the mammary gland was derived from an ancestral apocrine-like gland that was associated with hair follicles. The widely differing compositions of milk of different species is the outcome of selection pressures that are related to the protective and nutritional needs of the newborn and constraints on the mother by diet, and behavioral and environmental characteristics of individual species (Mepham, 1983).

Ideas on the evolution of the function of lactation also have been put forward. Unlike rigid calcified eggshells of birds, parchment-shelled eggs of the synapsids were soft and porous, and lost water very rapidly when exposed to dry air. The secretion of complex, nutrient-rich milk in mammaliaforms that existed about 200 million years ago allowed a progressive decline in egg size and an increasing immaturity of the young at hatching. Thus, Oftedal (2002b) proposed that milk underwent a gradual evolutionary transformation from supplying moisture to prevent dehydration and withering of parchment-shelled eggs, to nutrient supplementation of the egg, and finally to a complex secretion providing the hatchling with nourishment and protection against bacterial, viral, parasitic, and fungal infection (Oftedal, 2002b; Mete *et al.*, 2006). Indeed, milk may still accomplish all of these roles in monotremes, such as the platypus, with their cluster of mammo-pilo-sebaceous glands that secrete milk onto a mammary patch (areola). Nipples and teats developed from the mammary patch to replace the role of the mammary hairs in directing milk to the young.

Recently, Vorbach *et al.* (2006) postulated an intriguing alternative explanation for the functional and morphological evolution of the mammary gland. Whereas most explanations have centered on the development of the secretion of a complex nutritive fluid (milk) for nourishment of the young, this hypothesis focuses on the innate immune system and an inflammatory response in the skin providing rapid defense against pathogenic microorganisms for eggs, hatchlings, and the newborn. Innate immunity is mediated by various peptides, proteins, enzymes, and oligosaccharides that possess pattern recognition of microbial receptors, as well as the disruption of microbial cell walls by certain fatty acids and deprivation of nutrients to microorganisms by proteins that bind certain vitamins and minerals. All of these components of the innate immune system are present in milk, and thus milk has the dual role of immunological protection and nourishment of the mammalian newborn.

Vorbach *et al.* proposed that the crucial nutritional role of milk subsequently developed from the inflammatory response due to the contributions of two antimicrobial enzymes, xanthine oxidoreductase and lysozyme, facilitating the development of fat secretion and α-lactalbumin and lactose synthesis, respectively.

Xanthine oxidoreductase is involved in the synthesis of reactive oxygen species with antimicrobial actions either alone or through contribution to the lactoperoxidase system. However, xanthine oxidoreductase is also essential for the unique process of milk fat droplet envelopment and secretion by the lactocyte (mammary secretory epithelial cell). Therefore, xanthine oxidoreductase has a dual role in the lactating mammary gland: an antimicrobial function and a nutritional role by facilitation of milk fat droplet secretion (the major energy component of milk). Lactocytes also secrete the antimicrobial enzyme, lysozyme, and this protein over time evolved into α-lactalbumin. In addition to being a dietary protein with a very high biological value, α-lactalbumin together with β-1,4 galactosyltransferase constitute the unique enzyme complex, lactose synthase, that is responsible for the synthesis of the milk sugar– lactose, forms a complex (HAMLET) that induces apoptosis in tumor cells (Gustafsson *et al.*, 2005), and is bactericidal to *Streptococcus pneumoniae* (Hakansson, 2005). Lactose, through its osmotic influence, draws water into the Golgi-apparatus increasing milk volume and, in addition, makes a major contribution to the energy content of milk, provides galactose that is important for liver metabolism, and is a component of numerous oligosaccharides that inhibit pathogens and bacterial toxins.

Furthermore, lactation is regulated by molecules and signaling pathways that are central to the inflammatory response. For example, in the lactocyte, xanthine oxidoreductase is a direct downstream target of Tumour Necrosis Factor TNFα/NF-κ cellular pathway that normally plays a key role in the inflammatory response to infection in other cell types. NF-κB activation in turn is stimulated by RANKL (receptor activator of NF-κB ligand), and RANKL acts in conjunction with prolactin to stimulate the expression of the key milk protein, β-casein, in lactocytes. In addition, prolactin and interferon-γ are both known to activate cellular pathways that are required for the growth of the mammary parenchyma and for the regulation of xanthine oxidoreductase in the lactocytes (Vorbach *et al.*, 2006).

This new molecular evidence led Vorbach *et al.* to hypothesize that lactation evolved from an inflammatory response to tissue damage and infection and that inflammatory molecules became key regulators of lactation. Initially, small protective skin glands that secreted mucus containing a variety of antimicrobial molecules mediated the inflammatory response. Subsequently, two of the inflammatory molecules, xanthine oxidoreductase and lysozyme, facilitated the development of the key nutritional components of lactation. This hypothesis extends the initial hypothesis of Hayssen and Blackburn (1985) that the nutritional role of the mammary gland evolved subsequent to its protective function. This hypothesis is also largely compatible with Oftedal's focus on the parchment-shelled eggs, as this secretion would have protected both the egg surface and the newly hatched young. However, Vorbach *et al.* have argued convincingly that the primary driving force for the development of lactation was to provide a high level of innate immune protection for the young and that the nutritional value of milk evolved later.

The Vorbach *et al.* hypothesis emphasizes the metabolic "multi-tasking" that has been achieved during the evolution of the mammary gland with many molecules possessing species-specific protective and nutritional functions. In addition, it highlights the flawed concept in the provision of infant 'formula' as a substitute for breastmilk for human babies. These products are usually derived from modified cow's milk and are *not* formulated to meet the primary innate immune protective function of breastmilk, but rather only try to address the secondary nutritional role of human lactation. Even in this respect, it would appear that the milk of the mare is closer in macronutrient composition to human milk than that of the cow (**Table 1**). Perhaps our ancestors got it wrong and should have domesticated horses for milking and cattle for riding.

HUMAN LACTATION

While "natural" lactation can be defined within reasonably strict limits in terms of suckling behavior, feeding frequency, time of introduction of other foods, and length of lactation for most wild mammals, this is not possible for human lactation. For example, advice on the duration of lactation varies from exclusive bottle-feeding to breastfeeding for up to about six years, and from a strict schedule of breastfeeding at stated times of the day to child led breastfeeding when the infant indicates a desire to breastfeed. In Western countries, in particular, women receive varied advice on how to breastfeed and the choice of these options greatly influences the success of the breastfeeding period (Hartmann *et al.*, 1984). The function of human lactation can be considered in terms of optimizing innate immune protection, nutrition, and psychological development of the baby. However, compared to other mammals, it is very difficult to apply rational standards to infant nutrient intake and growth and, therefore, to determine an optimal strategy for human lactation. One possibility in determining what is "natural" is to observe lactation practices in traditional societies.

HUNTER-GATHERERS

The few hunting and gathering societies that have been studied are thought to rèpresent some aspects of the Pleistocene epoch of evolution (Konner & Worthman, 1980) in the period from 1.8 million to 11,500 years Before Present (BP). In these societies, breastfeeding was essential to ensure the survival of the newborn baby and, therefore, it is possible that hunting and gathering mothers may provide a model for "natural" human lactation. Konner and Worthman (1980) described breastfeeding in the !Kung hunter-gatherers in Botswana and Namibia from observations made between dawn and dusk. Infants were always within close physical proximity to their mothers, and breastfeeding occurred a few minutes at a time, several times an hour. We have observed a similar frequency of breastfeeding in village women in North Fore in the Highlands of Papua, New Guinea (**Figure 1**), and observations suggested that breastfeeding at night was also common. It was of interest that the number minutes spent breastfeeding during the day in North Fore was about the same as babies spent at the breast in Perth, Australia, where there were fewer, but longer breastfeeds. Australian Aboriginal children were also breastfed whenever they indicated they were hungry (Berndt & Berndt, 1974). In this context, it should be noted that if the average milk intake of an exclusively breastfed baby is approximately 750-800 mL/24 hours, then the average milk intake at a breastfeed for these babies would be less than 30 mL at a breastfeed. In contrast, Western babies breastfeeding less than six times each day would consume on average greater than 125 mL at each breastfeed and even more in the morning feed if the baby slept for more than six hours at night. The digestive and metabolic consequence for the infant of this higher intake of milk at each breastfeed, together with the impact of longer breastfeeds on nipple trauma, require further investigation.

The !Kung weaned their children at 3.5 years of age and had a long interval of 44 months between births. Aboriginal Australians breastfed their babies into their fourth to sixth year of life, often tandem breastfeeding with the arrival of a new baby. They also had a similar interval between births (Berndt & Berndt, 1974; Thomson, 1983). Extremes range from weaning at four months in Hottentots to fifteen years of age in some inhabitants of Greenland. However, Wickes (1953a) concluded that the average duration of lactation in traditional societies was between three and four years.

Australian Aboriginal languages lacked words that clearly distinguish work from play. Aboriginal children spent a lot of time either helping or imitating adults in everyday tasks, a learning process that probably

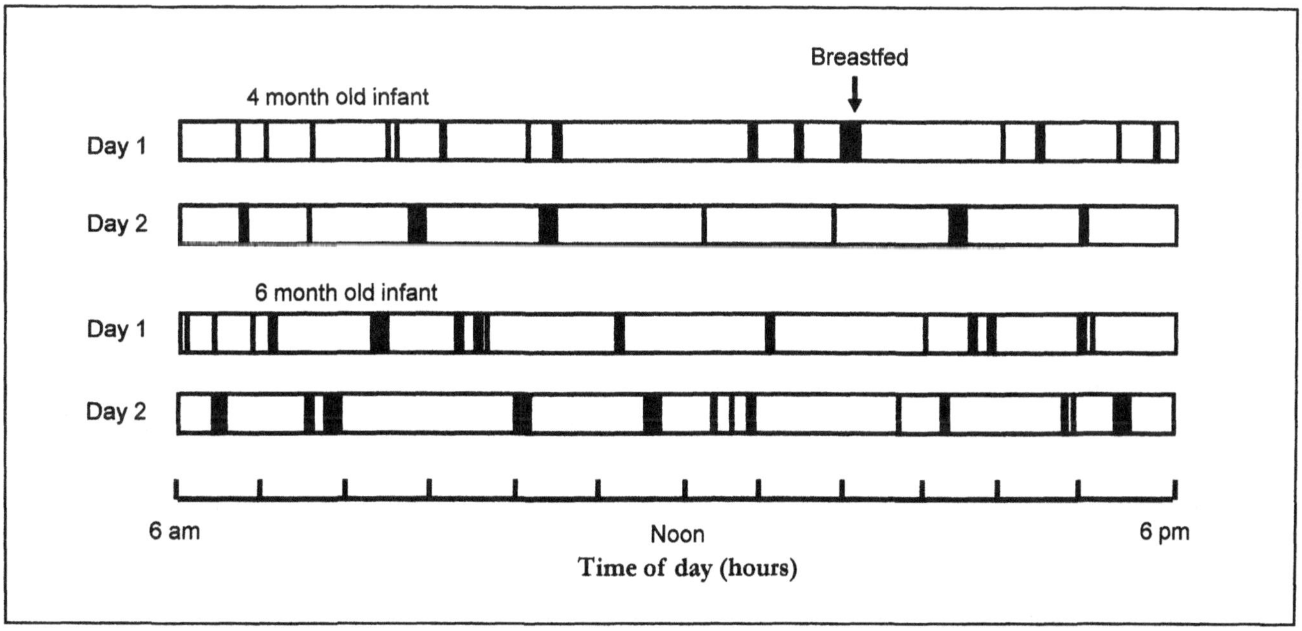

Figure 1. Frequency and duration of breastfeeding of four and six month old babies in North Fore, Papua New Guinea (Hewitt, 1978).

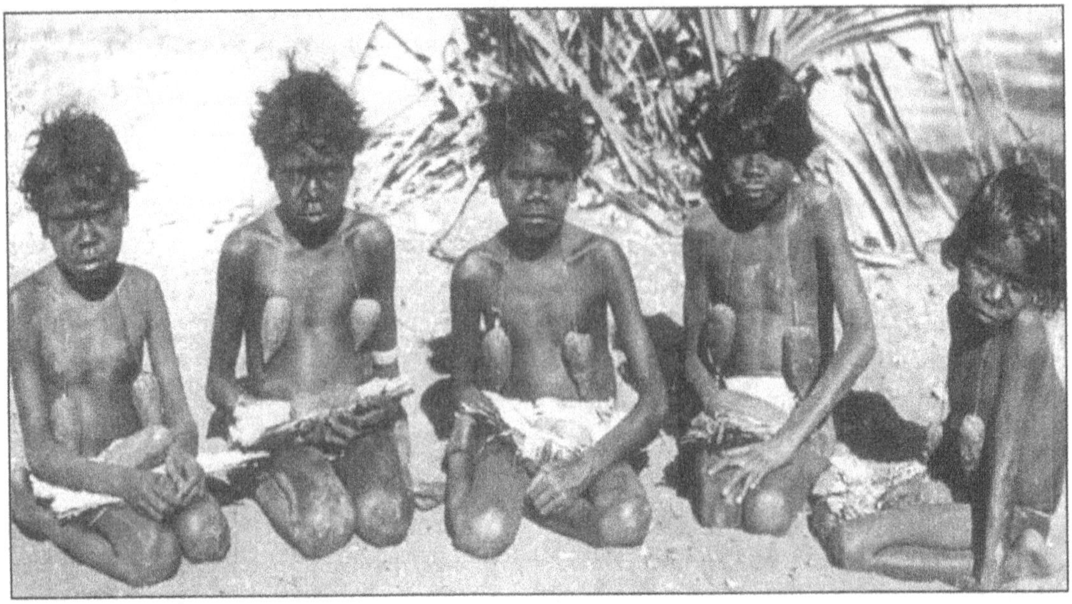

Figure 2. Australian aboriginal children learning to breastfeed by observation, imitation, and practice. (Source: Thomson, 1983)

involves the mirror neuron system that mediates a direct matching process in which observed actions are mapped onto motor representations of the action (Falck-Ytter *et al.*, 2006). As in other hunting and gathering societies, Aboriginal Australians had no formal education system. Their children learned by observing, imitating, and practising the activities of adults, accompanied by the strong reinforcement of their achievements by adults, resulting in efficient intergenerational transfer of knowledge (osmosis learning). For example, girls learned breastfeeding skills at a young age by observing and mimicking breastfeeding mothers in the camp (**Figure 2**) as noted by Thomson (1983):

'Little 'mothers,' each with a mud baby and clay breasts hung from the neck, at play after the arrival of a new baby in the camp."

Thomson also observed that a favorite 'game' of the Aboriginal children was 'mothers and fathers' and that often one of the babies in the camp would be 'borrowed' and carried by the small 'mother,' who might decorate herself with mock breasts.

Lactation in Aboriginal Australians was very resilient to harsh environmental conditions; indeed, Thomson commented that mothers who lived in the extremely arid Great Sandy Desert of Western Australia *"grow the fattest babies in the world."* He was puzzled about how the slim Aboriginal mothers were able to grow such fat babies and noted that *'whereas very fat babies in Western societies may grow into obese children and adults, there was no chance that this could happen in the traditional hunting and gathering life.'* Further confirmation of the capacity of the human breast to produce milk was observed in the Pygmies of the Ituri Forest in Zaire. The infants of these small women are relatively large and tend to follow Western infant growth standards. Breastfeeding was facilitated by identifying lactating mothers with red dye, providing them with food, and freeing them from all other duties until it was time for the baby to be weaned (Vis & Hennert, 1978).

It is of interest that in remote rural areas in Australia, Aboriginal women do not appear to experience common breastfeeding problems, such as positioning and attachment difficulties and mastitis (S. Roth, personal communication, 2002). Therefore, a more detailed understanding of breastfeeding management in traditional societies may allow the resolution of current management and social practices that are impeding 'natural' breastfeeding in Western societies. However, it would be incorrect to assume that 'natural' breastfeeding was perfected in hunter-gatherer societies as some traditional beliefs may also have adverse affects. For example, most traditional societies did not commence breastfeeding until after their milk 'came in' at about two to three days postpartum (Kulski *et al.*, 1981). In view of the current knowledge in regard to the high level of innate immune protection offered by colostrum, this was clearly an unwise practice.

WESTERN SOCIETIES

Yalom (1997) reviewed the earliest medical documents dating back to the Egyptian papyri from 3,500 BP that described methods of stimulating the flow of breastmilk and prized breastmilk for its healing powers. European medicine originated in Greece about 2,400 BP. Hippocrates considered that breastmilk was derived from menstrual blood, which was transferred to the breast in 'special vessels' after birth. The influential Galen of Pergamon (129-199) also promoted this view. Galen's authority dominated medical thinking for centuries. Indeed, Leonardo da Vinci (1452-1519) followed Galenic tradition mistakenly showing a 'vessel,' the *Vas menstrualis*, connecting the breast to the uterus in his drawing of coition (Calder, 1970). It is possible that the recognition of an association between the suckling stimulus and uterine activity may have, in part, promoted the longevity of the concept that milk was uterine in origin. Aristotle mistakenly believed that the milk produced in the first few days after birth was unsuitable for infants. The gynaecologist Soranus of Ephesus (98-138) supported wet nursing and dismissed the idea that a wet nurse for a male baby should have already given birth to a male baby, arguing that if twins of different sexes nursed from the same breast, the boy did not become more feminine nor the girl more masculine. He strongly advised against co-sleeping because he was concerned that the nurse might over-lay the baby.

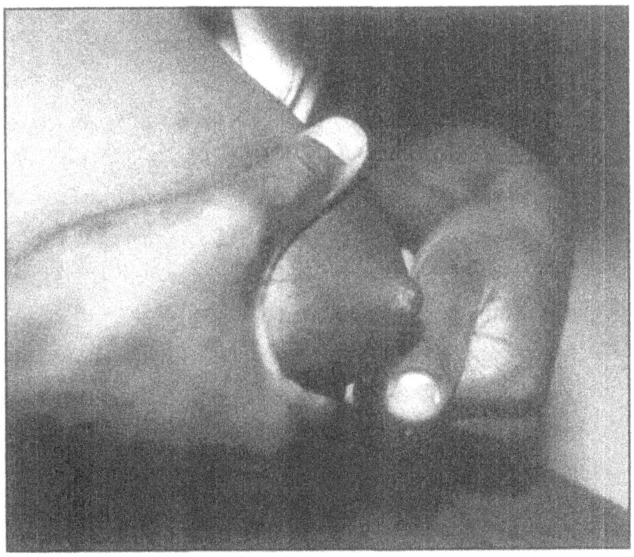

Figure 3. The 'nail test' - currently the only routine clinical pathology test available to assess the function of the lactating breast.

Soranus also advised that the milk from an ideal wet nurse should be white with no red or greenish tinge and have a pleasant odor, sweet taste, and medium consistency, the latter tested by expressing a drop of milk onto the finger nail (**Figure 3**) and observing if it held together without dispersing too rapidly (Yalom, 1997). This qualitative, clinical test was the first and remains the only routine pathological test of the function of the lactating breast. In stark contrast, the non-lactating breast and other equivalent organs in the human body have an ever-increasing battery of tests available for the diagnosis of dysfunction.

Science entered a transitional phase following the discovery of blood circulation by William Harvey in 1628 and the lymphatic system by Thomas Bartholm in 1652, with a gradual acceptance of cellular pathology in the nineteenth century (Yalom, 1997). In 1622, Gasparo Aselli discovered vessels draining the intestine of a dog and when he pricked one of the white cords a milk-like fluid gushed out. Thus, he concluded that milk was formed from chyle and carried to the breast by these (lymphatic) vessels. However, Astley Cooper (1840) rejected this suggestion when he demonstrated that fluid injected into the breast lymphatics always flowed away from the breast tissue. It then became generally accepted that milk was synthesized in the mammary gland from substrates transported to it in the blood, as expressed cogently by Foster in 1888 (Mepham, 1983):

'The secretion of milk appears to illustrate, even more fully and clearly than do other glands, the truth on which we have so often insisted, that a secretion is eminently the result of the metabolic activity of the secretory cell. The blood is the ultimate source of milk, but it becomes milk only through the activity of the cell, and that activity consists largely in a metabolic manufacture by the cell and in the cell of the common things brought by the blood into the special things present in milk.'

Scientific research on milk composition began to expand in the nineteenth century (Mayer & Klein, 1961). Cooper (1840) placed a container of breastmilk on the mantle and observed its changes over a period of six months. Donne, in 1844, carried out cytological studies of breastmilk and described colostrum corpuscles (the corpuscles of Donne). The introduction of the cell theory stimulated the histological and cytological examination of the mammary parenchyma. It was first thought that milk formation involved filtering off the necessary constituents from the blood. However, as chemical methods were developed, it became clear that active synthesis must occur in the mammary gland as some milk components were not present in the blood (Cowie, 1961). Little progress was made in understanding the physiological mechanisms controlling milk secretion for more than a century because of the erroneous belief that during suckling the 'let-down' of milk was the result of active milk synthesis.

In a comprehensive review of milk-ejection, Cowie, Forsyth, and Hart (1980) noted that despite numerous reviews on the subject, there was lingering confusion about the quite distinct processes of milk secretion and milk ejection up until the 1930s, however, this lingering confusion still exists today among some health practitioners. Milk ejection in domestic mammals was recognized as early as 5,000 BP, for example, in mural paintings in Egyptian temples and tombs (Cowie *et al.*, 1980). It was apparent then, as now, that the milker could experience problems in removing milk from the mammary glands of domestic animals. Despite vigorous milking, cows could 'hold up' their milk until the calf was allowed to suckle to induce a rapid 'let-down.' Furthermore, Cowie *et al.* suggest that lactating women must always have been aware of the occurrence of milk ejection ('the draught'). Soranus appeared to be aware of milk ejection because he wrote that it was unwise to allow an infant to fall asleep at the breast because milk might flow spontaneously and choke the infant. The occurrence of milk ejection was depicted by artists such as Tintoretto (1518-1594) and Rubens (1577-1640 (Folley, 1969). However, Cooper (1840) provided a classic description of milk ejection:

' ...the secretion of milk may be said to be constant or occasional; by the first, the milk tubes and reservoirs are constantly supplied by means of a slow and continued production of the fluid, so that milk is thus, in some degree, prepared for the child. By the occasional, is to be understood that secretion which is called by mothers and nurses, the draught of the breast, by which is meant a sudden rush of blood to the gland, during which the milk is so abundantly secreted, that if the nipple be not immediately caught by the child, the milk escapes from it, and the child when it receives the nipple is almost choked by the rapid and abundant flow of the fluid; if it lets go its hold, the milk spurts into the infant's eyes. Even the sight of the child will produce this draught, or sudden rush of blood and copious supply of milk, as the thought or sight of food occasions an abundant secretion of saliva. The draught is also greatly increased by the child pressing the breast with its little hands, or by its drawing out of the nipple by its tongue, lips, and gums, and by the presence of its head against the breast. In other mammalia, so far as we can judge, a similar process occurs, and the same effect is produced by the animal striking the udder with its head, and forcibly drawing out the teat.'

All of Cooper's observations were correct except the idea that there was a rapid increase in milk secretion at milk ejection; unfortunately, this idea became widely accepted. In 1910, Ott and Scott noted that when a posterior pituitary extract was injected into a lactating goat, it caused milk to flow from a cannulated teat. However, they thought that the extract stimulated milk secretion. Subsequently, Gaines, in 1915, carried out experiments that showed that milk synthesis and milk removal were separate processes and that the udder of the goat could contain the volume of milk obtained at a milking. He concluded that milk was actively ejected from the alveoli by a reflex contraction of gland musculature in response to the stimulus of milking. Unfortunately, other researchers ignored the extensive studies by Gaines (Cowie *et al.*, 1980). Evidence supporting the neuro-endocrine control of milk ejection was presented by Ely and Petersen (1941). They concluded from a study of the milk ejection response in dairy cows in which one-half of the udder had been denervated that:

'The letting down of milk is a conditioned reflex operated by sensory stimuli associated with milking. Afferent impulses reach the central nervous system and cause the release of oxytocin from the posterior pituitary, which in time causes a rise in milk pressure probably because of the contraction of muscular tissue which is believed to surround the alveoli and small ducts.'

They were quite innovative in designing an experiment to test the effects of stress on the ejection of milk as follows:

'(Cow) E307 was systematically frightened as the mechanical milker was attached. Frightening first consisted of placing a cat on the cow's back and exploding paper bags every ten seconds for two minutes. Later the cat was dispensed with as unnecessary.'

This experiment clearly demonstrated that stress inhibited milk ejection in the dairy cow.

Newton and Newton (1948) carried out studies that fully supported *'the idea that Petersen's theory of the mechanism of milk let-down in animals holds for the lactating woman'* including the effects of stress imposed as follows:

The nature of the distraction to be used presented some problems, since distraction of the baby from sucking was undesirable: also, the mother was not easily prevented from letting down her milk and tended to become accustomed to any particular distraction if used on two or more successive days. It was finally decided to use three distractions. They were: (1) immersion of feet alternatively for ten seconds out of every thirty in ice water (The subject stated that this was the worst distraction.); (2) a combination of electric shocks of moderate intensity with a rapid series of questions involving mathematical problems (The shock was given when an incorrect answer was returned or the subject delayed more than ten seconds before replying). This distraction was effective in disturbing the subject emotionally and making her angry, although the effect was diminished when the baby was seeking food at her breast. It was noted that she then tended to have difficulty hearing the questions and frequently delayed answering; (3) a length of surgical bandage was attached to each of the subjects big toes and pulled intermittently, causing sharp pain from the stretching and the tightness of the gauze around the toe.'

When the distraction was applied and the mother was injected with saline, 99 mL milk was removed, which was significantly less than for the control breastfeeds (168 mL) and the distraction plus the injection of oxytocin (158 mL). Perhaps the most important conclusion to be made from these studies is, in fact, the robustness of the milk ejection reflex, in that it was able to function in spite of these 'distractions.' In this connection, it is of interest that recent studies (Mitoulas *et al.*, 2002, Kent *et al.*, 2003) showed that prior to milk ejection a mean of <10 mL of milk could be removed from the breast with an electric breast pump. Thus, at least one milk ejection must have occurred for the mother to produce 99 mL of milk.

Identification of the substrates removed from the blood for milk synthesis was not achieved until the middle of the 20th century by the use of *in vivo*

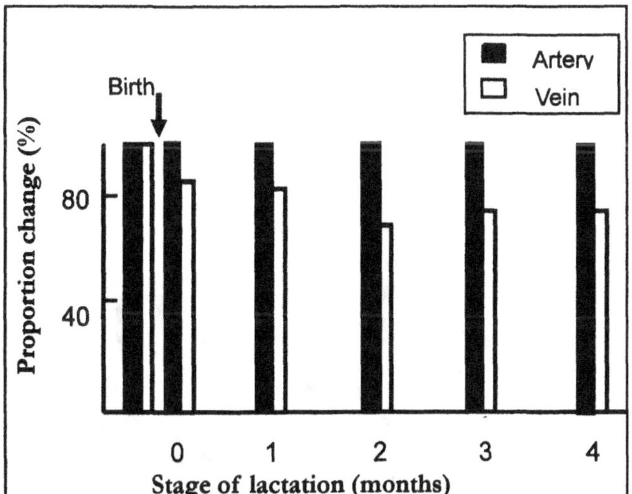

Figure 4. The proportional decrease (%) in the concentration of glucose from arterial (100%) to mammary venous blood during lactation in the cow. Source: Hartmann & Lascelles, 1964.

arteriovenous difference measurements (**Figure 4**) (Hartmann & Lascelles, 1964; Linzell, 1974) and the infusion of radioactively-labelled tracer substrates, and *in vitro* studies using isolated perfused mammary glands and tissue slices (Folley, 1956). Jim Linzell demonstrated the central role of glucose as a precursor for milk synthesis by demonstrating the inhibition of milk synthesis when glucose was removed from the perfusate of an isolated udder from the goat. He succinctly reported this finding as 'no milk without sugar' in a cable to his colleague, Derek Lindsay, who was on a voyage to Australia. Further artero-venous difference studies by Linzell's group identified the free amino acids that were required for protein synthesis, and Folley (1956) showed that acetate rather than glucose was required for *de novo* fatty acid synthesis in ruminants and that the reverse was true for monogastric animals. It was also demonstrated that long-chain fatty acids could be directly incorporated into milk triacylglycerols. An understanding of the endocrine control of milk secretion was facilitated by the isolation of ovarian hormones and the discovery that milk secretion was temporarily augmented by the injection of anterior pituitary extracts into the mammary glands of pseudo-pregnant rabbits. Five years later, in 1933, the principle that was responsible for this lactogenic response was extracted from the anterior pituitary glands, purified, and called "prolactin" (Cowie, 1961). These findings stimulated much research into the endocrine control of milk secretion (Cowie *et al.*, 1980).

The high metabolic demand of lactation was acknowledged, and it was realized that lactation was not simply a peripheral event, but involved a major re-orientation of the body's metabolic priorities (Mepham, 1983). Nevertheless, detailed knowledge of the milk composition is confined to relatively few species (<5%) (Oftedal & Iverson, 1995), and even in economically important mammals, such as the dairy cow, knowledge of the physiology of lactation is still incomplete. Compared to other organs, the lactating human breast has been almost completely ignored in medical research.

The management of breastfeeding has had a more problematical history than research into milk synthesis, secretion, and removal. William Cadogan (1711-1797) has been promoted as the 'father of childcare' (Rendle-Short & Rendle-Short, 1966) on the basis of his influential 'Essay upon the nursing and management of children from their birth to three years of age' written to the governors of the foundling hospital in London.

Cadogan encouraged breastfeeding from birth, but considered:

"Their meals, and in my opinion their sucking to, ought to be at stated times, and the same time every day.... Four times in four and twenty hours will be often enough to give suck; letting it have as much as it will take, out of both breast, at each time.... By night I would not have them fed or suckled at all, that they might at least be hungry in a morning. It is the night feeding that makes them so over-fat and bloated."

Cadogan was concerned that children in general were over-clothed and over-fed. He introduced the concept of scheduled breastfeeding because he considered that excessive breastfeeding, particularly at night, caused children to become obese – a valid concern but a remedy that has had negative implications for breastfeeding up to this day. Indeed, it would have been a better outcome if he had concentrated on their 'meals' rather than their 'sucking.' However, Cadogan started a new trend by addressing women directly, and women became accustomed to consulting male experts rather than midwives. These male experts continued to promote scheduled breastfeeding for the next 100 years by providing rules to be observed. For example, advice by Thomas Bull in 1848 (breastfeed from birth; demand feed for the first ten days: feed 4-hourly day and night for the first month; eliminate night feeds and feed 4-hourly during the day for six months giving no other fluid; commence weaning from six months and completely wean by 12-18 months) was similar to that of Truby King (1941).

Wickes (1953b) opposed scheduled breastfeeding stating that:

"Later the work of Aldrich and Hewitt (1947) did much to popularise the self-demand or self regulatory method (of breastfeeding.) When this regime becomes universally adopted, as it surely will, so the last chapter on the history of infant feeding will be concluded."

Wickes (1953c) also concluded that much of the advice that had been given by health professionals was not helpful, stating that:

"In some ways this historical review might be regarded as a chronicle of man-made errors, for many of the ideas in the writings that have been quoted were intended to be an improvement upon nature though few have succeeded. Those who have heeded nature anyway, namely the nursing mothers, have seldom found it necessary to put pen to paper."

These views are as valid today (Franz, 2007) as they were in 1953.

Statistics on the proportion of women breastfeeding that were collected for the first time in the UK in 1946 showed that the average duration of breastfeeding was only 4.2 months (Douglas, 1950a; 1950b) and only 53% of infants were breastfed at two months of age. In 1946, Bain (1948) found that only 38% of infants were exclusively breastfed at discharge from hospital. The widespread and prolonged decline in breastfeeding in industrialized countries was attributed to urbanization, change in the status of women, insufficient government support, negative inputs from health professionals, and marketing and promotion of breastmilk substitutes (Vahlquist, 1975; Jelliffe & Jelliffe, 1978).

The incidence of breastfeeding in Western countries (Australia, Sweden, Poland, USA, Canada, UK, and Denmark) reached a nadir in 1972 (Hartmann *et al.*, 1984), and then a resurgence in breastfeeding occurred over the next 30 years. As in the past, the choice to breastfeed was related to educational and socio-economic status. However, in contrast to prior to 1972, now it is the better-educated women of higher socio-economic status who choose to breastfeed their babies (**Figure 5**) (Hartmann *et al.*, 1985), finally adhering to Linnaeus's intention to encourage women of high socio-economic status to breastfeed their babies by selecting the term mammalia for classification of this group of animals.

The revival of breastfeeding in the 1970s caused renewed interest in human lactation, and it became apparent that there was a considerable lack of scientific

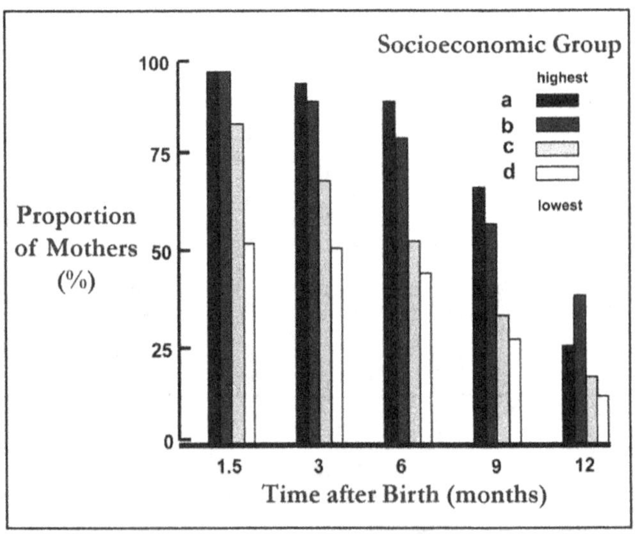

Figure 5. Time after birth and the proportion (%) of mothers breastfeeding in Australia in relation to maternal socioeconomic status. Source: Hitchcock, 1983.

knowledge of the physiology of the human breast (Jelliffe & Jelliffe, 1978; Whitehead *et al.*, 1978).

DEVELOPING COUNTRIES

In contrast to developed countries, there has been a decline in the proportion of women choosing to breastfeed their babies in developing countries, particularly in the last quarter of the 20th century (Hartmann *et al.*, 1984). This is in part due to increasing standards of living and urbanization in developing countries and in part to the aggressive promotion of breastmilk substitutes as the markets declined in the developed countries. The intrusion of this unnecessary technology into developing countries has had some highly insidious effects. Whereas breastfeeding ensured birth intervals of about three years in hunter-gatherer and traditional societies, the introduction of bottle-feeding to developing countries decreased the inter-birth interval (McCann *et al.*, 1981), placing mothers under greater physical and emotional stress. The cost of breastmilk substitutes often represents a large proportion of the family income and children are deprived of the primary function of breastmilk, that is, innate immune protection against a high pathogen burden. This situation is exacerbated by a lack of sterilization facilities and inappropriate storage time and temperatures, leading to spoilage due to the Maillard (protein-sugar) reaction.

Although poor water supplies have been considered to be the major cause of the high mortality from diarrhea in babies fed breastmilk substitutes in developing countries, research by Howie *et al.* (1990) suggests that breastmilk substitutes may be the primary cause of diarrhea. A similar high incidence of diarrhea (~20% in breastmilk substitute fed infants) was found in Dundee, Scotland, where there was a high quality water supply. However, the high quality health service in Dundee prevented a high infant mortality from diarrhea in Scotland. Although the cessation of breastfeeding by four months in HIV exposed infants is associated with reduced transmission of the virus, there is an increased infant mortality (especially from diarrhea) up to 24 months of age (WHO, 2006a), indicating again the importance of the innate immune protection from breastmilk. The relative risk of infant death from diarrhea was found to be 16.3 times higher in breastmilk substitute fed babies compared to babies fed breastmilk in Brazil (Victora, 1987). The magnitude of the problems associated with the early cessation of breastfeeding in developing countries has received considerable attention; however, decreased morbidity associated with breastfeeding in developed countries (Yeung & Peters, 2001) has not received equivalent acknowledgement. Furthermore, from an analysis of 1988 statistics in the USA on infant mortality, Chen and Rogan (2004) calculated that if 70% of infants were breastfed on discharge from maternity hospital and 33% were still breastfed at six months of age, then 720 postnatal deaths might be prevented each year if all children were breastfed.

PRESENT AND FUTURE

The evolution of the mammary gland holds a place of privilege in mammals because it is the site of an activity vital to the survival of the species. Similarly, the evolution of a large brain has given humankind a significant competitive advantage over other primates, and indeed over other mammals in general. An appreciation of the evolutionary importance of the human brain can be gauged by the fact that a large proportion of resting energy utilization (~23%) is required for the maintenance of brain function. However, it is not generally appreciated that metabolically the brain and the lactating human breast have much in common. The lactating breast, in fact, demands a higher proportion (~30%) of the resting energy (FAO, 2004) than the brain. Both organs have an obligatory requirement for glucose, do not store energy, and the blood/milk barrier has similarities to the blood/brain barrier. Furthermore, unlike other mammals, the human brain undergoes extensive growth and development of its dendritic network in the first two years of life, and its growth and development is facilitated by the supply of vital nutrients, such as docosohexanoic acid (DHA), cholesterol, choline, taurine, galactose, and oligosaccharides, as well as prolactin from breastmilk. Indeed, it is difficult to conceive how the human brain could have evolved in the absence of the specific nutrients provided from the lactating mammary gland. In addition, it is often overlooked that breastfeeding has positive outcomes for the mother, including more rapid uterine involution, reduced risk of obesity, suppression of maternal fertility, assistance in cholesterol clearance, association with a lower risk of some cancers, and improved spatial memory and learning. In addition, the function of the lactating breast is maintained under severe stress (e.g., in active war zones), and breastmilk production shows little down-regulation even under extreme dietary restriction (Hartmann *et al.*, 1984). And, contrary to common beliefs, breastmilk production is relatively independent of maternal water intake (Morrison, 1952). Clearly, a strong case can be made for the lactating breast to have a similar evolutionary status to that of the human brain. However, there is a stark difference in the medical appreciation of these two organs.

In contrast to neuroscience, the curricular of most medical faculties devote little time to instruction on human lactation. The fundamental reason for this does not lie with medical faculties, but rather with medical research priorities. While research into the function and dysfunction of the human brain clearly is commensurate with its metabolic status, there is not a similar recognition by medical scientists of the functional importance of the lactating breast. For example, tens of thousands of scientists attend annual neuroscience research conferences, whereas less than two hundred scientists attend the International Society for Research in Human Milk and Lactation conference held every other year. Thus, there is a large deficit in knowledge of the physiology and pathology of the lactating breast compared with other metabolically equivalent organs in the human body. Consequently, the lactating breast is the only significant organ in the human body without standard evidence-based diagnostic tests to assess its normality. Indeed, unlike the dairy industry, there are no standard assays for the measurement of the macronutrients (fat, protein, and lactose), in addition there are no agreed normal clinical ranges set for milk production, the content of both the macronutrients and micronutrients, or the concentration of metabolically active and innate immune factors in breastmilk. As a result, the effectiveness of breastfeeding is mostly judged on whether it is either exclusive or partial breastfeeding. In this context, it is surprising that so many positive outcomes for the infant have been observed. It is of concern that most national dietary guidelines (with the exception of Australia) do not provide guidelines for breastfeeding, although the infant's first food has considerable implications in relation to the developmental origins of health and disease. There is also a lack of clinical reference values for lactating mothers, for example, at least in Australia, there is no agreed normal range for blood prolactin for lactating women, yet the administration of drugs to increase the concentration of prolactin in women with perceived low milk supply is quite common. Fortunately, the formation of the Academy of Breastfeeding Medicine has provided an important beginning for the development of an evidence-based medical speciality in human lactation and has now published 15 clinical protocols for the diagnosis, treatment, and policies for breastfeeding management (http://www.bfmed.org/).

A major factor contributing to the reversal of the decline in breastfeeding in 1972 in developed countries was the practical promotion of breastfeeding by self-help mother's organizations, including La Leche League International (http://www.lalecheleague.org/fiftieth.html; founded in 1956) and the Australian Breastfeeding Association (http://www.breastfeeding.asn.au/; founded in 1964) that trained experienced mothers as counselors to assist other mothers with breastfeeding problems. Subsequently, health professionals supported the trend back to breastfeeding with the establishment of the International Board of Lactation Consultant Examiners (http://www.iblce.org/old/; founded in 1985) providing a specialist accreditation in lactation (Lactation Consultant) for health professionals, and belated but important support from the medical profession with the formation of the Academy of Breastfeeding Medicine (http://www.bfmed.org/) in 1995. As a result, the clinical support for human lactation is predominantly experience-based rather than evidence-based.

It is now clear that feeding babies breastmilk substitutes is inferior to breastfeeding (Yeung & Peters, 2001), and wide endorsement has been given by health authorities to the WHO statement on breastfeeding (Kramer & Kakuma, 2002):

"Breastfeeding is an unequalled way of providing ideal food for the healthy growth and development of infants; it is also an integral part of the reproductive process with important implications for the health of mothers. A recent review of evidence has shown that, on a population basis, exclusive breastfeeding for 6 months is the optimal way of feeding infants. Thereafter infants should receive complementary foods with continued breastfeeding up to 2 years of age or beyond."

Furthermore, healthy infants who are exclusively breastfed for six months under optimal conditions have different growth patterns to infants fed breastmilk substitutes (WHO, 2006b). Therefore, it has been necessary to develop new growth charts for breastfed babies.

In a number of countries, including Australia and Sweden, more than 90% of mothers choose to breastfeed their babies. Therefore, it is reasonable to conclude that all mothers in these countries now know that breastfeeding is best for their babies. However, many mothers experience difficulties in sustaining their lactation and about 40-50% cease breastfeeding by six months post-partum. Experience-based care for breastfeeding mothers is extremely important in Western countries where girls have not been given the opportunity to 'learn' to breastfeed by 'osmosis,' as in traditional societies. Since breastfeeding for the mother is an acquired skill, the challenge for self-help organizations and health professionals is to teach mothers in a few hours breastfeeding skills that would have been acquired over years in traditional societies. However, experiences vary and consequently mothers receive conflicting (different) advice that erodes confidence and consequently often impedes rather than facilitates lactation.

Now that health education programmes have been effective in increasing the proportion of mothers that breastfeed, there is an obligation for health authorities to support research directed towards the development of evidence-based diagnosis and treatment protocols for human lactation to ensure that the mothers who commence breastfeeding can receive appropriate support to enable them to have a sustained and successful breastfeeding experience. Then, this crucial and interesting organ that has been a key contributor to the success of mammalian evolution will be able to fulfill its current important physiological role of facilitating both infant and maternal development.

ACKNOWLEDGEMENT

Research funding from Medela AG.

References

Akers RM. *Lactation and the mammary gland.* Ames: Iowa State Press; 2002.

Berndt RM, Berndt CH. *The first Australians.* Sydney:Ure Smith; 1974.

Bain K. The incidence of breastfeeding in hospitals in the United States. *Pediatrics.* 1948; 2:313-20.

Calder R. *Leonardo & the age of the eye.* Milan: Amilcare Pizzi; 1970.

Chen A, Rogan WJ. Breastfeeding and the risk of postnatal death in the United States. *Pediatrics.* 2004; 113: e435-39.

Cooper A. *The anatomy of the breast.* London: Harrison & Co; 1840.

Cowie AT. The hormonal control of milk secretion. In Kon SK, Cowie AT (eds.). *Milk: the mammary gland and its secretion.* Vol 1. London: Academic Press; 1961. p. 163-203.

Cowie AT, Forsyth IA, Hart IC. *Hormonal control of lactation.* Berlin: Springer –Verlag; 1980.

Douglas JWB. The extent of breastfeeding in Great Britain in 1946, with special reference to the health and survival of children: 1. Duration of breastfeeding. *J Obstet Gynaecol.* 1950a; 57: 335-49.

Douglas JWB. The extent of breastfeeding in Great Britain in 1946, with special reference to the health and survival of children: 11. Infant feeding in relation to survival, health and development. *J Obstet Gynaecol.* 1950b; 57: 349-61.

Ely F, Petersen WE. Factors involved in the ejection of milk. *J Dairy Sci.* 1941; 24: 211-23.

FAO. Human energy requirements. Report of a Joint FAO/ WHO/UNU Expert Consultation. Rome: Food and Agriculture Organization of the United Nations; 2004. Available from: http://www.fao.org/docrep/007/ y5686e/y5686e00.htm.

Falck-Ytter T, Gredeback G, von Hofsten C. Infants predict other people's action goals. *Nature Neuroscience.* 2006; 9:878-79.

Fara P. *Sex, botany and empire: The story of Carl Linnaeus and Joseph Banks.* UK: Icon Books; 2003.

Folley SJ. *The physiology and biochemistry of lactation.* London: Oliver and Boyd; 1956.

Folley SJ. The milk-ejection reflex: a neuroendocrine theme in biology, myth and art. *J Endocrin.* 1969; 44(4):ix-xx.

Franz K. Doesn't the breast work anymore? A rant on the state of lactation advice today. *Essence.* 2007; 43:9-11.

Gustafsson L, Hallgren O, Mossberg A-K, Pettersson J, Fischer W, Aronsson A, *et al.* HAMLET kills tumor cells by apoptosis: Structure, cellular mechanisms, and therapy. *J Nutr.* 2005; 135:1299-1303.

Hakansson A, Svensson M, Mossberg A-K, Sabharwal H, Linse S, Lazou I, *et al.* A folding variant of α-lactalbumin with bactericidal activity against *Streptococcus pneumoniae. Mol Microbiol.* 2000; 35:589-600.

Hartmann PE, Lascelles AK. The uptake of plasma lipid and some non-lipid constituents by the mammary gland of the cow. *Australian Journal of Biological Science.* 1964; 17:935-44.

Hartmann PE, Rattigan S, Prosser CG, Saint L, Arthur PG. Human lactation: Back to nature. In: *Physiological Strategies in Lactation. Symposia of the Zoological Society of London.* 1984; 51:337-68.

Hartmann PE, Rattigan S, Saint L, Supriyana O. Variation in the yield and composition of human milk. In: Clarke E. (ed.). *Oxford reviews of reproductive biology.* 1985; 7:118-67.

Hayssen V, Blackburn DG. α-lactalbumin and the origins of lactation. *Evolution.* 1985; 39:1147-49.

Hewitt B. *The influence of diet on the fatty acid composition of breastmilk from North Fore women.* BMedSci Thesis: The University of Western Australia; 1978.

Hitchcock NE. *Feeding practices and growth of Australian infants.* MSc Thesis: The University of Western Australia; 1983.

Howie PW, Forsyth JS, Ogston SA, Clark A, Florey CD.) Protective effect of breastfeeding against infection. *Br Med J.* 1990; 300:11-16.

Jelliffe DB, Jelliffe EFP. *Human milk in the modern world: psychological, nutritional, and economic significance.* Oxford: Oxford University Press; 1978.

Kent JC, Ramsay DT, Doherty D, Larsson M, Hartmann PE. Response of breasts to different stimulation patterns of an electric breast pump. *J Hum Lact.* 2003; 19:179-86.

Konner M, Worthman C. Nursing frequency, gonadal function, and birth spacing among !Kung hunter-gatherers. *Science NY.* 1980; 207:788-91.

Kramer MS, Kakuma R. *The optimal duration of exclusive breastfeeding a systematic review.* Geneva: World Health Organization; 2002. Available from: www.who.int/child-adolescent-health/New_Publications/Nutrition/WHO_CAH_01_23.pdf .

Kulski JK, Smith M, Hartmann PE. Normal and caesarean section delivery and the initiation of lactation in women. *Aust J Exp Bio Med Sci.* 1981; 59:405-12.

Linzell JL. Mammary gland blood flow and methods of identifying and measuring precursors of milk. In: Larsen BL (ed.). *Lactation.* Vol 1. New York: Academic Press; 1974. p. 143-225.

Mayer G, Klein M. Histology and cytology of the mammary gland. In: Kon SK, Cowie AT (eds.). *Milk: the mammary gland and its secretion.* Vol 1. London: Academic Press; 1961. p. 47-126.

McCann MF, Liskin LS, Piotrow PT, Rinehart W, Fox G. Breastfeeding, fertility and family planning. *Population Reports.* 1981; 9:J525-75.

Mepham TB. Physiological aspects of lactation. In: Mepham TB (ed.). *Biochemistry of lactation.* Amsterdam: Elsevier Science Publishers; 1983.

Mete E, Bavbek N, Dayi A, Erkmen M, Andiran, F. In vitro antifungal effects of human milk. *Allergy Asthma Proc.* 2006; 27:412-14.

Mitoulas LR, Lai CT, Gurrin LC, Larsson M, Hartmann PE. Effect of vacuum profile on breast milk expression using an electric breast pump. *J Hum Lact.* 2002; 18:353-60.

Morrison SD. Human milk yield: proximate principles and inorganic constituents. In: *Technical Communication* No 18 *Commonwealth bureau of animal nutrition.* Bucksburn, Scotland: Rowett Research Institute; 1952.

Newton M, Newton NR. The let-down reflex in human lactation. *J Pediatr.* 1948; 33:698-704.

Oftedal OT. The mammary gland and its origin during Synapsid evolution. *J Mammary Gland Biol Neoplasia.* 2002a; 7:225-52.

Oftedal OT. The origin of lactation as a water source for parchment-shelled eggs. *J Mammary Gland BiolNeoplasia.* 2002b; 7:253-66.

Oftedal OT, Iverson SJ. Comparative analysis of nonhuman milks A. Phylogenetic variations in the gross composition of milks. In: Jensen RG (ed.). *Handbook of milk composition.* New York: Academic Press; 1995.

Pond CM. Physiological and ecological importance of energy storage in the evolution of lactation: Evidence for a common pattern of anatomical organization of adipose tissue in mammals. In: *Physiological Strategies in Lactation. Symposia of the Zoological Society of London.* 1984; 51:1-32.

Short RV. Foreword. In: Minchin MK (ed.). *Breastfeeding Matters.* Melbourne: Alma Publications; 1985.

Rendle-Short J, Rendle-Short M. *The father of child care. Life of William Cadogan (1711-1797).* Bristol: John Wright and Sons Ltd.; 1966.

Schiebinger L. Why Mammals are Called Mammals: Gender Politics in Eighteenth-Century Natural History. *The American Historical Review.* 1993; 98:382-411.

Truby King M. *Mothercraft.* Sydney: Whitcombe and Tombs Ltd.; 1941.

Thomson D. *Children of the wilderness.* Melbourne: Currey O'Neil Ross; 1983.

Vahlquist B. Evolution of breastfeeding in Europe. *J Trop Pediatr Environ Child Health.* 1975; 21:11-18.

Victora CG, Smith PG, Vaughan JP, Nobre LC, Lombardi C, Teixeira AM, *et al.* Evidence for protection by breast-feeding against infant deaths from infectious diseases in Brazil. *Lancet.* 1987; 2(8554):319-22.

Vis HL, Hennert P. Decline in breastfeeding: About some of its causes. *Acta Paediatrica Belgium.* 1978; 31:195-206.

Vorbach C, Capecchi MR, Penninger JM. Evolution of the mammary gland from the innate immune system. *BioEssays.* 2006; 28:606-16.

WHO. WHO HIV and infant Feeding Technical Consultation Held on behalf of the Inter-agency Task Team (IATT) on Prevention of HIV Infections in Pregnant Women, Mothers and their Infants. Geneva: World Health Organization; 2006a.

WHO. WHO Child growth standards: Methods and development. Geneva: World Health Organization; 2006b. Available from: http://www.who.int/childgrowth/mgrs/en/.

Wickes IG. A history of infant feeding. Part I: Primitive people, ancient works, renaissance writer. *Archives of Diseases in Childhood.* 1953a; 28:495-502.

Wickes IG. A history of infant feeding. Part III: Eighteenth and nineteenth century. *Archives of Diseases in Childhood.* 1953b; 28:332-40.

Wickes IG. A history of infant feeding. Part V: Nineteenth century concluded and twentieth century. *Archives of Diseases in Childhood.* 1953c; 28:495-502.

Whitehead RG, Hutton M, Muller E, Rowland MGM, Prentice AM, Paul A. Factors influencing lactation in rural Gambian mothers. *Lancet.* 1978; 22(2):178-81.

Yalom M. *A history of the breast.* London: HarperCollins; 1997.

Yeung DL, Peters CT. Functional foods: Implications for infant development and later health. *Heinz Sight.* 2001; 58:1-6.

SECTION I

ANATOMY AND BIOCHEMISTRY

Chapter 2

Gross Anatomy of the Lactating Breast

Donna T. Geddes

INTRODUCTION

The magnificent work *The Anatomy of the Breast* by Sir Astely Cooper (1840) has been the definitive reference for our knowledge of the gross anatomy of the breast to date. The stimulus for this investigation of the breast arose after Cooper had presented a paper entitled 'Diseases of the Breast' which he intended to follow-up with a written description 'Malignant Diseases of the Breast.' In attempting to write the paper, he discovered scant data and conflicting reports regarding the anatomy of the breast. His reaction was *'I felt that it was absolutely necessary to give an account of the natural structure of the Breast, before its morbid changes could be properly explained or understood.'* Thus, Cooper embarked on his research and produced a remarkably detailed description of the anatomical structures of the breast. Due to both the immense difficulty in procuring the breasts of women who had died during lactation and in performing the dissections themselves, little investigation has been performed since then. However, with the resurgence of breastfeeding, there has been renewed interest in the development and anatomy of the breast with regard to both lactation and pathological conditions.

DEVELOPMENT OF THE BREAST

Successful lactation is dependent upon the ability of the breast to synthesize, secrete, and release milk (milk ejection) for removal by the infant and, for increasing numbers of women, by the use of a breast pump. Unlike other organs of the body, the breast does not reach its full functional capacity until reaching maturity during pregnancy and childbirth. Thus, breast development occurs in distinct phases: fetal (**Table 1**), neonatal/prepubertal, and post-pubertal. Development of the breast can then proceed through a number of lactation cycles (pregnancy, lactogenesis I, lactogenesis II, galactopoiesis, involution, then finally to postmenopausal involution (**Table 2**).

Table 1. Fetal Development of the Female Human Breast

Gestational Stage	Stage of Development of the Breast
5-6 weeks	Appearance of ectodermal ridge (milk line)
7-8 weeks	Mammary disc appears Primitive blood vessels are formed
10-12 weeks	Formation of epithelial buds
16 weeks	Mammary vascular system completely formed
13-20 weeks	Parenchymal branching
20 weeks	15-20 solid cords (ductal structures) are formed
32 weeks	Canalization of the solid cords completed to form primary milk ducts
32 weeks - term	Some lobulo-alveolar development Increased periductal stroma Lobules have a single layer of epithelium

Table 2. Development of the Female Human Breast

Stage of Development	Characteristics of Development
Prepubertal	-Rudimentary ductal system -Symmetrical growth
Puberty	-Increased epithelial growth with each menstrual cycle -Differentiation of Terminal Ductule Units (TDLU) from Type 1 to Type 3 -Growth of the ductal system -Unsymmetrical growth of the epithelium and stroma
Pregnancy	
Mammogenesis First half of pregnancy	-Rapid ductal branching and lobular formation -Increase in epithelial cells -Differentiation of Type 3 lobules into Type 4 lobules
Lactogenesis I	-Differentiation of epithelial cells into lactocytes -Synthesis of milk specific components secreted into lobules and ducts
Term	
Lactogenesis II	-Closure of epithelial tight junctions -Onset of copious milk production
Post lactation involution	-Gradual weaning decreases milk production slowly -Apoptosis -Composition secretion is similar to colostrum
Postmenopausal involution	-Atrophy of the glandular tissue -Increase in adipose tissue -Decreased elasticity of supporting connective tissues

FETAL DEVELOPMENT

The human breast begins to develop by six weeks of gestation when a thickened ectodermal ridge situated along the anterior body wall from the groin to the axilla of the embryo becomes apparent (milk line). Eventual regression of this ridge occurs, except for the pectoral region (2nd-6th rib), to form the mammary gland. Supernumerary glands may develop anywhere along the ectodermal ridges and may either mature into mammary glands or remain as accessory nipples in 2-6% of women (Vorherr, 1974; Russo & Russo, 2004).

During the seventh and eighth week of gestation (embryo 10-11 mm), the mammary parenchyma invades the stroma and a raised portion, called the mammary disc, appears. Epithelial buds begin to form between ten and twelve weeks (embryo 30-68 mm) and parenchymal branching occurs during the 13th-20th week. Between the 12th and 16th week of gestation, the smooth musculature of areola and nipple are formed and, at approximately 20 weeks gestation (fetus=10 cm), 15-25 solid cords form in the subcutaneous tissue (Gould, 1983; Hovey *et al.*, 2002; Russo & Russo, 2004). Branching continues and canalization of the cords occurs by apoptosis of the central epithelial cells to become the primary milk ducts by 32 weeks gestation (Hovey *et al.*, 2002).

Mesenchymal cells differentiate into erythroblasts and primitive blood vessels at seven weeks gestation. Subsequently, small capillaries appear between nine and ten weeks gestation and, by 12-13 weeks gestation, a concentric vascular network has formed in the mammary gland. Development of the vascular system is complete by week 16 and blood begins circulating to the skin, secretory, adipose, and connective tissues of the mammary gland.

In the last eight weeks of gestation, there is little lobulo-alveolar development; however, the periductal stroma increases in density (Naccarato *et al.*, 2000). Also, at 32 weeks gestation, the ducts open onto an area which develops into the nipple (Tobon & Salazar, 1974). The ectoderm around the nipple becomes pigmented and Montgomery glands develop in this region. The adipose tissue of the mammary gland is assumed to be formed by connective tissue that has lost its capacity to form fibers and is considered essential as a medium for further growth of the parenchyma of the mammary gland (Vorherr, 1974).

Shortly after birth, colostrum ("witches milk") can

be expressed from the infant's mammary glands. This is thought to be due to the pro-lactation hormones present in fetal circulation at birth. Regression of the mammary gland usually occurs by four weeks postpartum and coincides with a decrease in the secretion of prolactin from the anterior pituitary gland of the infant (Vorherr, 1974; Russo *et al.*, 1982).

NEONATAL AND PRE-PUBERTAL DEVELOPMENT

The newborn breast consists only of rudimentary ducts that have small club-like ends that regress soon after birth. Prior to puberty, the growth of the breast is isometric and in proportion to the body (Russo & Russo, 2004). At puberty (eight to twelve years), allometric (unsymmetrical) growth of both the epithelium and stroma occurs. In ruminants, allometric growth begins before puberty (Hovey *et al.*, 2002). Impaired mammary development and subsequent lactation performance has been observed in ruminants that have a dietary intake in excess of their energy requirements (Sejrsen & Purup, 1997).

PUBERTY

At puberty, the human breast increases in size mainly due to increased deposition of adipose tissue within the gland (Russo & Russo, 1987). Epithelial proliferation also begins with elongation and branching of the ductal system to form a more extensive ductal network. Growth of the ends of the ducts into terminal ductle lobular units (TDLU/acini) occurs (Sternlicht *et al.*, 2006). The most rudimentary TDLU consist of approximately 11 ductules and are defined as Type 1. Type 2 TDLU consist of about 47 ductules, and Type 3 consist of approximately 80 ductules. Although the hormonal regulation of mammary growth during this period is not well understood in women, it has been associated with increased levels of estrogen, prolactin, lutenizing hormone, follicle stimulating hormone, and growth hormone (Lee *et al.*, 1976; Thorner *et al.*, 1977; Rose *et al.*, 1991; Ankarberg-Lindgren *et al.*, 2001). Epithelial growth continues with each successive menstrual cycle until the age of 35 years when growth of the breast diminishes (Vorherr, 1974). Development of the breast can then proceed through a number of lactation cycles (pregnancy, lactogenesis I, lactogenesis II, galactopoiesis, involution, and finally to postmenopausal involution).

GROSS ANATOMY OF THE MATURE NON-LACTATING BREAST

The current descriptions of the anatomy of the breast have changed little in the past 160 years and are based on Cooper's dissections of lactating breasts in 1840 (**Figure 1**). The breast is composed of glandular (secretory) and adipose (fatty) tissue and is supported by a loose framework of fibrous connective tissue called Cooper's ligaments. Apart from the external number, position, and appearance of the mammary glands, the internal structure (glandular tissue and supporting tissues) is similar in practically all species (Cowie, 1974). In women, the glandular tissue is composed of 15 20 lobes, comprised of lobules containing 10-100 alveoli that are approximately 0.12 mm in diameter (Hartmann, 1991). It is generally believed that each lobe of the breast exists as a single entity (Cooper, 1840; Love & Barsky, 2004; Going & Moffat, 2004), with just one study demonstrating connections between lobes on two occasions in the mastectomized breast of a 69-year-old woman. Three dimensional reconstructions of the entire ductal system (16 lobes) were made, and the connections were located more than 40 mm from the nipple (Ohtake *et al.*, 2001). The amount of tissue associated with each lobe within the breast is variable and may show 20-30 fold differences (Moffatt & Going, 1996).

Most of the descriptions of the ductal system of the breast are standardized and based on Cooper's dissections (**Figure 2**). The alveoli of the breast are drained by small ducts and these ducts coalesce into larger ducts (2 mm) that eventually converge into one main milk duct that dilates slightly to form what was termed the lactiferous sinus (2-4.5 mm) (Venta *et al.*, 1994) before narrowing as it passes through the nipple and opens onto the nipple surface (**Figure 2**). The nipple pores are 0.4-0.7 mm in diameter (Fawcett, 1986) and are surrounded by circular muscle fibers (Vorherr, 1974; Bannister *et al.*, 1995). There are a few conflicting reports stating that there are six to ten ductal openings at the nipple (Hicken, 1937; 1940; Lanfranchi, 2000), whereas, standard anatomy textbooks state that there are 15-20 (Bannister *et al.*, 1995). Three more recent studies have counted the number of ducts in histological sections of nipples and reported numbers that agree with the quoted 15-20 [mean=17 ducts (Going & Moffat, 2004); median=27 ducts (Taneri *et al.*, 2006); median=23 ducts (Rusby *et al.*, 2007)]. Histological sections of the nipple, however, allow the number of openings in the nipple to be counted, but do not allow one to determine if all of the ducts are connected to functional lobes within the breast (Love & Barsky, 2004). Indeed, in a mastectomy breast, Going and Moffat (2004) found of all the ducts identified, six that had large duct diameters drained lobes that accounted for 75% of the glandular portion of the breast, while the remaining smaller ducts drained only a small proportion of the glandular tissue, and four ducts ended blindly. In addition, Going and Moffat (2004) were unable to demonstrate merging of ducts within the nipple.

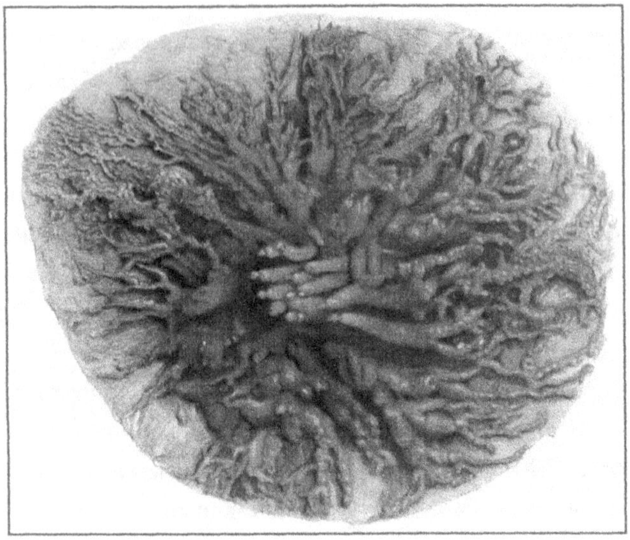

Figure 1. Artist's impression of the ductal system of the breast of a woman that died during lactation. The ductal system was injected with colored wax or glue (Cooper, 1840).

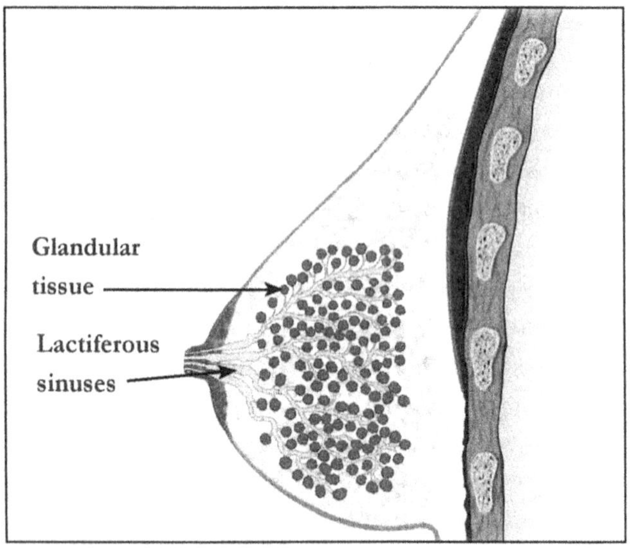

Figure 2. A schematic diagram of the anatomy of the breast representing conventional anatomy. (Reproduced with the permission, copyright Medela AG.)

Galactography is a procedure whereby the duct is cannulated through the nipple and radio-opaque contrast is injected in order to outline the ductal system on subsequent radiographs (Horatio *et al.*, 2001). Hicken (1937) used galactography and found that the ducts were relatively superficial in the breast. The main ducts of the breast are depicted as being regularly spaced around the nipple (Bannister, 1995; Moffatt & Going, 1996), despite observations that the lobes are difficult to separate on dissection (Bannister, 1995). In addition, one study of the breast of a 19-year-old cadaver showed that her ten main ducts branched within 4-28 mm of the nipple (Moffatt & Going, 1996).

The ratio of glandular to adipose tissue in the breasts of 30 to 80-year-old women was found to be on average 1:1 in Malaysian, Australian, and German women when measured by mammography (Heggie, 1996; Klein *et al.*, 2002; Jamal *et al.*, 2004). Furthermore, the proportion of glandular tissue decreases with advancing age (Soares *et al.*, 2002; Jamal *et al.*, 2004) and increasing breast size (Cruz-Korchin, 2002). Although quantitative measurements of the amount of tissue in the breast have not been made, one study has correlated mammographic images with the ultrasound parenchymal pattern of the non-lactating breast (Kaizer *et al.*, 1988).

The distribution of adipose tissue in the breast is highly variable and is situated beneath the skin (subcutaneous) between the glandular tissue (intra-glandular) (Cooper, 1840; Nickell & Skelton, 2005) and behind the breast (retromammary fat pad). The function of the adipose tissue of the mammary gland is not entirely clear or well studied. Cooper (1840) speculated both a protective function from trauma and a mechanism of temperature regulation. Currently, it is believed that the adipose tissue is necessary for proliferation of glandular tissue. In addition, there is evidence to suggest that both the long chain fatty acids and medium chain fatty acids synthesized in milk are in part imported or derived from adipose tissue stores (Davies *et al.*, 1983; Hachey *et al.*, 1987).

The tissues of the breast are supported by fibrous structures known as suspensory ligaments or Cooper's ligaments, so named after the discoverer himself. The ligaments emanate from the posterior fascia of the gland in an irregular fashion toward the anterior fascia of the gland. The ligaments are broad at the base converging to peaks at the extremity (Cooper, 1840).

ETHNICITY

Little literature exists with reference to differences in ethnic morphology of the breast. One study has shown that Asian-American women tend to have lower absolute mammographic density (a lesser proportion of glandular tissue) as measured by mammography than either African-American women or Caucasian women (Chen *et al.*, 2004).

Although differences in the external appearance of the breast may exist between different ethic groups, it is unlikely that the morphology of the breast varies dramatically (Heggie, 1996; Klein *et al.*, 2002; Jamal *et al.*, 2004). Furthermore, milk production of women in both developed and developing countries are not significantly different (Coward *et al.*, 1984), indicating that the function of the mammary gland is also unlikely to be affected by ethnicity.

PREGNANCY

At three to four weeks gestation, ductal branching and lobular formation (mammogenesis) escalates exceeding normal premenstrual changes, and often the increased breast tenderness associated with these changes is the first indicator of pregnancy. Mammogenesis is influenced by numerous hormones, such as estrogen, progesterone, prolactin, growth hormone, epidermal growth factor, fibroblast growth factor, insulin-like growth factor, human placental lactogen, and parathyroid hormone related protein (Oka *et al.*, 1991; Kelly *et al.*, 2002; Wysolmerski *et al.*, 1995), resulting in the differentiation of Type 3 lobules into Type 4 lobules (full differentiation). Some secretory development is evident by mid-pregnancy with colostrum present in the alveoli and milk ducts (Lactogenesis I). It is of note that mothers who deliver preterm (<28 weeks) may interrupt development of the breast, and this may impact lactation, resulting in delayed initiation of lactogenesis II and/or reduced volumes of milk produced in the first week postpartum (Henderson *et al.*, 2004). It appears that the glandular tissue grows by invading the fat lobules, hence decreasing the amount of adipose tissue relative to glandular tissue in the breast (Vorherr, 1974). This may be assisted by the hormone relaxin, which has been shown to be essential for mammary growth by causing both an increase in the amount of adipose tissue in the mammary gland and dilation of the mammary microvessels in rats (Bani, 1997). Prior to 16 weeks gestation, the alveoli and ducts have a two layer epithelial lining. After 16 weeks gestation, the superficial layer disappears in the alveoli, and this single layer persists for the rest of pregnancy and the duration of lactation (Vorherr, 1974). There is some secretory development (colostrum) by mid-pregnancy, with colostrum beginning to dilate both the alveolar and ductal lumina. In the last trimester, there is a further increase in lobular size associated with hypertrophy of the cells to twice their resting size and further accumulation of secretion in the lumen of the alveoli. These changes usually lead to a marked increase in breast size during pregnancy. However, breast growth during pregnancy varies greatly between women, ranging from either little or no increase to a considerable increase in size that can occur either rapidly during the first trimester or more gradually over the entire pregnancy (Cox *et al.*, 1999). While the major increase in breast size is usually completed by week 22 of pregnancy, it is clear that for some women significant breast growth occurs during the last trimester of pregnancy. The rate of growth of the mother's breast during pregnancy was correlated with the increase in the concentration of human placental lactogen in the mother's blood, suggesting that this hormone may stimulate breast growth in women as it does in some other mammals (Cox *et al.*, 1999).

The effect of nutrition on the development of the mammary gland during pregnancy has not been extensively studied in women; however, a recent study of rats has shown that the restriction of energy intake by 40% in the first part of pregnancy resulted in increased mammary cell proliferation (46%) and suppressed apoptosis, resulting in a 14% increase in milk yield (Kim & Park, 2004). In addition, an association between obesity and lactation failure in dairy cows, sows, and rats has been demonstrated. Studies of the effect of obesity on lactation in women have been difficult to perform due to influencing factors, such as the type of delivery and breastfeeding behavior; however, recent evidence suggests that women with a high pregnant body mass index are more likely to experience delayed lactogenesis II (Rasmussen *et al.*, 2001).

Currently, there is a growing interest in stem cell research from both a research and a commercial viewpoint, and the mammary gland is no exception.

The isolation and study of the behavior of mammary stem cells is providing us with a better understanding of mammary gland development and tissue stability. Although progress with human mammary stem cells has been limited by difficulties in isolation of the cells (Visvader & Lindeman, 2006), it has been shown that a single stem cell implanted into the cleared mammary fat pad of a mouse is able to develop into a fully differentiated (lactating) gland (Shackleton *et al.*, 2006). The ability of the structures of the human breast to proliferate and self-renew is characteristic of the presence of stem cells. Indeed, Cregan *et al.* (2007) have shown that putative stem cells are present in breastmilk. Breastmilk may well provide an alternative noninvasive source of stem cells compared to tissue obtained by biopsy or reduction mammoplasty, facilitating further study of mammary gland biology.

GROSS ANATOMY OF THE LACTATING BREAST

During lactation, the alveoli of the breast are lined with lactocytes that synthesize breastmilk. Little or no difference has been demonstrated in the structure of these cells between species (Cowie, 1974). Although the structure of the mammary parenchyma is remarkably similar in all mammals, including women, the arrangement of the ducts and the size of the storage spaces vary from species to species. For example, goats and cows have large cisterns that may store as much as 20% of the available milk and only one duct from the cistern to the surface of the teat. In contrast, the rabbit and bitch are similar to women in that they do not have cisterns and have multiple ducts leading to the nipple (Cooper, 1840). In general, in animals with no cisterns, almost all of the milk is stored in the alveolar portion of the gland and very little in the ductal system (Cowie, 1974).

Apart from Cooper's (1840) dissections of the breasts of women that had died during lactation, few other studies exist that examine the lactating breast, despite the abundance of literature showing both the nutritional and immunological benefits of breastmilk for the developing infant. However, there is renewed interest in breast anatomy with regard to breast cancer, but only one study included a group of lactating women. Love and colleagues (2004) examined 219 lactating women during breast expression with a pump. They observed an average of five (range 1-17) patent nipple openings, most frequently in the central portion of the nipple. This was confirmed by histology of ten mastectomy (non-lactating) nipples (5-7 patent ducts) in the same paper. Going and Moffat (2004) were able to procure a mastectomized lactating breast and found four ducts in the nipple that connected to functioning lobes. Similarly, Ramsay *et al.* (2005) have shown an average of nine main milk ducts (range 4-18) at the base of the nipple in the lactating breast. Indeed, although Cooper (1840) observed up to 22 ducts in some cadavers, more commonly seven to twelve were patent.

Nipple appearance and diameter varies between mothers. In addition, nipple size has been shown to increase during pregnancy and is related to plasma prolactin levels (Cox *et al.*, 1996). Ramsay *et al.* (2005) quoted an average of 16mm nipple diameter for both breasts. Other studies have noted that their populations have included larger proportions of mothers with nipple diameters greater than 16mm (and some greater than 23mm) (**Figure 3**) (Wilson-Clay & Hoover, 2005). Clinically, it is recognized that the size of the nipple may influence the attachment of the infant to the breast and subsequently milk removal.

The ducts of the lactating breast are relatively small (mean diameter 2mm) (Ramsay *et al.*, 2005) which is similar to the measurements quoted for non-lactating women (2-4.5mm) (Venta *et al.*, 1994). This is

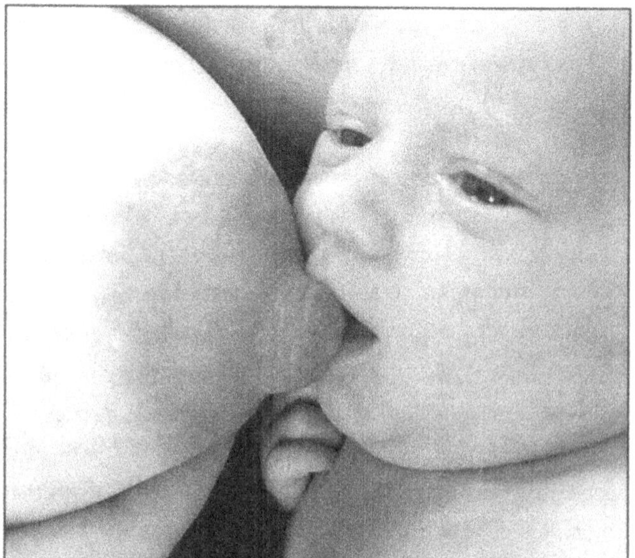

Figure 3. Nipple diameters vary between women. Large nipples, as pictured here, may be problematic for the infant to attain a good attachment to the breast. (Reproduced with permission; copyright Wilson-Clay and Hoover.)

in agreement with Cardenosa and Eklund (1996) who, using ductography in lactating women, concluded that the ducts do not necessarily enlarge during lactation. However, at milk ejection, intra-ductal pressure increases and the milk ducts dilate to accommodate milk flow. Unfortunately, the ejected milk is not stored in the main milk ducts, as reverse flow is observed as myoepithelial cell contraction relaxes (Ramsay *et al.*, 2004). Ramsay (2005), using high definition ultrasound, also showed that the ducts are often superficial; an observation also made by Hicken (1937) using ductography. In addition, the milk ducts are easily compressed, providing a possible explanation for milk stasis, which has been suggested as a cause for blocked ducts. The course of the ducts is erratic, even though the main ducts of the breast are depicted as regularly spaced around the nipple (Bannister, 1995; Moffatt & Going, 1996), despite observations that the lobes are difficult to separate on dissection (Bannister, 1995). Ramsay *et al.* (2005) found that the main milk ducts did not display the typical sac-like appearance of the 'lactiferous sinus.' Instead, the glandular tissue located directly beneath the nipple is drained by branches that merge into the main collecting duct very close to the nipple (**Figure 4a**).

Despite vast improvements in imaging techniques, the volume of glandular tissue in the breast has not been quantified. This is due to the intermingling of glandular and adipose tissue throughout the breast. Ramsay *et al.* (2005) used a semi-quantitative ultrasound measurement of both glandular and adipose tissue in 21 Caucasian mothers and found the ratio of glandular to adipose tissue to be approximately 2:1. There is, however, great variability in the proportion of glandular tissue in the breast, ranging from half of the breast to most of the breast comprised of this tissue, providing further evidence that breast size is not indicative of lactation potential. Furthermore, the amount of fat situated among the glandular tissues is also highly variable (**Figure 4b**). It is of interest that there is little subcutaneous fat in the nipple-areolar region, the area where the infant attaches to breastfeed.

Until recently, the understanding of the gross anatomy of the breast has not changed for some 160 years. Knowledge of the development and anatomy of the breast is integral to both understanding the normal development and function of the breast and breast pathology. New breast anatomy findings, such as lower numbers of patent ducts (9 compared to 15-25), superficial and compressible ducts that lack lactiferous sinuses, and ducts do not store a large amount of milk, impact upon our understanding of the process of lactation.

Summary Points

- Recent evidence suggests fewer milk ducts (5-9) in the breast on average. Although nipple specimens exhibit higher numbers (11-48), connection to lobes has not been established.
- Milk ducts in the lactating breast are small (2 mm), superficial, and compressible.

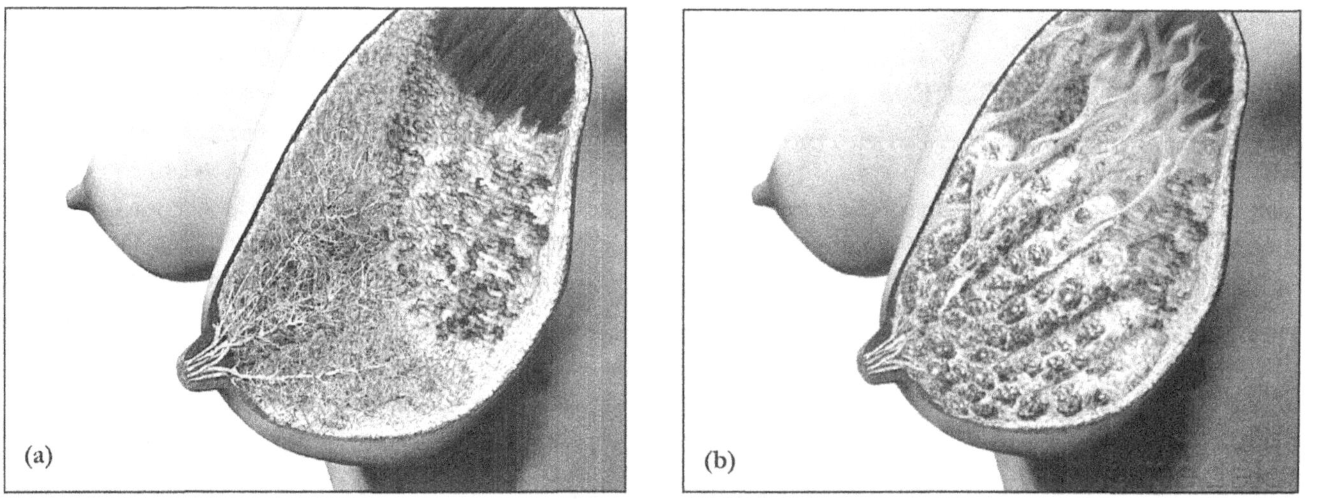

Figure 4. (a) 3-dimensional illustration of the ductal system of the lactating breast. Note the small ducts and early branching of the ducts below the nipple in addition to the system's complexity. (b) 3-dimensional illustration of the glandular and adipose tissues along with the Cooper's Ligaments. (Reproduced with the permission, copyright Medela AG.)

- Milk ducts do not display typical lactiferous sinuses (dilated portions beneath the nipple) and do not store large amounts of milk.
- The amount of adipose tissue in the breast is highly variable.

POST-LACTATION INVOLUTION

When suckling decreases and is discontinued, involution of the mammary gland occurs. The milk accumulates in the ducts causing atrophy of the lactocytes. If cessation of breastfeeding is abrupt, engorgement of the breast is more intense than a gradual weaning that decreases milk production slowly (Kent *et al.*, 1999; Lawrence & Lawrence, 1999). The secretions in the ducts and alveoli are absorbed, and the alveoli gradually collapse and undergo apoptosis (Vorherr, 1974). Also, there is an increase in the adipose and periareolar connective tissue. During the involution process, changes occur in milk composition with increased concentrations of sodium, potassium, and protein (lactoferrin, IgA, IgG, IgM, albumin, α-lactalbumin, and casein) and decreased concentrations of lactose and potassium. As a result, the composition of the involution secretion is not dissimilar to that of colostrum (Hartmann & Kulski, 1978). The breast does not, however, return to its pre-pregnancy state as some of the alveoli formed during pregnancy do not involute, but rather returns to a resting state, and the breast is again influenced by the hormonal changes of the menstrual cycle. Secretions may remain in the ducts for at least two months (Hartmann & Kulski, 1978; Fawcett, 1986).

POSTMENOPAUSAL INVOLUTION

After menopause, declining ovarian function is associated with diminishing levels of estrogen and progesterone, and involution of the breast. This involution is typified by the reduction and eventual atrophy of the glandular tissue of the breast, resulting in the ductules in the lobules decreasing by approximately a third (Tavassoli, 1992). Dilation of the ductules (cystic atrophy) may be present in some breasts. As the glandular tissue decreases, there is a concomitant increase in adipose tissue (Bannister, 1995), usually beginning at the periphery of the breast and progressing towards the nipple (Vorherr, 1974). This is clearly apparent on mammograms (Laya *et al*, 1995; Sterns & Zee, 2000), although there is a wide variation between women in the proportion of glandular and adipose tissue in the breast at this time (Bannister, 1995) and decreased elasticity of the supporting connective tissues of the breast is also obvious (Hutson *et al.*, 1985). Conversely, women taking combined hormone replacement therapy show increased mammographic density (glandular tissue) due to either epithelial or stromal proliferation (Greendale *et al.*, 2005).

BLOOD SUPPLY

Descriptions of the blood supply to the breast have been based on the classic dissections of lactating cadavers by Cooper (1840). Methods used to investigate the vasculature of the mammary gland in cadavers include injection of either colored wax or mercury into the vessels (Cooper, 1840), surgical dissection (Anson *et al.*, 1939), and injection of a suspension of fine lead and radiography of the blood supply in one non-lactating female cadaver (Salmon, 1939). The breast is supplied mainly by the anterior and posterior medial branches of the internal mammary artery (60%) and the lateral mammary branch of the lateral thoracic artery (30%) (Vorherr, 1974; Cunningham, 1977; Doughty *et al.*, 1996).

The limited number of studies performed since Cooper (1840) have highlighted the variation in blood supply to the breast between women. Cooper showed four anterior perforating branches of the IMA supplying the breast. Later, the perforating branch at the second intercostal space was considered to be the main source of blood due to its large size (Maliniak, 1934). Other studies have shown that two main anterior perforating branches supply the breast (Anson *et al.*, 1939). More recently Aljazaf (2005) has shown that more often there is one dominant artery with multiple arteries occurring less frequently. Although the lateral thoracic artery is considered to supply up to a third of the blood to the breast, a recent study has shown that the lateral thoracic artery does not supply any blood to the breast in as many as a third of women (Doughty *et al.*, 1996). Smaller sources of arterial blood also include the posterior intercostal arteries and the pectoral branch of the thoracoacromial artery (Freeman *et al.*, 1981; Bannister *et al.*, 1995). The internal mammary artery and lateral thoracic artery provide approximately 60% and 35% of the blood supply to the breast; however, there is wide variation in the proportion of blood supplied by each artery between women (Doughty *et al.*, 1996; Aljazaf, 2005) and little evidence of symmetry between breasts (Anson *et al.*, 1939; Aljazaf, 2005). Furthermore, the course of the arteries does not appear to be associated with the ductal system of the breast (Cooper, 1840).

During pregnancy, blood flow to the breast doubles by 24 weeks and then remains constant during lactation (Vorherr, 1974; Thoresen & Wesche, 1988). Whereas breast skin temperature increases by 1°C by week nine of pregnancy and then remains stable until two days postpartum when the temperature increases again (Burd *et al.*, 1977). As with the non-lactating breast, Aljazaf (2005) has shown that there is a wide variation between women in the proportion of blood supplied by each artery, and there is little evidence of symmetry between breasts. Along with an increase in blood flow, the superficial veins of the breast also become more prominent during pregnancy and lactation.

In general, there is a close relationship between blood flow and milk yield in animals (Prosser *et al.*, 1996), and the ratio of blood flow to milk yield is approximately 500:1 (Linzell, 1960; Christensen *et al.*, 1989). Aljazaf (2005) investigated the mammary blood flow in women and found that the ratio of blood flow to milk yield was also 500:1 in keeping with the animal model, but was unable to demonstrate a correlation between blood flow and milk yield.

During breastfeeding, Doppler ultrasound of the lateral thoracic artery of four women has shown that blood flow decreases by 40-50% just prior to milk ejection and then increases in the following one to two minutes. These blood flow changes are also observed after intravenous injections of oxytocin (Janbu *et al.*, 1985). Furthermore, a significant decrease in blood flow at milk ejection has been observed in other species (Pearl *et al.*, 1973; Davis *et al.*, 1995; Eriksson *et al.*, 1996). Although oxytocin has been shown to cause vasodilation, it is possible that the contraction of the alveoli may inhibit blood flow temporarily at milk ejection.

LYMPHATIC DRAINAGE

In 1622, Gasparo Aselli proposed that chyle was conveyed to the breast via the lymphatic vessels for the synthesis of milk. This theory persisted until 1840 when Cooper (1840) dissected and injected the lymphatic vessels of the lactating breast and concluded that fluid in the vessels flowed away from the breast. The drainage of lymph from the breast has been extensively investigated because of its importance in the spread of breast carcinoma. The lymph is drained by two main pathways: to the axillary nodes (Turner-Warwick, 1959) and to the internal mammary nodes (Hultborn *et al.*, 1955; Turner-Warwick, 1955; Vendrell-Torné *et al.*, 1972). The axillary nodes have been reported to receive more than 75% of the lymph from both the medial and lateral portions of the breast (Turner-Warwick, 1959; Borgstein *et al.*, 2000), whereas, the internal mammary nodes receive lymph from the deep portion of the breast (Aukland & Reed, 1993). However, there is wide variation in the drainage of lymph from the breast and less common pathways have been demonstrated. Lymph may occasionally pass through either the interpectoral nodes (Bannister, 1995) or lymph nodes in the breast parenchyma (Tanis *et al.*, 2001). Sometimes, direct drainage of lymph occurs to the supraclavicular nodes (Tanis *et al.*, 2001), and infrequently lymph may pass retrosternally into the contralateral internal mammary nodes. In addition, lymph has been shown to drain into the posterior (Turner-Warwick, 1959) and anterior intercostal nodes (Tanis *et al.*, 2001). Since Cooper's (1840) work, there has been no investigation of the lymphatic drainage of the lactating breast.

INNERVATION

Cooper (1840) showed that the second to sixth intercostal nerves supply the breast and that they have a relatively superficial course within the gland. Eckhard (1850) reported that the intercostal nerves divide into superficial and deep branches. The deep branches supply the nipple and glandular tissue while the superficial branches supply the nipple and areola. The distribution and course of the nerves innervating the nipple and areola are complex and frequently variable. However, the nipple and areola are always supplied by the anterior and lateral cutaneous branches of the third to fifth intercostal nerves (Craig & Sykes, 1970; Schlenz *et al.*, 2000). The anterior branches of the third to fifth intercostal nerves lie along the ducts to the nipple (Craig & Sykes, 1970). However, Sarhadi *et al.* (1996) found that the anterior branch of the second intercostal nerve also contributed to the innervation of the nipple and areola. The lateral supply of the nipple and areola is less variable than the medial supply. The lateral supply is provided by the fourth lateral cutaneous nerve (Farina, 1980; Schlenz *et al.*, 2000), and it most often takes a sub-glandular course within the pectoral fascia to the posterior aspect of the nipple (Craig & Sykes, 1970; Gonzalez *et al.*, 1993; Schlenz *et al.*, 2000). Less commonly, it takes a superficial course (Cooper, 1840; Farina, 1980; Sarhadie *et al.*, 1996). Detailed descriptions of the course of the anterior cutaneous branches are scant and conflicting. A deep course is described by Craig and Sykes (1970), whereas Sarhadi *et al.* (1996) and Schlenz *et al.* (2000) describe a superficial course.

Nerves have been demonstrated in association with the major duct system, but none have been identified near the smaller ducts (Linzell, 1971). The areola and nipple are sparsely innervated with all neural elements concentrated at the base of the nipple, with only a few at the side of the nipple and practically none in the areola (Montagna & MacPherson, 1974). These nerves are sensory nerves and, together with the lack of evidence of motor innervation of either the lactocytes or myoepithelial cells, suggest that both the synthesis and secretion of milk is independent of neural stimulation. Nevertheless, there is motor innervation of the smooth muscle of the areola and nipple (Courtiss & Goldwyn, 1976) and the arteries of the breast (Cowie, 1974). It is of note that the knowledge of the innervation of the breast is relatively limited compared to that of other major organs of the body. Indeed, it has come to light recently that the nerve supply to the lung is more abundant than previously thought (Sparrow & Lamb, 2003; Weichselbaum *et al.*, 2005).

Investigation of the innervation and sensitivity of the breast has predominantly focused on women that have undergone breast surgery, such as reduction mammoplasty. Only one study investigated the sensitivity of the breast during lactation. This study found that women displayed a marked increase in areola and nipple sensitivity within 24 hours postpartum (Robinson & Short, 1977), although this tends to decrease in the following days. In addition, Kent *et al.* (unpublished observations) have found that women in established lactation (one to six months) displayed limited sensory discrimination of the skin of the breast, areola, and nipple using the two-point discrimination method. Lack of sensitivity of the epidermis of the nipple has been noted previously (Vorherr, 1974). Clinical evidence supports the limited distribution of nerve fibers in the glandular tissue, in that, while women may recognize the overall fullness of a distended breast and pain associated with some abnormalities, they are often unable to accurately localize either sensation (Cowie *et al.*, 1980). Indeed, women often experience influenza-like symptoms associated with mastitis before they are aware of tenderness in their breasts.

CLINICAL IMPLICATIONS

Breast Surgery

The number of women having breast surgery is increasing annually. Disturbingly, two retrospective studies have shown that as many as 50% of women may experience low milk production after breast augmentation (Strom *et al.*, 1997; Hurst, 1996). Moreover, periareolar incisions were associated with an increased likelihood of lactation insufficiency (Hurst 1996; Neifert *et al.*, 1990). Several mechanisms may contribute to low milk production. Severing of ducts and glandular tissue, for instance, may diminish the volume of glandular tissue that can be drained through the nipple. In addition, the implant itself could compress ducts in the breast, particularly if the mother becomes overfull or engorged, thus obstructing milk flow. However, the reason the woman sought augmentation originally must be considered. It is possible that the mother had insufficient glandular tissue prior to lactation, and this can contribute to low milk production (Neifert *et al.*, 1985). In addition, damage to the nerve supply of the nipple may affect the milk ejection reflex.

Similarly, reduction mammoplasty may impact lactation with 0 to 82% of women able to breastfeed (at least partially), depending on the surgical technique used (Johansson *et al.*, 2003). The removal of a large quantity of glandular tissue may provide a possible explanation for why these mothers may have low milk production. Unfortunately, the co-distribution of glandular and fatty tissue demonstrated within both the lactating (Ramsay *et al.*, 2005) and non-lactating breast (Nickell & Skelton, 2005) would make it difficult to preferentially remove fatty tissue. In addition, it is possible that the surgery may impair the outflow of milk, especially since the breast has a lower number of patent ducts than previously thought (Love & Barsky, 2004; Moffat & Going, 2004; Ramsay *et al.*, 2005).

Pathology

Although many women experience breastfeeding difficulties, abnormalities of the lactating breast have not been extensively investigated in comparison to the pathologies of the non-lactating breast. Breast masses, such as galactoceles, are readily identifiable on ultrasound (Stavros, 2004); however, the effect on the ductal system is unknown with respect to either compression or removal of milk. Our laboratory has scanned several women with fibroadenomas and cysts during lactation. Of note was a case of a pregnant woman with focal dermal hypoplasia who presented with a mass in her right breast. The mass was well defined on ultrasound, and we were unable to trace milk ducts from the breast to the nipple as the mass obstructed the path of the ducts (**Figure 5**). Therefore, it was unlikely that the woman would be able to breastfeed successfully from the right breast due to the obstruction of milk flow. In this event, a successful strategy was devised to enhance milk production from the left breast in order to exclusively supply breastmilk to the infant.

Low Milk Production

The foremost reason for weaning an infant is perceived low milk supply (ABS, 2001; McCann & Bender, 2005). Unfortunately, there is little information regarding the incidence of verified low milk supply; however, it is certainly recognized as a significant problem, particularly for mothers of preterm infants that must express their milk to feed their baby and to maintain lactation (Morton, 2003). Clinically, pharmacological intervention (metoclopramide, domperidome) to increase prolactin levels and boost milk production may be trialed. This usually occurs without measurement of prolactin prior to the intervention and not unexpectedly provides varying success. Another reason for low milk production may be insufficient glandular tissue as discussed earlier. Quantification of the volume of glandular tissue in the breast (possibly by ultrasound, CT, or MRI) would be valuable to exclude a maternal, physiological cause for low milk production. Further investigation could then be directed towards the effectiveness of milk removal by either the infant or breast pump, or the management of breastfeeding/expressing. Finally, knowledge of the normal features of the ductal system is integral to diagnosing ductal abnormalities that may affect milk flow and drainage of the glandular tissue and manifest themselves as low milk production by local inhibition of milk secretion (Peaker *et al.*, 1998).

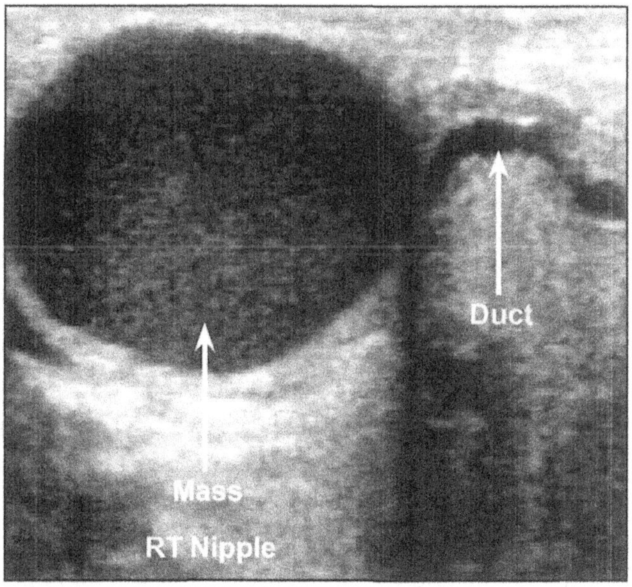

Figure 5. Ultrasound image of a mass beneath the nipple. The milk duct on the right cannot be traced past the mass to the nipple.

Milk Removal

Effective milk removal from the breast by either the infant or a breast pump is necessary to avoid down regulation of milk synthesis by local control mechanisms (Peaker *et al.*, 1998). The effect of breast anatomy on the expression of milk is largely unexplored; however, there is an indication that larger milk duct diameters are associated with longer milk ejection episodes and more of the available milk being expressed during pumping (Ramsay *et al.*, 2006). It is possible to image the milk ducts within the nipple with ultrasound (Stavros, 2004), and we have seen marked differences in duct size between women. It then follows that either milk duct size or nipple integrity may indeed affect milk flow during expression and breastfeeding. Since the ducts are superficial and compressible, it is possible that the breast shield used to apply vacuum to the breast may compress some ducts and thereby compromise milk flow. This emphasizes the need for the mother to use a correctly fitted breastshield during breast expression.

The absence of lactiferous sinuses (milk reservoirs) leads one to reconsider the mechanism by which the infant removes milk from the breast. It is commonly believed that the infant uses a peristaltic motion of the tongue to strip milk from the nipple (Woolridge, 1986). However, a recent study using ultrasound and intra-oral vacuum measurements has shown that milk flow into the infant's oral cavity occurs when the tongue is lowered and vacuum in the oral cavity is increased (Ramsay *et al.*, 2004). In addition, the absence of lactiferous sinuses further emphasizes the critical nature of milk ejection for successful milk transfer, as it is well documented that only small amounts of milk are available prior to the stimulation of milk ejection (Kent *et al.*, 2003; Ramsay *et al.*, 2004). Milk removal during a milk ejection period should be optimized, as milk ejection is a discrete event. Ultrasound imaging of both the non-suckled and the non-expressed breast has shown the milk duct to increase to accommodate milk flow, then reduce in diameter with the reversal of milk flow (back into the breast) (Ramsay *et al.*, 2004). Similarly, milk flow during pumping has been shown to increase to a peak and then decrease during milk ejection (Ramsay *et al.*, 2006). It then follows that interruption of milk removal during milk ejection will result in a reduction of the amount of milk removed. The reversal of milk flow within the breast in the second half of milk ejection has important implications with regard to mastitis, as any pathogens gaining access to the ducts in the nipple would be effectively distributed into the glandular tissue by this backward flow in the unsuckled breast. Therefore, the anatomical integrity of the opening of the ducts to the surface of the nipple must be of considerable importance in protecting against mastitis.

HISTOLOGY OF THE BREAST

The histology of the human lactating breast has not been studied in depth as evidenced by the scarcity of data compared to that of the non-lactating breast and animal models.

This is due to both ethical considerations and frequency in acquiring tissue from a lactating breast and is illustrated in Linzell's work on myoepithelial cells (1952) in which he was able to obtain only two tissue samples from lactating women as opposed to 26 samples from lactating cats.

Lactocyte

The alveolus consists of a continuous single layer of lactocytes (secretory epithelial cells) that secrete milk. The lactocytes are cuboidal/columnar in shape and are coupled by several specialized cell junctions, such as tight junctions. The tight junctions do not allow the passage of substances external to the alveolus during established lactation, but are 'leaky' in the non-lactating and pregnant breast (Peaker & Linzell, 1983). This is demonstrated by the low levels of lactose detected in colostrum during pregnancy and lactogenesis I compared to significantly higher levels during lactogenesis II. Thus, increased levels of lactose in the milk reflect tight junction closure (Arthur *et al.*, 1989). The portion of the lactocyte directed towards the lumen of the alveoli is termed apical and the outer portion, basal. Microvilli project from the apical surface of the cell into the alveolar lumen, presumably to increase surface area of the cell, although this has not been confirmed. Milk secretion occurs at the apical surface of the lactocyte where the basal surface is involved in the uptake of substrates from the blood that are necessary for the production of milk components (Pitelka & Hamamoto, 1983). Increased intra-alveolar pressure in goats has been shown to flatten lactocytes and decrease milk secretion. This decrease was reversible, but not attributable to other factors expected to decrease milk secretion, such as restricted blood flow, decreased suckling frequency, or the presence of a feed-back inhibitor in the milk (Fleet & Peaker, 1978; Peaker, 1980). One might speculate from these findings that women experiencing engorgement may exhibit a transient decrease in milk production.

Myoepithelial Cells

The monolayer of lactocytes that comprise the alveolus are surrounded by myoepithelial cells that also extend onto the milk ducts. These cells contain smooth muscle filaments and their appearance differs depending on their location. The myoepithelial cells that surround the alveoli are stellate shaped, where those associated with ducts are spindle shaped and aligned in a longitudinal manner (Richardson, 1948; Linzell, 1952). The first evidence that myoepithelial cells are contractile was provided by Richardson (1949) who showed structural differences in the cells when the alveoli and ducts were distended compared to when they were contracted. The myoepithelial cells are devoid of innervation and contraction is effected by the hormone oxytocin (Linzell, 1955). Stimulation of the nipple elicits neural impulses that cause oxytocin to be released from supraoptic and paraventricular nuclei of the hypothalamus into the blood stream. There is a rich vascular complex in close contact with the myoepithelial cells. Thus, it is assumed that oxytocin reaches most alveoli almost simultaneously (Linzell, 1952). The contraction of the myoepithelial cells forces milk into the ducts towards the nipple so that either the infant or the breast pump can easily remove the milk.

Oxytocin causes contraction of the alveoli by binding to a receptor (OTR) on the myoepithelial cell. While there is an increase in OTR in the uterus before birth, a parallel increase in the breast has not been clearly established in humans. On the other hand, the lactating breast is highly sensitive to oxytocin with only minute amounts (1 mU) required to elicit milk ejection (Cobo *et al.*, 1967). Interestingly, a recent study has found OTR in the ductal and glandular epithelium, leading to speculation that oxytocin may have multiple physiological effects in the breast other than myoepithelial cell contraction (Kimura *et al.*, 1998).

Basal Lamina

A thin smooth layer of epithelial secretions, termed the basal lamina, delineates the epithelium from the connective tissue matrix and appears to act as a boundary to all cells apart from leucocytes. It is comprised of substances that seem to assist morphogenesis of the breast and proliferation of the epithelial cells (Pitelka & Hamamoto, 1983).

Milk Ducts

The milk ducts form the pathway for milk to be transported to the nipple and do not actively participate in either the secretion or modification of milk. Ducts consist of an inner layer of epithelium, which is stratified squamous type in the nipple and cuboidal type within the gland. An outer layer of myoepithelial cells surrounds the epithelium, and the main ducts are supported further by fibrous connective tissue. As with the alveoli, the shape of the ducts varies according to the amount of milk, appearing more irregular when containing less milk (Pitelka & Hamamoto, 1983).

Adipose Cells

Study of the adipocytes (fat cells) of the breast has not been vigorously pursued despite an indication that changes in the cells during pregnancy and lactation may contribute nutrients to the lactocytes of the mammary glands of mice (Bartley *et al.*, 1981). Some remarkable research has shown that adipocytes are transformed into lactocytes during pregnancy in mice and these lactocytes revert back to adipocytes during the involution phase (Morroni *et al.*, 2004). These results further highlight the need for investigation into the function of the adipocyte in the mammary gland.

CONCLUSION

As recognized by Cooper (1840), a thorough understanding of both the anatomy, histology, and the physiology of the breast provides a solid foundation upon which to investigate and treat women and infants experiencing breastfeeding difficulties. In this vein, it is encouraging that more research into the anatomy of the breast is now being performed, thus increasing the body of knowledge upon which to practice.

ACKNOWLEDGEMENT

Research funding from Medela AG.

References

Aljazaf KMNH. *Ultrasound imaging in the analysis of the blood supply and blood flow in the human lactating breast.* Thesis: The University of Western Australia; 2005.

American Society of Plastic Surgeons. *Cosmetic surgery quick facts: 2005 ASAPS statistics.* January 3, 2000. Available from: http://www.smartplasticsurgery.com/surgery/statistics.html#STATS2005.

Anson BJ, Wright RR, Wolfer JA. Blood supply of the mammary gland. *Surg Gynecol Obstet.* 1939; 69:468-73.

Aukland K, Reed RK. Interstitial lymphatic mechanisms in the control of extracellular fluid volume. *Physiol Rev.* 1993; 73:1-78.

Arthur PG, Smith M, Hartmann PE. Milk lactose, citrate and glucose as markers of lactogenesis in normal and diabetic women. *J Pediatr Gastroenterol Nutr.* 1989; 9:488-96.

Australian Bureau of Statistics 2001. *Breastfeeding in Australia, 2001.* (Online) 2003. Available from: http://www.abs.gov.au/Ausstats/abs@.nsf525a1b9402141235ca25682000146ab8e65d6253e10f802ca256da40003a07c!OpenDocument#2.%20BREASTFEEDING%20PRACTICES%20IN%20AUS.

Bannister LH, Berry MM, Collins P, Dyson M, Dussek JE. *Gray's anatomy.* 38th Ed. New York: Churchill Livingston; 1995. p. 417-24.

Borgstein PJ, Meijer S, Pijpers R. Intradermal blue dye to identify the sentinel node biopsy in breast cancer: echoes from the past and the periareolar blue method. *Ann Surg.* 2000; 232:81-89.

Bartley JC, Emerman JT, Bissell MJ. Metabolic cooperativity between epithelial cells and adipocytes of mice. *Am J Physiol.* 1981; 241:c204-8.

Burd LI, Dorin M, Philipose V, Lemons J. The relationship of mammary temperature to parturition in human subjects. *Am J Obstet Gynecol.* 1977; 128:272-78.

Cardeonosa G, Eklund GW. Ductography. In: Dershaw DD. *Interventional breast procedures.* New York: Churchill Livingstone; 1996.

Chen Z, Wu AH, Gauderman J, Bernstein L, Ma H, Pike MC, *et al.* Does mammographic density reflect ethnic differences in breast cancer incidence rates? *Am J Epidem.* 2004; 159:140-47.

Christensen K, Nielsen MO, Bauer R, Hilden K. Evaluation of mammary blood flow measurements in lactating goats using the ultrasound Doppler principle. *Comp Biochem Physiol.* 1989; 92A:385-92.

Cooper AP. *Anatomy of the breast.* London: Longman, Orme, Green, Browne and Longmans; 1840.

Cosmetic Surgery Consultants. *Recent cosmetic surgery statistics 2005.* Available from: http://www.cosmeticsurgeryconsultants.co.uk/recent-surgery-of-2005.htm

Courtiss EH, Goldwyn RM. Breast sensation before and after plastic surgery. *Plast Reconstr Surg.* 1976; 58:1-13.

Coward WA, Paul AA, Prentice AM. The impact of malnutrition on human lactation: observations from community studies. *Fed Proc.* 1984; 43:2432-37.

Cowie AT. Overview of the mammary gland. *J Invest Dermatol.* 1974; 63:2-9.

Cowie AT, Forsyth IA, Hart IC. *Hormonal control of lactation.* New York: Springer-Verlag; 1980.

Cox DB, Kent JC, Casey TM, Owens RA, Hartmann PE. Breast growth and the urinary excretion of lactose during human pregnancy and early lactation: endocrine relationships. *Exp Physiol.* 1999; 84:421-34.

Craig RD, Sykes PA. Nipple sensitivity following reduction mammaplasty. *Br J Plast Surg.* 1970; 23:165.

Cregan MD, Fan YP, Appelbee A, Brown ML, Klopcic B, Koppen J, *et al.* Identification of nestin positive putative mammary stem cells in human breastmilk. *Cell Tissue Res.* 2007; [in press].

Cruz-Korchin N, Korchin L, Gonzalez-Keelan C, Climent C, Morales I. Macromastia. How much of it is fat? *Plas Reconstr Surg.* 2002; 109:64-68.

Cunningham L. The anatomy of the arteries and veins of the breast. *J Surg Oncol.* 1977; 9:71-85.

Davis SR, Garr VC, Prosser CG. Dose dependent effects of oxytocin on the microcirculation in the mammary gland in the rat. In: Wilde CJ, Peaker M, Knight CH (eds.). *Intercellular signalling in the mammary gland.* New York: Plenum Press; 1995.

Doughty JC, McCarter DHA, Kane E, Reid AW, Cooke TG, McArdle CS. Anatomical basis of intra-arterial chemotherapy for patients with locally advanced breast cancer. *Br J Surg.* 1996; 83:1128-30.

Elias JJ, Pitelka DR, Armstrong RC. Changes in fat cell morphology during lactation in the mouse. *Anat Rec.* 1973; 177:533-47.

Eriksson M, Lundeberg T, Uvnas-Moberg K. Studies on cutaneous blood flow in the mammary gland of lactating rats. *Acta Physiologic Scandinavica.* 1996; 158:1-6.

Farina, MA, Newby BG, Alani HM. Innervation of the nipple-areola complex. *Plast Reconstr Surg.* 1980; 66:497.

Fleet IR, Peaker M. Mammary function and its control at the cessation of lactation in the goat. *Journal of Physiology.* 1978; 279:491-507.

Freeman JL, Walker EP, Wilson JSP, Shaw HJ. The vascular anatomy of the pectoralis major myocutaneous flap. *Br J Plas Surg.* 1981; 34:3-10.

Going JJ, Moffat D. Escaping from Flatland: clinical and biological aspects of human mammary duct anatomy in three dimensions. *J Pathol.* 2004; 203:538-44.

Gonzalez F, Brown FE, Gold ME, Walton RL, Shafer B. Preoperative and postoperative nipple-areola sensibility in patients undergoing reduction mammaplasty. *Plast Reconstr Surg.* 1993; 92:809.

Greendale GA, Palla SL, Ursin G, Laughlin GA, Crandall C, Pike MC, *et al.* The association of endogenous sex steroids and sex steroid binding proteins with mammmographic density: results from the Postmenopausal Estrogen/Progestin Interventions Mammographic Density Study. *Am J Epidemol.* 2005; 162:826-34.

Hartmann PE, Kulski JK. Changes in the composition of the mammary secretion of women after abrupt termination of breast feeding. *J Physiol (Lond.).* 1978; 275:1-11.

Hartmann PE. The breast and breast-feeding In: Philipp EE, Setchell M, Ginsburg J. *Scientific foundations of obstetrics and gynaecology.* 4th Ed. Boston: Oxford:Butterworth Heinemann; 1991.

Hartmann PE, Ramsay DT. Mammary anatomy and physiology. In: Jones E. *Feeding and nutrition in the preterm infant.* London: Elsevier, Churchill and Livingston; 2005. p. 53 - 68.

Heggie JCP. Survey of doses in screening mammography. *Australas Phys Eng Sci Med.* 1996; 19:207-16.

Henderson JJ, Simmer K, Newnham JP, Doherty DA, Hartmann PE. Impact of very preterm delivery on the timing of lactogenesis II in women. *Proceedings of the 12th International Conference of the International Society for Research in Human Milk and Lactation (ISRHML).* September 10 - 14, 2004. Queens' College, Cambridge, UK; 2004. p.80.

Hovey RC, Trott JF, Vonderhaar BK. Establishing a framework for the functional mammary gland: from endocrinology to morphology. *J Mamm Gland Biol Neoplasia.* 2002; 7:7-37.

Hurst NM. Lactation after augmentation mammoplasty. *Obstet Gynecol.* 1996; 87:30-34.

Jamal N, Ng KH, McLean D, Looi LM, Moosa F. Mammographic breast glandularity in malaysian women: data derived from radiography. *Am J Roentgenol.* 2004; 182:713-17.

Janbu T, Koss KS, Thoresen M, Wesche J. Blood velocities to the female breast during lactation and following oxytocin injection. *J Dev Physiol.* 1985; 7:373-80.

Johansson AS, Wennborg H, Blomquist L, Isacson D, Kylberg E. Breastfeeding after mammaplasty and augmentation mammaplasty. *Epidemiology.* 2003; 14(1):127-29.

Kelly PA, Bachelot A, Kedzia C, Hennighausen L, Ormandy CJ, Kopchick JJ, *et al.* The role of prolactin and growth hormone in mammary development. *Mol Cell Endocrinol.* 2002; 197:127-31.

Kent JC, Mitoulas LR, Cox DB, Owens RA, Hartmann PE. Breast volume and milk production during extended lactation in women. *Exp Physiol.* 1999; 84: 435-47.

Kent JC, Ramsay DT, Doherty D, Larsson M, Hartmann PE. Response of breasts to different stimulation patterns of an electric breast pump. *J Hum Lact.* 2003; 19:179-87.

Klein R, Aichinger H, Dierker J, Jansen JT, Joite-Barfuss S, Sabel M, *et al.* Determination of average glandular dose with modern mammography units for two large groups of patients. *Phys Med Biol.* 1997; 42:651-71.

Lawrence RA, Lawrence RM. Weaning. In: Lawrence RA, Lawrence RM. *Breastfeeding: a guide for the medical profession.* Missouri, USA: Mosby Inc.; 1999. p. 341.

Linzell JL. Mammary gland blood flow and oxygen, glucose and volatile fatty acid uptake in the conscious goat. *J Physiol.* 1960; 153:492-509.

Linzell JL, Peaker M. The permability of mammary ducts. *J Physiol.* 1971; 216(3):701-16.

Linzell JL. Some observations of the contractile tissue of the mammary glands. *J Physiol.* 1955; 130:257-267.

Linzell JL. The silver staining of myoepithelial cells, particularly the mammary gland, and their relation to the ejection of milk. *J Anat.* 1952; 86:49-57.

Love SM, Barsky SH. Anatomy of the nipple and breast ducts revisited. *Cancer.* 2004; 101:1947-57.

Maliniac JW. Arterial blood supply of the breast: revised anatomic data relating to reconstructive surgery. *Arch Surg.* 1943; 47:329-43.

McCann MF, Bender DE. Perceived insufficient milk as a barrier to optimal infant feeding: examples from Bolivia. *J Biosoc Sci.* 2006; 38(3): 341-64.

Moffat DF, Going JJ. Three dimensional anatomy of complete duct systems in the human breast: pathological and developmental implications. *J Clin Pathol.* 1996; 49:48-52.

Montagna W, McPherson EE. Some neglected aspects of the anatomy of human breasts. *J Invest Dermatol.* 1974; 63:10.

Morroni M, Giordano A, Zingaretti MC, Boiani R, De Matteis R, Kahn BB, *et al.* Reversible transdifferentiation of secretory epithelial cells into adipocytes in the mammary gland. *Proc Natl Acad Sci USA.* 2004; 101:16801-6.

Morton JA. The role of the pediatrician in extended breastfeeding of the preterm infant. *Pediatr Ann.* 2003; 32:308-16.

Neifert M, Seacat J, Jobe W. Lactation failure due to inadequate glandular development of the breast. *Pediatrics.* 1985; 76:823-28.

Neifert M, DeMarzo S, Seacat J, Young D, Leff M, Orleans M. The influence of breast surgery, breast appearance and pregnancy-induced breast changes on lactation sufficiency as measured by infant weight gain. *BIRTH.* 1990; 17:31-38.

Nickell WB, Skelton J. Breast fat and fallacies: More than 100 years of anatomical fantasy. *J Hum Lact.* 2005; 21(2):126-30.

Ohtake T, Kimijima I, Fukushima T, Yasuda M, Sekikawa K, Takenoshita S, *et al.* Computer assisted complete three-dimensional reconstruction of the mammary ductal/lobular systems. Implications of ductal anastomoses for breast conserving surgery. *Cancer.* 2001; 91(12):2263–72.

Oka T, Yoshimura M, Lavandero S, Wada K, Ohba Y. Control of growth and differentiation of the mammary gland by growth factors. *J Dairy Sci.* 1991; 71:2788-2800.

Panaritis V, Despotidis P, Kyriadidis A. Diameter of mammary terminal ducts as an additional tool in evaluation of women with polycystic ovarium disease. *Arch Gynecol Obstet.* 2004; 270:252-54.

Peaker M. Wilde CJ. Knight CH. Local control of the mammary gland. *Biochem Soc Symp.* 1998; 63:71-79.

Peaker M. Secretion of ions and water. In: Mepham TB (ed.). *Biochemistry of lactation.* Amsterdam: Elsevier Science Publishers; 1983. p.285.

Peaker M. The effect of raised intramammary pressure on mammary function in the goat in relation to the cessation of lactation. *J Physiol.* 1980; 301:415-28.

Pearl SL, Downey HF, Lepper, TL. Intramammary pressure and mammary blood flow in lactating goats. *J Dairy Sci.* 1973; 56(10):1319-23.

Pitelka DR, Hamamoto ST. Ultrastructure of the mammary secretory cell. In: Mepham TB (ed.). *Biochemistry of lacation.* Amsterdam: Elsevier Science Publishers; 1983. p.29.

Prosser CG, Davis SR, Farr VC, Lacasse P. Regulation of blood flow in the mammary microvasculature. *J Dairy Sci.* 1996; 79:1184-97.

Ramsay DT, Mitoulas LR, Kent JC, Hartmann PE. Ultrasound imaging of the sucking mechanics of the breastfeeding infant. *Proceedings of the 12th International Conference of the International Society for Research in Human Milk and Lactation (ISRHML)*; September 10-14, 2004. Queens' College Cambridge, UK. p.53.

Ramsay DT, Kent JC, Owens RA, Hartmann PE. Ultrasound imaging of milk ejection in the breast of lactating women. *Pediatrics.* 2004; 113:361-67.

Ramsay DT, Kent JC, Hartmann RL, Hartmann PE. Anatomy of the lactating human breast redefined with ultrasound imaging. *J Anat.* 2005; 206: 525–34.

Ramsay DT, Mitoulas LR, Kent JC, Cregan MD, Doherty DA, Larsson M, *et al.* Milk flow rates can be used to identify and investigate milk ejection in women expressing breast milk using an electric breast pump. *Breastfeeding Medicine.* 2006; 1:14-23.

Rasmussen KM, Hilson JA, Kjolhede CL. Obesity may impair lactogenesis II. *J Nutr.* 2001; 131:3009S-11S.

Richardson KC. Contractile tissue in the mammary gland, with special reference to the myoepithelium in the goat. *Proc R Soc Biol Sci.* 1949; 136:30-34.

Robinson JE, Short RV. Changes in breast sensitivity at puberty, during the menstrual cycle, and at parturition. *Br Med J.* 1977; 1:1188-91.

Rusby JE, Brachtel EF, Michaelson JS, Koerner FC, Smith BL. Breast duct anatomy in the human nipple: three-dimensional patterns and clinical implications. *Breast Cancer Res Treat.* 2007; [Epub ahead of print].

Russo J, Russo IH. Development of the human breast. *Maturitas.* 2004; 49:2-15.

Russo J, Russo IH. Development of the human mammary gland. In: Neville MC, Daniel CW. *The mammary gland: Development, regulation and function.* New York: Plenum Press; 1987.

Salmon M. Les arteres de la glande mammaire. *Ann Anat Pathol.* 1939; 16:477-500.

Sarhadi NS, Dunn JS, Lee FD, Soutar DS. An anatomical study of the nerve supply of the breast, including the nipple and areola. *Br J Plast Surg.* 1996; 49:156.

Schlenz I, Kuzbari R, Gruber H, Holle J. The sensitivity of the nipple-areola complex: An anatomic study. *Plast Reconstr Surg.* 2000; 105:905-9.

Shackleton M, Vaillant F, Simpson KJ, Stingl J, Smyth GK, Asselin-Labat M, *et al.* Generation of a functional mammary gland from a single stem cell. *Nature.* 2006; 439:84-88.

Soares D, Reid M, James M. Age as a predictive factor of mammographic breast density in Jamaican women. *Clin Radiol.* 2002; 57:472-76.

Sparrow MP, Lamb JP. Ontogeny of airway smooth muscle: structure, innervation, myogenesis and function in the fetal lung. *Respir Physiol Neurobiol.* 2003; 137(2-3):361-72.

Stavros AT. *Breast ultrasound.* Philadelphia:Lippincott Williams and Wilkins; 2004.

Sternlicht MD, Kouros-Mer H, Lu P, Werb Z. Hormonal and local control of mammary branching morphogenesis. *Differentiation.* 2006; 74:365-81.

Strom SS, Baldwin BJ, Sigurdson AJ, Schusterman MA. Cosmetic saline breast implants: A survey of satisfaction, breast-feeding experience, cancer screening, and health. *Plas Reconstr Surg.* 1997; 100:1553-57.

Taneri F, Kurukahvecioglu O, Akyurek N, Tekin EH, Ilhan MN, Cifter C, *et al.* Microanatomy of milk ducts in the nipple. *Eur Surg Res.* 2006; 38:545-49.

Tanis PJ, Nieweg OE, Valdes Olmos RA, Kroon BBR. Anatomy and physiology of lymphatic drainage of the breast from the perspective of sentinel node biopsy. *J Am Coll Surg.* 2001; 192(3):399-409.

Thoresen M, Wesche J. Doppler measurements of changes in human mammary and uterine blood flow during pregnancy and lactation. *Acta Obstet Gynecol Scand.* 1988; 67:741-45.

Tobon H, Salazar H. Ultrastructure of the human mammary gland. II. Postpartum lactogenesis. *J Clin Endocrinol Metab.* 1975; 40:834-44.

Turner-Warwick, RT. The lymphatics of the breast. *Br J Surg.* 1959; 46:574-82.

Venta LA, Dudiak CM, Salomon CG, Flisak MI. Sonographic evaluation of the breast. *Radiographics.* 1994; 14:29-50.

Visvader JE, Lindeman GJ. Mammary stem cells and mammopoiesis. *Cancer Res.* 2006; 66:9798-801.

Vorherr H. *The breast: Morphology, physiology and lactation.* London: Academic Press; 1974.

Weichselbaum M, Sparrow MP, Hamilton EJ, Thompson PJ, Knight DA. A confocal microscopic study of solitary pulmonary neuroendocrine cells in human airway epithelium. *Respir Res.* 2005; 6:115.

Wilson-Clay B, Hoover K. *The breastfeeding atlas.* 3rd Ed. Manchaca, Texas, USA: LactNew Press; 2005. p. 102.

Woolridge MW. The 'anatomy' of infant sucking. *Midwifery.* 1986; 2(4):164-71.

Wysolmerski JJ, McCaughern-Carucc JF, Daifotis AJ, Broadus AE, Philbrick WM. Over expression of parathyroid hormone related protein and parathyroid hormone in transgenic mice impairs branching morphogenesis during mammary gland development. *Development.* 1995; 121:3530-47.

Chapter 3

The Histology and Cytology of the Human Mammary Gland and Breastmilk

Clare A. Berry, Elizabeth C. Thomas, Kristin M. E. Piper, and Mark D. Cregan

THE LACTATION CYCLE

In the sexually mature human female, the mammary gland is capable of undergoing repeated cycles of cellular proliferation, differentiation, and apoptosis (physiological cell death) for each pregnancy and subsequent lactation (Liu *et al.*, 2005). To this end, the human mammary gland comprises a range of cell types to meet the structural and synthetic capabilities of the organ. These cell types include cells of an epithelial lineage that constitute a branched ductal network (ductal epithelial cells) and the cells synthesizing and secreting breastmilk (lactocytes), in addition to the myoepithelial cells involved in milk ejection and the respective tissue-specific stem cells necessary for maintaining these cell populations. Depending upon the stage of the lactation cycle, the presence of each population differs, such that in the virgin and post-lactation gland, the ductal epithelial cells are the predominant cell types, whereas during lactation, the lactocytes and myoepithelial cells are more abundant.

MAMMARY GLAND GROWTH AND DEVELOPMENT

Mammogenesis refers to the development of the mammary gland, beginning in embryonic development and extending beyond the initiation of lactation. The developing embryo consists of three germ cell layers - the ectoderm (the outermost layer), mesoderm (the middle layer), and endoderm (the innermost layer), with the mammary gland evolving from the ectoderm and mesoderm (Hovey *et al.*, 2002). The structure of the mammary gland develops by the cells of the ectodermal area on the ventral surface multiplying and differentiating to form a ridge (four weeks gestation) that further develops into mammary discs (five weeks gestation), followed by the appearance of mammary

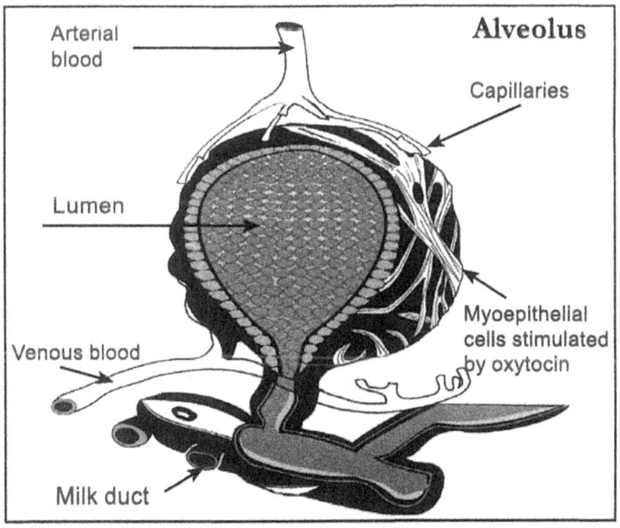

Figure 1. Structure of an alveolus. A layer of lactocytes line each alveolus before merging into the ducts. Also visible is a thin network of contractile myoepithelial cells surrounding each alveoli that upon stimulation by the hormone oxytocin contract to eject milk through the ducts to the suckling infant. The capillary network supplies nutrients and substrates to the lactocytes of the alveoli required for the synthesis of breastmilk. Adapted from Vorherr, 1974.

buds (eight weeks of gestation or when the embryo has a crown rump length of 31-42 mm) (Russo & Russo, 2004). Between weeks 13-20 in gestation, the parenchyma of the mammary buds branches giving rise to 15-25 solid cords (Hovey *et al.*, 2002). These structures will eventually become lactiferous ducts. The mass of luminal cells requires apoptosis in the center to give the ducts their hollow appearance, which is preceded by polarization of cellular compartments (Debnath *et al.*, 2002). It is hypothesized that the central luminal cells that lack the basement membrane contact cannot utilize Akt-mediated cell survival signal (Debnath *et al.*, 2002). It is also important to note that apoptosis in the center of these cords allows them to take on their hollowed feature that will ultimately be able to accommodate breastmilk.

In the newborn infant, hollowing of the ducts has been completed, except for a solid core of mammary stem cells at the terminal end bud that upon the hormonal stimulation of puberty and pregnancy will further grow and develop. Until puberty, growth of the mammary gland remains isometric (Lamote *et al.*, 2004).

At puberty, females release cyclical patterns of follicle stimulating hormone (FSH) and luteinizing hormone (LH) that act upon the ovaries to synthesize estrogen and progesterone, stimulating mammary gland proliferation. This development of the mammary gland occurs by the elongation and branching of the ductal system from the terminal end bud into the mammary fat pad. The primary hormone involved in mammary development during adolescent development is estrogen (Sternlicht *et al.*, 2006).

During pregnancy, the mammary gland enters the final phase of development under the control of hormones that accelerate the growth as pregnancy develops. During this stage of mammogenesis, numerous hormones are involved in the differentiation of the mammary gland to prepare it for lactation, including estrogen, progesterone, prolactin, growth hormone, epidermal growth factor, fibroblast growth factor, human placental lactogen, and parathyroid hormone related protein (Wysolmerski *et al.*, 1995; Horseman, 1999; Dunbar *et al.*, 2001; Kelly *et al.*, 2002; Lamote *et al.*, 2004). These hormones allow the extensive branching of ductal regions, the development of numerous alveoli, and the preparation and initiation of the secretory epithelial cells to produce and secrete milk components.

LOBULE DEVELOPMENT

The lobules are clusters of alveoli that comprise the lactocyte population which synthesize and secrete milk during lactation. The development of the lobules themselves can be broken down into four stages: lobule types 1-4. During puberty, hormonal increases of ovarian estrogen and progesterone target the mammary cells to initiate the formation of the terminal duct and the sprouting ductules that make up the first identifiable lobule, lobule type 1 (Lob 1) or the terminal ductule lobular unit (TDLU). Lob 1 is represented in highest proportions and remains constant throughout life in nulliparous women (Russo & Russo, 2004). Extra hormonal stimulation during estrus cycling in women results in the formation of more differentiated lobules. Lobules type 2 (Lob 2) are characterized by an increase in ductal sprouting and alveolar development, with lobules type 3 (Lob 3) showing even more development in the ductal and alveolar regions than Lob 2. Lob 1-3 are seen in normally cycling non-pregnant women with Lob 2 and Lob 3 containing approximately 47 and 80 lobules, respectively (Russo & Russo, 2004). During pregnancy, maximum development of the lobules takes place due to higher levels of circulating estrogen and progesterone, leading to increases in ductal branching and cellular proliferation, resulting in higher proportions of Lob 3. Once the alveolar epithelial cells become secretory, the mammary gland is at its most developed and Lobule type 4 (Lob 4) can be identified, which is characterized by high densities of alveolar structures and extensive ductal branching.

THE CELLS OF THE MAMMARY GLAND

Ductal Epithelial Cells

Ductal epithelial cells line the luminal interface of the ducts (**Figure 1**). These cells display a cuboidal morphology with an enlarged nucleus typical of epithelial lineages (Toban & Salazar, 1974) and are connected by intercellular tight junctions to form a continuous lining of the inner walls of the milk ducts (Brooker 1980). The ductal epithelium is the most common site of neoplastic transformation that leads to mammary carcinoma in situ (Sternlicht *et al.*, 2006).

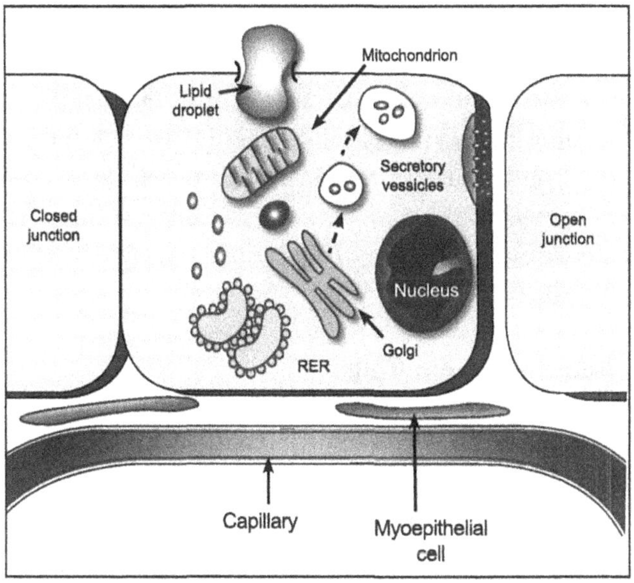

Figure 2. Illustration of a typical cuboidal lactocyte including large nuclei, rough endoplasmic reticulum, and other cellular components.

Alveoli and Secretory Epithelial Cells

The secretory epithelial cells that comprise the alveoli are also known as lactocytes as they have the ability to secrete milk components during lactation. Depending upon the fullness of the alveoli, lactocytes are cuboidal (in full alveoli) to columnar (in empty alveoli) in appearance and line the lumen of the alveoli (Toban & Salazar, 1974). During lactation, intercellular tight junctions connect adjacent lactocytes to form a continuous, selectively permeable epithelial layer (Nguyen & Neville, 1998) (**Figure 2**). The presence of tight junctions enables the lactocytes to actively regulate the composition of breastmilk, in that the constituents of breastmilk are synthesized and secreted by these cells or are selectively and actively transported into the lumen from the circulation.

Typical to all secretory epithelium, lactocytes are characterized by a polarized morphology. At the basal margin, these cells are attached to a laminin/integrin-rich extracellular matrix called the basement membrane. Internally, the basal pole of the lactocyte contains the nucleus and is also an area rich in rough endoplasmic reticulum (Flint & Gardner, 1994). Abundant secretory vesicles appear internally at the apical pole of the lumen, while microvilli and a high concentration of dispersed fat globules and protein aggregates are visible on the apical membrane (Brooker, 1980).

The interaction of lactocytes with the underlying extracellular matrix is an important factor regulating milk protein gene expression, acting concurrently with endocrine and autocrine mechanisms to regulate the synthesis and secretion of milk (Bawden & Nicholas, 1999; Streuli & Gilmore, 1999). This interaction with the extracellular matrix is dictated by the stresses placed upon the cytoskeleton of the lactocyte by the distension of the alveoli during milk accumulation. Indeed, in vitro studies of mice secretory epithelial cells have shown that the cell shape (dictated by the stresses placed upon the cytoskeleton) influences the ability of prolactin to activate milk protein gene expression (Streuli *et al.*, 1995). Where the adhesive substrata were similar to that of the basement membrane, normal milk protein gene expression was seen. However, on non-adhesive substrata, the morphology of the cells became rounded, resembling the cuboidal cells seen in distended alveoli, thereby indicating that the change in cell shape observed in full alveoli may be a consequence of a change in binding to the basement membrane.

Among the lactocyte population, the mechanism by which cell shape can influence the expression of milk protein genes has been suggested to involve integrins. Integrins are a family of heterodimeric transmembrane receptors that mediate interactions between cells and the extracellular matrix (Streuli & Edwards, 1998). One such adhesion complex involves laminin that is required for prolactin to induce phosphorylation of its receptor, which in turn triggers an intracellular signalling cascade that ultimately results in transcription of milk protein genes. The binding of laminin to integrin is dictated by the stresses placed upon the cytoskeleton, thereby providing a mechanism by which the cell shape and thus degree of alveolar fullness can control the synthesis of milk proteins (Streuli & Edwards, 1998).

Myoepithelial Cells

The myoepithelial cells form an irregular network surrounding the alveoli at the basement membrane interface. In response to the suckling infant activating mechanoreceptors in the nipple, the hormone oxytocin is released and acts upon the myoepithelial cells causing them to contract around the alveoli thereby ejecting milk out of the lumen and along the ducts to the feeding infant (Neville *et al.*, 1983). The myoepithelial cells are attached to the basement membrane by hemidesmosomes and to the apposing luminal epithelia by desmosomes (Flint & Gardner, 1994). They display an irregular smooth muscle-like morphology, with

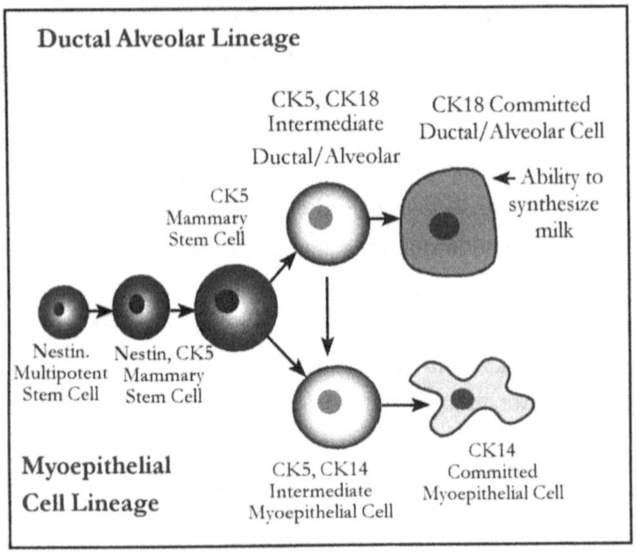

Figure 3. The expression of the intracellular markers found in mammary stem cells and terminally differentiated mammary epithelial cells. These markers can be used to identify the differentiation status of the various cells of the mammary gland.

characteristic pinocytic vesicles containing dense bodies and microfilaments (Lakhani & O'Hare, 2001).

Identifying Cells of the Mammary Gland: The Use of Intracellular Markers

Cytokeratins (CK) are intermediate filaments expressed in all epithelial tissues (Bosch *et al.*, 1988) and have been shown to be differentially expressed in mammary epithelia dependent upon the differentiation status of the cell (Lendahl *et al.*, 1990) (**Figure 3**). Expression of CK5 in the absence of other cytokeratins is indicative of mammary progenitor cells (Dahlstrand *et al.*, 1992; Sting *et al.*, 1998; Boecker & Buerger, 2003; Dontu *et al.*, 2003). Co-expression of CK5 with a mature epithelial cell marker, such as CK14 or CK18, has been characterized as an intermediary epithelial cell, with those co-expressing CK18 being intermediary epithelial cells of ductal and alveolar (glandular) lineage, while those co-expressing CK14 being intermediary cells of myoepithelial lineage (Boecker & Buerger, 2003). Further, cells expressing one of CK14, CK18, and CK19 are characteristic of mature, terminally differentiated mammary epithelial cells (Neville & Daniel, 1987; Toma *et al.*, 2001; Zulewski *et al.*, 2001; Gudjonsson *et al.*, 2002). Sole expression of CK14 is considered representative of a mature myoepithelial cell, and CK18 of a glandular cell. While CK19 is accepted to be expressed in the glandular compartment of the mammary epithelium, it remains to be determined whether CK19 is expressed solely in the intermediary or mature glandular cells or whether it is present throughout the stages of differentiation. Recently, the stem cell marker nestin has been utilized to identify putative mammary stem cells in human breastmilk (Cregan *et al.*, 2007) enabling a proposed differentiation pathway of mammary stem cells to be described.

Mammary Stem Cells

Stem cells are multipotent, cycling cells that divide to generate differentiated, functional tissues. Almost all adult tissues have been shown to have a committed stem cell population. Adult stem cells divide asymmetrically to give rise to two daughter cells, one that is committed to terminal differentiation and one that maintains the stem cell population. Most regenerating tissues are characterized by self-renewing cells at different stages of differentiation from stem cells to terminally differentiated, non-cycling cells. A stem cell population has been identified in the human mammary gland and has been shown to give rise to all three epithelial cell types characteristic of the fully differentiated gland (Shackleton *et al.*, 2006). The onset of gestation sees mass clonal expansion of the stem cell population of the resting gland, which respond to ovarian and lactogenic hormones to differentiate into the lobulo-alveolar units of the competent secretory tissue. As terminally differentiated cells have exited the cell-cycle and are by definition incapable of self-renewal, generation of healthy tissue relies on maintenance of the stem cell population. As the mammary gland undergoes massive proliferation and self-renewal during puberty, pregnancy, and lactation, it is logical to presume this process is mediated by mammary stem cells (Shackleton *et al.*, 2006).

Many studies have explored the notion of stem or progenitor cell populations within the mammary gland. This has been illustrated in studies involving mice, where a single mammary stem cell has been transplanted into the cleared fat pads of mice, producing a fully functional mammary gland (Shackleton *et al.*, 2006). A stem/progenitor cell population has also been examined via the use of mammary tissue sections (Dontu *et al.*, 2003), illustrating a side population of cells defined by the exclusion of Hoechst dye, as well as the ability of some cells to self-renew and undergo differentiation when stimulated appropriately. Human work on stem cells isolated from the mammary gland has been restricted to the use of biopsy tissue or that isolated from breast reduction mammoplasty. These studies utilized cytokeratin (CK) markers to identify mammary stem cells of different lineages. Consistent among all these studies on mammary stem cells is that when cultured a heterogenous population of stem and differentiated cells is observed, as defined by the CK markers.

Recent studies have utilized immunofluorescence and RT-PCR in the characterization of the presence of cytokeratins in cells isolated and cultured from human breastmilk (Cregan *et al.*, 2007). Primary monolayer cultures of cells isolated from human breastmilk have been shown to differentially express cytokeratins 5, 14, 18, and 19, in addition to the stem cell marker nestin, highlighting the heterogenous nature of the epithelial cells in the mammary gland and also in breastmilk (Cregan *et al.*, 2007). This study shows the presence of cells of myoepithelial lineage in primary culture, thus highlighting the ability of mammary progenitor cells to differentiate into both glandular and myoepithelial lineages, particularly as cells of myoepithelial lineage are located on the basal side of the gland (Flint & Gardner, 1994; Lakhani & O'Hare, 2001) and are thus highly unlikely to be exfoliated into breastmilk. This finding supports those of Pechoux *et al.* (1999) who show the ability of epithelial cells with glandular morphology to differentiate into cells exhibiting morphology of cells of myoepithelial origin when exposed to the appropriate environmental stimuli.

HISTOLOGY AND CYTOLOGY OF THE MAMMARY GLAND

The Virgin Mammary Gland

The virgin mammary gland is comprised of undifferentiated structures, Lob 1, and dependent upon the degree of hormonal stimulation during normal hormonal cycling, some individuals display mammary tissue with more differentiated lobular structures - Lob 2 and Lob 3. When viewed as a cross section under a microscope, the lobules in the mammary gland appear as dispersed structures, interwoven with surrounding connective and adipose tissue and lymph nodes (Sternlicht *et al.*, 2006).

The Lactating Mammary Gland

The proliferation of ductal, alveolar, and myoepithelial structures during pregnancy increases the density of mammary gland structures. Further, with the onset of colostrum production in the final trimester of pregnancy (Lactogenesis I), Lob 4 structures fill with milk and thus appear distended, and the alveoli appear as the most dominant structure of the mammary gland. Within these Lob 4 structures, the lactocytes in the mammary gland are present at a high density and produce and secrete milk components into the alveoli. Following the initiation of lactation (Lactogenesis II), these lactocytes secrete breastmilk components into the lumen of the alveoli in a process called exocytosis.

Synthesis and Exocytosis of Major Breastmilk Components

Breastmilk is comprised of a range of macro and micro constituents, including proteins, carbohydrates, lipids, metabolites, and elemental molecules. The primary mechanistic secretion of these constituents is by exocytosis, whereby the constituents are packaged into secretory vesicles and transported to the apical plasma membrane of the secretory cell where fusion takes place, resulting in the expulsion of the contents from the plasma membrane (McManaman & Neville, 2003).

The protein component of breastmilk is either transported from the circulation and secreted into the alveoli or synthesized by the lactocytes from amino acid precursors and exocytosed into the lumen. Proteins transported into breastmilk that derive from the circulation, such as intact immunoglobulins involved in infant immunity, hormones, and growth factors, are recognized by receptors on the basolateral surface of the lactocyte and are endocytosed (ingested) by the secretory cell. Following internalization of the receptor-protein complex, the receptor is cleaved and the protein is secreted into the lumen (Linzell & Peaker, 1971).

Lactose makes up approximately 98% of the carbohydrates in human breastmilk. Lactose is a disaccharide comprised of glucose and galactose joined by a 1,4 β-glycosidic bond that is synthesized in the Golgi secretory vesicle system (Neville *et al.*, 1983). The substrates for lactose synthesis, glucose and UDP-galactose, are transported into the Golgi secretory vesicle system of the lactocyte, and lactose is synthesized by the enzyme, lactose synthase (Neville *et al.*, 1983). Lactose synthase is an enzyme complex consisting of the membrane bound enzyme, β-1,4 galactosyl transferase, and the protein, α-lactalbumin (Nickerson & Akers, 1984). Under normal physiological conditions, galactosyl transferase has a low affinity for glucose; however, by binding α-lactalbumin, the K_m for glucose is lowered and thus the affinity increased, in turn permitting the formation of lactose (Neville *et al.*, 1983). Since the Golgi vesicle is impermeable to lactose, water is drawn in osmotically (Neville *et al.*, 1983), and thus in women, the amount of lactose synthesized largely determines the volume of milk produced (Arthur *et al.*, 1994). The secretory vesicles then migrate towards the apical membrane, facilitated by the presence of microtubules and microfilaments, and eject their contents into the lumen via exocytosis (Nickerson & Akers, 1984).

Apart from being the major osmole in human milk, lactose is a major source of energy for the infant. Indeed, lactose is broken down to glucose and galactose by the brush border enzyme lactase in the intestine that can then be used by the infant. Galactose can be utilized by the brain for energy and is used to make galactolipids (e.g., cerebroside), which are essential for the developing central nervous system (Lawrence & Lawrence, 2005). Furthermore, it has been suggested that lactose improves the absorption of calcium (Riordan & Auerbach, 1993).

The fat content of mature human milk is approximately 38 g/L (Mitoulas, 2000). Fat provides approximately 50% of the energy in milk and assists with the delivery of essential fatty acids and fat-soluble vitamins to the infant (Riordan & Auerbach, 1993). Triacylglycerols are the most abundant class of fat, representing 98-99% of total fat, with the remainder consisting of di- and mono-acylglycerols, free fatty acids, phospholipids, cholesterol, and cholesterol esters (Jensen *et al.*, 1995).

Milk lipids can either be synthesized within the gland or imported from the blood stream, where they are either derived from the immediate diet or from mobilized body fat (Davies *et al.*, 1986). Indeed, the majority of the lipids (80%) found in milk are long chain fatty acids that cannot be synthesized by the lactocytes and have to be imported from the blood (Thompson & Smith, 1985). It has been reported that the differences in fatty acid composition of milk between women from different cultures are due to differences in diet (Jensen, 1989). Therefore, given that the fatty acids of human milk are a very important source of both nutritional and developmental factors to the infant (Jensen, 1989), this output of the diet of the mother appears important in the development of the infant. In this connection, supplementation of the mother's diet with long-chain fatty acids increases these same fatty acids proportionally in the milk (Harris *et al.*, 1984; Makrides *et al.*, 1996). Although more recently, Mitoulas (2000) suggested that supplementation of a particular medium- or long-chain fatty acid may have deleterious affects on others, such that as the proportion of one increases, another decreases. Therefore, any targeted recommendation on dietary supplementation with either medium- or long-chain fatty acids should be undertaken with care.

The earliest intracellular precursors of milk lipid globules appear to form at focal points either in or on the endoplasmic reticulum of lactocytes. The first lipid globule precursors can be seen in the cytoplasm as small droplets (< 0.5 mm diameter) and grow by fusion with each other into cytoplasmic lipid droplets (diameters of >1 mm) (Patton & Keenan, 1975). Lipid droplets are secreted by fusion with the plasma membrane of the lactocyte, becoming surrounded by apical portions of the plasma membrane as they are budded from the cells (Ferguson & Anderson, 1983). This process results in large losses of surface membrane material, which must continually be replaced by the cell (Pitelka, 1988), probably by the Golgi secretory vesicles fusing with the apical membrane during the secretion of lactose and protein.

Metabolites are both intermediate and products of metabolism. Citrate is a metabolite that is synthesized within the mitochondria from glucose and translocated to the cytosol, where it is likely transported into the Golgi apparatus (Zulak & Keenan, 1983). Via exocytosis of the Golgi apparatus, citrate is finally secreted into the alveolar lumen together with lactose (Linzell *et al.*, 1975; Zulak & Keenan, 1983). The role for citrate in human milk remains uncertain. A relationship between citrate and calcium in the milk of women exists between days one and five postpartum (Kent *et al.*, 1992). A calcium concentration of 2-4 mM is required for lactose synthesis (Powell & Brew, 1976). Furthermore, it is suggested that low calcium concentration in the Golgi apparatus could limit the amount of lactose synthesized (Allen & Neville, 1983). Therefore, the role of citrate may be one of maintaining calcium concentration within the Golgi apparatus.

During established lactation, elemental molecules like sodium and potassium usually reach the alveolar lumen via the transcellular pathway. Across the basement membrane lies an active pump that acts to exclude sodium and accumulate potassium (Peaker, 1983). Both the Golgi membrane and the apical membrane are permeable for sodium and potassium (Peaker, 1983). Occasions when sodium and potassium movement into the lumen are not via the transcellular pathway occur during periods when the tight junctions between lactocytes are open, permitting movement of monovalent ions into milk. These include prior to lactogenesis II (Kulski & Hartmann, 1981), during episodes of mastitis (Peaker, 1983; Prosser & Hartmann, 1983), and when there is more than 24 hours of milk accumulation (Hartmann & Kulski, 1978).

The Involuting Mammary Gland

There are two stages of involution: post-lactational involution and involution associated with menopause. During post-lactational involution, the alveolar epithelial cells undergo apoptosis, a form of physiological cell death, and extracellular remodelling (Furth *et al.*, 1997; Sutherland *et al.*, 2007). The accumulation of milk in the alveolar lumen has an inhibitory affect on milk synthesis that results in the alveolar atrophy by the activation of apoptosis and the Janus kinase/signal transducer and activator of transcription (JAK/STAT) pathway (Philp *et al.*, 1996; Li *et al.*, 1997; Watson, 2006; Sutherland *et al.*, 2007). STAT5 is activated by prolactin, which returns to baseline levels at involution and, therefore, no longer provides stimulus for STAT5. Tyrosine phosphorylation of STAT5 isoforms is sharply decreased during involution, showing its potential role in the remodelling of the mammary gland following lactation (Lui *et al.*, 1996). Involution due to aging occurs in menopausal women as a result of declining ovarian function. Ovarian hormones, estrogen and progesterone, that previously targeted the alveolar and ductal cells to proliferate are decreased (Steiner *et al.*, 2003; Wu *et al.*, 2005), causing regression in both the epithelia and stroma (Walker & Martin, 2007). Morphometric studies have shown the amount of epithelial tissue present in the mammary gland to decline steadily from the third decade (Hudson *et al.*, 1985).

CELLS IN BREASTMILK

Human breastmilk has sometimes been referred to as a 'live fluid,' as it contains a heterogeneous population of living cells (**Table 1**). Breastmilk samples fractionated by centrifugation produce a cell isolate made up of immune cells (leukocytes), terminally differentiated ductal and secretory epithelial cells, putative mammary progenitor cells committed to epithelial lineage, and cell fragments. The cellular components of human breastmilk vary between individuals and also with the stage of lactation (Ho *et al.*, 1979; Pitt, 1979; Brooker, 1980; Buescher & Pickering, 1986). This cellular component comprises various types of immune cells that range from 99% of the total cell count at parturition and decrease to eight percent at six months postpartum (Ho *et al.*, 1979; Brooker, 1980). Meanwhile, the epithelial-derived proportion of cells in breastmilk rises from as little as one percent at birth to up to 85% at six months postpartum (Kordon & Smith, 1998). The leukocyte population that is involved in both protecting the breast from infection and passive immunity for the

Table 1. The Cell Types in Human Milk Before and During Lactation

Time	Total	Macrophages	Neutrophils	Lymphocytes	Epithelial
Pre-Partum	3430	2140	360	240	*
Post-Partum					
Days 0-4	2840	1490	1360	250	*
Days 5-8	450	320	93	27	10
Weeks 1-2	69	52	4	1	6
Weeks 2-4	51	4	3	1	8
Months 1-2	17	4	3	1	8
Months 2-4	16	3	2	1	10
Months 4-6	10	1	1	1	9

Adapted from Ho *et al.*, 1979; Pitt, 1979; Brooker, 1980; Hayward, 1983; Buescher & Pickering, 1986; Lawrence & Lawrence, 2005. All values given are cell per µL. *Indicates the content of this cell type in milk was below the detected threshold.

infant consists of approximately 80% neutrophils and 15% macrophages, with the remaining five percent a mixed population of lymphocytes, polymorphonuclear leukocytes, and monocytes (Mohr *et al.*, 1970).

Leukocyte Population

Leukocytes have been shown to be present in small lymphatic vessels surrounding the alveoli (Knight, 1995) and enter into the alveoli by passing between lactocytes via diapedesis (Seelig Jr. & Beer, 1981; Lin *et al.*, 1995). The leukocyte population is primed to play a protective role in the mammary gland (Fetherston *et al.*, 2001), although some of their activities, such as proliferation following stimulation and cytokine secretion, differ from those of blood leukocytes (Filteau, 2001)(**Table 2**). The leukocyte population is made up of lymphocytes, macrophages, and polymorphonuclear leukocytes (Mohr *et al.*, 1970).

Lymphocytes in human milk vary in size from 5-15 μm in diameter (cytospin smears) (Weiss, 1988). Small lymphocytes have a round or slightly indented nucleus without visible nucleoli and are surrounded by a very small rim of cytoplasm (Weiss, 1988). Large lymphocytes have a larger cytoplasm and may have a flattened nucleus (Weiss, 1988). Small quantities of lipids have been found to be present in milk lymphocytes (Richie, 1986; Lawrence & Lawrence, 2005). At all stages of lactation, lymphocytes make up less than 10% of total cell numbers (Richie, 1986; Lawrence & Lawrence, 2005).

Table 2. Proposed Functions of the Immune Cells in Human Breastmilk

Immune Cell	Functions
Macrophage	Kill microbes in baby's gastrointestinal tract. Manufactures lysozyme to destroy bacteria. Activates other immune components. Involved in phagocytosis. Recruits lymphocytes to site of infection.
Neutrophils	Ingests bacteria in baby's gastrointestinal tract. Involved in immune development. Protects mother.
B Lymphocytes	Gives rise to antibodies targeted against specific microbes.
T Lymphocytes	Activated in presence of organisms. Kills infected cells by activating chemical messengers to mobilize other defenses, strengthening the infant immune response.

Adapted from Newman (1995) and Ichikawa *et al.* (2003).

Macrophages have a granular cytoplasm filled with many lipid containing vacuoles and a round to oval nucleus with a distinct nuclear membrane (Papanicolaou *et al.*, 1958). They vary in size from 8-40 μm diameter (cytospin smears) and may have a characteristic foamy appearance due to the presence of large quantities of ingested material (Smith & Goldman, 1968; Lascelles *et al.*, 1969; Ho *et al.*, 1979).

Macrophages account for 30-60% of leukocytes in milk during early lactation (Lascelles *et al.*, 1969; Ho *et al.*, 1979; Pitt, 1979; Lawrence & Lawrence, 2005); however, numbers decrease markedly with progress through lactation (Ho *et al.*, 1979; Brooker, 1980). The milk macrophage is similar to those found in other tissues, in that it can phagocytose and kill bacteria, mediate lymphokine activity, and synthesize inflammatory proteins (Kleinman & Walker, 1979; Pitt, 1979). Macrophages synthesize both specific (e.g., IgA antibodies) and non-specific host resistance factors (e.g., lysozyme) (Ho *et al.*, 1979), and a number of studies have suggested that they may act as a vehicle of immunoglobulin transport into the neonate (Smith & Goldman, 1968; Ho *et al.*, 1979; Buescher & Pickering, 1986; Mandyla & Xanthou, 1986; Lawrence & Lawrence, 2005).

Neutrophils and eosinophils (polymorphonuclear leukocytes) contain multiple nuclear lobes, arranged in a circular fashion around the center of the cell or crowded in the center, and range in size from 12-15 μm (cytospin smears) (Papanicolaou *et al.*, 1958; Weiss, 1988). They often contain fat globules and large cytoplasmic vacuoles may be seen pushing the nucleus to the periphery of the cell (Holmquist & Papanicolaou, 1956; Smith & Goldman, 1968; Ho *et al.*, 1979; Richie, 1986). These cells are found in milk at times when risk of mammary gland infection is high, such as in early lactation, during episodes of mastitis, and during involution (Buescher & Pickering, 1986; Lawrence & Lawrence, 2005).

Epithelial-Derived Populations

The terminally differentiated epithelial population is believed to be derived from the lumen and ducts of the actively secreting gland and are exfoliated from the glandular walls as a result of tortional stress imposed by the constant expansion and contraction of the gland during the filling and emptying cycle associated with milk synthesis and milk removal (Thompson *et al.*, 1998). Secretory epithelial cells are identifiable by the presence of profuse cisternae and rough endoplasmic reticulum, lipid droplets, secretory vesicles, and protein aggregates. Ductal epithelial cells represent less than one percent of the total cell population and are identifiable by the abundant microvilli dispersed across their luminal surface membrane. In some cases, remnants of desmosome and tight junction proteins that connect ductal epithelium in vivo are visible in diametrically opposed positions along the perimeter of the cell (Brooker, 1980; Barraclough & Rudland, 1989). The dominant cellular entity in human breastmilk is cell fragments arising from secretory vesicles and as a product of cellular degradation (Brooker, 1980). In addition to protein aggregates, such as casein micelles, these fragments contribute to a complex environment of cell fragments that significantly confound gross morphological and molecular analysis of specific cell populations in breastmilk. However, recently human breastmilk cell isolates have been demonstrated as an effective, non-invasive source of human mammary epithelial cells for *in vitro* propagation of epithelial primary cultures (Cregan *et al.*, 2007). This represents a powerful tool for studying both lactation and mammary gland biology.

Using electron microscopy, freshly isolated lactocytes can be identified by the prescence of one to two large lipid droplets and a Golgi apparatus producing secretory vesicles containing casein micelles; they are circular with a centrally-offset, prominent nucleus (Brooker, 1980; Pitelka, 1988). Using cytospin smears, the size of lactocytes most commonly range from 15-20 μm (Ho *et al.*, 1979).

Throughout lactation in women, the lactocyte numbers in milk are fairly constant. However, during early lactation, other cell types are greatest in number. As lactation progresses, the numbers of other cell types decline, resulting in the proportion of lactocytes increasing, becoming the predominant cell type at two to three months postpartum (Ho *et al.*, 1979; Pitt, 1979; Brooker, 1980; Buescher & Pickering, 1986; Lawrence & Lawrence, 2005). There is, however, great variation between individuals in the proportion of total cells that are lactocytes, with studies reporting a range between

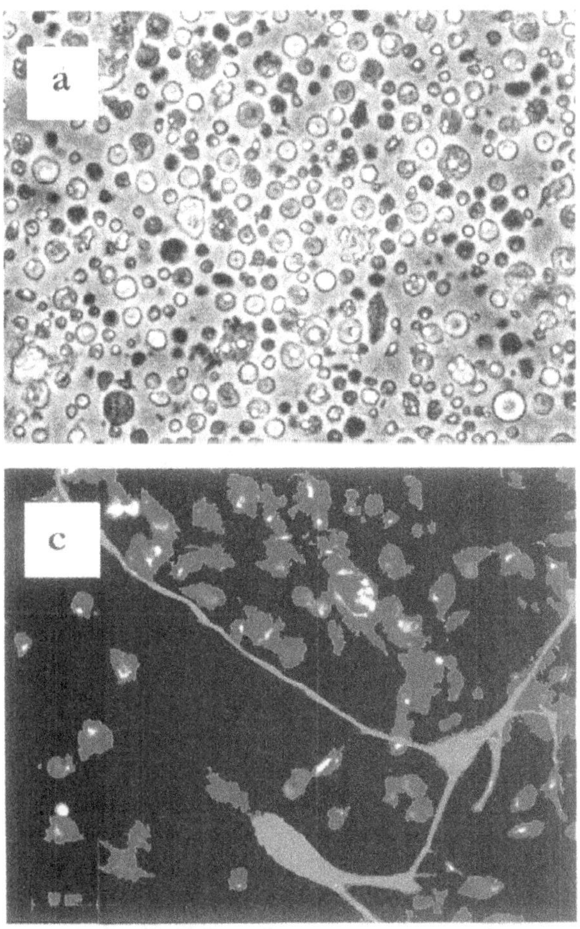

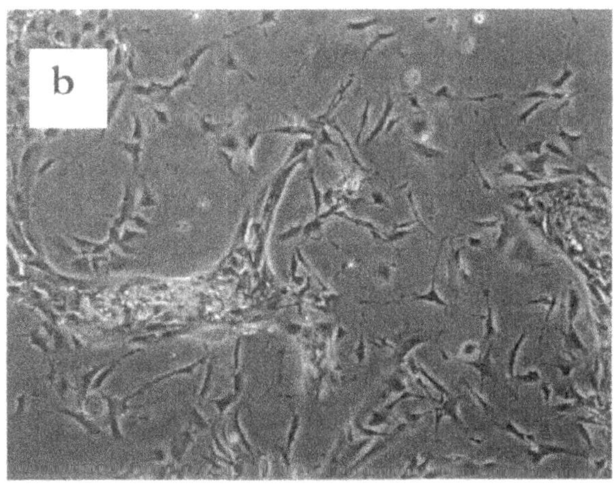

Figure 4. (a) Cell smear of the cells isolated from human breastmilk, (b) breastmilk cells grown in primary culture, and (c) mammary stem cells (Lt. blue/Dk. blue) and differentiated adult mammary cells (gray) isolated from human breastmilk

11% and 99% (Gaffney *et al.*, 1976; Ho *et al.*, 1979; Brooker, 1980).

Mammary Stem Cells From Breastmilk

Cregan *et al.* (2007) have identified that a heterogeneous population of progenitor/stem cells, as well as their differentiated progeny, can be isolated and propagated from expressed human breastmilk (**Figure 4**). By using the CK 5, CK14, CK18, and CK19 markers, in addition to the multipotent stem cell marker - nestin, Cregan *et al.* (2007) were able to show that the cells in breastmilk were positive for both CK5 and nestin, indicating the presence of a multipotent mammary stem cell in human breastmilk. Further, cells grown in culture from primary breastmilk cell isolates were also positive for these markers. Together, these findings indicate the presence of a putative mammary stem cell in breastmilk. Also described was the co-expression of CK5 and CK14, inferring the presence of an intermediate lineage of myoepithelial cells in breastmilk. This discovery of a plentiful source of nestin-positive stem cells from breastmilk provides a useful tool for future analysis of mammary gland development and lactation.

Benefits of the Cellular Components to Infants

Human breastmilk is a highly complex secretion composed of proteins, lipids, carbohydrates, metabolites, and elemental molecules that comprise the bioactive factors that are important for infant nutrition and development and the immune protection of the infant and mammary gland. However, until recently the role of the cellular components of breastmilk in mammary gland immunity and infant development has been overlooked. The role of immune cells in the protection of the mammary gland from infection has been suggested by the presence of activated immune cells in human breastmilk (Wirt *et al.*, 1992). Further, this work also suggests that these activated leukocytes may confer protection to the infant from the pathogens to which they are activated. Radiolabelled human breastmilk leukocytes have been shown to be detected in the circulating blood of infant baboons (Jain *et al.*, 1989). Studies on mice have shown that maternal cells of B-cell lineage can be detected in B-cell deficient offspring (Arvola *et al.*, 2000). These studies demonstrate the possibility that the leukocyte population in breastmilk can diapedese through the wall of the gastrointestinal tract of the infant and confer immune protection. Should such a mechanism be occurring in the human infant, it would clearly demonstrate a unique immunological interaction between the mother and the breastfed infant.

ACKNOWLEDGEMENT

Research funding from Medela AG.

References

Allen JC, Neville MC. Ionized calcium in human milk determined with a calcium-selective electrode. *Clin Chem.* 1983; 29:858-61.

Arthur PG, Kent JC, Hartmann PE. Lactose in blood in nonpregnant, pregnant, and lactating women. *J Pediatr Gastroenterol Nutr.* 1994; 13:254-59.

Arvola M, Gustafsson E, Svensson L, Jansson L, Holmdahl R, Heyman B, *et al.* Immunoglobulin-secreting cells of maternal origin can be detected in b-cell deficient mice. *Biol Reprod.* 2000; 63:1817-24.

Barraclough R, Rudland PS. Differentiation of mammary stem cells in vivo and in vitro. *Environ Health Perspect.* 1989; 80:39-48.

Bawden WS, Nicholas KR. *Molecular aspects of milk production.* New York: Cabi Publishing; 1999.

Boecker W, Buerger H. Evidence of progenitor cells of glandular and myoepithelial cell lineages in the human adult female breast epithelium: A new progenitor (adult stem) cell concept. *Cell Prolif.* 2003; 36(1):33-44.

Bosch FX, Leube RE, Achtstatter Moll R, Franke WW. Expression of simple epithelial type cytokeratins in stratified epithelia as detected by immunolocalization and hybridization in situ. *J Cell Biol.* 1988; 106:1635-48.

Brooker BE. The epithelial cells and cell fragments in human milk. *Cell Tissue Res.* 1980; 210(2):321-32.

Buescher ES, Pickering LK. *Human milk in infant nutrition and health.* Springfield, USA: Thomas Publisher; 1986.

Cregan MD, Applebee A, Brown ML, Klopcic B, Koppen J, Mitoulas LR, *et al.* Identification of nestin-positive putative mammary stem cells in human breastmilk. *Cell Tissue Res.* 2007; 329(1):129-36.

Dahlstrand J, Zimmerman LB, McKay RD. Characterization of the human nestin gene reveals a close revolutionary relationship to neurofilaments. *J Cell Sci.* 1992; 103:589-97.

Davies DT, Holt C, Christie WW. *The biochemistry of lactation.* Amsterdam: Elsevier Science Publishers; 1986.

Debnath J, Mills KR, Colins NL, Reginato MJ, Muthaswamy SK, Brugge JS. The role of apoptosis in creating and maintaining luminal space within normal and ocogene-expressing mammary acini. *Cell.* 2002; 111(4):29-40.

Dontu G, Al-Hajj M, Abdallah WM, Clarke MF, Wicha MS. Stem cells in normal breast development and breast cancer. *Cell Prolif.* 2003; 36 Suppl 1:59-72.

Dunbar ME, Dann P, Brown CW, Van Houton J, Dreyer B, Philbrick WP, *et al.* Temporally regulated overexpression of parathyroid hormone-related protein in the mammary gland reveals distinct fetal and pubertal phenotypes. *J Endocrinol.* 2001; 171:403-16.

Ferguson DJP, Anderson TJ. An ultrastructural study of lactation in the human breast. *Anat Embryol.* 1983; 168: 349-59.

Fetherston CM, Lee CS, Hartmann PE. Mammary gland defense: The role of colostrum, milk and involution secretion. In: *Advances in nutritional research.* New York: Plenum Publishers; 2001.

Filteau SM. Milk components with immunomodulatory potential. In: *Advances in nutritional research.* New York: Plenum Press; 2001.

Flint DJ, Gardner M. Evidence that growth hormone stimulates milk synthesis by direct action on the mammary gland and that prolactin exerts effects on milk secretion by maintenance of mammary deoxyribonucleic acid content and tight junction status. *Endocrinol.* 1994; 135:1119-24.

Furth PA, Bar-Peled U, Li M. Apoptosis and mammary gland involution: Reviewing the process. *Apoptosis.* 1997; 2:19-24.

Gaffney E, Polanowski FP, Blackburn SE, Lambiase JP. Origin, concentration and structural features of human mammary gland cells cultured from breast secretions. *Cell Tissue Res.* 1976; 172:269-79.

Gudjonsson T, Villadsen R, Nielsen HL, Ronnov-Jessen L, Bissell MJ, Petersen OW. Isolation, immortalization, and characterization of a human breast epithelial cell line with stem cell properties. *Genes Dev.* 2002; 16(6):693-706.

Harris WS, Connor WE, Lindsey S. Will dietary omega-3 fatty acids change the composition of human milk. *Am J Clin Nutr.* 1984; 40:780-85.

Hartmann PE, Kulski JK. Changes in the composition of the mammary secretion of women after abrupt termination of breast feeding. *J Physiol.* 1978; 275:1-11.

Hayward AR. *The immunology of human milk.* New York, USA: Plenam Press; 1983.

Ho FCS, Wong RLC, Lawton SWM. Human colostral and breast milk cells: a light and electron microscopic study. *Acta Paediatr Scand.* 1979; 68:389-96.

Holmquist DG, Papanicolaou GN. The exfoliative cytology of the mammary gland during pregnancy and lactation. *Ann NY Acad Sci.* 1956; 63:1409-21.

Horseman ND. Prolactin and mammary gland development. *J Mammary Gland Biol Neoplasia.* 1999; 4(1):79-88.

Hovey RC, Trott JF, Vonderhaar BK. Establishing a framework for the functional mammary gland: from endocrinology to morphology. *J Mammary Gland Biol Neoplasia.* 2002; 7(1):17-38.

Hudson SW, Cown PN, Bird CC. Morphometric studies of age related changes in normal human breast and their significance for evolution of mammary cancer. *J Clin Pathol.* 1985; 38:281-87.

Ichikawa M, Sugita M, Takahashi M, Satomi M, Takeshita T, Araki T, *et al.* Breast milk macrophages spontaneously produce granulocyte-macrophage colony-stimulating factor and differentiate into dendritic cells in the presence of exogenous interleukin-4 alone. *Immunology.* 2003; 108:189-95.

Jain L, Vidyasagar D, Xantaou M, Ghai V, Shimada S, Blend M. In vivo distribution of human milk leukocytes after ingestion by newborn baboons. *Arch Dis Child.* 1989; 64: 930-33.

Jensen RG. *The lipids of human milk.* Boca Raton, FL, USA: CRC Press; 1989.

Jensen RG, Bitman J, Carlson SE, Couch SC, Hamosh M, Newberg DS. *Handbook of milk composition.* San Diego, CA, USA: Academic Press; 1995.

Kelly PA, Bachelot A, Kedzia C, Hennighausen L, Ormandy CJ, Kopchick JJ, *et al.* The role of prolactin and growth hormone in mammary development. *Mol Cell Endocrinol.* 2002; 197:127-31.

Kent JC, Arthur PG, Retallack RW, Hartmann PE. Calcium, phosphate and citrate in human milk at initiation of lactation. *J Dairy Res.* 1992; 59:161-67.

Kleinman RE, Walker WA. The enteromammary immune system. An important new concept in breast milk host defense. *Dig Dis Sci.* 1979; 24:876-82.

Knight CH. *Intercellular signalling in the mammary gland.* New York: Plenum Press; 1995.

Kordon EC, Smith GH. An entire functional mammary gland may comprise the progeny from a single cell. *Development.* 1998; 125:1921-30.

Kulski JK, Hartmann PE. Changes in human milk composition during the initiation of lactation. *Aust J Exp Biol Med Sci.* 1981; 59:101-14.

Lakhani SR, O'Hare MJ. The mammary myoepithelial cell - Cinderella or ugly sister? *Breast Cancer Res.* 2001; 3:1-4.

Lamote I, Meyer E, Massart-Leen AM, Burvenich C. Sex steroids and growth factors in the regulation of mammary gland proliferation, differentiation, and involution. *Steroids.* 2004; 69:145-59.

Lascelles AK, Gurner BW, Coombs RRA. Some properties of human colostral cells. *Aust J Exp Biol Med Sci.* 1969; 47:349-60.

Lawrence RA, Lawrence RM. *Breastfeeding: A guide for the medical profession.* Philidelphia: Elsevier Mosby; 2005.

Lendahl U, Zimmerman LB, McKay RD. CNS stem cells express a new class of intermediate filament protein. *Cell.* 1990; 60:585-95.

Li M, Lui X, Robinson G, Bar-Peled U, Wagner K, Scott Young W, *et al.* Mammary-derived signals activate programmed cell death during the first stage of mammary gland involution. *Proc Natl Acad Sci.* 1997; 94:3425-30.

Lin Y, Xia L, Turner JD, Zhao X. Morphologic observation of neutrophil diapedesis across bovine mammary gland epithelium in vitro. *Am J Vet Res.* 1995; 56: 203-7.

Linzell JL, Peaker M. Mechanism of milk secretion. *Physiol Rev.* 1971; 51(3):564-97.

Linzell JL, Peaker M, Taylor JC. The effects of prolactin and oxytocin on milk secretion and on the permeability of the mammary epithelium in the rabbit. *J Physiol.* 1975; 253:547-63.

Liu S, Dontu G, Wicha MS. Mammary stem cells, self-renewal pathways, and carcinogenesis. *Breast Cancer Res.* 2005; 7(3):86-95.

Lui X, Robinson G, Hennighausen L. Activation of Stat5a and Stat5b by tyrosine phosphorylation is tightly linked to mammary gland differentiation. *Mol Endocrinol.* 1996; 10(12):1496-1506.

Makrides M, Neumann MA, Gibson RA. Effect of maternal docosahexaenoic acid (DHA) supplementation on breast milk composition. *Eur J Clin Nutr.* 1996; 50:352-57.

Mandyla H, Xanthou M. *Human lactation 2. Maternal and environmental factors.* New York, USA: Plenum Press; 1986.

McManaman JL, Neville MC. Mammary physiology and milk secretion. *Adv Drug Deliv Rev.* 2003; 55(5):629-41.

Mitoulas LR. Short- and long-term variation in the production and content and composition of human milk fat. *Biochemistry.* Perth: The University of Western Australia, PhD; 2000.

Mohr JA, Leu R, Mabry W. Colostral leukocytes. *J Surg Oncol.* 1970; 2(2):163-67.

Neville MC, Allen JC, Watters C. *The mechanisms of milk secretion.* New York: Plenum Press; 1983.

Neville MC, Daniel CW. *The mammary gland: Development, regulation, and function.* New York and London: Plenum Press; 1987.

Newman J. How breast milk protects newborns. *Sci Am.* 1995; 273(6):76-80.

Nguyen DD, Neville MC. Tight junction regulation in the mammary gland. *J Mammary Gland Biol Neoplasia.* 1998; 3(3):233-46.

Nickerson SC, Akers RM. Biochemical and ultrastructural aspects of milk synthesis and secretion. *Int J Biochem.* 1984; 16:855-65.

Papanicolaou GN, Holmquist DG, Bader GM, Falk EA. Exfoliative cytology of the mammary gland and its value on the diagnosis of cancer and other diseases of the breast. *Cancer.* 1958; 11:377-409.

Patton S, Keenan TW. The milk fat globule membrane. *Biocim Biophys Acta.* 1975; 415(3):273-309.

Peaker M. *Biochemistry of lactation.* New York, USA: Elsevier; 1983.

Pechoux C, Gudjonsson T, Ronnov-Jessen L, Bissell MJ, Petersen OW. Uman mammary luminal epithelial cells contain progenitors to myoepithelial cells. *Devel Biol.* 1999; 206:88-99.

Philp JAC, Burdon TG, Wastson CJ. Differential activation of Stats 3 and 5 during mammary gland development. *FEBS J.* 1996; 396:77-80.

Pitelka DL. *Cell and tissue biology.* Baltimore, USA: Urban and Schwatzenberg; 1988.

Pitt J. The milk mononuclear phagocyte. *Pediatrics.* 1979; 64:745-49.

Powell JT, Brew K. Metal ion activation of galactosyltransferase. *J Biol Chem.* 1976; 251:3645-52.

Prosser CG, Hartmann PE. Comparison of mammary gland function during the ovulatory menstrual cycle and acute breast inflammation in women. *Aust J Exp Biol Med Sci.* 1983; 61:277-86.

Richie ER. *Human milk in infant nutrition and health.* Springfield, USA: Thomas Publisher; 1986.

Riordan J, Auerbach KG. *Breastfeeding and human lactation.* Boston, USA: Jones and Bartlett Publishers; 1993.

Russo J, Russo IH. *Molecular basis of breast cancer: Prevention and treatment.* New York: Springer; 2004.

Seelig Jr LL, Beer AE. Intraepithelial leukocytes in the human mammary gland. *Biol Reprod.* 1981; 24:1157-63.

Shackleton M, Vaillant F, Simpson KJ, Stingl J, Smyth GK, Asselin-Labat ML, *et al.* Generation of a functional mammary gland from a single stem cell. *Nature.* 2006; 439(7072):84-88.

Smith CW, Goldman AS. The cells of human colostrum: In vitro studies of morphology and function. *Pediatr Res.* 1968; 2:103-9.

Steiner M, Dunn E, Born L. Hormones and mood: From menarche to menopause and beyond. *J Affect Disord.* 2003; 74:67-83.

Sternlicht MD, Kouros-Mehr H, Lu P, Werb Z. Hormonal and local control of mammary branching morphogenesis. *Differentiation.* 2006; 74(7):365-81.

Sting L, Eaves CJ, Kuusk U. Phenotypic and functional characterization in vitro of a multipotent epithelial cell present in the normal adult human breast. *Differentiation.* 1998; 63:201-13.

Streuli CH, Edwards GM. Control of the normal mammary epithelial phenotype by intergins. *Journal Mammary Gland Biol Neoplasia.* 1998; 3:151-63.

Streuli CH, Edwards GM, Delcommenne M, Whitelaw CBA, Burdon TG, Schindler C, *et al.* Stat5 as a target for regulation by extracellular matrix. *J Biol Chem.* 1995; 270:21639-44.

Streuli CH, Gilmore AP. Adhesion-mediated signalling in the regulation of mammary epithelial cell survival. *J Mammary Gland Biol Neoplasia.* 1999; 4:183-91.

Sutherland KD, Lindeman GJ, Visvader JE. The molecular culprits underlying precocious mammary gland involution. *J Mammary Gland Biol Neoplasia.* 2007; 12:15-23.

Thompson BJ, Smith S. Biosynthesis of fatty acids by lactating human breast epithelial cells: An evaluation of the contribution to the overall composition of human milk fat. *Pediatr Res.* 1985; 19:139-43.

Thompson PA, Kadlubar FF, Vena SM, Hill HL, McClure GHY, McDaniel LP, *et al.* Exfoliative ductal epithelial cells in human breast milk: A source of target tissue DNA for molecular epidemiologic studies of breast cancer. *Cancer Epidemiol Biomarkers Prev.* 1998; 7:37-42.

Toban H, Salazar H. Ultrastructure of the human mammary gland. II. Postpartum lactogenesis. *J Endocrinol Metab.* 1974; 40:834-43.

Toma JG, Akhavan M, Fernandes KJ, Barnabe-Heider F, Sadikot A, Kaplan DR, *et al.* Isolation of multipotent adult stem cells from the dermis of mammalian skin. *Nat Cell Biol.* 2001; 3:778-84.

Vorherr H. *The breast: Morphology, physiology and lactation.* New York: Academic Press; 1974.

Walker RA, Martin CV. The aged breast. *J Pathol.* 2007; 211:232-40.

Watson CJ. Post-lactational mammary gland regression: Molecular basis and implications for breast cancer. *Expert Rev Mol Med.* 2006; 8(32):1-15.

Weiss L. *Cell and tissue biology. A textbook of histology.* Baltimore, USA: Urban and Schwarzenberg; 1988.

Wirt DP, Adkins LT, Palkowetz KH, Achmalstieg FC, Goldman AS. Activated and memory T lymphocytes in human milk. *Cytometry.* 1992; 13:282-90.

Wu JM, Zelinski MB, Ingram DK, Ottinger MA. Ovarian aging and menopause: Current theories, hypotheses, and research models. *Exp Biol Med.* 2005; 230:818-28.

Wysolmerski JJ, McCaughern-Carucci JF, Dalfotis AG, Broadus AE, Philbrick WM. Overexpression of parathyroid hormone-related protein or parathyroid hormone in transgenic mice impairs branching morphogenesis during mammary gland development. *Development.* 1995; 121:3539-47.

Zulak IM, Keenan TW. Citrate accumulation by a golgi apparatus-rich fraction from lactating bovine mammary gland. *Int J Biochem.* 1983; 15:747-50.

Zulewski H, Abraham EJ, Gerlach MJ, Daniel PB, Moritz W, Muller B, *et al.* Multipotential nestin-positive stem cells isolated from adult pancreatic islets differentiate ex vivo into pancreatic endocrine, exocrine, and hepatic phenotypes. *Diabetes.* 2001; 50:521-33.

Chapter 4

Human Milk Composition - Fat

Charles Czank, Leon R. Mitoulas, and Peter E. Hartmann

INTRODUCTION

"...even modern formulas are only superficially similar to breastmilk. Fundamentally, they are inexact copies based on outdated and incomplete knowledge of what breastmilk is. Formulas contain no antibodies, no living cells, no enzymes, no hormones. They contain much more aluminium, manganese, cadmium, and iron than breastmilk. They contain significantly more protein than breastmilk. The proteins and fats are fundamentally different from those in breastmilk. Formulas do not vary from the beginning of the feed to the end of the feed, or from day 1 to day 7 to day 30, or from woman to woman, or from baby to baby." - Dr Jack Newman (1997)

As described in chapter one, lactation is common to all mammals, indeed the class *Mammalia* was so coined by Carl Linnaeus due to the presence of mammary glands and the ability of mammals to provide milk to feed their own young. The significance of lactation to mammals cannot be understated for it is believed that the ability to provide nutrients to the newborn, regardless of the status of appropriate food in the environment, is one of the major evolutionary adaptations which have allowed mammals to prosper in many and varied habitats (Pond, 1984).

Pond's commentary places emphasis on nutrition and is in keeping with current opinion that nutrition is the major function of human milk with respect to the needs of the developing infant. However, it is interesting to note that Vorbach and colleagues (Vorbach *et al.*, 2006) argue that mammary secretions and the mammary gland itself evolved as part of the innate immune system and that the nutritional function of lactation was subsequent to the protective function.

While the biological imperatives that drove the evolution of lactation are still being uncovered, it is clear that milk from all species of mammals is an incredibly complex mixture of components which provide energy and nutrients (fats, lactose, proteins) together with developmental (e.g., LCPUFA, growth factors, cytokines, oligosaccharides, and enzymes) and protective (secretory IgA, lysozyme, lactoferrin, etc.) factors, and many of the milk components are multifunctional with nutritional and protective functions (e.g., α-lactalalbumin, casein, and lactoferrin). Milk also contains vitamins and minerals in concentrations and forms that are tailored to the specific needs of the neonate of each species. In addition to this level of complexity, it is important to reiterate that the composition of milk is not uniform and that it does differ significantly from species to species, but it also differs within species - with changes with the stage of lactation (to reflect the needs of the infant, e.g., high IgA levels in colostrum compared to established milk), with time of day, and over the course of a feed.

The chemistry of breastmilk, like its components, is also complex. Generally, milk can be described in three ways:

1) An oil in water emulsion with the fat suspended in a continuous serum phase,

2) A colloidal suspension of casein micelles, globular proteins, and lipoprotein particles, and
3) A solution of lactose, soluble proteins, minerals, and vitamins (Goff, 1995).

These three descriptions illustrate the compartmentalization of milk components based on their chemical composition. However, it is clear that these descriptions are but overviews of the final complexity of breastmilk composition. The following sections describe the various macronutrients in milk. It is the authors' intent to outline the major components of human milk and discuss the significance of these components to the lactation process. However, for a more detailed account of all possible milk components, we highly recommend the *Handbook of Milk Composition* (Jensen, 1995).

FAT CONTENT OF HUMAN MILK

Milk is an emulsion of fat globules suspended in an aqueous phase. The milk fat globule (MFG) is essentially a triacylglycerol core surrounded by a coating of phospholipids, proteins, cholesterol, and enzymes, collectively known as the milk fat globule membrane (MFGM) (Jensen *et al.*, 1995) (see Figure 6 in Chapter 6). The MFGM originates from the phospholipid membrane of the lactocyte during secretion of the MFG. The size of the fat globule in human milk varies from less than 1 micron to 12 microns. Around 70-90% of the total number of fat globules are in the sub-micron size range, but they contribute just a few percent of the total fat volume. The majority of the fat volume is made up of globules around 4 microns. A third of the population of globules are greater than 8 microns and contribute just 0.01% of total fat volume (Ruegg & Blanc, 1981). In comparison, the average fat globule size of infant formulas ranges from 0.3–1.1 microns (Michalski *et al.*, 2005b; Simonin *et al.*, 1984), unhomogenized bovine milk ranges from 2.5-4.6 microns, and homogenized bovine milk ranges from 0.13-1.7 microns (Michalski *et al.*, 2002a; Michalski *et al.*, 2002b; Ruegg & Blanc, 1981; Thiebaud *et al.*, 2003; Walstra, 1969; Wiking *et al.*, 2004). It has been suggested that the disparity between the fat globule sizes of human milk, bovine milk, and infant formula could influence fat absorption by the infant gut. In adult humans and small animal models, ingestion of large native fat globules results in faster gastric emptying and fat metabolization compared to small homogenized fat globules (Armand *et al.*, 1999; Michalski *et al.*, 2005b; Borel *et al.*, 1994; Michalski *et al.*, 2005a). However, the effect in the infant is confounding, with studies either demonstrating slower gastric emptying (Cavell, 1981) or no significant difference (Armand *et al.*, 1996) when infant formula is ingested (Michalski *et al.*, 2005b).

The fat content of mature human milk is approximately 40 g/L (Jensen *et al.*, 1995). However, fat is the most variable component of human milk and the content changes within a feed, over the course of the day, with stage of lactation, between breasts, with parity, with age, and between women (Nims *et al.*, 1932; Hytten, 1954; Hall, 1979; Prentice *et al.*, 1981; Jackson *et al.*, 1988a; Jackson *et al.*, 1988b; Daly *et al.*, 1993a; Lawrence, 1995; Emmett & Rogers, 1997). Despite these degrees in variation, the fat in milk is very important to the newborn infant. Fat provides approximately 50% of the energy in milk and essential fatty acids (EFA), and serves as a vehicle for the delivery of fat soluble vitamins to the infant (Riordan, 1993).

Variation in Total Fat Content of Human Milk

It is generally accepted that there is little difference in total fat content between breasts. However, a significant difference in total fat content between women occurs throughout the course of the day (Mitoulas *et al.*, 2002), which in turn influences the amount of energy the infant receives. Differences in the fat content from before (foremilk) to after (hindmilk) a breastfeed (nipple-alveoli gradient) are evident from writings as old as those of Metlinger (1473), where he advised that "*...the wet nurse should first milk the breast so that the watery parts run from it, and then give the child to suck*" (Hytten, 1954). Hytten showed that there was considerable variation in both the regularity and the degree of the rise in milk fat during a breastfeed. Prentice *et al.* (1981) and Jackson *et al.* (1988a) found that the degree of increase of fat could be predicted by the amount of milk removed by the infant. However, Dorea *et al.* (1982) and Hartmann *et al.* (1986) failed to find a similar relationship. Furthermore, it has been established that the increase in fat content over the course of a feed is not linear and increases more steeply as the breast is emptied (Watson *et al.*, 1982).

Jackson *et al.* (1988a) determined that the length of time between feeds was the best single predictor of foremilk fat content, explaining 26% of the observed variation. Daly and coworkers (Daly *et al.*, 1993a) determined that 69% of the variation in milk fat content within women was explained by the 'degree of breast fullness' or the amount of milk held in the breast at that time (Cox *et al.*, 1996). These two theories complement one another in that the longer the interval between feeds, the more milk synthesized, the greater the 'degree of fullness,' and therefore, the lower the fat content of the subsequent foremilk sample. Furthermore, when looking at the change in fat content over the course of the feed, as milk is removed, the 'degree of fullness' is decreased and the fat content increases.

Several theories have been put forward to explain the observed nipple-alveoli gradient of the fat content of milk. Whittlestone (1953) proposed a fat globule filtration effect whereby fat globules cluster in the lumen of the alveolus and are removed only towards the end of the feed. Hytten (1954) suggested that the increase was a result of fat globules adsorbing to the large alveolar and ductal surface of the full alveolus, only being removed towards the end of the feed. Atwood and Hartmann (1992) postulated that the removal of adsorbed fat globules was the result of the changing morphology of the lactocyte and the shape of the alveolus. When the lumen is full, lactocytes are squamous in shape, providing maximal surface area for the fat globules to adsorb. As the lumen drains, the lactocytes change from squamous to columnar and the lumen of the alveolus becomes more convoluted. This subsequent decrease in luminal surface area together with mechanical shearing forces generated by the convolution of the alveolus displaces the adsorbed fat globules, facilitating their removal. This theory would also explain the previously noted rapid rise in fat content as more milk was removed from the gland.

Table 1. Lipid Composition (wt%) of Human Milk in Two Studies

Lipid	Total Lipids (%, w/w)	
Hydrocarbons	Trace	NR
Sterol Esters	Trace	NR
Triacylglycerols	98.1	98.76
Diacylglycerols	0.7	0.01
Monoacylglycerols	Trace	0.0
Nonesterified Fatty Acids	0.4	0.08
Sterols (cholesterol)	0.25	0.34
Phospholipids	0.3	0.81

From: Jensen, 1989. Reprinted with permission.
NR: not reported

Composition of Human Milk Fat

The fat fraction of human milk consists of several different classes. Triacylglycerols are the most abundant, representing 98-99% of total fat. The remaining one to two percent consists of di- and monoacylglycerols, nonesterified fatty acids (NEFA), phospholipids, cholesterol, and cholesterol esters. The relative proportion of the fat classes changes slightly over the course of lactation, for example, levels of cholesterol and cholesterol esters decrease (Bitman *et al.*, 1983) and triacylglycerols increase (**Table 1**).

Triacylglycerols

The composition of triacylglycerols in human milk is usually given in terms of types and amounts of fatty acids (FA) present. However, it is also important to consider structure (Jensen *et al.*, 1995). Triacylglycerols consist of three FA bound to a glycerol molecule. The location of the FA on the glycerol backbone can be identified by stereospecific numbering (*sn*). With this nomenclature if either the hydroxyl or substituent group on the triacylglycerol is drawn to the left, the group above is numbered *sn*-1 and the group below *sn*-3 (Jensen *et al.*, 1995) (**Figure 1-f**).

Due to the nature of the structure of the triacylglycerol and the fact that breastmilk contains seven FA in amounts greater than one percent, it could be expected that 7^3 (i.e., 343) types of triacylglycerols exist (Jensen, 1989). However, Jensen *et al.* (1995) state that the distribution of FA on the glycerol backbone is not random and that certain FA have a preference for certain positions.

The conservation of the positional distribution of certain FA has been well documented (Breckenridge *et al.*, 1969; Watts & Dils, 1968; Hundrieser *et al.*, 1984; Myher *et al.*, 1994; Martin *et al.*, 1993a). From these studies, it has become apparent that most of the palmitate (16:0; 70%) is located at the *sn*-2 position, with laurate (12:0) at *sn*-3, stearate (18:0) at *sn*-1, and both oleate (18:1n9) and linoleate (18:2n6) at *sn*-1 or -3 (Jensen *et al.*, 1995). Furthermore, Martin *et al.* (1993a) found that the very long chain polyunsaturated fatty acids (VLCPUFA) were primarily found at the *sn*-2 and *sn*-3 positions.

The specific positional distribution demonstrated by the FA on the glycerol backbone may indicate that the structure influences the metabolic fate of the component FA in the infant intestine (Martin *et al.*, 1993a). The presence of VLCPUFA in the outer positions (*sn*-1 and

-3) can induce resistance to pancreatic lipase *in vitro* (Martin *et al.*, 1993a). Furthermore, the distribution of FA between the outer *sn*-1 and -3 positions and the inner *sn*-2 position determines the luminal partition of non-esterified fatty acids (NEFA) to 2-monoacyl-*sn*-glycerols (Martin *et al.*, 1993a) as pancreatic lipase hydrolyzes at the *sn*-1 and -3 positions (Innis *et al.*, 1994). This has implications regarding the efficiency of absorption of FA from the infant intestine. Palmitate, mostly found at the *sn*-2 position, is relatively poorly absorbed as a NEFA due to a melting point above body temperature and a tendency to form hydrated FA soaps at intestinal pH (Innis *et al.*, 1994). Infants fed triacylglycerols with palmitate at the *sn*-2 position have shown higher

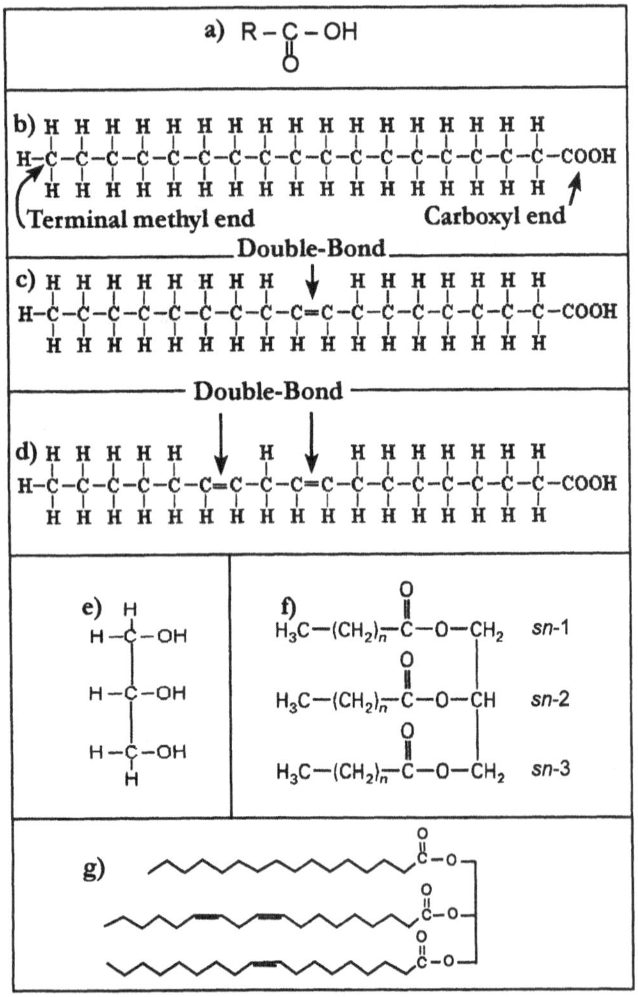

Figure 1. a) Generic chemical formula structure of fatty acids where R represents a long chain carbon, b) stearic acid (18:0) – a saturated fatty acid, c) oleic acid (18:1) – a monounsaturated fatty acid, d) linoleic acid (18:2n6) – a polyunsaturated fatty acid, e) glycerol, f) generic structure of triacylglycerol, g) example of triacylglycerol with palmitic acid (16:0) at the sn-1 position, linoleic acid (18:2n6) at the sn-2 position, and oleic acid (18:1) at the sn-3 position.

fat absorption (Filer *et al.*, 1969; Fomon *et al.*, 1970). Indeed, a recent analysis of 28 different infant formulas found that a majority of formulas contained oleic acid at the *sn*-2 position, which is likely to be responsible for the higher number of instances of constipation commonly observed in formula-fed infants than in breastmilk-fed infants (Straarup *et al.*, 2006). This supports the view that palmitate is positioned at the *sn*-2 position of the triacylglycerol to promote fat absorption in the infant intestine (Innis *et al.*, 1995) (**Figure 1**).

Fatty Acids

The FA of human milk are a major component of the fat fraction and comprise 85% of the triacylglycerols (Jensen, 1989). Over 200 different types of FA, including saturated, mono- and polyunsaturated, branched and cyclic FA, have been described for human milk, most of these in quantities of less than one percent (Jensen, 1999). Due to this wide variety of FA, it is necessary to establish a suitable nomenclature. In the past, the more common FA were identified by generic names, for example, laurate, myristate, palmitate, oleate, linoleate, etc. However, these names provided no information regarding structure. Fatty acids can be structurally identified by their true chemical name, for example, laurate becomes dodecanoate. While this method is technically correct, it becomes cumbersome when dealing with LCPUFA, for example, linoleate becomes 9-12 octadecadienoate.

To overcome these problems, a shorthand notation has been devised to easily identify the structure of the FA while also being able to account for subtle differences between FA (Jensen, 1989). For example, laurate becomes 12:0 and linoleate, 18:2n6. The figure before the colon signifies the number of carbon atoms (chain length), while the figure immediately after the colon denotes the number of double bonds. The 'n6' tells the reader that the first double bond is 6 carbon atoms from the terminal methyl group. As FA in human milk are nearly always the *cis* isomer, they are not explicitly defined. However, the *trans* isomer is identified by the addition of a 't' after the position of the double bonds, for example, 18:1n9t. In addition, *trans* FA isomers can be differentiated by the identification of the position of the *trans* double bond, e.g., 18:2Δ9t, 12t.

Human milk fat contains medium chain fatty acids (MCFA; 10:0 – 14:0) and long chain fatty acids (LCFA; 16:0 – 24:0), including the long chain polyunsaturated fatty acids (LCPUFA) (e.g., 20:4n6, 22:6n3). In comparison, bovine milk fat contains short chain fatty acids (SCFA) (4:0 – 8:0), MCFA (10:0 – 14:0) and some LCFA (16:0 – 20:0), but very few LCPUFA. Human milk has few if any SCFA, with the shortest reported usually being 6:0 or 8:0. In most human milk, there are only seven to nine FA with proportions greater than one percent (**Table 2**). MCFA are synthesized within the gland (*de novo* synthesis) and represent approximately 15% of the FA of mature milk. Mammary gland lactocytes contain a unique thioesterase (thioesterase II) which catalyses the termination of FA synthesis at the 14th carbon and not the 16th, as is the case in all other tissues (Thompson & Smith, 1985). The major FA of human milk are 16:0 and 18:1n9, together representing over 50% of the total FA. As the FA longer than that 14:0 are derived from blood, it seems likely that the abundance of these two FA is due to their high concentration in maternal blood. The LCPUFA account for approximately 12% of the total FA in mature milk. However, this amount and the constituent FA are all very much dependent on maternal diet (**Table 2**).

Significantly, it is the LCPUFA present in human milk that are believed to help in the development of the infant's central nervous and immune systems, and affect growth. Indeed, 22:6n3, existing predominantly as phosphatidlyethanolamine and phosphatdylserine, and 20:4n6, existing as phosphatidylcholine, are the most abundant LCPUFA in cellular membranes of the brain and retina (Jumpsen *et al.*, 1997b; Jumpsen *et al.*, 1997a). Makrides and coworkers (1994) found that the amount of 22:6n3 in the frontal lobes of breastfed infants increased with age, whereas there was no change with age in infants fed formula. This improved 22:6n3 status of the brain of the breastfed infant provides a possible explanation for the increases in infant neurological function (Lanting *et al.*, 1994) and later cognitive ability (Horwood & Fergusson, 1998) of breastfed infants and highlights the findings of Lucas *et al.* (1992) that preterm infants who were fed mother's milk had an 8.3 IQ unit advantage at seven to eight years of age over those who were fed formula.

It is likely that modification of the PUFA content in the diet influences membrane structure and the function of associated proteins, as well as the production of second messengers, such as eicosanoids, that affect cell function. This is supported by dietary PUFA studies using peripheral nerves, which demonstrated that PUFA intake affects FA composition of neuronal membranes, myelin, and neurotransmission properties of norepinephrine-containing sympathetic neurons (Fernstrom, 1999). In addition, studies on the visual transduction system have demonstrated that G protein signalling is compromised in membranes with reduced n-3 FA, which occurs as a result of impeded binding of rhodopsin to the G protein and lower phosphodiesterase activity (Mitchell *et al.*, 2003). Thus, it is probable that the physiological effect of LCPUFA on the central nervous and visual systems is mediated by molecular interactions between LCPUFA and membrane proteins which regulate important processes, such as signal transduction, cell signalling, receptor function, and ion transport, and in turn, cell function.

While LCPUFA appear to positively contribute to the maturation of the infant's central nervous system, the effect on growth is confounding. Several studies involving the addition of LCPUFA to formula have shown either a positive effect (Innis *et al.*, 2002), no effect (Carnielli *et al.*, 1998; Boehm *et al.*, 1997; Uauy *et al.*, 1994; Makrides *et al.*, 1999), little effect (Vanderhoof *et al.*, 2000; O'Connor *et al.*, 2001) or a negative effect (Carlson *et al.*, 1993; Carlson *et al.*, 1996; Ryan *et al.*, 1999; Carlson *et al.*, 1992; Fewtrell *et al.*, 2002) on growth characteristics, in comparison to infants fed a non-supplemented diet (Lapillonne *et al.*, 2003). Suggested mechanisms for such effects include altered nutrient intake, absorption and/or utilization of low plasma and tissue contents of 20:4n6, imbalance between n3 and n6 LCPUFA eiconasoid precursors, and altered membrane characteristics and effects on gene expression (Lapillonne *et al.*, 2003). Though it remains to be determined whether the LCPUFA present in mother's own milk has similar effects, such evidence reflects the complexity of biological functions that LCPUFA has on the developing infant.

In addition, studies have shown increases in immune function (Lopez-Alarcon *et al.*, 1997; Oddy *et al.*, 1999) between infants fed breastmilk and those fed artificial formula. Indeed, some of the non-esterified fatty acids (8:0-12:0 and 18:2n6) and their monoacylglycerols released by hydrolysis of milk triacylglycerols in the infant's gut have been shown to disrupt enveloped viruses (Issacs *et al.*, 1986; Thormar *et al.*, 1987) and kill parasitic protozoa (Gillin *et al.*, 1985) *in vitro*. Apart from these directly attributable effects, the LCPUFA may also provide modulation of the immune system. Miles and

Table 2. Fatty Acid Composition (wt%) of Human Milk from 15 Different Countries

	America				Europe			
Fatty acid	USA [d]	Canada [d]	Mexico [d]	Chile [d]	Germany [a]	UK [d]	Spain [f]	Netherlands [g]
6:0	N.D	N.D	N.D	N.D	N.D	N.D	N.D	0.28
8:0	0.16	0.17	0.19	0.20	N.D	0.20	0.13	0.66
10:0	1.50	1.66	1.46	1.87	0.71	1.84	1.32	3.00
12:0	4.40	5.25	4.97	6.15	4.41	4.99	5.9	9.78
14:0	4.91	5.84	5.57	6.80	6.73	5.87	6.25	7.89
15:0	0.29	0.33	0.32	0.30	0.46	0.36	0.3	N.D
16:0	19.26	18.67	19.91	18.79	21.83	22.59	19.45	23.21
17:0	0.32	0.32	0.33	0.35	0.57	0.29	0.36	N.D
18:0	6.21	5.83	6.07	5.77	8.15	6.25	6.85	7.18
20:0	0.19	0.20	0.18	0.21	0.22	0.20	0.23	0.21
22:0	0.09	0.10	0.08	0.09	0.09	0.08	N.D	0.10
24:0	0.06	0.06	0.05	0.08	N.D -	0.06	N.D	0.07
14:1 n 9	N.D	N.D	N.D	N.D	0.29	N.D	0.21	N.D
16:1 n 7	2.64	2.79	2.64	2.70	2.68	2.85	2.07	2.33
18:1 n 9	32.77	35.18	30.79	26.19	34.31	32.77	38.39	26.5
20:1 n 9	0.39	0.52	0.42	0.55	-	0.39	0.51	0.35
22:1 n 9	0.08	0.11	0.08	0.14	0.08	0.08	N.D	N.D
18:1 n 9 *t*	N.D	N.D	N.D	N.D	3.12	N.D	N.D	N.D
18:2 n 6 *tt*	N.D	0.25	0.20	0.16	0.14	0.09	N.D	N.D
18:2 n 6	14.78	11.48	16.05	17.75	10.76	10.45	12.02	12.84
18:3 n 6	0.17	0.16	0.15	0.15	0.16	0.17	-	0.09
20:2 n 6	0.27	0.21	0.34	0.54	0.34	0.22	0.41	0.31
20:3 n 6	0.35	0.27	0.33	0.44	0.26	0.33	0.5	0.33
20:4 n 6	0.45	0.37	0.42	0.42	0.36	0.36	0.5	0.37
22:4 n 6	0.11	0.04	0.11	0.04	0.08	0.08	0.17	0.07
18:3 n 3	1.05	1.22	1.05	1.14	0.81	1.22	0.78	1.02
20:5 n 3	0.07	0.08	0.07	0.09	0.04	0.11	0.14	0.05
22:5 n 3	0.14	0.16	0.16	0.22	0.17	0.18	0.12	0.12
22:6 n 3	0.17	0.17	0.26	0.43	0.22	0.24	0.34	0.19
Total %	89.48	91.44	92.2	91.6	97.7	92.27	97.0	97.25
Medium chain sat	10.96	12.95	12.19	15.02	11.8	12.9	13.6	19.8
Odd chain sat	0.61	0.61	0.65	0.65	1.03	1.03	0.66	N.D
Long chain sat	26.13	25.18	26.62	25.29	30.3	29.47	26.89	30.7
Saturated	37.39	38.43	39.13	40.61	43.2	42.73	40.79	52.1
Monunsat	33.24	35.81	31.29	26.88	37.3	33.24	40.97	27.36
Trans	N.D	0.25	0.20	0.16	3.26	0.09	N.D	N.D
Polyunsat	17.56	14.16	18.94	21.22	13.2	13.36	14.98	15.39
Polyunsat/sat	0.46	0.36	0.48	0.54	0.30	0.31	0.36	0.37
n6	16.13	12.53	17.4	19.34	11.9	11.96	13.6	14.01
n3	1.43	1.63	1.54	1.88	1.24	1.75	1.38	1.38
n6/n3	11.36	7.86	11.29	10.28	9.64	6.83	9.86	10.15

N.D denotes no data available a - Koletzko *et al.*, 1988, b - Spear *et al.*, 1992, c - Kneebone *et al.*, 1985, d - Yuhas *et al.*, 2006, e - Mitoulas *et al.*, 2000, f - de la Presa-Owens *et al.*, 1996, g - Smit *et al.*, 2002

Asia					Other		
Malaysia [c]	China [d]	Japan [d]	Phillipines [d]	Pakistan [g]	Carribean [g]	Australia [d]	Australia [e]
N.D	N.D	N.D	N.D	0.32	0.17	N.D	N.D
N.D	0.17	0.22	0.28	0.46	0.67	0.20	N.D
0.9	1.67	2.00	2.35	2.28	3.62	1.62	1.16
8.86	4.24	5.86	13.82	10.03	13.82	5.49	5.27
10.05	3.61	6.11	12.12	10.99	11.54	6.28	7.27
0.16	0.12	0.29	0.21	N.D	N.D	0.39	0.47
26.86	18.62	20.20	23.02	27.94	20.89	22.26	24.50
0.27	0.22	0.32	0.24	N.D	N.D	0.41	0.418
4.09	6.13	6.14	4.75	5.20	5.45	6.77	7.88
0.19	0.20	0.20	0.13	0.17	0.2	0.20	0.67
0.09	0.09	0.09	0.06	0.07	0.09	0.08	0.07
0.16	0.05	0.05	0.05	0.06	0.07	0.06	0.07
0.33	N.D	N.D	N.D	N.D	N.D	N.D	0.41
4.17	1.88	2.56	4.59	2.23	2.58	2.97	2.60
30.82	36.49	31.43	21.85	24.2	21.4	32.23	32.27
0.51	1.25	0.52	0.28	0.25	0.38	0.38	0.27
0.20	1.21	0.13	0.07	N.D	N.D	0.08	0.05
N.D	N.D	N.D	N.D	N.D	N.D	N.D	1.00
N.D	0.09	0.12	0.06	N.D	N.D	0.09	0.31
8.84	14.88	12.66	7.90	12.47	11.26	10.66	9.19
Trace	0.15	0.13	0.10	0.05	0.09	0.17	0.15
0.29	0.39	0.25	0.23	0.16	0.32	0.20	0.120
0.27	0.28	0.25	0.31	0.21	0.38	0.31	0.27
0.47	0.49	0.40	0.39	0.26	0.50	0.38	0.37
N.D	0.11	0.08	0.11	0.06	0.12	0.09	0.08
0.30	2.02	1.33	0.43	0.34	0.67	0.90	0.76
N.D	0.07	0.26	0.15	0.02	0.06	0.10	0.08
0.21	0.18	0.29	0.23	0.05	0.11	0.18	0.17
0.90	0.35	0.99	0.74	0.06	0.33	0.23	0.20
98.9	95.0	92.88	94.47	98.5	94.55	93.17	97.75
21.33	9.69	14.19	28.57	13.73	29.65	13.39	13.69
0.43	0.43	0.61	0.45	N.D	N.D	N.D	0.882
31.4	25.31	27	28.25	33.44	26.7	29.78	33.06
51.6	35.12	41.26	56.75	57.2	56.35	43.63	47.22
36.0	38.95	32.08	22.2	24.45	21.78	32.69	37.4
N.D	0.09	0.12	0.06	N.D	N.D	0.09	1.31
11.3	18.92	16.64	10.59	13.68	13.84	13.22	11.39
0.22	0.53	0.40	0.18	0.24	0.25	0.30	0.22
9.87	16.3	13.77	9.04	13.21	12.67	11.81	10.24
1.41	2.62	2.87	1.55	0.47	1.17	1.41	1.05
7.42	6.22	4.79	5.83	28.11	10.83	8.38	9.07

Calder (1998) have reviewed the effects of the amount and type of fat in the diet on immune cell function and documented the suppression of lymphocyte function by the n3 family of LCPUFA, in particular. Furthermore, it has been demonstrated that supplementation of the maternal diet with fish oil leads to a decrease in neonatal pro-inflammatory cytokines, such as IL-13, and a potential reduction in infant allergy (Dunstan *et al.*, 2003a; Dunstan *et al.*, 2003b). Perhaps, the enhanced vaccine responses and the down regulation of other immune reactions, such as transplant rejection (Hanson *et al.*, 1996) and atopy (Saarinen & Kajosari, 1995) in breastfed compared to non-breastfed infants, is related to n3 LCPUFA in breastmilk initiating programmed immune modulation.

It is this level of complexity coupled with the different sources of the FA that makes the composition remarkably variable. While not affected by all the factors that can alter total content of fat in milk, the FA composition is affected by stage of lactation, gestational age, parity, individuality, and diet (Jensen *et al.*, 1995). Furthermore, in contrast to total fat content, it is diet that has the greatest effect on FA composition (**Table 2**).

Factors Affecting Fatty Acid Composition

Stage of Lactation

Few studies have comprehensively investigated longitudinal changes of individual FA over the first year of lactation. However, it has been shown that FA composition can change with stage of lactation, from both colostrum to mature milk (Gibson & Kneebone, 1981; Bitman *et al.*, 1983; Martin *et al.*, 1993b) and during established lactation (Bitman *et al.*, 1983; Harzer *et al.*, 1983; Idota *et al.*, 1991; Lukkainen *et al.*, 1994; Makrides *et al.*, 1995; Huisman *et al.*, 1996). Gibson and Kneebone (1981) found that although the difference between total saturated and unsaturated FA were minor, there were larger changes observed for individual FA. They found that both 10:0 and 12:0 increased from colostrum to mature milk, while Martin *et al.* (1993b) found the LCPUFA to decrease. Harzer *et al.* (1983) noted an increase in 12:0 and 14:0 as lactation progressed. These results led Gibson and Kneebone (1981) and Harzer *et al.* (1983) to speculate that increases in the MCFA was an indication of the maturation of the gland, while Martin *et al.* (1993b) concluded that LCPUFA variation was due to the maternal mobilization (and perhaps depletion) of a preformed LCPUFA pool during early lactation. Similarly, Harzer *et al.* (1983) noted that the major LCFA - 16:0, 18:0, and 18:1n9, decreased as lactation progressed. Studies from our laboratory that followed the FA composition over the first year of lactation have demonstrated that 16:0 and 18:0 concentrations decrease towards six to nine months of lactation and 18:1n9 concentrations decrease between six and 12 months (Mitoulas *et al.*, 1999; Mitoulas *et al.*, 2000).

In general, PUFA concentrations tend to change over time in a manner similar to 18:1n9, with the essential FA 18:2n6 and 18:3n3 concentrations increasing up to six to nine months, followed by a decrease towards 12 months (Mitoulas *et al.*, 1999; Mitoulas *et al.*, 2000). Similar trends were observed by other researchers up to three months (Huisman *et al.*, 1996), six months (Lukkainen *et al.*, 1994), and eight months of lactation (Idota *et al.*, 1991), though one study demonstrated no such change over 7.5 months (Makrides *et al.*, 1995). All the above studies demonstrated a decrease in LCPUFA, namely 20:4n6, 20:5n3, and 22:6n3, over the specified time periods, though our results demonstrated a slight increase in 22:6n3 between two to six months before decreasing again towards twelve months. This lack of consistency demonstrates the reliance of 22:6n3 on maternal dietary intake, while 20:4n6 and 20:5n3, as well as PUFA, may preferentially come from adipose stores (Cheruku *et al.*, 1999; Fidler *et al.*, 1999; Del Prado *et al.*, 2000). Altogether these results are consistent with the mobilization and gradual depletion of body fat stores over the first six months of lactation, the minimum period of breastfeeding suggested to maximize fat loss during lactation (Hartmann *et al.*, 1998; Sadurkis *et al.*, 1988).

Gestational Age

It is well established that milk from mothers of term infants can vary in FA composition from that of mothers of preterm infants (Bitman *et al.*, 1983; Butte *et al.*, 1984; Jensen, 1989; Lukkainen *et al.*, 1994; Beijers & Schaaffsma, 1996; Genzel *et al.*, 1997). Watts and Dils (1968) found that milk from mothers who delivered preterm contained 22% MCFA. This is in contrast to the 10-15% reported for milk from mothers delivering at term (Jensen, 1989). Bitman *et al.* (1983) showed similar results in milk collected at day 42 of lactation from mothers who delivered very preterm, preterm, and term infants, with the MCFA representing 15.7% for both the very preterm and preterm groups, compared to 9.8% for the term group.

It is tempting to speculate that the differences between these groups may be an adaptation to the immaturity of the infant's digestive tract (Bitman *et al.*, 1983). The shorter chain, saturated FA are more readily absorbed, an obvious advantage for the preterm infant (Jensen, 1999). However, the preterm infant also has a high need for long chain polyunsaturated fatty acids to match the high interuterine accretion rates that would have otherwise occurred had the infant been delivered at term (Clandinin, 1999). Thus, it is unlikely that this is an evolutionary adaptation, as a preterm birth is an anomalous event (Jensen, 1999), and as insufficient milk production is common to the preterm mother (Lawrence & Lawrence, 1999), delivery of FA to the infant is reduced when compared to the term infant. It is more likely that the higher proportion of MCFA in milk of mothers who deliver preterm is due to either the immaturity of the gland with regard to FA incorporation from the blood (Bitman *et al.*, 1983) or the decreased preparedness of maternal fat metabolism to provide the LCFA compared to that of a mother giving birth at term.

Circadian Rhythm

In a review of the literature, Jensen (1989) found that several studies provided no evidence of the existence of either diurnal or circadian rhythms in FA composition. Studies conducted by Hall (1979), Harzer *et al.* (1983), and Gibson and Kneebone (1981) failed to find either diurnal or circadian variations in FA composition. Indeed, the study conducted by Hall (1979) has been cited as evidence of the lack of a diurnal rhythm in FA composition for the justification of sampling procedures (Borschel *et al.*, 1986).

Closer inspection of the data presented by Hall (1979) show some FA with coefficients of variation of up to 40%, indicating a high degree of variability around the mean. Furthermore, Daly *et al.* (1993b) found that the FA composition of milk did change over the course of the day, with MCFA reciprocally related to the LCFA over the course of the day, and that the same relationship was observed for each mother on two separate occasions, three days apart. Similarly, we found no evidence for a circadian rhythm, as well as an inverse relationship between MCFA and LCFA concentrations throughout the day, though this relationship was not conserved within or between women (Mitoulas *et al.*, 2000; Mitoulas *et al.*, 1999). Despite an absence of a circadian rhythm, the variation in FA composition is not random, indicating that it is unlikely that endocrine factors (prolactin, growth hormone, insulin) regulate these changes. Perhaps this non-circadian, non-random daily FA composition pattern arises as a result of a feedback loop, given the evidence that FA themselves can regulate synthesis and import FA into the lactocyte (Neville & Picciano, 1997).

In contrast to the above, a recent study from Lubetzky *et al.* (2006) claimed that total human milk fat concentrations of preterm infant mothers do follow a circadian rhythm with fat content significantly higher in the evening, supposedly after three daily meals. In a follow-up study, this was also demonstrated to occur over the entire first seven weeks of lactation (Lubetzky *et al.*, 2007). Though the authors do demonstrate a significant difference between fat content in the morning and evening, the actual difference is small and is inconsistent with the evidence that adipose stores are used as a source of some FA, and knowledge of rates of triacylglycerol biosynthesis and their secretion into the breastmilk. Furthermore, differences between morning and evening fat concentrations can be accounted for by differences in breast fullness at these time periods. In the morning period, the breast would be at its fullest due to fact that this is the longest period without any draining, in turn decreasing the total content of fat. Therefore, any clinical or health management implications based on this data should be taken with caution until further studies support these results.

Nonetheless, the importance of determining whether a circadian rhythm exists cannot be understated. The regulated entry of FA into the mammary gland could allow for optimized supplementation routines, maximizing the increase in proportions of desirable FA in breastmilk and avoiding wasteful supplementation. Clearly, with the current discrepancies in the literature, this is an area requiring further investigation.

Diet

The FA of human milk are the most responsive component to diet (Jensen *et al.*, 1995). Furthermore, as approximately 85% of the FA of mature milk are ultimately derived from the diet, the scope for dietary intervention is enormous. The first indication that diet affected FA composition was from Thiemich in 1899. He noted that the unsaturated FA content of milk increased when mothers were fed increased amounts of unsaturated fat (Jensen, 1989).

It is now well understood that dietary fat plays a major role in the FA composition of human milk. From the first dietary manipulation studies (Insull & Ahrens, 1959), it was evident that the composition was easily altered. Furthermore, from these studies, it was evident that a lack of dietary fat also affected milk FA composition. Insull and Ahrens (1959) showed that when energy and fat intake were decreased, milk FA resembled those of fat stores. Then, by increasing energy intake and carbohydrate intake, the FA synthesized in the breast (MCFA from glucose) increased. Finally, FA in milk were made to resemble the dietary FA profile by increasing maternal fat intake.

The differences in FA composition between women from different cultures (**Table 2**) (Read *et al.*, 1965; Finley & Lonnerdal, 1985; Kneebone *et al.*, 1985; Borschel *et al.*, 1986; Innis & Kuhnleim, 1988; Ruan *et al.*, 1995; Spear *et al.*, 1992; Mitoulas *et al.*, 2000; Yuhas *et al.*, 2006; de la Presa-Owens *et al.*, 1996; Smit *et al.*, 2002) is almost certainly due to differences in diet (Jensen, 1989). Kneebone *et al.* (1985) found differences in the FA composition between women from three racial groups living in the same city, Penang, Malaysia. Furthermore, Finley and Lonnerdal (1985) showed differences between vegetarians and non-vegetarians living in the Northern California area. Although Finley and Lonnerdal found differences in the n-6/n-3 ratio of breastmilk between diets, neither was found to be deficient with respect to FA composition.

Most investigations examining the effect of diet have looked at long term maternal intake, whereas few have been concerned with acute effects (Francois *et al.*, 1998). Hachey *et al.* (1987) showed that dietary FA peak in milk approximately six hours after the blood peak time of two to four hours. Francois *et al.* (1998) found the time to peak in milk to differ between FA, with the range being seven to 15 hours after ingestion. They found that a single meal could affect milk FA composition for as long as three days, with the maximum affect occurring in the first 24 hours. However, not all FA entered the milk at the same rate. The FA that were less affected by dietary sources were those with a large body pool size, e.g., 16:0 and 18:1n9 (Francois *et al.*, 1998).

With the discovery of the importance of particular LCFA to the development of the infant, the desire to increase the proportion of individual FA arose, in spite of the lack of information regarding required and actual infant intakes. Supplementation in pregnancy studies by our research group using fish oil significantly increased concentrations of 20:4n6, 20:5n3, 22:5n3, and 22:6n3 in breastmilk collected three days postpartum (Dunstan *et al.*, 2004). Similarly, Harris *et al.* (1984) showed that dietary supplementation with fish oil capsules was able to increase the proportion of both 20:5n3 and 22:6n3 in the milk, while Makrides *et al.* (1996) were able to show the same effect in a dose dependent manner using supplements derived from unicellular algae. These studies along with others indicate the possibility of selective FA enhancement through dietary intervention to meet the infant's needs.

Other Fat Classes

The phospholipid concentration of human milk is 20-40 mg/dL or 0.5 to 1% of total fat, depending on the stage of lactation (Jensen, 1989) (**Figure 2**). They originate from the membranes of the secretory cells and are mainly associated with the milk fat globule membrane (Jensen, 1989). Phospholipids (sphingomyelin, phosphotidylcholine, phosphotidylethanolamine, phosphotidylserine, and phosphotidylinositol) are believed to play vital roles in the myelinization of the CNS and also in the development of the retina (Harzer *et al.*, 1983).

Human milk also contains small quantities of sphingomyelins, neutral glycosylceramides, and gangliosides (Jensen, 1996). These complex lipids are derived from mammary gland secretory cell membranes and, as such, occur as components of the fat globule membrane (Bouhours & Bouhours, 1981). Sphingomyelin represents 29% of the phospholipid fraction of whole milk, with the same proportions in both the fat and skim fractions (Bouhours & Bouhours, 1981). It is believed to provide the newborn infant with a supply of FA and additional choline for CNS myelination (Zeisel *et al.*, 1986). Neutral glycosylceramides are believed to play a role in the non-specific protection of the infant (Newburg & Chaturvedi, 1992). The gangliosides of human milk are also believed to have non-specific antimicrobial actions (Jensen *et al.*, 1995), as well as promoting the fusion of microdroplets of fat in the globules (Keenan & Patton, 1995).

Phospholipid content varies during lactation and with gestational age. A recent study of Japanese preterm and term mothers' milk has demonstrated that human milk phospholipid content is significantly higher in colostrum compared to mature milk for both term and preterm mothers (Shoji *et al.*, 2006), with preterm mature milk containing significantly more phospholipids than term mature milk. There are also differences in specific phospholipids during different stages of lactation and gestational age. Phosphoethanolamine concentrations are similar in the colostrum of preterm and term mothers, as well as in mature milk, but are higher in the transitional milk of the preterm mother. Phosphatidylserine concentrations are lower in the colostrum of the term mother compared to preterm mothers, but are similar in transitional milk. Phosphoinositol concentrations are higher in preterm mothers' colostrum, similar in transitional milk, and less in mature milk compared with term mothers. Though the content of specific phospholipids changes during lactation, the concomitant decrease in total phospholipid content over the course of lactation supports evidence that the biosynthesis of phospholipids decreases in the later stages of lactation (Bitman *et al.*, 1984), leading to a decrease in the thickness of the milk fat globule membrane (Ruegg & Blanc, 1981).

The sterol content of human milk varies from 100-200 mg/L with cholesterol representing 90.1% of total sterols (Jensen, 1996). In general, it is believed that the content of cholesterol in milk is not affected by either diet or maternal blood levels (Jensen *et al.*, 1995). Indeed, milk may provide the mother with a physiological means of lowering blood cholesterol. Human milk also contains measurable quantities of (in descending order) squalene, demosterol, lanosterol, methostenol, dimethylsterol, and lathosterol (Jensen *et al.*, 1995). Most of the cholesterol is associated with the lipid globule membrane, except the 15% that is present as the ester and is found in the triacylglycerol fraction of the lipid

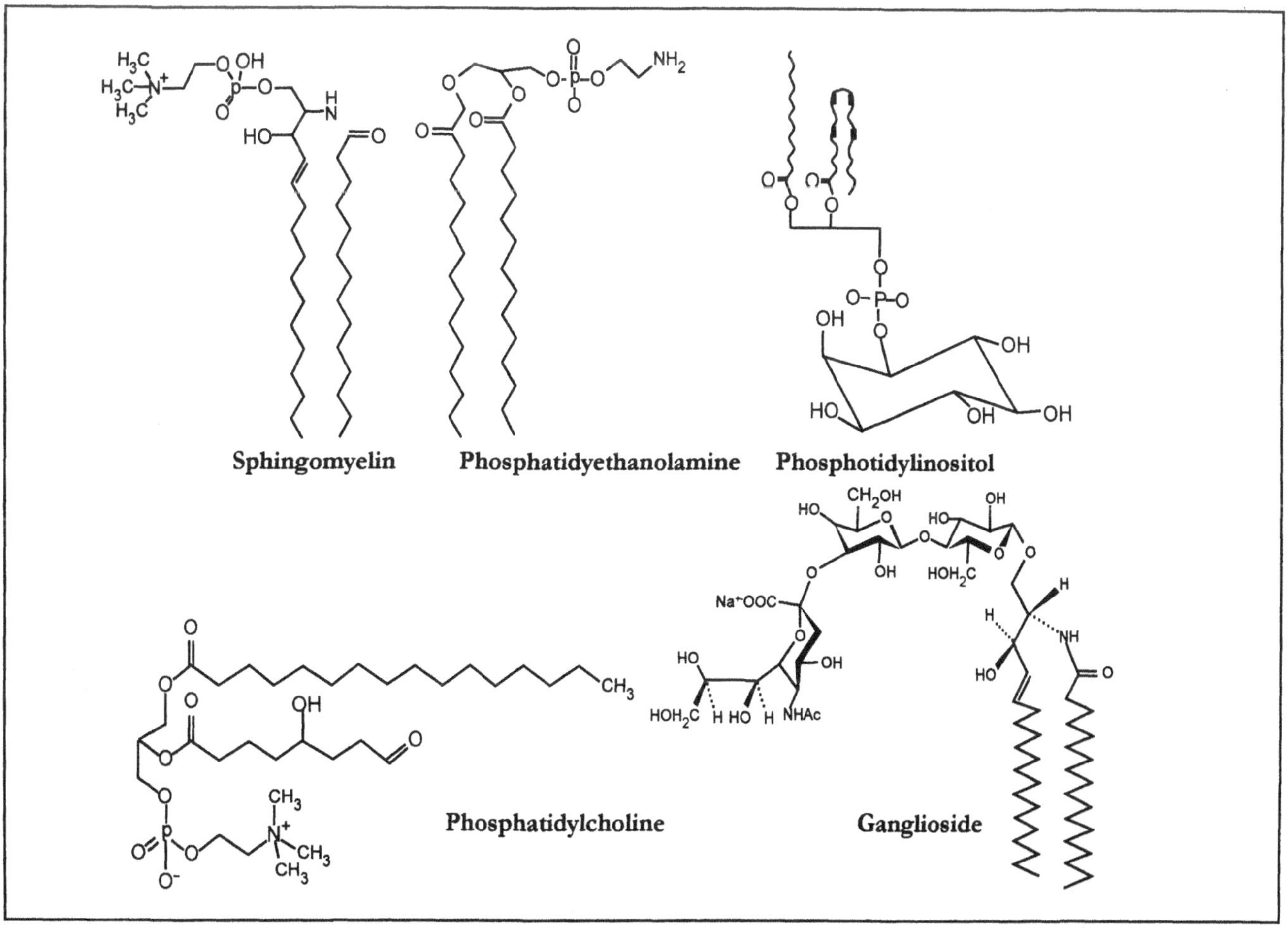

Figure 2. Chemical structures of some of the other lipids found in human milk

globule (Jensen, 1996). Although the cholesterol content of milk is not high, infant consumption as compared to the adult is elevated (Jensen, 1996). It is believed that this 'high' level of cholesterol contributes to its homeostasis in the adult who was breastfed as an infant (Reiser *et al.*, 1979).

HUMAN MILK FAT SYNTHESIS AND SECRETION

Fat Synthesis

The fats in human milk are derived from two sources: *de novo* synthesis and blood lipids (Davies *et al.*, 1983) (Figure 2, Chapter 3). The blood lipids themselves can arise from three areas: tissue synthesis and mobilization of adipose tissue, as very low density lipoproteins (VLDL) and NEFA, and the immediate diet, as chylomicrons. Indeed, Hachey *et al.* (1987) determined that VLDL and chylomicrons were the primary sources of milk fat.

De Novo Synthesis of Fatty Acids

The overall contribution of the human lactocyte derived FA to total FA is quite low, less than 20% by weight (Thompson & Smith, 1985). The mammary gland synthesizes mainly MCFA, such as 12:0 and 14:0. The FA are synthesized using acetyl-CoA derived from glucose and reducing equivalents (NADPH) from the pentose phosphate pathway (Neville *et al.*, 1983), via the reactions of acetyl-CoA carboxylase (1) and the fatty acid synthase complex (2).

Acetyl-CoA + CO_2 + ATP -----(1)--->
Malonyl-CoA + ADP + Pi
Acetyl-CoA + 7malonyl-CoA + 14 NADPH + 14 H^+----(2)--->
Palmitic acid + $7CO_2$ + 8CoA + 14NADPH + $6H_2O$.

Figure 3. First steps in FA synthesis.

The first and committed step in FA synthesis is the conversion of acetyl-CoA to malonyl-CoA by acetyl-CoA carboxylase (EC 6.4.1.2) (**Figure 3**). The fatty acid synthase complex then carries out a series of several reactions that have the net effect of adding a two carbon unit derived from malonyl-CoA to a fatty acyl chain. This chain remains covalently attached to the enzyme complex for successive additions of two carbons units from malonyl-CoA. In the mammary gland, thioesterase II stops FA elongation once the chain is 8 to 14 carbon atoms in length by the hydrolysis of the thioester bond between the complete FA and the enzyme complex (Neville *et al.*, 1983).

Blood Derived Fatty Acids

Long chain fatty acids are imported from the blood, where they are either released from circulating chylomicrons or very low density lipoproteins (VLDL) under the action of a very active lipoprotein lipase within the capillary lumen. Fatty acids can also be derived from NEFA circulating in the blood bound to albumin (Neville & Picciano, 1997). The mechanism of transfer of FA to the alveolar cell basal membrane is unclear (Neville & Picciano, 1997). However, once at the lactocyte cell membrane, they can either enter by diffusion or by a membrane transport system (Barber *et al.*, 1997; Neville & Picciano, 1997). Fatty acid binding proteins (FABP) on the plasma membrane have been implicated in the translocation of FA into the cell (Barber *et al.*, 1997). Once in the cell, FA can be either activated by the addition of CoA and bound to acyl-CoA binding proteins or they can bind to one of the abundant cytosolic FABP (Neville & Picciano, 1997). These bound FA form a pool, readily available for incorporation into triacylglycerol (Neville & Picciano, 1997) (**Figure 4**).

Chylomicron Derived Fatty Acids

Triacylglycerol and cholesterol are absorbed and re-esterified in the cells of the intestinal wall and then secreted as chylomicrons via the lymphatic system into the circulation (Frayn, 1996). Hachey *et al.* (1987) reported that 10–12% of 16:0, 18:1n9, and 18:2n6 originated from the immediate diet via chylomicrons. Francois *et al.* (1998) found that transfer of FA from the diet to milk occurred within six hours of consumption, with maximum levels of incorporation occurring 10 to 24 hours after consumption, depending on the source of the FA. Hachey *et al.* (1987) found that peak FA incorporation into milk was delayed by 6.0 ± 1.9 hours from peak FA levels in blood, but attributed this delay to time needed for lipolysis of chylomicrons by lipoprotein lipase in the mammary gland and re-synthesis into triacylglycerol in the mammary secretory cell, and then extrusion of the milk fat globule into the alveolar lumen.

Tissue Derived Fatty Acids

In contrast to the lipogenic state of pregnancy, lactation is characterized as a period of net lipolysis. In this regard, *de novo* fat synthesis in adipose tissue is decreased during lactation (Williamson & Lund, 1994). Although glucose utilization of adipose tissue was no different in the lactating compared to the non-lactating rat (Burnol *et al.*, 1987), conversion of glucose to FA was decreased in isolated adipocytes from lactating rats, whereas synthesis of glycerol was not affected (Burnol *et al.*, 1986). This inhibition of lipogenesis is due to decreased activity of pyruvate dehydrogenase and acetyl-CoA carboxylase (Williamson & Lund, 1994).

Fatty acids are also released by the liver, packaged as triacylglycerol in the form of VLDL. These FA are either synthesized *de novo* in the liver or incorporated from FA released from adipose tissue circulating in the blood. The liver also has the capacity to modify FA through the use of elongation and desaturation enzymes. Indeed, Calabro *et al.* (1982) found increased stearoyl-CoA desaturase activity in the liver of lactating rats. These results suggest that the liver may serve as an important source of 18:1n9 during lactation. Whether this increase in stearoyl-CoA desaturase can be extended to include other hepatic FA modifying enzymes and delivery of LCPUFA to the lactating mammary gland is unclear. Indeed, regulation of the enzymes involved in LCPUFA synthesis is not well defined (Cook, 1996) and, as such, constitutes an area requiring further research.

Triacylglycerol Synthesis

The precursors for triacylglycerol are glycerol-3-phosphate and fatty acyl CoA. Glycerol-3-phosphate is derived from either glycolysis by the reduction of dihydroxyacetone phosphate or from

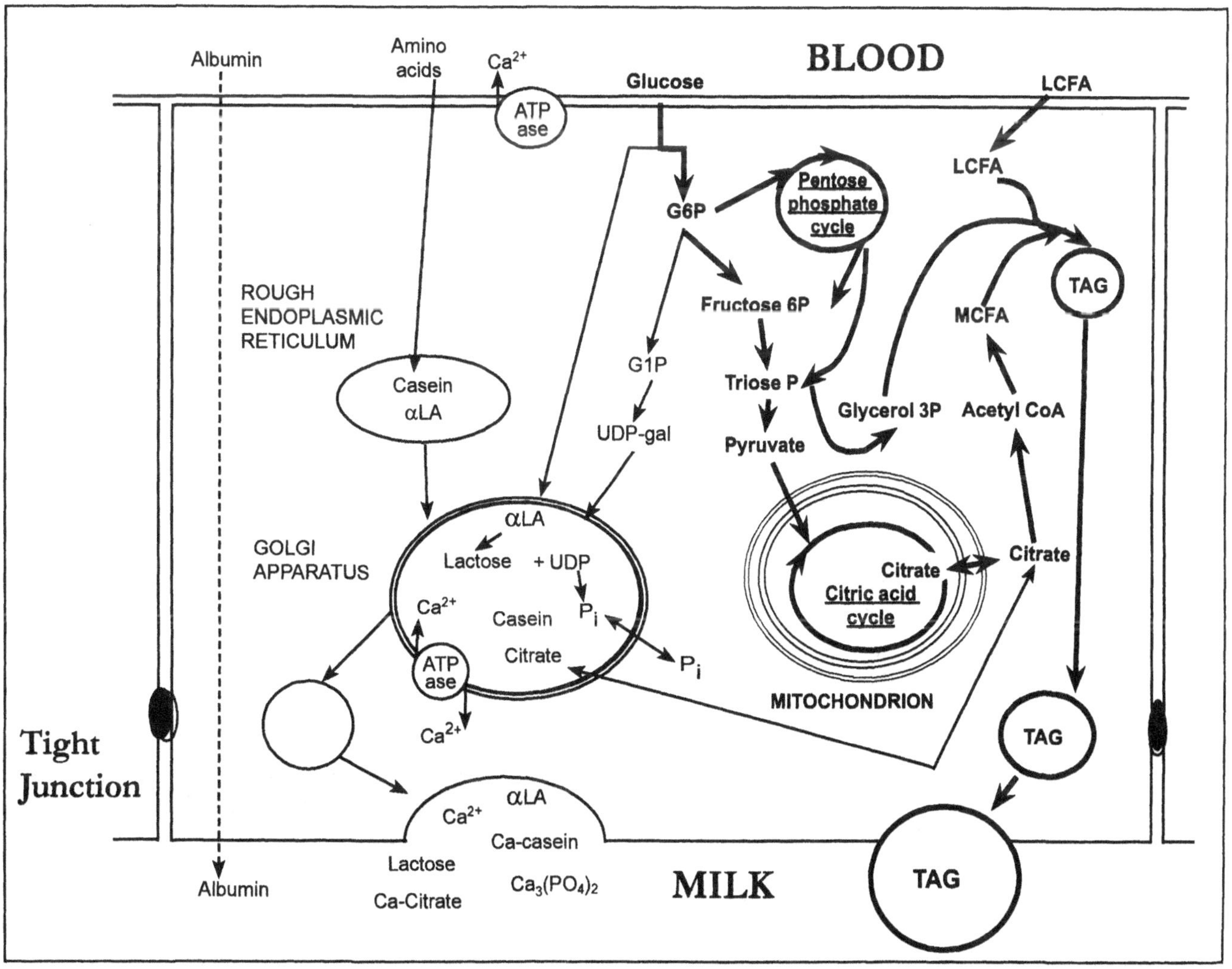

Figure 4. Biosynthetic pathways in the lactocyte highlighting pathways involved in fat synthesis. Abbreviations: G6P - glucose 6 phosphate, Pi - phosphate, MCFA - medium chain fatty acids, LCFA - long chain fatty acids, TAG - triacylglycerol, ATP - adenosine triphosphate, UDPgal - uridine diphosphate galactose, αLA - α-lactalbumin. Adapted from Hartmann, 1986.

the phosphorylation of glycerol. The first step in triacylglycerol formation is acylation of the free hydroxyl groups on glycerol-3 phosphate with two fatty acyl molecules. This results in phosphatidic acid which is dephosphorylated to give diacylglycerol. This can then combine with a third fatty acyl-CoA to give a triacylglycerol (Neville *et al.*, 1983).

Fat Secretion

The complex nature of milk requires an equally complex secretory system. Lactocytes have been described as 'stunningly beautiful' with regard to their organization (Mather & Keenan, 1998). Secretory cells are polarized with the basal area dominated by the nucleus, parallel cisternae of rough endoplasmic reticulum (Nickerson & Akers, 1984), and a supra-nuclear Golgi complex bordering the apical cytoplasm (Mather & Keenan, 1998) (Figure 2, Chapter 3). The apical cytoplasm is characterized by the presence of fat droplets and secretory vesicles with microtubules, orientated perpendicular to the apical membrane (Nickerson & Akers, 1984). Mitochondria and free ribosomes are found throughout the cytoplasm (Nickerson & Akers, 1984).

The polarization of these cells has developed a flow through synthetic process from basal to apical membrane. Precursors derived from blood capillaries are transported across the endothelial lining and basal lamina and through the plasma membrane (Nickerson & Akers, 1984). Indeed, experiments conducted by Jim Linzell in the 1970s showed that milk was made from a relatively simple mixture of blood-borne substrates: glucose, amino acids, FA, glycerol, and minerals (Linzell, 1974). These substrates are sequentially processed into a range of diverse substances, moving further from the basal membrane until a secretory product is released from the apical membrane (Mather & Keenan, 1998).

The method of fat secretion is unique to the mammary gland secretory cell and has been reviewed extensively by Mather and Keenan (1998). Fat droplets originate in the rough endoplasmic reticulum and are released into the cytoplasm coated with proteins and polar lipids derived from the endoplasmic reticulum (Mather & Keenan, 1998). These droplets ($\leq$ 0.5 μm in diameter) accumulate inside and between the cisternae of the rough endoplasmic reticulum; several cisternae may produce and harbor one fat droplet (Vorherr, 1974). The regulation of droplet fusion, whether it is a controlled or a random process, is unknown (Mather & Keenan, 1998). The fat droplets formed in the basal area of the cell then migrate to the apical membrane by an unknown process.

Secretion of the fat globule requires the binding of the cellular membrane to the fat globule followed by actual secretion. Binding of the cell membrane to the fat globule to form the MFGM is likely mediated by the butrophylin/xanthine oxidoreductase complex, which binds the cell membrane to the fat droplet (Keenan & Patton, 1995). The fat droplets are secreted through two possible mechanisms. The first, and most widely accepted method involves the protruding droplet slowly being enveloped with apical plasma membrane until the membranes at the neck of the extruding droplet meet, fuse together and release the membrane-coated fat droplet in the alveolar lumen. The second and more controversial method involves the association of Golgi derived secretory vesicles with fat droplets. In this instance, the progressive fusion of secretory vesicles on the surface of the fat droplet leads to the formation of an intracytoplasmic vacuole that contains both casein and fat within a secretory vesicle membrane. The contents of these vesicles would then be released into the lumen by exocytosis such that the casein would be free in the lumen, but the fat droplet would be enclosed by a layer of secretory vesicle membrane. While it is possible that both methods may be occurring simultaneously, it is believed that the former of these two theories is the predominant route for fat secretion. However, the latter method may explain the relatively strong coupling between lactose and protein secretion with that of fat globule secretion with regard to autocrine control mechanisms.

ACKNOWLEDGEMENT

Research funding from Medela AG.

References

Armand M, Hamosh M, Mehta NR, Angelus PA, Philpott JR, Henderson TR, *et al.* Effect of human milk or formula on gastric function and fat digestion in the premature infant. *Pediatr Res.* 1996; 40: 429-37.

Armand M, Pasquier B, Andre M, Borel P, Senft M, Peyrot J, *et al.* Digestion and absorption of 2 fat emulsions with different droplet sizes in the human digestive tract. *Am J Clin Nutr.* 1999; 70:1096-106.

Atwood CS, Hartmann PE. Collection of fore and hind milk from the sow and the changes in milk composition during suckling. *J Dairy Res.* 1992; 59:287-98.

Barber MC, Clegg RA, Travers MT, Vernon RG. Lipid metabolism in the lactating mammary gland. *Biochimica et Biophysica Acta.* 1997; 1347:101-26.

Beijers RJ, Schaaffsma A. Long-chain polyunsaturated fatty acid content in Dutch preterm breast milk: Differences in concentrations of docohexaenoic acid and arachadonic acid due to length of gestation. *Early Hum Dev.* 1996; 44:215-23.

Bitman J, Wood DL, Mehta NR, Hamosh P, Hamosh M. Comparison of the phospholipid composition of breast milk from mothers of term and preterm infants during lactation. *Am J Clin Nutr.* 1984; 40:1103-19.

Bitman J, Wood L, Hamosh M, Hamosh P, Mehta NR. Comparison of the lipid composition of breast milk from mothers of term and preterm infants. *Am J Clin Nutr.* 1983; 38:300-12.

Boehm G, Muller G, Kohn G, Moro G, Minoli I, Bohles HJ. Docosahexaenoic and arachidonic acid absorption in preterm infants fed LCP-free or LCP-supplemented formula in comparison to infants fed fortified breast milk. *Annual Nutrition Metabolism.* 1997; 41:235-41.

Borel P, Armand M, Pasquier B, Senft M, Dutot G, Melin C, *et al.* Digestion and absorption of tube-feeding emulsions with different droplet sizes and compositions in the rat. *J Parenter Enteral Nutr.* 1994; 18:534-43.

Borschel MW, Elkin RG, Kirksey A, Story JA, Galal O, Harrison GG, *et al.* Fatty acid composition of mature human milk of Egyptian and American women. *Am J Clin Nutr.* 1986; 44:330-35.

Bouhours JF, Bouhours D. Ceramide structure of sphigomyelin from human milk fat globule membrane. *Lipids.* 1981; 16:726-31.

Breckenridge WC, Marai L, Kuksis A. Triglyceride structure of human milk fat. *Can J Biochem.* 1969; 47:761-69.

Burnol AF, Ferre P, Leturque A, Girard J. Effect of insulin on in vivo glucose utilization in individual tissues of anesthetized lactating rats. *Am J Physiol.* 1987; 252:E183-88.

Burnol AF, Guerre-Millo M, Lavau M, Girard J. Effect of lactation on insulin sensitivity of glucose metabolism in rat adipocytes. *FEBS Letters.* 1986; 194:292-96.

Butte NF, Garza C, Smith EO, Nichols BL. Human milk intake and growth in exclusively breast fed infants. *J Pediatr.* 1984; 104:187-95.

Calabro MA, Prasad MR, Wakil SJ, Joshi VC. Steroyl-coenzyme A desaturase activity in the mammary gland and liver of lactating rats. *Lipids.* 1982; 17:397-402.

Carlson SE, Cooke RJ, Werkman SH, Tolley EA. First year growth of preterm infants fed standard compared to marine oil n-3 supplemented formula. *Lipids.* 1992; 27:901-7.

Carlson SE, Werkman SH, Peeples JM, Cooke RJ, Tolley EA. Arachidonic acid status correlates with first year growth in preterm infants. *Proc Natl Acad Sci USA.* 1993; 90:1073–77.

Carlson SE, Werkman SH, Tolley EA. Effect of long-chain n-3 fatty acid supplementation on visual acuity and growth of preterm infants with and without bronchopulmonary dysplasia. *Am J Clin Nutr.* 1996; 63(5):687-97.

Carnielli VP, Verlato G, Pederzini F, Luijendijk I, Boerlage A, Pedrotti D. Intestinal absorption of long chain polyunsaturated fatty acids in preterm infants fed breast milk or formula. *Am J Clin Nutr.* 1998; 67:97-103.

Cavell B. Gastric emptying in infants fed human milk or infant formula. *Acta Paediatr Scand.* 1981; 70:639-41.

Cheruku S, Ohajunwa U, Wijendran V, Lammi-Keefe CJ. Dichotomy in relationship of infant n-6 vs n-3 long chain polyunsaturated fatty acids (LCPUFA) to breast milk and maternal dietary LCPUFA. *9th International Conference for the International Society for Research in Human Milk and Lactation.* Bavaria, Germany: Kloster Irsee; 1999.

Clandinin MT. Brain development and assessing the supply of polyunsaturated fatty acid. *Lipids.* 1999; 34:131-37.

Cook HW. Fatty acid desaturation and chain length elongation in eukaryotes. In: Vance DE, Vance JE (eds.) *Biochemistry of lipids, lipoproteins and membranes.* Amsterdam: Elsevier; 1996.

Cox DB, Owens RA, Hartmann PE. Blood and milk prolactin and the rate of milk synthesis in women. *Exp Physiol.* 1996; 81:1007-20.

Daly SE, Di Rosso A, Owens RA, Hartmann PE. Degree of breast emptying explains changes in the fat content, but not fatty acid composition of human milk. *Exp Physiol.* 1993a; 78: 741-55.

Daly SE, Owens RA, Hartmann PE. The short-term synthesis and infant-regulated removal of milk in lactating women. *Exp Physiol.* 1993b; 78:209-20.

Davies DT, Holt C, Christie WW. The composition of milk. In: Mepham TB (ed.). *The Biochemistry of Lactation.* Amsterdam: Elsevier Science Publishers; 1983.

De La Presa-Owens S, Lopez-Sabater MC, Rivero-Urgell M. Fatty acid composition of human milk in Spain. *J Pediatr Gastroenterol Nutr.* 1996; 22:180-85.

Del Prado M, Villalpando S, Lance A, Alfonso E, Demmelmair H, Kolestzko B. Contribution of dietary and newly formed arachidonic acid to milk secretion in women on low fat diets. In: Kolestzko B, Michaelsen KF, Hernell O (eds.). *Short and long term effects of breast feeding on child health.* New York: Kluwer Academic/Plenum Publishers; 2000.

Dorea JG, Horner MR, Bezerra VLVA. Correlation between changeable human milk constituents and milk intake in breast-fed babies. *J Pediatr.* 1982; 101:80-83.

Dunstan JA, Mori TA, Barden A, Beilin LJ, Taylor AL, Holt PG, *et al.* Fish oil supplementation in pregnancy modifies neonatal allergen-specific immune responses and clinical outcomes in infants at high risk of atopy: A randomized, controlled trial. *J Allergy Clin Immunol.* 2003a; 112:1178-84.

Dunstan JA, Mori TA, Barden A, Beilin LJ, Taylor AL, Holt PG, *et al.* Maternal fish oil supplementation in pregnancy reduces interleukin-13 levels in cord blood of infants at high risk of atopy. *Clin Exp Allergy.* 2003b; 33:442-48.

Dunstan JA, Roper J, Mitoulas L, Hartmann PE, Simmer K, Prescott SL. The effect of supplementation with fish oil during pregnancy on breast milk immunoglobulin A, soluble CD14, cytokine levels and fatty acid composition. *Clin Exp Allergy.* 2004; 34:1237-42.

Emmett PM, Rogers IS. Properties of human milk and their relationship with maternal nutrition. *Early Hum Dev.* 1997; 49 Suppl:S7-28.

Fernstrom JD. Effects of dietary polyunsaturated fatty acids on neuronal function. *Lipids.* 1999; 34:161-69.

Fewtrell MS, Morley R, Abbott RA, Singhal A, Isaacs EB, Stephenson T. Double-blind, randomized trial of long-chain polyunsaturated fatty acid supplementation in formula fed to preterm infants. *Pediatrics.* 2002; 110:73-82.

Fidler N, Sauerwalkd TU, Demmelmair H, Pohl A, Kolestzko B. Docahexonoic acid (DHA) transfer into human milk after dietary DHA supplementation. *9th International Conference for the Internation Society for Research in Human Milk and Lactation.* Bavaria, Germany: Kloster Irsee; 1999.

Filer LJ Jr, Mattson FH, Fomon SJ. Triglyceride configuration and fat absorption by the human infant. *J Nutr.* 1969; 99:293-98.

Finley DC, Lonnerdall B. Fatty acid composition of breast milk from vegetarian and non vegetarian lactating women. In: Schaub J (ed.). *Composition and physiological properties of human milk.* Amsterdam: Elsevier Science Publishers; 1985.

Fomon S J, Ziegler EE, Thomas LN, Jensen RL, Filer LJ Jr. Excretion of fat by normal full-term infants fed various milks and formulas. *Am J Clin Nutr.* 1970; 23:1299-313.

Francois CA, Connor SL, Wander RC, Connor WE. Acute effects of dietary fatty acids on the fatty acids of human milk. *Am J Clin Nutr.* 1998; 67:301-8.

Frayn K. *Metabolic regulation: A human perspective.* London: Portland Press; 1996.

Genzel BO, Wahle J, Kolestzko B. Fatty acid composition of human milk during the 1st month after term and preterm delivery. *Eur J Pediatr.* 1997; 156:142-47.

Gibson RA, Kneebone GM. Fatty acid compostion of human colostrum. *Am J Clin Nutr.* 1981; 34(2):252-57.

Gillin FD, Reiner DS, Gault MJ. Cholate dependent killing of Giardia lamblia by human milk. *Infect Immun.* 1985; 47:619-22.

Goff D. Dairy chemistry and physics. University of Guelph; 1995. Available at: http://www.foodsci.uoguelph.ca/dairyedu/chem.html.

Hachey DL, Thomas MR, Emken EA, Garza C, Brown BL, Adlof RO, *et al.* Human lactation: Maternal transfer of dietary triglycerides labeled with stable isotopes. *J Lipid Res.* 1987; 28:1185-92.

Hall B. Uniformity of human milk. *Am J Clin Nutr.* 1979; 32:304-12.

Hanson LA, Wiedernmann U, Ashraf R, Zaman S, Adeleberth I, Dahgren U, *et al.* Effects of breastfeeding on the baby and on its immune system. *Food Nutr Bull.* 1996; 17:384-89.

Harris WS, Connor WE, Lindsey S. Will dietary omega 3 fatty acids change the composition of human milk? *Am J Clin Nutr.* 1984; 40(4):780-85.

Hartmann PE. The breast and breast feeding. In: Philipp E, Setchell M, Ginsburg M (eds.). *Scientific foundations of obstetrics and gynaecology.* Oxford: Butterworth Heinemann; 1986.

Hartmann PE, Morgan SEG, Arthur PG. Milk let-down and the concentration of fat in breast milk. In: Hamosh M, Goldman AS (eds.). *Human lactation 2: Maternal and environmental factors.* New York: Plenum Press; 1986.

Hartmann PE, Sherriff JL, Mitoulas LR. Homeostatic mechanisms that regulate lactation during energetic stress. *J Nutr.* 1998; 128:394S-99S.

Harzer G, Haug M, Dieterich I, Gentner PR. Changing patterns of human milk lipids in the course of the lactation and during the day. *Am J Clin Nutr.* 1983; 37:612-21.

Horwood LJ, Fergusson DM. Breastfeeding and later cognitive and academic outcomes. *Pediatrics* 1998; 101:E9.

Huisman M, Lanting CI, Nijeboer HJ, Muskiet FA, Boersma ER. Triglycerides, fatty acids, sterols, mono- and dissacharides and sugar alcohols in human milk and current types of infant formula. *Eur J Clin Nutr.* 1996; 50: 255-60.

Hundrieser KE, Clark RM, Jensen RG. A comparison of methods for determination of total lipids in human milk. *Nutr Res.* 1984; 4:21-26.

Hytten FE. Clinical and chemical studies in human lactation: 1. Collection of milk samples. II. Variation in major constituents during feeding. III. Diurnal variation in major constituents in milk. *Br Med J.* 1954; 1: 249-55.

Idota T, Sakurai M, Sagawara Y, Ishiyama Y, Murakami Y, Moriguchi H, *et al.* The latest survey for the composition of milk obtained from Japanese mothers. Part II. Changes of fatty acid composition, phospholipid and cholesterol contents during lactation. *Japan Journal of Pediatric Gastroenterology and Nutrition.* 1991;5.

Innis SM, Adamkin AH, Hall RT, Kalhan SC, Lair C, Lim M. Docosahexaenoic acid and arachidonic acid enhance growth with no adverse effects in preterm infants fed formula. *J Pediatr.* 2002; 140:547-54.

Innis SM, Dyer R, Nelson CM. Evidence that palmitic acid is absorbed as sn-2 monoacylglycerol from human milk by breast-fed infants. *Lipids.* 1994; 29:541-45.

Innis SM, Dyer R, Quinlan P, Diersen-Schade D. Palmitic acid is absorbed as sn-2 monopalmitin from milk and formula with rearranged triacylglycerols and results in increased plasma triglyceride sn-2 and cholesteryl ester palmitate in piglets. *J Nutr.* 1995; 125:73-81.

Innis SM, Kuhnleim HV. Long chain n-3 fatty acids in breast milk of inuit women consuming traditional foods. *Early Hum Dev.* 1988; 18:185-89.

Insull WJ, Ahrens EHJ. The fatty acids of human milk from mothers on diets taken ad libitum. *Biochem J.* 1959; 72:27-33.

Issacs CE, Thormar H, Pessolano T. Membrane-disruptive effect on human milk: Inactivation of enveloped viruses. *J Infect Dis.* 1986; 154:966-71.

Jackson DA, Imong SM, Silprasert A, Preunglumpoo S, Leelapat P, Yootabootr Y, *et al.* Estimation of 24 h breast-milk fat concentration and fat intake in rural northern Thailand. *Br J Nutr.* 1988a; 59:365-71.

Jackson DA, Imong SM, Silprasert A, Ruckphaopunt S, Woolridge MW, Baum JD, *et al.* Circadian variation in fat concentration of breast-milk in a rural northern Thai population. *Br J Nutr.* 1988b; 59:349-63.

Jensen R (ed.). *Handbook of milk composition.* San Diego: Academic Press; 1995.

Jensen RG. *The lipids of human milk.* Boca Raton: CRC press; 1989.

Jensen RG. The lipids in human milk. *Prog Lipid Res.* 1996; 35:53-92.

Jensen RG. Lipids in human milk. *Lipids.* 1999; 34:1243-71.

Jensen RG, Bitman J, Carlson SE, Couch SC, Hamosh M, Newburg DS. A. Human milk lipids. In: Jensen RG (ed.). *Handbook of milk composition.* London: Academic Press Inc; 1995.

Jumpsen J, Lien EL, Goh YK, Clandinin MT. Small changes of dietary (n-6) and (n-3) fatty acid content ratio alter phosphatidylethanolamine and phosphatidylcholine fatty acid composition during development of neuronal and glial cells in rats. *J Nutr.* 1997a; 127:724-31.

Jumpsen JA, Lien EL, Goh YK, Clandinin MT. During neuronal and glial cell development diet n - 6 to n - 3 fatty acid ratio alters the fatty acid composition of phosphatidylinositol and phosphatidylserine. *Biochimt Biophys Acta.* 1997b; 1347:40-50.

Keenan TW, Patton S. The structure of milk: Implications for sampling and storage. A. The milk lipid globule membrane. In: Jensen RG (ed.). *Handbook of milk composition.* California: Academic Press, Inc.; 1995.

Kneebone GM, Kneebone R, Gibson RA. Fatty acid composition of breast milk from three racial groups from Penang, Malaysia. *Am J Clin Nutr.* 1985; 41:765-69.

Koletzko B, Mrotzek M, Bremer HJ. Fatty acid composition of mature human milk in Germany. *Am J Clin Nutr.* 1988; 47:954-59.

Lanting CI, Fidler V, Huisman M, Touwen BC, Boersma ER. Neurological differences between 9-year-old children fed breast-milk or formula-milk as babies. *Lancet.* 1994; 344:1319-22.

Lapillonne A, Clarke SD, Heird WC. Plausible mechanisms for effects of long-chain polyunsaturated fatty acids on growth. *J Pediatr.* 2003; 143:S9-16.

Lawrence RA, Lawrence RM. *Breastfeeding: A guide for the medical profession.* St. Louis: Mosby; 1999.

Linzell JL. Mammary blood flow and methods of idenifying and measuring precursors of milk. In: Larson BL, Smith VR (eds.). *Lactation: A comprehensive treatise.* New York: Academic Press; 1974.

Lopez-Alarcon M, Villalpando S, Fajardo A. Breast-feeding lowers the frequency and duration of acute respiratory infection and diarrhea in infants under six months of age. *J Nutr.* 1997; 127:436-43.

Lubetzky R, Littner Y, Mimouni FB, Dollberg S, Mandel D. Circadian variations in fat content of expressed breast milk from mothers of preterm infants. *J Am Coll Nutr.* 2006; 25:151-54.

Lubetzky R, Mimouni FB, Dollberg S, Salomon M, Mandel D. Consistent circadian variations in creamatocrit over the first 7 weeks of lactation: A longitudinal study. *Breastfeeding Medicine* 2007; 2:15-18.

Lucas A, Morley R, Cole TJ, Lister G, Leeson-Payne C. Breast milk and subsequent intelligence quotient in children born preterm. *Lancet.* 1992; 339:261-64.

Lukkainen P, Salo MK, Nikkari T. Changes in the fatty acid composition of preterm and term human milk from 1 week to 6 months of lactation. *J Pediatr Gastroenterol Nutr.* 1994; 18:355-60.

Makrides M, Neumann MA, Byard RW, Simmer K, Gibson RA. Fatty acid composition of brain, retina, and erythrocytes in breast- and formula-fed infants. *Am J Clin Nutr.* 1994; 60:189-94.

Makrides M, Neumann MA, Gibson RA. Effect of maternal docosahexanoic acid (DHA) supplementation on breast milk composition. *Eur J Clin Nutr.* 1996; 50:352-57.

Makrides M, Neumann MA, Simmer K, Gibson RA. Dietary long-chain polyunsaturated fatty acids do not influence growth of term infants: A randomized clinical trial. *Pediatrics.* 1999; 104:468-75.

Makrides M, Simmer K, Neumann MA, Gibson RA. Changes in the polyunsaturated fatty acids of breast milk from mothers of full term infants over 30 wk of lactation. *Am J Clin Nutr.* 1995; 61(6):1231-33.

Martin JC, Bougnoux P, Antoine JM, Lanson M, Couet C. Triacylglycerol structure of human colostrum and mature milk. *Lipids.* 1993a; 28:637-43.

Martin JC, Bougnoux P, Fignon A, Theret V, Antoine JM, Lamisse F, *et al.* Dependence of human milk essential fatty acids on adipose stores during lactation. *Am J Clin Nutr.* 1993b; 58:653-59.

Mather IH, Keenan TW. The cell biology of milk secretion: Historical notes. *J Mammary Gland Biol Neoplasia.* 1998; 3:227-32.

McManaman JL, Neville MC. Mammary physiology and milk secretion. *Adv Drug Deliv Rev.* 2003; 55:629-41.

Michalski MC, Briard V, Desage M, Geloen A. The dispersion state of milk fat influences triglyceride digestibility in the rate: a 13CO2 breath test study. *Eur J Nutr.* 2005a; 44(7):436-44.

Michalski MC, Briard V, Michel F, Tasson F, Poulain P. Size distribution of fat globules in human colostrum, breast milk, and infant formula. *J Dairy Sci.* 2005b; 88:1927-40.

Michalski MC, Cariou R, Michel F, Garnier C. Native vs. damaged milk fat globules: Membrane properties affect the viscoelasticity of milk gels. *J Dairy Sci.* 2002a; 85:2451-61.

Michalski MC, Michel F, Geneste C. On the size distribution and zeta - potential of homogenized milk fat globules. In:

Anton M (ed.). *Food emulsions and dispersions.* Kerala, India: Research Signpost; 2002b.

Miles CA, Calder PC. Modulation of immune function by dietary fatty acids. *Proceedings of the National Society.* 1998; 57:277-92.

Mitchell DC, Niu SL, Litman BJ. DHA-rich phospholipids optimize G-protein-coupled signalling. *J Pediatr.* 2003; 143:80-86.

Mitoulas LR, Kent JC, Cox DB, Owens RA, Sherriff JL, Hartmann PE. Variation in fat, lactose and protein in human milk over 24 h and throughout the first year of lactation. *Br J Nutr.* 2002; 88:29-37.

Mitoulas LR, Sherriff JL, Hartmann PE. Short and long term variation in the production, content and composition of human milk lipids. In: Kolestzko B, Michaelsen KF, Hernell O (eds.). *Short and long term effect of breast feeding on child health.* London: Kluwer Academic/Plenum Publishers; 1999.

Mitoulas LR, Sherriff JL, Hartmann PE. Short-and long term variation in the production, content, and composition of human milk fat. *Adv Exp Med Biol.* 2000; 478:401-2.

Myher JJ, Kuksis A, Tilden C, Oftedal OT. A cross-species comparison of neutral lipid composition of milk fat of prosimian primates. *Lipids.* 1994; 29: 411-9.

Neville MC, Allen JC, Watters C. The mechanisms of milk secretion. In: Neville MC, Neifert MR (eds.). *Lactation: Physiology, nutrition and breastfeeding.* New York, Plenum Press; 1983.

Neville MC, Picciano MF. Regulation of milk lipid secretion and composition. *Annu Rev Nutr.* 1997; 17:159-83.

Newburg DS, Chaturvedi P. Neutral glycolipids of human and bovine milk. *Lipids.* 1992; 27:923-27.

Nickerson SC, Akers RM. Biochemical and ultrastructural aspects of milk synthesis and secretion. *Int J Biochem.* 1984; 16:855-65.

Nims B, Macy I, Brown M, Hunscher H. Human milk studies. Variations in the composition of milk at four hour intervals during the day and night. *Am J Dis Child.* 1932; 828-44.

O'Connor DL, Hall R, Adamkin D, Auestad N, Castillo M, Connor WE, *et al.* Growth and development in preterm infants fed long-chain polyunsaturated fatty acids: A prospective, randomized controlled trial. *Pediatrics.* 2001; 108:359-71.

Oddy WH, Holt PG, Sly PD, Read AW, Landau LI, Stanley FJ, *et al.* Association between breast feeding and asthma in 6 year old children: Findings of a prospective birth cohort study. *BMJ.* 1999; 319:815-19.

Pond C. Physiological and ecological importance of energy storage in the evolution of lactation: Evidence for a common pattern of anatomical organization of adipose tissues in mammals. In: Peaker M, Vernon R, Knight C (eds.). *Physiological strategies in lactation.* Symposia of the Zoological Society of London. London: Academic Press; 1984.

Prentice A, Prentice AM, Whitehead RG. Breast-milk fat concentrations of rural African women. 2. Long-term variations within a community. *Br J Nutr.* 1981; 45:495-503.

Read WW, Lutz PG, Tashjian A. Human milk lipids. II. The influence of dietary carbohydrates and fat on the fatty acids of mature milk. A study in four ethnic groups. *Am J Clin Nutr.* 1965; 17:180-83.

Reiser R, O'Brien B, Henderson G, Moore G. Studies on the possible function of cholesterol in milk. *Nutr Rep Int.* 1979; 19:835.

Riordan J. The biological specificity of breastmilk. In: Riordan J, Auerback K (eds.). *Breastfeeding and human lactation.* Boston: Jones and Bartlett; 1993.

Ruan C, Liu X, Man H, Ma X, Lu G, Duan G, *et al.* Milk composition in women from five different regions of China: The great diversity of milk fatty acids. *J Nutr.* 1995; 125:2993-98.

Ruegg M, Blanc B. The fat globule size distribution in human milk. *Biochim Biophys Acta.* 1981; 666:7-14.

Ryan AS, Montalto MB, Groh-Wargo S, Mimouni F, Sentipal-Walerius J, Doyle J, *et al.* Effect of DHA-containing formula on growth of preterm infants to 59 weeks postmenstrual age. *Am J Human Biol.* 1999; 11:457-67.

Saarinen UM, Kajosaari M. Breastfeeding as prophylaxis against atopic disease: Prospective follow-up study until 17 years old. *Lancet.* 1995; 346:1065-69.

Sadurskis A, Kabir N, Wager J, Forsum E. Energy metabolism, body composition, and milk production in healthy Swedish women during lactation. *Am J Clin Nutr.* 1988; 48:44-49.

Shoji H, Shimizu T, Kaneko N, Shinohara K, Shiga S, Saito M, *et al.* Comparison of the phospholipid classes in human milk in Japanese mothers of term and preterm infants. *Acta Paediatr.* 2006; 95:996-1000.

Simonin C, Ruegg M, Sidiropoulos D. Comparison of the fat content and fat globule size distribution of breast milk from mothers delivering term and preterm. *Am J Clin Nutr.* 1984; 40:820-26.

Smit EN, Martini IA, Mulder H, Boersma ER, Muskiet FA. Estimated biological variation of the mature human milk fatty acid composition. *Prostaglandins Leukot Essent Fatty Acids.* 2002; 66:549-55.

Smith J. Human milk supply in Australia. *Food Policy.* 1999; 24:71-91.

Spear ML, Bitman J, Hamosh M, Wood DL, Gavula D, Hamosh P. Human mammary gland function at the onset of lactation: Medium-chain fatty acid synthesis. *Lipids.* 1992; 27:908-11.

Straarup EM, Lauritzen L, Faerk J, Hoy Deceased CE, Michaelsen KF. The stereospecific triacylglycerol structures and fatty acid profiles of human milk and infant formulas. *J Pediatr Gastroenterol Nutr.* 2006; 42:293-99.

Thiebaud M, Dumay E, Picart L, Guiraud J, Cheftel J. High pressure homogenization of raw bovine milk. *Int Dairy J.* 2003; 13:427-39.

Thompson BJ, Smith S. Biosynthesis of fatty acids by lactating human breast epithelial cells: An evaluation of the contribution to the overall composition of human milk fat. *Pediatr Res.* 1985; 19:139-43.

Thormar H, Isaacs CE, Brown HR, Barshatzky MR, Pessolano T. Inactivation of enveloped viruses and killing of cells by fatty acids and monoglycerides. *Antimicrob Agents Chemother.* 1987; 31:27-31.

Uauy R, Hoffman DR, Birch EE, Birch DG, Jameson DM, Tyson J. Safety and efficacy of omega-3 fatty acids in the nutrition of very low birth weight infants: Soy oil and marine oil supplementation of formula. *J Pediatr.* 1994; 124:612-20.

Vanderhoof J, Gross S, Hegyi T. A multicenter long-term safety and efficacy trial of preterm formula supplemented with long-chain polyunsaturated fatty acids. *J Pediatr Gastroenterol Nutr.* 2000; 31:121-27.

Vorherr H. *The breast: Morphology, physiology and lactation.* New York: Academic Press; 1974.

Walstra P. Studies on milk fat dispersion II. The globule size distribution of a cow's milk. *Neth Milk Dairy J.* 1969; 23:99-110.

Watson M, Alford E, Dill CW. Richter R, Garza C. Compositional changes during sequential sampling of human milk. *Nutr Rep Int.* 1982; 26:1105-11.

Watts R, Dils R. Human milk: Quantitative gas-liquid chromatographic analysis of triclyceride and cholesterol content during lactation. *Lipids.* 1968; 3:471-76.

Whittlestone W. Variations in the fat content of milk throughout the milking process. *J Dairy Res.* 1953; 20:146-53.

Wiking L, Stagsted L, Bjorck L, Nielson J. Milk fat globule size is affected by fat production in dairy cows. *Int Dairy J.* 2004; 14:909-13.

Williamson D, Lund P. Cellular mechanism for the regulation of adipose tissue lipid metabolism in pregnancy and lactation. In: Allen L, King J, Lonnerdal B (eds.). *Nutrient regulation during pregnancy.* New York: Plenum Press; 1994.

Yuhas R, Pramuk K, Lien EL. Human milk fatty acid composition from nine countries varies most in DHA. *Lipids.* 2006; 41:851-58.

Zeisel SH, Char D, Sheard NF. Choline, phosphatidylcholine and sphingomyelin in human and bovine milk and infant formulas. *J Nutr.* 1986; 116:50-8.

Chapter 5

Human Milk Composition - Carbohydrates

Charles Czank, Leon R. Mitoulas, and Peter E. Hartmann

INTRODUCTION

The major carbohydrate in human milk is the disaccharide lactose. In addition to lactose, human milk also contains monosaccharides (mainly glucose and galactose) and over 130 different oligosaccharides (McVeagh & Miller, 1997). Lactose is the major osmole of human milk, and in most terrestrial species, the rate of lactose synthesis is strongly related to the volume of milk produced (Neville *et al.*, 1983).

LACTOSE

Lactose is a disaccharide comprised of galactose and glucose joined by a 1,4 β-glycosidic bond (**Figure 1**). Glucose and UDP-galactose are transported into the Golgi secretory vesicle system of the lactocyte, and lactose is formed by way of lactose synthase (Neville *et al.*, 1983). This enzyme complex consists of a membrane bound enzyme, galactosyl transferase, and a regulatory protein, α-lactalbumin. The binding of α-lactalbumin to galactosyl transferase increases the affinity of glucose to the latter and allows the formation of lactose rather than N-acetyllactosamine under physiological conditions (Ebner & Schanbacher, 1974).

Human milk contains one of the highest lactose concentrations of any species, contributing approximately 40% of the energy delivered to the infant (Hambraeus, 1984). Lactose is hydrolyzed to the monosaccharides, galactose and glucose, by the brush border enzyme, lactase, in the small intestine and then delivered to the liver via the portal vein (Kliegman & Sparks, 1985).

Glucose transportation into the liver is mediated by phosphorylation to glucose 6-phosphate by glucokinase and hexokinase. Glucokinase has a significantly higher Michaelis-Menten rate constant (K_m) compared to hexokinase. Thus, hepatic glucokinase can phosphorylate glucose at the high concentrations delivered to the liver in the portal vein following absorption of glucose from the small intestine. However, newborn infants have low glucokinase activity (Walker & Holland, 1965; Kliegman *et al.*, 1983), and as hexokinase has a low K_m, they are not able to augment hepatic phosphorylation of glucose, therefore leading to a reduced uptake of glucose by the liver and an increase in the proportion of glucose entering the peripheral circulation in these infants. Thus, low birth weight infants develop diabetic-like glucose tolerance curves, and it has been demonstrated that glucose intolerance is a contributing factor to higher infant mortality rates in preterm infants (Zarif *et al.*, 1976). Fortunately, the galactose derived from the hydrolysis of lactose in the small intestine is phosphorylated to galactose 1-phosphate by galactokinase, which has a high activity in the liver of the newborn infant. This facilitates the rapid phosphorylation of galactose by the liver (Meloncelli, 2007; Kliegman *et al.*, 1983; Kliegman & Sparks, 1985; Walker & Khan, 1968) to glucose 1-phosphate, ensuring that 50% of the hexose (glucose 1 phosphate) obtained

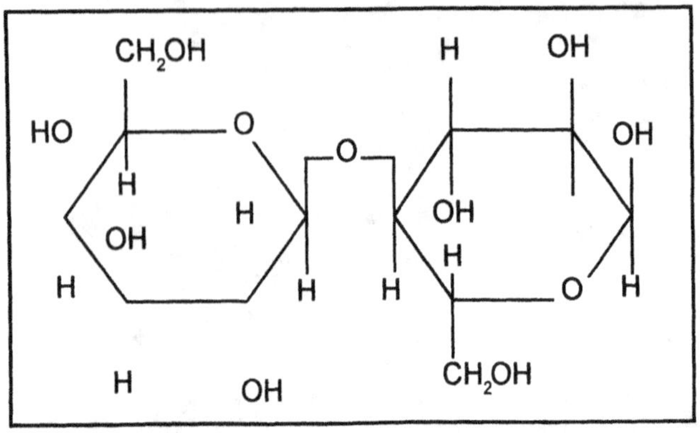

Figure 1. Structure of lactose

from lactose digestion is available to replenish liver glycogen stores (**Figure 2**).

Although both galactose and glucose can be used by the brain for energy, galactose is also used to make galactolipids (e.g., cerebroside) that are essential for the developing central nervous system (Lawrence, 1995). In addition, lactose has also been shown to improve the absorption of calcium by the infant (Riordan, 1993).

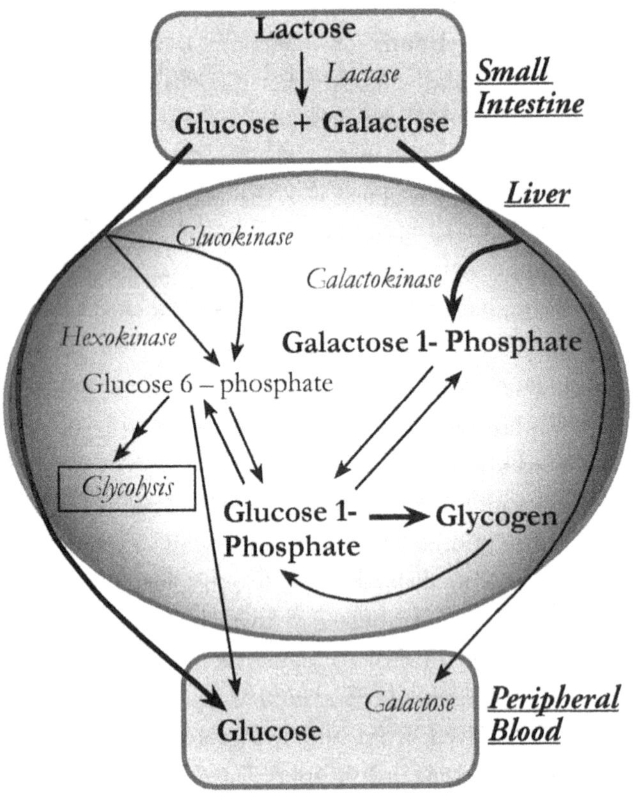

Figure 2. Simplified biochemical pathways illustrating the metabolization of lactose in the small intestine and initial stages of glucose and galactose uptake in the liver. The relative size of the arrows and text represent the pathways that are utilized in the infant as a result of low glucokinase activity and low K_m of hexokinase affecting the glucose phosphorylation pathway.

Synthesis And Secretion Of Lactose

Lactose is synthesized in the Golgi secretory vesicle system (**Figure 3**) (Neville *et al.*, 1983). α–Lactalbumin is glycosylated as it moves through the Golgi where it combines with the membrane-bound galactosyl transferase to produce the functional lactose synthase complex (Nickerson & Akers, 1984). The Golgi membrane is impermeable to the newly formed larger lactose molecule, and therefore lactose is trapped in the luminal spaces of the Golgi complex and secretory vesicles (Mather & Keenan, 1998). Consequently, water is drawn in to maintain osmotic equilibrium (Neville *et al.*, 1983). The secretory vesicles migrate toward the apical membrane, facilitated by the presence of microtubules and microfilaments, the majority of which are found in the apical and paranuclear cytoplasm, in particular around the Golgi (Nickerson & Akers, 1984). Once at the apical membrane, they eject their contents by exocytosis, thus accounting for the secretion of water (therefore exerting major control over milk yield), water soluble components, casein micelles, and some monovalent ions (Mather & Keenan, 1998).

Oligosaccharides

In 1933, a non-lactose fraction of milk was identified by Polonovsky and Lespagnol (Newburg & Neubauer, 1995). It is now understood that this fraction is not a single carbohydrate, but a complex mixture of approximately 130 different oligosaccharides (McVeagh & Miller, 1997). Furthermore, this fraction is a major component of human milk present at levels comparable to that of protein. Coppa and coworkers (1993) found the concentration of oligosaccharides in colostrum and mature milk to be 20.9 ± 4.81 and 12.9 ± 3.30 g/L (mean ± SD), respectively. Small quantities have been found in the milks of other eutherian mammals; however, not only do they lack in total amount, but they also lack in diversity (McVeagh & Miller, 1997).

Oligosaccharides are complex carbohydrates consisting of glucose, galactose, *N*-acetylglucosamine, fucose, and sialic acid (Coppa *et al.*, 1993), with lactose usually found at the reducing end (McVeagh & Miller, 1997). They are synthesized in the Golgi vesicles and range from three to ten monosaccharide units in length (McVeagh & Miller, 1997). Unlike lactose, oligosaccharides are not believed to provide a major proportion of the energy requirements of the infant, as they are not readily digested in the small intestine

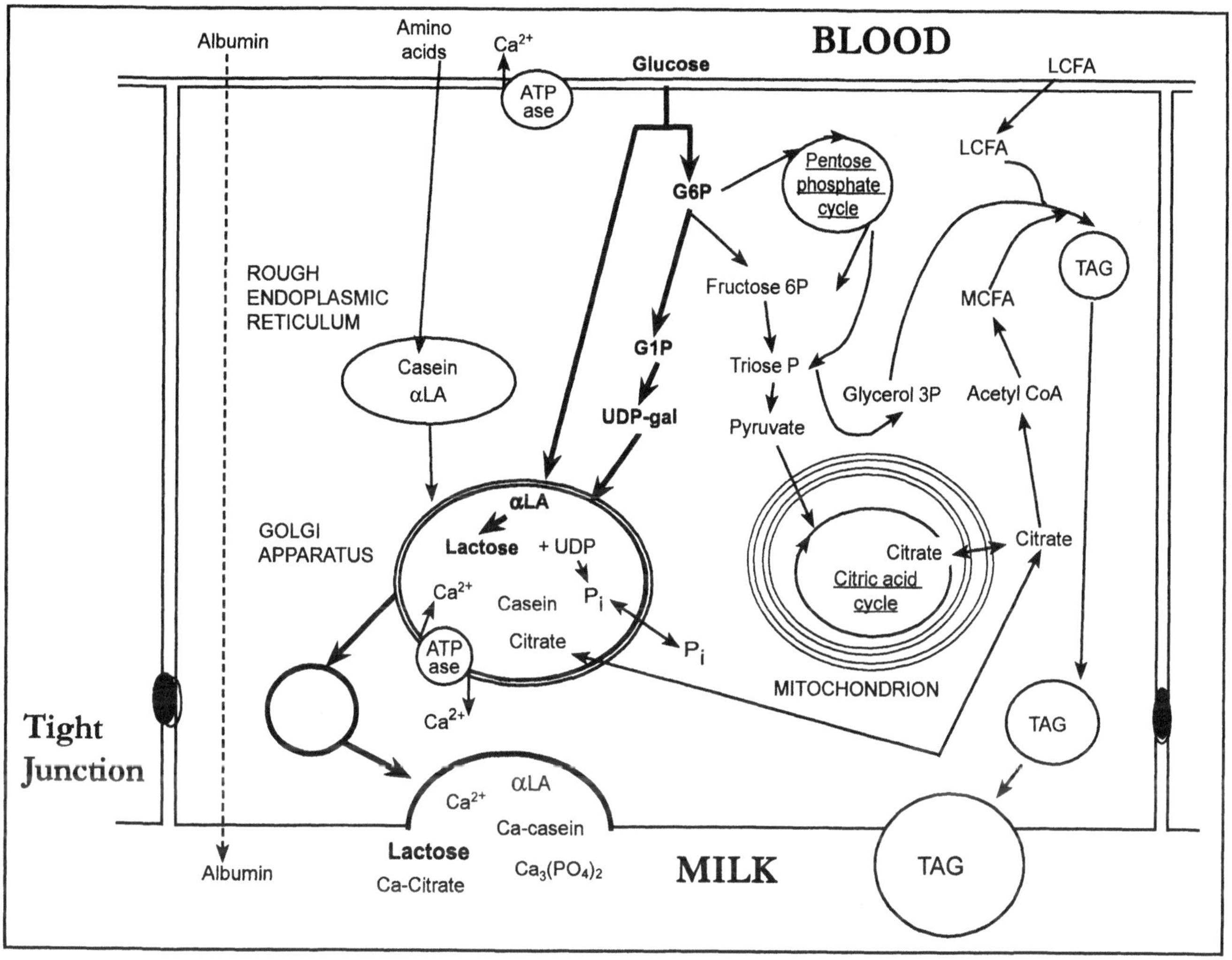

Figure 3. Biosynthetic pathways in the lactocyte highlighting pathways involved in lactose synthesis. Abbreviations: G6P - glucose 6 phosphate, Pi - phosphate, MCFA - medium chain fatty acids, LCFA - long chain fatty acids, TAG - triacylglycerol, ATP - adenosine triphosphate, UDPgal - uridine diphosphate galactose, αLA - α-lactalbumin. Adapted from Hartmann, 1986.

(McVeagh & Miller, 1997) and appear to, instead, have probiotic activities that promote growth of the harmless bacteria, *Bifidobacterium bifidum* (McVeagh & Miller, 1997), as well as various anti-infective properties (Coppa *et al.*, 1993). Bacterial adhesion to the host's epithelial cells is the first stage of infection, which is mediated by carbohydrate binding proteins present on the surface of bacteria that bind to oligosaccharides on the epithelial cell surface (Sharon, 1996). Many of the oligosaccharides present in human milk are structurally identical to epithelial cell surface oligosaccharides and, therefore, function as alternate binding sites for bacteria, in turn preventing bacteria from binding to the epithelial cell surface and initiating infection (Bode, 2006). For example, *Campylobacter jejuni,* one of the most common causes of diarrhea, binds to the intestinal 2-fucosyllactosamine, which is also found in human milk (Ruiz-Palacios *et al.*, 2003) and, indeed, the incidence of *Campylobacter* related infantile diarrhea is less in breastfed infants as a result (Morrow *et al.*, 2004).

While ligand mimicry and probiotic activity appear to be the main function of human milk oligosaccharides, they may also alter the glycome of the intestinal epithelial cells. *In vitro* glycan micro array studies of Caco-2 cells exposed to 3-sialyllactose, a common human milk oligosaccharide, show evidence of altered glycosyltransferase expression, leading to lower amounts of cell surface sialic acid, fucose, and galactose (Angeloni *et al.*, 2005). The end result being the production of altered surface antigens that are not recognized by invading bacteria, therefore preventing infection. Indeed, the above study demonstrated a 50% reduction in adhesion of enteropathogenic *E. coli* (Angeloni *et al.*, 2005). Similar mechanisms may also contribute to reduced pathogen adhesion in the upper respiratory tract, as human milk has been shown to reduce the adherence of *Haemophilus influenzae* and *Streptococcus pneumoniae* to human pharangeal and buccal cells (Andersson *et al.*, 1986).

Given that human milk oligosaccharides are able to withstand digestion and are also partially absorbed by the infant intestine and secreted in the urine of breastfed infants (Obermeier *et al.*, 1999; Rudloff *et al.*, 1996; Gnoth *et al.*, 2001), it is possible that they may be able to exert their effects systemically; however, human milk derived oligosaccharides have not yet been detected in blood. Based on the assumption that human milk oligosaccharides do make it into systemic circulation, a wide range of protein-carbohydrate interactions may be altered by their effect. For instance, alterations to the composition of selectins, which mediate cell-cell interactions in the immune system (Springer, 1994), could potentially effect the inflammatory response (Bode, 2006) because P and E selectins mediate leukocyte deceleration (rolling) on activated epithelial cells and initiate leukocyte extravasation at sites of inflammation (Springer, 1994). Another important target may be DC-SIGN, which mediates capture and the escape of several important human pathogens, including HIV-1, hepatitis C, Ebola, Dengue virus, and cytomegalovirus (van Kooyk & Geijtenbeek, 2003), thus alterations to the structure of DC-SIGN would significantly affect the infectivity of such pathogens. In addition, the presence of oligosaccharides in the urine of breastfed infants suggests they may also protect against infection from urinary pathogens (Bode, 2006). Finally, while human milk oligosaccharides play mainly a protective role, they are also are an important source of sialic acids that, in turn, are an integral part of the gangliosides found in the infant cerebral and cerebellar grey matter (McVeagh & Miller, 1997).

ACKNOWLEDGEMENT

Research funding from Medela AG.

References

Andersson B, Porras O, Hanson LA, Lagergard T, Svanborg-Eden C. Inhibition of attachment of Streptococcus pneumoniae and Haemophilus influenzae by human milk and receptor oligosaccharides. *J Infect Dis.* 1986; 153:232-37.

Angeloni S, Ridet JL, Kusy N, Gao H, Crevoisier F, Guinchard S, *et al.* Glycoprofiling with micro-arrays of glycoconjugates and lectins. *Glycobiology.* 2005; 15:31-41.

Bode L. Recent advances on structure, metabolism, and function of human milk oligosaccharides. *J Nutr.* 2006; 136:2127-30.

Coppa GV, Gabrielli O, Pierani P, Catassi C, Carlucci A, Giorgi PL. Changes in carbohydrate composition in human milk over 4 months of lactation. *Pediatrics.* 1993; 91:637-41.

Ebner K, Schanbacher F. Biochemistry of lactose and related carbohydrates. In: Larson BL, Smith V (eds.). *Lactation.* 2nd Ed. New York: Academic Press; 1974.

Gnoth MJ, Rudloff S, Kunz C, Kinne RK. Investigations of the in vitro transport of human milk oligosaccharides by a Caco-2 monolayer using a novel high performance liquid chromatography-mass spectrometry technique. *J Biol Chem.* 2001; 276:34363-70.

Hambraeus L. Composition of human milk: Nutritional aspects. *Bibl Nutr Dieta.* 1996; 37-44.

Hartmann P. The breast and feeding. In: Philipp E, Setchell M, Ginsburg M (eds.). *Scientific foundations of obstetrics and gynaecology.* Oxford: Butterworth Heinemann; 1986.

Kliegman RM, Miettinen EL, Morton S. Potential role of galactokinase in neonatal carbohydrate assimilation. *Science.* 1983; 220:302-4.

Kliegman RM, Sparks JW. Perinatal galactose metabolism. *J Pediatr.* 1985; 107:831-41.

Lawrence R. *Breastfeeding: A guide for the medical profession.* St. Louis: Mosby; 1995.

Mather IH, Keenan TW. The cell biology of milk secretion: Historical notes. Introduction. *J Mammary Gland Biol Neoplasia.* 1998; 3:227-32.

McVeagh P, Miller JB. Human milk oligosaccharides: Only the breast. *J Paediatr Child Health.* 1997; 33:281-86.

Meloncelli P. *Development of an alternative carbohydrate source for pre-term infants.* Department of Chemistry, School of Biomedical, Biomolecular and Chemical Science. Perth, Western Australia: University of Western Australia; 2007.

Morrow AL, Ruiz-Palacios GM, Altaye M, Jiang X, Guerrero ML, Meinzen-Derr JK, *et al.* Human milk oligosaccharides are associated with protection against diarrhea in breast-fed infants. *J Pediatr.* 2004; 145:297-303.

Neville M, Allen J, Watters C. The mechanisms of milk secretion. In: Neville MC, Neifert MR (eds.). *Lactation: Physiology, nutrition and breastfeeding.* New York: Plenum Press; 1983.

Newburg D, Neubauer S. Carbohydrates in milks: analysis, quantities and significance. In: Jensen R (ed.). *Handbook of milk composition.* San Diego: Academic Press; 1995.

Nickerson SC, Akers RM. Biochemical and ultrastructural aspects of milk synthesis and secretion. *Int J Biochem.* 1984; 16:855-65.

Obermeier S, Rudloff S, Pohlentz G, Lentze MJ, Kunz C. Secretion of 13C-labelled oligosaccharides into human milk and infant's urine after an oral [13C]galactose load. *Isotopes Environ Health Stud.* 1999; 35:119-25.

Riordan J. The biological specificity of breastmilk. In: Riordan J, Auerbach K (eds.). *Breastfeeding and human lactation.* Boston: Jones and Bartlett; 1993.

Rudloff S, Pohlentz G, Diekmann L, Egge H, Kunz C. Urinary excretion of lactose and oligosaccharides in preterm infants fed human milk or infant formula. *Acta Paediatr.* 1996; 85:598-603.

Ruiz-Palacios GM, Cervantes LE, Ramos P, Chavez-Munguia B, Newburg DS. Campylobacter jejuni binds intestinal H(O) antigen (Fuc alpha 1, 2Gal beta 1, 4GlcNAc), and fucosyloligosaccharides of human milk inhibit its binding and infection. *J Biol Chem.* 2003; 278:14112-20.

Sharon N. Carbohydrate-lectin interactions in infectious disease. *Adv Exp Med Biol.* 1996; 408:1-8.

Springer TA. Traffic signals for lymphocyte recirculation and leukocyte emigration: The multistep paradigm. *Cell.* 1994; 76:301-14.

van Kooyk Y, Geitjenbeek TB. DC-SIGN: Escape mechanism for pathogens. *Nat Rev Immunol.* 2003; 3:697-709.

Walker DG, Holland G. The development of hepatic glucokinase in the neonatal rat. *Biochem J.* 1965; 97:845-54.

Walker DG, Khan HH. Some properties of galactokinase in developing rat liver. *Biochem J.* 1968; 108:169-75.

Zarif M, Pildes RS, Vidyasagar D. Insulin and growth-hormone responses in neonatal hyperglycemia. *Diabetes.* 1976; 25:428-33.

Chapter 6

Human Milk Composition - Nitrogen and Energy Content

Charles Czank, Leon R. Mitoulas, and Peter E. Hartmann

INTRODUCTION

The nitrogen concentration of mature human milk is approximately 1.71 ± 0.31 g/L (mean ± SD) (Hambraeus *et al.*, 1978). Nitrogen in human milk is derived from two sources, protein and other non-protein components. The non-protein nitrogen constitutes approximately 25% of the total nitrogen in mature human milk (Hambraeus, 1984) and remains relatively constant in concentration (0.45 ± 0.05 g/L; mean ± SD) throughout lactation (Hambraeus, 1984; Lonnerdal & Atkinson, 1995).

NON-PROTEIN NITROGEN

Non-protein nitrogen is derived from free amino acids, peptides, nucleic acids and nucleotides, creatine and creatinine, urea, uric acid, ammonia, amino sugars, polyamines, carnitine, and other biologically active compounds (Atkinson, 1989) (**Figure 1**). Many of these components are thought to be either metabolic breakdown products filtered directly from the maternal blood or derived from the mammary gland itself (Atkinson, 1989). In general, however, the contribution each component plays in either the nutritional (e.g., energy) or developmental value of breastmilk remains to be fully explained.

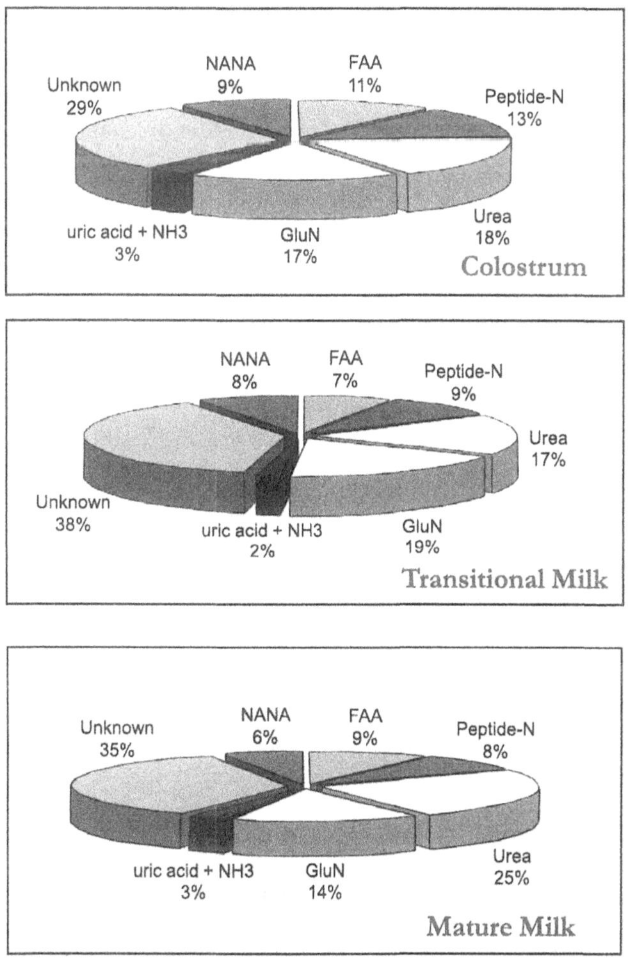

Figure 1. Representation of non-protein nitrogen components of human milk during different lactation stages, illustrating relative percentage of free amino acids (FAA), glutamine/glutamic acid (GluN), N-acetyl-nuramic acid (NANA), and uric acid + NH3. Adapted from Atkinson & Lonnerdal, 1995a.

NUCLEOTIDES AND NUCLEOSIDES

Nucleotides are comprised of a nitrogenous base, a 5-carbon sugar (deoxyribose or ribose), and 1-3 phosphate groups (**Figure 2**) and are generally found at concentrations of around 50-150 µmol/L in human milk. The nitrogenous bases are derivatives of purines (adenine, guanine) or pyrimidines (cytosine, thymine, or uracil), and ribonucleotides and deoxyribonucleotides are the monomeric precursors of RNA and DNA, respectively (Yu, 2002). Nucleotides are synthesized *de novo*, as well as being derived from the protease and nuclease degradation of nucleoproteins. Nucleosides are considered to be metabolic products, as they formed as a result of alkaline phosphatase metabolism of nucleotides (Yu, 2002).

Given that the nucleotides are synthesized by the infant, it remains uncertain what contribution dietary-derived nucleotides have on the infant's nutrition (Quan & Barness, 1990). However, assuming that under certain physiological conditions where demand for nucleotides outweighs the capacity of *de novo* synthesis and endogenous salvage (Quan & Barness, 1990), they are therefore classified as either semi-essential or conditionally essential vitamins. Semi-essential vitamins become essential during times of insufficient intake, during a high rate of physiological growth, and in the presence of disease, which are circumstances that are faced by the premature or small-for-gestational-size infant (Yu, 2002).

Though the nutritional contribution of human milk-derived-nucleotides remains unclear, there is evidence that suggests that nucleotides regulate several key functions in the body (Carver, 1994; Carver, 1999). A putative immunomodulatory function has been suggested as animal studies have shown incidences of enhanced lymphocyte proliferation in animals fed nucleotide-supplemented diets (Cohen *et al.*, 1984; Perignon *et al.*, 1987; Marijnen *et al.*, 1989). Similarly, animal studies have demonstrated a potential role for nucleotides in regulating the development of the gastrointestinal system, though the mechanisms for both of these putative functions remain to be determined (Uauy *et al.*, 1990; Carver, 1994; Bueno *et al.*, 1994; Lopez-Navarro *et al.*, 1996; Sato *et al.*, 1999).

Nucleotides are known to have several non-nutritive effects in the infant, hence its inclusion in many modern formulas. Nucleotides appear to stimulate the growth of beneficial bacteria, such *Bifidobacteria,* that lower the pH of intestinal contents and impair growth of pathogenic bacteria (Yu, 2002). Additionally, in a large randomized controlled study (n=194) comparing nucleotide and non-nucleotide supplemented diets, the incidence of first episodes of diarrhea was significantly lower in the supplemented group (Brunser *et al.*, 1994). Though there have been very few clinical studies on the effect of dietary nucleotides on the infant immune system, one study has shown an increase in IgM and IgA in the nucleotide supplemented group, suggesting that nucleotides may act upon the lymphocytes to

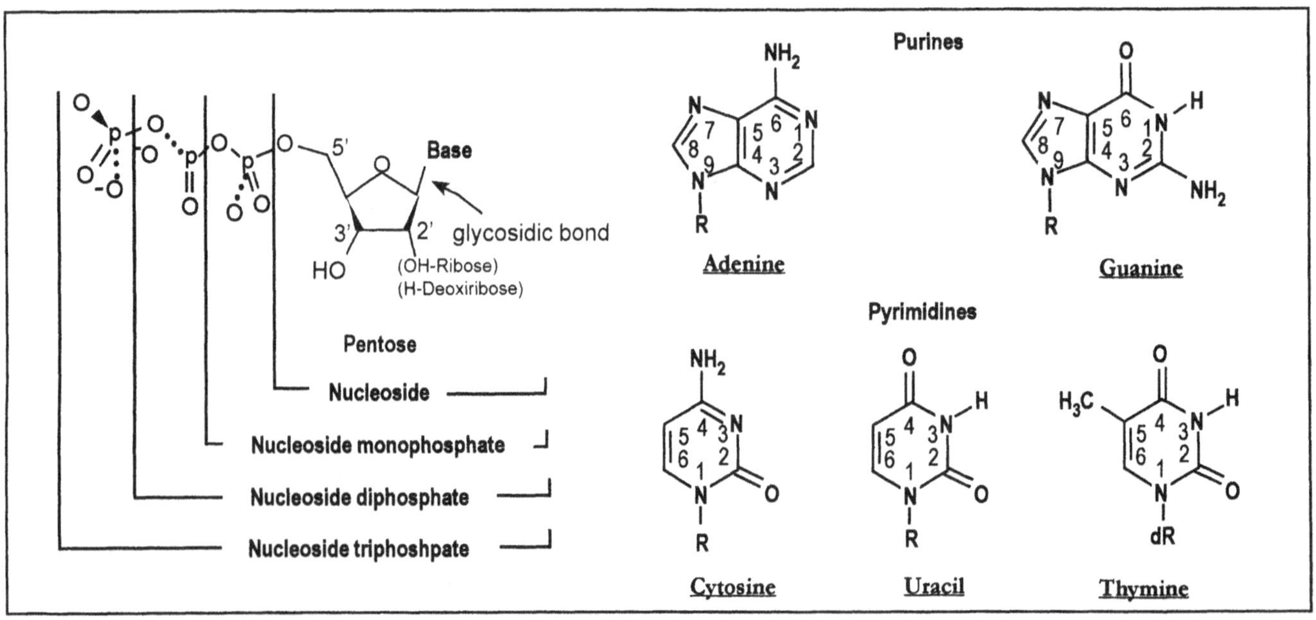

Figure 2. Structural characteristics of nucleotides, nucleosides, and nitrogenous bases that form the overall structure.

enhance the production of immunoglobulins (Navarro *et al.*, 1999). A putative effect on lipid metabolism has also been suggested as several studies found that the relative amount of n3 and n6 LCPUFA decreased in non-nucleotide supplemented infant diets (DeLucchi *et al.*, 1987; Pita *et al.*, 1988). Interestingly, many studies have shown no effect on the growth of appropriate-for-gestational-age infants fed nucleotide supplemented diets; however, faster catch up growth is seen in small-for-gestational-age infants fed supplemented diets (Cosgrove *et al.*, 1996). It is obvious that dietary nucleotides have many beneficial effects on the infants; however, more research is required to elucidate the mechanisms by which they act.

CARNITINE

Carnitine is a quaternary amine that is functionally essential in fatty acid metabolism as it is involved in the transport machinery that transfers fatty acids into the matrix of the mitochondrian for β-oxidation (Borum, 1985) (**Figure 3**). Fatty acids are an important fuel source for the developing neonate, and utilization of long chain fatty acids is dependent on the concentration of carnitine present. Carnitine is involved in several critical physiological processes that ensure the survival of the neonate, such as lipolysis, thermogenesis, and ketogenesis (Borum, 1985). Though the infant has the ability to synthesize carnitine, it is often at inadequate concentrations, and as such, carnitine can be considered as conditionally essential. Human milk carnitine concentrations are not subject to variations in either maternal diet or time of day (Atkinson & Lonnerdal, 1995a).

UREA (CARBAMIDE)

The urea content of human milk is particularly high, contributing around 30-50% of the total nitrogen present and is known to fluctuate with stage of lactation

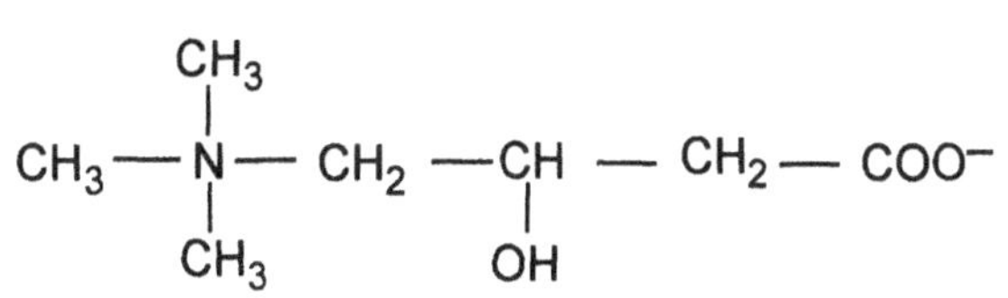

Carnitine

Figure 3. Structure of carnitine

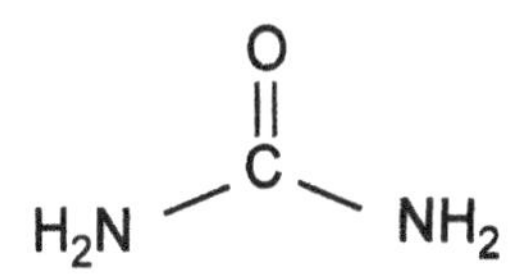

Figure 4. Structure of urea (carbamide)

(Atkinson & Lonnerdal, 1995a) (**Figure 4**). The amount of urea present in human milk increases during the stages of lactation and averages around 100-118 mg/L in colostrum, 119-133 mg/L in transitional milk, and 120-217 mg/L in mature milk (Atkinson *et al.*, 1980; Erickson *et al.*, 1934; Atkinson *et al.*, 1989; Atkinson & Lonnerdal, 1995a). Several studies have demonstrated a correlation between plasma urea concentrations, which range from 7-25 mg per 100 ml of blood, and breastmilk concentrations, suggesting that passive diffusion determines the concentration of urea in breastmilk (Denis & Talbot, 1919; Erickson *et al.*, 1934; Svanberg *et al.*, 1977). However, this does not support the evidence that urea concentration in breastmilk increases with stage of lactation, and it is therefore likely that another mechanism is involved.

FREE AMINO ACIDS

Free amino acids are well characterized components of human milk and represent around 3-5% of total amino acids or 18-24% of total nitrogen present (Atkinson & Lonnerdal, 1995a). Free amino acid concentrations in human milk are greatly influenced by diet as demonstrated by restricted protein diet studies (Forsum & Lonnerdal, 1980; Lindblad & Rahimtoola, 1974; Wurtman & Funstrom, 1979). In general, the relative concentration of free amino acids is highest in colostrum and decreases throughout lactation. The exception, however, appears to be glutamate/glutamic acid, which has been found by most studies to increase in concentration during lactation (Atkinson *et al.*, 1980). In addition, the free amino acid content of preterm colostrum, transitional, and mature milk is significantly higher than term mothers' milk of the same stage (Chuang *et al.*, 2005) (**Table 1**).

For all stages of lactation, the most abundant free amino acids tend to be taurine and glutamic acid. The role of taurine as a conditionally essentially nutrient continues to be debated. However, there is evidence that taurine insufficiency in both term and preterm

Table 1. **Average Concentrations of Free Amino Acids in Full Term and Preterm Milk during Stage of Lactation**

	Full term human milk			Preterm human milk		
Amino acid (μmol/L)	Colostral	Transitional	Mature	Colostral	Transitional	Mature
Essential						
Leucine	80	60	61	1933	37	52
Threonine	124	88	116	593	76	93
Valine	110	96	102	1223	61	109
Lysine	156	99	90	1395	76	128
Isoleucine	30	23	24	20	3	10
Phenylalanine	27	22	22	303	15	29
Histidine	33	32	32	241	33	20
Cysteine	24	19	31	47	18	24
Tryptophan	19	23	11	33	39	9
Non-essential						
Glutamine	4	5	51	3	3	1
Glutamic acid	1225	1086	881	1208	1839	1611
Aspartic acid	205	118	128	7078	160	109
Asparagine	1	1	0	4	0	0
Serine	120	84	167	545	112	122
Proline	85	57	28	3190	36	38
Alanine	245	224	384	1286	258	247
Glycine	87	67	155	331	133	92
Arginine	65	33	27	402	45	59
Tyrosine	36	25	31	725	19	42
Other						
Taurine	6751	563	491	844	845	388
Phosphoserine	161	97	95	243	101	115
Ethanolamine	82	41	35	166	88	43
Phosphoenthanolamine	135	121	130	121	138	73
Ornithine	36	23	13	172	13	9
Total	3831	3065	3492	16722	4196	3500

Adapted from Chuang *et al.*, 2005.

infants results in impaired fat absorption, bile acid secretion, retinal function, and hepatic function, which can easily be reversed via taurine supplementation (Chesney *et al.*, 1998). Similarly, the fact that glutamic acid concentrations increase over lactation while total nitrogen concentration falls, suggests that this free amino acid does indeed have an important nutritive function. This temporal change in concentration and the ability of glutamic acid to protect the enteral mucosa, act as a neurotransmitter, and as a source of nitrogen (Agostoni *et al.*, 2000) may mediate some aspects of infant development while the child is breastfed.

PROTEIN

The protein content of human milk is approximately 9 g/L, but decreases as lactation progresses (Riordan, 1993). Compared with bovine milk, human milk contains less total protein, but it is of a higher biological value. From providing amino acids and nitrogen for protein synthesis and energy production to intact proteins to assist infant development (e.g., sIgA, bile salt stimulated lipase), the proteins of human milk support the growth and development of the infant in a variety of ways. They are present in micelles, bound to the milk fat globule membrane, or in free solution in the whey fraction (Kunz & Lonnerdal, 1989).

Caseins

Casein is the protein component that gives milk its characteristic white color, and in most species, except humans, is the most abundant class of proteins (Lonnerdal & Atkinson, 1995). Caseins are classified into different subunits, with β-casein (24 kDa) and κ-casein (19 kDa) present in human milk, and bovine milk containing an additional two subtypes of α-casein (23 kDa) (α_{S1} and α_{S2}). Caseins exist as micelles composing different subunits, which are complexed with calcium phosphate in the center of the micelle. Micelle formation is a complex process that is thought to be mediated by the attraction between phosphorylated serine residues on the β-casein subunit and charged sialic acid residues on the highly glycosylated κ-casein subunit. One model proposed by Schmidt and then modified by van Dijk proposes that in bovine milk, the α_{S1}-, β-, κ-casein associate to form submicelles with a hydrophobic core and hydrophilic κ-casein and phosphate-rich N-terminals of the β- casein on the surface. In this model, as calcium phosphate is deposited on the submicelles, they shrink then aggregate to form micelles, with submicelles on the outside containing κ-casein (Kent, 1999; Schmidt, 1982; van Dijk, 1992). *In vitro* studies have demonstrated that human casein micelles form under lower calcium concentrations than bovine casein micelles, which is likely to be responsible for the lower calcium concentrations exhibited in human milk (Lonnerdal & Atkinson, 1995).

The κ-casein subunit is particularly susceptible to proteolytic cleavage at Ile 105 and Met 106 peptide bond, leading to destabilization of the casein micelle. Further cleavage of casein subunits by other enzymes results in the release of amino acids and small peptides for absorption by the infant intestine. Thus, the casein micelle is the main nutritional mechanism for delivering calcium and phosphorous to the infant, both of which are essential for bone mineralization, as well as essential amino acids which cannot be synthesized by the infant.

In general, casein has a mainly nutritive function of providing essential minerals and amino acids to the infant. In addition to this primary role, casein is also a source of peptides with a multitude of functions. Casein-derived peptides are formed in the milk itself (Ferranti *et al.*, 2004) due to intrinsic protease activity and from the activity of proteases in the stomach, such as trypsin (Fiat *et al.*, 1993). A major class of these peptides are caseinphosphatepeptides (CPP) derived from β-casein. CPP are able to resist enzymatic hydrolysis and remain complexed with calcium phosphate, and exhibit increased solubility compared to casein alone. *In vitro* studies in small animal models have demonstrated that the CPP - calcium phosphate complex exhibits enhanced absorption by the small intestine (Clare & Swaisgood, 2000). In addition, casein-derived peptides with antimicrobial, antihypertensive, antithrombotic, opioid, immunomodulating, and gastrointestinal functions have been discovered (Clare & Swaisgood, 2000). For instance, chymotrypsin degradation of κ-casein releases a 4000-6000 kDa peptide known as casecidin, which exhibits potent antibacterial action against a range of gram positive and negative bacteria (Lahov & Regelson, 1996). Antihypertensive peptides derived from human milk caseins include a tripeptide derived from κ-casein and decapeptide derived from β-casein, which both inhibit angiotensin I converting enzyme (ACE) to inhibit the angiotensin pathway responsible for vasoconstriction. Casopiastrin and several κ-caseinglycopeptides demonstrate antithrombotic activity by inhibiting platelet aggregation (Clare & Swaisgood, 2000; Clare *et al.*, 2003; Ferranti *et al.*, 2004; Fiat *et al.*, 1993). β-Casomorphins, as the name suggests, are β-casein-derived peptides with opioid-like activity. These peptides function as ligands for the opioid receptor that modulate a very large number of biological functions, such as social behavior, analgesic behavior, and gastrointestinal and endocrine function. The above examples of casein-derived peptides are not exhaustive and new peptides continue to be discovered. However, it is evident that the combined function of such peptides contributes to the unique qualities of human milk and the benefits conferred upon the infant. Furthermore, with the advent of protein-based pharmaceuticals, the potential to utilize such peptides for therapeutic reasons is also becoming evident. Further research is required to unlock the full potential of these molecules and the benefits they can deliver.

Lysozyme

Lysozyme, a 15 kDa protein, is one of the major whey proteins, and along with lactoferrin and secretory IgA, is considered to be one of the "big three" that contribute to the bacteriostatic and bactericidal properties of human milk. Lysozyme catalyses the hydrolysis of β-1,4 linkages between *N*-acetylmuramic acid and 2-acetylamino-2-deoxy-D-glucose in the cell walls of gram positive bacteria, resulting in lysis (Chipman & Sharon, 1969). *In vitro* studies have shown that lysozyme can kill gram negative bacteria in the presence of lactoferrin, which binds to and removes the lipopolysaccharide on the outer membrane, allowing lysozyme to enter the bacteria and degrade the proteoglycan matrix of the membrane (Lonnerdal & Atkinson, 1995; Ellison & Giehl, 1991).

Lysozyme has been shown to inhibit growth of both amoeba (Leon-Sicairos *et al.*, 2006) and HIV (Lee-Huang *et al.*, 1999). Interestingly, a nona-peptide (HL9) corresponding to 107-115 amino acid residues of lysozyme has been shown to have full anti-HIV activity (Lee-Huang *et al.*, 2005), compared against the whole enzyme. However, HL-9 does not lyse bacterial cells, instead blocking viral entry, replication, and modulating several cellular signal pathways of HIV cells, including p53, TGFβ, PKC, and NF-κB. Thus, there exists the potential for lysozyme and lysozyme derivatives to be developed as therapeutics in the future.

Current research on lysozyme is focused on producing recombinant lysozyme as a food additive, so that formula-fed infants may also receive the protective benefits conferred by the enzyme. Lysozyme has been expressed in rice, allowing lysozyme to be directly incorporated in infant formulas (Lonnerdal, 2006). Another approach involves the modification of mammary-specific genes such that human milk proteins will be expressed in non-human animals. Recently, human lysozyme has been successfully expressed in the milk of transgenic mice (Yu *et al.*, 2006). Ultimately, the aim of such research will be to produce transgenic cattle capable of expressing human lysozyme into milk at levels seen in human milk (Wall *et al.*, 1997). Thus, this could serve both as a means of producing commercial quantities of lysozyme for supplementation into infant formula and as a means of delivering lysozyme-fortified bovine milk direct to the public. Unfortunately, though the technology and methods to achieve this currently exist, many hurdles remain to be conquered. More research is required into the safety and efficacy of fortifying food with human lysozyme, as well as the need to educate the general public and disseminate negative attitudes toward genetic modification.

Lactoferrin

Traditionally, lactoferrin is classified as an iron-binding protein which mediates iron absorption (Lonnerdal & Atkinson, 1995) via a lactoferrin receptor found on the cell membrane of enterocytes (Suzuki *et al.*, 2001). Structurally, lactoferrin is a 78-80 kDa single peptide consisting of two lobes, each of which binds one Fe^{3+} molecule, connected by an α-helix. Lactoferrin contributes to the bacteriostatic properties of human milk by withholding Fe^{3+} from iron-requiring pathogens, therefore preventing their growth. In addition to iron absorption and host defense functions, lactoferrin has been demonstrated to have other functions. These include cell growth regulation (Zimecki *et al.*, 1995), DNA binding and transcriptional activation of specific DNA sequences (Fleet, 1995; He & Furmanski, 1995), natural killer cell activation (Mantel *et al.*, 1994), antitumor activity (Bezault *et al.*, 1994). Lactoferrin also has multiple enzyme activities, such as protease (Hendrixson *et al.*, 2003), deoxyribonuclease, ribonuclease, ATPase, phosphatase, and oligosaccharide hydrolysis (Kanyshkova *et al.*, 2003). Though many of the above functions of lactoferrin have been demonstrated *in vitro* using murine cell lines, given the obvious restrictions with determining these activities *in vivo*, it is possible that these functions also contribute to the antimicrobial properties of lactoferrin. For instance, the deoxyribonuclease, ribonuclease activity may function to digest viral DNA, while protease and oligosaccharide hydrolysis may digest bacterial surface attachment proteins, therefore preventing infection. While the biochemical basis that allows lactoferrin to be so functionally diverse has yet to be discovered, it has been proposed that conformational flexibility of the polypeptide and the ability to oligomerize with other lactoferrin molecules in the presence of ATP may result in different catalytic isoforms being formed, each with quite different catalytic domains (Semenov *et al.*, 1999; Semenov *et al.*, 1998).

It is no surprise then that when lactoferrin is subjected to proteolysis by pepsin in the stomach, the release of polypeptides known as lactoferricins (Lfcin) also have multiple biological functions. The most studied Lfcins derived from human lactoferritin (LfcinH) and bovine milk (LfcinB) have been shown to have antimicrobial, antiviral, antitumor, and immunological functions (Gifford *et al.*, 2005). LfcinB is a 25 amino acid polypeptide derived from the 17-41 region of bovine lactoferrin that forms a looped structure via an intramolecular disulphide bond (Bellamy *et al.*, 1992). The exact size and structure of LfcinH remains controversial, though studies have demonstrated that it is a 47-49 amino acid polypeptide with a similar looped structure to that of LfcinB (Bellamy *et al.*, 1992; Hunter *et al.*, 2005). The three dimensional structures of LfcinH and LfcinB have slight differences and greatly differ structurally from their parent molecule,

```
MRFFVPLFLVGILFPAILAKQFTKCELSQLLK--DIDGYGGIALPELICTMFHTSGYDTQ
-------------------KVFERCELARTLKRLGMDGYRGISLANWMCLAKWESGYNTR
                   * * :***:: **  .:*** **:* ..:*     ***:*:

AIVENN--ESTEYGLFQISNKLWCKSSQVPQSRNICDISCDKFLDDDITDDIMCAKKIL
ATNYNAGDRSTDYGIFQINSRYWCNDGKTPGAVNACHLSCSALLQDNIADAVACAKRVVR
*   *   .**:**:***..: **:..:.* : * *.:**. :*:*:*:* : ***:::

DIKGIDYWLAHKALCTEKLEQWLCEKL--
DPQGIRAWVAWRNRCQNRDVRQYVQGCGV
* :**  *:* :  * ::  :   :
```

Figure 5. Sequence alignment of human α-lactalbumin (top sequence) and lysozyme (bottom sequence) demonstrating high sequence homology.
*** denotes full conservation of amino acid residues.**
: and . denote partial conservation of amino acid residues.

which is likely to account for the difference in activities and microbial specificities (Gifford *et al.*, 2005). Given the wide variety of functions that lactoferritin and lactoferricin can perform, the potential use of these proteins as pharmaceuticals continues to be an exciting and continuously growing area of study.

α-Lactalbumin

One of the major whey proteins, α-lactalbumin is present in the milk of all species studied to date and constitutes 10-20% of total protein in human milk (Atkinson & Lonnerdal, 1995b). α-Lactalbumin and lactoferrin share approximately 40% of the same gene homology (**Figure 5**). It is believed that the α-lactalbumin gene evolved from the lysozyme gene as a result of gene sharing during the evolution of the mammary gland from the innate immune system (Vorbach *et al.*, 2006).

α-Lactalbumin consists of a single unglycosylated and unphosphorylated polypeptide chain of 123 amino acids. α-Lactalbumin binds Ca^{2+} and Zn^{2+}. However, it is unlikely that α-lactalbumin has a significant role in calcium transport and absorption, as only about 1% of the calcium present in milk is bound to protein (Lonnerdal & Glazier, 1985). Owing to its high nutritional value, the major role of α-lactalbumin appears to be nutritive, as its amino acid composition appears to be similar to the amino acid requirement of newborn infants (Forsum, 1974). In addition, α-lactalbumin-derived-peptides formed during digestion also appear to have antibacterial and immunostimulatory functions, while a novel folding variant that results in a multimeric α-lactalbumin complex has anti-infective properties and enhances apoptosis and, therefore, may possibly affect mucosal cell turnover and proliferation (Lonnerdal & Lien, 2003).

Apart from the important roles above, α-lactalbumin is involved in lactose synthesis in the mammary gland. Lactose synthase, the enzyme that catalyses the production of lactose, comprised of α-lactalbumin and galactosyltransferase, which when paired, catalyze the binding of glucose to UDP-galactose. In this complex, α-lactalbumin acts to lower the K_m of glucose for the enzyme, therefore allowing lactose synthesis to occur at physiological concentrations (Brew & Hill, 1975).

Immunoglobulins

Immunoglobulins are the mother's means of passing immunity against foreign bodies, usually invading pathogens, to the infant (Chapter 10). Several immunoglobulins are present in breastmilk, with sIgA being the most abundant at concentrations of 1-2 g/L early in lactation and 0.5-1 g/L later in lactation (Goldman, 1993). Secretory IgA, which is ubiquitously found in all human secretions, is secreted as a dimer linked via a secretory chain, and confers resistance against intestinal proteolysis (Goldman, 1993). The transfer of the mother's acquired immunity to the infant, via the enteromammary pathway, assists in protecting the infant's immature immune system (Lonnerdal, 2003). In addition to providing such protection, recent evidence suggests that sIgA has enzyme-like activity and is able to catalyze the phosphorylation of oligo- and polysaccharides (Karataeva *et al.*, 2006) and hydrolyze casein (Odintsova *et al.*, 2005). Though the biological significance of such activities remains to be established, it may be possible that such activities contribute to the overall immunological properties of human milk. For instance, phosphorylation of oligo- and polysaccharides could produce novel substrates that prevent binding of invading pathogens to the intestinal wall, and the hydrolysis of caseins may result in casein-derived-peptides with immunological and immunomodulating functions.

Milk Fat Globule Membrane Proteins

The proteins of the milk fat globule membrane only represent 0.3 to 0.4 g/L of human milk (4% of total protein). Furthermore, they only represent 1% of fat globule mass (Keenan & Patton, 1995). These proteins can either be associated with the outer surface of the globule, integrated in the membrane, or associated with cytoplasmic surface (Patton & Huston, 1989).

Traditionally, the study of milk fat globule membrane proteins was limited due to the difficulties associated with obtaining pure fractions. However, the advent of proteomic technologies has allowed the unprecedented characterization of these proteins. Butyrophilin is the most abundant protein in the milk fat globule membrane (Patton & Huston, 1989), followed by xanthine oxidoreductase. In addition, some 20 or more other proteins have been identified, including carbonic anyhydrase, apololipoproteins AI, AIV, E, and C, mucin 1, lactadherin, adipophilin, CD36, fatty acid binding protein, cellular retinoic acid binding protein, GTP binding protein, polymeric Ig receptor, CD59, clusterin, lactoferrin, and secretory IgA (Cavaletto *et al.*, 2004; Charlwood *et al.*, 2002). As the milk fat globule membrane is acquired from the phospholipid membrane of the lactocyte, it is likely that proteins associated with the phosphoplipid membrane are incorporated into the membrane of the milk fat globule during secretion of the fat droplet (**Figure 6**). Thus, there are likely to be significantly more proteins associated with the milk fat globule than have been characterized so far.

The functional significance of many of the proteins associated with the milk fat globule membrane is unknown. However, it is thought that the interaction between xanthine oxidoreductase and butyrophilin is responsible for the structural characteristics of the milk fat globule membrane and its association

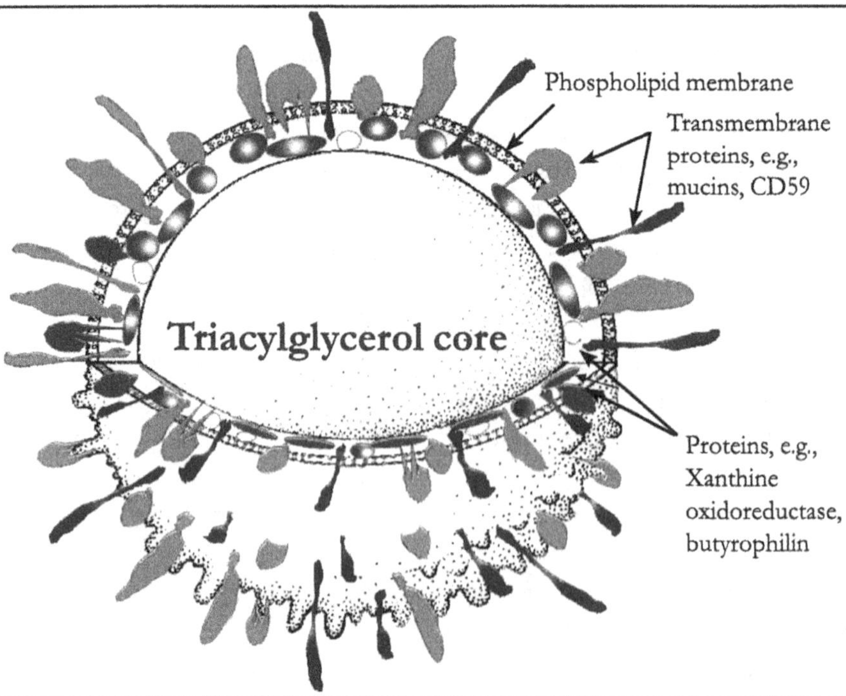

Figure 6. Putative structure of the human fat globule. The human fat globule is comprised of a triacylglycerol core surrounded by a phospholipid membrane and various proteins, including xanthine oxidoreductase, butyrophilin, carbonic anhydrase, apololipoproteins AI, AIV, E, and C, mucin 1, lactadherin, adipophilin, CD36, fatty acid binding protein, cellular retinoic acid binding protein, GTP binding protein, polymeric Ig receptor, CD59, clusterin, lactoferrin, and secretory IgA (Cavaletto *et al.*, 2004; Charlwood *et al.*, 2002).

with triacylglycerol core which forms the milk fat globule. Strong evidence exists to support this theory, in particular, the milk of xanthine oxidoreductase knockout mice (+/-) contains either partially enveloped or unenveloped milk fat globules. Furthermore, these mice were unable to maintain lactation, demonstrating that xanthine oxidoreductase is not only essential for milk fat globule membrane formation, but is also critical to lactation in general (Vorbach *et al.*, 2002). While xanthine oxidoreductase is almost ubiquitously expressed in nearly all cells, butyrophilin is exclusively associated with lactation, as it is only expressed in mammary tissue during lactation (Keenan & Patton, 1995). Butyrophilin is a classical integral transmembrane protein with a single transmembrane domain and cytoplasmic tail that interacts with xanthine oxidoreductase to form a complex that assists in the formation of the milk fat globule membrane around the milk fat globule. The acylation of this complex with long chain fatty acids (Keenan *et al.*, 1982) is believed to enhance the hydrophobic affinity of the proteins for the triacylglycerol core, therefore allowing the xanthine oxidoreductase/butyrophilin complex the ability to mediate fat globule enveloping by binding of the membrane to the droplet (Keenan & Patton, 1995).

Despite the fact that the function of many of the proteins associated with the milk fat globule membrane have not yet been studied, some do have putative functions based on previous studies. For instance, carbonic anhydrase is able to resist digestion in the infant stomach and may act as a trophic growth factor in the alimentary tract (Karhumaa *et al.*, 2001). Glycoproteins, such as mucin and lactadherin, also survive degradation in the stomach of the infant due to high levels of glycosylation and may also have immunological functions by acting as ligands for bacteria and viruses. For example, rotavirus is the most common cause of infantile gastroenteritis, and while easily treated in the developed world, is a major cause of mortality in developing countries. The lactadherin present in human milk prevents rotavirus from binding to the intestinal mucosa and initiating an infection by binding to the virus via a glycol moiety (Peterson *et al.*, 1998). While these proteins act to directly prevent infection, proteins, such as lactoferrin, clusterin, and CD59, act directly upon the immune system to inhibit the cytolytic activity of the complement pathway associated with the inflammatory response (Ogundele, 1999), thus reducing the risk of inflammation in the fragile infant while still allowing the benefits of the complement system to be received. When the immunomodulating proteins associated with the milk fat globule membrane and the anti-infective properties of the free fatty acids derived from lypolysis of the triacylglycerols core are combined, the result is a potent mixture that confers greater protective value upon the infant than any commercially available feed substitute. Despite this obvious benefit, further research is required to understand the function of many of the milk fat globule membrane proteins.

Bile stimulated lipase

Human milk bile stimulated lipase is a 90 kDa glycoprotein which aids in the formation of absorbable monoglycerides. Bile stimulated lipase is responsible for the efficient lipid digestion in breastmilk-fed infants due to its wide substrate specificity by catalyzing the hydrolysis of mono-, di-, triacylyglycerols, cholesterol esters, and diacylphosphatidylglycerols (Lonnerdal, 2003; Hernell & Blackberg, 1983). Unfortunately, human milk bile stimulated lipase is very heat labile (deactivated at 45°C) and, therefore, poses a problem in milk banks where human milk is stored and pasteurized prior to feeding (Tully *et al.*, 2001).

Amylase

Though human milk does not contain the substrate for amylase, it is present at physiological concentrations. Its purpose in human milk has yet to be established; however, it has been suggested that its presence may compensate for low salivary and pancreatic amylase activity and aid in the digestion of complex carbohydrates when complementary foods are fed alongside breastfeeding (Lonnerdal, 2003).

Growth factors

Several families of growth factors, such as epidermal growth factor (EGF), insulin-like growth factor (IGF), and transforming growth factor (TGF), that are present in human milk are believed to promote gastrointestinal maturation in the infant through their mitogenic activities. For instance, human milk EGF promotes DNA synthesis in cultured cells that have had their growth arrested (Carpenter, 1980). Furthermore, the observation that EGF concentrations are significantly higher in mothers of extremely premature infants (Dvorak *et al.*, 2003) and that this may act to reduce the incidence of necrotizing enterocolitis and intestinal inflammation (Dvorak, 2004) suggests that EGF is likely to have protective and developmental properties in the extremely premature infant.

Similarly, it has been demonstrated that the mothers' IGF concentrations are at their highest pre-partum and postpartum, which coincides with maximal proliferation of mammary cells and when the infant gut is least mature. This suggests that the IGFs have a dual function; first to promote the establishment and maintenance of the mammary system, and secondly, after secretion into the milk and ingestion by the infant, to support gastrointestinal development in the infant (Prosser, 1996). IGF's, their receptors, and binding proteins form a complex network known as the IGF axis. Given that the IGF family is able to affect the growth of such a wide range of cells, it is thought that any perturbance to the IGF axis may predispose certain alternatives in body metabolism, such as adipocity (obesity) and pathological states, like cancer, later in life. Hence, IGF's originating from human milk may play a role in "early life programming" which states that the adult individual's body physiology and potential morbidity is predetermined early in life (Schack-Nielsen & Michaelsen, 2006). However, confounding variables, such as socio-economic factors, makes it difficult to differentiate between what effects arise as a result of such pre-programming and the effects seen as a result of the environment the individual lives in (Ben-Shlomo *et al.*, 2005). Nonetheless, the effect that breastmilk

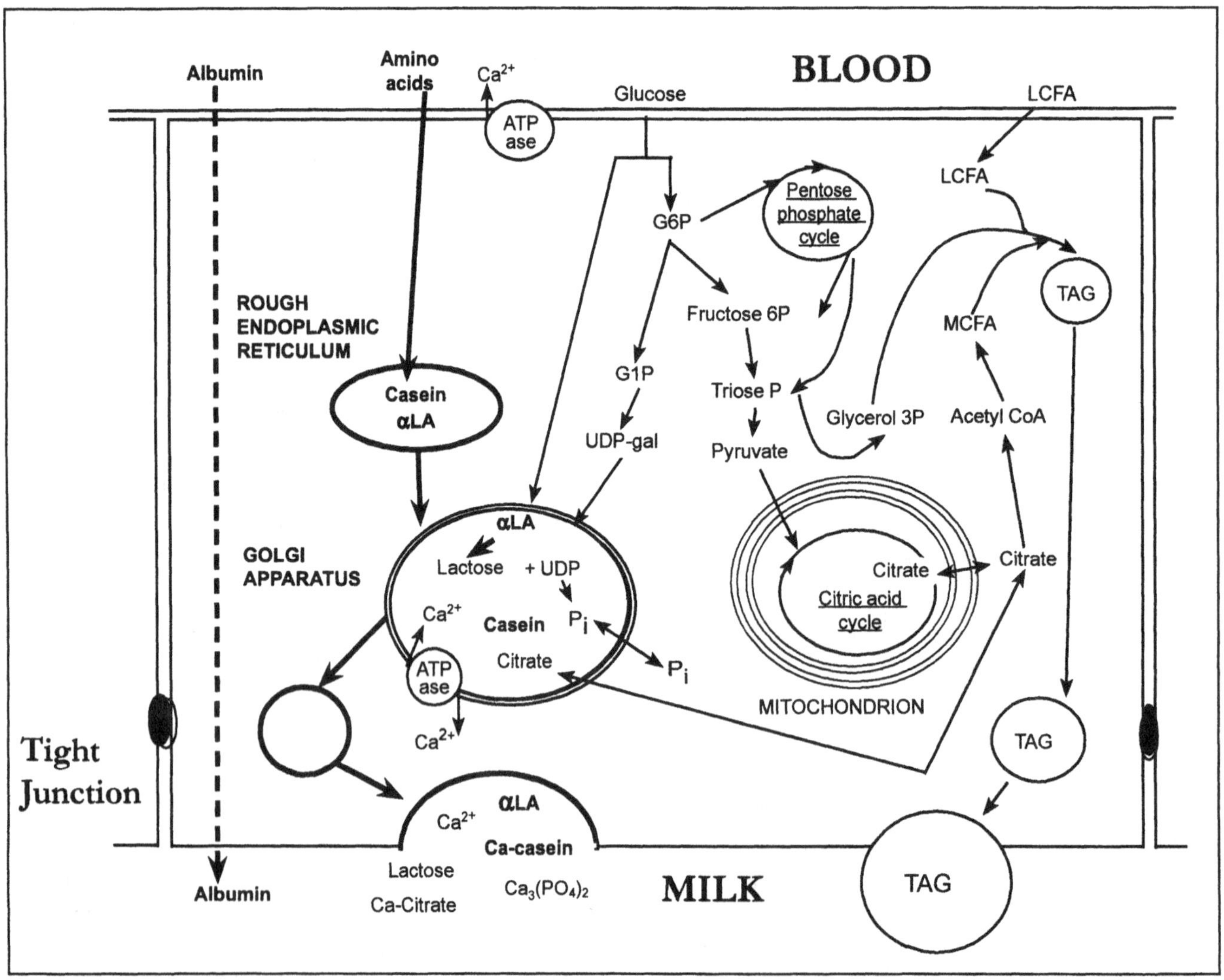

Figure 7. Biosynthetic pathways in the lactocyte highlighting pathways involved in protein synthesis. Abbreviations: G6P - glucose 6 phosphate, Pi - phosphate, MCFA - medium chain fatty acids, LCFA - long chain fatty acid, TAG - triacylglycerol, ATP - adenosine triphosphate, UDPgal - uridine diphosphate galactose, αLA - α-lactalbumin. Adapted from Hartmann, 1986.

nutrients in general have on the individual's future health remains an interesting area of study.

Synthesis and Secretion of Human Milk Proteins

A summary of the biosynthetic pathways associated with protein synthesis in the lactocyte are shown in **Figure 7**. The majority of milk proteins are synthesized within the secretory cell from imported amino acids (Nickerson & Akers, 1984). Proteins in human milk synthesized within the mammary secretory epithelial cell (lactocyte) by the rough endoplasmic reticulum from free amino acids (Lawrence, 1995) include caseins, lactoferrin, α-lactalbumin, whey acidic proteins, and protein associated with the fat globule membrane (Burgoyne & Duncan, 1998; Mather & Keenan, 1998). These proteins are then packaged into secretory vesicles and their contents released into the alveolar lumen by exocytosis (Neville *et al.*, 1983).

Additional milk proteins are derived from extracellular fluid, and these include albumin and transferrin (Burgoyne & Duncan, 1998). These proteins are taken up by endocytosis at the basolateral membrane, transported through the cell, and either released directly into the alveolar lumen or secreted by exocytosis with other milk proteins (Mather & Keenan, 1983). Immunoglobulins also follow a transcellular route across the epithelium (Mather & Keenan, 1998). The secretory component of IgA (synthesized in the gland) moves to the basolateral membrane and acts as a surface receptor for dimeric IgA. The receptor-ligand complex then enters the cell by endocytosis and moves towards the apical membrane where the complex is cleaved such that IgA is secreted into milk as sIgA with a portion of the receptor (the secretory component) still attached (Burgoyne & Duncan, 1998).

ENERGY CONTENT OF HUMAN MILK

The energy content of human milk over the first 12 months of lactation was found to range from 309-331 kJ/100 mL (74-79 kcal/100 mL) (Dewey & Lonnerdal, 1983). However, Whitehead (1995), in a review of the literature, found there to be marked variance around a mean value of 293 kJ/100 mL (70 kcal/100 mL) with the distribution ranging ± 50%. An analysis of milk energy content over the first 12 months performed in our laboratory demonstrated slightly lower results, ranging from 250-281 kJ/100ml (Mitoulas *et al.*, 2002). In all cases, these values represent the gross energy content of milk, of which approximately 92% is metabolizable energy (Butte *et al.*, 1984).

The energy content of milk can be determined by either bomb calorimetry (Butte *et al.*, 1984) or by summing the contribution to total energy from each of the major components of milk (Dewey & Lonnerdal, 1983; Garza *et al.*, 1985; Nommsen *et al.*, 1991). Garza *et al.* (1985) found the contributions of fat, lactose, and protein to be 38.7, 16.5, and 23.7 kJ/g, respectively (9.25, 3.95, and 5.65 kcal/g, respectively). Butte *et al.* (1984) found close agreement between bomb calorimetry and calculated energy content using conversion factors.

Energy Intake and Infant Growth

The high variability in the energy content of human milk (Whitehead, 1995) combined with the wide range of daily milk intake (600-900 g/day) (Butte *et al.*, 1984) between infants allows for great variability in energy intake between infants of the same age. However, it is important that energy intake is calculated correctly. First, this relies on the accurate measurement of milk intake. The test weighing of the infant is the most commonly used procedure to determine milk intake. Values obtained agree with volume estimates determined by the transfer of deuterium in human milk from mother to infant after the administration of labeled water to the mother, providing reliability in both methods (Garza & Butte, 1990). Secondly, and perhaps more importantly, a sample of milk representative of the daily intake must be obtained for analysis. This is much more problematic due to the high degree of variability of the fat content of milk (Garza & Butte, 1990).

As fat represents approximately 50% of the energy content of milk and has been shown to vary over the course of a feed (Hytten, 1954), between breasts (Jensen *et al.*, 1997), and with time of day (Nims *et al.*, 1932; Hytten, 1954; Hall, 1979; Prentice *et al.*, 1981; Jackson *et al.*, 1988; Daly *et al.*, 1993), it is imperative that sampling methods for the determination of energy intake account for most, if not all, of these levels of variability or they may not be considered representative (in terms of energy content) of milk consumed throughout the day (Garza & Butte, 1990). For example, to ensure that the variability in results arises due to the composition of milk and not the sampling procedure, we employ a sampling method that samples milk independently from each breast over 24 hours at specific time points that do not disrupt the feeding of the infant (Hartmann *et al.*, 1986).

Recommended energy intakes for breastfed infants have continually been amended since the first international publication in 1950 recommended a constant 420 kJ/kg/day (100 kcal/kg/day) for the first year of life (Davies, 1998). Subsequent studies led to the Food and Agriculture Organization, World Health Organization, and United Nations Expert Consultation (1985) report outlining a curvilinear relationship between energy intake and infant age, with intake up to 0.5 months of age being 519 kJ/kg/day (124 kcal/kg/day) compared to intake at five to six months of age being 402 kJ/kg/day (96 kcal/kg/day). This curvilinear relationship is best explained by the high demand for energy for growth (as much as one-third) by the newborn infant (Davies, 1998). The demand for energy for growth drops quickly, so that by six months of age, only 6% of energy intake is used for growth; however, at this age energy intake begins to increase again as the increased mobility of the infant has a greater energy cost (Davies, 1998).

The energy intake of breastfed infants has been found to be less than that of formula-fed infants (Garza & Butte, 1990; Heinig *et al.*, 1993). However, this is more noticeable after the introduction of solids, where the intake of milk by breastfed infants decreases, but the intake of formula by formula-fed infants does not (Garza & Butte, 1990). Furthermore, breastfed infants were consistently found to consume less than the recommended dietary allowance of energy over the first year of life (Heinig *et al.*, 1993). In this connection, longitudinal data suggests that National Child Health Services weight-for-age and weight-for-length percentiles (determined from formula-fed infants) are not maintained for the exclusively breastfed infant (Garza & Butte, 1990). These findings indicate the need for continued investigation into the determination of the energy content of human milk (accounting for all levels of variation in fat content of milk) and the establishment of new dietary recommendations and growth charts based on the requirements of the exclusively breastfed infant.

ACKNOWLEDGEMENT

Research funding from Medela AG.

References

Agostoni C, Carratu B, Boniglia C, Lammardo AM, Riva E, Sanzini E. Free glutamine and glutamic acid increase in human milk through a three-month lactation period. *J Pediatr Gastroenterol Nutr.* 2000; 31:508-12.

Atkinson S. *Protein and non-protein nitrogen in human milk.* Boca Raton: CRC Press; 1989.

Atkinson S, Lonnerdal B. Nitrogenous components of milk. A. Human milk proteins. In: Jensen R (ed.). *Handbook of milk composition.* London: Academic Press; 1995a.

Atkinson S, Lonnerdal B. Nonprotein nitrogen fractions of human milk. In: Jensen R (ed.). *Handbook of milk composition.* London: Academic Press; 1995b.

Atkinson S, Schnurr C, Donovan S, Lonnerdal B. The non-protein nitrogen components in human milk: Biochemistry and potential functional roles. In: Atkinson S, Lonnerdal B (eds.). *Protein and non-protein nitrogen in human milk.* Boca Raton: CRC Press; 1989.

Atkinson SA, Anderson GH, Bryan MH. Human milk: comparison of the nitrogen composition in milk from mothers of premature and full-term infants. *Am J Clin Nutr.* 1980; 33:811-15.

Bellamy W, Takase M, Yamauchi K, Wakabayashi H, Kawase K, Tomita M. Identification of the bactericidal domain of lactoferrin. *Biochim Biophys Acta.* 1992; 1121:130-36.

Ben-Shlomo Y, Holly J, McCarthy A, Savage P, Davies D, Davey SG. Prenatal and postnatal milk supplementation and adult insulin-like growth factor I: long-term follow-up of a randomized controlled trial. *Cancer Epidemiol Biomarkers Prev.* 2005; 14:1336-39.

Bezault J, Bhimani R, Wiprovnick J, Furmanski P. Human lactoferrin inhibits growth of solid tumors and development of experimental metastases in mice. *Cancer Res.* 1994; 54:2310-12.

Borum PR. Role of carnitine during development. *Can J Physiol Pharmacol.* 1985; 63:571-76.

Brew K, Hill RL. Lactose biosynthesis. *Rev Physiol Biochem Pharmacol.* 1975; 72:105-58.

Brunser O, Espinoza J, Araya M, Cruchet S, Gil A. Effect of dietary nucleotide supplementation on diarrhoeal disease in infants. *Acta Paediatr.* 1994; 83:188-91.

Bueno J, Torres M, Almendros A, Carmona R, Nunez MC, Rios A, *et al.* Effect of dietary nucleotides on small intestinal repair after diarrhoea. Histological and ultrastructural changes. *Gut.* 1994; 35:926-33.

Burgoyne RD, Duncan JS. Secretion of milk proteins. *J Mammary Gland Biol Neoplasia.* 1998; 3:275-86.

Butte NF, Garza C, Smith EO, Nichols BL. Human milk intake and growth in exclusively breast-fed infants. *J Pediatr.* 1984; 104:187-95.

Carpenter G. Epidermal growth factor is a major growth-promoting agent in human milk. *Science.* 1980; 210:198-99.

Carver JD. Dietary nucleotides: cellular immune, intestinal and hepatic system effects. *J Nutr.* 1994; 124:144S-48S.

Carver JD. Dietary nucleotides: effects on the immune and gastrointestinal systems. *Acta Paediatr Suppl.* 1999; 88:83-88.

Cavaletto M, Giuffrida MG, Conti A. The proteomic approach to analysis of human milk fat globule membrane. *Clin Chim Acta.* 2004; 347:41-48.

Charlwood J, Hanrahan S, Tyldesley R, Langridge J, Dwek M, Camilleri P. Use of proteomic methodology for the characterization of human milk fat globular membrane proteins. *Anal Biochem.* 2002; 301:314-24.

Chesney RW, Helms RA, Christensen M, Budreau AM, Han X, Sturman JA. The role of taurine in infant nutrition. *Adv Exp Med Biol.* 1998; 442:463-76.

Chipman DM, Sharon N. Mechanism of lysozyme action. *Science.* 1969; 165:454-65.

Chuang CK, Lin SP, Lee HC, Wang TJ, Shih YS, Huang FY, *et al.* Free amino acids in full-term and pre-term human milk and infant formula. *J Pediatr Gastroenterol Nutr.* 2005; 40:496-500.

Clare DA, Catignani GL, Swaisgood HE. Biodefense properties of milk: the role of antimicrobial proteins and peptides. *Curr Pharm Des.* 2003; 9:1239-55.

Clare DA, Swaisgood HE. Bioactive milk peptides: a prospectus. *J Dairy Sci.* 2000; 83:1187-95.

Cohen A, Barankiewicz J, Lederman HM, Gelfand EW. Purine metabolism in human T lymphocytes: role of the purine nucleoside cycle. *Can J Biochem Cell Biol.* 1984; 62:577-83.

Cosgrove M, Davies DP, Jenkins HR. Nucleotide supplementation and the growth of term small for gestational age infants. *Arch Dis Child Fetal Neonatal Ed.* 1996; 74:F122-25.

Daly SE, Di RA, Owens RA, Hartmann PE. Degree of breast emptying explains changes in the fat content, but not fatty acid composition, of human milk. *Exp Physiol.* 1993; 78:741-55.

Davies PS. Energy requirements for growth and development in infancy. *Am J Clin Nutr.* 1998; 68:939S-43S.

DeLucchi C, Pita ML, Faus MJ, Molina JA, Uauy R, Gil A. Effects of dietary nucleotides on the fatty acid composition of erythrocyte membrane lipids in term infants. *J Pediatr Gastroenterol Nutr.* 1987; 6:568-74.

Denis W, Talbot F. Non protein nitrogenous constituents of human milk. *J Biol Chem.* 1919; 39:47-51.

Dewey KG, Lonnerdal B. Milk and nutrient intake of breast-fed infants from 1 to 6 months: relation to growth and fatness. *J Pediatr Gastroenterol Nutr.* 1983; 2:497-506.

Dvorak B. Epidermal growth factor and necrotizing enterocolitis. *Clin Perinatol.* 2004; 31:183-92.

Dvorak B, Fituch CC, Williams CS, Hurst NM, Schanler RJ. Increased epidermal growth factor levels in human milk of mothers with extremely premature infants. *Pediatr Res.* 2003; 54:15-19.

Ellison RT III, Giehl TJ. Killing of gram-negative bacteria by lactoferrin and lysozyme. *J Clin Invest.* 1991; 88:1080-91.

Erickson B, Gulick M, Hunscher H, Macy I. Human milk studies XV: The non protein nitrogen constituents. *J Biol Chem.* 1934; 106:145-59.

Ferranti P, Traisci MV, Picariello G, Nasi A, Boschi V, Siervo M, *et al.* Casein proteolysis in human milk: tracing the pattern of casein breakdown and the formation of potential bioactive peptides. *J Dairy Res.* 2004; 71:74-87.

Fiat AM, Migliore-Samour D, Jolles P, Drouet L, Bal dlt SC, Caen J. Biologically active peptides from milk proteins with emphasis on two examples concerning antithrombotic and immunomodulating activities. *J Dairy Sci.* 1993; 76:301-10.

Fleet JC. A new role for lactoferrin: DNA binding and transcription activation. *Nutr Rev.* 1995; 53:226-27.

Forsum E. Nutritional evaluation of whey protein concentrates and their fractions. *J Dairy Sci.* 1974; 57:665-70.

Forsum E, Lonnerdal B. Effect of protein intake on protein and nitrogen composition of breast milk. *Am J Clin Nutr.* 1980; 33:1809-13.

Garza C, Butte NF. Energy intakes of human milk-fed infants during the first year. *J Pediatr.* 1990; 117:S124-31.

Garza C, Butte NF, Dewey KG. Determination of energy content of human milk. In: Human lactation 1: Milk components and methodologies. New York: Plenum Press; 1985.

Gifford JL, Hunter HN, Vogel HJ. Lactoferricin: a lactoferrin-derived peptide with antimicrobial, antiviral, antitumor and immunological properties. *Cell Mol Life Sci.* 2005; 62:2588-98.

Goldman AS. The immune system of human milk: antimicrobial, antiinflammatory and immunomodulating properties. *Pediatr Infect Dis J.* 1993; 12:664-71.

Hall B. Uniformity of human milk. *Am J Clin Nutr.* 1979; 32:304-12.

Hambraeus L. Human milk composition. *Nutrition Abstracts and Reviews in Clin Nut.* 1984; 54:219-36.

Hambraeus L, Lonnerdal B, Forsum E, Gebre-Medhin M. Nitrogen and protein components of human milk. *Acta Paediatr Scand.* 1978; 67:561-65.

Hartmann PE. The breast and breast feeding. In: Philipp E, Setchell M, Ginsburg M, (eds.). *Scientific foundations of obstetrics and gynaecology.* Oxford: Butterworth Heinemann; 1986.

Hartmann PE, Morgan S, Arthur P. Milk let-down and the concentration of fat in breast milk. In: Hamosh M, Goldman A (eds.). *Human lactation 2: Maternal and environmental factors.* New York: Plenum Press; 1986.

Semenov DV, Kanyshkova TG, Akimzhanov AM, Buneva VN, Nevinsky GA. Interaction of human milk lactoferrin with ATP. *Biochemistry (Mosc).* 1998; 63:944-51.

Semenov DV, Kanyshkova TG, Buneva VN, Nevinsky GA. Human milk lactoferrin binds ATP and dissociates into monomers. *Biochem Mol Biol Int.* 1999; 47:177-84.

Suzuki YA, Shin K, Lonnerdal B. Molecular cloning and functional expression of a human intestinal lactoferrin receptor. *Biochemistry.* 2001; 40:15771-79.

Svanberg U, Gebre-Medhin M, Ljungqvist B, Olsson M. Breast milk composition in Ethiopian and Swedish mothers. III. Amino acids and other nitrogenous substances. *Am J Clin Nutr.* 1977; 30:499-507.

Tully DB, Jones F, Tully MR. Donor milk: what's in it and what's not. *J Hum Lact.* 2001; 17:152-55.

Uauy R, Stringel G, Thomas R, Quan R. Effect of dietary nucleosides on growth and maturation of the developing gut in the rat. *J Pediatr Gastroenterol Nutr.* 1990; 10:497-503.

Van Dijk H. The properties of casein micelles. 6. Behaviour above pH9 and implications for the micelle model. *Neth Milk Dairy J.* 1992; 101-13.

Vorbach C, Capecchi MR, Penninger JM. Evolution of the mammary gland from the innate immune system? *Bioessays.* 2006; 28:606-16.

Wall R, Kerr D, Bondioli K. Transgenic dairy cattle: genetic engineering on a large scale. *J Dairy Sci.* 1997; 80:2213-24.

Whitehead RG. For how long is exclusive breast-feeding adequate to satisfy the dietary energy needs of the average young baby? *Pediatr Res.* 1995; 37:239-43.

Wurtman JJ, Fernstrom JD. Free amino acid, protein, and fat contents of breast milk from Guatemalan mothers consuming a corn-based diet. *Early Hum Dev.* 1979; 3:67-77.

Yu VY. Scientific rationale and benefits of nucleotide supplementation of infant formula. *J Paediatr Child Health.* 2002; 38:543-49.

Yu Z, Meng Q, Yu H, Fan B, Yu S, Fei J, *et al.* Expression and bioactivity of recombinant human lysozyme in the milk of transgenic mice. *J Dairy Sci.* 2006; 89:2911-18.

Zimecki M, Mazurier J, Spik G, Kapp JA. Human lactoferrin induces phenotypic and functional changes in murine splenic B cells. *Immunology.* 1995; 86:122-27.

Chapter 7

Hormonal Control of the Lactation Cycle

Charles Czank, Jennifer J. Henderson, Jacqueline C. Kent, Ching Tat Lai, and Peter E. Hartmann

INTRODUCTION

Before milk synthesis can occur, the breast must develop via a series of stages. The development of the breast begins in the fetus where the formation of rudimentary mammary structures occurs. After the initial fetal development, few changes to the mammary gland occur until puberty when breast growth is accelerated with each menstrual cycle until the woman becomes pregnant. Therefore, conception marks the beginning of the lactation cycle. Indeed, changes in the breast, such as breast tenderness, can be one of the earliest signs of pregnancy.

Lactation is an intermittent cyclical process of growth (mammogenesis and lactogenesis), secretion (lactation phase), and involution (weaning). The breast progresses from an undifferentiated pre-pregnancy state to full functional differentiation shortly after parturition, to involution and loss of differentiated tissue during weaning. The endocrine system has a major role in synchronizing this process either by acting directly on the mammary gland or indirectly by coordinating metabolic changes to facilitate the additional energy demands of providing milk for the offspring. Lactogenesis is defined as the initiation of milk secretion and is generally accepted to occur in two stages, lactogenesis I (secretory differentiation) and lactogenesis II (secretory activation) (Hartmann, 1973).

LACTATION CYCLE

Development During Pregnancy – Mammogenesis and Lactogenesis I

During pregnancy, histological and biochemical changes occur within the mammary tissue that prepare the breasts for synthesis and secretion of milk when the infant is born. Two distinct phases exist during pregnancy which are defined as mammogenesis and lactogenesis I. Mammogenesis (developmental differentiation), occurring early in pregnancy, involves the proliferation of distal components of the ductal tree which results in the formation of multiple alveoli. During lactogenesis I, occurring mid-to late pregnancy, the differentiation of the mammary epithelial cells into lactocytes in the alveoli occurs, conferring the ability to synthesize and secrete the unique fats, proteins, and carbohydrates that are present in human milk.

Mammogenesis

Mammogenesis involves the development of the mammary ducto-alveolar tissues that are generally associated with an increase in breast size. The Computerized Breast Measurement (CBM) system is a recent, accurate, noninvasive technology that has been used to determine changes in the size of the human breast. A longitudinal study using this system measured the size of breasts before conception and throughout pregnancy and lactation. An increase in breast size as a result of the increased growth and differentiation of the mammary tissue commenced at week ten of pregnancy (Cox *et al.*, 1999). The breasts of seven of the eight mothers studied increased by about 170 mL during pregnancy. However, there was considerable variation between women, with some women showing a gradual increase in breast size throughout pregnancy and others showing rapid growth in the first trimester (Cox *et al.*, 1999; Hytten, 1954). One mother, who did not show any substantial change in breast size during pregnancy, showed compensatory growth of 200 mL after birth. By one month postpartum, the average increase in breast size for all the mothers was 211 mL. This indicated that the breasts grow and develop during pregnancy, and this growth may continue during lactation (Cox *et al.*, 1999). Comparison of the increase in breast size during pregnancy with changes in hormones in the blood showed that breast growth (and areolar size) was associated with an increase in the concentration of placental lactogen in the blood (**Figure 1**).

LACTOGENESIS I

Lactogenesis I involves the differentiation of the alveolar epithelial cells into lactocytes (mammary alveolar secretory epithelial cells). During pregnancy, differentiated lactocytes are able to produce small quantities of mammary secretion containing milk specific compounds. This early milk secretion, known as colostrum, is detected in the second half of gestation in women and most species (Arthur *et al.*, 1991; Cowie, 1980). It is thick and yellowish and contains high concentrations of sodium, chloride, and total protein, including the immunoprotective proteins - secretory IgA and lactoferrin. These proteins provide protection for the newborn against pathogenic organisms present in the birth canal and associated with other human and environmental contact. Lower concentrations of lactose, citrate, and potassium are found in colostrum compared with mature milk (Cowie, 1980; Neville *et al.*, 2001). Because tight junctions between lactocytes remain open during pregnancy, these components, especially lactose, can escape into the bloodstream through the paracellular pathway (Neville & Allen, 1983; Neville & Casey, 1986). Lactose in the blood cannot be metabolized and is excreted in the urine. Hence, by measuring the lactose level in urine, Cox *et al.* (1999) were able to determine that lactogenesis I occurred about mid-pregnancy in women (Cox *et al.*, 1999) and calculated that in late pregnancy the mother produced about 30 ml colostrum each day. Comparison of the increase in lactose excretion in the urine during pregnancy with changes in hormones in the blood showed that the increase in lactose excretion (and nipple size) was associated with the increase in the concentration of prolactin in the blood (**Figure 2**). An increase in nipple size was also associated with an increase in prolactin.

The hormones required for lactogenesis I are depicted in **Figure 3**. In all species, the reproductive hormones - estrogen, progesterone, and prolactin - are required for alveolar growth and development (Neville

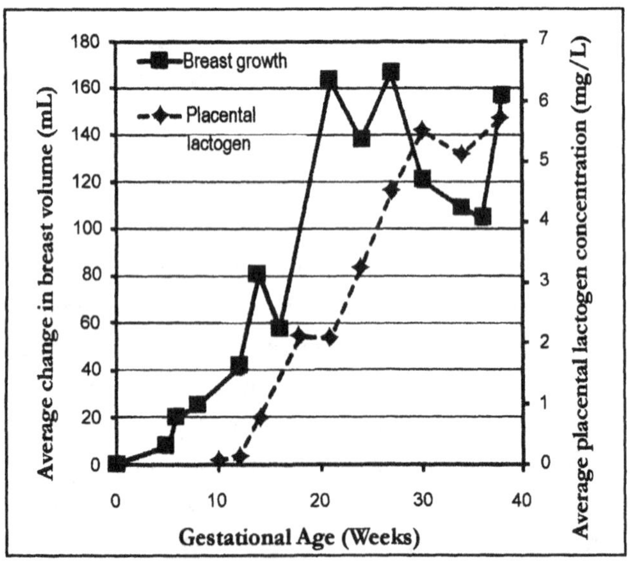

Figure 1. Breast growth and placental growth are closely associated. Adapted from Cox *et al.*, 1999.

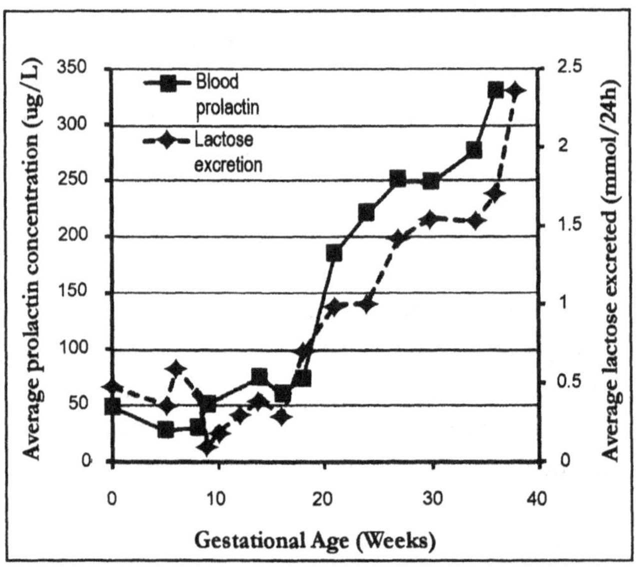

Figure 2. Relationship between lactose excretion into urine and prolactin concentration in the blood during pregnancy. Adapted from Cox *et al.*, 1999.

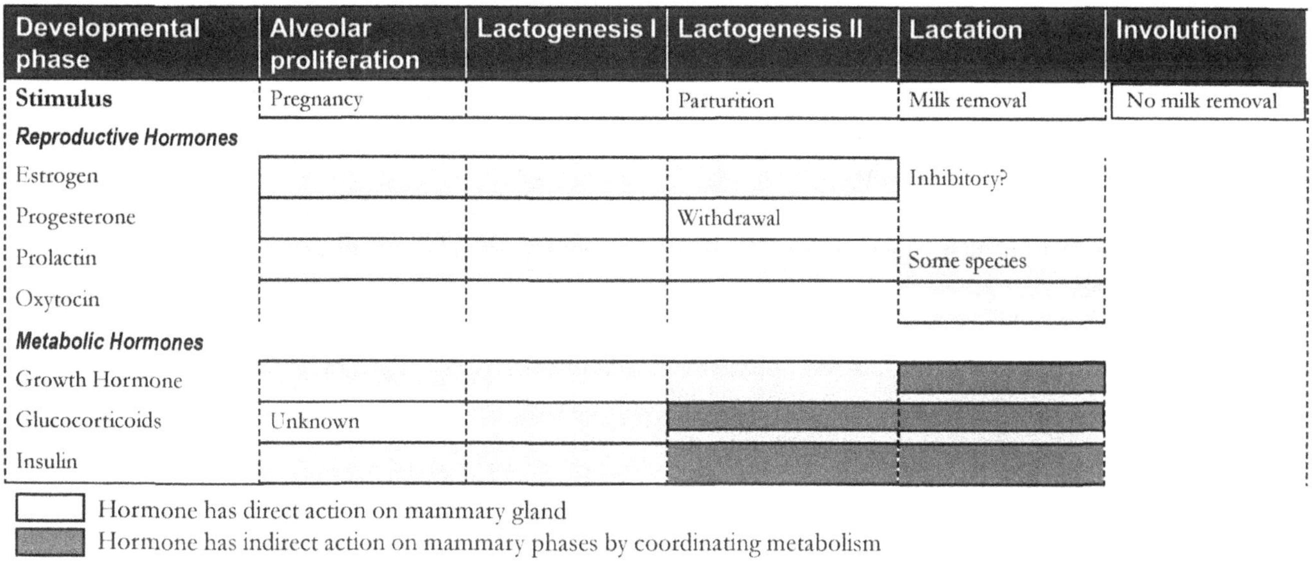

Figure 3. Hormonal action necessary for phases of the lactation cycle. Adapted from Neville *et al.*, 2002.

et al., 2002). Increasing concentrations of progesterone during pregnancy act to inhibit the onset of copious milk secretion (Kuhn, 1969; Hartmann *et al.*, 1973). Glucocorticoids also have an essential action on the developing mammary parenchyma. This has been demonstrated by mammary tissue culture experiments where the addition of cortisone is mandatory for the survival of cells *in vitro* (Cowie, 1980).

LACTOGENESIS II

Lactogenesis II is defined as the initiation of copious milk secretion and nearly always occurs after parturition, regardless of whether milk removal occurs (Neville *et al.*, 2001; Kulski & Hartmann, 1981). It is sensed by women as a sudden feeling of breast fullness, and their milk supply is said to be "coming in." The hormones active in lactogenesis II are shown in **Figure 3.**

While some hormones act directly on the mammary gland, other metabolic hormones are necessary to coordinate the body's response to the metabolic changes of lactation. In all species, lactogenesis II is triggered by the withdrawal of progesterone in the presence of high circulating concentrations of prolactin (Kuhn, 1969; Hartmann *et al.*, 1973; Turkington & Hill, 1969). The timing of lactogenesis II is species specific. In women, where the sudden drop in the concentration of progesterone occurs with the removal of the placenta, the onset of copious milk secretion does not occur until 30-40 hours after the birth (Kulski *et al.*, 1977) (**Figure** 4). Studies have shown that lactogenesis II is delayed in women who have retained placental products after birth (Neifert *et al.*, 1981). The capacity of the remaining placental fragments to secrete progesterone prolongs the inhibition of milk secretion in these women.

A decrease in permeability (closure) of the tight junctions between lactocytes accompanies the increase in the rate of milk secretion at the time of lactogenesis II (Linzell & Peaker, 1974). Before lactogenesis II, there is leakage of interstitial fluid between the lactocytes and milk products are able to move out of the alveoli

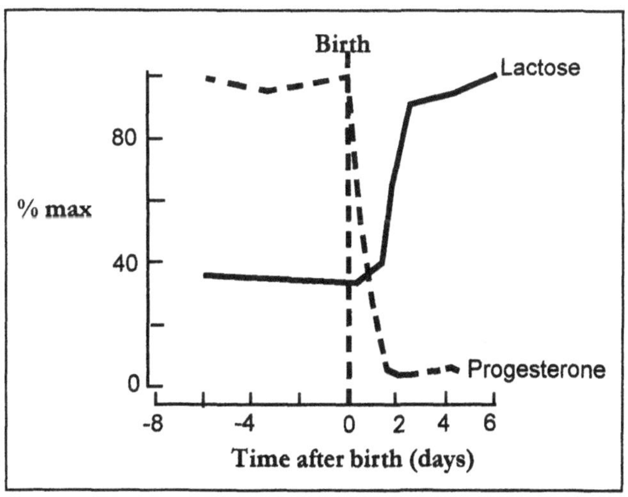

Figure 4. Progesterone withdrawal initiates lactogenesis II in women. The increase in lactose concentrations associated with increased synthesis of milk components coincides with a rapid decrease in progesterone concentration when the placenta is removed at parturition. Modified from Kulski *et al.*, 1978.

through paracellular pathways. The tight junctions close with lactogenesis II under the influence of glucocorticoids and the withdrawal of progesterone at parturition (Nguyen *et al.*, 2001). Due to the closure of the tight junctions, milk components that are synthesized in the lactocytes are then predominantly retained in the alveolar lumen before they are transferred to the nipple during either a breastfeed or breast expression during milk ejection (Neville & Allen, 1983). Therefore, measurements of milk components (lactose, fat, citrate, sodium, potassium, and protein), as well as the daily milk production are a means of determining the time of lactogenesis II in lactating women (Arthur *et al.*, 1989; Hartmann & Arthur, 1986) (**Figure 5**).

Studies of milk transfer in women breastfeeding their term infants have demonstrated rapid increases in milk volume from 36 to 96 hours postpartum, after which volumes stabilize at an average volume of 750-800ml/24 hours by one month postpartum (Saint *et al.*, 1984; Neville *et al.*, 1991). However, changes in milk composition commence before increases in volume are noted. At about one to two days after birth after lactogenesis II, the milk becomes thinner with a pale bluish color as the result of a 'fully' productive breast. The concentration of protein (particularly the immunoprotective proteins), sodium, and chloride decreases, while the concentration of fat, lactose, citrate, and potassium (Kulski & Hartmann, 1981; Neville *et al.*, 1991) increases. As stated previously, the early changes in sodium and lactose concentration are attributed to closure of tight junctions between lactocytes which prevent movement of constituents through the paracellular pathway of the lactocytes (Nguyen *et al.*, 2001; Nguyen & Neville, 1998).

MILK SYNTHESIS AND SECRETION

Although the rapid onset of copious secretion soon after parturition is independent of milk removal, sustained lactation requires regular emptying of the mammary gland (**Figure 3**) (Neville *et al.*, 2002). Once lactation is established, milk secretion is regulated by either the

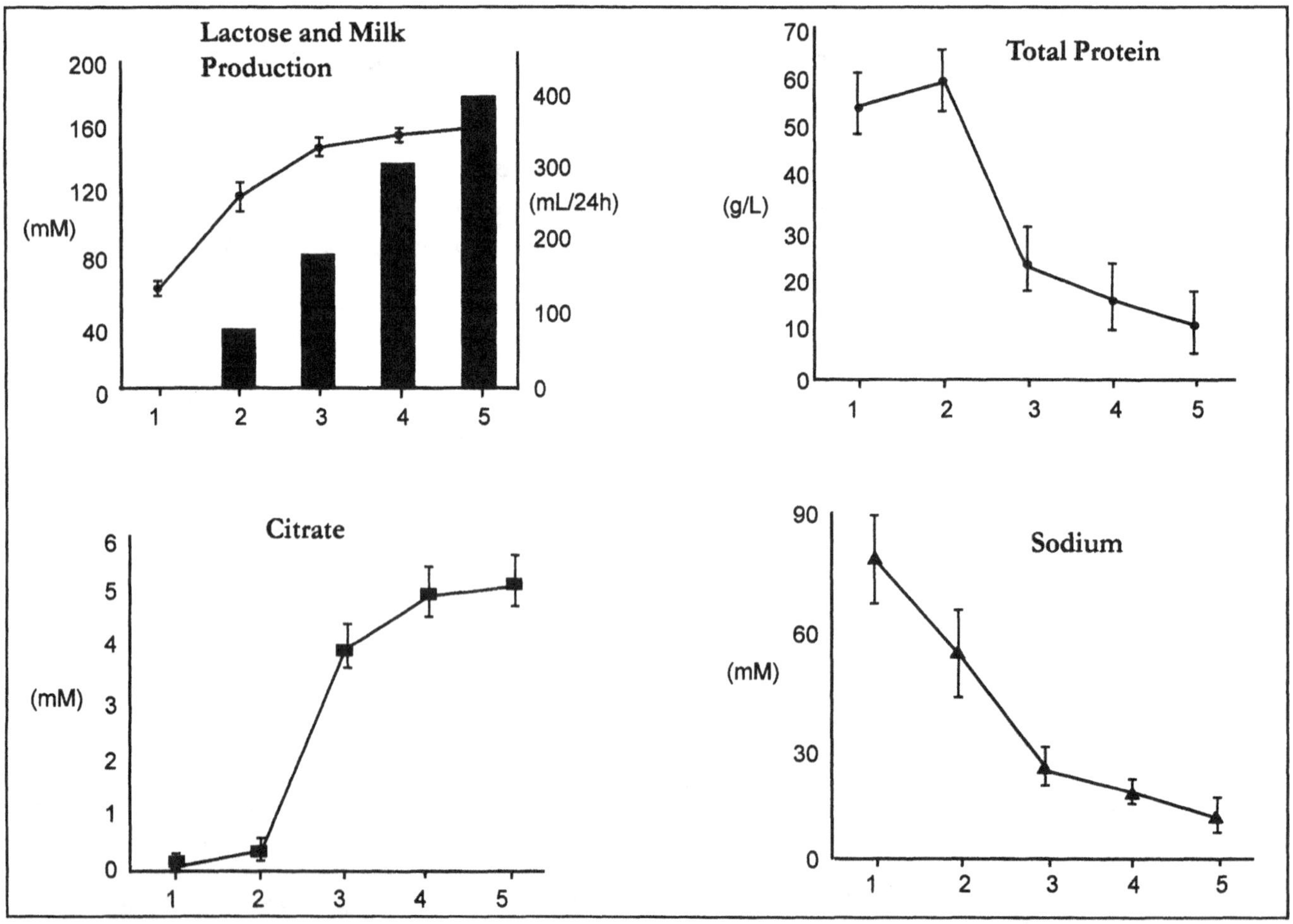

Figure 5. Relative concentrations of lactogenic markers found in human milk during the first five days following birth. Adapted from Cregan *et al.*, 2002.

demands of the suckling offspring or by expression and the associated hormone release, as well as the removal of autocrine inhibitory factors. Suckling stimulates release from the posterior pituitary of the hormone oxytocin, which acts on the myoepithelial cells of the mammary gland to cause milk ejection (Neville, 2001). The changes that occur in the alveoli during one cycle of milk removal and refilling are shown in **Figure 6.** After either a breastfeed or expression, milk synthesis is stimulated by prolactin. Initially, there is increased expression of milk proteins, such as α-lactalbumin and casein. It has been shown in domestic species that as the alveoli become more distended, the milk becomes fattier, expression of α-lactalbumin is down-regulated, and lactoferrin is up-regulated. At either the next feed or expression, oxytocin aids milk ejection and the emptying of the alveolus again.

INVOLUTION

Involution of the mammary gland commences when emptying of the gland by either suckling or expression ceases. The trigger for involution is mechanical pressure from the distended gland coupled with the cessation of stimulation of the gland (Marti *et al.*, 1997; Akers, 2002). Milk stasis in the distended gland initiates a cascade of signals, leading to apoptosis of the lactocytes and, in mice, restructuring of the gland (see Chapter 8). Li *et al.* demonstrated that local signals of milk stasis are sufficient to induce apoptosis in mice, even in the presence of systemic lactogenic hormones, including exogenous glucocorticoids (Li *et al.*, 1997). A number of studies have shown that the initiation of apoptosis at involution is multifactorial and requires both the activation of a wide number of signaling triggers, including milk stasis, α-lactalbumin, and STAT3, as well as the inactivation of a wide number of survival factors, including glucocorticoids, integrins, laminin, and STAT5 (Green & Streuli, 2004).

The lack of stimulation via either suckling or mechanical expression is hypothesized to lead to a drop in the lactogenic hormones prolactin and glucocorticoids (Baik *et al.*, 1998), which in turn leads to a decrease in the synthesis of milk proteins. In ewes, the expression of α-lactalbumin mRNA, a milk protein which is required for the synthesis of lactose, is markedly reduced in alveoli distended with fatty milk, whereas lactoferrin, a milk protein accepted to be a marker for involution, is highly expressed in lactocytes in distended alveoli (Molenaar *et al.*, 1996; Molenaar *et al.*, 1992). This process is depicted in **Figure 6.**

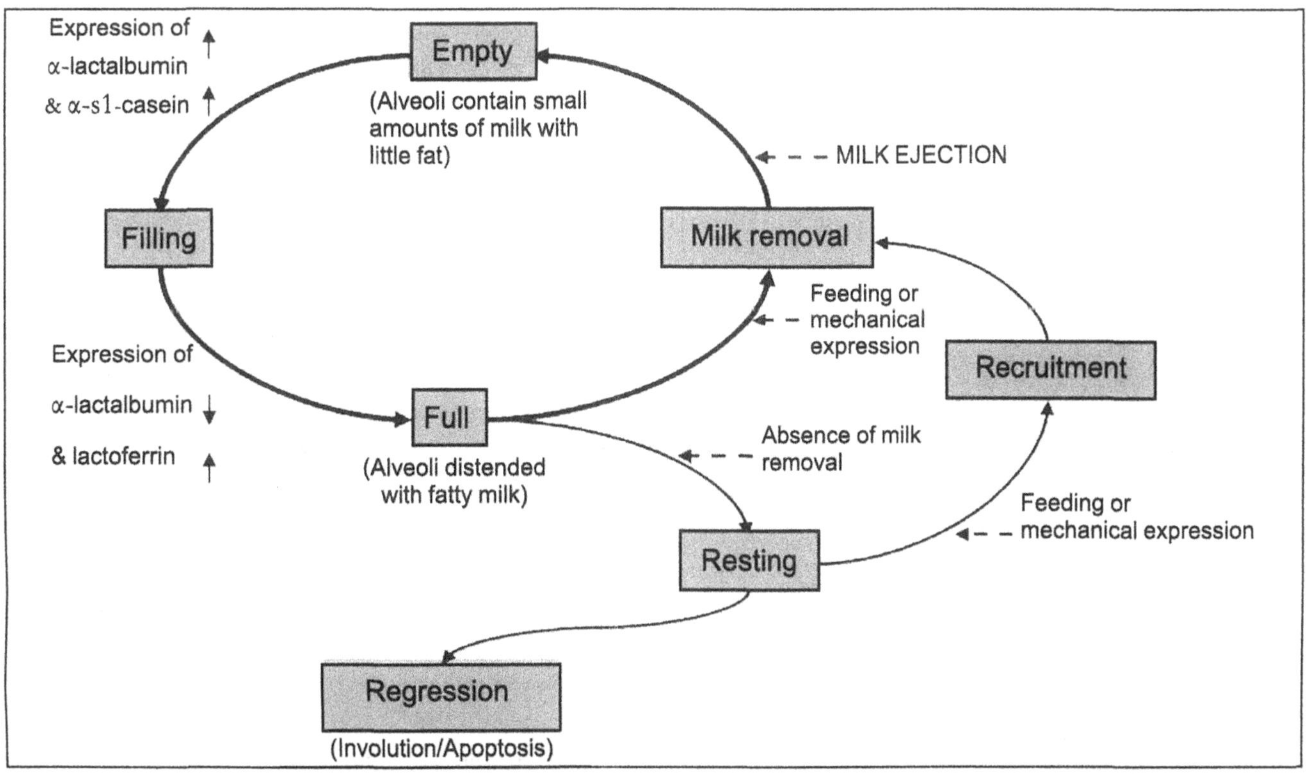

Figure 6. Cyclic changes in lactocytes during lactation. Adapted from Molenaar *et al.*, 1992.

ENDOCRINOLOGY OF LACTATION

The hormones regulating lactation are well conserved between species (**Figure 3**). As described above, prolactin, estrogen, placental lactogen, and glucocorticoids promote mammary growth and differentiation during pregnancy and are essential for lactogenesis II and maintenance of lactation. Oxytocin causes milk ejection by stimulating contraction of the myoepithelial cells of the mammary gland. Progesterone is active in the development of the mammary gland during pregnancy, but its withdrawal triggers the onset of lactogenesis II.

Prolactin

Due to structural similarities with growth hormone, which is present in the pituitary at levels 100 times greater than that of prolactin, it was originally thought that women lacked prolactin (Lawrence & Lawrence, 1999). It is now recognized that prolactin is a 23 kDa peptide, mainly synthesized in lactotrophic cells of the anterior pituitary (Henninghausen & Robinson, 1997). Prolactin is critical for the establishment and maintenance of lactation in women and other mammals (Ostrom, 1990). This has been clearly illustrated by the immediate fall in milk production in rabbits after the administration of the ergot alkaloid bromocryptine, an inhibitor of prolactin release from the anterior pituitary (Cowie *et al.*, 1980) and the suppression of the initiation of lactation by bromocryptine in women (Kulski *et al.*, 1978) (**Figure 7**). Once lactation is established, however, high basal levels are not required in most species. Secretion of prolactin by the anterior pituitary gland for ongoing lactogenic activity is dependent on a positive feedback loop (Cowie, 1980). The suckling stimulus, in addition to regular emptying of the gland, is essential to promote prolactin secretion. Conversely, prolactin release is inhibited by alveolar distension.

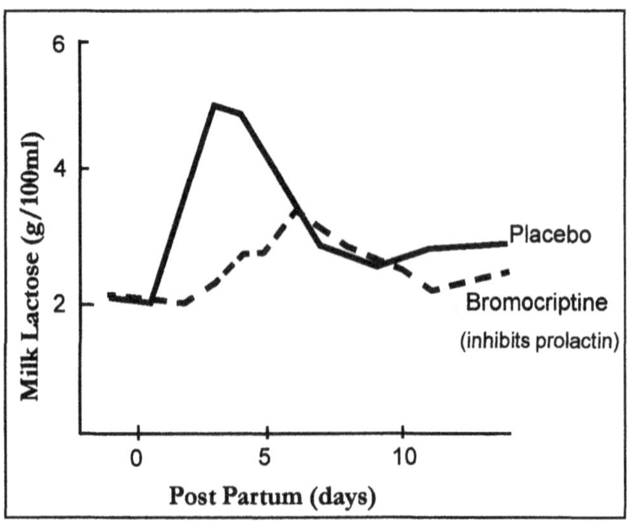

Figure 7. Bromocryptine inhibition of prolactin release results in suppression of lactogenesis II as demonstrated by reduced lactose production. Adapted from Kulski, 1978.

Levels of prolactin in the blood are highest in early lactation (Jacobs, 1977) and decline as lactation progresses (Cox *et al.*, 1996). This observation suggests that the function of prolactin may differ during the course of lactation. Prolactin concentration in the blood has been found to follow a circadian rhythm, being higher at night when compared to day (Neville, 1999). In addition, prolactin is secreted in response to suckling, peaking 45 minutes after the start of the feed (Noel *et al.*, 1974). It has been shown that nipple stimulation in the absence of breastfeeding will result in the release of prolactin in lactating and non-lactating women (Frantz, 1977). Prolactin has also been found in breastmilk (Cox *et al.*, 1996). Prolactin binds to an integral membrane receptor on epithelial cells before being transported into the milk through the lactocyte (Ollivier-Bousquet *et al.*, 1993).

In women, mammary engorgement, milk ejection, and an increase in milk fat content have all been observed with increased prolactin levels in blood (Tyson *et al.*, 1975). Prolactin stimulates lipogenic activity in the mammary gland (Martyn & Falconer, 1985) by increasing the rate of synthesis of key lipogenic enzymes (Ros *et al.*, 1990). In addition, it is believed to play a key role in the coordination of fat metabolism between adipose tissue and the mammary gland (Ros *et al.*, 1990). Studies have shown that the administration of drugs that increase prolactin levels can increase milk synthesis in women in the declining phase of lactation and stimulate milk production in women suffering lactational insufficiency. However, even in these cases, prolactin has not always proven to be very successful (Tyson *et al.*, 1975). In this regard, Cox *et al.* (1996) determined that prolactin in the blood did not regulate the short- or long-term rates of milk synthesis, leading to the conclusion that the requirement for blood prolactin for lactation was permissive rather than regulatory (Neville, 1999; Cregan & Hartmann, 1999).

With the advent of biotechnology, recombinant human prolactin (rhPRL) is becoming available as a potential therapeutic for the treatment of prolactin deficiency in women to help establish or maintain lactation. Detailed studies are required to determine the effect of rhPRL on lactation and currently there are several clinical trials in progress (US National Library of Medicine, 2006a; US National Library of Medicine, 2006b; US National Library of Medicine, 2006c). In particular, it is essential that such studies establish the need for supplementation by assessing the basal and stimulated prolactin concentrations in the blood. Prolactin concentrations peak at approximately 45 minutes after infant attachment or initiation of pumping (Cox *et al.*, 1996), and therefore this time point should be used as common protocol. In addition, the decrease in prolactin response with stage of lactation should be considered.

Prolactin Receptor

Prolactin binds to specific prolactin receptors (PrlR) on the surface of lactocytes, inducing a lactogenic signaling pathway that leads to the switching on of the transcription of genes that regulate the secretion of milk proteins, such as casein and α-lactalbumin (**Figure 8**) (Tucker, 2000; Rosen *et al.*, 1999). PrlR is a member of the cytokine receptor family, which is up-regulated in the lactocytes at the time of parturition and the occurrence of lactogenesis II (Liu *et al.*, 1996).

The coordination of the large number of mRNAs promoting synthesis of milk proteins is regulated by PrlR and amplified by the glucocorticoid receptor at a transcriptional level (Mepham, 1983). This process is depicted in **Figure 9**. In brief, binding of prolactin to PrlR induces dimerization of the receptor, which activates Janus Kinase 2 (JAK2). JAK2 then induces phosphorylation and activation of transcription factors, STAT5a and STAT5b. STAT5s are members of the signal transducer and activator of transcription (STAT) protein family and are major transducers in cytokine receptor signaling. Phosphorylated STAT5s then dissociate from the PrlR, dimerize with other STAT

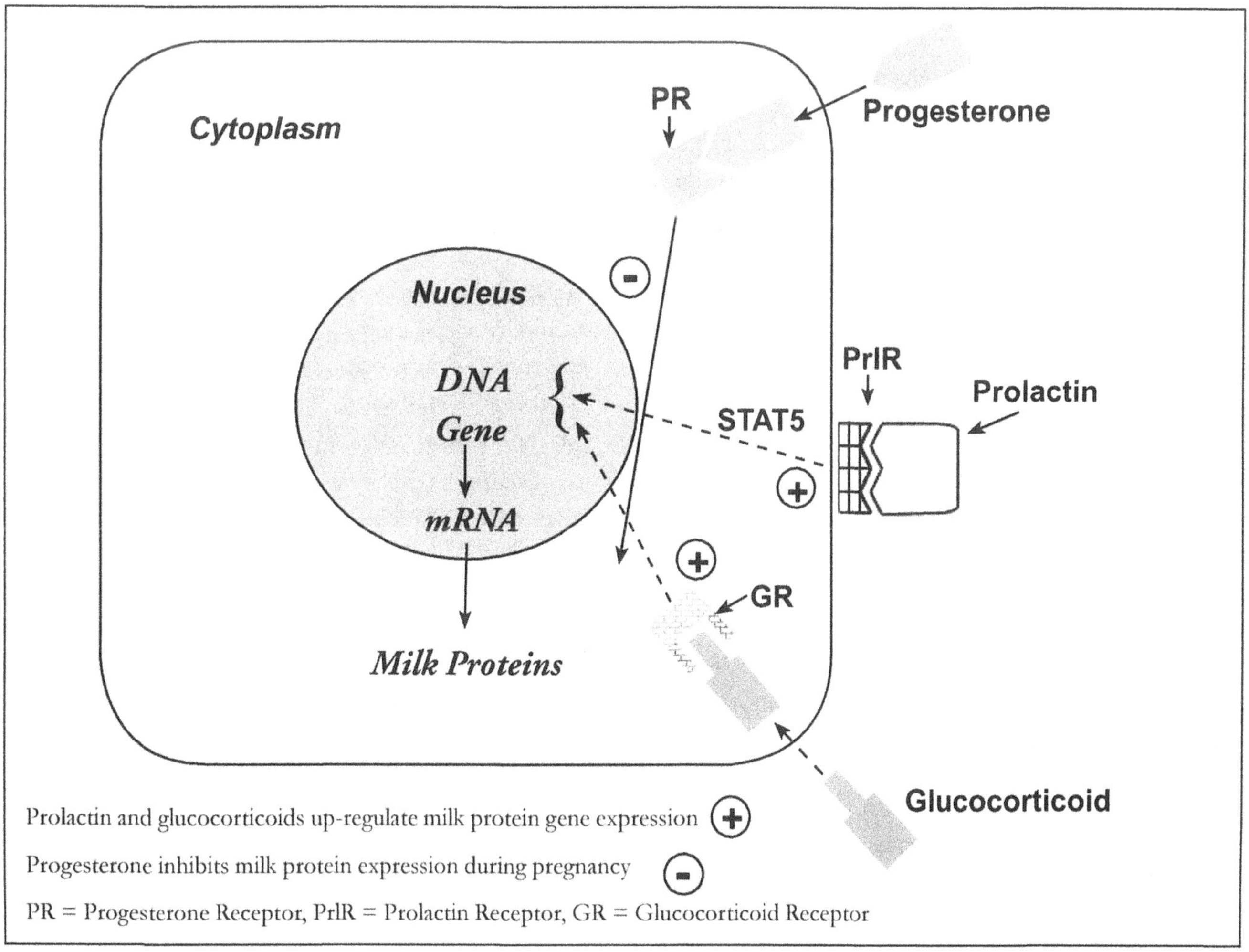

Figure 8. Intracellular hormonal signaling in the lactocyte during lactation. Adapted from Mercier & Gaye, 1983.

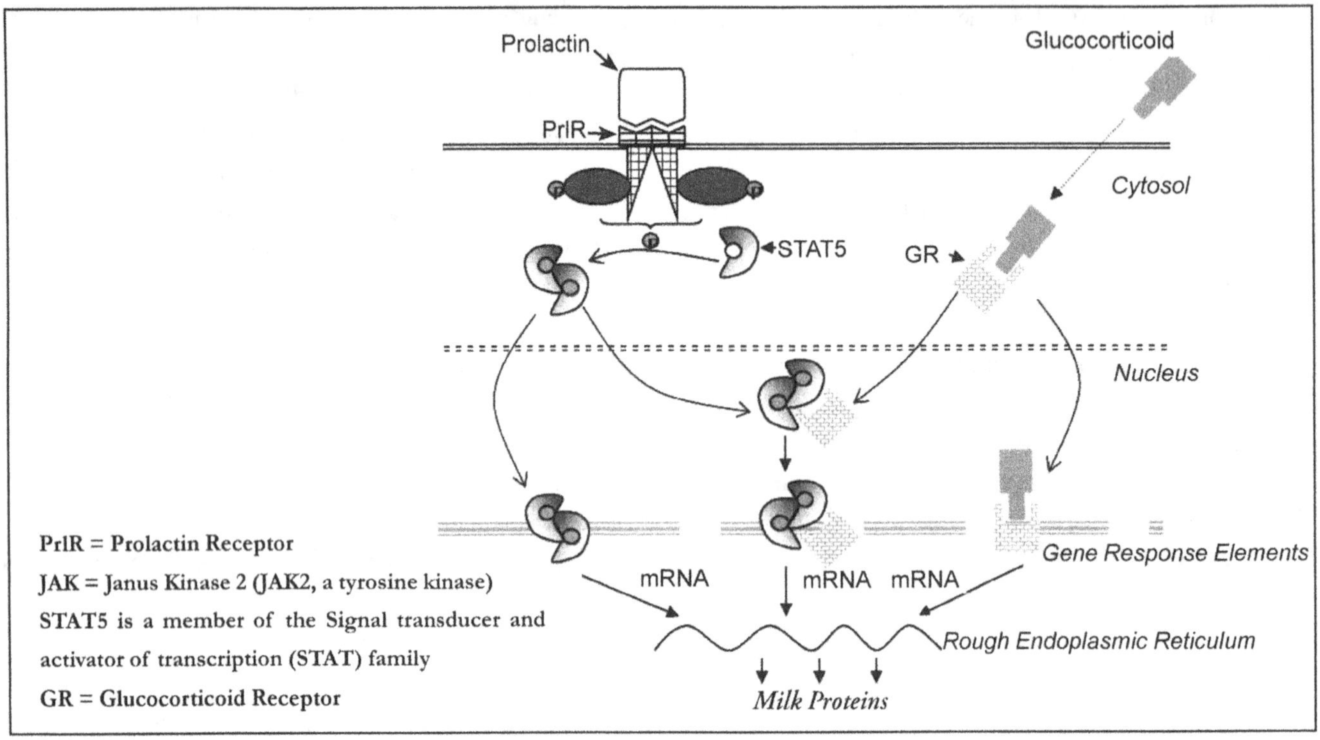

Figure 9. Signal transduction pathways in the lactocyte during lactation. Modified and simplified from Stoecklin *et al.*, 1997 and Freeman *et al.*, 2000.

molecules, and translocate to the nucleus. STAT5s then activate specific STAT DNA-binding motifs in the promoter of a target gene (GAS) (γ-interferon activated sequence), thereby promoting expression of specific genes regulating milk protein synthesis (Tucker, 2000; Freeman *et al.*, 2000) (**Figure 9**). In addition, STAT5 synergizes with activated glucocorticoid receptor in the transcription of these genes (Rosen *et al.*, 1999; Stocklin *et al.*, 1997). Milk protein genes promote synthesis of milk proteins from amino acids on the rough endoplasmic reticulum (Cowie, 1984).

Integrity of the extracellular matrix is also required for continued activity of PrlR in the lactocyte (Zoubiane *et al.*, 2003; Edwards *et al.*, 1998). Cellular interaction with extracellular matrix proteins (chiefly laminin), transduced via β1 integrins, controls the ability of prolactin to activate PrlR, thereby initiating the JAK/STAT pathway. This pathway is therefore interrupted by milk stasis, which leads to apoptosis of lactocytes.

Glucocorticoids

Glucocorticoids (GC) are essential for mammary alveolar development during pregnancy and for maintenance of lactation, as well as being critical for the onset of lactogenesis II (Neville *et al.*, 2002; Tucker, 2000). In the dairy industry, it has long been known that administration of exogenous glucocorticoids, prolactin, and estrogen can initiate lactation when the lobulo-alveolar system of mammary glands is well-developed. This observation raises the possibility that glucocorticoid (e.g., betamethasone) administration to women with high prolactin and estrogen levels could stimulate breast secretion. Fortunately, the human mammary gland appears to be much less sensitive to exogenous glucocorticoids than dairy animals, such as sheep (Henderson, 2007). Glucocorticoids also play an indirect role in lactation through their roles in energy homeostasis, immune system regulation, organ development, stress adaptation, and behavior modification (Reichardt *et al.*, 2001).

In the rat, glucocorticoids have been shown to play a regulatory role in the synthesis of fat, lactose, and protein (Horsrud & Baldwin, 1972a; Korsrud & Baldwin, 1972b; Korsrud & Baldwin, 1972c). Experiments using adrenalectomized rats deprived of the foetoplacental unit showed that without corticosteroids in late pregnancy, the concentration of lactose in the mammary tissue and the total wet weight of mammary tissue were significantly decreased. When these rats were treated with corticosteroids, milk secretion was restored (Nicholas & Hartmann, 1981). Furthermore, in mice corticosterone has been shown to increase the ability of the lactocytes to bind prolactin (Sakai *et al.*, 1979) and that without corticosterone, the expression of messenger RNA for the prolactin receptor within the lactocytes is low (Mizoguchi *et al.*, 1997).

In ruminants and humans, cortisol is the main endogenous glucocorticoid, whereas corticosterone is predominant in species such as mice and rats. In sheep, mice, and rats, maternal plasma concentrations of glucocorticoids remain relatively low during pregnancy (around 10 ng/mL) but rise to a peak just before parturition (Neville *et al.*, 2002; Tucker, 2000; Young, 2001). In sheep, the source of the rise of cortisol has been attributed to a surge in secretion of fetal cortisol in late gestation, which increases maternal levels, inducing labor and stimulating lactogenesis II in conjunction with a withdrawal of progesterone (Young, 2001; Whittle *et al.*, 2001). The basal maternal concentration of cortisol in plasma is higher in humans and increases by a factor of five during pregnancy (above 200 ng/mL) (Neville *et al.*, 2002). In maternal circulation, cortisol is bound to corticosteroid binding globulin (CBG) thereby inactivating its lactogenic effects. Levels of CBG reduce during the peri-parturient period, increasing the availability of cortisol for uptake and binding in mammary tissue during lactogenesis II (Akers, 2002; Tucker, 2000).

In dairy species, such as sheep, maternal glucocorticoid levels often increase during mature lactation, as they are required to maintain blood glucose in a time of relative nutrient starvation (Neville *et al.*, 2002). In contrast, cortisol levels in women are reduced in mature lactation compared with pregnancy levels (urine 24 hour cortisol 270 $\pm$ 67 nmol/day at three months postpartum compared with 747 $\pm$ 213 nmol/day in pregnancy) (Butte *et al.*, 1999).

One mechanism for the lactogenic effects of glucocorticoids on mammary development and lactation is indirectly via body metabolism. Glucocorticoids are essential for the maintenance of glucose homeostasis. Direct actions of glucocorticoids on lactation include the regulation of tight junction permeability, as well as prevention of involution and apoptosis of mammary tissue during established lactation (Nguyen & Neville, 1998; Berg *et al.*, 2002; Feng *et al.*, 1995). Glucocorticoids are also required to assist the synthesis of milk proteins, such as casein and α-lactalbumin.

Glucocorticoid Receptor

Glucocorticoid receptors (GR) were first identified in the cytoplasm of mammary cells in the 1970s (Gardner & Wittliff, 1973). After binding with glucocorticoids, activated receptors translocate to the nucleus where they act synergistically with prolactin-activated transcription factors to enable synthesis of milk proteins, such as casein and α-lactalbumin (**Figures 8, 9**) (Rosen *et al.*, 1999; Stocklin *et al.*, 1997; Stocklin *et al.*, 1996).

Progesterone also binds to GR in the mammary cytoplasm, possibly explaining the inhibitory action of progesterone during pregnancy (Collier & Tucker, 1978; Maki *et al.*, 1980). Progesterone does not translocate to the nucleus after binding, thus preventing GR from reaching sites where transcription of milk protein genes occurs (Forsyth, 1983). Although the affinity of progesterone to GR is lower than that of glucocorticoids, the concentration of progesterone is much higher during pregnancy, thus displacing glucocorticoid binding until GC concentrations increase dramatically in the peri-parturient period (Mesiano, 2001), and the concentration of progesterone declines with the delivery of the placenta.

Human Growth Hormone

Human growth hormone (hGH) is a 23 kDa single chain polypeptide secreted from the eosinophilic cells of the anterior pituitary (Lawrence & Lawrence, 1999). Clinical trials have proven the efficacy of hGH as a means of increasing milk production in healthy women (Milsom *et al.*, 1992), women with lactational insufficiency (Milsom *et al.*, 1998), and women of preterm infants (Gunn *et al.*, 1996). The role of hGH in established lactation in women is not well defined, but it is thought to work synergistically with prolactin and glucocorticoids (Lawrence & Lawrence, 1999). In lactating women, both high and low levels of hGH have been observed. Normal lactation in ateliotic dwarf women who are deficient in hGH has shown that lactation is possible in its absence (Rimoin & Holzman, 1968). Furthermore, acute interruption of hGH secretion does not interfere with milk secretion (Lawrence & Lawrence, 1999).

As discussed previously in ruminants, high levels of prolactin are not essential to maintain lactation after lactogenesis II. In contrast, milk production was stimulated in cows treated with either recombinant growth hormone (Oldenbroek *et al.*, 1993) or bovine growth hormone (McCutcheon & Bauman, 1986;

Sechen *et al.*, 1990). In ruminants such as sheep, growth hormone (GH) plays a more important role in the maintenance of lactation (Forsyth, 1986). Sheep demonstrate increased yields of milk and lactose when treated with bovine GH (Min *et al.*, 1997) or GH releasing factor (Kann, 1997).

It appears that in most mammals the principal action of GH in lactation is by regulation of metabolism. It has been shown that GH partitions glucose away from body tissues and towards milk secretion (Forsyth, 1986). Treatment of lactating ruminants with GH has marked coordinated effects on glucose metabolism in a number of tissues, including liver, adipose tissue, and the mammary gland (Bell & Bauman, 1997).

Placental Lactogen

Placental lactogen is a hormone produced in the placenta in many species, including sheep and women, that has prolactin-like activity (Forsyth, 1986). During pregnancy it stimulates growth and development of the mammary gland (Cox, 1996). The lactogenic activity of placental lactogen occurs only during pregnancy, and exogenous treatment during lactation has not been shown to have any effect on milk yield in sheep (Min *et al.*, 1997). Moreover, a role for human placental lactogen either in lactogenesis I or II has not been found in women (Neville *et al.*, 2002).

Oxytocin

The role of oxytocin in milk ejection and its physiological significance is discussed in detail in Chapter 9.

It has also been suggested that oxytocin may possess some galactopoietic effects as Bencini (1993) showed increased rates of milk secretion in ewes that were injected with oxytocin after milking. This galactopoietic effect has also been observed in cows (Nostrand *et al.*, 1991) and goats (Linzell & Peaker, 1971). Ballou *et al.* (1993) found equal increases in milk yield with oxytocin injections both before and after milking in cows, suggesting that the increase in milk yield is due to increased gland output, the mechanism of which is unknown. However, Knight (1994) found increased milk output only in the gland injected with oxytocin prior to milking, supporting the established view that the galactopoietic effects of oxytocin are mediated indirectly through the removal of an inhibitor of milk production from the gland.

Progesterone

It has long been known that administration of progesterone in pregnancy prevents normal initiation of synthesis of α-lactalbumin, lactose, and casein. Lactogenesis II in rats was first shown to be triggered by the withdrawal of progesterone (Kuhn, 1969) and a similar control mechanism occurs in other mammals, including women (Kuhn, 1969; Turkington & Hill, 1969; Hartmann *et al.*, 1995). It was later shown that artificially maintaining high levels of progesterone after parturition blocks lactogenesis II in the ewe (Hartmann *et al.*, 1973). In women, the retention of placental fragments after delivery was observed to inhibit lactogenesis II, suggesting the progesterone synthesized by the placenta inhibits lactogenesis II during pregnancy (Neifert *et al.*, 1981). Hence the delivery of the placenta at parturition in women leads to the reduction of progesterone in maternal blood, which in turn triggers the synthesis of lactose in lactocytes (Cox *et al.*, 1999; Neville, 1999; Kulski *et al.*, 1977). Since it is the delivery of the placenta that initiates the fall in progesterone, lactogenesis II is therefore delayed until progesterone clears from the circulation, some 30 to 40 hours postpartum.

In species such as mice and rats, the corpus luteum in the ovary secretes progesterone throughout pregnancy, whereas the placenta is the principal source of progesterone in women and sheep (Forsyth, 1983). In the ewe, the concentration of progesterone increases steadily throughout pregnancy to a peak of 3–10 ng/mL at about day 120 to 140 of pregnancy (Cowie *et al.*, 1980). There is a wide variation of values reported by different investigators and within individual ewes, and early studies used questionable methodology to determine progesterone concentration. Most studies show declining levels in the last two weeks of gestation, although this may only occur on the day of lambing.

The concentration of plasma progesterone in pregnant women is much higher than in sheep, increasing 100-fold above non-pregnant levels and nearing 200 ng/mL before parturition (Heap & Flint, 1984). In many species including humans, progesterone is rapidly metabolized and removed from the blood stream (Heap & Flint, 1984). However, progesterone is a fat soluble hormone, and it is possible that there may be a delay in the clearance of progesterone in obese mothers, although this was not observed by previous studies (Rasmussen & Kjolhede, 2004). Measurement of the concentration of the urinary metabolite, pregnanediol glucuronide (PdG), by immunoassay is therefore a good indicator of plasma progesterone levels with high sensitivity and specificity observed in several studies (Brown *et al.*, 1988; Brown *et al.*, 1989; Sauer & Paulson, 1991). In the non-pregnant woman, daily urinary PdG levels rise from below 1 mg/24 hours pre-ovulation to up to 6 mg/24 hours in the second half of the menstrual cycle (Brown *et al.*, 1989). These levels are vastly increased during both ovarian hyperstimulation for fertility treatments and also pregnancy.

The presence of progesterone is required to maintain uterine quiescence during pregnancy (Challis *et al.*, 2000). Progesterone withdrawal at the end of pregnancy triggers the onset of parturition in many species including sheep, but not women (Challis *et al.*, 2000; Heap *et al.*, 1977). In contrast with most other species, progesterone is maintained during parturition in women (Challis *et al.*, 2000) and is withdrawn only after birth with the delivery of the placenta. In all species, however, progesterone withdrawal is essential for the initiation of lactation.

Increasing concentrations of progesterone during pregnancy inhibit lactogenesis II by suppressing the up-regulation of prolactin receptors in the lactocytes (Djiane & Durand, 1977). In addition, progesterone competes with glucocorticoids for binding to glucocorticoid receptors in mammary epithelial cells, thus suppressing the lactogenic activity of endogenous glucocorticoids (Collier & Tucker, 1978). Once lactation is established, however, exogenous progesterone has been shown to have little or no effect on milk supply, allowing women to use either the progesterone-only mini pill or depo provera (medroxyprogesterone acetate) as effective contraceptive agents during lactation (Danli *et al.*, 2000; Hale, 2006). Furthermore, milk production is not suppressed when menstrual cycles return.

Insulin

The role of insulin in the development of the breast during pregnancy and in the functioning of the breast during lactation remains poorly understood. Insulin is required in *in vitro* systems to maintain mammary epithelium functionality (Neville & Picciano, 1997). However, although insulin is required for the development of the breast during pregnancy, it is not required for either ductal or alveolar growth (Topper & Freeman, 1980). Despite insulin levels being generally decreased in lactating compared to non-lactating women (Neville *et al.*, 1993), it has been shown to affect several enzymes involved in carbohydrate and lipid metabolism (Neville & Picciano, 1997) during established lactation. It has been hypothesized that a major role for insulin in lactating woman is in the regulation of nutrient partitioning, and that these effects may either act directly on the mammary gland or provide systemic homeorhetic adaptations to support the dominant status of lactation (Hartmann *et al.*, 1998).

AUTOCRINE CONTROL

It is well known that milking a cow three times a day produces more milk than milking only twice daily (Wilde *et al.*, 1987). This response to more frequent milking is rapid and lasts for as long as the pattern is continued (Wilde & Peaker, 1990). Henderson and Peaker (1984) found that if only one udder half in the goat was milked three times a day, milk production from the other udder half did not increase. This finding demonstrated that there was a degree of local (autocrine) control of milk synthesis in each udder half.

Originally, it was thought that the local mechanism of control was due to an increase in physical pressure as milk accumulated in the mammary gland. However, Henderson and Peaker (1984) found that the rates of milk synthesis in glands in which the expressed milk was replaced by a similar volume of iso-osmotic sucrose was similar to that of thrice milked udders. This indicated that physical distension was not the inhibiting factor. This was further reinforced by the finding that diluting the milk in the udder with an inert isotonic solution increased the rate of secretion (Wilde *et al.*, 1987). These results suggested that it was the removal of a factor in the milk which caused the increase in milk synthesis and led to the isolation of a protein called Feedback Inhibitor of Lactation (FIL).

Feedback Inhibitor of Lactation

FIL is a 7.5 kDa acidic whey protein (or perhaps peptide) produced by the lactocytes that has been shown to acutely regulate milk synthesis and secretion in a dose dependent manner (Wilde *et al.*, 1995) in laboratory and domestic mammals. Rennison *et al.* (1992) showed FIL decreased protein synthesis and Wilde *et al.* (1995)

showed FIL decreased lactose and casein synthesis. Experiments using Pulse-chase radiolabeling of milk proteins showed that the inhibition by FIL was at the early stages of the secretory pathway, that is, at the level of protein transport from endoplasmic reticulum to Golgi vesicle (Rennison *et al.*, 1993). The inhibition by FIL became apparent when milk had accumulated in the mammary gland, and its effect on secretion could be detected in as little as one hour (Rennison *et al.*, 1993). These effects were mediated by the disruption of the endoplasmic reticulum and the *trans*-Golgi network (Rennison *et al.*, 1992) and were specific to FIL (Wilde *et al.*, 1998).

FIL has been identified in the milk of goats (Wilde *et al.*, 1995), women, and cows (Wilde *et al.*, 1998). However, it is uncertain whether the inhibitor is secreted into the milk in an active form or if it is secreted as a proinhibitor. The concentration-dependent nature of the inhibition suggests an increase in FIL occurs as milk accumulates in the gland, and it is relieved upon milk removal. However, this model does not allow for increased rate of milk synthesis after the gland is milked, as the residual milk would still contain elevated concentrations of FIL (Wilde *et al.*, 1995). One possibility that has gained favor is that the active inhibitor is secreted into the milk from the gland and is inactivated in a first order process by an enzyme in the milk. With the continuous secretion of inhibitor, the degradation process is saturated and active inhibitor levels increase and produce their effects (Wilde & Peaker, 1990), which may be mediated by receptors on the apical membrane of the lactocytes (Wilde *et al.*, 1987). Although there is good evidence for the local control of milk synthesis and secretion and these effects are consistent with the presence of FIL, the purification sequence data and mechanism of action still remain unclear. Unfortunately, intellectual property considerations and the recent closure of the principal research laboratory has restricted the progress of this research.

Daly *et al.* (1996) observed that significant changes in the rate of milk synthesis occurred in women from one breastfeed to the next and that these changes depended on whether the breast was either full (low rate of synthesis) or drained (high rate of synthesis) of milk. An autocrine inhibitory control mechanism could explain the breast-specific, short-term regulation of milk synthesis observed from breastfeed to breastfeed by Daly *et al.* because milk secretion would have been inhibited as the breasts filled with milk over longer suckling intervals (> six hours). On the other hand, such a response would not be expected to occur with either frequent (every hour) breastfeeding or pumping sessions because only relatively small volumes of newly synthesized milk could accumulate in the gland, and this would not be sufficient to invoke the autocrine inhibitory response.

The response time for changes in milk synthesis appears to be longer than those for milk secretion. Radioactive tracer studies in goats showed that it took at least 1.5 hours for milk casein to be synthesized in the mammary gland. Barry (1952) and Popjak *et al.* (1950) found that the complete synthesis of milk fat in the mammary gland took approximately four to six hours. It is clear from a number of studies in dairy animals that increasing the frequency of milking from two to four times per day increases milk production and that the response is observed in six to twelve hours (Wilde *et al.*, 1987). Furthermore, compensatory changes in milk production have been documented in goats, cows, sheep, rabbits, and mice (Knight *et al.*, 1998). For example, if a goat was milked four times per day and then one gland was milked twice per day, milk yield dropped in that gland, but a compensatory increase in yield occurred in the gland that continued to be milked four times per day (Wilde *et al.*, 1987). These findings strongly suggest that milk synthesis responds to a systemic effector. Furthermore, Dewey and Lonnerdal (1986) found that milk production increased by an average of 124 ml/24-hour when women expressed their breasts after each breastfeed for a period of two weeks. This response was obtained by ensuring the breasts were drained of milk by expressing the remaining milk after each breastfeed, rather than by increasing the frequency of breastfeeding. These considerations suggest that when milk accumulates in the mammary gland, local factors inhibit milk secretion, and when the gland is released from this inhibitory effect, separate systemic factors can stimulate an increase in milk synthesis. Indeed, Wilde *et al.* (1987) reported that there was a significant increase in activity of several key enzymes required for milk synthesis within two weeks of the start of thrice daily milking. These findings suggest that it is first necessary to reduce the effects of the local inhibitory factor before an increase in the activity of key enzymes involved in milk synthesis can occur. It is of interest that if increased stimulatory pressure (increased frequency of removal of breastmilk by either the baby sucking or breast expression) is maintained over a longer period of time, it can lead to increased cell division and growth of mammary secretory tissue (Wilde *et al.*, 1987; Knight *et al.*, 1998). Indeed, suckling pressure is able to induce lactation in non-pregnant, non-lactating women (Kolodny *et al.*, 1972). It can be concluded that increasing the stimulatory pressure on the mammary gland by increasing the frequency of breastfeeding/ breast expression mediates a series of responses that first decreases local inhibition, then stimulates metabolic activity, and finally causes proliferation of the mammary parenchyma, leading to progressive increases in milk secretion and then synthesis. If these considerations are correct, the longest interval between breastfeeds/breast expressions may be a more important determinant of milk production than the total number of breastfeeds/ breast expressions per day.

ASSESSING THE FUNCTION OF THE BREAST DURING LACTATION

Breast size

The increase in the size of the breast during pregnancy and lactation is an obvious sign of an increase in the secretory tissue and physiological activity of the breasts. The Computerized Breast Measurement system provides an objective, quantitative measurement of the growth of the breast, and mothers can be reassured that, irrespective of the size of their breasts prior to conception, an increase of 200 mL (or one brassiere size) during pregnancy or up to one month after birth is an indication of sufficient proliferation of secretory tissue for adequate milk production. In addition, the volume of breast tissue has been shown to decrease before there is a decrease in the 24-hour milk production, and significant milk production continues after the breasts have returned to their pre-conception size by 15 months of lactation (Knight *et al.*, 1998).

Furthermore, measurement of the decrease in breast size from before to after a breastfeed correlates well with the volume of milk removed from the breast during that breastfeed (Dewey & Lonnerdal, 1986). Therefore, measurement of the increase in volume of the breast from immediately after a breastfeed to immediately before the next breastfeed provides a measure of the short-term rate of milk synthesis (Daly *et al.*, 1993). In addition, the difference between the maximum and minimum breast volume measured over a period of 24 hours of breastfeeding is the storage capacity of the breast (the demonstrated capacity of the breast to store milk that is available to the infant) (Dewey & Lonnerdal, 1986).

Hormones

The association of the concentration of placental lactogen with the growth of breast tissue and the areola during pregnancy, and the concentration of prolactin with the growth of the nipple and the secretory activity of the breast means that measurement of the concentrations of these hormones can provide an assessment of the development of the breast (Hartmann *et al.*, 1973; Cox *et al.*, 1996). After birth, if milk production is low, measurement of the concentration of progesterone provides an indication of retained placental fragments, and if the concentration of prolactin is low, treatment to increase prolactin may be effective. Finally, given the importance of the milk ejection reflex for adequate milk removal, an objective measurement of oxytocin is important. However, oxytocin has a short half-life, thus frequent, invasive sampling of blood and milk is needed in order to obtain a precise assessment. Therefore, objective measures, such as dilation of the milk ducts viewed using ultrasound and increases in milk flow during breast expression, are more practical.

Initiation of milk synthesis

If lactogenesis I has occurred, the lactose synthesized by the lactocytes is not secreted, but is reabsorbed, appears in the blood, and is cleared in the urine. As very little lactose is normally present in the non-pregnant circulation, it is presumed that lactose in the blood has originated from the mammary gland. Thus, measurement of plasma lactose and/or the rate of lactose excretion in urine accurately reflects the synthesis of lactose and is therefore a useful indicator of lactogenesis I (Turkington & Hill, 1969). In studies using CBM, a mother who showed no breast growth during pregnancy also had no increase in urinary lactose during pregnancy, indicating that lactogenesis I had not occurred (Kulski & Hartmann, 1981).

Measurement of milk volume is the most direct method for determining the onset of copious milk secretion, but accurate measurement is often difficult to achieve. Milk volume can be easily measured when mothers are expressing for infants who are sick or preterm. However, the effect of frequency of expression on milk production during initiation of lactation is not known (Hartmann *et al.*, 2003; Neville & Morton, 2001). In mothers who are breastfeeding their term infants, test weighing of the infant before and after all feeds is the most reliable method of determining milk transfer from mother to infant (Schanlon *et al.*, 2002; Arthur *et al.*, 1987). However, this method is a demanding procedure for new mothers and may not accurately determine synthesis if milk production exceeds demand for milk by the infant or the infant is not feeding effectively.

Maternal perception of breast fullness is frequently used to quantify timing of the onset of lactogenesis II in studies of women (Pérez-Escamilla & Chapman, 2001; Chapman & Pérez-Escamilla, 2000). This marker is less reliable than either biochemical markers or milk volume because of its subjective nature. It may also be associated with transient edema. Therefore, the level of synthetic activity of the breast has been determined by either measuring the concentration of the substrates that have been taken up, the conversion rate of the substrates, or concentration of the synthesized milk components (Arthur *et al.*, 1989). The latter was proved to be the most non-invasive method and provided equally as precise information on synthetic activity of the breast as the first two methods (Nicholas & Hartmann, 1981).

Lactose, sodium, citrate, and protein are known as markers of lactogenesis (Arthur *et al.*, 1991; Kent *et al.*, 1992). The concentrations of these milk components change rapidly during lactogenesis II (Hartmann, 1973; Kuhn, 1969; Kulski & Hartmann, 1981). Lactose is the most widely used component in determining the initiation of lactation because it is unique to milk. In most species, it is the major osmotic component of milk, and therefore as lactose is synthesized, water is drawn into the Golgi vesicles to maintain osmotic equilibrium. Furthermore, the measurement of lactose is relatively simple and accurate (Baik *et al.*, 1998). Therefore, during the initiation of lactation, the increase in the concentration of lactose in milk is closely related to an increase in the volume of milk produced (**Figure 5**). The mother who showed no increase in breast volume or urinary lactose during pregnancy, but increased breast volume after birth showed an increase in milk lactose during the first few days of lactation and went on to produce over 700 mL of milk per day at one month of lactation (Kulski & Hartmann, 1981). Measurement of milk lactose is also useful at times when either milk is not being completely removed from the breast (e.g., if positioning and attachment is poor) (Arthur *et al.*, 1991; Cox *et al.*, 1999; McNeill *et al.*, 1998) or when breast permeability is increased (e.g., during mastitis) (Fetherston, 2006).

Therefore, lactose is used as a marker of lactogenesis II. In addition, sodium, chloride, citrate, and protein are also used as markers (Kent *et al.*, 1992). Rapid decreases in sodium and chloride concentrations in milk occur with the closure of tight junctions (Neville *et al.*, 2001; Neville

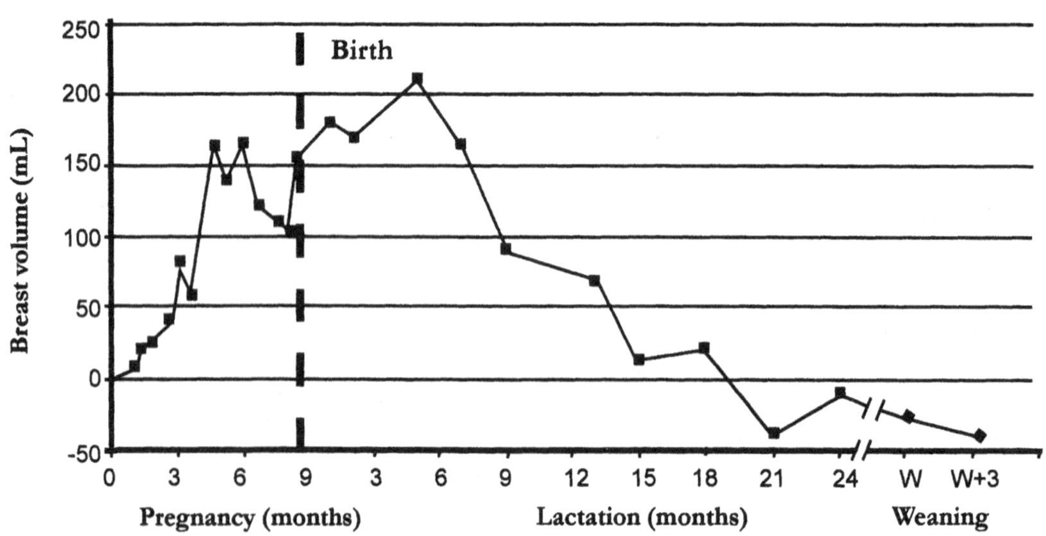

Figure 10. Average change in breast volume during pregnancy, lactation, and after weaning (w) compared to preconception breast volume. Adapted from Kent *et al.*, 1999.

et al., 1991), while citrate is secreted into milk together with lactose and protein by exocytosis from the Golgi apparatus. Similar to lactose, citrate rapidly increases in concentration during initiation of lactation. Protein, on the other hand, has been found to be significantly reduced during the initiation of lactation (Kulski & Hartmann, 1981).

Using these measurements, Arthur *et al.* (1989) defined the normal range for women with exclusively breastfed term babies. In addition, Cregan *et al.* (2002) showed that 82% of women who deliver prematurely had an impaired initiation of lactation (lower milk production at day five) if the concentration of at least one of these markers is outside the normal range.

OVERVIEW OF THE LACTATION CYCLE

The average changes in breast volume throughout the lactation cycle are shown in **Figure 10**. It should be noted that there will be differences between individual mothers and may be differences between breasts. The hormonal changes of pregnancy cause proliferation of the mammary secretory tissue and an increase in breast size. After birth, further increase in breast size may be partly due to further proliferation of secretory tissue and most noticeably due to a sudden increase in the milk in the breast, as lactogenesis II occurs after the withdrawal of progesterone. Changes in breast size within a day can vary from 74 mL to 382 mL as the breast fills with milk and is drained during either breastfeeding or breast expressing (Kent *et al.*, 2006). Milk production in response to milk removal is relatively constant during exclusive breastfeeding from one to six months after birth, and the amount of breast tissue remains constant, as filled alveoli are emptied and synthesis of milk components begins again. A decrease in breast size occurs after six months. This may be due to mobilization of fat from the breast since it occurs prior to a significant reduction in milk production. As complementary foods are introduced, milk production decreases accompanied by a decrease in breast size, as apoptosis of the lactocytes occurs. However, even when the breasts return to pre-conception size, significant milk production continues while the infant is breastfeeding. This size is maintained after weaning, so there is no net gain or loss of breast tissue over the lactation cycle (that is from preconception to post weaning).

FACTORS ASSOCIATED WITH LACTATION PROBLEMS AND FAILURE

In mothers of term infants, the timing of lactogenesis II has been shown to influence the success of breastfeeding. Women who experience delayed lactogenesis II are more likely to have shorter durations of breastfeeding, regardless of their original intentions (Chapman & Pérez-Escamilla, 1999). Moreover, subsequent milk transfer is strongly influenced by maternal milk yield in the first weeks of lactation (Neville *et al.*, 1988). Hence, lactogenesis II is a critical event in the breastfeeding experience in mothers of term infants. The evidence is less clear for mothers who deliver before term. Although the necessary conditions for lactogenesis II to occur (fully-developed lactocytes, raised plasma concentration of prolactin, and a sharp decrease in progesterone concentration) are present in most women after birth, a number of factors can cause delay of lactogenesis II (Neville *et al.*, 2001).

Parity

Parity influences the timing of lactogenesis II, with studies showing that postnatal increases in milk volume occur later in primiparous women compared with multiparous women (Chen *et al.*, 1998; Dewey *et al.*, 2003). A study which used maternal report of increased breast fullness to define onset of lactation found that primiparous women were more likely to perceive delayed onset (Dewey *et al.*, 2003). In this study of middle-class American mothers, primiparas were also more likely to experience early breastfeeding failure.

Mode of Delivery

The literature is inconsistent about the effects of mode of delivery on timing of lactogenesis II in women who deliver at term. However, studies that examined the effect of emergency (non-elective) cesarean section were more likely to find adverse effects on onset of lactation than those which investigated elective cesarean section alone. Kulski and associates found no effect of elective cesarean section on changes in milk composition indicating lactogenesis II in a sample of women who were highly motivated to breastfeed (Kulski *et al.*, 1981). Chapman *et al.* (1999) found no effect of elective cesarean section on maternal perception of timing of onset of lactation compared with vaginal delivery (Chapman *et al.*, 1999). In contrast, the authors found that unplanned cesarean section was significantly associated with perceived delay of onset of lactation.

Dewey *et al.* (2003) found that maternal report of breast fullness was delayed in mothers having a cesarean section (Dewey *et al.*, 2003). This study, which did not specify whether the operative delivery was elective or emergency, suggested a delay in lactogenesis II in women delivering by cesarean section for any reason. In another study that did not discriminate between elective and non-elective cesarean section, milk transfer was reduced in women who delivered by cesarean section on days two to five compared with vaginal delivery, but no difference was observed after that time (Evans *et al.*, 2003). Healthy women who delivered a term infant weighed their infants before and after each feed (test weighing) for up to six days postpartum in that study of breastmilk transfer. However, test weighing has limitations when used as a marker of lactogenesis, as it only measures the infant's capacity to remove milk from the breast and hence may underestimate potential milk production in women who are able to produce more than their infants' need.

A study which sampled blood for hormonal analysis during breastfeeding on day two postpartum found different patterns of hormone release according to mode of delivery, suggesting a delay in onset of lactation after emergency cesarean section (Nissen *et al.*, 1996). Compared with normal vaginal delivery, women who delivered by emergency cesarean section demonstrated fewer pulses in oxytocin and lower prolactin concentration in blood samples taken while they were breastfeeding their term infants, suggesting less effective lactation in the early postnatal period. The mode and nature of anesthesia is an additional complicating factor that requires further research.

Maternal Diabetes

Several studies have shown that lactogenesis II is delayed in mothers with type 1 diabetes mellitus (previously know as insulin-dependent diabetes mellitus) (Arthur *et al.*, 1989; Ferris *et al.*, 1988; Ferris *et al.*, 1993; Neubauer *et al.*, 1993). Arthur *et al.* (1989) used the milk constituents, lactose and citrate, as markers of lactogenesis II to demonstrate a delay of 15 to 28 hours in women with type 1 diabetes. These findings were consistent with those of Neubauer *et al.* (1993). This study of 33 women with type 1 diabetes and 33 matched controls found significantly lower lactose and higher nitrogen concentrations in milk on postnatal days two, three, and seven and lower milk transfer on day seven, suggesting less effective lactation in the first postnatal week. This delay was more marked in women with less stable plasma glucose. The cause of this delay is unclear. The issue of metabolic control during lactation has not been defined, but episodes of hypoglycemia may influence the uptake of glucose by the lactocytes, decreasing the synthesis of lactose and thus the ability to successfully initiate and maintain lactation.

Type 1 diabetes also generally results in a high risk pregnancy with a higher risk of cesarean section delivery. Delivery, postnatal, and neonatal management protocols tend to delay early breastfeeding events with fewer opportunities to breastfeed in the first postpartum day than for the non-diabetic women. Neonates of diabetic mothers also frequently have hypoglycemia and are more likely to be offered supplementary feeds. Ferris *et al.* (1993) demonstrated that women with type 1 diabetes spent less time with their term infant, the first breastfeed was later, and frequency of breastfeeding was reduced in the first week, regardless of mode of delivery. The majority of infants of type 1 diabetic mothers were admitted to the neonatal nursery within the first day, and this early separation was correlated significantly with the time the mothers perceived their breasts commencing to fill.

Compared with type 1 diabetes, there is a paucity of research about the effects of either type 2 diabetes or gestational diabetes on lactation. A retrospective New Zealand study found that mothers with type 2 diabetes were less likely to breastfeed than mothers with gestational diabetes (Simmons *et al.*, 2005). In this study, mothers were more likely to be breastfeeding on discharge from the hospital when the first feed was a breastfeed or if delivery was not by cesarean section.

It is interesting that even a short period of lactation has a beneficial effect on glucose metabolism in women who have gestational diabetes (McManus *et al.*, 2001; Kjos *et al.*, 1993). Moreover, longer duration of breastfeeding has been found to reduce the incidence of type 2 diabetes later in life in women who had gestational diabetes during pregnancy (Stuebe *et al.*, 2005).

Maternal Obesity

Several studies have suggested an association between maternal obesity and reduced initiation and duration of lactation (Rasmussen *et al.*, 2001; Hilson *et al.*, 1997;

Lovelady, 2005). In a study of 40 mothers where blood samples were taken before and after breastfeeds, mothers who were obese before the pregnancy were less likely to have increased prolactin concentration after breastfeeding at two and seven days postpartum than those of normal weight (Rasmussen & Kjolhede, 2004). These results suggest a hormonal cause of the potential negative impact of maternal body mass index on lactogenesis II and breastfeeding duration. Other studies have shown sub-optimal breastfeeding behaviors and delayed lactogenesis II in mothers with raised body mass index (BMI) (Dewey *et al.*, 2003; Hilson *et al.*, 1997).

Retained Products of Conception

Delayed lactogenesis II resulting from placental fragments retained after birth was first reported in 1981 (Neifert *et al.*, 1981). In this case series, breast engorgement indicating onset of lactation only commenced after surgical removal of the retained products of conception. The cause of this delay is hypothesized to be the continued secretion of progesterone by the placental fragments, which inhibits the onset of copious milk secretion.

Stress in Labor and Delivery

High levels of stress during labor and delivery have

Table 1. Factors, Possible Causes, and Potential Treatments Associated with Delayed or Inhibited Lactogenesis II in Term Mothers

Factor	Cause	Treatment
Retained placental fragments	Elevated progesterone	Dilatation and curettage
Previous surgery or radiation treatment	Distortion/severing of innervations and ducts	?
Inadequate stimulation	Absence of milk ejection	Use gentle hand massage, pump near baby, double pump
Cesarean delivery	No labor, disturbed endocrine balance?	Informed support
Anesthetic agents	Poorly researched	?
Maternal obesity	Delayed progesterone withdrawal	Progesterone antagonist?
Type 1 diabetes	Intracellular signaling?	Informed support
Prolactin deficiency	Prolactin activates milk genes	Domperidone, metoclpramide
Drugs/hormones	Milk ejection and milk synthesis inhibited	Reduce exposure Oxytocin?
Colostrum/milk not removed	Autocrine inhibition due to milk stasis	Commence breastfeeding and/or breast expression
Glandular insufficiency	Unknown	?

Adapted from Hartmann & Ramsay, 2005.

Table 2. Additional Factors, Possible Causes, and Potential Treatments Associated with Delayed or Inhibited Lactogenesis II in Preterm Mothers

Factor	Cause	Treatment
Poor breast development	Shortened gestation	Increase frequency of pumping
Stress, fatigue	Inhibition of milk ejection	Stress management and relaxation techniques
Maternal-infant separation	Inadequate stimulation for milk ejection leading to ineffective pumping	Pump near baby and practice kangaroo care
Inadequate frequency of pumping	Autocrine inhibition due to milk stasis	Increase frequency of pumping, double pumping

Adapted from Hartmann & Ramsay, 2005.

been found to be associated with delayed onset of lactation in some women (Chen *et al.*, 1998; Grajeda & Pérez-Escamilla, 2002). In a study that measured salivary cortisol during labor and defined lactogenesis II according to women's perception, multiparous women with high salivary cortisol levels had significantly delayed onset compared with multiparous women without high levels. In this study, primiparous women were more likely to have high antenatal and postnatal cortisol levels than multiparas. Furthermore, compared to multiparas, primiparas who had an emergency cesarean delivery had later onset of lactation (Grajeda & Pérez-Escamilla, 2002). Dewey and associates have also demonstrated an association between stress in the postnatal period and delayed perception of onset of lactation (Dewey, 2001); however, the authors qualified their findings by speculating about the causation of the postnatal stress and suggesting that delayed lactogenesis II could in fact be a causative factor.

Delay in Commencement of Breast Emptying

Early milk removal either by breastfeeding or expression is hypothesized to promote early onset of lactation, although the evidence for this is inconsistent. A randomized controlled trial of women at risk of delayed lactogenesis II after cesarean section delivery found that early breast pumping was not effective in improving the volume of breastmilk produced in the first 72 hours postpartum (Chapman *et al.*, 2001). In addition, early milk expression was thought to have a potential negative impact on breastfeeding duration in this study.

Delayed Lactogenesis II and Lactation Failure

A number of studies have shown a strong association between delayed onset of lactogenesis II or low supply in the first postnatal week and early unplanned cessation of breastfeeding in term infants (Chapman & Perez Escamilla, 1999; Neville *et al.*, 1988; Hruschka *et al.*, 2003; Sievers *et al.*, 2003; Ingram *et al.*, 1999; Houston *et al.*, 1983). These findings were unrelated to the mothers' motivation to successfully breastfeed. The evidence is less clear for mothers of preterm infants.

Potential causes of delayed initiation of lactation in term and preterm mothers are presented in **Tables 1** and **2**.

ACKNOWLEDGEMENT

Research funding from Medela AG.

References

Akers RM. *Lactation and the mammary gland.* Ames, IA: Iowa State Press; 2002.

Arthur PG, Hartmann PE, Smith M. Measurement of the milk intake of breast-fed infants. *J Pediatr Gastroenterol Nutr.* 1987; 6(5):758-63.

Arthur PG, Kent JC, Potter JM, Hartmann PE. Lactose in blood in nonpregnant, pregnant, and lactating women. *J Pediatr Gastroenterol Nutr.* 1991; 13:254-59.

Arthur PG, Smith M, Hartmann PE. Milk lactose, citrate, and glucose as markers of lactogenesis in normal and diabetic women. *J Pediatr Gastroenterol Nutr.* 1989; 9(4):488-96.

Baik MG, Lee MJ, Choi YJ. Gene expression during involution of mammary gland. *Int J Mol Med.* 1998; 2:39-44.

Ballou LU, Bleck JL, Bleck GT, Bremel RD. The effects of daily oxytocin injections before and after milking on milk production, milk plasmin, and milk composition. *J Dairy Sci.* 1993;7 6(6):1544-49.

Barry JM. The source of lysine, tyrosine, and phosphorus for casein synthesis. *J Biol Chem.* 1952; 195(2):795-803.

Bell AW, Bauman DE. Adaptations of glucose metabolism during pregnancy and lactation. *J Mammary Gland Biol Neoplasia.* 1997; 2(3):265-78.

Bencini R. The sheep as a dairy animal: Lactation, production of milk and its suitability for cheese making. Crawley: The University of Western Australia; 1993.

Berg MN, Dharmarajan AM, Waddell BJ. Glucocorticoids and progesterone prevent apoptosis in the lactating rat mammary gland. *Endocrinology.* 2002; 143(1):222-27.

Brown JB, Blackwell LF, Cox RI, Holmes JM, Smith MA. Chemical and homogeneous enzyme immunoassay methods for the measurement of estrogens and pregnanediol and their glucuronides in urine. *Prog Biol Clin Res.* 1988; 285:119-38.

Brown JB, Blackwell LF, Holmes J, Smyth K. New assays for identifying the fertile period. *Int J Gynecol Obstet.* 1989; Supplement 1:111-22.

Butte NF, Hopkinson JM, Mehta N, Moon JK, O'Brien Smith E. Adjustments in energy expenditure and substrate utilization during late pregnancy and lactation. *Am J Clin Nutr.* 1999; 69:299-307.

Challis JRG, Matthews SG, Gibb W, Lye SJ. Endocrine and paracrine regulation of birth at term and preterm. *Endocr Rev.* 2000; 21(5):514-50.

Chapman DJ, Pérez-Escamilla R. Does delayed perception of the onset of lactation shorten breastfeeding duration? *J Hum Lact.* 1999; 15(2):107-11.

Chapman DJ, Pérez-Escamilla R. Identification of risk factors for delayed onset of lactation. *J Am Diet Assoc.* 1999; 99:450-4.

Chapman DJ, Pérez-Escamilla R. Maternal perception of the onset of lactation: A valid indicator of lactogenesis stage II? *Adv Exp Med Biol.* 2000; 478:423-24.

Chapman DJ, Young S, Ferris AM, Pérez-Escamilla R. Impact of breast pumping on lactogenesis stage II after cesarean delivery: A randomized clinical trial. *Pediatrics.* 2001; 107(6):e94.

Chen DC, Nommsen-Rivers L, Dewey KG, Lönnerdal B. Stress during labor and delivery and early lactation performance. *Am J Clin Nutr.* 1998; 68:335-44.

Collier RJ, Tucker HA. Regulation of cortisol uptake in mammary tissue of cows. *J Dairy Sci.* 1978; 61:1709-14.

Cowie AT, Forsyth IA, Hart IC. *Hormonal control of lactation.* Berlin: Springer-Verlag; 1980.

Cowie AT, Forsyth IA, Hart IC. *Hormonal control of lactation. Monographs on Endocrinology.* 1980; 15:I-XIV.

Cowie AT. Lactation. In: Austin CR, Short RV (eds.). *Hormonal control of reproduction.* 2nd Ed. Cambridge: Cambridge University Press; 1984. p. 195-231.

Cox DB, Kent JC, Casey TM, Owens RA, Hartmann PE. Breast growth and the urinary excretion of lactose during human pregnancy and early lactation: endocrine relationships. *Exp Physiol.* 1999; 84(2):421-34.

Cox DB, Kent JC, Casey TM, Owens RA, Hartmann PE. Breast growth and the urinary excretion of lactose during human pregnancy and early lactation: Endocrine relationships. *Exp Physiol.* 1999; 84:421-34.

Cox DB, Owens RA, Hartmann PE. Blood and milk prolactin and the rate of milk synthesis in women. *Exp Physiol.* 1996; 81(6):1007-20.

Cox DB. *The morphological and functional development of the human breast during pregnancy and lactation.* Perth, Western Australia: University of Western Australia; 1996.

Cregan MD, De Mello TR, Kershaw D, McDougall K, Hartmann PE. Initiation of lactation in women after preterm delivery. *Acta Obstet Gynecol Scand.* 2002; 81(9):870-77.

Cregan MD, Hartmann PE. Computerized breast measurement from conception to weaning: clinical implications. *J Hum Lact.* 1999; 15(2):89-96.

Daly SE, Owens RA, Hartmann PE. The short-term synthesis and infant-regulated removal of milk in lactating women. *Exp Physiol.* 1993; 78(2):209-20.

Danli S, Qingxiang S, Guowei S. A multicentered clinical trial of the long-acting injectable contraceptive Depo Provera in Chinese women. *Contraception.* 2000; 62:15-18.

Dewey KG, Lonnerdal B. Infant self-regulation of breast milk intake. *Acta Paediatr Scand.* 1986; 75(6):893-98.

Dewey KG, Nommsen-Rivers LA, Heinig MJ, Cohen RJ. Risk factors for suboptimal infant breastfeeding behavior, delayed onset of lactation, and excess neonatal weight loss. *Pediatrics.* 2003; 112:607-19.

Dewey KG. Maternal and fetal stress are associated with impaired lactogenesis in humans. *J Nutr.* 2001; 131:3012S-5S.

Djiane J, Durand P. Prolactin-progesterone antagonism in self regulation of prolactin receptors in the mammary gland. *Nature.* 1977; 266:641-43.

Edwards GM, Wilford FH, Liu X, Hennighausen L, Djiane J, Streuli CH. Regulation of mammary differentiation by extracellular matrix involves protein-tyrosine phosphatases. *J Biol Chem.* 1998; 273(16):9495-500.

Evans KC, Evans RG, Royal R, Esterman AJ, James SL. Effect of caesarean section on breast milk transfer to the normal term newborn over the first week of life. *Arch Dis Child Fetal Neonatal Ed.* 2003; 88(5):F380-F2.

Feng Z, Marti A, Jehn B, Altermatt HJ, Chicaiza G, Jaggi R. Glucocorticoid and progesterone inhibit involution and programmed cell death in the mouse mammary gland. *J Cell Biol.* 1995; 131(4):1095-103.

Ferris AM, Dalidowitz CK, Ingardia CM, Reece EA, Fumia FD, Jensen RG, *et al.* Lactation outcome in insulin-dependent diabetic women. *J Am Diet Assoc.* 1988; 88:317-22.

Ferris AM, Neubauer SH, Bendel RB, Green KW, Ingardia CM, Reece EA. Perinatal lactation protocol and outcome in mothers with and without insulin-dependent diabetes mellitus. *Am J Clin Nutr.* 1993; 58:43-48.

Fetherston C. Excretion of lactose in urine as a measurement of increased permeability of the lactating breast during inflammation. *Acta Obstet Gynecol Scand.* 2006; 85:20-25.

Forsyth IA. The endocrinology of lactation. In: Mepham TB (ed.). *Biochemistry of lactation.* Amsterdam: Elsevier; 1983.

Forsyth IA. Variation among species in the endocrine control of mammary growth and function: The roles of prolactin, growth hormone, and placental lactogen. *J Dairy Sci.* 1986; 69:886-903.

Frantz AG. The assay and regulation of prolactin in humans. *Adv Exp Med Biol.* 1977; 80:95-133.

Freeman ME, Kanyickska B, Lerant A, Nagy G. Prolactin: structure, function, and regulation of secretion. *Physiol Rev.* 2000; 80(4):1523-631.

Gardner DG, Wittliff JL. Characterization of a distinct glucocorticoid-binding protein in the lactating mammary gland of the rat. *Biochim Biophys Acta.* 1973; 320:617-27.

Grajeda R, Pérez-Escamilla R. Stress during labor and delivery is associated with delayed onset of lactation among urban Guatemalan women. *J Nutr.* 2002; 132:3055-60.

Green KA, Streuli CH. Apoptosis regulation in the mammary gland. *Cell Mol Life Sci.* 2004; 61:1867-83.

Gunn A, Gunn T, Rabone D, Breier B, Blum W, Gluckman P. Growth hormone increases breast milk volumes in mothers of preterm infants. *Pediatrics.* 1996; 98(2):978.

Hale TW. *Medications and mother's milk.* 12th Ed. Amarillo, TX: Hale Publishing; 2006.

Hartmann P, Ramsay D. Mammary anatomy and physiology. In: Jones E, King C (eds.). *Feeding and nutrition in the preterm infant.* London: Elsevier; 2005.

Hartmann PE, Arthur PG. Assessment of lactation performance in women. In: Hamosh M, Goldman AS (eds.). *Human lactation 2: maternal and environmental factors.* New York: Plenum; 1986:215-30.

Hartmann PE, Cregan MD, Ramsay DT, Simmer K, Kent JC. Physiology of lactation in preterm mothers: Initiation and maintenance. *Pediatr Ann.* 2003; 32(5):351-55.

Hartmann PE, Sherriff J, Kent J. Maternal nutrition and the regulation of milk synthesis. *Proc Nutr Soc.* 1995; 54:379-89.

Hartmann PE, Sherriff JL, Mitoulas LR. Homeostatic mechanisms that regulate lactation during energetic stress. *J Nutr.* 1998; 128(2 Suppl):394S-99S.

Hartmann PE, Trevethan P, Shelton JN. Progesterone and oestrogen and the initiation of lactation in ewes. *J Endocr.* 1973; 59:249-59.

Hartmann PE. Changes in milk composition and yield of the secretion of cows during the initiation of lactation. *J Endocrinol.* 1973; 59:231-47.

Hartmann PE. Changes in the composition and yield of the mammary secretion of cows during the initiation of lactation. *J Endocrinol.* 1973; 59:231-47.

Heap RB, Flint AP. Pregnancy. In: Austin CR, Short RV (eds.). *Hormonal control of reproduction.* 2nd Ed. Cambridge: Cambridge University Press; 1984:153-94.

Heap RB, Galil A, Harrison FA, Jenkin G, Perry JS. Progesterone and oestrogen in pregnancy and parturition: comparative aspects and hierarchical control. In: Foundation C (ed.). *The fetus and birth.* Amsterdam: Elsevier; 1977:127-50.

Henderson AJ, Peaker M. Feed-back control of milk secretion in the goat by a chemical in milk. *J Physiol.* 1984; 351:39-45.

Henderson J. *The effects of antenatal glucocorticoid treatment on lactogenesis II in ewes and women.* Perth, Western Australia: University of Western Australia; 2007.

Henninghausen L, Robinson GW. Development and differentiation of the mammary gland from the prespective of prolactin. In: Wilde CJ, Peaker M, Taylor E (eds.). *Biological signalling and the mammary gland.* Ayr: Hannah Research Institute; 1997.

Hilson JA, Rasmussen KM, Kjolhede CL. Maternal obesity and breast-feeding success in a rural population of white women. *Am J Clin Nutr.* 1997; 66:1371-78.

Houston MJ, Howie PW, McNeilly AS. Factors affecting the duration of breast feeding: 1. Measurement of breast milk intake in the first week of life. *Early Hum Dev.* 1983; 8:49-54.

Hruschka DJ, Sellen DW, Stein AD, Martorell R. Delayed onset of lactation and risk of ending full breast-feeding early in rural Guatemala. *J Nutr.* 2003; 133:2592-99.

Hytten F. Clinical and chemical studies in human lactation. VII. The effect of difference in yield and composition of milk on the infant's weight gain and the duration of breast-feeding. *Br Med J.* 1954; 1:912-15.

Ingram JC, Woolridge MW, Greenwood RJ, McGrath L. Maternal predictors of early breast milk output. *Acta Paediatr Scand.* 1999; 88:493-99.

Jacobs LS. The role of prolactin in mammogenesis and lactogenesis. *Adv Exp Med Biol.* 1977; 80:173-91.

Kann G. Evidence for a mammogenic role of growth hormone in ewes: Effects of growth hormone-releasing factor during artificial induction of laction. *J Anim Sci.* 1997; 75:2541-49.

Kent J, Mitoulas L, Cregan M, Ramsay D, Doherty D, Hartmann P. Volume and frequency of breastfeeds and fat content of breastmilk throughout the day. *Pediatrics.* 2006; 117:e387-e95.

Kent JC, Arthur PG, Retallack RW, Hartmann PE. Calcium, phosphate and citrate in human milk at initiation of lactation. *J Dairy Res.* 1992; 59(2):161-67.

Kent JC, Mitoulas L, Cox DB, Owens RA, Hartmann PE. Breast volume and milk production during extended lactation in women. *Exp Physiol.* 1999; 84(2):435-47.

Kjos SL, Henry O, Lee RM, Buchanan TA, Mishell DRJ. The effect of lactation on glucose and lipid metabolism in women with recent gestational diabetes. *Obstet Gynecol.* 1993; 82(3):451-55.

Knight CH, Peaker M, Wilde CJ. Local control of mammary development and function. *Rev Reprod.* 1998; 3(2):104-12.

Knight CH. Short-term oxytocin treatment increases bovine milk yield by enhancing milk removal without any direct action on mammary metabolism. *J Endocrinol.* 1994; 142(3):471-73.

Kolodny RC, Jacobs LS, Daughaday WH. Mammary stimulation causes prolactin secretion in non-lactating women. *Nature.* 1972; 238(5362):284-86.

Korsrud GO, Baldwin RL. Effects of adrenalectomy, adrenalectomy--ovariectomy, and cortisol and estrogen therapies upon enzyme activities in lactating rat mammary glands. *Can J Biochem.* 1972; 50(4):366-76.

Korsrud GO, Baldwin RL. Estimations of rates of synthesis and degradation of several rat mammary gland enzymes from changes in enzyme activities. *Can J Biochem.* 1972; 50(4):386-91.

Korsrud GO, Baldwin RL. Hormonal regulation of rat mammary gland enzyme activities and metabolite patterns. *Can J Biochem.* 1972; 50(4):377-85.

Kuhn NJ. Progesterone withdrawal as the lactogenic trigger in the rat. *J Endocr.* 1969; 44:39-54.

Kulski JK, Hartmann PE, Martin JD, Smith M. Effects of bromocriptine mesylate on the composition of the mammary secretion in non-breast-feeding women. *Obstetr Gynecol.* 1978; 52(1):38-42.

Kulski JK, Hartmann PE. Changes in human milk composition during the initiation of lactation. *Aust J Exp Biol Med Sci.* 1981; 59(1):101-14.

Kulski JK, Smith M, Hartmann PE. Normal and caesarean section delivery and the initiation of lactation in women. *AJEBAK.* 1981; 59(4):405-12.

Kulski JK, Smith M, Hartmann PE. Perinatal concentrations of progesterone, lactose and a-lactalbumin in the mammary secretion of women. *J Endocr.* 1977; 74:509-10.

Lawrence RA, Lawrence RM. *Breastfeeding: A guide for the medical profession.* 5th Ed. St. Louis: Mosby; 1999.

Li M, Liu X, Robinson G, Bar-Peled U, Wagner K-U, Young WS, *et al.* Mammary-derived signals activate programmed cell death during the first stage of mammary gland involution. *Proc Natl Acad Sci USA.* 1997; 94(7):3425-30.

Linzell JL, Peaker M. Changes in colostrum composition and in the permeability of the mammary epithelium at about the time of parturition in the goat. *J Physiol.* 1974; 243:129-51.

Linzell JL, Peaker M. The effects of oxytocin and milk removal on milk secretion in the goat. *J Physiol.* 1971; 216(3):717-34.

Liu X, Robinson GW, Hennighausen L. Activation of stat5a and stat5b by tyrosine phosphorylation is tightly linked to mammary gland differentiation. *Mol Endocrin.* 1996; 10:1496-506.

Lovelady CA. Is maternal obesity a cause of poor lactation performance? *Nutr Rev.* 2005; 63(10):352-5.

Maki M, Hirose M, Chiba H. Occurrence of common binding sites for progestin and glucocorticoid in the lactating mammary gland of the rat. *J Biochem.* 1980; 88:1845-54.

Marti A, Feng Z, Altermatt HJ, Jaggi R. Milk accumulation triggers apoptosis of mammary epithelial cells. *Eur J Cell Biol.* 1977; 73:158-65.

Martyn P, Falconer IR. The effect of progesterone on prolactin stimulation of fatty acid synthesis, glycerolipid synthesis and lipogenic-enzyme activities in mammary glands of pseudopregnant rabbits, after explant culture or intraductal injection. *Biochem J.* 1985; 231(2):321-28.

McCutcheon SN, Bauman DE. Effect of chronic growth hormone treatment on responses to epinephrine and thyrotropin-releasing hormone in lactating cows. *J Dairy Sci.* 1986; 69(1):44-51.

McManus RM, Cunningham I, Watson A, Harker L, Finegood DT. Beta-cell function and visceral fat in lactating women with a history of gestational diabetes. *Metab Clin Exp.* 2001; 50(6):715-19.

McNeill DM, Murphy PM, Lindsay DR. Blood lactose v. milk lactose as a monitor of lactogenesis and colostrum production in Merino ewes. *Aust J Agric Res.* 1998; 49:581-87.

Mepham TB (ed.). *Biochemistry of lactation.* Amsterdam: Elsevier; 1983.

Mercier J-C, Gaye P. Milk protein synthesis. In: Mepham TB (ed.). *Biochemistry of lactation.* Amsterdam: Elsevier; 1983.

Mesiano S. Roles of estrogen and progesterone in human parturition. In: Smith R (ed.). *The endocrinology of parturition.* London: Karger; 2001:86-104.

Milsom S, Breier B, Gallaher B, Cox V, Gunn A, Gluckman P. Growth hormone stimulates galactopoeis in healthy lactating women. *Acta Endocrinol.* 1992; 127:337-43.

Milsom S, Rabone D, Gunn A, Gluckman P. Potential role for growth hormone in human lactation insufficiency. *Horm Res.* 1998; 50:147-50.

Min SH, Mackenzie DDS, McCutcheon SN, Breier BH, Gluckman PD. Comparative effects of recombinant ovine placental lactogen and bovine growth hormone on galactopoiesis in ewes. *J Dairy Sci.* 1997; 80:640-45.

Mizoguchi Y, Yamaguchi H, Aoki F, Enami J, Sakai S. Corticosterone is required for the prolactin receptor gene expression in the late pregnant mouse mammary gland. *Mol Cell Endocrinol.* 1997; 132(1-2):177-83.

Molenaar AJ, Davis SR, Wilkins RJ. Expression of α-lactalbumin, α-S1-casein, and lactoferrin genes is heterogeneous in sheep and cattle mammary tissue. *J Histochem Cytochem.* 1992; 40(5):611-18.

Molenaar AJ, Kuys YM, Davis SR, Wilkins RJ, Mead PE, Tweedie JW. Elevation of lactoferrin gene expression in developing, ductal, resting, and regressing parenchymal epithelium of the ruminant mammary gland. *J Dairy Sci.* 1996; 79:1198-208.

Neifert MR, McDonough SL, Neville MC. Failure of lactogenesis associated with placental retention. *Am J Obstet Gynecol.* 1981; 140(4):477-78.

Neubauer SH, Ferris AM, Chase CG, Fanelli J, Thompson CA, Lammi-Keefe CJ, *et al.* Delayed lactogenesis in women with insulin-dependent diabetes mellitus. *Am J Clin Nutr.* 1993; 58:54-60.

Neville MC, Allen JC, Archer PC, Casey CE, Seacat J, Keller RP, *et al.* Studies in human lactation: milk volume and nutrient composition during weaning and lactogenesis. *Am J Clin Nutr.* 1991; 54:81-92.

Neville MC, Allen JC. The mechanisms of milk secretion. In: Neville MC, Neifert MR (eds.). *Lactation: Physiology, nutrition and breast-feeding.* New York: Plenum Press; 1983.

Neville MC, Casey CE. Changes in milk composition after six months of lactation. In: Hamosh M, Goldman AS (eds.). *Human lactation 2: Maternal and environmental factors.* New York: Plenum Press; 1986:141-54.

Neville MC, Keller RP, Seacat J, Lutes V, Neifert M, Casey C, *et al.* Studies in human lactation: Milk volumes in lactating women during the onset of lactation and full lactation. *Am J Clin Nutr.* 1988; 48:1375-86.

Neville MC, McFaddin TB, Forsyth I. Hormonal regulation of mammary differentiation and milk secretion. *J Mammary Gland Biol Neoplasia.* 2002; 7(1):49-66.

Neville MC, Morton J, Umemura S. Lactogenesis. The transition from pregnancy to lactation. *Pediatr Clin North Am.* 2001; 48(1):35-52.

Neville MC, Morton J. Physiology and endocrine changes underlying human lactogenesis II. *J Nutr.* 2001; 131(11):3005S-8S.

Neville MC, Picciano MF. Regulation of milk lipid secretion and composition. *Annu Rev Nutr.* 1997; 17:159-83.

Neville MC, Sawicki VS, Hay WW, Jr. Effects of fasting, elevated plasma glucose and plasma insulin concentrations on milk secretion in women. *J Endocrinol.* 1993; 139(1):165-73.

Neville MC. Anatomy and physiology of lactation. *Pediatr Clin North Am.* 2001; 48(1):13-34.

Neville MC. Physiology of lactation. *Clin Perinatol.* 1999; 26(2):251-79.

Nguyen D-A, Neville MC. Tight junction regulation in the mammary gland. *J Mammary Gland Biol Neoplasia.* 1998; 3(3):233-46.

Nguyen D-A, Parlow AF, Neville MC. Hormonal regulation of tight junction closure in the mouse mammary epithelium during the transition from pregnancy to lactation. *J Endocr.* 2001; 170:347-56.

Nicholas KR, Hartmann PE. Progressive changes in plasma progesterone, prolactin and corticosteroid levels during late pregnancy and the initiation of lactose synthesis in the rat. *Aust J Biol Sci.* 1981; 34(4):445-54.

Nissen E, Uvnäs-Moberg K, Svensson K, Stock S, Widström A-M, Winberg J. Different patterns of oxytocin, prolactin but not cortisol release during breastfeeding in women delivered by caesarean section or by the vaginal route. *Early Hum Dev.* 1996; 45:103-18.

Noel GL, Suh HK, Frantz AG. Prolactin release during nursing and breast stimulation in postpartum and nonpostpartum subjects. *J Clin Endocrinol Metab.* 1974; 38(3):413-23.

Nostrand SD, Galton DM, Erb HN, Bauman DE. Effects of daily exogenous oxytocin on lactation milk yield and composition. *J Dairy Sci.* 1991; 74(7):2119-27.

Oldenbroek JK, Garssen GJ, Jonker LJ, Wilkinson JI. Effects of treatment of dairy cows with recombinant bovine somatotropin over three or four lactations. *J Dairy Sci.* 1993; 76(2):453-67.

Ollivier-Bousquet M, Guesnet P, Seddiki T, Durand G. Deficiency of (n-6) but not (n-3) polyunsaturated fatty acids inhibits the secretagogue effect of prolactin in lactating rat mammary epithelial cells. *J Nutr.* 1993; 123(12):2090-100.

Ostrom KM. A review of the hormone prolactin during lactation. *Prog Food Nutr Sci.* 1990; 14(1):1-43.

Pérez-Escamilla R, Chapman DJ. Validity and public health implications of maternal perception of the onset of lactation: An international analytical overview. *J Nutr.* 2001; 131:3021S-4S.

Popjak G, French TH, Folley SJ. Utilization of acetate in milk-fat synthesis in the lactating goat. *Process Biochem.* 1950; 2:28-29.

Rasmussen KM, Hilson JA, Kjolhede CL. Obesity may impair lactogenesis II. *J Nutr.* 2001; 131:3009S-11S.

Rasmussen KM, Kjolhede CL. Prepregnant overweight and obesity diminish the prolactin response to suckling in the first week postpartum. *Pediatrics.* 2004; 113:e465-71.

Reichardt HM, Horsch K, Gröne H-J, Kolbus A, Beug H, Hynes N, *et al.* Mammary gland development and lactation are controlled by different glucocorticoid receptor activities. *Eur J Endocrinol.* 2001; 145:519-27.

Rennison ME, Handel SE, Wilde CJ, Burgoyne RD. Investigation of the role of microtubules in protein secretion from lactating mouse mammary epithelial cells. *J Cell Sci.* 1992; 102(Pt 2):239-47.

Rennison ME, Kerr M, Addey CV, Handel SE, Turner MD, Wilde CJ, *et al.* Inhibition of constitutive protein secretion from lactating mouse mammary epithelial cells by FIL (feedback inhibitor of lactation), a secreted milk protein. *J Cell Sci.* 1993; 106(Pt 2):641-48.

Rimoin DL, Holzman GB. Lactation in the absence of human growth hormone. *J Clin Endocrinol Metab.* 1968; 28(8):1183-88.

Ros M, Lobato MF, Garcia-Ruiz JP, Moreno FJ. Integration of lipid metabolism in the mammary gland and adipose tissue by prolactin during lactation. *Mol Cell Biochem.* 1990; 93(2):185-94.

Rosen JM, Wyszomierski SL, Hadsell D. Regulation of milk protein gene expression. *Annu Rev Nutr.* 1999; 19:407-36.

Saint L, Smith M, Hartmann PE. The yield and nutrient content of colostrum and milk of women from giving birth to 1 month post-partum. *Br J Nutr.* 1984; 52:87-95.

Sakai S, Bowman PD, Yang J, McCormick K, Nandi S. Glucocorticoid regulation of prolactin receptors on mammary cells in culture. *Endocrinology.* 1979; 104(5):1447-49.

Sauer MV, Paulson RJ. Utility and predictive value of a rapid measurement of urinary pregnanediol glucuronide by enzyme immunoassay in an infertility practice. *Fertil Steril.* 1991; 56(5):823-26.

Scanlon KS, Alexander MP, Serdula MK, Davis MK, Bowman BA. Assessment of infant feeding: The validity of measuring milk intake. *Nutr Rev.* 2002; 60(8):235-51.

Sechen SJ, Dunshea FR, Bauman DE. Somatotropin in lactating cows: Effect on response to epinephrine and insulin. *Am J Physiol.* 1990; 258(4 Pt 1):E582-88.

Sievers E, Haase S, Oldigs H-D, Schaub J. The impact of peripartum factors on the onset and duration of lactation. *Biol Neonate.* 2003; 83:246-52.

Simmons D, Conroy C, Thompson CF. In-hospital breast feeding rates among women with gestational diabetes and pregestational Type 2 diabetes in South Auckland. *Diabet Med.* 2005; 22:177-81.

Stöcklin E, Wissler M, Gouilleux F, Groner B. Functional interactions between stat5 and the glucocorticoid receptor. *Nature.* 1996; 383:726-28.

Stocklin E, Wissler M, Moriggl R, Groner B. Specific DNA binding of stat5 but not of glucocorticoid receptor is required for their functional cooperation in the regulation of gene transcription. *Mol Cell Biol.* 1997; 17(11):6708-16.

Stuebe AM, Rich-Edwards JW, Willet WC, Manson JE, Michels KB. Duration of lactation and incidence of type 2 diabetes. *JAMA.* 2005; 294:2601-10.

Topper YJ, Freeman CS. Multiple hormone interactions in the developmental biology of the mammary gland. *Physiol Rev.* 1980; 60(4):1049-106.

Tucker HA. Hormones, mammary growth, and lactation: A 41-year perspective. *J Dairy Sci.* 2000; 83:874-84.

Turkington RW, Hill RL. Lactose synthetase: Progesterone inhibition of the induction of α-lactalbumin. *Science.* 1969; 163(3874):1458-60.

Tyson JE, Khojandi M, Huth J, Andreassen B. The influence of prolactin secretion on human lactation. *J Clin Endocrinol Metab.* 1975; 40(5):764-73.

US National Library of Medicine. Recombinant human prolactin for lactation induction in adoptive mothers (NCT00181649). 2006a. [Cited 2007 14 June]. Available from: http://clinicaltrials.gov/ct/show/NCT00181649?order=1.

US National Library of Medicine. Recombinant human prolactin for lactation induction in mothers of premature infants (NCT0018160). 2006b. [Cited 2007 14 June]. Available from: http://clinicaltrials.gov/ct/show/NCT00181610?order=1.

US National Library of Medicine. Recombinant human prolactin for lactation induction in prolactin deficient mothers (NCT00181623). 2006c. [Cited 2007 14 June]. Available from: http://clinicaltrials.gov/ct/show/NCT00181623?order=1.

Whittle WL, Patel FA, Alfaidy N, Holloway AC, Fraser M, Gyomorey S, *et al.* Glucocorticoid regulation of human and ovine parturition: The relationship between fetal hypothalamic-pituitary-adrenal axis activation and intrauterine prostaglandin production. *Biol Reprod.* 2001; 64:1019-32.

Wilde CJ, Addey CV, Boddy LM, Peaker M. Autocrine regulation of milk secretion by a protein in milk. *Biochem J.* 1995; 305(Pt 1):51-58.

Wilde CJ, Addey CV, Bryson JM, Finch LM, Knight CH, Peaker M. Autocrine regulation of milk secretion. *Biochem Soc Symposia.* 1998; 63:81-90.

Wilde CJ, Calvert DT, Daly A, Peaker M. The effect of goat milk fractions on synthesis of milk constituents by rabbit mammary explants and on milk yield in vivo. Evidence for autocrine control of milk secretion. *Biochem J.* 1987; 242(1):285-88.

Wilde CJ, Henderson AJ, Knight CH, Blatchford DR, Faulkner A, Vernon RG. Effects of long-term thrice-daily milking on mammary enzyme activity, cell population and milk yield in the goat. *J Anim Sci.* 1987; 64(2):533-39.

Wilde CJ, Peaker M. Autocrine control in milk secretion. A review. *J Agric Sci.* 1990; 114:235-38.

Young I. The comparative physiology of parturition in mammals. In: Smith R (ed.). *The endocrinology of parturition.* London: Karger; 2001:86-104.

Zoubiane GS, Valentijn A, Lowe ET, Akhtar N, Bagley S, Gilmore AP, *et al.* A role for the cytoskeleton in prolactin-dependent mammary epithelial cell differentiation. *J Cell Sci.* 2003; 117(2):271-80.

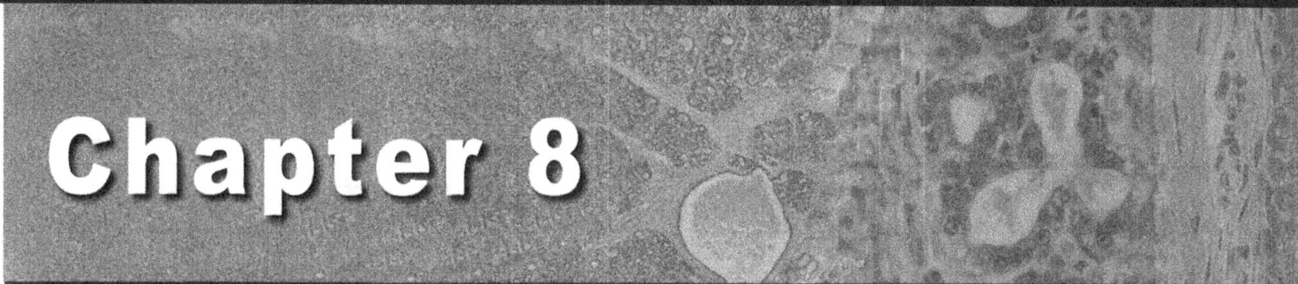

Chapter 8

Molecular Aspects of Mammary Gland Development

Thomas Martin and Charles Czank

INTRODUCTION

During the past 100 years, extensive efforts have been made to understand the structural and functional development of the mammary gland. Progress in the understanding of the molecular biochemistry and physiology of the mammary gland was greatly assisted by the realization that milk was synthesized in the mammary gland from substances that were removed from the arterial blood supply to the gland. The second major advance is based on studies by Ely and Petersen (1941) correctly identifying that milk ejection was the removal of stored milk from the mammary gland and that it was not the result of rapid synthesis of milk. Subsequent biochemical studies identified the substrates removed from the blood for the synthesis of milk (Linzell, 1974) and the intracellular metabolic pathways, enzymes, and intermediate metabolites (Mepham, 1983) leading to the synthesis of the proteins, fats, and carbohydrates in milk. Furthermore, hormones involved in the growth and functional development of the mammary gland have been identified (Cowie *et al.*, 1980).

Progress in the understanding of the molecular biochemistry and physiology of the mammary gland was greatly assisted by the realization that milk was synthesized in the mammary gland from substances that were removed from the arterial blood supply to the gland. It was revealed that a number of these genes encode for components which are part of intricate intracellular signaling pathways. The gradual elucidation, an ongoing process, revealed complex interactions of signaling molecules with epigenetic factors that interact at the level of gene expression to fine tune the readout of the genetic information and ultimately are responsible for the physiological outcome of lactation in each individual. The majority of knowledge in this field has arisen from studies performed on small animal models and *in vitro* studies of human mammary epithelial carcinomas, where such pathways are usually malfunctioning. Given these factors, there are still considerable gaps in the understanding of intracellular signaling during normal human mammary development.

The basic features of this area of research are identification of the cell surface and intracellular receptors for extracellular signals (mostly hormones, autocrine and paracrine factors), the chain of reactions that convey the signal to a site of action (mostly a gene(s) or regulation of another signaling pathway) and a class of compounds that regulate gene expression (e.g., transcription factors) depending upon modification to their structures and the nature of their binding to the genetic material (**Table 1**).

Unfortunately, the language describing these mechanisms is generally coded and not necessarily intuitive. This can easily confuse both the unacquainted reader as well as the experienced molecular biologist. To date, the genes and gene products involved in intracellular signaling in mammary development have not been systemized in the same manner as, for example, the nomenclature for enzymes. In particular,

Table 1. List of Known Proteins and Genes Involved in Intracellular Signaling during Particular Stages of Mammary Development

Abbreviation	Full Name	Stage of Mammary Development	References
Hormone/Ligand			
Nrg3	Neuregelin 3	Embryonic	Zhang *et al.*, 1997
PTHrP	Parathyroid related peptide	Embryonic	Jüppner *et al.*, 1991; Lanske *et al.*, 1996; Dunbar *et al.*, 1999; Foley *et al.*, 2001
FGF10	Follicular growth factor 10	Embryonic	Mailleux *et al.*, 2002; Takeuchi *et al.*, 2003; Eblaghie *et al.*, 2004
RANKL(TNFS11)	Receptor Activator of Nuclear Factor Kappa	Pregnancy	Yasuda et al., 1998; Hsu *et al.*, 1999; Cao et al., 2001
IGF-I	Insulin-like growth factor I	Involution	Tonner *et al.*, 1995; Hadsell *et al.*, 1996; Moorehead *et al.*, 2001; Tonner *et al.*, 2002
IGF-II	Insulin-like growth factor II	Involution	
PRL	Prolactin	Pregnancy/Lactation	Ormandy *et al.*, 1997; Freeman *et al.*, 2000; Gallego *et al.*, 2001; Kelly *et al.*, 2002
Kinases			
Erbb4	Erb-erythroblastic	Embryonic	Anton *et al.*, 2004; Gordon-Thomson *et al.*, 2005; Ghashghaei *et al.*, 2006
PI3K	Phosphotidylinositol 3 kinase	Involution	Moorehead *et al.*, 2001; Schwertfeger *et al.*, 2001; Ackler *et al.*, 2002
Jak2	Janus Kinase 2	Pregnancy	See Stat 5 refs
PKB (Akt)	Protein Kinase B	Involution	Moorehead *et al.*, 2001
Transcription Factor			
Tbx3	T-box 3	Embryonic	Bamshad *et al.*, 1997; Davenport *et al.*, 2003; Eblaghie *et al.*, 2004; Jerome-Majewska *et al.*, 2005
WNT10	Wingless-type protein	Embryonic	Akiyama, 2000; Durmowicz *et al.*, 2002; Miller, 2002; Turashvili *et al.*, 2006
Lef1	Lymphoid enhancer-binding factor 1	Embryonic	Boras-Granic *et al.*, 2006
Stat 5	Signal transducer and activator of transcription 5	Pregnancy/Lactation	Liu *et al.*, 1997; Gallego *et al.*, 2001; Miyoshi *et al.*, 2001
Stat 3	Signal transducer and activator of transcription 3	Involution	Chapman *et al.*, 1999; Humphreys *et al.*, 2002; Kritikou *et al.*, 2003
SRC-1	Steroid receptor coactivator 1	Puberty	Xu *et al.*, 1998; Xu *et al.*, 2000; Liao *et al.*, 2002; Xu & Li, 2003
SRC-2 (GRIP1)	Steroid receptor coactivator 2	Puberty	
SRC-3 (p/CIP)	Steroid receptor coactivator 3	Puberty	
Msx1	MSH homeobox homolog 1	Embryonic/Puberty	Friedmann & Daniel, 1996; Phippard *et al.*, 1996; Satoh *et al.*, 2004; Satoh *et al.*, 2007
Msx2	MSH homeobox homolog 2	Embryonic/Puberty	
c/EBPβ	CCAAT enhancer binding protein	Pregnancy	Robinson *et al.*, 1998; Seagroves *et al.*, 1998; Grimm & Rosen, 2003
Receptor			
PTHR1	Parathyroid receptor 1	Embryonic	Lanske *et al.*, 1996
PRLR	Prolactin receptor	Pregnancy/Lactation	Horseman *et al.*, 1997; Ormandy *et al.*, 1997; Freeman *et al.*, 2000; Gallego *et al.*, 2001; Kelly *et al.*, 2002
RANK	Tumor necrosis factor receptor superfamily	Pregnancy	Yasuda *et al.*, 1998; Hsu *et al.*, 1999; Cao *et al.*, 2001
Others			
Eda	Ectodysplasin A	Embryonic	Laurikkala *et al.*, 2001; Durmowicz *et al.*, 2002
Id2	Inhibitor of DNA binding 2	Pregnancy	Mori *et al.*, 2000
Cyclin D1	Cyclin D1	Pregnancy	Fantl *et al.*, 1995; Sicinski *et al.*, 1995; Hu *et al.*, 2001; Muraoka *et al.*, 2001

the method for labeling genes and proteins has not been standardized like it has for other organisms, such as *Arabidopsis thaliana*. For the purpose of this chapter, proteins will be referred to in capitals (e.g., WNT), genes with a capital followed by lower case (e.g., Wnt), and mutants in lower case (e.g., ska); however, it is important that the reader is aware that this nomenclature varies throughout the literature. It is the authors' intent that this chapter focus on the current knowledge in the field of intracellular signaling during mammary development. For an overview on the functional aspects of lactation and specifically the hormonal control of the lactation cycle, refer to chapter 7.

MAMMARY GLAND DEVELOPMENT – A STRUCTURAL OVERVIEW

Based on recent research, it is now clear that the mammary gland has its evolutionary origin in skin glands (Oftedal, 2002). For example, molecular studies have revealed that mammary gland development shares a great number of signaling and regulatory factors with the development of other skin appendages, such as hair, whiskers, feathers, and teeth (Oftedal, 2002; Hennighausen & Robinson, 2005). Apart from identifying the same set of developmental factors, it was shown in numerous experiments that manipulation of these factors by molecular, biochemical, or genetic means often impacts formation and function of several epidermal appendages. A further developmental feature shared by the mammary gland and other skin appendages is reciprocal signaling as a way of communication between epidermal and mesenchymal cells (Robinson *et al.*, 1999; Hennighausen & Robinson, 2001). Despite the many shared factors, individual developmental, structural, and functional features of the various skin appendages strongly imply appendage specific molecular events, most likely at the level of individual cell types and at the end of molecular signaling and response events.

Molecular analysis has further led to the hypothesis that the milk gland and lactation originated from the innate immune system. This hypothesis is supported by common regulatory molecules acting during development of the mammary gland, as well as in inflammatory responses, e.g., tissue damage (Vorbach *et al.*, 2006).

The process of mammary gland development can be divided into six distinct stages (**Figure 1**): embryonic stage, prepubescent stage, pubescent stage, pregnancy, lactation, and involution. However, it has to be kept in mind that mammary gland development is mostly a continuous process which is initiated during early embryogenesis in both female and male embryos. During late embryogenesis, male and female specific hormones cause the gland either to arrest and partially deteriorate, as is seen in male embryos, or to continue along the developmental path until birth when development comes to an arrest. The hormones involved in embryonic development act via receptor proteins by initiating intracellular signaling events which ultimately either lead to the production of other intra- or intercellular signaling molecules or changes in cell metabolism leading to structural or functional changes of the cell. In any case, the changes initiated occur at either the protein and/or gene level.

During prepubescent life, the gland is developmentally quiescent, but continues to grow with the animal. There are indications that estrogen and its receptor are required for growth of the epithelium during this period (Wiesen *et al.*, 1999; Bocchinfuso *et al.*, 2000). Growth continues until hormones trigger further development, resulting in rapid ductal elongation and side branching with the onset of puberty. During puberty, ovarian sex hormones initiate major changes in the structure and size of the female mammary tissue, inducing and promoting changes such as growth, extension, and branching of the mammary duct system. Secondary and tertiary ducts develop from the primary ducts. This duct system penetrates the entire fat pad in the mature animal at around ten weeks of age. Sequential changes in estrogen and progesterone levels during each estrous cycle induce continual structural changes in the mammary tissue. With each cycle, a peak in cell proliferation leads to formation of small ductal side branches during the late proestrus phase. These small branches degenerate by apoptotic cell death in the diestrus phase until new growth is initiated with the next cycle. This process continues within each menstrual cycle until pregnancy.

Throughout pregnancy, the mammary gland undergoes massive developmental changes in order to prepare for its secretory role during lactation. Characteristic for this developmental stage is a massive proliferation and differentiation of the alveolar epithelium triggered by hormones with a prominent role played by the cytokine hormone, prolactin (PRL).

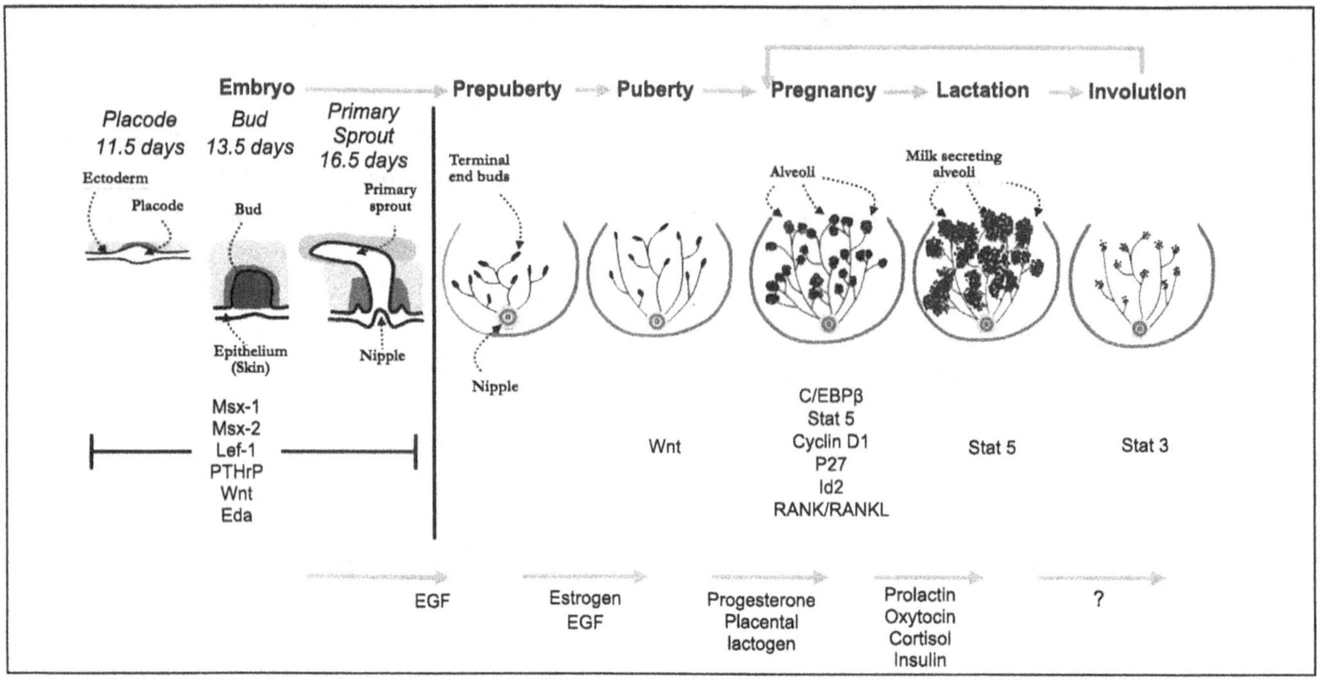

Figure 1. Schematic diagram illustrating the major stages of mammary development, including the lactation cycle. The specific genes involved in each stage are shown, as well as the hormones required for the transition between stages and maintenance of each mammary development stage. During embrogenesis, the mammary gland develops from a small placode within the ectoderm (11.5 days) into a mammary epithelial bud (blue) that forms within the dermal mesencyme (intermediate gray, at 13.5 days). Cell proliferation at the base of the bud results in the formation of an elongated duct, known as the primary sprout (16.5 days), that grows towards the fat pad (light gray) and forms the beginnings of the mammary ductule system. The placode, bud, and primary sprout are partly surrounded by the mammary mesenchyme (dark gray), which contributes to the formation of the nipple. Epidermal growth factor (EGF) controls mammary growth up until and during puberty. Estrogen and EGF promote ductule elongation and branching. During pregnancy and lactation, progesterone, placental lactogen, prolactin, oxytocin, cortisol, and insulin regulate secretory differentiation, secretory and synthesis activation, and actual secretion and synthesis of milk (chapter 7). General mammary growth is controlled by the wnt gene during puberty, mass alveolar proliferation during pregnancy by C/EBPβ, Stat5, RANKL, cyclin D1, P27 and Id2, while maintenance of lactation is regulated by prolactin via stat5. Involution is characterized by apoptosis and tissue remodeling associated with stat3, bax, and bcl-x. Adapted from Henninghausen & Robinson (2001) and Robinson (2004).

Continuing cell proliferation in ducts and alveoli will last into early lactation, leading to mammary fat pads filled with a dense epithelial compartment. In this compartment, alveolar lobules are lined with secretory epithelial cells which at term actively secrete milk proteins and lipid droplets into the luminal space. Synthesis of milk proteins begins at mid gestation. WDMN1 is one of the first such proteins expressed, followed by β–casein, with appearance of Whey acidic protein and α-lactalbumin shortly before birth (Robinson *et al.*, 1995).

After lactation, the mammary gland undergoes massive restructuring to revert to a near pre-pregnancy state. This restructuring and remodeling of the mammary tissue involves a number of factors associated with organized cell death (apoptosis).

EMBRYONIC DEVELOPMENT

The progression of mammary gland development follows similar patterns in all mammals. Best understood so far is the milk gland development in mice, which serves as a model system and as the basis for discussion of molecular events presented here (Veltmaat *et al.*, 2003). Embryonic development of the mammary gland is a two step process (Sakakura, 1987). The first step involves the manifestation of two milk lines (mammary ridges) during embryonic life and ends with bud-like invaginations of epidermal cells into the underlying mesenchyme at characteristic locations along the milk line. Milk lines consist of bands of raised epidermal tissue appearing on both sides of the ventral midline. Between embryonic days 10 and 11, cells collect at centers of concentration within each milk line, forming small lens-shaped structures called placodes. Placodes are areas of thickening in the embryonic epithelial layer, slightly protruding from the body wall. They can be considered as a basal unit of ectodermal organogenesis. Placodes give rise to the mammary anlagen between embryonic day 11.5 and 13.5 by first growing into bulb-shaped epithelial buds that invaginate the dermal mesenchyme (Turner & Gomez, 1933; Veltmaat *et al.*, 2003). In mice, five pairs of mammary buds (Mb1 anterior to Mb5 posterior) form along the two milk lines (Turner & Gomez, 1933). Location of the buds depends on the species, they are either found in the thoracic region in primates, in the inguinal area in ungulates, or along the entire length of the trunk in rodents and pigs.

The primary duct is formed during the second step. On day 15 of embryonic development, rapid epithelial cell development at the bud tip is initiated, leading to outgrowth of a primary epithelial sprout or mammary cord that grows towards the fat pad. The epithelial sprout elongates and bifurcates creating a small ductal tree that is connected to the skin. Later, the cord opens at the skin end forming the nipple. The other end of the chord branches out and grows into the mammary fat pad where ten to fifteen embryonic, secondary ducts are formed. The nipple sheath forms as a skin modification in the immediate vicinity of the duct. Here development of the mammary tissue arrests until puberty (Veltmaat *et al.*, 2003).

Interestingly, development of the mammary tissue in male mice embryos is identical to that in female embryos until days 13-15 of gestation. At this time, a change in hormones takes place in male embryos and testosterone prevents further development of mammary glands. Instead, the mesenchyme around the center of the mammary bud condenses and causes the cells of the epithelial cord to undergo apoptosis. As a result, the mammary gland in male embryos is disconnected from the skin and does not extend to the surface. The involvement of testosterone in the decision-making process towards cell death was shown by studying a developmental mutation in mice, which also exists in humans, called androgen insensitivity syndrome. This mutation causes the loss of a functional testosterone receptor and individuals are unable to respond to testosterone. As one consequence, individuals with such mutation develop female-type breasts. These experiments further showed that the target for testosterone is the mesenchyme, not the epithelium (Kratochwil, 1971; Kratochwil & Schwartz, 1976).

MOLECULAR ASPECTS OF EMBRYONIC MAMMARY DEVELOPMENT

Although the morphological and histological aspects of mouse mammary gland formation during embryonic development are very well described, this is not matched by descriptions on the molecular level. However, good progress was made in recent times employing approaches such as mutant analysis, overexpression of genes in stable and transient systems, promoter/reporter gene analysis, and tissue transplantation to name a few (Howard & Ashworth, 2006; Robinson, 2004; Hennighausen & Robinson, 2001; Hennighausen & Robinson, 2005). Further important data are obtained from research into mammary tumor formation. The following section overviews some of the key genes and molecular players involved in embryonic mammary gland formation. These can be basically classified into (a) hormones and messenger molecules which transfer information between cells, (b) receptors receiving the signaling molecules on the outside or inside of the cell and initiating a signaling event inside the cell, (c) modifying proteins, such as protein kinases, which are part of intracellular signaling cascades, and (d) transcriptional regulators which can either inhibit or promote expression of target genes (**Table 1**).

It was shown that the initial stages of embryonic mammary development during gestation are independent of systemic signals, but require reciprocal signaling between the epithelium and the mesenchyme (Kratochwil, 1971; Kratochwil & Schwartz, 1976; Howard & Ashworth, 2006). These signaling events beginning with mesenchymal signals appear to cause local migration of pluripotent epidermal cells along specific lineages thereby forming the mammary anlage (Propper, 1978; Fuchs & Raghavan, 2002; Pispa & Thesleff, 2003).

Formation of the mammary gland in the embryo depends on signaling molecules, such as Neuregulin growth factor 3, wingless-type proteins, parathyroid hormone-related protein and its receptor PTHR1, fibroblast growth factors, their receptors (e.g., Erbb), and transcription factor/regulators, such as the T-box transcriptional regulator. A model has emerged whereby complex interactions of these factors and signaling pathways initiate, maintain, and further the formation and development of the mammary gland during embryonic development until birth, when further development comes to a resting stage. The following section gives a brief outline of our current knowledge of these factors, summarizing some of the experimental evidence for their involvement in embryonic mammary gland development and exemplifying potential interactions between them.

The First Step of Embryonic Mammary Gland Development

As outlined above, the first step in mammary gland development begins with the manifestation of two milk lines (mammary ridges) leading up to the formation of bud-like invaginations of epidermal cells into the underlying mesenchyme. Early molecular markers for this stage of mammary gland development include genes encoding for wingless type proteins, T-box transcriptional regulator, fibroblast growth factors, and neuregulin 3. It can be assumed that these genes or their gene products are involved in early mammary gland development and that potential interactions between at least some of these factors contribute to gland initiation and the early stages of its formation.

The wingless-type (wnt) signaling pathway is central in embryonic mammary gland development (Miller, 2002). The key proteins involved in this pathway are Wingless-type (Wnt) proteins, a class of cysteine-rich, secreted glycoproteins which bind to co-receptors on the surface of target cells. Wnts are encoded by gene families which in mammals consist of approximately 20 members. The genes are highly conserved in evolution and depending on the activated signaling pathway fall into two classes, classical Wnts or non-classical Wnts. Classical Wnts act via the so called canonical or Wnt/β-catenin pathway, while non-classical Wnts act by one of several non-canonical pathways (Akiyama, 2000; Miller, 2002; Turashvili *et al.*, 2006). The best studied 'canonical' pathway involves binding of Wnt to a member of the seven transmembrane domains Frizzled (FZ) receptor family. The canonical pathway furthermore requires action of co-receptors belonging to the single transmembrane domain lipoprotein receptor-related protein (LRP) family. In the canonical signaling pathway, binding of WNT to its receptor/co-receptor leads to inactivation of proteins that degrade cytoplasmic β-catenin. As a result, β-catenin accumulates in the cytoplasm, translocates to the nucleus, and forms active transcriptional complexes with members of the LEF/TCF transcription factor family (Huelsken & Birchmeier, 2001). Non-canonical WNT pathways require 'frizzled' receptors, but are independent of other typical canonical factors (Niehrs, 2001).

In general, action of WNT proteins regulates cell fate decisions, cell proliferation, morphology, migration, apoptosis, differentiation, and self-renewal of stem cells (Akiyama, 2000; Miller, 2002). During embryonic mammary gland development, WNT proteins are involved in the dorso-ventricular development of the mesoderm. In mammary gland development, Wnts are critical for the induction of the gland. This was elegantly demonstrated in mice ectopically expressing the secreted Wnt antagonist Dickkopf1 (DKK1, D47). DKK1 acts rapidly by removing LRP from the plasma membrane (Zorn, 2001; Mao *et al.*, 2002). Mice expressing this inhibitor failed to produce mammary buds in developing epithelia, demonstrating activity of the Wnt/canonical pathway during mammary gland development (Andl *et al.*, 2002; Chu *et al.*, 2004).

Based on observations in rabbit embryos, it was suggested that placodes form as a result of migration and accumulation of motile cells at defined locations along the mammary lines (Propper, 1978). Interestingly, Wnt expression patterns appear to reflect such migration. During embryonic development at around embryonic day 11.25, wnt6, wnt10a, and wnt10b start to be expressed in the surface ectoderm, preceding the appearance of mammary placodes. Initially, expression is found along a concise line that defines the border between the dorsal and the ventral body walls. This expression pattern changes within 1.5 days, when expression of these genes becomes restricted to the placodes, possibly reflecting migration of Wnt-expressing cells during placode formation (Veltmaat *et al.*, 2004).

The ectodysplasin A (Eda) gene is one of the known targets of Wnt signaling during embryonic mammary gland development. The Eda gene product is critical for interaction between the embryonic ectoderm and mesoderm cell layers (Mikkola & Thesleff, 2003; Pispa & Thesleff, 2003). Ectoderm-mesoderm interactions are essential for the formation of several structures that arise from the ectoderm, including the skin, hair, nails, teeth, and sweat glands. Eda and its cell surface receptor (Edar) are members of the tumor necrosis factor (TNF) superfamily. Many TNF family members play a role in host defence and immune response and often mediate cell death by apoptosis or cell survival. However, the mouse Eda gene does not seem to be involved in such events. Instead, this Eda gene appears to promote cell adhesion to the extracellular matrix, which is consistent with a role of this protein in epithelial-mesenchymal interactions (Mikkola *et al.*, 1999). Eda is required for the initiation, morphogenesis, and differentiation of several ectodermally-derived organs in humans and mice and is an early and necessary signal required for placode formation (Mikkola & Thesleff, 2003; Pispa & Thesleff, 2003). The developmental impact of Eda was demonstrated by ectopic expression of the Eda gene under the control of the keratin 14 promoter. Mice expressing this construct developed supernumerary nipples along the presumptive milk line (Mustonen *et al.*, 2003).

The Eda gene is expressed in the ectoderm (Laurikkala *et al.*, 2001; Laurikkala *et al.*, 2002) and may be under control of the canonical pathway via the lymphocyte enhancer factor 1 (Lef-1). This transcription factor was found to specifically bind to the Eda promoter thereby increasing Eda transcription (Durmowicz *et al.*, 2002).

The lymphocyte enhancer factor 1 (Lef1) belongs to a class of TCF/LEF transcription factors which mediate Wnt signals, further demonstrating the relationship between Eda and Wnt signaling pathways. Lef-1 is initially expressed in the area of placode formation from embryonic day 11.5 onwards. However, during later development, Lef-1 expression is also found in the mesenchyme. Lef1 plays a role in early specification of placodes 2 and 3 and in progression of placode development 1, 4, and 5 (Boras-Granic *et al.*, 2006). Deletions within the Lef1 gene do not affect early placode development, but lead to an arrest at the early bud stage (van Genderen *et al.*, 1994). It was shown that induction of Lef1 requires paracrine signals from the mammary epithelium involving the parathyroid hormone-related protein (PTHrP) and its receptor PTHR1. Lef1 induction by PTHrP is possibly the way cells in the developing gland becomes susceptible to Wnt signaling (van Genderen *et al.*, 1994).

The T-box transcriptional regulator 3 (Tbx3) is a transcriptional repressor belonging to the family of T-box transcriptional regulators (Papaioannou, 2001; Mailleux *et al.*, 2002). Tbx proteins are characterized by a highly conserved DNA-binding domain, called the T-domain, that binds specific sequences in the promoters of target genes (Bollag *et al.*, 1994). Crystal structure analysis of TBX3 complexed with DNA suggests that TBX3 binds these target sequences as a monomer (Coll *et al.*, 2002). It acts as a transcriptional repressor and may negatively regulate cell cycle control genes (He *et al.*, 1999; Carlson *et al.*, 2001). Recently, it was demonstrated that Tbx3 promotes growth of mammary epithelial cells via repression of p19ARF, also known as cyclin-dependent kinase inhibitor 2A (CDKN2A) (Platonova *et al.*, 2007).

The developmental impact of Tbx3 is best known by a mutation in the human TBX3 gene, causing the human disorder Ulmar-Mammary Syndrome, a disruption of apocrine gland and limb development, sometimes also leading to a complete lack of mammary glands (Bamshad *et al.*, 1997). Expression of Tbx3 is required for mammary bud initiation, as demonstrated by the lack of such initiation in Tbx3 knockout mice. Furthermore, tbx3 homozygous knock-out mutations are lethal (Davenport *et al.*, 2003).

Before formation of the mammary anlagen, Tbx3 expression is localized in the mesenchyme along the presumptive mammary line, but shifts to the epithelial component once the anlagen become visible (Eblaghie *et al.*, 2004; Jerome-Majewska *et al.*, 2005). Tbx3 is one of the earliest expressed genes in developing mammary buds. Its expression precedes the expression of other genes known to be involved in mammary bud formation, such as Lef1 (Eblaghie *et al.*, 2004). During limb initiation, Tbx3 is known to act in concert with Wnt and fibroblast growth factor (FGF) signals in both mesenchyme and ectoderm (Takeuchi *et al.*, 2003). A similar interaction was assumed for mammary gland development. First reports showed that Tbx3 activity occurs upstream of both Wnt and FGF signaling in mammary gland initiation (Eblaghie *et al.*, 2004). This was supported by the lack of Lef1 and Wnt10b expression in Tbx3 knockout mice (Davenport *et al.*, 2003). However, Wnt and FGF signaling appear to be involved in induction and/or maintenance of Tbx3 expression (Eblaghie *et al.*, 2004). Furthermore, ectopic expression of the Wnt inhibitor, Dkk1, blocks localized epithelial expression of Tbx3. Thus, it is likely that WNT signaling lies both upstream and downstream of Tbx3 in mammary placode development (Chu *et al.*, 2004).

The fibroblast growth factor (FGF) family comprises at least 22 members with roles in multiple developmental processes (Ornitz & Itoh, 2001). FGF receptors are encoded by four genes, Fgfr1 to Fgfr4 which, due to alternative splicing of the messenger RNA, give rise to at least seven receptor protein isoforms (Ornitz *et al.*, 1996). The receptor isoform, FGFR2b, is mainly found in epithelia and binds four of the primarily mesenchymal expressed FGFs: FGF1, FGF3, FGF7, and FGF10. FGF10 has been associated with mesenchymal-epithelial interactions, as they occur during branching morphogenesis (Mailleux *et al.*, 2002). FGF10 signaling through the receptor FGFR2b is required for mammary bud initiation with the exception of mammary bud 4, which can form in the absence of either the ligand or its receptor (Mailleux *et al.*, 2002). Interestingly, in the receptor null mutant, the bud is formed and regresses by apoptosis, while in FGF10-deficient embryos, it is maintained, but fails to undergo branching. This difference in phenotype could be due to expression of another FGF (FGF7) during early stages of embryonic development, possibly compensating for a loss of FGF10. FGF signaling through another FGF receptor (FGFR1) has been implicated in the induction of Tbx3 expression (Eblaghie et al., 2004).

Is the Neuregulin Dependent Signaling Pathway Bringing it all Together?

A better understanding of the events associated with very early mammary gland development came from studies of the scaramanga (ska) mutation in mice. This mutation leads to defects in shape, size, and position of the mammary anlagen, failure of bud 3 formation, and development of ectopic mammary buds adjacent to bud 4. Thus, the ska mutation disturbs the inductive effects leading to normal morphology of the mammary bud (Howard & Gusterson, 2000; Howard & Ashworth, 2006). The gene affected in the ska mutation encodes for the growth factor, Neuregulin3 (Nrg3) (Howard *et al.*, 2005). Nrg3 binds to the Erbb4 tyrosine kinase receptor (**Figure 2**) (Zhang *et al.*, 1997) and thereby initiates signaling events which trigger cell proliferation and terminal differentiation of the mammary gland (Zhang *et al.*, 1997; Sartor *et al.*, 2001; Tidcombe *et al.*, 2003). Based on the ability of Erbb4 to modulate cell migration in a number of systems (Luo & Miller, 2000; Anton *et al.*, 2004; Gambarotta *et al.*, 2004; Gordon-Thomson *et al.*, 2005; Ghashghaei *et al.*, 2006) and in analogy to the ability of another Erbb4 ligand, Nrg1, to induce migration of breast cancer and melanoma cells (Luo & Miller, 2000; Gordon-Thomson *et al.*, 2005), it was proposed that Nrg3/Erbb4 interaction controls migration of mammary epithelial precursor cells during formation of the anlagen (Howard & Ashworth, 2006).

The suggestion that Nrg3 acts as a specification signal for mammary glands in mice (Howard *et al.*, 2005) is further strongly supported by observations showing that mammary anlagen appear along the mammary line at sites where Nrg3 and Erbb4 expression is co-localized. The appearance of mammary anlagen additionally requires expression of other genes involved in mammary gland development, such as FGF10, Wnt, and Tbx3. In the embryonic mesenchyme, such co-localized expression with Nrg3 occurs shortly before the determination of the embryonic ectoderm to develop into mammary epithelial tissue (Howard *et al.*, 2005). Furthermore, ectopic mammary placodes and expression of the early mammary bud marker, Lef1, can be artificially induced in mesenchyme cells by the addition of recombinant NRG3. However, this induction requires that the mesenchyme cells express other embryonic mammary markers, such as FGF10, Tbx3, and Wnts (Howard *et al.*, 2005).

A model of mammary anlagen formation appears to crystallize in which the various factors form complex interactive networks (**Figure 2**) (Howard & Ashworth, 2006). Simplified, this model suggests that the inductive mammary line mesenchyme expressing Tbx3, FGF10, and Nrg3 initiate mammary gland development when combined with epithelia expressing Fgfr2B and Erbb receptors. It is still unknown how signals from FGF10 and Tbx3 are transmitted from the lateral plate mesoderm to the precursor epithelial population. Based on expression patterns and localization of Nrg3 expression, it was suggested that Nrg3 may mediate such signals downstream of FGF10 and Tbx3 to the overlying epithelia expressing Wnt genes. This could initiate local aggregation of epithelial cells leading to formation of the mammary anlagen (Howard & Ashworth, 2006).

This is certainly a simplified view of the complex interactions occurring during mammary anlagen formation. As discussed above, the effects of deficiencies on mammary anlage and ductal development is well established for some genes, such as FGF10, Lef1, and Tbx3. However, it is far from understandable how these and other genes contribute to the formation of

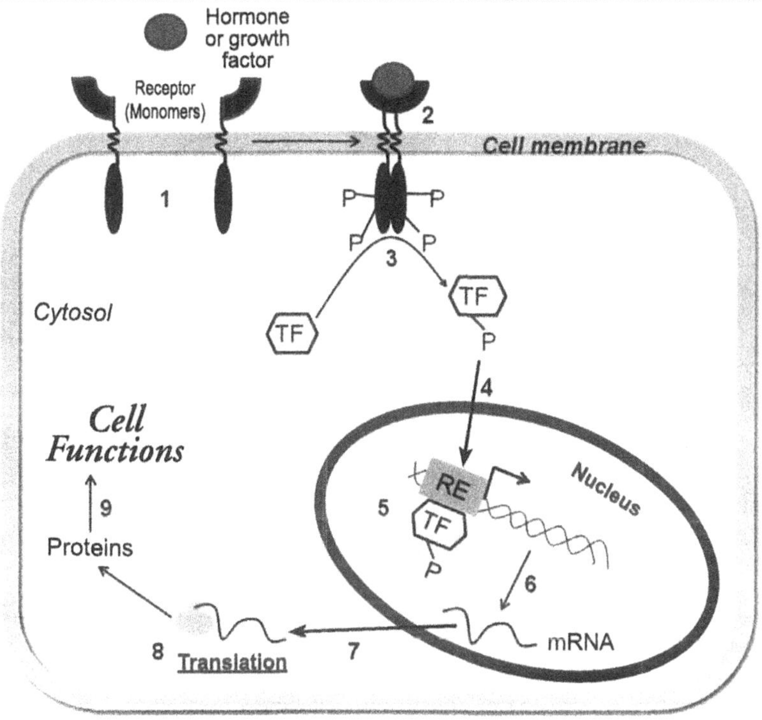

Figure 2. Schematic diagram of tyrosine kinase receptor function. Tyrosine kinase receptors consist (1) of an extracellular hormone binding domain, a transmembrane domain anchoring the receptor in the cell membrane, and an intracellular protein kinase domain, which when activated can phosphorylate tyrosine amino acid residues in its target proteins. Binding of hormones (2) and growth factors to such receptors will firstly initiate activation of the kinase domain leading to autophosphorylation of the receptor molecule (3) thereby stabilizing its active state. Secondly, the activated kinase domain will phosphorylate intracellular target proteins, such as other protein kinases and/or transcriptional factors (TF) (3). Activated transcription regulators localize to the nucleus (4) and bind to regulatory elements (5) within promoter regions (gene switches) finally leading to changes in gene expression (6-8). These changes can consist of reduced expression caused by transcriptional inhibitors or promotion of gene expression via transcriptional activators. Alterations in gene expression may produce other signaling molecules, sensitize the cell to new signals, or change the cells metabolic state, proliferation, or differentiation state (9).

specific anlagen along the body axis. It also has to be kept in mind that formation of individual placodes is likely to require individual expression patterns or combinations of the genes and factors described in **Figure 3**.

The Second Step of Embryonic Mammary Gland Development

This part of mammary gland development begins with the formation of the primary duct and ends with formation of the secondary ducts and the nipple. This developmental stage requires a different set of regulatory proteins, including the parathyroid hormone-related protein and Msx homeodomain proteins.

The parathyroid hormone-related protein PTHrP is a small peptide hormone involved in calcium homeostasis (Lanske *et al.*, 1996; Weir *et al.*, 1996). One role for PTHR1P was already discussed in the induction of Lef-1. Additionally, but not less important, this hormone is crucial for the formation of mammary ducts and the nipple. The importance of this hormone and the related signaling mechanisms can be seen in humans where a loss-of-function mutation of the PTHrP receptor (PTHR1) causes a lethal form of dwarfism with defects in endochondral bone formation and the absence of nipples and breasts (Wysolmerski *et al.*, 2001). In mammary glands of mice, expression of the hormone and its receptor are clearly separated. While the PTHrP gene is expressed in epithelial cells of the mammary bud, its G protein-coupled receptor (PTHR1) is expressed in the surrounding ventral dermal mesenchymal cells (Jüppner *et al.*, 1991; Dunbar *et al.*, 1999). Interfering with normal expression patterns causes abnormal developmental features. For example, misexpression of PTHrP in developing skin transformed the ventral dermis into mammary mesenchyme and the entire

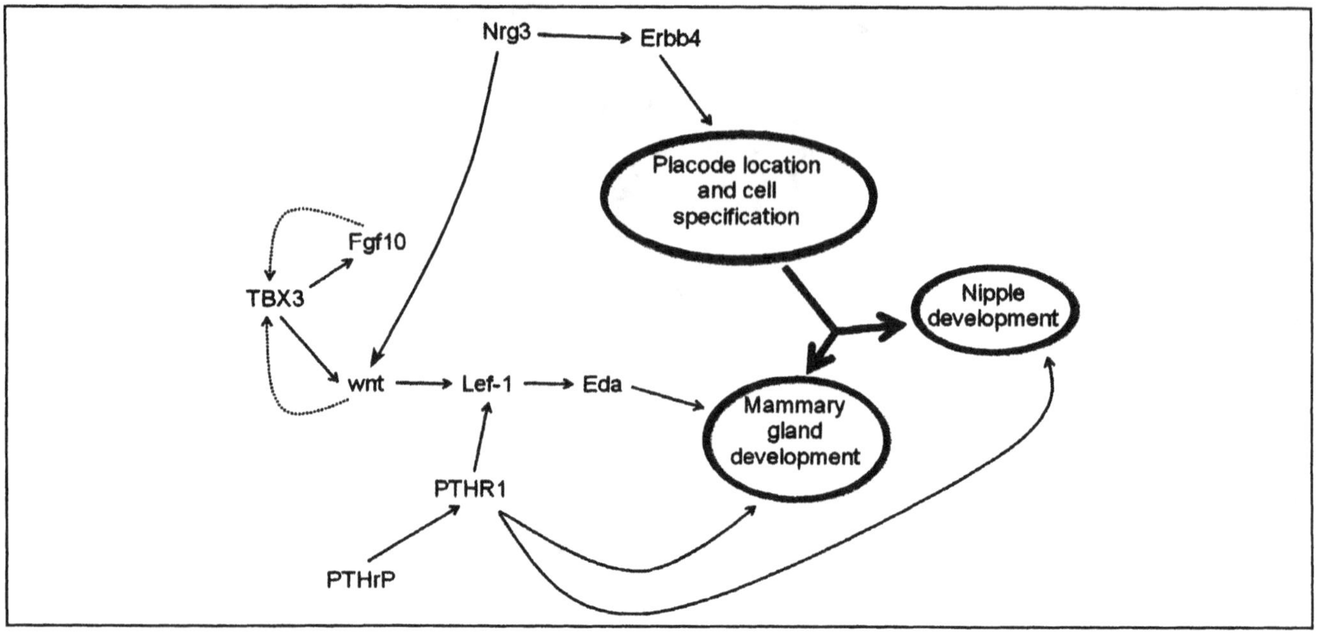

Figure 3. Simplified model of signal transduction pathways involved in early mammary gland development during embryogenesis.

ventral epidermis formed nipple skin (Foley *et al.*, 2001). Furthermore, the critical role of this protein and its receptor in mammary development is exemplified by the fact that deletion of the PTHrP or PTHR1 gene causes an arrest of mammary gland development and a failure to form mammary ducts and the nipple (Wysolmerski *et al.*, 2001). The roles of PTHrP in mammary development were confirmed by reintroducing the PTHrP transgene into PTHrP knock-out mice, thereby restoring normal development (Wysolmerski *et al.*, 2001).

A model was proposed in which PTHrP secretion from epithelial cells of the bud induces, in a paracrine manner, the surrounding mesenchymal cells to differentiate into mammary-specific mesenchyme. In turn, the mammary mesenchyme causes the mammary fate of the epithelial cells and triggers ductal morphogenesis. Additionally, the mammary mesenchyme initiates the overlying epidermis to develop into nipple skin (Foley *et al.*, 2001).

PTHrP is also involved in the events leading to apoptosis of mammary gland tissue and prevention of further mammary gland development in male embryos. Here PTHrP signaling induces the synthesis of androgen hormone receptors in the mammary mesenchyme, making cells susceptible to testosterone signaling. In male embryos, testosterone production then causes the developmental changes which, for the first time, lead to differences in male and female mammary gland development (Dunbar *et al.*, 1999; Foley *et al.*, 2001).

Other Genes and Factors Involved in Embryonic Mammary Gland Development

The complex development of the mammary gland during embryogenesis requires a great number of other genes and proteins and only a selection of the key players were discussed in this chapter. Several of the genes involved in embryonic gland development will also play roles during other stages of mammary gland development. One class of genes with a large impact on the morphological development of a variety of organs are the homeobox genes. Each organ expresses a specific set of homeobox genes which will act in combination to regulate aspects of the organ's development. During embryo development, such factors are involved in specifying cell identity and positioning. Expression of homeobox genes is often found in sites where mesenchymal and epithelial tissues interact and in regions of cellular proliferation. Homeobox genes encode for proteins characterized by a conserved 61-long amino acid motif, the homeodomain. Homeobox genes can be divided into two classes, class I genes sharing a high degree of amino acid identity (>80%) in their homeodomains and class II genes with less than 50% identity (Chen & Sukumar, 2003). Based on additional conserved amino acid sequence motifs, homeodomain proteins can be further subdivided into subclasses. The Msx subclass of class II homeobox genes has great impact on mammary gland development. This gene family composed of three members, Msx-1,

Msx-2, and Msx-3, is related to the *Drosophila* (fruit fly) muscle segment homeobox gene msh (Lewis, 1978; Jowett *et al.*, 1993; Wang & Sassoon, 1995; Satoh *et al.*, 2004; Howard & Ashworth, 2006; Satoh *et al.*, 2007). In the mammary gland, only Msx-1 and Msx-2 expression have been reported so far (Friedmann & Daniel, 1996; Phippard *et al.*, 1996). Msx expression is found throughout mammary gland development, but appears to be stage-dependent. Glands of embryonic, neonatal, pubescent, and mature nulliparous animals express Msx mRNAs which are down-regulated during pregnancy. Expression during lactation and involution is not clear yet, as contrasting results were described by various research laboratories (Satoh *et al.*, 2004). Msx-2 transcription is found in epithelial and mesenchymal cells during fetal development. After birth, expression of this gene is restricted to mesenchymal cells neighboring the mammary ducts (Friedmann & Daniel, 1996; Phippard *et al.*, 1996). Msx-2 expression in nulliparous adult and in pregnant mice is mostly localized to the stromal cells surrounding branching ducts and those associated with secretory alveolar structures. The Msx-1 and Msx-2 genes share a high level of homology, which may suggest a degree of functional redundancy as observed in mutant analysis. While female Msx-1 null mice show no defects of mammary gland development at birth, Msx-2 null mice had abnormal gland development due to an arrest at the embryonic mammary sprout stage. Double Msx-1/Msx-2 null mice showed the strongest effect with a lack of epithelial invaginations and regression, resulting in the absence of the anlagen (Satokata & Maas, 1994; Phippard *et al.*, 1996; Satokata *et al.*, 2000). Further experiments revealed potential roles for both Msx-1 and Msx-2. Targeting Msx-1 expression to mice mammary glands caused strong inhibition of functional gland differentiation during pregnancy and decreased levels of casein through mid-pregnancy (Hu *et al.*, 2001). Thus, Msx-1 appears to be a negative regulator of functional differentiation with enhancing cellular proliferation with roles during late pregnancy and lactation. Removal of the epithelium from fat pads of prepubescent animals caused disappearance of Msx-2 expression, demonstrating a dependence of its expression on the presence of epithelial cells (Friedmann & Daniel, 1996). Transfection of a normal mouse mammary cell line with Msx-2 led to formation of ducts even under absence of a growth factor (hepatocyte growth factor, HGF) normally required for duct formation in such cells (Satoh *et al.*, 2004). Mutant analysis, expression pattern, and transfection experiments have implicated Msx-2 in branching morphogenesis. Like Msx-2, progesterone is required for tertiary branching, possibly also involving paracrine stimulation of Wnt-4 pathways (Atwood *et al.*, 2000; Brisken *et al.*, 2000), indicating a potential link of the two factors. In this context, it is interesting to note that Msx-2 expression and the progesterone receptor have a similar distribution pattern (Atwood *et al.*, 2000). Further evidence for a link between Msx-2 expression and progesterone was obtained from ovary-ectomized mice and mice with a knock-out mutation in the progesterone receptor gene. Both types of mice had very low levels of Msx-2 transcript in the mammary gland (Satoh *et al.*, 2004). However, progesterone treatment alone did not restore Msx-2 expression in ovary-ectomized mice, while estrogen treatment partially restored expression (Friedmann & Daniel, 1996; Satoh *et al.*, 2004). Full restoration of Msx-2 expression required a combination of progesterone and estrogen treatment, possibly reflecting induction of the progesterone receptor by estrogens (Haslam, 1988). Estrogen and progesterone receptors, in addition to their hormone binding activity, also play a crucial role as transcription factors. Thus, in theory, these receptors may directly impact Msx expression by modulating the expression of these genes. However, a direct interaction of these receptor/transcription factor molecules with the Msx-2 promoter is unlikely, as this promoter lacks known estrogen or progesterone receptor binding sites. However, the Msx-2 promoter contains binding sites for the Sp1 transcription factor (Satoh *et al.*, 2004). In analogy to other systems (Owen *et al.*, 1998; Qin *et al.*, 1999), Sp1 could mediate binding of the steroid hormone receptors to Msx-2 promoters thereby facilitating regulation of Msx-2 expression by these hormones.

MOLECULAR MECHANISMS LEADING TO CHANGES IN MAMMARY DEVELOPMENT DURING PUBERTY

During postnatal growth, the mammary gland grows proportionally to the body, but is developmentally quiescent until the onset of puberty. As previously mentioned, growth of the epithelium during this developmentally inactive period may involve estrogen and the estrogen receptor (Wiesen *et al.*, 1999;

Bocchinfuso *et al.*, 2000). Growth continues until ovarian sex hormones trigger further development, resulting in rapid ductal elongation and side branching with the onset of puberty. Action of these hormones leads to major changes in the structure and size of the female mammary tissue, preparing the gland further for the metabolic tasks in upcoming pregnancies and lactations. Repeated changes in progesterone and estrogen levels are reflected in cyclic changes of tissue build-up and degradation continuing until pregnancy.

The roles of Msx genes, as well as of the hormones estrogen and progesterone and their receptors were already mentioned in the previous sections of this chapter. Here we discuss in more depth the involvement of steroid sex hormones in mammary gland development. Discussion of apoptotic mechanisms will follow in the section discussing involution.

Progesterone and Estrogen Receptor Proteins

From puberty onwards, further development of the mammary gland becomes more dependent on the presence and action of systemic hormones, such as systemic steroid hormones. This is reflected in high expression of estrogen (ER) and progesterone receptor (PR) genes in the mammary gland tissue which during puberty can reach levels similar to those found in the ovary (Imagawa *et al.*, 1994). Progesterone and estrogen receptors have specific and overlapping functions during the developmental process in the mammary gland. The primary role of the steroid hormones, estrogen and progesterone, is binding to their receptor proteins. These steroid receptor proteins are, in contrast to other hormone receptors, localized in the cytosol where they interact with the hormone. Binding of steroid hormones to the receptor releases an inhibitory protein from the receptor allowing the hormone/receptor complex to enter the nucleus and bind to hormone-specific response elements within target gene promoters. This interaction may involve other co-activator proteins and transcription factors.

The mammary tissue expresses two progesterone receptor proteins, PR-A and PR-B. These belong to the nuclear receptor superfamily of transcription factors (Lydon *et al.*, 1995). Both proteins are encoded by the same gene using two distinct promoters and translation initiation at two alternative AUG translational start codons (Conneely *et al.*, 1989; Kastner *et al.*, 1990). PR-B, the longer of the two proteins is essentially a 165 amino acid N-terminal extended version of the shorter PR-A. Progesterone binding causes the formation of active progesterone receptor dimers which can be homo- (PR-A/PR-A and PR-B/PR-B) or heterodimers (PR-A/PR-B). These three dimers are likely to contribute to the diverse physiological activities of progesterone. Absence of PR-A and PR-B causes severely limited mammary gland development in mice (Lydon *et al.*, 1995). The phenotypic expression of these mutations becomes most obvious during later development when in pregnancy alveolar development does not occur as a consequence of the mutation. Isoform-specific functional analysis became possible using mice in which the translational ATG start codon used for correct PR-A expression was mutated (Mulac-Jericevic *et al.*, 2000). As these mice still express the correct PR-B isoform, it became feasible to analyze PR-B function in a PR-A null background. The PR-A mutant mice are infertile, but still respond to estrogen and progesterone stimulation by ductal branching and alveolar budding. These results indicated that PR-B alone is sufficient for ductal outgrowth, branching, and formation of alveolar lobules. Generation of a mouse line without PR-B expression confirmed functional specificities of the two receptors. Such mouse lines showed no effect on ovarian or uterine responses to progesterone compared to wild type animals, but had significantly reduced mammary ductal side branching and alveologenesis during pregnancy (Mulac-Jericevic *et al.*, 2003). Moreover this study revealed that PR-B absence causes diminished receptor activator of nuclear factor κB ligand (RANKL) signaling. (For more details on RANKL, see pregnancy section.)

The significance of the estrogen receptor, ERα, for mammary gland development was studied using ERα null mutants of mice (Bocchinfuso *et al.*, 2000). These mutants are characterized by a mammary tissue phenotype with severely reduced ductal development. The gland of such ERα null mutant mice resembled the phenotype of mice with failures in estrogen signaling. More far reaching, ERα null mutants cause reduced levels of the signaling molecule prolactin with impact on later stages of mammary development, such as pregnancy and lactational stages. Reduced prolactin levels as a consequence of a loss of ERα lead to formation of a non-functional corpus luteum (Bocchinfuso *et al.*, 2000). Furthermore, synthesis of progesterone in ERα knockout mice is insufficient to maintain pregnancies and to successfully execute mammary ductal development during pregnancy.

Investigations into the roles of estrogen and progesterone receptor function revealed hormone specific as well as overlapping roles in mammary gland development. To date, the regulatory pathways of progesterone signaling in mammary development are still poorly understood. However, as discussed earlier, it appears that cell proliferation induced by progesterone requires wnt signaling pathways and that such signaling involves a paracrine mechanism (Qin *et al.*, 1999).

Steroid Receptor Co-activators (SRCs)

Steroid hormone receptors are bifunctional. They act as hormone receptors and as transcriptional regulators. The DNA binding properties of steroid hormone receptors can be modified by so called co-activators. Several such co-activators belonging to the Steroid Receptor Co-activator (SRC) family were identified, namely SRC-1, SRC-2 (GRIP1), and SRC-3 (p/CIP) (Xu & Li, 2003).

Possible mechanisms by which these SRC's impact on steroid hormone signaling involve interaction with other transcription factors and with ligand bound nuclear receptors, interaction with common transcriptional co-ordinators, or a potential involvement in chromatin remodeling causing conformational changes of DNA. Indeed, it was demonstrated that SRCs have intrinsic acetyltransferase activity which could be involved in remodeling chromatin structure (Ratajczak, 2001; Xu & Li, 2003).

The involvement of SRC's in steroid hormone mediated mammary gland development was demonstrated by investigating SRC mutants. Deletion mutants of the SRC-1 gene are partially estrogen and progesterone resistant and mammary gland development is slightly reduced (Xu *et al.*, 1998). However, this effect may be indirect, as it could mostly be explained by insufficient steroid signaling via the ovary. SRC-3 mutants display a more severe phenotype with retarded outgrowth of mammary ducts during puberty and a decreased level of systemic estrogen (Xu *et al.*, 2000). Sexual maturation is delayed in SRC-3 mutants and may account at least partially for the ductal outgrowth defects and the general impact on female reproduction observed in such mice mutants. The SCR-3 mutant phenotype can be partially overcome by application of estrogen and progesterone, indicating a reduced sensitivity and or production of these hormones in those mutants. However, hormone application cannot completely rescue branching of the mammary epithelium, which will remain reduced compared to non-mutant controls (Xu *et al.*, 2000). Thus, reduced steroid hormone production or sensitivity in SRC-3 mutants can only explain part of the mutant phenotype. Despite some progress, investigating the involvement of SRCs in steroid hormone signaling is hindered by the functional redundancy of these co-activators. Further difficulties are associated with their overall broad impact on general sexual development, with potential indirect consequences for mammary gland development.

PREGNANCY AND LACTATION – A ROLE FOR PROLACTIN

During pregnancy, the mammary gland undergoes massive changes in order to prepare for its secretory role during lactation. The mammary ductal system grows to the full extent of the mammary fat pad until mid-pregnancy via ductal elongation and branching. Characteristic for this developmental stage is a massive proliferation and differentiation of the alveolar epithelium. The lobulo-alveolar epithelium gives rise to the secretory form at parturition and the breast synthesizes all required milk components, including milk proteins and lactogen. Development of the mammary tissue during pregnancy is triggered by hormones, such as estrogen, progesterone, placental lactogen, and/or prolactin (Lydon *et al.*, 1995; Korach *et al.*, 1996; Kelly *et al.*, 2002), with prolactin (PRL) playing a prominent role (Freeman *et al.*, 2000; Kelly *et al.*, 2002). Most of the prolactin is produced in the anterior pituitary gland, with a small local contribution by the mammary epithelium. Prolactin has important roles in maintaining the corpus luteum during early stages of pregnancy and in inducing further mammary gland development. Female mice lacking the prolactin receptor (PRLR) also lack a functional corpus luteum. A functional corpus luteum is required for secretion of the steroid hormones, estrogen and progesterone, which are required for ductal and alveolar development. Mammary development is basically completely prevented in homozygous prolactin and in prolactin receptor mice mutants (Horseman *et al.*, 1997; Ormandy *et al.*, 1997; Gallego *et al.*, 2001; Kelly *et al.*, 2002). Despite the absolute requirement of epithelial PRLR for lobulo-alveolar development, it seems that virgin ductal tissue and alveolar bud formation is independent of this receptor (Horseman *et al.*, 1997; Ormandy *et al.*, 1997; Gallego *et al.*, 2001). Presence of only one prolactin receptor gene in mice led to a failure to produce sufficient milk to guarantee survival of the offspring (Ormandy *et al.*, 1997). Furthermore, such homozygous mutations blocked proliferation and differentiation of the mammary tissue during the second half of pregnancy, indicating PRL dose dependent development of the mammary tissue. This demonstrates that the degree of epithelial cell proliferation during pregnancy and the postpartum period depends on a threshold of PRLR expression.

Between mid-pregnancy and birth, placental lactogen takes over the role of prolactin. After birth, prolactin becomes once again essential, this time for the maintenance of lactation.

Jak2 – Stat5 Signaling

The cytokine hormone, prolactin, binds to the extracellular binding domain of the PRL receptor (PRLR). This triggers gene activation via the Jak2/Stat5 pathway, thereby initiating changes in cell proliferation and differentiation (**Figure 4**). During later developmental stages, i.e., during lactation, prolactin also activates the synthesis of milk proteins via the Jak/Stat signaling pathway (chapter 7).

The transcription factors, Stat5a and 5b, are 92% to 95% identical on the amino acid level (Hennighausen & Robinson, 2001), suggesting possible functional redundancy. Such redundancy can be observed in Stat5 mutants. Mutant analysis has further shown that action of Stat5s is dosage dependent. For example, Stat5a null mice have reduced epithelium with an impaired differentiation during pregnancy. Consequently, Stat5a null mice fail to develop functional mammary tissue during pregnancy (Liu *et al.*, 1997). However, some functional mammary tissue in Stat5a null mice can be obtained after several pregnancies (Liu *et al.*, 1998). This partial restoration coincides with an increased expression of Stat5b, showing partial rescue by compensation and partial functional redundancy of the Stat5 transcription factors. In contrast, Stat5a/5b double knock out mutants have a non-functional corpus luteum (Teglund *et al.*, 1998). In addition, such mice are infertile, demonstrating the wider consequences of Stat5 action on normal sexual development and function. Transplantation experiments have further helped to elucidate the combined contribution of Stat5a and 5b mutations on mammary development. Mammary epithelium transplanted from Stat 5 double null mice into wild type mammary epithelium showed that Stat5a/b null epithelia are able to develop ducts (Miyoshi *et al.*, 2001). This result suggests that Stat5a/b null tissue is reacting to factors produced by the wild type tissue or to other forms of interaction with the wild type tissue. However, the transplanted Stat5a/b null tissue was unable to develop alveoli during pregnancy, demonstrating that Stat5 function cannot be completely compensated for by external factors or interaction with normal tissue (Miyoshi *et al.*, 2001). It further demonstrates the various regulatory roles of Stat5 transcription factors in determination, proliferation, and differentiation of mammary alveoli during pregnancy.

Despite well described mutant phenotypes, target genes of Stat5 signaling in mammary epithelium are so far still unknown (Hennighausen & Robinson, 2001). A potential Stat5 target gene encodes for Id2, a member of the Id family, encoding for negative modulators of the basic helix-loop-helix family of transcription factors. Members of the Id protein family have important roles in cell proliferation and development in many tissues (Mori *et al.*, 2000). Indications for a possible connection between Stat5s and Id2 came from findings showing that expression of Id2 in mammary epithelial cells coincides with Stat5 activation by prolactin signaling. Furthermore, Id2 null mutants show mammary phenotypes resembling changes observed in Stat5 mutants (Mori *et al.*, 2000). This includes reduced proliferation of the mammary epithelium during early pregnancy followed by a lack of functional differentiation and increased rates of apoptosis during late pregnancy.

Another class of proteins implicated as targets of the JAK/STAT signaling pathways belong to the suppressor of cytokine signaling (SOCS) family. These proteins were shown to down-regulate the prolactin signaling pathway (Tomic *et al.*, 1999; Barkai *et al.*, 2000). The mechanism of SOCS action is still unknown.

As discussed, Stat5 activity is crucial for normal development and function of the mammary gland throughout pregnancy and lactation. During involution, the developmental phase following lactation, Stat5 gene expression is down-regulated and STAT5 activity diminishes.

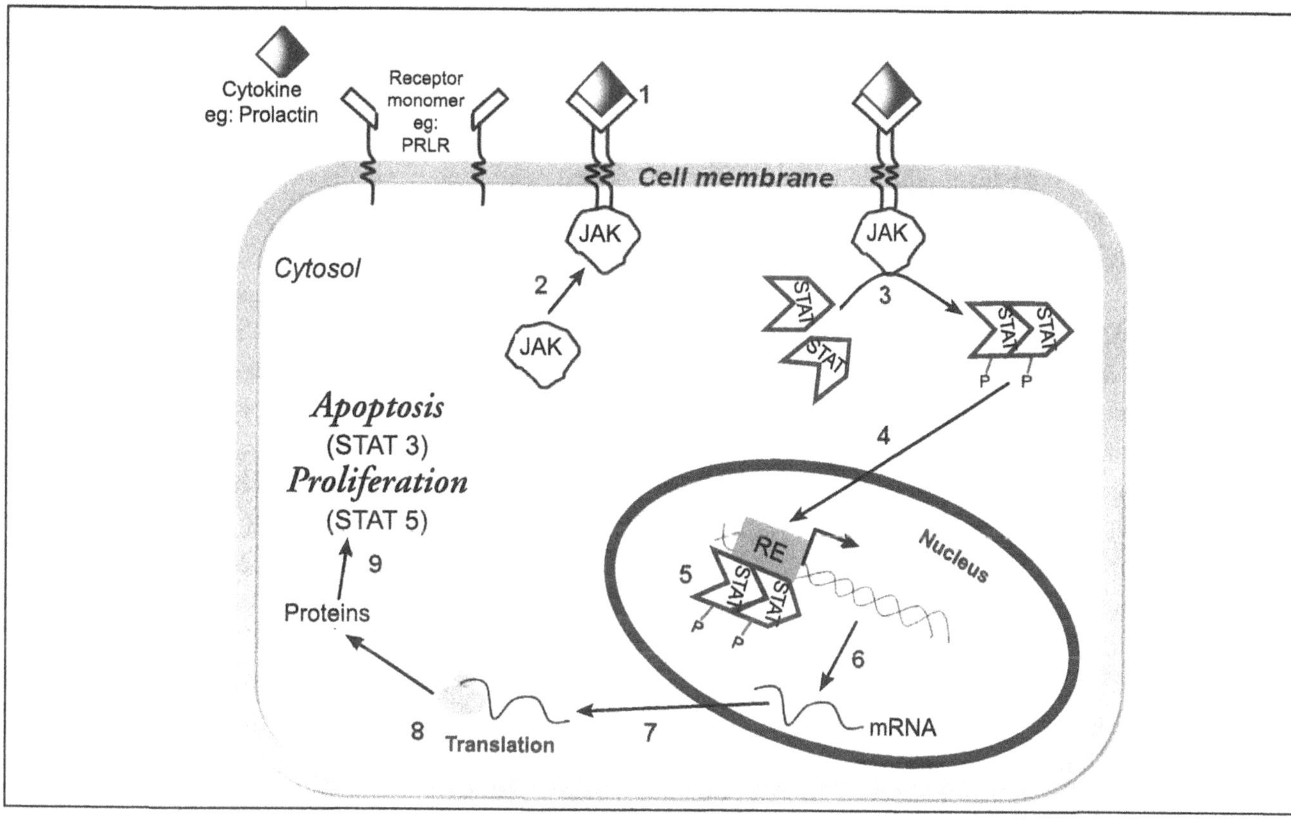

Figure 4. Schematic diagram of Jak/Stat signalling pathway associated with many cytokines. Cytokine (eg: Prolactin). Cytokine (prolactin) binding to receptor (PRL) causes receptor dimerisation (1) and conformational changes of the cytosolic domains that expose specific tyrosine residues to phosphorylation by the receptor associated kinase Jak2 (2). Jak2 kinase is activated via this interaction and phosphorylates downstream target proteins, such as the signal transducers and activators of transcription (Stat) proteins. Inactive Stats are non-phosphorylated monomeric proteins which, upon phosphorylation, form homodimers (3). Activated Stat5 dimers are able to cross the nuclear envelope (4) and bind to specific DNA sequences in the regulatory promoter (RE) regions of their target genes, such as CyclinD1 and Id2 (5). This triggers gene activation (6), thereby initiating changes in cell proliferation and differentiation (or apoptosis in the case of stat 3 during involution-see Figure 6) (7-9).

Cell Cycle Regulators

Normal development and function of the mammary tissue depends strongly on a functioning cell cycle. Cyclins, such as D1, D2, and D3, are expressed during the G1 phase of the cell cycle and contribute to substrate specificity of cyclin-dependent protein kinase involved in cell cycle regulation. Regulation of the cyclin D1 gene by prolactin signaling pathways shows a connection between the hormone and cell cycle regulation. This regulation occurs via activation involving STAT5 signaling and can also involve the RANK NFκB signaling pathway (see below) (Hinz *et al.*, 1999; Cao *et al.*, 2001).

Mouse mutants with deletions of the cell cycle protein D1 failed to develop normal mammary tissue during pregnancy (Fantl *et al.*, 1995; Sicinski *et al.*, 1995). Cyclin-dependent kinase inhibitors, such as p27, impact on proliferation of mammary tissue during pregnancy (Sherr & Roberts, 1999). This was shown using a p27 null mutant. This mutant has a decreased proliferation rate and delayed differentiation of the mammary epithelium (Muraoka *et al.*, 2001). Surprisingly, double mutants in which both cyclin D1 and p27 are non-functional develop normal mammary tissue (Geng *et al.*, 2001). This result points to antagonistic functions of the two proteins. Nevertheless, given the strong impact of the two mutations in isolation on mammary development, it is still surprising to see normal development in the double mutant. It was suggested that normal development in double mutants is possible due to activation of, so far unknown, secondary signaling pathways. A speculative secondary signaling pathway compensating for cyclin D1 and p27 double mutations is the prolactin pathway. A connection between cyclin and prolactin signaling was revealed in Id2 null mutant analysis (Mori *et al.*, 2000). These mutants show increased expression of the two cyclin-dependent kinase inhibitors, p27 and p21. However, further experiments are required to establish whether prolactin signaling compensates for the double mutation or if the connection between prolactin Id2 and cyclin-dependent kinases is of a different nature.

The RANK/RANKL Pathway

In mammals, sex and pregnancy hormones control mammary gland morphogenesis and formation of a lactating mammary gland. During pregnancy, ductal side branching increases and expansion and proliferation of ductal and alveolar epithelium causes further development of lobulo-alveolar structures (Neville, 1999; Robinson *et al.*, 2000). Formation of a lactating mammary gland is essential for providing newborns with nutrient-rich milk. Additionally, milk supplies neonates with calcium. Two essential mechanisms are in place to help mothers to cope with the increased demand for calcium during pregnancy and lactation (Kovacs & Kronenberg, 1997). The first is an increase in the mother's intestinal calcium absorption. The second mechanism involves demineralizing and recycling of calcium from the mother's skeleton via activation of bone-resorbing osteoclasts (Kovacs & Kronenberg, 1997). A key-regulator of skeletal calcium release is RANKL, the Receptor Activator of Nuclear Factor Kappa B (NFκB) Ligand (Lacey *et al.*, 1998; Hsu *et al.*, 1999). Severe osteopetrosis is one of the consequences of RANKL gene inactivation (Anderson *et al.*, 1997; Wong *et al.*, 1997; Lacey *et al.*, 1998; Yasuda *et al.*, 1998). RANKL, also known as Osteoprotegerin ligand (OPGL), is a member of the tumor necrosis factor (TNF) family of cytokines (Yasuda *et al.*, 1998). Induction of osteoclast differentiation and activation is triggered upon RANKL binding to RANK, a member of the Tumor Necrosis Factor/cytokine receptor family (Hsu *et al.*, 1999).

Recently, it was shown that RANKL and RANK are also essential for the formation of the lactating mammary gland, the organ required for transmission of maternal calcium to neonates in mammalian species (Fata *et al.*, 2000). Mice lacking RANKL or RANK have, as could be expected, severe osteoporosis. More surprising was the finding that such mutants show undeveloped lobulo-alveolar buds and fail to express β–casein (Fata *et al.*, 2000). The mammary gland defect in female RANKL mutants is further characterized by enhanced apoptosis. Thus, RANKL signaling can act as a survival factor by activating AKT-mediated pathways (Fata *et al.*, 2000). Local recombinant RANKL application allowed restoration of lobulo-alveolar defects and β–casein expression in pregnant mice. These results clearly demonstrated a role for the RANKL signaling in mammary gland development. Transplantation experiments and RANKL rescue experiments have further shown that RANKL acts directly on RANK-expressing mammary epithelial cells (Fata *et al.*, 2000).

Osteoprotegerin (OPG) a soluble protein competes with RANK for binding to RANKL, thereby acting as a decoy receptor (Lacey *et al.*, 1998). RANKL expression in the mammary gland is under developmental and hormonal regulation. On the other hand, expression of RANK and OPG are constitutively expressed (Srivastava *et al.*, 2003). This shifts the balance between RANKL and OPG in a developmental fashion, determining the activation capability of RANKL (Srivastava *et al.*, 2003). RANKL expression levels are regulated by hormones and cytokine growth factors, including the female sex hormones, estrogen and progesterone, as well as reproductive and lactation hormones, such as prolactin and parathyroid hormone-related peptide (Karsenty, 1999; Ross, 2000; Srivastava *et al.*, 2003). Similarities between RANKL and prolactin signaling are known as both are involved in the activation of ß-casein expression and bone formation (Clement-Lacroix *et al.*, 1999; Fata *et al.*, 2000). The connection between RANKL and prolactin became clearer with the discovery that the RANKL promoter contains a γ–interferon activation sequence (GAS) which can confer prolactin responses (Srivastava *et al.*, 2003). This led to a number of experiments finally indicating that RANKL induction by prolactin in the mammary gland requires functional JAK2 and STAT5. This clearly demonstrated a direct connection between prolactin and RANKL signaling in lobulo-alveolar development (Srivastava *et al.*, 2003). Despite this recent progress, it is still unknown how RANKL/RANK signaling supports lobulo-alveologenesis. What confuses the situation is that RANKL appears to act via a number of pathways. For example, RANKL can regulate β–casein expression in a JAK/STAT independent way via the transcription factor C/EBP (Kim *et al.*, 2000), a factor critical for proliferation and differentiation of epithelial cells and alveologenesis (Seagroves *et al.*, 1998) (see also C/EBP discussion further below). Furthermore, RANKL can impact cell proliferation by affecting G1/S transition during the cell cycle. This is achieved by RANKL activation of NF-κB signaling and activation of Cyclin D1 (Hinz *et al.*, 1999; Cao *et al.*, 2001). Thus, it appears that prolactin, in addition to JAK/STAT signaling, requires other factors to maintain correct alveolar morphogenesis. RANKL could have the role of a local prolactin mediator, facilitating the activation of pathways acting via NF-κB, AKT, and C/EBP.

c/EBP Transcription Factors

The involvement of a CCAAT/enhancer binding protein (c/EBP) in RANKL regulated β–casein expression was already introduced in the previous section. Originally, a C/EBP isoform (C/EBPC) was thought to be mainly involved in regulating milk protein gene expression (Rosen *et al.*, 1998; Rosen *et al.*, 1999). In addition to the regulation of ß-casein gene expression via a glucocorticoid receptor (GR) and Stat5 dependent mechanism, C/EBPβ may indirectly impact on the regulation of the whey acidic protein (WAP) gene (Robinson *et al.*, 1998; Seagroves *et al.*, 1998; Zahnow *et al.*, 2001). However, recently it became apparent that C/EBPβ also plays an important role in mammary gland development (Grimm & Rosen, 2003). Major developmental roles of members of the c/EBP transcription factor family, such as regulators of cell proliferation and differentiation, were described for a great number of tissues (Ramji & Foka, 2002; Grimm & Rosen, 2003). These transcription factors contain a highly conserved basic leucine zipper (bZIP) motif within the C-terminal end which enables interaction with other proteins and the formation of protein dimers. These dimers include c/EBP homodimers and heterodimers in which one c/EBP interacts with another member of the c/EBP family (Osada *et al.*, 1996). Heterodimers consisting of c/EBPβ and a member of the larger bZIP protein family were also described (Yeh *et al.*, 1995). However, such heterodimers bind to non-canonical binding sequences (Takiguchi, 1998). Furthermore, c/EBP's are able to interact with a great number of other transcription factors and co-activators accounting for the wide spectrum of developmental processes c/EBP's are involved in (Takiguchi, 1998; Zahnow *et al.*, 2001; Ramji & Foka, 2002; Lekstrom-Himes & Xanthopoulos, 1998; McKnight, 2001). A DNA binding domain adjacent to the bZIP domain mediates binding of c/EBPs to dyad symmetrical DNA repeats (PuGTTGCGPyrAAPyr) within target gene promoters (Osada *et al.*, 1996). In contrast to the C-terminus, the N-terminal amino acid sequence is highly variable between individual c/EBP protein members, but may contain one or two conserved transactivation domains. Protein phosphorylation, in addition to autoregulation, plays a key role in the modulation of c/EBP activity (Takiguchi, 1998; Ramji & Foka, 2002). A number of protein kinases, including mitogen activated protein kinases (MAPK), protein kinases A and C (PKA, PKC), and calcium calmodulin-dependent protein kinase (CaMK) can phosphorylate c/EBP at serine and threonine residues (Kowenz-Leutz *et al.*, 1994; Ramji & Foka, 2002).

In the context of mammary gland development, c/EBPs are required for ductal growth and morphogenesis during pregnancy (Grimm & Rosen, 2003). The best characterized c/EBP with an involvement in ductal growth and morphogenesis is c/EBPβ. The genomes of mice, humans, and other mammals contain only a single c/EBPβ gene from which a sole mRNA is derived (Hendricks-Taylor *et al.*, 1992; Jenkins *et al.*, 1995). However, translation of the single mRNA can occur from alternative translation start sites leading to the expression of at least three distinct c/EBPβ-derived protein isoforms (**Figure 5**) (Descombes & Schibler, 1991; Ossipow *et al.*, 1993; Welm *et al.*, 1999). These isoforms are the Liver-enriched activating proteins (LAP and LAP2) and the Liver-enriched inhibitory protein (LIP). In mice, the LAP isoform (38kDa) is the largest c/EBPβ isoform derived by translation from the first translational start site. It contains two regulatory domains (RD1 and RD2), a protein interaction domain, and three N-terminal transactivation domains, in addition to DNA binding domains. The regulatory domains interact with and inhibit the transactivation and the DNA binding domains (Kowenz-Leutz *et al.*, 1994; Williams *et al.*, 1995). The second largest isoform LAP2 (35kDa) lacks the first 21 amino acids of LAP, but contains the same interaction and regulatory domains. Despite the high similarity between LAP and LAP2, they are functionally distinct proteins (Grimm & Rosen, 2003). The shorter LIP isoform (21kDa) is translated from a third translational start codon and lacks the N-terminal transactivation domains found in LAP and LAP2. However, LIP still contains the DNA and protein dimerisation domain found in LAP and LAP2. LIP is

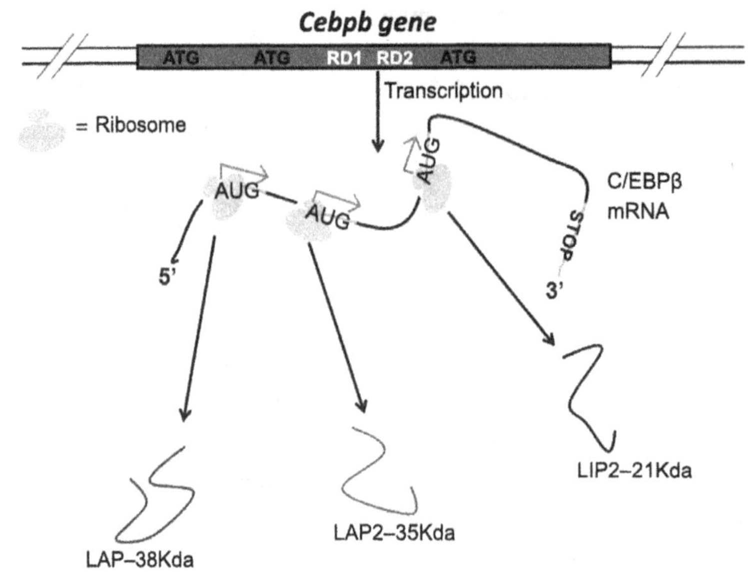

Figure 5. Schematic diagram illustrating the generation of three different c/EBPβ isoforms from the one cebpb gene. The transcribed c/EBPβ mRNA has three translational start sites (AUG) from which three different proteins can be translated. This results in the production of LAP (38Kda - liver-enriched activating protein) from the first translational start site, LAP2 (31Kda) from the second translational start site, and LIP (21Kda - liver-enriched inhibitory protein) from the third translational start site. Furthermore, proteolytic cleavage of LAP can result in the production of LIP and a 14Kda protein. The cebpb gene contains two regulatory domains (RD1, RD2) between the second and third translation site. As a result, LAP and LAP2 contain domains that are able to participate in transcriptional regulation via these DNA binding sites and, as LIP does not contain these domains, it therefore lacks such activity (Grimm & Rosen, 2003).

assumed to act as a dominant negative c/EBP isoform (Descombes & Schibler, 1991), as it has a higher DNA binding affinity than LAP. In addition to the direct action on DNA levels, LIP may act directly by inhibiting LAP function.

The biological importance of c/EBPβ for mammary gland development during pregnancy was shown using mice carrying a deletion which eliminates expression of all three c/EBPβ protein isoforms (Robinson *et al.*, 1998; Seagroves *et al.*, 1998). Lobulo-alveolar development and functional development of the gland are severely inhibited in such mutants with additional subtle changes in ductal morphogenesis. The impaired lobulo-alveolar phenotype of the c/EBPβ mutation is similar to phenotypes observed in mutants with defects in other core genes of mammary gland development, such as knock-outs of Stat5a/b, the prolactin receptor, or CyclinD1 (Hennighausen & Robinson, 2001; Shillingford & Hennighausen, 2001).

Transcription of c/EBPβ is already detectable at low levels in pubescent mice and increases during pregnancy (Gigliotti & DeWille, 1998; Robinson *et al.*, 1998; Sabatakos *et al.*, 1998). A minor decrease in c/EBPβ mRNAs occurs during lactation, followed by another induction within 48 hours after the onset of involution. More significant than transcriptional regulation of the c/EBPβ gene is the ratio of the individual c/EBPβ protein isoforms. Both the LAP and LIP isoform are expressed at low levels in virgin mice. Expression of the two isoforms increases during pregnancy, reflecting increased mRNA expression (Raught *et al.*, 1995; Seagroves *et al.*, 1998; Dearth *et al.*, 2001). However, while LAP protein expression increases three-fold, LIP protein expression increases more than 100-fold. LIP expression decreases at parturition to almost undetectable levels and remains low during the following stages of mammary gland development. On the other hand, LAP protein expression decreases only marginally at parturition and remains well detectable during lactation and involution.

The shifts in LAP to LIP protein ratios are crucial in understanding their regulatory role in mammary gland development. This is due to the role of LIP as a dominant negative regulator of LAP function. For example, during pregnancy, a high LIP to LAP ratio may prevent LAP-dependent activation of ß-casein expression. Down-regulation of LIP protein expression with only marginal changes in LAP protein expression shifts the isoform ratio in favor of LAP, allowing for LAP mediated activation of β-casein expression. At the same time, action of progesterone, prolactin, and the Jak2/Stat5 signaling pathway would allow for further promotion of β-casein gene expression and the expression of other milk proteins at the onset of lactation (Wyszomierski & Rosen, 2001). Similarly, changes in LIP to LAP ratio may regulate morphological processes during mammary gland development, especially during pregnancy. Furthermore, a hypothesis was recently introduced suggesting that c/EBPβ plays a role in the specification of progenitor cell fate in a number of tissues and cell types (Sterneck *et al.*, 1997; Darlington *et al.*, 1998; Maytin & Habener, 1998; Cortes-Canteli *et al.*, 2002) and therefore may play a greater role in tissue development than previously thought.

APOPTOSIS AND INVOLUTION

Apoptosis plays an important role in mammary gland development and function during embryonic and ductal mammary development and after pregnancy and lactation (Green & Streuli, 2004). For example, in mice, both male and female embryos develop initial mammary gland tissue with epithelial buds emerging from the ectoderm into the mammary mesenchyme. While in female embryos, this is the starting point for further development of the mammary anlagen, development comes to an arrest in male embryos. Formation of testes and subsequent testosterone production in male embryos trigger inhibition of further gland development and apoptosis of epithelial buds (Nguyen & Pollard, 2000). In female mice, apoptosis leads to cell removal from the mammary ducts within the terminal endbud during puberty. It is believed that this prepares the gland for the passage of milk to the nipple and/or serves to remove excess cells at the highly proliferative endbud.

Apoptosis is also crucial for epithelial homeostasis during estrous/menstrual cycles (Potten *et al.*, 1988; Andres & Strange, 1999; Metcalfe *et al.*, 1999). Here apoptosis occurs within the ductal tissue and is regulated by estrogen and progesterone. After weaning, apoptotic cell death removes milk-secreting alveolar epithelial cells to remodel the structure of the gland to pre-pregnancy status and prepare the gland for future reproductive development.

The full picture of apoptotic processes involved in the diverse stages of mammary gland development is far from understood. It appears that two basic mechanisms are in place, active induction of apoptosis and inactivation of apoptotic inhibitors (**Figure 6**). Best known and investigated are apoptotic events involved in remodeling the mammary gland during post-lactational involution. Involution or rebuilding of the gland to a pre-pregnancy state involves apoptotic and tissue remodeling events. Forced involution and gene deletion studies have been used to synchronize and study this process in laboratory animals, such as mice (Lund *et al.*, 1996; Li *et al.*, 1997). Post-lactational involution is triggered when suckling ceases after lactation. Characteristic apoptotic markers, such as DNA laddering, changes in epithelial cell morphology, and activation of apoptosis specific caspases can be observed within two days of the onset of weaning (Walker *et al.*, 1989; Strange *et al.*, 1992; Lund *et al.*, 1996; Metcalfe *et al.*, 1999; Prince *et al.*, 2002). Forced weaning has shown that this is a two-step process, an initial apoptotic step and a second step involving a continuation of apoptosis together with matrix degradation and remodeling of the gland (Martinez-Hernandez *et al.*, 1976; Lund *et al.*, 1996; Li *et al.*, 1997). Mammary-derived signals are activated upon milk accumulation in the gland. It is believed that components within milk, such as α-lactalbumin, are potential apoptotic triggers, as they can be used to artificially initiate apoptosis (Hakansson *et al.*, 1995; Hakansson *et al.*, 1999). A second potential pro-apoptotic signal under discussion involves the activation of stretch induced receptors by accumulating volumes of milk during milk stasis (Wernig *et al.*, 2003). It is reasonable to assume that the switch from lactation and active milk production to involution, apoptosis, and mammary gland remodeling may require more than just a simple or single signaling pathway. This appears the case, as no single currently known pathway involved in triggering involution appears to be sufficient to initiate and maintain apoptosis on its own. This can clearly be seen in the fact that losing one of the apoptotic signaling pathways can, at best, delay but not prevent apoptosis completely (Green & Streuli, 2004) (**Figure 6**).

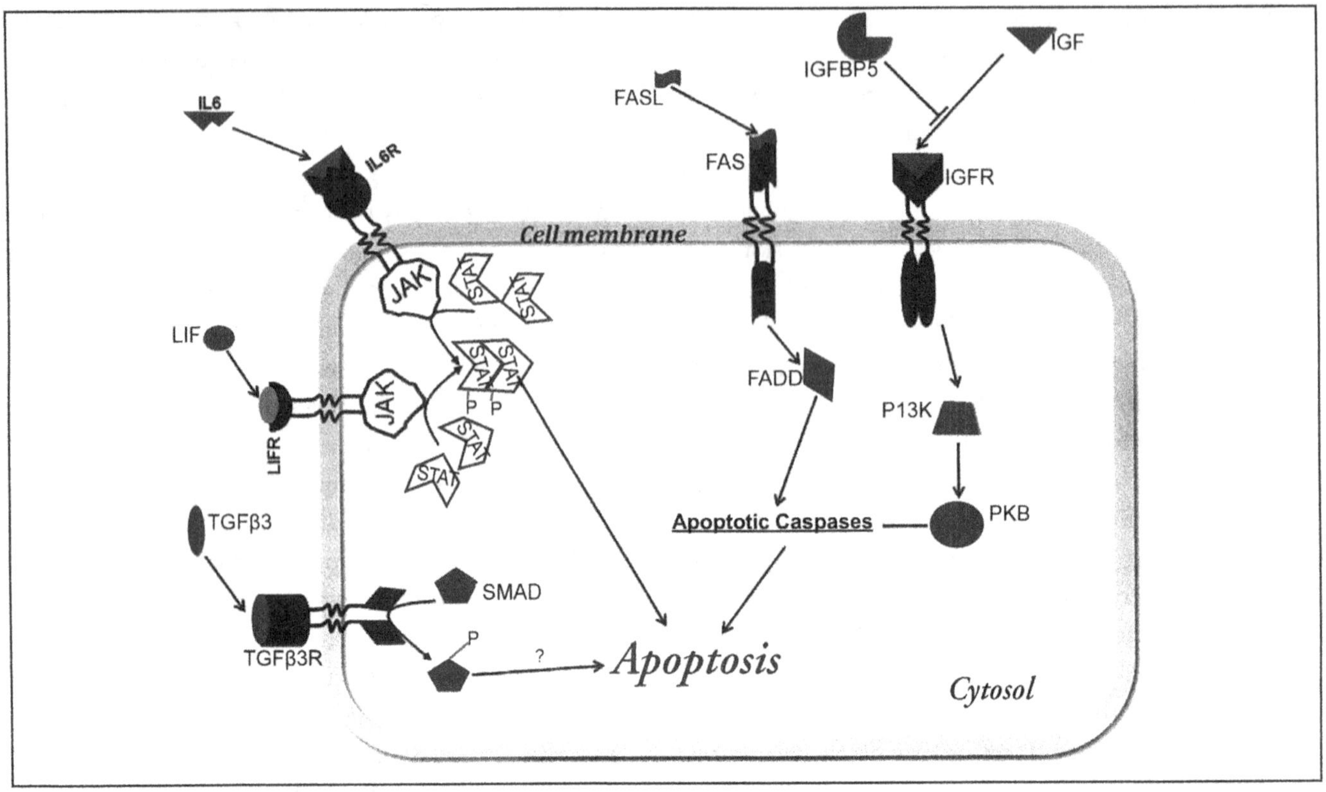

Figure 6. Schematic diagram illustrating the multiple pathways associated with apoptosis occurring during involution as a result of prolonged milk stasis. Apoptosis is induced through two general schemes. The inhibition of the anti-apoptotic regulators (e.g., increase in IGFBP5 inhibits anti-apoptotic effects of IGF) and general apoptotic pathway activation (e.g., TGFβ3, FAS/FASL, LIF, and IL6 via JAK/STAT3 signaling). Importantly, Stat3 is up-regulated during involution while Stat5 is down-regulated.

The Insulin-like Growth Factor – Protein Kinase B (IGF-PKB) Signaling Pathway

It is well established that insulin-like growth factors (IGFs) stimulate cell survival in the mammary gland via the IGF-PKB signaling pathway. This pathway is activated by IGF binding to its receptor, triggering a kinase signaling pathway involving phosphatidylinositol-3'-kinase (P13K) and PKB (also known as Akt), ultimately resulting in phosphorylation and activation of PKB (Moorehead *et al.*, 2001; Schwertfeger *et al.*, 2001; Ackler *et al.*, 2002; Dupont *et al.*, 2002; Li *et al.*, 2002).

Inhibition of IGF signaling and/or IGF production is a possible mechanism involved in triggering apoptosis in the gland. The IGF signaling inhibitor protein, IGFBP-5, may play an important role in this. IGFBP-5 mRNA and protein expression levels increase considerably within 24 hours of the onset of involution (Tonner *et al.*, 1995; Tonner *et al.*, 1997). Application of IGFBP-5 inhibits IGF-1 signaling and further promotes apoptosis in mammary epithelial cell cultures (Marshman *et al.*, 2003). Premature apoptosis was also induced in transgenic mice overexpressing IGFBP-5 under control of the β–lactoglobulin promoter (Tonner *et al.*, 2002).

IGFBP-5 may act by preventing IGF receptor activation and thus circumventing the generation of IGF-dependent anti-apoptotic signals. In agreement with its potential role in triggering apoptosis, expression of IGFBP-5 is inhibited by prolactin, one of the major hormones acting during pregnancy and lactation, and stimulated by milk stasis, as found after weaning (Tonner *et al.*, 1997). The inhibitory role of the IGF-PKB pathway on apoptosis was further demonstrated using transgenic mice overexpressing an IGF-I isoform with reduced affinity for IGFBP in the mammary gland. This resulted in incomplete involution of the gland with a lack of remodeling features on the cellular level (Hadsell *et al.*, 1996). Expressing IGF-II under a mouse mammary tumor virus (MMTV) promoter, thereby directing expression to mammary cells, led to delayed involution of the mammary gland (Moorehead *et al.*, 2001). These mammary glands showed increased phosphorylation due to PKB activity. The involvement of PKB in preventing mammary involution was confirmed by ectopic expression of the PKB gene under the control of the MMTV promoter which led to delayed involution (Schwertfeger *et al.*, 2001; Ackler *et al.*, 2002). Involution was also delayed by conditional deletion of PTEN, a negative regulator of PI3K (Dupont *et al.*, 2002; Li *et al.*, 2002). Together, these results clearly demonstrate the inhibitory role of the IGF-PKB signaling pathway on mammary gland apoptosis and involution.

Regulation of the IGF-PKB signaling pathway and thereby the onset of involution and apoptosis appear to require the correct cellular context (Lee & Streuli, 1999). Using mammary cell culture experiments, it was shown that IGF-I mediated signaling and cell survival depends on contact of primary cells with a basement membrane (BM), while contact with collagen I contained *in vivo* in the stromal extracellular matrix (ECM), leads to weak IGF signaling and occurrence of apoptosis (Lee & Streuli, 1999). Inefficient signal transduction from the type I IGF receptor is involved in triggering apoptosis under such conditions. It is possible that mammary epithelial cells survive during lactation because the BM separates these cells from the collagen I containing stromal ECM. The molecular basis for such altered responses to BM and collagen I could be the interaction of growth factor receptors, such as the IGF receptor, with various integrins (Green & Streuli, 2004). It is known that different integrins are used in adhesion of mammary cells to BM proteins and to collagen I, thus, different integrins may cause a different response of the IGF pathway.

Switching from Stat5 to Stat3

A second important signaling pathway regulating apoptosis in the mammary gland involves the transcription factor Stat3 (**Figures 4 and 6**). As for Stat5, Stat3 belongs to the Stat family of transcription factors. Stat5, as discussed above, is crucial for mammary gland function and development during pregnancy and lactation. At the onset of involution, Stat5 activity is down-regulated as a necessity for the successful onset of the involution program (Philp *et al.*, 1996). The role of Stat3 is opposite of Stat5, as its expression is required for progression of involution. This was demonstrated using two different transgenic mice mutants - mice in which Stat3 was non-functional due to a knock-out mutation and mice overexpressing STAT5 (Chapman *et al.*, 1999; Humphreys *et al.*, 2002; Iavnilovitch *et al.*, 2002). Both types of manipulation led to delayed involution. Thus, Stat3 is clearly a promoter of involution and stimulator of the apoptotic events involved in reorganization of the mammary tissue.

The Leukemia inhibitory factor (LIF) appears to be a central factor of STAT3 activation in the mammary gland (Kritikou *et al.*, 2003; Schere-Levy *et al.*, 2003). STAT3 is non-phosphorylated in mice lacking LIF and involution following weaning is delayed. Moreover, artificial application of LIF to lactating mammary glands of wild-type mice increases apoptosis. How STAT3 triggers apoptosis is unknown, but it may involve changes in the expression of genes that are either directly or indirectly involved in apoptotic events. Another potential activator of STAT3 is the cytokine, Interleukin (IL)-6 (Zhao *et al.*, 2002). IL-6 mRNA expression increases strongly after weaning, and ablation of IL-6 leads to delayed involution. A potential mechanism by which IL-6 could trigger involution was revealed by its ability to strongly activate STAT3. These results point to a potentially important role of IL-6 for the onset of involution.

Further Potential Regulators of Mammary Gland Apoptosis and Involution

A number of other genes and proteins are described in the literature as being rapidly induced in mammary tissue at the onset of involution (Green & Streuli, 2004). This includes a member of the transforming growth factors β (TGFβs) proteins known to act as apoptotic regulators in a number of tissues. Expression of TGFβ3 mRNA and protein are rapidly up-regulated at the onset of involution (Nguyen & Pollard, 2000). Experiments in which TGFβ3 was expressed in lactating epithelial cells showed that this factor is able to stimulate apoptosis (Nguyen & Pollard, 2000). TGFβ3 appears to be a specifically recruited TGFβ member in mammary gland involution, as none of the other TGFβ family members appears to be involved in apoptosis during this developmental stage (Green & Streuli, 2004). How TGFβ3 could act in mammary involution is unclear and existing models of TGFβ3 action are currently based on signaling pathways involving other TGFβ members. It was suggested that TGFβ3 regulation of involution may involve transcription factors, such as RUNX and members of the Smad gene family (Green & Streuli, 2004).

An elegant model describing the potential regulation of apoptotic events during involution is based on the interaction of so called death ligands and their receptor proteins (Green & Streuli, 2004). One such death ligand, FasL, triggers a signaling cascade that leads to activation of apoptosis via caspase activation (Green & Streuli, 2004). FasL is expressed in mammary gland tissue during pregnancy and lactation (Green & Streuli, 2004). However, the FasL receptor, Fas, is absent in mammary tissue during these developmental stages, but expressed in virgin mammary tissue (Green & Streuli, 2004). The exclusive expression of the two proteins during these stages prevents activation of the FasL–Fas signaling pathway, leading normally to apoptosis of a cell. A rapid increase of Fas and FasL expression during the onset of involution allows for interaction of the two proteins and is likely to be the event leading to FasL-mediated apoptosis.

In the previous sections, we have given an overview of some of the molecular factors and mechanisms involved in the regulation of mammary gland development from embryo development to involution. The use of molecular techniques, generation of mutant animals, and transgenic technology have contributed substantially to our current knowledge. It is already obvious that the regulation of mammary gland development is dependent on a great number of factors, including various hormones, their receptors, and signaling proteins, such as protein kinases, transcription factors, and other DNA binding proteins. Several of these factors impact on the formation of the mammary gland during more than one developmental stage, while others appear so far to be restricted to a short period of time. A great deficit of current knowledge is that many signaling pathways are only known in fragments, and target genes of many regulatory pathways are often unknown. However, given the fact that this field of research is still very young, the rapid progress seen so far is promising.

ACKNOWLEDGEMENT

Research funding from Medela AG.

References

Ackler S, Ahmad S, Tobias C, Johnson M, Glazer R. Delayed mammary gland involution in MMTVAKT1 transgenic mice. *Oncogene.* 2002; 21:198–206.

Akiyama T. Wnt/b-catenin signaling. *Cytokine Growth Factor Rev.* 2000; 11:273–82.

Anderson D, Maraskovsky E, Billingsley W, Dougall W, Tometsko M, Roux E, *et al.* A homologue of the TNF receptor and its ligand enhance T-cell growth and dendritic-cell function. *Nature.* 1997; 390:175–79.

Andl T, Reddy S, Gaddapara T, Millar S. WNT signals are required for the initiation of hair follicle development. *Dev Cell.* 2002; 2:643–53.

Andres A, Strange R. Apoptosis in the estrous and menstrual cycles. *J Mammary Gland Biol Neoplasia.* 1999; 4:221–28.

Anton E, Ghashghaei H, Weber J, McCann C, Fischer T. Receptor tyrosine kinase ErbB4 modulates neuroblast migration and placement in the adult forebrain. *Nat Neurosci.* 2004; 7:1319–28.

Atwood C, Hovey R, Glover J, Chepko G, Ginsburg E, Robison W, *et al.* Progesterone induces side-branching of the ductal epithelium in the mammary glands of peripubertal mice. *J Endocrinol.* 2000; 167:39-52.

Bamshad M, Lin R, Law D, Watkins W, Krakowiak P, Me M. Mutations in human TBX3 alter limb, apocrine and genital development in ulnar–mammary syndrome. *Nat Genet.* 1997; 16:311–15.

Barkai U, Prigent-Tessier A, Tessier C, Gibori G, Gibori G. Involvement of SOCS-1, the suppressor of cytokine signaling, in the prevention of prolactin-responsive gene expression in decidual cells. *Mol Endocrinol.* 2000; 14(4):554-63.

Bocchinfuso W, Lindzey J, Hewitt S, Clark J, Myers P, Cooper R, *et al.* Induction of mammary gland development in estrogen receptor-alpha knockout mice. *Endocrinology.* 2000; 141: 2982-94.

Bollag R, Siegfried Z, Cebra-Thomas J, Garvey N, Davison E, Silver L. An ancient family of embryonically expressed mouse genes sharing a conserved protein motif with the T locus. *Nat Genet.* 1994; 7:383-89.

Boras-Granic K, Chang H, Grosschedl R, Hamel P. Lef1 is required for the transition of Wnt signaling from mesenchymal to epithelial cells in the mouse embryonic mammary gland. *Dev Biol.* 2006; 295:219–31.

Brisken C, Heineman A, Chavarria T, Elenbaas B, Tan J, Dey S, *et al.* Essential function of Wnt-4 in mammary gland development downstream of progesterone signaling. *Genes Dev.* 2000; 14:650-54.

Cao Y, Bonizzi G, Seagroves T, Greten F, Johnson R, Schmidt E, *et al.* IKKalpha provides an essential link between RANK signaling and cyclin D1 expression during mammary gland development. *Cell.* 2001; 107:763–75.

Carlson H, Ota S, Campbell C, Hurlin P. A dominant repression domain in Tbx3 mediates transcriptional repression and cell immortalization: relevance to mutations in Tbx3 that cause ulnar-mammary syndrome. *Hum Mol Genet.* 2001; 10:2403-13.

Chapman R, Lourenco P, Tonner E, Flint D, Selbert S, Takeda K. Suppression of epithelial apoptosis and delayed mammary gland involution in mice with a conditional knockout of Stat3. *Genes Dev.* 1999; 13:2604–16.

Chen H, Sukumar S. Role of homeobox genes in normal mammary gland development and breast tumorigenesis. *J Mammary Gland Biol Neoplasia.* 2003; 8:159-75.

Chu E, Hens J, Andl T, Kairo A, Yamaguchi T, Brisken C, *et al.* Canonical WNT signaling promotes mammary placode development and is essential for initiation of mammary gland morphogenesis. *Development.* 2004; 131:4819–29.

Clement-Lacroix P, Ormandy C, Lepescheux L, Ammann P, Damotte D, Goffin V, *et al.* Osteoblasts are a new target for prolactin: analysis of bone formation in prolactin receptor knockout mice. *Endocrinology.* 1999; 140:96–105.

Coll M, Seidman J, Muller C. Structure of the DNA bound T-box domain of human TBX3, a transcription factor responsible for ulnar-mammary syndrome. *Structure.* 2002; 10:343-56.

Conneely O, Kettelberger D, Tsai M, Schrader W, O'Malley B. The chicken progesterone receptor A and B isoforms are products of an alternate translation initiation event. *J Biol Chem.* 1989; 264:14062–64.

Cortes-Canteli M, Pignatelli M, Santos A, Perez-Castillo A. CCAAT/enhancer-binding protein beta plays a regulatory role in differentiation and apoptosis of neuroblastoma cells. *J Biol Chem.* 2002; 277:5460–67.

Cowie AT, Forsyth I, Hart IC. *Hormonal control of lactation. Monographs of endocrinology.* Berlin: Springer-Verlag; 1980.

Darlington G, Ross S, MacDougald O. The role of C/EBP genes in adipocyte differentiation. *J Biol Chem.* 1998; 273:30057–60.

Davenport T, Jerome-Majewska L, Papaioannou V. Mammary gland, limb and yolk sac defects in mice lacking Tbx3, the gene mutated in human ulnar mammary syndrome. *Development.* 2003; 130:2263–73.

Dearth L, Hutt J, Sattler A, Gigliotti A, DeWille J. Expression and function of CCAAT/enhancer binding proteinbeta (C/EBPbeta) LAP and LIP isoforms in mouse mammary gland, tumors and cultured mammary epithelial cells. *J Cell Biochem.* 2001; 82:357–70.

Descombes P, Schibler U. A liver-enriched transcriptional activator protein, LAP, and a transcriptional inhibitory protein, LIP, are translated from the same mRNA. *Cell.* 1991; 67:569–79.

Dunbar M, Dann P, Robinson G, Hennighausen L, Zhang J, Wysolmerski J. Parathyroid hormone-related protein signalling is necessary for sexual dimorphism during embryonic mammary gland development. *Development.* 1999; 126:3485-93.

Dupont J, Renou J, Shani M, Hennighausen L, LeRoith D. PTEN overexpression suppresses proliferation and differentiation and enhances apoptosis of the mouse mammary epithelium. *J Clin Invest.* 2002; 110:815–25.

Durmowicz M, Cui C, Schlessinger D. The EDA gene is a target of, but does not regulate, Wnt signaling. *Gene.* 2002; 285:203–11.

Eblaghie M, Song S, Kim J, Akita K, Tickle C, Jung H. Interactions between FGF and Wnt signals and Tbx3 gene expression in mammary gland initiation in mouse embryos. *J Anat.* 2004; 205:1–13.

Ely F, Petersen W. Factors involved in the ejection of milk. *J Dairy Sci.* 1941; 24:211-23.

Fantl V, Stamp G, Andrews A, Rosewell I, Dickson C. Mice lacking cyclin D1 are small and show defects in eye and mammary gland development. *Genes Dev.* 1995; 9:2364–72.

Fata J, Kong Y, Li J, Sasaki T, Sasaki J, Moorehead R, *et al.* The osteoclast differentiation factor osteoprotegerin-ligand is essential for mammary gland development. *Cell.* 2000;103:41–50.

Foley J, Dann P, Hong J, Cosgrove J, Dreyer B, Rimm D, *et al.* Parathyroid hormone related protein maintains mammary epithelial fate and triggers nipple skin differentiation during embryonic breast development. *Development.* 2001; 128:513-25.

Freeman M, Kanyicska B, Lerant A, Nagy G. Prolactin: Structure, function, and regulation of secretion. *Phys Rev.* 2000; 80:1523-1631.

Friedmann Y, Daniel C. Regulated expression of homeobox genes Msx-1 and Msx-2 in mouse mammary gland development suggests a role in hormone action and epithelial-stromal interactions. *Dev Biol.* 1996; 177:347-55.

Fuchs E, Raghavan S. Getting under the skin of epidermal morphogenesis. *Nat Rev Genet.* 2002; 3:199–209.

Gallego M, Binart N, Robinson G, Okagaki R, Coschigano K, Perry J, *et al.* Prolactin, growth hormone and epidermal growth factor activate Stat5 in different compartments of mammary tissue and exert different and overlapping developmental effects. *Dev Biol.* 2001; 229:163-75.

Gambarotta G, Garzotto D, Destro E, Mautino B, Giampietro C. ErbB4 expression in neural progenitor cells (ST14A) is necessary to mediate neuregulin-1beta1-induced migration. *J Biol Chem.* 2004; 279:48808–16.

Geng Y, Yu Q, Sicinska E, Das M, Bronson R, Sicinski P. Deletion of the p27Kip1 gene restores normal development in cyclin D1-deficient mice. *Proc Natl Acad Sci USA.* 2001; 98:194–99.

Ghashghaei H, Weber J, Pevny L, Schmid R, Schwab M. The role of neuregulin-ErbB4 interactions on the proliferation and organization of cells in the subventricular zone. *Proc Natl Acad Sci USA.* 2006; 103:1930–35.

Gigliotti A, DeWille J. Lactation status influences expression of CCAAT/enhancer binding protein isoform mRNA in the mouse mammary gland. *J Cell Physiol.* 1998; 174:232–39.

Gordon-Thomson C, Jones J, Mason R, Moore G. ErbB receptors mediate both migratory and proliferative activities in human melanocytes and melanoma cells. *Melanoma Res.* 2005; 15:21–28.

Green K, Streuli C. Apoptosis regulation in the mammary gland. *Cell Mol Life Sci.* 2004; 61:1867–83.

Grimm S, Rosen J. The role of C/EBPß in mammary gland development and breast cancer. *J Mammary Gland Biol Neoplasia.* 2003; 8:191-204.

Hadsell D, Greenberg N, Fligger J, Baumrucker C, Rosen J. Targeted expression of des(1-3) human insulin-like growth factor I in transgenic mice influences mammary gland development and IGF-binding protein expression. *Endocrinology.* 1996; 137:321–30.

Hakansson A, Andreasson J, Zhivotovsky B, Karpman D, Orrenius S, Svanborg C. Multimeric alpha-lactalbumin from human milk induces apoptosis through a direct effect on cell nuclei. *Exp Cell Res.* 1999; 246:451–60.

Hakansson A, Zhivotovsky B, Orrenius S, Sabharwal H, Svanborg C. Apoptosis induced by a human milk protein. *Proc Natl Acad Sci USA.* 1995; 92:8064–68.

Haslam S. Progesterone effects on deoxyribonucleic acid synthesis in normal mouse mammary glands. *Endocrinology.* 1988; 122:464-70.

He M, Wen L, Campbell C, Wu J, Rao Y. Transcription repression by Xenopus ET and its human ortholog TBX3, a gene involved in ulnar-mammary syndrome. *Proc Natl Acad Sci USA.* 1999; 96:10212-217.

Hendricks-Taylor L, Bachinski L, Siciliano M, Fertitta A, Trask A, de Jong P. The CCAAT/enhancer binding protein (C/EBP alpha) gene (CEBPA) maps to human chromosome 19q13.1 and the related nuclear factor NF-IL6 (C/EBP beta) gene (CEBPB) maps to human chromosome 20q13.1. *Genomics.* 1992; 14:12–17.

Hennighausen L, Robinson G. Signaling pathways in mammary gland development. *Dev Cell.* 2001; 1(4):467-75.

Hennighausen L, Robinson G. Information networks in the mammary gland. *Nat Rev Mol Cell Biol.* 2005; 6:715-25.

Hinz M, Krappmann D, Eichten A, Heder A, Scheidereit C, Strauss M. NF-KB function in growth control: Regulation of cyclin D1 expression and G0/G1-to-S-phase transition. *Mol Cell Biol.* 1999; 19:2690–98.

Horseman N, Zhao W, Montecino-Rodriguez E, Tanaka M, Nakashima K, Engle S, *et al.* Defective mammopoiesis, but normal hematopoiesis, in mice with a targeted disruption of the prolactin gene. *EMBO J.* 1997; 16:6926-35.

Howard B, Ashworth A. Signalling pathways implicated in early mammary gland morphogenesis and breast cancer. *PLoS Genetics.* 2006; 2:1121-30.

Howard B, Gusterson B. The characterization of a mouse mutant that displays abnormal mammary gland development. *Mamm Genome.* 2000; 11:234–37.

Howard B, Gusterson B. Mammary gland patterning in the AXB/ BXA recombinant inbred strains of mouse. *Mech Dev.* 2000; 91(1-2):305–9.

Howard B, Panchal H, McCarthy A, Ashworth A. Identification of the scaramanga gene implicates Neuregulin3 in mammary gland specification. *Genes Dev.* 2005; 19:2078–90.

Hsu H, Lacey D, Dunstan C, Solovyev I, Colombero A, Timms E, *et al.* Tumor necrosis factor receptor family member RANK mediates osteoclast differentiation and activation induced by osteoprotegerin ligand. *Proc Natl Acad Sci USA.* 1999; 96:3540–45.

Hu G, Lee H, Price S, Shen M, Abate-Shen C. Msx homeobox genes inhibit differentiation through upregulation of cyclin D1. *Development.* 2001; 128:2373-84.

Huelsken J, Birchmeier W. New aspects of Wnt signaling pathways in higher vertebrates. *Curr Opin Genet Dev.* 2001; 11:547-53.

Humphreys R, Bierie B, Zhao L, Raz R, Levy D, Hennighausen L. Deletion of Stat3 blocks mammary gland involution and extends functional competence of the secretory epithelium in the absence of lactogenic stimuli. *Endocrinology.* 2002; 143:3641–50.

Iavnilovitch E, Groner B, Barash I. Overexpression and forced activation of stat5 in mammary gland of transgenic mice promotes cellular proliferation, enhances differentiation and delays postlactational apoptosis. *Mol Cancer Res.* 2002; 1:32–47.

Imagawa W, Yang J, Guzman R, Nandi S. Control of mammary gland development. In: Knobil E, Neil J. *The physiology of reproduction.* New York, Raven Press; 1994.

Jenkins N, Gilbert D, Cho B, Strobel M, Williams S, Copeland N. Mouse chromosomal location of the CCAAT/ enhancer binding proteins C/EBP beta (Cebpb), C/EBP delta (Cebpd), and CRP1 (Cebpe). *Genomics.* 1995; 28:333–36.

Jerome-Majewska L, Jenkins G, Ernstoff E, Zindy F, Sherr C, Papaioannou V. Tbx3, the ulnar-mammary syndrome gene, and Tbx2 interact in mammary gland development through a p19Arf/p53-independent pathway. *Dev Dyn.* 2005; 234:922–33.

Jowett A, Vainio S, Ferguson M, Sharpe P, Thesleff I. Epithelial-mesenchymal interactions are required for msx 1 and msx 2 gene expression in the developing murine molar tooth. *Development.* 1993; 117:461-70.

Jüppner H, Abou-Samra A, Freeman M, Kong X, Schipani E, Richards J, *et al.* A G protein-linked receptor for parathyroid hormone and parathyroid hormone-related peptide. *Science.* 1991; 254:1024-26.

Karsenty G. The genetic transformation of bone biology. *Genes Dev.* 1999; 13:3037–51.

Kastner P, Krust A, Turcotte B, Strupp U, Tora L, Gronemeyer H, *et al.* Two distinct estrogen-regulated promoters generate transcripts encoding the two functionally different human progesterone receptor forms A and B. *EMBO J.* 1990; 9:1603–14.

Kelly, P, Bachelot A, Kedzia C, Hennighausen L, Ormandy CJ, Kopchick JJ, *et al.* The role of prolactin and growth hormone in mammary gland development. *Mol Cell Endocrinol.* 2002; 197:127-31.

Kim H, Yoon M, Lee J, Penninger J, Kong Y. Osteoprotegerin ligand induces beta-casein gene expression through the transcription factor CCAAT/enhancer-binding protein beta. *J Biol Chem.* 2000; 277:5339–44.

Korach K, Couse J, Curtis S, Washburn T, Lindzey J, Kimbro K, *et al.* Estrogen receptor gene disruption: molecular characterization and experimental and clinical phenotypes. *Recent Progr Horm Res.* 1996; 51:159-86.

Kovacs C, Kronenberg H. Maternal-fetal calcium and bone metabolism during pregnancy, puerperium, and lactation. *Endocr Rev.* 1997; 18:832–72.

Kowenz-Leutz E, Twamley G, Ansieau S, Leutz A. Novel mechanism of C/EBP beta (NF-M) transcriptional control: Activation through derepression. *Genes Dev.* 1994; 8: 2781–91.

Kratochwil K. In vitro analysis of the hormonal basis for sexual dimorphism in the embryonic development of the mouse mammary gland. *J Embryol Exp Morphol.* 1971; 25:141-53.

Kratochwil K, Schwartz P. Tissue interaction in androgen response of embryonic mammary rudiment of mouse: Identification of target tissue for testosterone. *Proc Natl Acad Sci USA*. 1976; 73:4041-44.

Kritikou E, Sharkey A, Abell K, Came P, Anderson E, Clarkson R. A dual, non-redundant, role for LIF as a regulator of development and STAT3-mediated cell death in mammary gland. *Development.* 2003; 130:3459–68.

Lacey D, Timms E, Tan H, Kelley M, Dunstan C, Burgess T, *et al.* Osteoprotegerin ligand is a cytokine that regulates osteoclast differentiation and activation. *Cell.* 1998; 93:165–76.

Lanske B, Karaplis A, Lee K, Luz A, Vortkamp A, Pirro A, *et al.* PTH/PTHrP receptor in early development and Indian hedgehog-regulated bone growth. *Science.* 1996; 273:663-66.

Laurikkala J, Mikkola M, Mustonen T, Åberg T, Koppinen P, Pispa J, *et al.* TNF signaling via the ligand-receptor pair ectodysplasin and edar controls the function of epithelial signaling centers and is regulated by Wnt and activin during tooth organogenesis. *Dev Biol.* 2001; 229:443-55.

Laurikkala J, Pispa J, Jung H, Nieminen P, Mikkola M, Wang X, *et al.* Regulation of hair follicle development by the TNF signal ectodysplasin and its receptor Edar. *Development.* 2002; 129(10): 2541-53.

Lee Y, Streuli C. Extracellular matrix selectively modulates the response of mammary epithelial cells to different soluble signaling ligands. *J Biol Chem.* 1999; 274:22401–8.

Lekstrom-Himes J, Xanthopoulos K. Biological role of the CCAAT/enhancer-binding protein family of transcription factors. *J Biol Chem.* 1998; 273:28545–48.

Lewis E. A gene complex controlling segmentation in Drosophila. *Nature.* 1978; 276:565-70.

Li G, Robinson G, Lesche R, Martinez-Diaz H, Jiang Z, Rozengurt N. Conditional loss of PTEN leads to precocious development and neoplasia in the mammary gland. *Development.* 2002; 129:4159–70.

Li M, Liu X, Robinson G, Bar-Peled U, Wagner K, Young W. Mammary-derived signals activate programmed cell death during the first stage of mammary gland involution. *Proc Natl Acad Sci USA*. 1997; 94:3425–30.

Liao L, Kuang S-Q, Yuan Y, Gonzalez SM, O'Malley BW, Xu J. Molecular structure and biological function of the cancer-amplified nuclear receptor coactivator SRC-3/AIB1. *J Steroid Biochem Mol Biol.* 2002; 83(1-5):3-14.

Linzell J. Mammary gland blood flow and methods of identifying and measuring precursors of milk. In: Larsen B (ed.). *Lactation.* New York: Academic Press; 1974. p.143-225.

Liu X, Gallego M, Smith G, Robinson G, Hennighausen L. Functional rescue of Stat5a-null mammary tissue through the activation of compensating signals including Stat5b. *Cell Growth Differ.* 1998; 9:795–803.

Liu X, Robinson G, Wagner K, Garrett L, Wynshaw-Boris A, Hennighausen L. Stat5a is mandatory for adult mammary gland development and lactogenesis. *Genes Dev.* 1997; 11:179–86.

Lund L, Romer J, Thomasset N, Solberg H, Pyke C, Bissell M. Two distinct phases of apoptosis in mammary gland involution: proteinase-independent and –dependent pathways. *Development.* 1996; 122:181–93.

Luo J, Miller M. Ethanol enhances erbB-mediated migration of human breast cancer cells in culture. *Breast Cancer Res Treat.* 2000; 63:61–69.

Lydon J, DeMayo F, Funk C, Mani S, Hughes A, Montgomery C, *et al.* Mice lacking progesterone receptor exhibit pleiotropic reproductive abnormalities. *Genes Dev.* 1995; 9:2266–78.

Mailleux A, Spencer-Dene B, Dillon C, Ndiaye D, Savona-Baron C. Role of FGF10/FGFR2b signaling during mammary gland development in the mouse embryo. *Development.* 2002; 129:53–60.

Mao B, Wu W, Davidson G, Marhold J, Li M, Mechler B, *et al.* Kremen proteins are Dickkopf receptors that regulate Wnt/beta-catenin signalling. *Nature.* 2002; 417:664-67.

Marshman E, Green K, Flint D, White A, Streuli C, Westwood M. Insulin-like growth factor binding protein 5 and apoptosis in mammary epithelial cells. *J Cell Sci.* 2003; 116:675–82.

Martinez-Hernandez A, Fink L, Pierce G. Removal of basement membrane in the involuting breast. *Lab Invest.* 1976; 34:455–62.

Maytin E, Habener J. Transcription factors C/EBP alpha, C/EBP beta, and CHOP (Gadd153) expressed during the differentiation program of keratinocytes in vitro and in vivo. *J Invest Dermatol.* 1998; 110:238–46.

McKnight S. McBindall—A better name for CCAAT/enhancer binding proteins? *Cell.* 2001; 107:259–61.

Mepham TB (ed.). *Biochemistry of lactation.* Amsterdam: Elsevier; 1983.

Metcalfe A, Gilmore A, Klinowska T, Oliver J, Valentijn A, Brown R. Developmental regulation of Bcl-2 family protein expression in the involuting mammary gland. *J Cell Sci.* 1999; 112:1771–83.

Mikkola M, Pispa J, Pekkanen M, Paulin L, Nieminen P, Kere J, *et al.* Ectodysplasin, a protein required for epithelial morphogenesis, is a novel TNF homologue and promotes cell-matrix adhesion. *Mech Dev.* 1999; 88:133-46.

Mikkola M, Thesleff I. Ectodysplasin signaling in development. *Cytokine Growth Factor Rev.* 2003; 14:211-24.

Miller J. The Wnts. *Genome Biol.* 2002; 3:3001.1–1.15.

Miyoshi K, Shillingford J, Smith G, Grimm S, Wagner K, Oka T, *et al.* Signal transducer and activator transcription 5 (Stat5) controls the specification and proliferation of mammary alveolar epithelium. *J Cell Biol.* 2001; 155:531-42.

Moorehead R, Fata J, Johnson M, Khokha R. Inhibition of mammary epithelial apoptosis and sustained phosphorylation of Akt/PKB in MMTV-IGF-II transgenic mice. *Cell Death Differ.* 2001; 8:16–29.

Mori S, Nishikawa S, Yokota Y. Lactation defect in mice lacking the helix-loop-helix inhibitor Id2. L *EMBO J.* 2000; 19:5772–81.

Mulac-Jericevic B, Lydon J, DeMayo F, Conneely O. Defective mammary gland morphogenesis in mice lacking the progesterone receptor B isoform. *Proc Natl Acad Sci USA.* 2003; 100: 9744–49.

Mulac-Jericevic B, Mullinax R, DeMayo F, Lydon J, Conneely O. Subgroup of reproductive functions of progesterone mediated by progesterone receptor-B isoform. *Science.* 2000; 289:1751–54.

Muraoka R, Lenferink A, Simpson J, Brantley D, Roebuck L, Yakes F, *et al.* Cyclin-dependent kinase inhibitor p27(Kip1) is required for mouse mammary gland morphogenesis and function. *J Cell Biol.* 2001; 153:917–32.

Mustonen T, Pispa J, Mikkola M, Pummila M, Kangas A, Pakkasjarv L, *et al.* Stimulation of ectodermal organ development by Ectodysplasin A1. *Dev Biol.* 2003; 259:123-36.

Neville M. Physiology of lactation. *Clin Perinatol.* 1999; 26:251–79.

Nguyen A, Pollard J. Transforming growth factor beta3 induces cell death during the first stage of mammary gland involution. *Development.* 2000; 127:3107–18.

Niehrs C. Solving a sticky problem. *Nature.* 2001; 413:787-88.

Oftedal O. The mammary gland and its origin during synapsid evolution. *J Mammary Gland Biol Neoplasia.* 2002; 7:225-52.

Ormandy C, Camus A, Barra J, Damotte J, Lucas B, Buteau H, *et al.* Null mutation of the prolactin receptor gene produces multiple reproductive defects in the mouse. *Genes Dev.* 1997; 11:167–78.

Ornitz D, Itoh N. Fibroblast growth factors. *Genome Biology.* 2001; 2:1-12.

Ornitz D, Xu J, Colvin J, McEwen D, MacArthur C, Coulier F, *et al.* Receptor specificity of the fibroblast growth factor family. *J Biol Chem.* 1996; 271:15292-97.

Osada S, Yamamoto H, Nishihara T, Imagawa M. DNA binding specificity of the CCAAT/enhancer-binding protein transcription factor family. *J Biol Chem.* 1996; 271:3891–96.

Ossipow V, Descombes P, Schibler U. CCAAT/enhancer-binding protein mRNA is translated into multiple proteins with different transcription activation potentials. *Proc Natl Acad Sci USA.* 1993; 90:8219–23.

Owen G, Richer J, Tung L, Takimoto G, Horwitz K. Progesterone regulates transcription of the p21(WAF1) cyclin dependent kinase inhibitor gene through Sp1 and CBP/p300. *J Biol Chem.* 1998; 273:10696-701.

Papaioannou V. T-box genes in development: from hydra to humans. *Int Rev Cytol.* 2001; 207:1–70.

Philp J, Burdon T, Watson C. Differential regulation of members of the family of signal transducers and activators of transcription during mammary gland development. *Biochem Soc Trans.* 1996; 24:370S.

Phippard D, Weber-Hall S, Sharpe P, Naylor M, Jayatalake H, Maas R, *et al.* Regulation of Msx-1, Msx-2, Bmp-2 and Bmp-4 during foetal and postnatal mammary gland development. *Development.* 1996; 122:2729-37.

Pispa J, Thesleff I. Mechanisms of ectodermal organogenesis. *Dev Biol.* 2003; 262:195–205.

Platonova N, Scotti M, Babich P, Bertoli G, Mento E, Meneghini V, *et al.* TBX3, the gene mutated in ulnar-mammary syndrome, promotes growth of mammary epithelial cells via repression of p19ARF, independently of p53. *Cell Tissue Res.* 2007; 328:301–16.

Potten C, Watson R, Williams G, Tickle S, Roberts S, Harris M. The effect of age and menstrual cycle upon proliferative activity of the normal human breast. *Br J Cancer.* 1988; 58:163–70.

Prince J, Klinowska T, Marshman E, Lowe E, Mayer U, Miner J. Cell-matrix interactions during development and apoptosis of the mouse mammary gland in vivo. *Dev Dyn.* 2002; 223:497–516.

Propper A. Wandering epithelial cells in the rabbit embryo milk line. A preliminary scanning electron microscope study. *Dev Biol.* 1978; 67:225-31.

Qin C, Singh P, Safe S. Transcriptional activation of insulin like growth factor-binding protein-4 by 17beta-estradiol in MCF-7 cells: role of estrogen receptor-Sp1 complexes. *Endocrinology.* 1999; 140:2501-8.

Ramji D, Foka P. CCAAT/enhancer-binding proteins: Structure, function and regulation. *Biochem J.* 2002; 365:561–75.

Ratajczak T. Protein coregulators that mediate estrogen receptor function. *Reprod Fertil Dev.* 2001; 13(4):221-29.

Raught B, Liao W, Rosen J. Developmentally and hormonally regulated CCAAT/enhancer-binding protein isoforms influence beta-casein gene expression. *Mol Endocrinol.* 1995; 9:1223–32.

Robinson G. Identification of signalling pathways in early mammary gland development by mouse genetics. *Breast Cancer Res.* 2004; 6:105-8.

Robinson G, Hennighausen L, Johnson P. Side-branching in the mammary gland: the progesterone-Wnt connection. *Genes Dev.* 2000; 14:889–94.

Robinson G, Johnson P, Hennighausen L, Sterneck E. The C/EBPbeta transcription factor regulates epithelial cell proliferation and differentiation in the mammary gland. *Genes Dev.* 1998; 12:1907–16.

Robinson G, Karpf A, Kratochwil K. Regulation of mammary gland development by tissue interaction. *J Mammary Gland Biol Neoplasia.* 1999; 4:9-19.

Robinson G, McKnight R, Smith G, Hennighausen L. Mammary epithelial cells undergo secretory differentiation in cycling virgins but require pregnancy for the establishment of terminal differentiation. *Development.* 1995; 121:2079-90.

Rosen J, Wyszomierski S, Hadsell D. Regulation of milk protein gene expression. *Annu Rev Nutr.* 1999; 19:407–36.

Rosen J, Zahnow C, Kazansky A, Raught B. Composite response elements mediate hormonal and developmental regulation of milk protein gene expression. *Biochem Soc Symp.* 1998; 63:101–13.

Ross F. RANKing the importance of measles virus in Paget's disease. *J Clin Invest.* 2000; 105:555-58.

Sabatakos G, Davies G, Grosse M, Cryer A, Ramji D. Expression of the genes encoding CCAAT-enhancer binding protein isoforms in the mouse mammary gland during lactation and involution. *Biochem J.* 1998; 334:205–10.

Sakakura T. Mammary embryogenesis. In: Neville M, Daniel C. *The mammary gland, development, regulation and function.* New York: Plenum Press; 1987. p. 37-65.

Sartor C, Zhou H, Kozlowska E, Guttridge K, Kawata E. Her4 mediates ligand-dependent antiproliferative and differentiation responses in human breast cancer cells. *Mol Cell Biol.* 2001; 21:4265–75.

Satoh K, Ginsburg J, Vonderhaar B. Msx-1 and Msx-2 in mammary gland development. *J Mammary Gland Biol Neoplasia.* 2004; 9:195-205.

Satoh K, Hovey R, Malewski T, Warri A, Saito K, Goldhar A, *et al.* Progesterone enhances branching morphogenesis in the mouse mammary gland by increased expression of Msx2. *Oncogene.* 2007; in press.

Satokata I, Ma L, Ohshima H, Bei M, Woo I, Nishizawa K, *et al.* Msx2 deficiency in mice causes pleiotropic defects in bone growth and ectodermal organ formation. *Nat Genet.* 2000; 24:391-95.

Satokata I, Maas R. Msx1 deficient mice exhibit cleft palate and abnormalities of craniofacial and tooth development. *Nat Genet.* 1994; 6:348-56.

Schere-Levy C, Buggiano V, Quaglino A, Gattelli A, Cirio M, Piazzon I. Leukemia inhibitory factor induces apoptosis of the mammary epithelial cells and participates in mouse mammary gland involution. *Exp Cell Res.* 2003; 282:35–47.

Schwertfeger K, Richert M, Anderson S. Mammary gland involution is delayed by activated Akt in transgenic mice. *Mol Endocrinol.* 2001; 15:867–81.

Seagroves T, Krnacik S, Raught B, Gay J, Burgess-Beusse B, Darlington G, *et al.* C/EBPβ, but not C/EBPα, is essential for ductal morphogenesis, lobuloalveolar proliferation, and functional differentiation in the mouse mammary gland. *Genes Dev.* 1998; 12:1917–28.

Sherr C, Roberts J. CDK inhibitors: positive and negative regulators of G1-phase progression. *Genes Dev.* 1999; 13:1501–12.

Shillingford J, Hennighausen L. Experimental mouse genetics—Answering fundamental questions about mammary gland biology. *Trends Endocrinol Metab.* 2001; 12:402–8.

Sicinski P, Donaher J, Parker S, Li T, Fazeli A, Gardner H, *et al.* Cyclin D1 provides a link between development and oncogenesis in the retina and breast. *Cell.* 1995; 82:621–30.

Srivastava S, Matsuda M, Hou Z, Bailey J, Kitazawa R, Herbst M, *et al.* Receptor activator of NF-κB ligand induction via Jak2 and Stat5a in mammary epithelial cells. *J Biol Chem.* 2003; 278:46171–78.

Sterneck E, Tessarollo L, Johnson P. An essential role for C/EBPbeta in female reproduction. *Genes Dev.* 1997; 11:2153–62.

Strange R, Li F, Saurer S, Burkhardt A, Friis R. Apoptotic cell death and tissue remodelling during mouse mammary gland involution. *Development.* 1992; 115:49–58.

Takeuchi J, Koshiba-Takeuchi K, Suzuki T, Kamimura M, Ogura K, Ogura T. Tbx5 and Tbx4 trigger limb initiation through activation of the Wnt/Fgf signaling cascade. *Development.* 2003; 130(12): 2729–39.

Takiguchi M. The C/EBP family of transcription factors in the liver and other organs. *Int J Exp Pathol.* 1998; 79:369–91.

Teglund S, McKay C, Schuetz E, van Deursen J, Stravopodis D, Wang D, *et al.* Stat5a and Stat5b proteins have essential and nonessential, or redundant, roles in cytokine responses. *Cell Growth Differ.* 1998; 93:841 50.

Tidcombe H, Jackson-Fisher A, Mathers K, Stern D, Gassmann M. Neural and mammary gland defects in ErbB4 knockout mice genetically rescued from embryonic lethality. *Proc Natl Acad Sci USA.* 2003; 100:8281–86.

Tomic S, Chughtai N, Ali S. SOCS-1, -2, -3: selective targets and functions downstream of the prolactin receptor. *Mol Cell Endocrinol.* 1999; 158:45-54.

Tonner E, Barber M, Allan G, Beattie J, Webster J, Whitelaw C. Insulin-like growth factor binding protein-5 (IGFBP-5) induces premature cell death in the mammary glands of transgenic mice. *Development.* 2002; 129:4547–57.

Tonner E, Barber M, Travers M, Logan A, Flint D. Hormonal control of insulin-like growth factor-binding protein-5 production in the involuting mammary gland of the rat. *Endocrinology.* 1997; 138:5101–7.

Tonner E, Quarrie L, Travers M, Barber M, Logan A, Wilde C. Does an IGF-binding protein (IGFBP) present in involuting rat mammary gland regulate apoptosis? *Prog Growth Factor Res.* 1995; 6:409–14.

Turashvili G, Bouchal J, Burkadze G, Kolar Z. Wnt signaling pathway in mammary gland development and carcinogenesis. *Pathobiology.* 2006; 73:213–23.

Turner C, Gomez E. The normal development of the mammary gland of the male and female albino mouse. I. Intrauterine. *Mo Agric Exp Stn Res Bull.* 1933; 182:3–20.

van Genderen C, Okumura R, Farina, I, Quo R, Parslow T, Bruhn L, *et al.* Development of several organs that require inductive epithelial–mesenchymal interactions is impaired in LEF-1-deficient mice. *Genes Dev.* 1994; 8(22):2691-2703.

Veltmaat J, Mailleux A, Thiery J, Bellusci S. Mouse embryonic mammogenesis as a model for the molecular regulation of pattern formation. *Differentiation.* 2003; 71:1-17.

Veltmaat J, Van Veelen W, Thiery J, Bellusci S. Identification of the mammary line in mouse by Wnt10b expression. *Dev Dyn.* 2004; 229(2):349-56.

Vorbach C, Capecchi MR, Penninger JM. Evolution of the mammary gland from the innate immune system? *Bioessays.* 2006; 28:606-16.

Walker N, Bennett R, Kerr J. Cell death by apoptosis during involution of the lactating breast in mice and rats. *Am J Anat.* 1989; 185:19–32.

Wang Y, Sassoon D. Ectoderm-mesenchyme and mesenchyme-mesenchyme interactions regulate Msx-1 expression and cellular differentiation in the murine limb bud. *Dev Biol.* 1995; 168:374-82.

Weir E, Philbrick W, Amling M, Neff L, Baron R, Broadus A. Targeted overexpression of parathyroid hormone related peptide in chondrocytes causes chondrodysplasia and delayed endochondral bone formation. *Proc Natl Acad Sci USA.* 1996; 93:10240-45.

Welm A, Timchenko N, Darlington G. C/EBPalpha regulates generation of C/EBPbeta isoforms through activation of specific proteolytic cleavage. *Mol Cell Biol.* 1999; 19:1695–1704.

Wernig F, Mayr M, Xu Q. Mechanical stretch-induced apoptosis in smooth muscle cells is mediated by beta1-integrin signaling pathways. *Hypertension.* 2003; 41:903–11.

Wiesen J, Young P, Werb Z, Cunha G. Signaling through the stromal epidermal growth factor receptor is necessary for mammary ductal development. *Development.* 1999; 126:335-44.

Williams S, Baer M, Dillner J, Johnson P. CRP2 (C/EBP beta) contains a bipartite regulatory domain that controls transcriptional activation, DNA binding and cell specificity. *Embo J.* 1995; 14:3170–83.

Wong B, Rho J, Arron J, Robinson E, Orlinick J, Chao M, *et al.* TRANCE is a novel ligand of the tumor necrosis factor receptor family that activates c-Jun N-terminal kinase in T cells. *J Biol Chem.* 1997; 272:25190–94.

Wysolmerski J, Cormier S, Philbrick W, Dann P, Zhang J, Roume J, *et al.* Absence of functional type 1 parathyroid hormone (PTH)/PTH-related protein receptors in humans is associated with abnormal breast development and tooth impaction. *J Clin Endocrinol Metab.* 2001; 86:1788-94.

Wyszomierski S, Rosen J. Cooperative effects of STAT5 (signal transducer and activator of transcription 5) and C/EBPbeta (CCAAT/enhancer-binding protein-beta) on beta-casein gene transcription are mediated by the glucocorticoid receptor. *Mol Endocrinol.* 2001; 15:228–40.

Xu J, Li Q. Review of the in vivo functions of the p160 steroid receptor coactivator family. *Mol Endocrinol.* 2003; 17(9):1681-92.

Xu J, Liao L, Ning G, Yoshida-Komiya H, Deng C, O'Malley BW. The steroid receptor coactivator SRC-3 (p/CIP/ RAC3/ AIB1/ACTR/TRAM-1) is required for normal growth, puberty, female reproductive function, and mammary gland development. *Proc Natl Acad Sci USA.* 2000; 97:6379–84.

Xu J, Qiu Y, DeMayo F, Tsai S, Tsai M, O'Malley B. Partial hormone resistance in mice with disruption of the steroid receptor coactivator-1 (SRC-1) gene. *Science.* 1998; 279:1922–25.

Yasuda H, Shima N, Nakagawa N, Yamaguchi K, Kinosaki M, Mochizuki S, *et al.* Osteoclast differentiation factor is a ligand for osteoprotegerin/osteoclastogenesis-inhibitory factor and is identical to TRANCE/RANKL. *Proc Natl Acad Sci USA.* 1998; 95:3597–3602.

Yeh W, Cao Z, Classon M, McKnight S. Cascade regulation of terminal adipocyte differentiation by three members of the C/EBP family of leucine zipper proteins. *Genes Dev.* 1995; 9:168–81.

Zahnow C, Cardiff R, Laucirica R, Medina D, Rosen J. A role for CCAAT/enhancer binding protein beta-liver-enriched inhibitory protein in mammary epithelial cell proliferation. *Cancer Res.* 2001; 61:261–69.

Zhang, D, Sliwkowski M, Mark M, Frantz G, Akita R. Neuregulin-3 (NRG3): A novel neural tissue-enriched protein that binds and activates ErbB4. *Proc Natl Acad Sci USA.* 1997; 94: 9562–67.

Zhao L, Melenhorst J, Hennighausen L. Loss of interleukin 6 results in delayed mammary gland involution: a possible role for mitogen-activated protein kinase and not signal transducer and activator of transcription 3. *Mol Endocrinol.* 2002; 16:2902–12.

Zorn A. Wnt signalling: antagonistic Dickkopfs. *Curr Biol.* 2001; 11:R592-95.

Chapter 9

Oxytocin: Milk Ejection and Maternal-Infant Well-being

Danielle K. Prime, Donna T. Geddes, and Peter E. Hartmann

INTRODUCTION

The fundamental neurohormonal nature of the milk ejection reflex was not defined until 1941 (Ely *et al.*, 1941). Initially, it was thought that the period of milk ejection was the rapid and simultaneous synthesis and removal of milk, and that only a small amount was stored in the mammary gland. It is now understood that this is not the case. Milk is continuously synthesized within the lactating gland. If milk is not actively expelled by the process of milk ejection, the gland will undergo involution. For a more detailed representation of important research that has elucidated how we now understand milk secretion and milk removal, see Chapter 1.

Oxytocin is the key hormone involved in the process of milk ejection [also known as the draught (in women) or let-down (in cows) reflex]. A functioning milk ejection reflex is essential for successful lactation in women. Without it, milk is not removed from the gland, the infant is not satiated, and milk synthesis is inhibited (Peaker *et al.*, 1996). Furthermore, milk accumulating in the breast over extended periods of time may lead to engorgement and predispose the mother to nipple damage, mastitis, and breast abscess (Wilson-Clay *et al.*, 2002).

This chapter will discuss the hormone oxytocin, the milk ejection reflex, the effect this reflex has on the mammary gland, and the stimuli that cause both the release and inhibition of oxytocin. Further, the involvement of oxytocin in a broad range of physiological effects in both women and men has stimulated intense research of this hormone, thus, the final part of this chapter will examine current knowledge in this rapidly expanding area of interest.

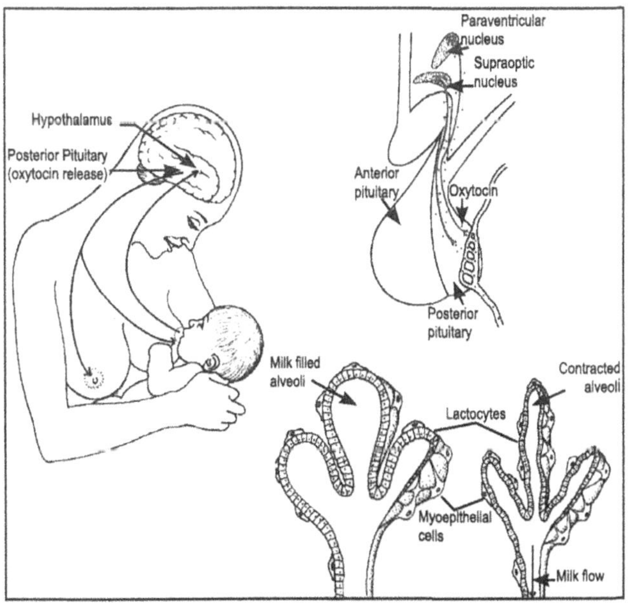

Figure 1. The milk ejection reflex. The neurohormonal reflex is initiated by stimulation of the nipple, sending neural impulses to the hypothalamus and the consequent release of oxytocin from the posterior pituitary into the maternal circulation. Oxytocin causes the contraction of the myoepithelial cells surrounding the milk filled alveoli in the breasts. Contraction of the alveoli moves milk into the collecting ducts and milk flows forward to the nipple.

MILK EJECTION REFLEX

The milk ejection reflex is defined as a neurohormonal reflex which is primarily triggered by the tactile stimulation of the nipple, resulting in neural impulses being transmitted to the hypothalamus, and the neurohypophysial release of oxytocin into the systemic circulation. Oxytocin then causes the contraction of myoepithelial cells surrounding the alveoli in the breast, moving milk into the collecting ducts, and expanding these ducts as milk moves forward to the nipple (**Figure 1**) (Ramsay *et al.*, 2004).

The milk ejection reflex has two components, neural and hormonal. The neural component involves stimuli, such as tactile stimulation of the nipple, and the sensory nerves of the nipple that transmit impulses via the spinothalamic tract to the brain stem. These nerves synapse at the hypothalamus, then travel down the hypothalamo-neurohypophysial tract to the posterior lobe of the pituitary where the hormone oxytocin is released into the maternal circulation (Crowley *et al.*, 1992). It is important to note that the reflex can be triggered by conditioned responses in the absence of suckling. For example, the milk ejection reflex may be stimulated by the emotional response of the mother to her baby's cry.

Oxytocin is a small peptide hormone of nine amino acids (**Figure 2**) and is produced by cleaving a 30 kD preprohormone that is synthesized in the magnocellular neurons of the supraoptic and paraventricular nuclei of the hypothalamus. The preprohormone, which consists of neurophysin, a signal peptide, and the oxytocin component, undergoes cleavage and modification steps whereby it is converted to secretory granules which are then transported down the magnocellular neurons to the posterior pituitary where the completed form of oxytocin can be released (Brownstein *et al.*, 1980; Mohr *et al.*, 1992).

The posterior pituitary stores of oxytocin are well in excess of that physiologically required for milk ejection (Lincoln *et al.*, 1982; Lincoln, 1984). When the neural pathway is triggered, oxytocin is released from the posterior pituitary into the maternal circulation. The hormone then binds to the appropriate receptors which, in the case of milk ejection, are located on both the ductal epithelium and the myoepithelial cells surrounding the milk-filled alveoli of the lactating mammary gland (Kimura *et al.*, 1998).

The binding of oxytocin to the receptors on the myoepithelial cells causes the contraction of these cells which surround the alveoli and contain the synthesized milk (**Figure 3**). This contraction forces the milk from the alveoli toward the nipple. As the milk enters the collecting ducts, it causes the intra-ductal pressure (Cobo *et al.*, 1967) to increase and the ducts to expand in diameter (**Figure 4**) (Ramsay *et al.*, 2004).

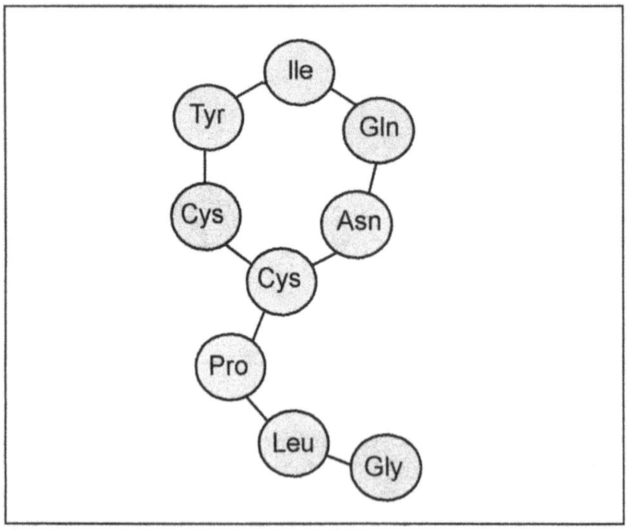

Figure 2. The molecular structure of oxytocin. Oxytocin is comprised of nine amino acids (Cysteine, Tyrosine, Isoleucine, Glutamine, Asparagine, Cysteine, Proline, Leucine, Glycine).

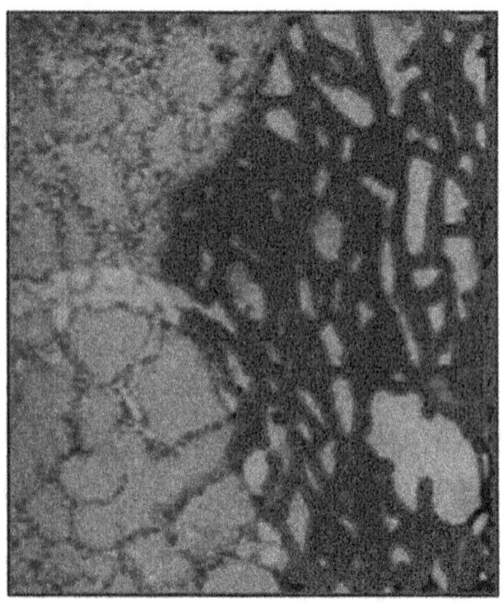

Figure 3. A section of rat mammary gland demonstrating full alveoli on the left and contracted alveoli on the right. Contraction of the alveoli was achieved by local injection of oxytocin (Molenaar *et al.*, 1992).

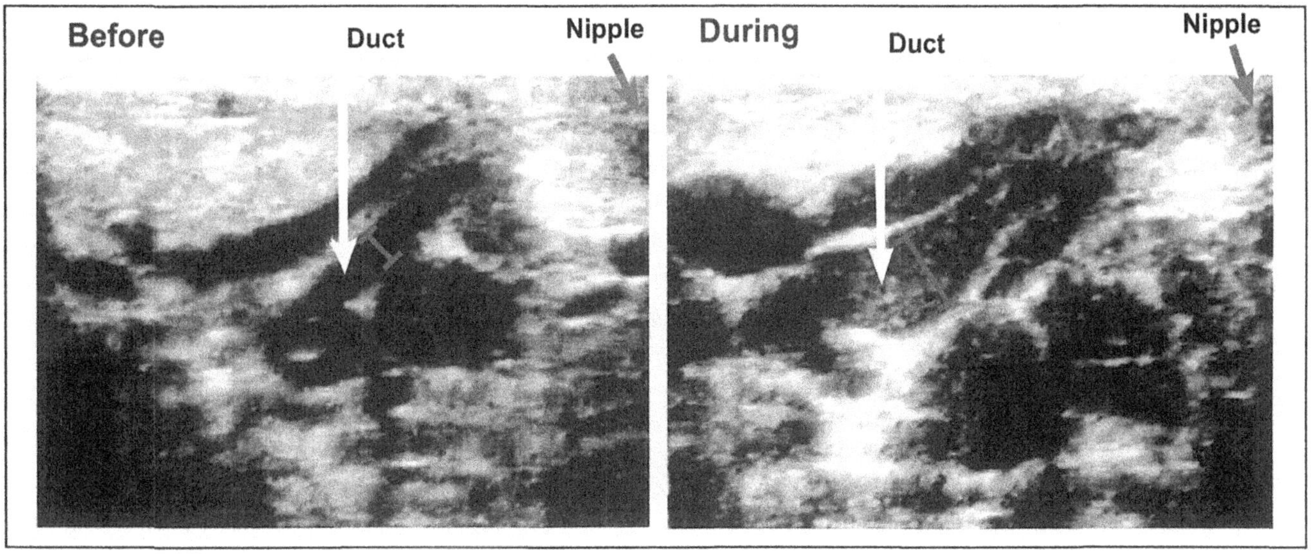

Figure 4. **Milk duct diameter before and at milk ejection as imaged by ultrasound. The ducts are shown as black tubular structures within the breast. At milk ejection, the milk duct expands and milk flows towards the nipple. White flecks within the duct represent fat globules in the milk (Ramsay *et al.*, 2004).**

MILK EJECTION

Milk ejection is referred to as the period of time when there is an increase in the availability of milk from the nipple as a result of stimulation of the milk ejection reflex. Milk ejection can sometimes be observed in women as milk 'dripping' or 'squirting' from the nipple. A milk ejection episode lasts for approximately two minutes, and multiple milk ejections during milk removal are common (Cobo, 1993; Ramsay *et al.*, 2004).

In women expressing their milk with a breast pump, milk ejection can easily be observed and measured by discrete increases in the rate of flow of milk from the nipple (**Figure 5**). It is not possible to measure this flow rate increase during breastfeeding; however, infant behavior can alter the milk ejection episode in that the frequency of audible 'swallowing' increases in response to increased milk flow rate. There is wide variation in the milk flow rate, timing, and pattern of milk ejections between mothers. It is interesting that the infant is generally able to adapt to both variable milk flow rates and timing of milk ejection during breastfeeding.

The intensity of the sensation of milk ejection varies dramatically between women, with some experiencing strong pain while others feel nothing. Clinical observations have described the sensation of milk ejection as tingling, pins and needles, a 'drawing' feeling, a 'rushing down' feeling, and a kind of pain that will begin sharply and then gradually decrease. Furthermore, feelings of nausea, intestinal colic, and vaginal bleeding have been associated with the sensation. The sensation of milk ejection tends to coincide with lactogenesis II (Secretory Activation) and becomes more regular in the month after birth. Occasionally, a mother may sense more than one milk ejection during the period of milk removal (Isbister, 1954).

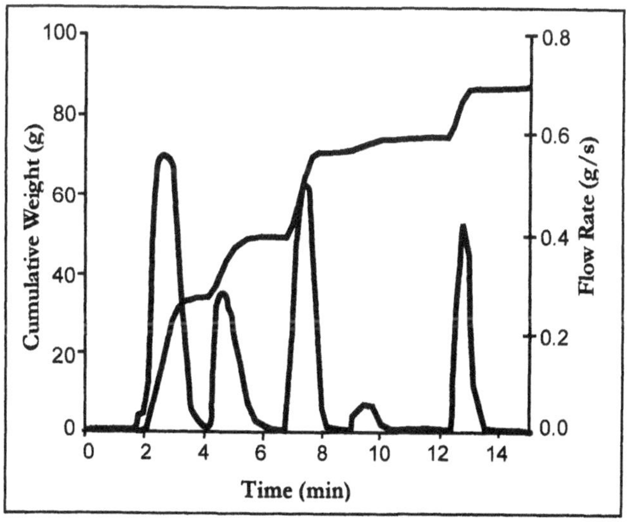

Figure 5. **Graph demonstrating milk flow from the right breast during expression. The black line represents the cumulative weight of the milk. Acute changes in the slope of this line are representative of milk ejection. The blue line is the derivative of the cumulative weight measurement. The derivative clearly demonstrates the increase and decrease in milk flow rate associated with milk ejection.**

EFFECTS ON THE MAMMARY GLAND

The human mammary gland consists of an average of nine milk ducts which rapidly branch under the areola and into the breast tissue, which consists of both glandular and adipose tissues (Ramsay *et al.*, 2005) (Chapter 2). These ducts continue to branch and get progressively smaller until they connect to alveoli which are surrounded by a basket-like mesh of myoepithelial cells. The alveoli contain lactocytes (mammary secretory epithelial cells) that synthesize breastmilk.

During a milk ejection episode, the contraction of myoepithelial cells increases the pressure within the ducts, causing them to distend. Various peptides have been identified in the nerves of the mammary gland which promote relaxation and contraction of the ducts. These peptides may allow some local control of the milk ejection reflex, facilitating some milk transfer, even in stressful situations (Eriksson *et al.*, 1996; Uvnas-Moberg *et al.*, 1996).

Many studies have measured oxytocin levels in blood, but this technique is difficult as oxytocin has a short half-life of approximately two minutes, is inactivated in the blood by oxytocinases, and is released in sporadic bursts. Therefore, to accurately measure oxytocin during both breastfeeding and breast expression, serial blood sampling at short intervals is necessary. Furthermore, the concentration of the hormone is dependent upon the site of blood sampling. For example, oxytocin is found in higher concentrations in the jugular vein compared to the peripheral circulation (Newton, 1978; Schams, 1983; Robinson, 1985).

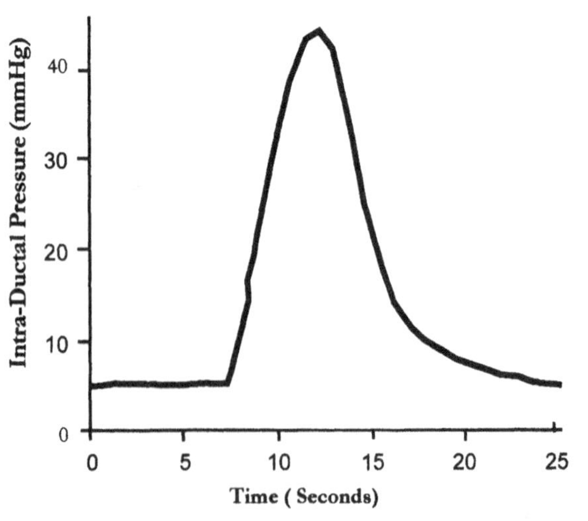

Figure 6. The increase and decrease in intra-ductal (intra-mammary) pressure associated with milk ejection in the sow (J Kent, personal communication).

Researchers have utilized the change in intra-ductal pressure (also known as intra-mammary pressure) to monitor milk ejection and oxytocin release with a methodology involving catherterization of one or more nipple ducts (Cobo *et al.*, 1967; Cobo, 1968; Alekseev *et al.*, 1998). There is a transient increase and decrease in pressure that lasts for the duration of a milk ejection episode (**Figure 6**) (Kent *et al.*, 2003). This technique is not widely employed as it is invasive and carries the risk of infection. Since the milk ejection reflex can be inhibited by stressors, it is possible that measurements of both intra-ductal pressure and oxytocin blood levels may be influenced in both this method and blood sampling.

Recently, a method that utilizes the noninvasive technique of ultrasound has been developed to measure milk ejection by monitoring milk duct diameter changes in the breast that is not suckled (Ramsay *et al.*, 2004). During milk ejection, duct diameter increases as the pressure in the duct rises, and subsequently, the duct decreases in size as the pressure reduces at the end of a milk ejection episode. As with the intra-ductal pressure measurements, defined peaks in duct diameter are observed which have been characterized as milk ejections (**Figure 4**).

It was further found that during expression with an electric breast pump, intermittent periods of increased milk flow from the nipple were observed. It is therefore logical to assume that as intra-ductal pressure increases at milk ejection, duct diameter will increase in response, and milk flow from the nipple will increase. Indeed, it has been demonstrated that there is a correlation between an increase in duct diameter and an increase in milk flow from the nipple (Ramsay *et al.*, 2006). Therefore, this is a noninvasive methodology that can be used to measure milk ejection episodes in women expressing milk (**Figure 5**).

The studies to date have assumed that measurement of the unsuckled or non-expressed breast is representative of milk ejection in the opposite breast. Indeed, using the milk flow technique, preliminary results (n=10) confirm that synchrony of milk ejection in both breasts occurs 92% of the time during double pumping (Prime *et al.*, 2006) (**Figure 7**). In addition, mothers (n=13) chose similar vacuum settings for both breasts and milk was removed from the left and right

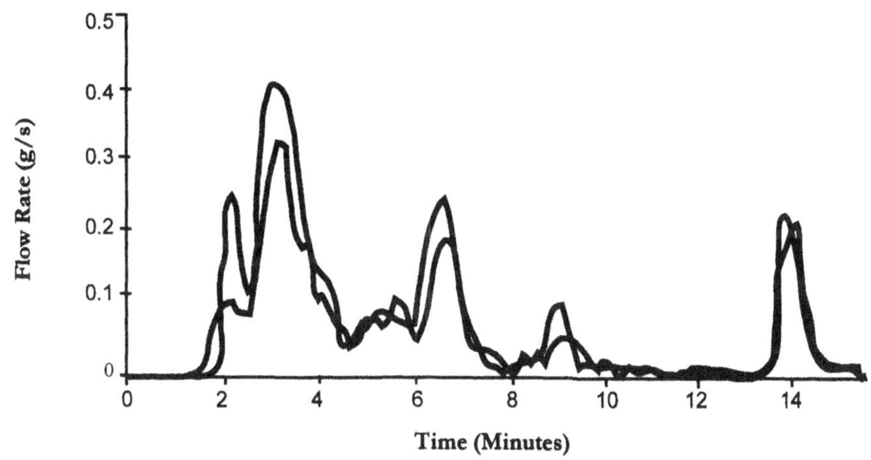

Figure 7. Graph demonstrating the rate of milk flow from the left (blue) and right (black) breasts during simultaneous breast expression. Peaks in milk flow rate associated with milk ejection, and occur simultaneously in both breasts (Prime *et al.*, 2006).

breasts at a similar rate during simultaneous expression (Prime *et al.*, 2007). These results indicate that the left and right breasts respond in a comparable manner and therefore the measurement of one breast can indeed be a good indicator of how both breasts are functioning.

In conclusion, the measurement of milk flow rate during expression can be used as a valid and inexpensive method for identifying milk ejection. In addition, the technique enables the investigation of the patterns of milk ejection and milk removal in pump-dependent mothers. This is of particular interest for mothers of premature infants where effective milk removal is imperative to maintain lactation.

Table 1. Location of Oxytocin Receptors in Human Tissues as Determined by Oxytocin Binding

Female reproductive system	Myometrium, endometrium, amnion, chorion, decidua, ovary, corpus luteum
Male reproductive system	Testis, epididymis, prostate gland
Central nervous system	Olfactory and limbic system, cortical areas, basal ganglia, thalamus, hypothalamus, brain stem, pituitary gland
Organs and cells	Kidney, heart, vascular endothelium, mammary gland, thymus, adiposites, pancreas, adrenal gland, osteoblasts, breast cancer cell lines

Adapted from Gimpl *et al.*, 2001

THE OXYTOCIN RECEPTOR

The oxytocin receptor is a 388-amino-acid polypeptide belonging to the G-protein-coupled seven transmembrane receptor superfamily (Kimura *et al.*, 1992; Kimura *et al.*, 2003). Oxytocin receptors have been found on both the myoepithelial cells and the ductal/glandular epithelium in the mammary gland (Kimura *et al.*, 1998) and in numerous places throughout the human body as shown in **Table 1**, illustrating the numerous possible effects of the hormone.

The presence of oxytocin receptors throughout the male and female body, as well as in the developing fetus, suggests that oxytocin has the potential to play a role in a vast range of physiological functions, in addition to the two well known functions of uterine and myoepithelial cell contraction. It has been hypothesized that the oxytocin receptors may play a role in switching on and off oxytocin target organs, depending on their relative concentration and that these concentrations are regulated by steroids (Soloff, 1985).

The human mammary gland has a very high sensitivity to oxytocin, with as little as 1 mU of intravenous oxytocin producing an intra-ductal pressure response typical of milk ejection (Cobo *et al.*, 1967). At parturition, oxytocin receptors in the uterus are massively up-regulated (Fuchs *et al.*, 1995; Kimura *et al.*, 1996). In the mammary gland of the rat, there is a gradual receptor up-regulation that reaches its maximum during lactation

(Soloff *et al.*, 1979). As yet, this change in oxytocin receptor concentration has not been demonstrated in humans. One study found no significant elevation of receptors when comparing non-lactating to lactating human mammary gland tissue specimens (Kimura *et al.*, 1998); however, the synthesis of milk proteins at the onset of lactation may have diluted the effect of the receptor up-regulation.

CIRCULATING OXYTOCIN AND PARTURITION

Once released into the circulation, little oxytocin can cross to the brain due to the blood-brain barrier; however, oxytocin can be directly released into the brain structures. The oxytocin release pattern can be different between the plasma and the different brain structures and plays a role in mediating certain behavioral characteristics in rats (Engelmann *et al.*, 2000). The basal levels of oxytocin (quantitated by radioimmunoassay) do not vary between men (1.5 ± 0.2 μU/mL), non-pregnant women (1.4 ± 0.2 μU/mL), and pregnant women before labor (1.3 ± 0.1 μU/mL), but do rise to 4.2 ± 1.1 μU/mL upon visualization of the fetal head at parturition (Leake *et al.*, 1981).

There is evidence that oxytocin is not the driving force for parturition in both humans and animals, but rather plays a role late in the second stage of labor. As is the case with milk ejection, there is an interaction between the mother and child during parturition. The fetal head dilating the cervix would most likely trigger the Ferguson reflex stimulating the mother to produce more oxytocin and facilitate expulsive contractions.

Although the role of oxytocin in the maternal circulation is greater in the late stages of labor, oxytocin is commonly used as an effective pharmacologic agent for the induction and augmentation of labor due to its uterotonic properties. The dramatic change in the uterus at parturition is still not well understood, but it is now known that oxytocin can be produced locally in tissues, such as the uterus and fetal membranes, and it may be these local interactions that are important for initiation of labor, rather than the circulating maternal oxytocin pulses (Smith *et al.*, 2006).

The uterus is most sensitive to oxytocin at parturition in all species, especially during the second stage of labor (Fuchs, 1985). However, the development of this sensitivity is different between species. Hormones, such as estrogen and progesterone, have been shown to regulate uterine sensitivity in a species dependent manner (Fuchs, 1985 {human}; Russell *et al.*, 2003 {rat}).

In this connection, it has been shown that women who deliver vaginally have more oxytocin pulses and a significant rise in prolactin compared to women delivering by cesarean section. Therefore, the second stage of labor may be important in coordinating these oxytocin pulses, which may also be influenced by the timing of the infant's first breastfeed, an event that is often delayed at a cesarean birth (Nissen *et al.*, 1996). It is now becoming more widely recognized that the interaction of mother and baby soon after birth can be very important for the regulation of infant physiology and behavior, such as infant crying, temperature, respiration, as well as the initiation and maintenance of breastfeeding (Winberg, 2005).

PATTERNS OF OXYTOCIN RELEASE AND MILK EJECTION

Oxytocin release has been well studied in the rat using intra-ductal pressure measurements. The rat pups will suckle the nipple for two to three hours, while the mother rat releases her milk in a pulsatile fashion to her pups every five to 15 minutes (Dyball *et al.*, 1986). During suckling, the rat pups undergo typical body movements termed the stretch reaction, elongating their bodies when the milk is made available to them. This pulsatile release, however, only occurs once the mother rat has fallen asleep (Wakerley *et al.*, 1973; Voloschin *et al.*, 1979; Voloschin *et al.*, 1984; Riggs *et al.*, 1985). Interestingly, a supraphysiological dose of oxytocin to the rat can depress the milk ejection reflex (Mena *et al.*, 1974).

The dairy industry has carried out extensive research in order to understand and maximize milk output of the dairy cow. Less than 20% of milk yield is available in cows before milk ejection, and this is stored in the milk cistern. In addition, continuously elevated oxytocin concentrations throughout the milking period are required for efficient milk removal. Two milk removal patterns have been characterized. The first is a bimodal milk flow where the cisternal milk is removed, and there is a delay until the ejection of the alveolar fraction. The second is a consistent flow without a delay between the two compartments (cisternal and alveolar), and this is achieved by pre-stimulation of the teat (Bruckmaier, 2005).

The sow has an enormous amount of control over the release of milk. Piglets suckle every 40 to 60 minutes, and only when the majority of piglets are attached does the milk ejection occur (Hartmann *et al.*, 1997). Milk ejection lasts between 4.8 and 11.8 seconds, and no milk can be removed from the sow outside of this short window of time (Kent *et al.*, 2003). Therefore, the pattern of oxytocin release is diverse between species, making it difficult to relate animal studies to women.

In women, oxytocin release has a circadian rhythm, more is released during the day compared to night (Forsling, 2000). Both significant milk ejecting activity post labor (Cobo, 1968), and spontaneous milk ejection between breastfeeds have been observed (Isbister, 1954; McNeilly *et al.*, 1978; Cobo, 1993). Suckling and expression induced oxytocin release have been described as uncoordinated and pulsatile, with discrete, short pulses (Cobo *et al.*, 1967; Ueda *et al.*, 1994). Intra ductal pressure recordings have demonstrated that it takes approximately 60 seconds of infant suckling before a rise in pressure (a milk ejection) is recorded. Multiple milk ejections have been reported, with one paper reporting a range of 1 to 17 contractions over a maximum duration of 25 minutes (Cobo, 1993), and another reporting 4 to 10 contractions per 10 minutes, with a single contraction having a duration of 50 to 150 seconds (Caldeyro-Barcia, 1968).

Ultrasound imaging has been used to monitor duct diameter during breastfeeding. The initial increase in duct diameter (milk ejection) was recorded within 56 seconds of the initiation of breastfeeding, and there were between 0 to 9 dilations (mean 2.5) detected during a breastfeed from a single breast (mean breastfeed duration: 6 minutes 40 seconds) (Ramsay *et al.*, 2004). Using an electric breast pump, the first milk ejection was stimulated on average after 90 seconds, and an average of 4.4 milk ejections were detected using ultrasound during 15 minutes of expression (Ramsay *et al.*, 2006).

The accuracy of mothers identifying milk ejection by the sensations they experience appears to decline after the initial milk ejection. In a study of mothers (n=28) who expressed milk with an electric breast pump for a total of 130 expression sessions, milk ejection was measured by ultrasound monitoring of the non-expressed breast. Overall, 79% of the initial milk ejections were felt by the mothers (Kent *et al.*, 2003). Interestingly, 50% of the mothers accurately sensed their first milk ejection at all visits, 11% did not sense milk ejection at any study visits, and 39% sometimes sensed their first milk ejection. In the 39% group, there were occasions of false positives where the mother communicated that she sensed milk ejection, but this was not observed by ultrasound (Kent, 2007, unpublished observations). Further, another study of 24 breastfeeding women found that 21 women sensed the first milk ejection, but none detected multiple milk ejection episodes which were observed using the ultrasound technique (Ramsay *et al.*, 2004).

OXYTOCIN RELEASE STIMULI

Touch

The tactile sensitivity of the human breast increases significantly at parturition (Robinson *et al.*, 1977), allowing mechanical stimulation of the breast - touch, suckling, or vacuum from a breast pump - to be an appropriate stimulus for triggering the milk ejection response (Sala *et al.*, 1974; Lincoln, 1984). In addition, manual breast massage by a trained nurse has been shown to stimulate oxytocin release (Yokoyama *et al.*, 1994). After birth, infants use their hands in a massage-like motion on the mothers' breasts during skin-to-skin contact which stimulates the mother to release oxytocin (Matthieson *et al.*, 2001). Furthermore, mothers who have skin-to-skin contact with their infant early after birth breastfeed longer (Uvnas-Moberg, 1998).

It is often observed in farm animals that the young bunt and nudge the gland before attaching to the teat to suckle. A similar event occurs among litters of piglets that scramble to find their position at the teat. Mechanical stimuli of the mammary gland such as this may play a role in initiating the milk ejection reflex. It has been shown in the rabbit that a 'tap' directly upon the lactating gland can stimulate the mammary myoepithelium, and it is suggested that this response may assist milk ejection, as well as allow some milk transfer during periods of inhibition (Cross, 1954).

The milk ejection reflex can be easily conditioned. Many women experience spontaneous milk ejections between feeds (Cobo, 1993). The sight, thought, sound, and smell of their infant will often cause the sensation of milk ejection and dripping of milk from the nipples (Newton, 1978). Similar responses have been reported in pump-dependent mothers who undergo milk ejection at the thought or sight of the breast pump. The psychological and conditioned component of the milk ejection has indeed been utilized by tetraplegic mothers to successfully breastfeed their infants by the implementation of mental imaging and relaxation techniques (Cowley, 2005).

Ferguson Reflex

Spontaneous uterine contractions can be stimulated by both an intravenous injection of oxytocin, as well as by inflating and deflating balloons in the vagina, cervix, and uterus, causing distension and relaxation of the reproductive tract, an event that is also observed at parturition (Ferguson, 1941). This neuro-hormonal reflex is called the Ferguson reflex. It often occurs close to parturition, but not in early pregnancy, and explains why human plasma oxytocin levels increase during the female sexual response (Carmichael *et al.*, 1987).

Measurements of intra-ductal pressure (which increases when oxytocin is released) during farrowing in the sow are indicative of oxytocin pulses with regard to the timing of the birth process. Only 12% of the sows (n=13) released oxytocin one minute prior to or as the piglet was delivered, whereas all sows had an increase in intra-ductal pressure after the piglet was expelled. Therefore, it is more likely that the release of a stretch stimulus causes oxytocin release rather than the initial stretch stimuli (Smith, 1994) (**Figure 8**). Although the Ferguson reflex is not fully understood, traditional societies have evoked the reflex by stimulating the reproductive tract of refractory dairy animals to prompt the release of oxytocin and initiate milk ejection (Cowie *et al.*, 1980).

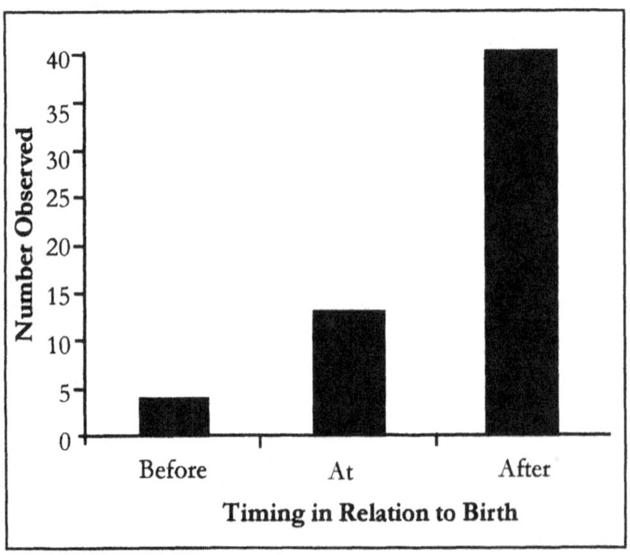

Figure 8. Frequency of intra-ductal pressure peaks measured during farrowing in the sow (Smith, 1994).

Food on the Brain

Both suckling and consuming food prompt the release of oxytocin. The digestive hormone, cholecystokinin, is released when foods, especially those of high fat and protein content, pass into the upper part of the small intestine. Cholecystokinin has been shown to stimulate oxytocin release via the afferent vagal nerves (Rehfeld *et al.*, 1984) in many species, including women (Verbalis *et al.*, 1986; Linden, 1989; Ohlsson *et al.*, 2002; Ohlsson *et al.*, 2004). Cholecystokinin is also synthesized by the pituitary neurons (Rehfeld *et al.*, 1984; Uvnas-Moberg, 1994).

It has been documented that oxytocin plays a role in appetite and metabolic and digestive processes. In animals, oxytocin given acutely will decrease appetite; however, when oxytocin is given over a longer period of time, appetite is increased, especially in nursing females. Oxytocin can also stimulate the release of gastric secretions and digestive hormones, allowing the body to adapt to different scenarios (Uvnas-Moberg, 2000). When animals are not hungry, oxytocin will promote increased digestive activity and nutrient storage. Conversely, when animals' appetites are increased, there will be inhibition of the digestive processes. Thus, suckling has been shown to promote digestion and energy storage through stimulation of anabolic metabolism (Uvnas-Moberg, 1994; Uvnas-Moberg, 1996a; Uvnas-Moberg *et al.*, 1996b; Uvnas-Moberg, 2000).

Suckling soon after birth is important not only for nutrition, but also to facilitate emotional bonding. It has been found in sheep that the digestive hormone cholecystokinin is integral for mother recognition and preference of the lambs. If the action of cholecystokinin is inhibited in the first few hours following birth, the formation of a preferential relationship between mother and lamb is prevented (Nowak *et al.*, 1997; Nowak *et al.*, 2001). Further, oxytocin levels are higher in calves that suckle compared to calves that drink from a bucket, demonstrating that the act of suckling itself is of importance, not only the transfer of nutrients (Lupoli *et al.*, 2001).

Oxytocin Nasal Spray

It has been shown that intravenous and intranasal administration of oxytocin produces a typical milk ejection reflex as measured by intra-ductal pressure (Sandholm, 1968). Therefore, it was assumed that the milk ejection reflex stimulated by use of a self-administered oxytocin nasal spray would improve milk yield in mothers. However, studies of intranasal oxytocin are varied. In term mothers, it was found that mothers had a higher milk yield when an oxytocin-covered cotton bud was placed in the nose for the entire expression period. Mothers were expressed initially for five minutes without intervention, then five minutes later were expressed once again for five minutes with intervention (Newton *et al.*, 1958).

Others have found that mothers given a sublingual tablet form of oxytocin had no effect on either infant weight gain or total milk yield. However, it was speculated that milk was made available to the infant (Friedman *et al.*, 1961). Another study compared a control group and a group receiving oxytocin. The study group had a lower frequency of suppressed lactation and less need for breastfeeding supervision during the successful establishment of lactation. Furthermore, the infants in the study group had higher average feed volumes and less weight loss compared to the control group. It is possible that oxytocin may facilitate emptying of the breast by the infant, but not necessarily increase the secretion of milk (Huntingford, 1961).

Using an oxytocin spray in the treatment of engorgement has also been of interest clinically. A large study of 500 participants found that when mothers used the oxytocin spray, the frequency of engorgement decreased (Ingerslev *et al.*, 1962), but there was no increase in infant weight gain. Furthermore, babies weighing less than 2500 grams grew well when fed breastmilk exclusively, suggesting again that the use of oxytocin allowed these babies to transfer milk with greater ease. Conversely, Huntingford (1961), with a smaller sample of women, did not find oxytocin to be of any benefit to engorgement.

In preterm mothers, the research has produced varying results. One paper recorded the cumulative volumes of milk obtained by eight primigravid women using a breast pump between the third and fifth days after delivery and found a 3.5-fold increase in the milk yield of the oxytocin nasal spray treated group. It was concluded that oxytocin nasal spray was an effective means of enhancing lactation despite the low number of women in the study (Ruis *et al.*, 1981).

Recently, a larger cohort of preterm mothers has been studied to determine the effects of oxytocin nasal spray. Total milk production did not differ with or without oxytocin treatment, but there were different patterns of production initially. With oxytocin nasal spray, there was a faster rate of milk removal initially, but then the two groups converged (Fewtrell *et al.*, 2006).

From these studies, it is difficult to determine how advantageous the application of oxytocin is in improving milk removal and establishing lactation. The studies discussed may have a placebo effect that has been overlooked, and more importantly, the long-term effectiveness of the administration of exogenous oxytocin has not been studied. Hence, the regular use of oxytocin has not been embraced clinically.

INHIBITION OF THE MILK EJECTION REFLEX

When discussing factors that inhibit milk ejection, it is important to consider the strong emotional/psychological component of the reflex. Events such as fright, unusual surroundings, and stress have been shown to inhibit the efficacy of the reflex. In dairy cows, milk yields were reduced when the milking process was interrupted by exploding paper bags filled with air or when a cat was placed on the cow's back (Ely *et al.*, 1941).

In women, a similar decrease in milk yield was observed when the breastfeeding mother was distracted (distractions included mathematical questions, moderate electric shocks, pain, and immersion of feet in ice-cold water). The average volume of milk transferred to the infant was 99 mL compared to 168 mL without distraction, and application of the distraction plus an injection of oxytocin resulted in a yield of 158 mL of milk (Newton *et al.*, 1948). It is important to note, however, the robustness of the milk ejection reflex. Despite the invasive distractions, infant intake was still 59% of that without distraction. Since the human mammary gland does not contain milk cisterns, less than 10 mL is available to the infant prior to milk ejection, thus the milk ejection reflex was partially inhibited by stress in this study (Mitoulas *et al.*, 2002; Kent *et al.*, 2003).

Further studies are required to understand the type of stress and its consequent effect on milk ejection. The distractions used by Newton (1948) could be considered severe, but did not completely inhibit the milk ejection reflex. Recent research into the mechanisms behind stress are indicating that different types of stress may alter the release of oxytocin via different pathways.

Therefore, the milk ejection reflex may be more efficient in overcoming one such pathway than another (Onaka, 2004). Newton and Newton (1948) also noted that certain distractions became ineffective over time as the mother became conditioned to those particular stimuli. This is also the case for dairy animals, new surroundings and different milkers will lead to less milk yield, but over time the dairy animals become tolerant of these new conditions (Bruckmaier *et al.*, 1998).

The milk ejection reflex is also inhibited by adrenaline (Cross, 1953; Cross, 1955). It is well known that hormonal systems in the body balance one another. Oxytocin is a prominent hormone involved in controlling 'calm and connecting reactions' and opposing the 'fight or flight reactions' that are primarily controlled by adrenaline (Uvnas-Moberg, 1998b; Uvnas-Moberg, 2000). It makes evolutionary sense that stressors inhibit the milk ejection reflex and minimize the release of oxytocin, so that if a 'fight or flight reaction' is required, the body can quickly and easily respond.

FURTHER EFFECTS OF OXYTOCIN

The central effects of oxytocin have been extensively reviewed (Argiolas *et al.*, 1990; Richard *et al.*, 1991; Crowley *et al.*, 1992; Evans, 1997; Leng *et al.*, 2005), and three primarily mammalian traits - parturition, copulation, and lactation - have all been linked by oxytocin. Therefore, it has been suggested that perhaps oxytocin is the factor involved in activating the rewarding properties of social interaction (Insel, 2003). The broad-ranging physiological, maternal, and social behaviors of oxytocin are well reviewed in the publication *The Oxytocin Factor - Tapping the Hormone of Calm, Love and Healing* (Uvnas-Moberg, 2000), with interesting speculations on potential effects.

Oxytocin has been shown to induce an anti-stress pattern. In rats, small doses induce anxiolytic-like effects, whereas large doses induce a sedative effect (Uvnas-Moberg *et al.*, 1994). Furthermore, oxytocin reduces blood pressure, decreases cortisol levels, decreases aggression, increases one's pain threshold, stimulates prolactin release, enhances wound healing, and has an effect on metabolic function (Uvnas-Moberg *et al.*, 1996; Uvnas-Moberg, 1996a; Uvnas-Moberg, 1998; Uvnas-Moberg, 1998a). In addition, oxytocin is a key hormone in sexual behavior and pair-bond formation (Insel *et al.*, 1997).

Maternal behavior is also influenced by oxytocin. A dose of oxytocin (0.4 μg) given to virgin rats induces maternal behavior, such as nesting, interest in pups, and increased grooming. The presence of oxytocin in breastmilk has been implicated as an olfactory cue to the young for nipple location (Pedersen *et al.*, 1979; Insel, 1992; Insel *et al.*, 1997). The calming and anti-stress patterns of oxytocin secretion are conducive to successful breastfeeding, as is the increased blood flow to the chest and nipple during oxytocin secretion. This increases the temperature of the skin area creating a nurturing environment for the infant (Uvnas-Moberg *et al.*, 1996; Uvnas-Moberg, 1996a).

Women who breastfeed for more than eight weeks are more relaxed, have a higher tolerance to monotony, and score higher on a socialization index (Sjogren *et al.*, 2000). Positive social feelings post-partum are correlated to the level of oxytocin in women. These levels are enhanced further in natural delivery compared to cesarean. Oxytocin may also play a role in the formation of olfactory memory in the mother, allowing her to recognize her young (Kendrick, 2000).

Alterations in the structure of the female mammal's brain associated with pregnancy and breastfeeding have been shown to make mothers more vigilant and nurturing and to improve their social memory and learning, suggesting that motherhood may make you smarter (Kinsley *et al.*, 2006). Magnetic resonance imaging of rats has shown that areas of the brain associated with olfaction, emotions, and reward are activated during pup suckling and oxytocin administration (Febo *et al.*, 2005). Interestingly, the amount of maternal care that mother rats give to their pups alters the expression of oxytocin and vasopressin receptors in the rat pups' brains (Francis *et al.*, 2002).

Oxytocin has been shown to modulate human social cognition and fear. The hormone seems to play a role in controlling the amygdala of the brain, a structure which has been implicated in social phobias and autism (Kirsch *et al.*, 2005). Autistic children show alterations in the oxytocin system. They have lower plasma oxytocin concentrations and different proportions of an extended form of the oxytocin peptide (Green *et al.*, 2001). From animal models, oxytocin seems to play a role in mediating the rewarding nature of social interactions and is therefore likely to play a role in social disorders, such as autism (Young, 2001).

Recently, oxytocin has been implicated in a human's ability to trust. In a series of trust games, researchers found that those participants who had received an intranasal oxytocin dose were more trusting of others compared to those who received a placebo. Researchers determined that this increased level of trust was not due to the participants' willingness to take risks (Kosfeld *et al.*, 2005).

Oxytocin also plays a role in the male. It is synthesized in the male reproductive tract which contains many oxytocin receptors. A burst of oxytocin is released in the male at ejaculation which facilitates the male reproductive tract to contract and release sperm. Furthermore, oxytocin is now being viewed as a potential therapeutic target since it has been found to effect the growth of the prostate gland, with one study finding oxytocin expression to be reduced with tumor progression (Whittington *et al.*, 2004; Thackare *et al.*, 2006). Oxytocin also plays an important role in male sexual arousal and penile erection (Uckert *et al.*, 2003).

Finally, many studies have used knockout mice that are deficient in either the oxytocin gene or receptor. The results of these studies have shown interesting and complex effects. Some of these effects include social amnesia, with oxytocin seemingly critical for the acquisition of social memory (Ferguson *et al.*, 2002; Winslow *et al.*, 2004). Mice pups vocalize less when separated from their mother, suggesting that they are less sensitive to maternal separation, and as adults these mice are more aggressive in nature (Winslow *et al.*, 2002; Takayanagi *et al.*, 2005).

In addition, oxytocin knockout mice are often infanticidal toward their young and commonly become the alpha female in a group (Ragnauth *et al.*, 2005). These mice, however, are still fertile, able to mate, and deliver live litters, but they do lack one fundamental function - the ability to eject milk. The young cannot remove the milk that is present and hence the litter dies (Young *et al.*, 1996; Takayanagi *et al.*, 2005).

CONCLUSIONS

Oxytocin is a molecule that is increasingly being implicated in central processes in the human body. Researchers are only just beginning to understand the full range of responses to oxytocin in both the systemic circulation and the central nervous system. Future therapeutic applications of oxytocin could include the therapeutic treatment of social disorders and other conditions that implicate oxytocin or oxytocin receptor abnormalities.

However, while animal models demonstrate the importance of the hormone to normal function, the key finding is that oxytocin is critical for milk ejection. In the absence of oxytocin, a mother rat can successfully give birth, but cannot nurse her young. This exemplifies the critical nature of milk ejection in initiating and maintaining a successful breastfeeding relationship between mother and infant. In this context, there is a need for further investigation of the physiology of oxytocin during pregnancy and lactation.

ACKNOWLEDGEMENT

Research funding from Medela AG.

References

Alekseev NP, Ilyin VI, Yaroslavski VK, Gaidukov SN, Tikhonova TK, Specivcev YA, *et al.* Compression stimuli increase the efficacy of breast pump function. *Eur J Obstet Gynecol Reprod Biol.* 1998; 77:131-39.

Argiolas A, Gessa GL. Central functions of oxytocin. *Neurosci Biobehav Rev.* 1990; 15(2):217-31.

Brownstein MJ, Russell JT, Gainer H. Synthesis, transport, and release of posterior pituitary hormones. *Science.* 1980; 207(4429):373-78.

Bruckmaier RM. Normal and disturbed milk ejection in dairy cows. *Domest Anim Endocrinol.* 2005; 29:268-73.

Caldeyro-Barcia R.. *Milk ejection in women.* Satellite Symposium to the XXIV International Congress of Physiological Sciences, University of Pennsylvania. Philadelphia: University of Pennsylvania Press; 1968.

Carmichael MS, Humbert R, Dixen J, Palmisano G, Greeleaf W, Davidson JM. Plasma oxytocin increases in human sexual response. *Journal of Endocrinology and Metabolism.* 1987; 64:27-31.

Cobo E. Uterine and milk-ejecting activities during human labor. *J Applied Physiol.* 1968; 24(3):317-23.Cobo E. Characteristics of the spontaneous milk ejecting activity occurring during human lactation. *J Perinat Med.* 1993; 21:77-85.

Cobo E, DeBernal MM, Gaitan E, Quintero CA. Neurohypophyseal hormone release in the human. II. Experimental study during lactation. *Am J Obstet Gynecol.* 1967; 97(4):519-29.

Cowie AT, Forsyth IA, Hart IC. *Hormonal control of lactation.* New York: Springer-Verlag; 1980.

Cowley KC. Psychogenic and pharmacologic induction of the let-down reflex can facilitate breastfeeding by tetraplegic women: A report of 3 cases. *Arch Phys Med Rehabil.* 2005; 86:1261-64.

Cross BA. Sympathetico-adrenal inhibition of the neurohypophysial milk-ejection mechanism. *Journal of Endocrinology.* 1953; 9:7-18.

Cross BA. Milk ejection resulting from mechanical stimulation of mammary myoepithelium in the rabbit. *Nature.* 1954; 173:450.

Cross BA. The hypothalamus and the mechanism of sympathetico-adrenal inhibition of milk ejection. *Journal of Endocrinology.* 1955; 12:15-28.

Crowley WR, Armstrong WE. Neurochemical regulation of oxytocin secretion in lactation. *Endocr Rev.* 1992; 13:33-65.

Dyball REJ, Leng G. Regulation of the milk ejection reflex in the rat. *J Physiol.* 1986; 380:239-56.

Ely F, Petersen WE. Factors involved in the ejection of milk. *J Dairy Sci.* 1941; 24:211-23.

Engelmann M, Wotjak CT, Ebner K, Landgraf R. Behavioural impact of intraseptally released vasopressin and oxytocin in rats. *Exp Physiol.* 2000; 85S:125S-30S.

Eriksson M, Lindh B, Uvnas-Moberg K, Hokfelt T. Distribution and origin of peptide-containing nerve fibres in the rat and human mammary gland. *Neuroscience.* 1996; 70(1): 227-45.

Evans JJ. Oxytocin in the human - regulation of derivations and destinations. *European J Endocrinol.* 1997; 137:559-71.

Febo M, Numan M, Ferris C. Functional magnetic resonance imaging shows oxytocin activates brain regions associated with mother-pup bonding during suckling. *J Neurosci.* 2005; 25(50):11637-44.

Ferguson JKW. A study of the motility of the intact uterus at term. *Surgery, Gynecology and Obstetrics.* 1941; 73:359-66.

Ferguson JN, Young LJ, Insel TR. The neuroendocrine basis of social recognition. *Front Neuroendocrinol.* 2002; 23:200-24.

Fewtrell MS, Loh KL, Blake A, Ridout DA, Hawdon J. Randomised, double blind trial of oxytocin nasal spray in mothers expressing breast milk for preterm infants. *Arch Dis Child Fetal and Neonat Ed.* 2006; 91(3):F169-74.

Forsling ML. Diurnal rhythms in neurohypophysial function. *Exp Physiol.* 2000; 85S: 179S-86S.

Francis DD, Young LJ, Meaney MJ, Insel TR. Naturally occurring differences in maternal care are associated with the expression of oxytocin and vasopressin (V1a) receptors: Gender differences. *J Neuroendocrinol.* 2002; 14:349-53.

Friedman EA, Sachtleben MR. Oxytocin in lactation. *Am J Obstet Gynecol.* 1961; 82(4):846-55.

Fuchs AR. Oxytocin in animal parturition. In: Amico JA, Robinson AG (eds.). *Oxytocin: Clinical and laboratory studies.* Amsterdam: Elsevier (Excerpta Medica International Congress Series No. 666); 1985. p. 259-76.

Fuchs AR, Fields MJ, Freidman S. Oxytocin and the timing of parturition. *Adv Exp Med Biol.* 1995; 395:405-20.

Fuchs F. Role of maternal and fetal oxytocin in human parturition. In: Amico JA, Robinson AG (eds.). *Oxytocin: Clinical and laboratory studies.* Amsterdam: Elsevier (Excerpta Medica International Congress Series No. 666); 1985. p. 236-56.

Gimpl G, Fahrenholz F. The oxytocin receptor system: Structure, function and regulation. *Physiol Rev.* 2001; 81(2):629-83.

Green L, Fein D, Modahl C, Feinstein C, Waterhouse L, Morris M. Oxytocin and autistic disorder: Alterations in peptide forms. *Society of Biological Psychiatry.* 2001; 50:609-13.

Hartmann PE, Smith NA, Thompson MJ, Wakeford CM, Arthur PG. The lactation cycle in the sow: Physiological and management contradictions. In: Tucker HA, Petitclerc D, Knight C, Sejrsen K (eds.). *Livestock production science: Third international workshop on the biology of lactation in farm animals.* Elsevier; 1997. 50:75-87.

Huntingford PJ. Intranasal use of synthetic oxytocin in management of breast-feeding. *Br Med J.* 1961; 1(5227):709-11.

Ingerslev M, Pinholt K. Oxytocin treatment during the establishment of lactation. *Acta Obstet Gynecol Scand.* 1962; 41:159-68.

Insel TR. Oxytocin - A neuropeptide for affiliation: Evidence from behavioral, receptor autoradiographic, and comparative studies. *Psychoneuroendocrinology.* 1992; 17(1):3-35.

Insel TR. Is social attachment an addictive disorder? *Physiol Behav.* 2003; 79:351-57.

Insel TR, Young LJ, Wang Z. Central oxytocin and reproductive behaviours. *Rev Reprod.* 1997; 2:28-37.

Isbister C. A clinical study of the draught reflex in human lactation. *Arch Dis Child.* 1954; 29(143):66-72.

Kendrick KM. Oxytocin, motherhood and bonding. *Exp Physiol.* 2000; 85S:111S-24S.

Kent JC, Kennaugh LM, Hartmann PE. Intramammary pressure in the lactating sow in response to oxytocin and during natural milk ejections throughout lactation. *J Dairy Res.* 2003; 70:131-38.

Kent JC, Ramsay DT, Doherty DA, Larsson M, Hartmann PE. Response of breasts to different stimulation patterns of an electric breast pump. *J Hum Lact.* 2003; 19(2):179-87.

Kimura T, Ito Y, Einspanier A, Tohya K, Nobunaga T, Tokugawa Y, *et al.* Expression and immunolocalization of the oxytocin receptor in human lactating and non-lactating mammary glands. *Hum Reprod.* 1998; 13(9):2645-53.

Kimura T, Saji F, Nishimori K, Ogita K, Nakamura H, Koyama M, *et al.* G-protein-coupled receptor signalling in neuroendocrine systems. *J Mol Endocrinol.* 2003; 30:109-15.

Kimura T, Takemura M, Nomura S, Nobunaga S, Kubota Y, Inoue T, *et al.* Expression of oxytocin receptor in human pregnant myometrium. *Endocrinology.* 1996; 137(2):780-85.

Kimura T, Tanizawa O, Mori K, Brownstein MJ, Okayama H. Structure and expression of a human oxytocin receptor. *Nature.* 1992; 356:526-29.

Kinsley CH, Lambert KG. The maternal brain. *Scientific American.* 2006; 294(1):58-65.

Kirsch P, Esslinger C, Chen Q, Mier D, Lis S, Siddhanti S, *et al.* Oxytocin modulates neural circuitry for social cognition and fear in humans. *J Neurosci.* 2005; 25(49):11489-93.

Kosfeld M, Heinrichs M, Zak PJ, Fischbacker U, Fehr E. Oxytocin increases trust in humans. *Nature.* 2005; 435:673-76.

Leake RD, Weitzman RE, Glatz TH, Fisher DA. Plasma oxytocin concentrations in men, nonpregnant women, and pregnant women before and during spontaneous labor. *J Clin Endocrinol Metab.* 1981; 53(4):730-33.

Leng G, Caquineau C, Sabatier N. Regulation of oxytocin secretion. *Vitam Horm.* 2005; 71:27-58.

Lincoln DW. The posterior pituitary. In: Austin CR, Short RV (eds.). *Hormonal control of reproduction.* Cambridge: Cambridge University Press; 1984. p. 21-51.

Lincoln DW, Paisley AC. Neuroendocrine control of milk ejection. *J Reprod Fertil.* 1982; 65:571-86.

Linden A. Role of cholecystokinin in feeding and lactation. *Acta Physiol Scand Suppl.* 1989; 585(i-vii):1-49.

Lupoli B, Johansson B, Uvnas-Moberg K, Svennersten-Sjauna K. Effect of suckling on the release of oxytocin, prolactin, cortisol, gastrin, cholecystokinin, somatostatin and insulin in dairy cows and their calves. *J Dairy Res.* 2001; 68:175-87.

Matthieson AS, Ransjo-Arvidson AB, Nissen E, Uvnas-Moberg K. Postpartum maternal oxytocin release by newborns: effects of infant hand massage and sucking. *Birth.* 2001; 28(1):13-19.

McNeilly AS, McNeilly JR. Spontaneous milk ejection during lactation and its possible relevance to success of breast-feeding. *Br Med J.* 1978; 2:466-68.

Mena F, Beyer C, Grosvenor CE. On the mechanism by which oxytocin depresses milk ejection and milk secretion in rats. *Am J Physiol.* 1974; 227(6):1249-54.

Mitoulas LR, Lai CT, Gurrin LC, Larsson M, Hartmann PE. Efficacy of breast milk expression using an electric breast pump. *J Hum Lact.* 2002; 18(4):344-52.

Mohr E, Meyerhof W, Richter D. The hypothalamic hormone oxytocin: from gene expression to signal transduction. *Rev Physiol Biochem Pharmacol.* 1992; 121:31-48.

Molenaar A J, Davis SR, Wilkins RJ. Expression of a-lactalbumin, a-S1-casein, and lactoferrin genes is heterogeneous in sheep and cattle mammary tissue. *J Histochem Cytochem.* 1992. 40(5):611-618.

Newton M, Egli GE. The effect of intranasal administration of oxytocin on the let-down of milk in lactating women. *Am J Obstet Gynecol.* 1958; 76(1):103-7.

Newton M, Newton N. The let-down reflex in human lactation. *J Pediatr.* 1948; 33(6):698-704.

Newton N. The role of the oxytocin reflexes in three interpersonal reproductive acts: coitus, birth and breastfeeding. In: Carenza L, Pancheri P, Zichella L (eds.). *Clinical psychoneuroendocrinology in reproduction - Proceedings of the Serono Symposia.* London: Academic Press; 1978. 22:411-18.

Nissen E, Uvnas-Moberg K, Svensson K, Stock S, Widstrom AM, Winberg J. Different patterns of oxytocin, prolactin but not cortisol release during breastfeeding in women delivered by caesarean section or by the vaginal route. *Early Hum Dev.* 1996; 45:103-18.

Nowak R, Breton G, Mellot E. CCK and development of mother preference in sheep: a neonatal time course study. *Peptides.* 2001; 22(8):1309-16.

Nowak R, Murphy TM, Lindsay DR, Alster P, Andersson R, Uvnas-Moberg K. Development of a preferential relationship with the mother by the newborn lamb: importance of sucking activity. *Physiol Behav.* 1997; 62(4):681-88.

Ohlsson B, Forsling ML, Rehfeld JF, Sjolund K. Cholecystokinin stimulation leads to increased oxytocin secretion in women. *Eur J Surg.* 2002; 168(2):114-18.

Ohlsson B, Rehfeld JF, Forsling ML. Oxytocin and cholecystokinin secretion in women with colectomy. *BMC Gastroenterol.* 2004; 4(25).

Onaka T. Neural pathways controlling central and peripheral oxytocin release during stress. *J Neuroendocrinol.* 2004; 16:308-12.

Peaker M, Wilde CJ. Feedback control of milk secretion from milk. *J Mammary Gland Biol Neoplasia.* 1996; 1(3):307-15.

Pedersen CA, Prange AJ. Induction of maternal behavior in virgin rats after intracerebroventricular administration of oxytocin. *Proc Natl Acad Sci USA.* 1979; 76(12):6661-65.

Prime DK, Trengove NJ, Larsson M, Doherty DA, Kent JC, Hartmann PE. *Comparison of milk ejection between the left and right breasts using changes in milk flow rates.* 13th ISRHML International Conference, Niagara-on-the-Lake, Ontario, Canada; 2006.

Prime DK, Trengove NJ, Larsson M, Hartmann PE. *Comparison of the milk removal characteristics of the left and right breasts during simultaneous breast expression.* Perinatal Society of Australia and New Zealand. 11th Annual Congress. Melbourne, Victoria, Australia; 2007.

Ragnauth AK, Devidze N, Moy V, Finley K, Goodwillie A, Kow LM, *et al.* Female oxytocin gene-knockout mice, in a semi-natural environment, display exaggerated aggressive behaviour. *Genes Brain Behav.* 2005; 4:229-39.

Ramsay DT, Kent JC, Owens RA, Hartmann PE. Ultrasound imaging of milk ejection in the breast of lactating women. *Pediatrics.* 2004; 113(2):361-67.

Ramsay DT, Mitoulas LR, Kent JC, Cregan MD, Doherty DA, Larsson M, *et al.* Milk flow rates can be used to identify and investigate milk ejection in women expressing breast milk using and electric breast pump. *Breastfeeding Medicine.* 2006; 1(1):14-23.

Ramsay DT, Mitoulas LR, Kent JC, Larsson M, Hartmann PE. The use of ultrasound to characterize milk ejection in women using an electric breast pump. *J Hum Lact.* 2005; 21(4):421-28.

Rehfeld JF, Hansen HF, Larsson LI, Stengaard-Pedersen K, Thorn NA. Gastrin and cholecystokinin in pituitary neurons. *Proc Natl Acad Sci USA.* 1984; 81(6):1902-5.

Richard P, Moos F, Freund-Mercier M. Central effects of oxytocin. *Physiol Rev.* 1991; 71(2):331-70.

Riggs CM, Sutherland RC, Wakerley JB. Reappraisal of the influence of mammary distension on the frequency of milk ejection in the rat. *Journal of Endocrinology.* 1985; 105:127-32.

Robinson ICAF. Radioimmunoassay of oxytocin: The standard. In: Amico JA, Robinson AG (eds.). *Oxytocin: Clinical and laboratory studies.* Amsterdam: Elsevier; 1985. (Excerpta Medica International Congress Series No. 666: 24-30.)

Robinson JE, Short RV. Changes in breast sensitivity at puberty, during the menstrual cycle, and at parturition. *Br Med J.* 1977; 1(6070):1188-94.

Ruis H, Rolland R, Doesburg W, Broeders G, Corbey R. Oxytocin enhances onset of lactation among mothers delivering prematurely. *Br Med J.* 1981; 283:340-42.

Russell JA, Leng G, Douglas AJ.. The magnocellular oxytocin system, the fount of maternity: adaptations in pregnancy. *Front Neuroendocrinol.* 2003; 24:27-61.

Sala NL, Luther EC, Arballo JC, Cordero Funes J. Roles of temperature, pressure, and touch in reflex milk ejection in lactating women. *J Applied Physiol.* 1974; 37(6):840-43.

Sandholm LE. The effect of intravenous and intranasal oxytocin on intramammary pressure during early lactation. *Acta Obstet Gynecol Scand.* 1968; 47:145-54.

Schams D. Oxytocin determination by radioimmunoassay III. Improvement to subpicogram sensitivity and application to blood levels in cyclic cattle. *Acta Endocrinol.* 1983; 103:180-83.

Sjogren B, Widstrom AM, Edman G, Uvnas-Moberg K. Changes in personality pattern during the first pregancy and lactation. *J Psychosom Obstet Gynecol.* 2000; 21(1):31-38.

Smith JG, Merrill DC. Oxytocin for induction of labor. *Clin Obstet Gynecol.* 2006; 49(3):594-608.

Smith NA. *Biochemical and physiological investigations of parturition and lactation in the pig.* PhD Thesis, Department of Biochemistry. Crawley: The University of Western Australia; 1994.

Soloff MS. Oxytocin receptors and mechanisms of oxytocin actions. In: Amico JA, Robinson AG (eds.). *Oxytocin: Clinical and laboratory studies.* Amsterdam: Elsevier (Excerpta Medica International Congress Series No. 666); 1985. p. 259-76.

Soloff MS, Alexandrova M, Fernstrom MJ. Oxytocin receptors: Triggers for parturition and lactation? *Science.* 1979; 204(4399):1313.

Takayanagi Y, Yoshida M, Bielsky IF, Ross HE, Kawamata M, Onaka T, *et al.* Pervasive social deficits, but normal parturition, in oxytocin receptor-deficient mice. *Proc Natl Acad Sci USA.* 2005; 102(44):16096-16101.

Thackare H, Nicholson HD, Whittington K. Oxytocin - Its role in male reproduction and new potential therapeutic uses. *Hum Reprod Update.* 2006; 12(4):437-48.

Uckert S, Becker AJ, Ness BO, Steif CG, Scheller F, Knapp WH, *et al.* Oxytocin plasma levels in the systemic and cavernous blood of healthy males during different penile conditions. *World J Urol.* 2003; 20:323-26.

Ueda T, Yokoyama Y, Irahara M, Aono T. Influence of psychological stress on suckling-induced pulsatile oxytocin release. *Obstet Gynecol.* 1994; 84(2):259-62.

Uvnas-Moberg K. Role of efferent and afferent vagal nerve activity during reproduction: integrating function of oxytocin on metabolism and behaviour. *Psychoneuroendocrinology.* 1994; 19(5-7):687-95.

Uvnas-Moberg K. Neuroendocrinology of the mother-child interaction. *Trends Endocrinol Metab.* 1996a; 7:126-31.

Uvnas-Moberg K. Oxytocin may mediate the benefits of positive social interactions and emotions. *Psychoneuroendocrinology.* 1998; 23(8):819-35.

Uvnas-Moberg K. Antistress pattern induced by oxytocin. *News Physiol Sci.* 1998a; 13:22-26.

Uvnas-Moberg K. Oxytocin may mediate the benefits of positive social interactions and emotions. *Psychoneuroendocrinology.* 1998b; 23(8):819-35.

Uvnas-Moberg K. *The oxytocin factor - tapping the hormone of calm, love and healing.* New York: Da Capo Press; 2000.

Uvnas-Moberg K, Ahlenius S, Hillegaart V, Alster P. High doses of oxytocin cause sedation and low doses cause an anxiolytic-like effect in male rats. *Pharmacol Biochem Behav.* 1994; 49(1):101-6.

Uvnas-Moberg K, Eriksson M. Breastfeeding: Physiological, endocrine and behavioural adaptations caused by oxytocin and local neurogenic activity in the nipple and mammary gland. *Acta Paediatr.* 1996; 85:525-30.

Uvnas-Moberg K, Eriksson M. Breastfeeding: Physiological, endocrine and behavioural adaptations caused by oxytocin and local neurogenic activity in the nipple and mammary gland. *Acta Paediatr.* 1996b; 85:525-30.

Verbalis JG, McCann MJ, McHale CM, Stricker EM. Oxytocin secretion in response to cholecystokinin and food: differentiation of nausea from satiety. *Science.* 1986; 232(4756):1417-19.

Voloschin LM, Tramezzani JH.. Milk ejection reflex linked to slow wave sleep in nursing rats. *Endocrinology.* 1979; 105(5):1202-7.

Voloschin LM, Tramezzani JH. Relationship of prolactin release in lactating rats to milk ejection, sleep state, and ultrasonic vocalization by the pups. *Endocrinology.* 1984; 114(2):618-23.

Wakerley JB, Dyball REJ, Lincoln DW. Milk ejection in the rat: the result of a selective release of oxytocin. *Journal of Endocrinology.* 1973; 57:557-58.

Whittington K, Assinder S, Gould M, Nicholson H. Oxytocin, oxytocin-associated neurophysin and the oxytocin receptor in the human prostate. *Cell Tissue Res.* 2004; 318(2):375-82.

Wilson-Clay B, Hoover K. *The breastfeeding atlas.* 2nd Ed. Austin, Texas: LactNews Press; 2002.

Winberg J. Mother and newborn baby: mutual regulation of physiology and behavior - a selective review. *Dev Psychobiol.* 2005; 47:217-29.

Winslow JT, Insel TR. The social deficits of the oxytocin knockout mouse. *Neuropeptides.* 2002; 36(2-3):221-29.

Winslow JT, Insel TR. Neuroendocrine basis of social recognition. *Curr Opin Neurobiol.* 2004; 14:248-53.

Yokoyama Y, Ueda T, Irahara M,Aono T. Releases of oxytocin and prolactin during breast massage and suckling in puerperal women. *Eur J Obstet Gynecol Reprod Biol.* 1994; 53(1):17-20.

Young LJ. Oxytocin and vasopressin as candidate genes for psychiatric disorder: lessons from animal models. *Am J Med Genet.* 2001; 105:53-54.

Young WSI, Shepard E, Amico J, Hennighausen L, Wagner K, Lamarca ME, *et al.* Deficiency in mouse oxytocin prevents milk ejection, but not fertility or parturition. *J Neuroendocrinol.* 1996; 8:847-53.

SECTION II

IMMUNOBIOLOGY

Chapter 10

The Role of Breastfeeding in the Defense of the Infant

Lars A. Hanson

INTRODUCTION

The newborn is in a very special situation when leaving the sterile and protected environment of the mother's uterus. The infant has to handle many new demands. Besides taking in food, the infant also has to meet a new environment which includes the presence of a multitude of microbes. Without an adequate defense against infectious agents, the neonate runs a very high risk of acquiring threatening infections. From this point of view, the neonatal period and the first year of life are the most dangerous times in man's life.

Our understanding of how we defend ourselves against infections has grown tremendously in recent decades, especially the defense of the infant, which is much more complex than later in life. This is mainly due to the fact that the infant's immune system must be built up and expanded so that the child can take over its own defense as soon as possible. The mother supports the host defense of the infant in two ways. One is via the antibodies from her blood which are actively transported over the placenta to the infant's circulation during fetal life. These antibodies are ready for use from birth on. The other is due to the numerous and complex defense factors provided via the mother's milk available directly after delivery.

This chapter describes the risks from and advantages of exposure to microbes directly from birth for the newborn and growing infant. It will illustrate how this exposure can be a threat, but also how it regularly induces the necessary build-up of the infant's immune system.

The initial deficiencies of the infant's immune system are related to the supportive role of the antibodies transferred via the placenta and, especially, to the numerous host defense factors in human milk. The complexity and considerable amounts of the many defense components in the milk delivered to the offspring illustrates the likely importance of this form of protection for the infant. Not only are there numerous milk factors which have direct capacity to protect the infant, but there is also a general principle in their function: they all act without causing inflammation and tissue damage which, in contrast, is the consistent mode of function for blood and tissue-mediated defense. These milk-mediated forms of defense are perfect for the growing child: defense without inducing inflammation means optimal conditions for normal growth and development.

Furthermore, human milk contains numerous substances that function as signals to the infant which may explain why there is growing evidence that the protection against certain infections noted during breastfeeding may remain at enhanced levels for some years after the termination of breastfeeding. Such long-term protective effects may also be provided against some inflammatory diseases, like celiac disease. For a recent, more complete review of this field, see Hanson, 2004b.

THE NEWBORN NEEDS AN IMMEDIATE DEFENSE AGAINST MICROBES: THE MICROBIAL FLORA AROUND THE INFANT

Man is constantly exposed to bacteria, but most are totally harmless. Starting from delivery, the newborn is colonized by such bacteria on the skin, in the upper respiratory tract, and in the gut, as well as in the vagina and the lowest part of the urethra. An adult normally carries around 1 kg of bacteria in the large intestine. The great majority of these bacteria are strict anaerobes, which cannot live in the presence of oxygen. They use up space and nutrients available in the bowel, so it becomes difficult for oxygen-requiring aerobic or facultative anaerobic bacteria to settle and grow. This competition is called "colonization resistance" and is a very important defense mechanism functioning against most potentially dangerous bacteria which try to infect humans via the gut. The common potential pathogens are almost exclusively found among the aerobic and facultatively anaerobic bacteria.

All mammals deliver next to the anus of the mother. This enables the offspring to receive the least dangerous bacteria around. As will be illustrated later, the mother provides special milk antibodies to protect against any danger involved with the baby taking up the mother's gut bacteria. Some of the strict anaerobic bacteria, like *Bacteroides thetaiotamicron,* may also have an anti-inflammatory effect in the gut (Kelly *et al.*, 2004). Others, like *Lactobacilli* and *Bifidobacteria* strains, may have antibacterial capacity directed against potential pathogens (Coconnier *et al.*, 1993; Lievin *et al.*, 2000; Coconnier *et al.*, 2000).

If this normal colonization at delivery is hindered, the infant will be colonized in an uncontrolled manner from hospital material or staff. The infant may pick up bacteria with increased resistance against antibiotics and with increased virulence. This can be seen when the baby is delivered by cesarean section or when misplaced hygiene practices try to prevent exposure to the mother's feces at delivery.

Within 48 hours of vaginal delivery, the baby's intestine already contains $10^{10\text{-}11}$ bacteria per gram of stool. Bacteria, like *Escherichia coli* and *enterococci*, which grow well in the presence of oxygen, can colonize the intestine of the newborn early. When these bacteria have consumed the oxygen, strictly anaerobic bacteria, like various *Bacteroides* and *Bifidobacterium* species, start to appear.

Breastfeeding influences the colonization process, but the results vary greatly between studies. Many early studies reported a pronounced influence by feeding mode on the microflora, but in modern Western societies, there seems to be less difference between breastfed and bottle-fed infants. Mata *et al.* investigated the intestinal microflora of breastfed indigenous Guatemalan neonates and found that *E. coli*, Enterococci, Clostridia, and *Bacteroides* were all present in high counts during the first days after birth (Mata *et al.*, 1969). But by the end of the first week of life, the microflora was completely dominated by *bifidobacteria.* Bullen investigated English infants in the early 1970s and saw a clear dominance of bifidobacteria in breastfed neonates, whereas in bottle-fed infants, bifidobacteria were present in lower numbers and were outnumbered by *Bacteroides, E. coli, Clostridia*, and *Enterococci* (Bullen & Tearle, 1976).

Many more recent studies reported similar and sometimes very low counts of *Bifidobacteria* in both breastfed and bottle-fed infants (Lundequist *et al.*, 1985; Balmer & Wharton, 1989; Kleessen, 1995), and only some investigators found more *Bacteroides* in bottle-fed than breastfed infants (Bullen & Tearle, 1976; Benno *et al.*, 1984). More persistent differences included lower counts of Clostridia and enterococci in breastfed than bottle-fed infants (Balmer & Warton, 1989; Stark & Lee, 1995). Also, bottle-fed infants commonly had a more diverse enterobacterial flora, with more *Klebsiella, Enterobacter,* and various *E. coli* strains (Bullen & Tearle, 1975; Adlerberth *et al.*, 1991).

Among these latter microbes are some potentially dangerous bacteria which may reach such high numbers that the risk of infection in the infant is increased. Bacteria, like *Klebsiella* and *E. coli,* may then succeed to translocate, i.e., to attach to and penetrate the gut wall, causing very dangerous infections, such as neonatal septicemia and meningitis, as well as necrotizing enterocolitis (NEC). The risk of such conditions is usually linked to prematurity and an immature immune system. The protective capacity of breastfeeding against these conditions will be discussed later. The number/gram feces of *E. coli,* as well as of *Clostridia*, was significantly lower in the gut of breastfed than formula-fed infants, possibly diminishing the risk of infections with these bacteria (Penders *et al.*, 2005). In this study, there was no difference in the number of *Bifidobacteria* comparing formula and breastfed infants.

After delivery, there is an early period in the infant's gut when there are high numbers of aerobic and facultatively anaerobic bacteria that can live in the presence of some oxygen. At that time, they can reach such high numbers that they will be able to cause infections. Gradually, the strict anaerobes, which are harmless, take over and reduce by competition for space and nutrients the numbers of other potentially pathogenic bacteria (Adlerberth, 1999).

Today, *Staphylococcus aureus* has become a common finding in the stool of Swedish infants. From the age of three days, *S. aureus* was found in the stool of 16% of the infants studied and was present in up to 73% of the infants by the age of two to six months (Lindberg *et al.*, 2000). These bacteria seemed to originate from the mother's breast, nose, and skin, but were also found in the father's skin flora. None of these infants showed any symptoms from the presence of these bacteria (Lindberg *et al.*, 2004). The fact that such potentially pathogenic bacteria are present in the gut of infants so early in life may indicate a changed microbial ecology. This may be due to reduced competition from the totally apathogenic anaerobic microbial flora normally seen in infancy to take over in numbers and successfully compete with and reduce the number of the aerobic and facultative anaerobic bacteria.

A prospective follow-up until 12 months of age of the gut microflora in Swedish infants has illustrated that those delivered vaginally more often had *E. coli* in the gut, whereas those delivered by cesarean section more often carried other *Enterobacteria*, such as *Klebsiella* and *Enterobacter* (Adlerberth *et al.*, 2006). From day three, both groups were colonized with *S. aureus* and not *Enterobacteria* as has been common previously. Colonization with the anaerobic *Bacteroides* was clearly delayed among those delivered by cesarean section compared with vaginal delivery.

Early breastfeeding helps the normal intestinal flora get settled and, in a number of ways, counteracts potential pathogens (Adlerberth *et al.*, 1999). Human milk seems to promote the growth of certain bacteria in the infant's gut, like lactobacilli, especially *Lactobacillus rhamnosus* (Ahrne *et al.*, 2005). Such harmless bacteria may compete with other potentially more dangerous bacteria, supporting the protective role of breastfeeding. Certain *Bifidobacterial* species have also been reported to be more frequent in the gut of breastfed than non-breastfed infants (Salminen *et al.*, 2005). Bacteria may increase their chance of remaining as colonizers in the gut by adhesins, which are small structures sticking out from the microbial surface that help the microbes attach to the gut wall. Human milk seems to favor the production of adhesins by *E. coli*, a capacity that may be linked to low virulence (Nowrouzian *et al.*, 2005).

INFANT'S OWN HOST DEFENSE COMPARED TO THAT OF THE ADULT

A full-term neonate has a more or less complete and competent immune system, but at delivery, it is still quite limited. This is due to the fact that although all cellular components are present, they are present in low numbers. Upon exposure after birth to all the microbes acquired from the mother, hospital staff, and family members, the infant's immune system starts to expand. Its priority is to be able to take over its own host defense, permitting normal growth and development unhampered by the burden of microbial onslaught (Hanson, 2004b).

Host Defense Consists of Three Cooperating Parts:

1) the **non-specific** part functions very broadly against infecting agents,
2) the **pattern-specific** part is directed against groups of structurally related microorganisms, and
3) the highly **specific** part reacts separately against various structures of each potentially dangerous microbe, be it a virus, a bacterium, or a large parasite.

The efficiency of the various host defense mechanisms in the young infant is compared to that of the adult (**Table 1**).

1. Non-Specific Defense

Non-specific mechanical defense against infections includes skin and mucosal membranes which prevent most microorganisms from entering the underlying tissues. The flow of saliva and urine, the presence of mucus on the mucosal membranes, the upward movement of cilia in the respiratory tract, and the continuous movement downwards of the gut content all help protect us against microbes trying to enter our tissues to establish themselves by causing an infection. The significance of such simple mechanisms is clearly illustrated by the fact that deficient ciliary function or impaired urinary flow brings a high risk of respiratory or urinary tract infections, respectively. A runny nose, cough, and diarrhea are other mechanical ways to dilute and eliminate unwanted microbes. At the same time, a normal bacterial flora in the upper respiratory tract and especially in the gut do, as discussed in the previous section, play a major role in preventing new, potentially pathogenic invaders from settling in those sites or, at least, in limiting their numbers which may be enough to prevent or at least ameliorate symptoms of infection.

Chemical and biochemical defense is exemplified by the low pH in the stomach which kills many, but not all, bacteria and by numerous additional components in blood, tissues, and secretions.

The neonate and young infant is somewhat deficient in some of the mentioned parameters (**Table 1**): the gastric pH is not as low in early life, the microbial killing by fatty acids in sweat is of reduced efficiency, and coughing may be inadequate. This is especially true in premature infants in whom most defense functions are more or less reduced.

2. Pattern-Specific Defense

The pattern-specific or group-specific defense acts most importantly via white blood cells, leukocytes, which can engulf and kill microbes by phagocytosis (Hanson, 2004b). They have receptors for certain surface structures on microbes and are called Toll-like receptors (TLRs). These are specific for groups of bacteria and function as "stranger signals" in the tissues (Bendelac & Medzhitov, 2002) (**Table 1**). The receptor TLR number 2 (TLR2), for instance, recognizes all gram-positive bacteria, including staphylococci and streptococci, while TLR4 recognizes gram-negative bacteria, like *E. coli* and *Klebsiella.* There are numerous additional receptors for other groups of microbes.

As soon as phagocytes with the help of the TLRs recognize any microbes in our tissues, these leukocytes, whether neutrophilic granulocytes, monocytes, or macrophages, increase their metabolism and via a transcription factor, NFκB, start producing a cascade of signals, or cytokines (**Figure 1A**). They also strongly activate other phagocytes in the vicinity to increase phagocytic activity. But the multiple cytokines produced have many more functions, coming together as the tissue reaction that we call inflammation (Janeway *et al.*, 2005). Cytokines cause local swelling, tenderness, redness, increased heat, and general symptoms like tiredness, pain, and loss of appetite. The most well

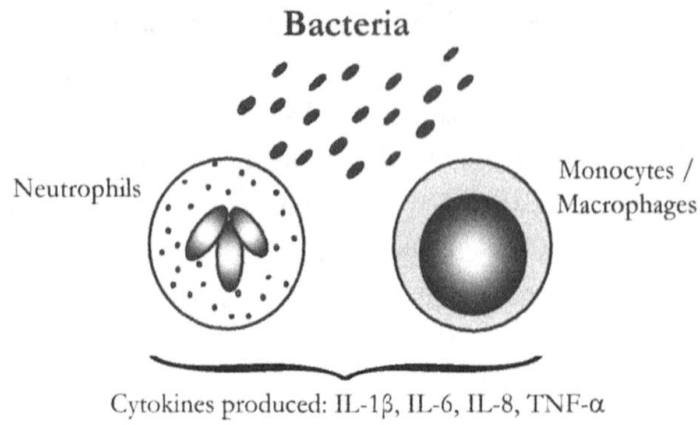

Figure 1A. Whenever microbes reach tissues in and under skin and mucosal membranes, they meet the leukocytes, or the white blood cells. These neutrophils, monocytes, and macrophages are capable of taking up and engulfing such microbes and often kill them. Their surface receptors, the TLRs, initially bind the microbes, thereby activating the leukocytes and producing a number of cytokines, which as part of the defense induce inflammation in surrounding tissues. They also efficiently activate the Antigen Presenting Cells, the APCs.

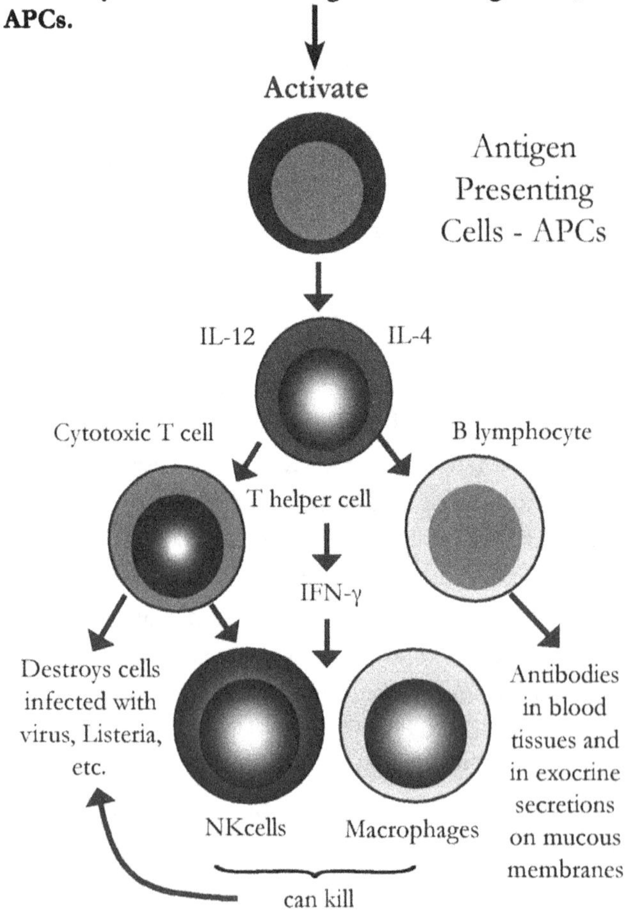

Figure 1B. The APCs present the antigens from the infecting microbe to the specific immune system, consisting of lymphocytes. The B lymphocytes respond by producing antibodies specifically directed against the invading microbes. The T lymphocytes provide cell-mediated immunity against the invaders.

Table 1. Host Defense in the Adult *with Functions Deficient in the Neonate-Young Infant (in italics)*

1. Non-specific Host Defense	
Mechanical, chemical, biochemical defense	Skin, mucosal membranes, mucus secretions
	Flow of saliva, urine, nasal discharge, *cough, gut peristalsis*, diarrhea
	Ciliary functions in the respiratory tract
	Fatty acids in sweat, low gastric pH
	Complement system
	Defensins
2. Pattern-specific Host Defense	
Phagocytes	Important cells in host defense, able to take up and kill many forms of microbes. They carry Toll-like receptors (TLRs) specific for groups of microbes, such as Gram-negative or Gram-positive bacteria. The TLRs present as "stranger signals," alarming host defense via production of numerous signals: the cytokines.
	The TLR receptors of the phagocytes in the neonate may react adequately, but in some studies, they react less efficiently in the presence of microbes, resulting in reduced production of regulating cytokines.
A. Neutrophils	*Fewer in bone marrow, reduced production, fewer migrating to infected sites because of limited complement function.*
	Good killing capacity, *but not in prematurity, during sepsis, pneumonia, and respiratory distress*
	Poor response to activating signals
B. Monocytes/macrophages	*Reduced response to IFN g, less efficient killing of Candida, less production of IFN g and TNF-a in the neonate. Production in monocytes and lymphocytes of the down-regulating cytokines IL-10 and TGF-b reduced in term and preterm infants.*
	Exposure to normal intestinal commensal bacteria, like Bifidobacteria and Lactobacilli, induces adequate cytokine responses also in neonatal monocytes
3. Specific Host Defense	
Antigen-presenting cells (APCs)	Cells which take up microbes and break them down, presenting small parts to lymphocytes in the specific immune system.
	Reduced specific immune responses because neonatal APCs produce fewer stimulating cytokines and carry fewer T cell stimulating surface receptors.
Thymus	Central organ in the immune system controlling the specificity of the T lymphocytes, eliminating auto-reactive ones.
	Small thymus in the newborn is linked to increased mortality.
	Non-breastfeeding is linked to a smaller thymus.
Specific immunity	Host defense via a lymphocyte-based system which attacks infecting agents with high specificity and capacity to increase the strength of the attack with more exposure to the agent. In addition, this response has an immunological memory with protective capacity that may remain through life. It works via special cytotoxic or killer T cells and via antibodies.
A. Antibody-mediated immunity	Antibodies are proteins with antigen binding sites in one end which fit well to a structure on part of a bacterium or a virus. There are different forms of these antibodies called IgG, IgM, and IgA. In secretions like milk and saliva, SIgA (secretory IgA) dominates.
	The newborn has a full setup of maternal IgG obtained via placenta during pregnancy. These are degraded and reach very low levels after a few months, while the IgM and IgG antibodies produced by the infant slowly take over in response to the microbes encountered from the environment. The SIgA antibodies remain at levels quite low initially in the secretions of the young infant, but increase with exposure.
B. Cell-mediated immunity	Consists of T lymphocytes with specific receptors for parts of an infecting virus expressed on the surface of an infected cell. The killer T cells also produce IFN-γ which activates other cells, like macrophages, to become capable of killing viruses and certain bacteria, like *Listeria* or *Mycobacteria*, which try to hide from the defense inside various cells.
	In early life, the killer T cells produce less cytokines, like IL-4, IL-10, and IFN-γ, but increased amounts of IL-13, resulting in somewhat reduced cell-mediated immune capacity.

known cytokines are Interleukin (IL)-1β, IL-6, IL-8, and Tumor Necrosis Factor (TNF)-α. Of these, IL-8 brings in more phagocytes to try to assure that all the infecting microbes really are taken up and killed. TNF-α adds to the inflammation and also causes tiredness, possibly making the infected individual rest more, concentrating his/her capacities on defense. IL-β, IL-6, and TNF-α increase the level of the hormone leptin which causes loss of appetite during the infection. The important protective mechanism of phagocytosis that we need for defense clearly has effects that can become problematic. For example, with repeated infections in a child in a poor community, the continued loss of appetite can add to undernutrition, and long-term continued tiredness can impair normal development.

In early infancy, there are fewer neutrophils in their depot or the bone marrow, where their production is reduced, and they respond poorly to activating cytokine signals (Schelonka & Infante, 1998). Their capacity to adhere and change shape when meeting microbes is decreased. In severe prematurity, on-going sepsis, pneumonia, or respiratory distress, the phagocytic capacity is reduced. In the blood, there is a series of components, the complement system, which strongly potentiates bacterial killing by phagocytosis. But, complement is low in the blood in the first three months of life, so the neutrophils aggregate less efficiently at the site of an infection, although their killing capacity is adequate (**Table 1**).

Monocytes/macrophages are just like the neutrophils in their efficiency in taking up and killing invading microbes. The monocytes are present in the circulation and the macrophages are present in tissues. However, in the neonate/young infant, there is a reduced capacity for these cells to respond to some activating signals, like interferon (IFN)-γ, and they show reduced capacity to kill *Candida* (Marodi, 2002). Neonatal monocytes in the term infant produce less of the pro-inflammatory cytokines TNF-α and IFN-γ (Levy, 2005). On the other hand, exposure of neonatal monocytes to bacteria from normal intestinal flora mainly induce via their TLR receptors at least as efficient a cytokine production as in adults (Karlsson *et al.*, 2002) (**Table 1**).

The monocytes and lymphocytes in term and preterm neonates show less efficient regulation of the pro-inflammatory cytokines IL-1β, IL-6, IL-8, and TNF-α and much more inhibition of the production of the down-regulating IL-10 and TGF-β. The latter two are important in controlling inflammatory processes. Therefore, a neonate with an infection may have stronger inflammatory reactivity than an older infant, causing more tissue damage (Schultz *et al.*, 2004). When the neutrophils/monocytes/macrophages meet invading bacteria via their TLR receptors, they fight them by phagocytosis, trying to kill them. Their production of the pro-inflammatory cytokines mentioned above engage surrounding tissues bringing about inflammation which is a sign of an extended defense reaction. That activation also includes "antigen-presenting cells" (APCs) (**Figure 1B**), usually called dendritic cells, which get very stimulated, take up the bacteria, break them down, and present portions of their foreign structures, called antigens (antibody generators), on their surface. These antigen-presenting cells and the cytokines they produce meet with activated lymphocytes which help develop an immune response highly specific for the presented antigen (**Figure 1B**). But in early life, the APCs produce less of the cytokines needed for a fully balanced and effective specific immune response to occur (Langrish *et al.*, 2002). The neonate´s dendritic cells also show reduced expression of some surface receptors which may be linked to a depressed capacity to stimulate the neonate's antigen-responding T cells (Liu *et al.*, 2001) (**Table 1**).

3. Specific Defense

The special lymphocytes which respond to the presented antigen are called T helper cells and represent the next step in the defense reaction serving to stop an ongoing infection (**Table 1, Figures 1A, B**). These cells are born in the bone-marrow, but they mature in the thymus, explaining their designation as T cells. The thymus is a central organ in the specific immune system. It helps eliminate T lymphocytes which have receptors of high binding-capacity for one's own tissues and therefore can be damaging. Only T cells which are tolerant to one's own tissues can be permitted in the circulation, otherwise, autoimmune diseases like rheumatoid arthritis and ulcerative colitis may occur (Högquist *et al.*, 2005). To further secure prevention of auto-immune reactivity, special regulatory T lymphocytes appear in the circulation and seem to play a major role in preventing immunological diseases like autoimmune diseases and allergies (Janeway *et al.*, 2005). It is of considerable interest that the intestinal microbial flora in early life plays an important role in inducing immunological tolerance. In an animal model, colonization with both lactobacilli and *E. coli,* not just one or the other, were needed to induce a soluble factor promoting such tolerance (Rask *et al.*, 2005).

The size of the thymus is strongly correlated to health. The larger the thymus in early life, the lower the infant mortality (Aaby *et al.*, 2002). Breastfeeding doubles the size of the thymus, which may be due to the presence of the cytokine IL-7 and possibly other factors in the milk (Ngom *et al.*, 2004).

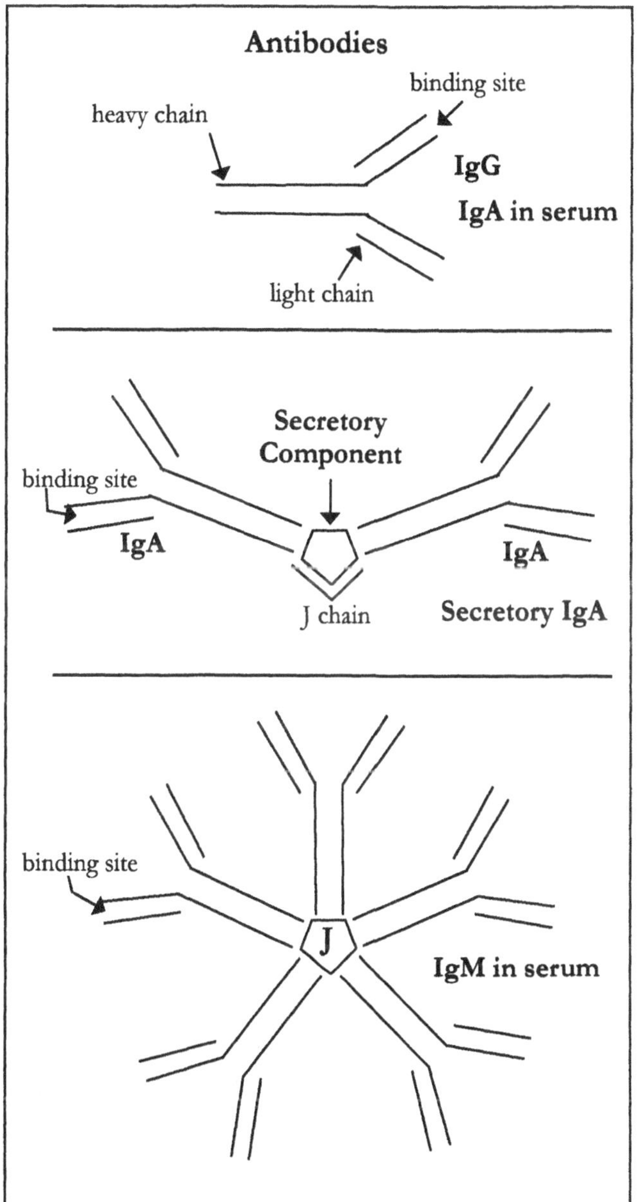

Figure 2. The structures of antibodies are illustrated. They consist of heavy and light polypeptide chains which form binding sites as indicated in the figures. The antibodies produced in response to a certain microbe have a structure of their binding sites that makes them fit perfectly to parts of the microbe; thus each antibody is specific for one part of the invading microbe and can recognize and bind to that microbe. The binding sites are in principle identical for the different types of antibodies, the IgG and IgA, as well as the larger IgM. The secretory IgA (SIgA) antibodies are found in different secretions like milk, saliva, etc.

The T helper cells, with receptors that fit to the antigens presented by the APCs, are already present in the neonate. Lymphocytes of numerous specificities are inborn and inherited in the immune system. They are present from fetal life with a limited number of cells of each specificity. There are already lymphocytes with receptors covering a broad range of different antigens. Their numbers expand after birth as they meet various antigens to which their receptors fit. The T helper cells provide cytokines which direct the continued immune response specific for a presented antigen, be it against a part of a virus, a bacterium, or a food stuff. The immune response becomes more and more specific for the antigen it is directed against. For instance, a bacterial toxin will become more and more efficiently neutralized.

The APC will present the antigen to B lymphocytes, which come from the bone marrow, and produce antibodies called immunoglobulins, Ig (**Figure 2**). They contain structures which form "binding sites" that fit perfectly to parts of the presented antigen. The antibodies appear in different forms called IgG, IgM, and IgA and are present in blood and tissues. IgA also appears as a larger, more complex molecule called secretory IgA (SIgA) which predominates in all secretions, like saliva, gut secretions, and milk (**Figure 2**). There are also IgE antibodies which are normally formed to provide defense against large parasites, like roundworm (*Ascaris)* and others, but may also cause certain forms of allergy.

Antibodies protect us by binding and neutralizing bacterial toxins and viruses. The IgG antibodies are especially effective in this function. The IgG and, even more efficiently, the IgM antibodies function by activating the complement system when they bind to microbes. As a consequence, phagocytes, like neutrophils and monocytes, are brought into the site of the infection in larger numbers and are activated to efficiently take up, phagocytize the microbes, and kill them. These antibodies function in tissues by activating leukocytes. Cytokines are then produced and inflammation follows, bringing more or less typical symptoms.

The infant starts producing antibodies against the microbes it meets following delivery. It initially produces IgM antibodies and then IgG antibodies upon exposure

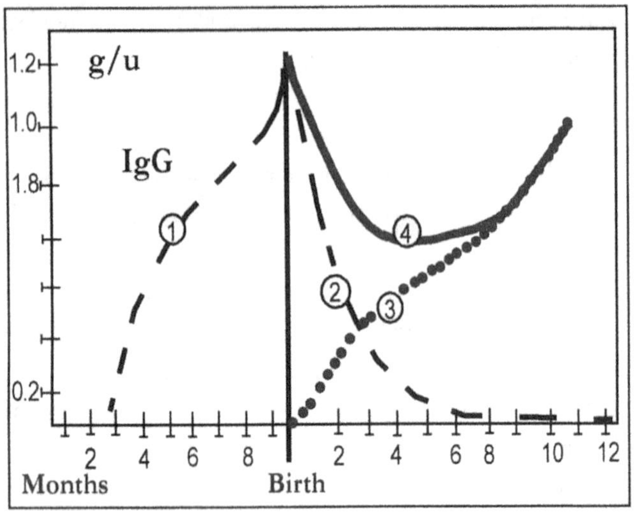

Figure 3. (1) Via the placenta, IgG antibodies are actively transported from the mother's circulation to that of the fetus. (2) From birth on, these IgG antibodies are degraded and slowly vanish during the first year of life. (3) The infant starts to produce IgG at birth, taking over as the placentally transferred IgG antibodies are metabolized and vanish. (4) The resulting level of IgG antibodies in the circulation of the infant is shown as (4). Also IgM is being produced.

to all antigens. The infant's antibody levels in the blood slowly increase during the first year, taking over from the maternal IgG transferred via the placenta during the pregnancy (**Figure 3**).

SIgA antibodies are present in various secretions and are especially high in milk. They function primarily by binding invading microbes, preventing them from reaching the mucosal membranes. Thus, microbes do not get a chance to attach to the mucosa, preventing them from entering the tissues where they might cause an infection. Tissue defense in the form of IgM and IgG antibodies will, therefore, not be stimulated and activate the complement system. Thus, phagocytes are not activated and no inflammation is induced.

For a young, growing infant, it is obvious that the SIgA mediated defense brings considerable advantages. But during the first ten days of life, neonates have no or very few IgA-producing lymphocytes in the gut mucosa (Brandtzaeg, 2001). Cells producing IgM and IgA increase rapidly two to four weeks after birth. Four to eight weeks after birth, the IgA-producing cells providing SIgA in the infant's gut predominate; they peak at about 12 months.

The IgE antibodies are attached to mast cells in tissues. When they react with their antigen, they bring in eosinophilic granulocytes. The mast cells and the eosinophils release a number of active substances which work together to cause an inflammatory reaction. This special reaction is mostly seen as inflammation causing allergic disease, but is normally targeted against larger parasites like helminths.

In the immune response to various microbes, cytotoxic T lymphocytes develop in addition to specific antibodies and are called killer T cells (Janeway *et al.*, 2005). T cells specific for a certain virus can attack and destroy a virus-infected tissue cell because that tissue cell expresses antigens from the infecting virus on its surface. The specific cytotoxic T cell recognizes the viral antigens and destroys the infected cell. Viruses are released, but are neutralized by the antibodies present in blood and tissues. Tissue cells infected by bacteria, like *Listeria* and *Mycobacteria*, may also be attacked and destroyed in a similar fashion by cytotoxic T cells. These cells produce IFN-γ which kill viruses and activate phagocytes, like macrophages, to kill pathogens like *Listeria*, a dangerous microbe in infants and pregnant women. In early infancy, the cytotoxic T cells produce lower levels of several cytokines, like IL-4, IL-10, and IFN-γ, but higher levels of IL-13 (Ribeiro-do-Couto *et al.*, 2001). There are suggestions that these observations are linked to immaturity and that the IL-7 present in human milk contributes to the maturation (Marshall-Clarke *et al.*, 2000).

Elaborate mechanisms have been developed for the immune system to be able to avoid reacting against its own tissues, food, and other environmental factors against which we do not need immunological defense. Such immunological tolerance is due to several mechanisms, one of which is the elimination in the thymus of lymphocytes which carry receptors against one's own tissues. Another mechanism is the regulatory T cells as mentioned above. A third mechanism is the exposure in the gut of the infant to certain bacteria which induce production of factors that may down-regulate or prevent unwanted immune reactivity (Rask *et al.*, 2005).

VIA THE PLACENTA

Throughout pregnancy, the fetus receives maternal IgG antibodies from the mother's blood circulation via an active transport over the placenta (Hanson, 2004b; Ribeiro-do-Couto *et al.*, 2001) (**Figure 3**). These antibodies are present at 90-150% of maternal blood levels at delivery and are then slowly degraded with a half life of 21-30 days. The IgG antibodies help

Table 2. Components in Human Milk with Likely Immunobiological Effects
Antibodies, especially SIgA
Lactoferrin
α-Lactalbumin
Carbohydrate components
Anti-secretory factor
Cytokines, growth factors and other signals from mother to infant
Fat
Defensins and cathelicidin
Lysozyme
Lactadherin
Leukocytes, etc

protect the fetus and young infant against infectious agents, primarily in blood and tissues. They are capable of neutralizing certain viruses and bacterial toxins and inducing phagocytosis, complement, and phagocyte-mediated inflammation.

Trace amounts of the maternal IgG antibodies may remain towards the end of the first year. These antibodies can inhibit the infant's new antibody responses, such as against the measles vaccine. That is why the measles vaccine is usually given after the first year of life (Sigrist, 2003).

VIA THE MILK

Components of Potential Protective Capacity

Human milk contains numerous components that may support the defense of the breastfed infant (**Table 2**).

These components range widely from large proteins, like antibodies, to lipids and carbohydrates to numerous signals from the mother to the offspring, such as ytokines, chemokines, hormones, anti-oxidants, growth factors, enzymes, and, finally, to cells, like lymphocytes and phagocytes (Hanson, 2004b). The major ones will be described below, and, when known, their possible role for the breastfed infant will be mentioned (**Table 3**).

Antibodies

Human milk, especially colostrum, is rich in antibodies. The predominant antibody is SIgA (**Figure 2**), making up 80-90% of the antibodies in colostrum and mature milk. There is a decrease from the high concentrations in colostrum, up to 12 g/L, to around 0.5-1.0 g/L in mature milk. The increase in daily milk volume from early colostrum to mature milk largely compensates for the initial decrease in concentration of SIgA. Infants receive about 125 mg of SIgA/kg/day at one month of age and about 40 mg/kg/day by four months of age (Butte *et al.*, 1984). SIgA levels are higher in milk from mothers with premature delivery than in milk from mothers with full-term babies (Goldblum *et al.*, 1982).

As mentioned previously, the SIgA antibodies function primarily by binding the microbes they are specifically directed against, preventing them from reaching the mucosal membranes, such as in the respiratory and gastrointestinal tracts (**Figures 4A, 4B**). Recently, it was shown that colostrum from mothers vaccinated against pneumococci prevented such bacteria from attaching to epithelial cells (Deubzer *et al.*, 2004). Such attachment is the first step in an infection.

The milk antibodies also neutralize viruses and bacterial toxins. The milk SIgA antibodies are supported in these functions by being quite resistant against degradation by proteolytic enzymes in the gastrointestinal tract. In addition, some of the milk SIgA antibodies together with their antigen are directed against bacterial enzymes which they neutralize (Gilbert *et al.*, 1983). A recent study suggests an additional mode of function of SIgA: such antibodies, together with their antigen, seem to be taken up by the mucosal M cells covering the Peyer patches shown in **Figure 4A** and stimulate

Table 3. Signals in Milk with Possible Short/Long Term Effects on the Offspring	
Cytokines, chemokines and colony-stimulating factors	TGF-β (Transforming Growth Factor-β) , IL-1β (Interleukin-1β), IL-2, IL-4, IL-5, IL-6, IL-7, IL-8, IL-10, IL-12, IL-13, IL-16, IFN-γ, TNF-α (Tumor Necrosis Factor-α), G-CSF(Granulocyte-Colony Stimulating Factor), M-CSF (Macrophage-Colony Stimulating Factor), MIF (Macrophage Migratory Inhibitory Factor), Eotaxin, etc.
Hormones and growth factors	EGF, FGF, IGF-1, VEGF, GH-releasing factor, HGF, erythropoietin, prolactin, thyroid hormone, leptin, TGF, etc.
Factors with anti-inflammatory capacity	SIgA, IL-10, TGF-β, IL-1β Receptor Antagonist, TNF-α soluble receptors I and II, Lactoferrin, Complement inhibiting factors, Prostaglandins which inhibit neutrophil enzymes, Anti-proteases which block enzymes which may be tissue-damaging, etc.

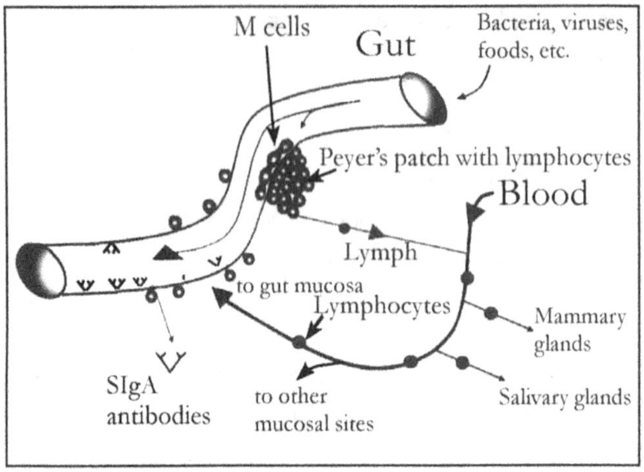

Figure 4A. The M cells covering the Peyer's patches in the gut take up bacteria, viruses, food, and other antigenic material from the gut. This material is presented to lymphocytes in the Peyer's patches which are directed to produce IgA dimers and J chains. These cells migrate via the lymph and blood to other mucosal sites and to exocrine glands. There, the SIgA antibodies are produced. As a result, protection against the microbes present or passing through the gut is spread to other sites. Human milk contains large amounts of SIgA antibodies against the microbes in the mother's gut, which the baby is normally colonized with at delivery and thereafter, and may need defense against. Source: Hanson, 2004b.

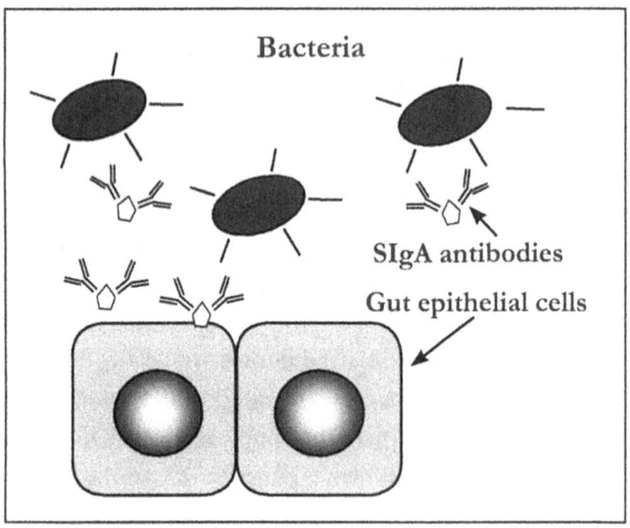

Figure 4B. Bacteria infect humans mostly via the mucosal membranes. They must attach to the mucosal cells to reach and infect the host's tissues. If SIgA antibodies are present in the baby, either from mother's milk, or later from its own production, the invading bacteria are bound by the SIgA antibodies and thereby prevented from reaching the baby's mucosa, for instance, in the respiratory or gastrointestinal tract. Thus, infection is prevented. In the breastfed baby, this is efficient since the mother's milk contains SIgA antibodies against the microbes in the mother's and infant's surroundings as shown in Figure 4A.

antigen-presenting cells there (Favre *et al.*, 2005). This could mean that SIgA antibodies from the mother's milk might both protect in the gut of the breastfed baby and stimulate the infant's own mucosal immune response against bacteria from its gut.

It seemed surprising that human milk SIgA antibodies often are directed against just about any bacteria present in the gut (Hanson *et al.*, 2004a). This was explained when it was discovered that lactogenic hormones important for the development of the mammary glands towards the end of pregnancy directly influence the migration of lymphocytes from the aggregates of lymphocytes in the gut to the mammary glands (Weisz-Carrington *et al.*, 1978). This is called the entero-mammaric link and results in SIgA antibodies in the milk being directed against bacteria in the mother's gut and bacteria arriving there from her upper respiratory tract secretions (**Figure 4A**). The breastfed infant is provided protection via the milk against the mother's intestinal bacterial flora to which it is normally exposed at delivery. At the same time, the baby builds up its own normal intestinal defense against the microbes it gets exposed to. This makes it obvious that breastfeeding should be initiated directly after birth to help the neonate handle exposure to microbes from birth on. As discussed further below, this can save lives, especially in poor areas (Edmond *et al.*, 2006).

The maternal lymphocytes in the mammary glands produce SIgA antibodies against quite a wide range of microbes (Hanson *et al.*, 2004b). The original observation of the efficiency of the protection provided via the milk was made in a Guatemalan village where mothers sick with dysentery caused by *Shigella* bacteria protected their breastfed babies from symptoms by breastfeeding, although the babies excreted the bacteria (Mata *et al.*, 1969). In exposed areas, the milk SIgA will also be directed against antigens, such as those from *Giardia* parasites (Tellez *et al.*, 2005). Vaccination of pregnant women against pneumococci increased the SIgA antibody levels to pneumococci in their colostrum and milk (Obaro *et al.*, 2004).

Several publications show that the specific milk SIgA antibodies protect against infections from *Vibrio cholerae, Campylobacter, Shigella*, enterotoxin-producing *E. coli*, and *Giardia lamblia* (Glass *et al.*, 1983; Ruiz-Palacios *et al.*, 1990; Hayani *et al.*, 1992; Cruz *et al.*, 1988; Waterspiel *et al.*, 1994).

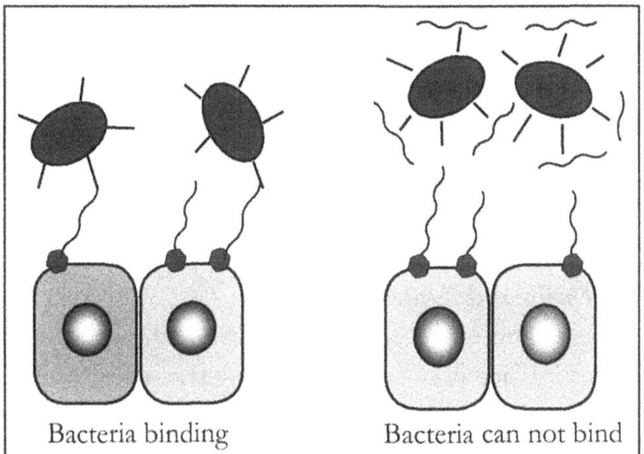

Figure 4C. This figure shows how bacteria attach to epithelial cells. The bacteria may carry specific structures called adhesins, or pili, for that purpose. They attach to specific structures on the epithelial cells, usually oligosaccharide side chains of glycoproteins or glycolipids, as indicated in the left part of this figure. To the right can be seen structures in milk similar to the cellular receptor blocking the bacterial attachment.

The protection against infections provided by breastfeeding has the advantage of preventing all tissue engagement, like inflammation and loss of appetite, because the infecting agents are kept away from the baby's tissues by the SIgA antibodies (Carbonare *et al.*, 2005). As will be seen below, numerous other defense mechanisms provided via the milk act in similar ways: defending without causing inflammation as tissue immunity does.

There are smaller amounts of IgM and IgG antibodies in the milk. Their protective capacity is not known in this setting.

Lactoferrin (LF)

This is another milk protein, the major value of which may not be for nutrition, but for defense like SIgA. This seems remarkable because human milk is relatively low in protein content compared to other species' milk. In colostrum, there is as much as 5-7 g/L of LF. In mature milk, there is about 1-3 g/L. The increase in milk volume during early lactation partly compensates for this decrease.

LF is a glycoprotein which binds iron. It is present in granulocytes. LF and some of its fragments can kill bacteria, certain viruses, and *Candida* (Ellison, 1994; Nikawa *et al.*, 1994). In an animal model, LF and certain LF fragments protected against experimental urinary tract infections caused by *E. coli* in mice (Håversen *et al.*, 2000). The human LF given perorally was taken up by a special receptor in the gut and excreted in the urine where it was protective. LF also has the capacity to enter the nuclei of leukocytes and block their capacity to induce inflammation by binding to the transcription factor NFκB (Håversen *et al.*, 2002). This effect may explain the anti-inflammatory effect of LF shown in an animal model of colitis (Håversen *et al.*, 2003).

Lactalbumin

This is also a major milk protein, but little is known about its functions with a remarkable exception. It has recently been found to have anti-tumor effects. When exposed to low pH, as in the stomach, the protein unfolds and binds oleic acid, formed when triglycerides are degraded in the stomach. Then, this complex attains the capacity to kill human tumor cells. In this form, it has been labeled human α-lactalbumin made lethal to tumor cells, or HAMLET (Håkansson *et al.*, 1995). This molecule kills numerous human tumor cell lines. It induces apoptosis and human studies give evidence for effects against skin papilloma (Gustafsson *et al.*, 2004; Gustafsson *et al.*, 2005).

Carbohydrate Components

Human milk contains numerous oligosaccharides, glycoproteins, and glycolipids. The oligosaccharides make up the third largest solid fraction in milk, next to lactose and fat. More than 130 different oligosaccharides have been isolated from human milk. They are not absorbed. Instead, they promote the growth of a specific microbial flora in the colon (Uauy *et al.*, 2004). They have been found to play an important role in protection against infections by preventing various forms of microbes from attaching to mucosal membranes as their initial step in starting an infection. Both microbes and microbial toxins bind to specific carbohydrate structures on mucosal cells which function as their receptors when they try to get into our tissues. The milk carbohydrates contain these structures used as receptors by the microbes and can thus block the attachment (Newburg *et al.*, 2005). Milk oligosaccharides were shown to prevent adhesion not only of enteropathogenic *E. coli*, but also of *Vibrio cholerae* and a *Salmonella* strain (Coppa *et al.*, 2006). The end result is the same as when the milk SIgA antibodies keep microbes and their toxins away from mucosal membranes preventing infections (**Figures 4B, 4C**).

Anti-secretory Factor

This protein is normally present in various tissues, blood, and secretions, like milk, after exposure to bacterial enterotoxins or after eating a specially treated cereal. It is anti-secretory (Lange & Lonnroth, 2001). Recently, it was found to protect against acute mastitis and also against acute and prolonged diarrhea in infants and children (Svensson *et al.*, 2004; Zaman *et al.*, 2007). It seems that inducing this component in milk may reduce the risk of mastitis in the mother and diarrhea in the infant.

Cytokines, Growth Factors, and Other Signals from Mother to Infant

Mother's milk contains numerous components which may function as signals from the mother to her infant, possibly helping various organs and functions to mature (**Table 3**) (Field, 2005). Little is known about such functions, but breastfeeding seems to have some long-term protective effects against certain infections and some diseases, like obesity, that remain after lactation has ceased.

For instance, it has been noted that blood lymphocytes of infants breastfed for six months had fewer receptors for cellular signaling, fewer of one T lymphocyte population, and more NK (natural killer) cells than nonbreastfed infants (Hawkes *et al.*, 1999; Böttcher *et al.*, 2000).

Another example is the observation that IL-7 in milk seems to be linked to an increased size of the thymus in breastfed infants (Ngom *et al.*, 2004). This could be one reason why the thymus, the central organ in the immune system, is twice as large in breastfed than in non-breastfed infants (Ngom *et al.*, 2004). Furthermore, IL-7 seems to have an important role in promoting the production of B lymphocytes, the antibody producing cells (Dias *et al.*, 2005).

The appetite-regulating hormone leptin present in milk has the structure of a cytokine and binds to cytokine receptors, illustrating cooperation between the neuroendocrine and immune systems (Lord, 2002). The many anti-inflammatory components in human milk may help protect normal growth and development of the infant. Breastfeeding seems, for instance, to have an anti-inflammatory effect on infants with respiratory syncytial virus infection (Roine *et al.*, 2005). Further examples of such biological effects are given in Hanson, 2004b.

Milk Fat

After enzymatic degradation, human milk lipids provide fatty acids which can attack certain bacteria and viruses as well as the parasite *Giardia liamblia.* They can also neutralize certain bacterial toxins (Hernell *et al.*, 1986; Herrera-Insua *et al.*, 2001; Isaacs, 2005).

Defensins and Cathelicidin

Several anti-microbial defensins and cathelicidin anti-microbial peptides have been demonstrated in human milk (Armogida *et al.*, 2001; Murakami *et al.*, 2005). The β-defensin-1 found in milk acts, for instance, against *E. coli* (Jia *et al.*, 2001).

Lysozyme

This enzyme can cleave peptidoglycans in the cell walls of potential bacterial pathogens, like *E. coli,* in cooperation with lactoferrin and SIgA (Adinolfi *et al.*, 1966). Its protective role has not been determined.

Lactadherin

The human milk-fat globule protein lactadherin inhibits rotavirus which is an important pathogen that causes severe dehydrating diarrhea in infants (Newburg *et al.*, 1998). Bovine milk lactadherin does not have this protective effect in humans (Kvistgaard *et al.*, 2004).

Leukocytes in Human Milk

During the first days of lactation, there are approximately 1-3 x 10^6 leukocytes/mL in milk. Two to three months later, there are fewer than 1 x 10^6 cells/mL. About 4% of them are lymphocytes (Goldblum *et al.*, 1982). The rest are neutrophils and macrophages. The primary role of the neutrophils and macrophages present in milk may be to protect the mammary glands against infections.

The role of lymphocytes in milk is not clear, but they seem to be a selected population (Lindstrand *et al.*, 1997). Surprisingly, there is some experimental evidence that they may be taken up by the offspring. There are findings to show that the breastfed offspring becomes tolerant to the mother's HLA, her tissue type antigens. That would permit her milk cells to be taken up undamaged by her breastfed infant. As another consequence, a renal transplant from a mother to her offspring gives better results if the infant has been breastfed and has been tolerized to her HLA (Campbell *et al.*, 1984).

The possible function of the NK cells in milk is unknown.

Breastfeeding and Protection Against Infections

To prove the presence of protective effects of breastfeeding against various infections and other diseases in a mode that agrees with the demands of today's evidence-based medicine would require randomized double-blind placebo-controlled trials. It is obvious that this is difficult to accomplish in studies of the effects of breastfeeding for ethical reasons; one cannot tell one mother to breastfeed her baby and another not. It is also important to realize that variations in living conditions, exposure to infectious agents, dietary intake, etc. between populations add to the problems of interpreting and evaluating reported results. These facts are important to keep in mind when reading the following review of published studies (**Table 4**). More and better controlled studies are needed in this area.

Breastfeeding, Infant Mortality, and Episodes of Illness

Mortality during the first year of life varies from three per 1000 in a country such as Sweden to around 100 deaths per 1000 in poor populations (Costello & White, 2001). Several studies from developing countries show strong reduction of infant mortality by breastfeeding. As many as 1.3 million children could be saved each year by optimal breastfeeding, i.e., six months of exclusive breastfeeding followed by partial breastfeeding for another six months (Labbok *et al.*, 2004). Part of this

Table 4. Breastfeeding May Protect Against

Acute Infections	
	Neonatal septicemia and meningitis
	Necrotizing enterocolitis
	Diarrhea
	Respiratory tract infections
	Urinary tract infections
	Sudden infant death syndrome
Likely Long Term Effects	
	Otitis media
	Upper and lower respiratory tract infections
	Urinary tract infections
	Invasive *H.influenzae* type b infections
	Severe manifestations of measles
Likely, or Possible Effects Against Inflammatory Diseases	
	Allergies (debated)
	Autoimmune and other inflammatory diseases
	Diabetes type 1 and 2, rheumatoid arthritis, celiac disease, ulcerous colitis, Crohn's disease, obesity, cardiovascular disease (hypertension, arteriosclerosis, dyslipidemia, insulin resistance)
Likely, or Possible Effects Against Certain Tumors	
In children:	Acute lymphoblastic leukemia
	Hodgkin's disease
	Neuroblastoma
In adults:	Breast cancer
	(*H. Pylori*-induced gastric cancer)

protection is due to the quite strong contraceptive effect of breastfeeding in poor populations with high fertility (Labbok *et al.*, 1997). A spacing of less than two years between births increases the risk of dying by 50% before the age of five years (Hobcraft *et al.*, 1985). It should be realized that approximately 97% of births take place in regions with the highest infant mortality and the worst poverty (Hanson *et al.*, 1994). In a controlled study from Brazil, it was found that the risk of dying from diarrhea was 4.2 times higher in those fed formula or cow's milk compared to those partially breastfed and 14.2 times higher compared with those exclusively breastfed (Victora *et al.*, 1987).

A WHO (2000) review by a collaborative team showed, with pooled odds ratios from a number of large studies in the world, significant protection, from 5.8 for infants younger than 2 months to 1.4 for those 9 to 11 months old. The first half year protection was better against diarrhea than against acute respiratory infections, with OR=6.1 compared to 2.4. For the second half year, the corresponding figures were 1.9 and 2.5. The figures ranged from OR=1.6 – 2.1 during the second year of life. A recent WHO report based on studies in Ghana, India, and Peru showed that there was no significant difference in risk of deaths between exclusively and predominantly breastfed (Bahl *et al.*, 2005). But, the hazard ratio for those not breastfed compared with those predominantly breastfed was 10.5 ($p<0.001$). When compared with those partially breastfed, it was 2.46 ($p<0.001$).

A recent statistically robust study of a representative sample of cases of postneonatal deaths claimed that promoting breastfeeding may prevent as many as 720 such deaths in the USA per year (Chen & Rogan, 2004). Several studies illustrate that breastfeeding reduces the number of episodes of illness as well as mortality (Labbok *et al.*, 2004). There are three randomized controlled trials in preterm infants indicating the protective capacity of breastfeeding against early infections. In a recent review, it was claimed, however, that these, as well as many other studies on this topic, do not fulfill the strict criteria that are needed for critical evaluation (de Silva *et al.*, 2004).

Breastfeeding and Protection Against Neonatal Infections (Table 4)

The effects on the early microbial flora colonizing the newborn probably are an important factor behind the observations that breastfeeding may protect against dangerous infections, like neonatal septicemia and meningitis (Winberg & Wessner, 1971; Ashraf *et al.*, 1991; Bhutta & Yusuf, 1997; Hylander *et al.*, 1998). Feeding low birth weight babies expressed human milk in a planned prospective study was significantly protective compared to feeding formula ($p<0.001$) (Narayanan *et al.*, 1982). A recent study of the neonatal morbidity in very low birth weight infants showed that 50 mL/kg daily of maternal milk decreased the rate of sepsis (Furman *et al.*, 2003). Obviously, mother's milk provides numerous components that can help protect the neonate who still has several limitations in its own immune capacity, even if it is full term.

One of the important principle functions for the protective milk components is to keep microbes from attaching to the mucosal membranes in the respiratory and gastrointestinal tracts. This initial step is needed for the microbe to be able to initiate an infection and is prevented by major milk components like SIgA antibodies and the numerous carbohydrate components as discussed above (**Figures 4B, 4C**). The milk SIgA antibodies, as illustrated in (**Figure 4A**), are directed against the microorganisms present in the mother's surroundings and those that pass through her gut, presently or previously. The milk carbohydrates cover a very broad range of microbes in their function as blocking receptor analogues. A recent study showed that cases of moderate-to-severe diarrhea, including those caused by *Campylobacter* and calicivirus, occurred significantly less often among infants fed mother's milk high in 2-linked fucosylated oligosaccharides (Morrow *et al.*, 2004). Breastfeeding may also protect the neonate against hypoglycemia and hypothermia, thus supporting its host defense (Huffman *et al.*, 2001).

A recent large study from Norway of the effect of very early full human milk feeding on late-onset septicemia showed a significantly reduced relative risk of 3.7 for septicemia if the human milk feeding was started within the second week of life (Ronnestad, 2005). An unmatched nested case-control study indicated that breastfeeding provided significant protection against neonatal respiratory infections in girls, but not in boys (Sinha *et al.*, 2003).

An important investigation from Ghana demonstrated that the risk of neonatal deaths was four times higher among infants given milk-based fluids or solids in addition to breastmilk. The study also illustrated the importance of starting breastfeeding early: late start, i.e., after day one, was linked to a 2.4-fold increase in risk of neonatal mortality. If all infants were breastfed from day one, neonatal deaths were reduced by 16%; if breastfeeding was started within the first hour, the reduction was 22% (Edmond *et al.*, 2006). This effect can be expected considering the lack in the neonate of an established protective normal microbial flora on the mucosal membranes in the respiratory and gastrointestinal tracts, the many limitations of the host defense systems at that age, and the many protective components provided by the mother's milk.

A recent policy statement from the American Academy of Pediatrics entitled *Breastfeeding and the Use of Human Milk* summarizes the studies, describing the child health benefits of breastfeeding, including protection against infections (Gartner *et al.*, 2005).

Breastfeeding and Necrotizing Enterocolitis (NEC)

This severe condition appears mainly in very low birth weight infants and may be an illustration of how early colonizing bacteria reach the intestinal mucosa of an individual with limited and poorly controlled defense mechanisms. The lack of defense factors like SIgA antibodies and carbohydrate analogues that prevent the potential invaders from attaching to the mucosa allow these microbes to reach gut tissues. For instance, Clostridia may be involved (de la Cochetiere *et al.*, 2004). In the gut tissues, the microbes can induce an unbalanced and damaging inflammatory reaction (Halpern *et al.*, 2002). Human milk has been shown to be protective against NEC (Lucas *et al.*, 1990; McGuire *et al.*, 2003; Schanler *et al.*, 1999).

Human milk contains an enzyme which degrades the released and damaging Platelet Activating Factor, PAF, and that may be one reason why milk is protective (Furukawa, 1993). Other protective factors include defensins which are locally produced in the intestinal epithelium (Salzman *et al.*, 1998). The anti-inflammatory IL-10 in human milk may also help protect against NEC by down-regulating the damaging inflammatory reaction (Fituch *et al.*, 2004). Probiotics, presumably protective bacteria which may be promoted by breastfeeding, could possibly also be preventive (Bell, 2005).

Sudden Infant Death syndrome (SIDS) and Breastfeeding

This syndrome is not fully understood. Recently, it has been realized that letting the baby sleep on its stomach is a significant risk factor. Taking this as well as other risk factors in regard in a collaborative Scandinavian study, it was found that breastfeeding had a weak, but significant protective effect (Alm *et al.*, 2002). Maternal smoking was shown to be another important risk factor, as well as bottle feeding (Chong *et al.*, 2004; Fleming *et al.*, 2003). Recently, a debate has started based on reports that pacifier use may decrease the risk of SIDS. At the same time, pacifier use has been negatively associated with breastfeeding, even with a dose-response effect noted (Nelson *et al.*, 2005). As to the use of pacifiers, parents need to be given full information about possible advantages and disadvantages.

It is unknown how breastfeeding helps protect against SIDS, but one study suggests that milk SIgA antibodies may block certain bacterial toxins involved in the pathogenesis (Gordon *et al.*, 1999).

Breastfeeding and Diarrhea

There are several studies that show that breastfeeding protects against diarrhea. This effect is a substantial reason why breastfeeding significantly reduces infant mortality, especially in poor areas. Critical studies have confirmed that such protection occurs in both poor and developed areas (Victora, 1990; Glass & Stoll, 1989; Howie *et al.*, 1990).

The protection often seems to be due to the presence in milk of SIgA antibodies directed against diarrhea-causing bacteria or their toxins, like enterotoxin-producing *E. coli* (ETEC), *Shigella, V. cholerae,* and *G. lamblia* (Glass *et al.*, 1983; Fuiz-Palacios, 1990; Hayani *et al.*, 1992; Cruz *et al.*, 1988; Long *et al.*, 1999). A recent randomized double blind study showed that the anti-secretory factor which can be induced in mother's milk (Svensson *et al.*, 2004) gave significant protection against acute as well as prolonged diarrhea (Zaman *et al.*, 2007). It is relevant to mention that a fully breastfed baby in a hot climate does not need any extra water. This often increases the risk of diarrheal infections if the water is not clean, besides potentially interfering with breastfeeding (Ashraf *et al.*, 1993).

In a large randomized study of breastfeeding and diarrhea in Belarus, it was found that breastfeeding protected against gastroenteritis during the first year of life (Kramer *et al.*, 2001). Exclusive breastfeeding for six months resulted in significantly fewer cases of gastroenteritis at ages three to six months than exclusive breastfeeding for three months (Kramer *et al.*, 2003). A case-control study in England showed that, after adjusting for confounders, breastfeeding protected against diarrhea comparing no breastmilk to any breastmilk, or not exclusive to exclusive breastfeeding ($p<0.005$, OR=2.74 and $p<0.006$, OR=3.62) (Quigley *et al.*, 2005). In less privileged areas, the protection reached OR=5 for the comparison of no breastmilk to any breastmilk and OR=17.66 when comparing no breastmilk to exclusive breastfeeding.

A study in Mexico demonstrated a five times lower risk of diarrhea caused by *Giardia lamblia* in breastfed compared to non-breastfed and a 1.8 times reduced risk comparing partially breastfed with not breastfed (Morrow *et al.*, 1992). Breastfeeding did not prevent chronic carriage of remaining parasites.

Rotavirus causes many cases of diarrhea, resulting in high mortality. Some studies show that breastfeeding does not provide efficient protection or results in postponement of the disease (Duffy *et al.*, 1986; Clemens *et al.*, 1993). Higher levels of SIgA antibodies in milk related to later appearance of the virus in the stool (Espinoza *et al.*, 1997). Longer breastfeeding tended to relate to asymptomatic infections. However, a more recent study of nosocomial rotavirus infections showed a significant protection by breastfeeding and none of those breastfed, but carrying the virus, showed any symptoms (Gianino *et al.*, 2002).

Breastfeeding and Respiratory Tract Infections

Middle ear infections (otitis media) are common in infancy. Several studies have investigated whether or not breastfeeding protects. Although there are some discrepant results (Kero & Piekkala, 1987; Sipila *et al.*, 1988), several studies support that breastfeeding, especially prolonged breastfeeding (>4 months), protects against acute and prolonged ear infections (Duncan *et al.*, 1993; Dewey *et al.*, 1995; Cushing *et al.*, 1998).

A common pathogen in the respiratory tract is *Haemophilus influenzae*. Breastfeeding prevents the microbes from settling in the nose and mouth of the infant (Harabuchi *et al.*, 1994), presumably via the mechanisms illustrated in **Figures 4B** and **C**. Colonization by such bacteria correlated to the risk of attracting otitis media. On the other hand, colonization of the respiratory tract with pneumococci, another common cause of respiratory infections, does not seem to be prevented by breastfeeding (Rosen *et al.*, 1996). Some studies, but not others, show that breastfeeding can protect against upper respiratory tract infections (Howie *et al.*, 1990).

Pneumonia together with diarrhea is a major cause of infant mortality in poor regions. In such areas, breastfeeding is strongly protective against lower respiratory infections (Victora *et al.*, 1987; Cesar *et al.*, 1999). A well controlled study in Belarus did not show any difference in the prevalence of respiratory infections comparing three and six months of exclusive breastfeeding (Kramer *et al.*, 2003). A large study in the USA showed that breastfeeding provided some protection against pneumonia and middle ear infections (Ford & Labbok, 1993). An additional large USA study demonstrated protection by breastfeeding against wheezing respiratory tract infections during the first four months of life (Wright *et al.*, 1989). Such wheezing infections are often of viral origin. Protection by breastfeeding against lower respiratory tract infections was more evident if the mother smoked (Nafstad *et al.*, 1996). In an Australian study, it was found that predominant breastfeeding for at least six months and partial breastfeeding for up to a year significantly reduced respiratory infections in infancy (Oddy *et al.*, 2003).

In a Navajo population in the USA, increasing rates of breastfeeding related to a 32.2% reduction in the prevalence of pneumonia and a 14.6% reduction in gastroenteritis (Wright *et al.*, 1989). Those fed formula from birth had increased prevalence of croup and bronchiolitis, possibly originating from an ongoing viral epidemic that did not affect those exclusively breastfed.

Based on the WHO recommendation of exclusive breastfeeding for the first six months of life, as also stated by the American Academy of Pediatrics, a large study was performed in the USA. Compared with full breastfeeding for four to up to six months, it was found that full breastfeeding for six months resulted in significantly smaller risk for pneumonia and repeated attacks of otitis media (Chantry *et al.*, 2006)

Breastfeeding and Protection Against Urinary Tract Infections

Urinary tract infections are mostly caused by bacteria originating from the stool, usually infecting from below via the urethra. Thus, it is not unreasonable that breastfeeding might prevent such infections since bacteria in the gut of breastfed infants often come from the mother and her surroundings. As a consequence of the entero-mammaric link illustrated in **Figure 4A**, the bacteria in the infant's gut will meet the milk SIgA antibodies directed against them. These antibodies may prevent them from ascending the urinary tract and attaching to the epithelium causing infection (**Figure 4B**).

The lactoferrin (LF) of human milk and fragments thereof are taken up in the gut and excreted in the urine. In a mouse model of urinary tract infection, we could show that orally given human LF and certain LF fragments were excreted via the kidneys and prevented experimental urinary tract infections (Håversen *et al.*, 2000). In addition to the bacterial killing, LF is anti-inflammatory and may help reduce pro-inflammatory reactivity induced by infectious agents in the breastfed infant which would cause symptoms such as pain, fever, loss of appetite, and listlessness (Håversen *et al.*, 2002; Håversen *et al.*, 2003).

Clinical studies have indicated that breastfeeding may prevent urinary tract infections (Pisacane *et al.*, 1992; Pisacane *et al.*, 1996). A recent more extensive prospective case-control study showed that ongoing breastfeeding provided significant protection (Mårild *et al.*, 2004). Longer duration of exclusive breastfeeding significantly reduced the risk of urinary tract infections in girls, with a similar trend in boys. The better protection in girls than boys might possibly be explained by the anatomical differences of the lower urinary tracts. Breastfeeding until seven months gave enhanced protection until two years of age. Such long-term protective effects of breastfeeding are further discussed below.

Breastfeeding and proposed protection against other infections

There have been suggestions that breastfeeding may protect against botulism, acute appendicitis, and hypertrophic pyloric stenosis and may prevent the need for a tonsillectomy (Arnon *et al.*, 1982; Pisacane *et al.*, 1995; Pisacane *et al.*, 1996; Pisacane *et al.*, 1996). All these reports need confirmation.

Enhancing and long-term effects on the infant's immune system by breastfeeding

Breastfeeding and vaccinations

Increased antibody responses in blood and secretions were reported among breastfed compared to non-breastfed infants given vaccines against tetanus, diphtheria, and poliovirus. The latter was a live poliovirus vaccine (Hahn-Zoric *et al.*, 1990). The increases included IgG antibodies in serum, IgM antibodies in stool, and SIgA antibodies in saliva indicating enhanced serum as well as secretory responses. Similar increases remained one to two years later. A comparable enhancement by breastfeeding was seen using *H. influenzae* type b (Hib) polysaccharide-conjugate vaccine (Pabst *et al.*, 1990). The enhancing effect was also present when vaccinating months after breastfeeding had been terminated.

Other studies using test vaccines with live viruses have not seen any enhancing effects of breastfeeding. This may be due to differences in the prevalence of these agents in the environment. The mother's immune response to them may differ, both as IgG antibodies transferred via the placenta and SIgA antibodies via the milk, affecting the vaccine response.

Live oral poliovirus vaccines can, if given too close to a breastmilk meal, be neutralized by the milk SIgA antibodies and become ineffective as noted by Sabin and confirmed by WHO (1995). It is not safe to breastfeed within half an hour before or after giving the live oral vaccine. This problem is avoided if inactivated killed poliovirus vaccine is used. There are also studies of tetanus toxoid and Hib vaccines not showing any enhancing effects because of breastfeeding (Stephens *et al.*, 1984; Watemberg *et al.*, 1991; Decker *et al.*, 1992). Again, transplacentally transferred maternal IgG antibodies may affect these vaccine responses. Recent studies of the antibody responses to Hib and pneumococcal conjugate vaccines showed that children breastfed exclusively for 90 days or more had a higher proportion of antibody responses with antibody levels against both vaccines above protective levels compared with the responses in those breastfed less (Silfverdal *et al.*, 2007a).

Breastfeeding and long term protection against infections

In a study in Finland of the protection against otitis media by breastfeeding, it was noted that the improved protection not only lasted during the period of breastfeeding, but also during a three year follow-up (Saarinen *et al.*, 1982). Breastfeeding for more than 13 weeks reduced the number of attacks of gastroenteritis through the first year of life in an investigation in Dundee (Howie *et al.*, 1990). Follow-up of these children suggested a reduced risk of respiratory tract infections at the age of seven years. An ecologic Swedish study showed that breastfeeding was followed by enhanced protection against invasive Hib (*H. influenzae* type b) infections, like meningitis during the first ten years of life (Silfverdal *et al.*, 1999). These results agreed with the findings in a case-control study (Silfverdal *et al.*, 1997). The long-term protective effect by breastfeeding may at least partly be explained by the fact that breastfeeding showed long-term enhancement of the production of the protective anti-Hib antibodies of the IgG subclass 2 (Silfverdal *et al.*, 2002). The duration of breastfeeding related to the level of anti-Hib antibodies up to school age. A Dutch study of breastfeeding through six months of age claimed better protection against respiratory tract infections, diarrhea, skin infections, and urinary tract infections during the first three years of life (van den Bogaard *et al.*, 1991).

A recent critical review of the results reported above gave support to the existence of long-term protective effects by breastfeeding against gastrointestinal and respiratory tract infections (Chien & Howie, 2001). A careful analysis of a well defined clinical material supports the concept that breastfeeding up to seven months of age enhances protection against urinary tract infections in girls through the second year of life (Mårild *et al.*, 2004).

An analysis of the very large 1970 British cohort supported the presence of a long-lasting protective effect by breastfeeding up to the age of ten years against more severe manifestations of measles infections (Silfverdal *et al.*, 2007b).

Breastfeeding for at least one month was suggested to reduce the risk of respiratory tract infections causing wheezing during the first two years (Porro *et al.*, 1993). It is important to distinguish between wheezing caused by infections as mainly seen during the early part of the first year of life and wheezing at higher ages caused by asthma as discussed in the following section.

Effects of Breastfeeding on Inflammatory Diseases and Tumors in the Infant

The immune system defends firstly via the mucosal defense by keeping infectious agents from entering our tissues. If that fails, it defends tissues against infections by inducing inflammation (**Table 4**). The inflammatory reaction can take different forms.

It can be dominated by 1) IgM and IgG antibodies which, when reacting, activate the complement system bringing in stimulated aggressive neutrophils. These add to the inflammation by releasing numerous substances, including cytokines, that damage the tissues.

The inflammation can also be dominated by 2) T lymphocytes which, when reacting with their specific antigens, start a reaction via stimulated aggressive monocytes and/or macrophages, again with the release of tissue-damaging components.

The inflammatory reaction may also be initiated by 3) IgE antibodies which via mast cells and eosinophils cause a special inflammation through a number of released mediators (histamine, prostaglandins, leukotrienes, etc.) to defend us against large parasites, but this reaction is mostly seen in patients with allergic reactivity.

It is quite clear that the various forms of inflammation may cause disease if not properly controlled. Allergy is a typical example. This special form of inflammation which, if it appears without normal control as in the allergic patient, can be induced by harmless materials, such as certain food, pollen, etc., to which the individual produces IgE antibodies. It will give rise to one or several forms of allergic diseases, like asthma, hay fever, eczema, food allergy, etc., often summarized as atopic diseases.

Since human milk contains numerous components with immunological activity, such as antibodies, lymphocytes, cytokines, chemokines, etc., it might be expected that breastfeeding could affect, for good or bad, untoward immunological reactivity, such as seen in allergic or autoimmune diseases. The data suggesting that such effects may appear in the breastfed baby are summarized below and will also include diseases which we now recognize as having immunological components, such as obesity, diabetes, and arteriosclerosis.

Breastfeeding and Allergy

Allergic diseases in childhood often start as food allergies with symptoms from the gastrointestinal tract and skin (eczema) which may vanish spontaneously. The allergy may continue into airway diseases like hay fever and asthma. This sequence is called "the allergy march" (Bergmann *et al.*, 1998). For some years, there has been a striking increase in allergic diseases, but there are now some signs that this may start to taper off (Cole, 2005).

Whether or not breastfeeding protects or increases the risk of allergic disease in the offspring is a very complex question. There is no simple answer for several reasons. One reason is that allergy is a group of diseases with involvement of many different genetic and environmental factors (Hanson, 2003). Also, it is difficult to perform studies which are adequate as to size of groups and characteristics of included individuals, definitions of exposure, details about diet, medications, exposures, and comparison with relevant controls. There are numerous studies in the field but, for the complex reasons mentioned, they do not always provide clear answers.

Basically, it can be said that allergic diseases, like autoimmune diseases, are mostly examples of disease states which result from the fact that the immune system has not developed the capacity to respond with adequate immunological tolerance against the component inducing the allergic reaction, be it a certain food, pollen, drug, or the fur of cats. Presently, it is being investigated whether exposure to certain microbes during the early intestinal colonization in the first year of life may induce regulatory T cells supporting development of tolerance. Tolerance may reduce the risk of allergic diseases to appear. No tolerogenic factor was produced in germ-free mice when colonized with either *E. coli* or *Lactobacillus plantarum*, but a full intestinal flora induced such a transferable tolerance-inducing factor in conventional mice (Rask *et al.*, 2005). In agreement with this, regulatory T cells appeared in the circulation of children in conjunction with their recovery from cow's milk allergy (Karlsson *et al.*, 2004). The role of the bacterial colonization, which induces regulatory T cells, is in agreement with the "hygiene or microflora hypothesis" for allergic diseases (Noverr & Huffnagle, 2005).

A recent critical review summarizes studies of breastfeeding and the risk for allergic diseases, dividing the reports into those supporting significant protection results and those which show no effect or increased risk (Friedman & Zeiger, 2005). Several studies are listed which show protection including the large randomized study from Belarus which reported a 46% reduction of atopic dermatitis in the group of mothers who had been educated as to breastfeeding and its effects and, therefore, breastfed more often (Kramer *et al.*, 2003). They were compared with a group of mothers not specifically educated. Some other sizable and well designed studies showing protection are also mentioned (Laubereau *et al.*, 2004; Oddy *et al.*, 2003; Kull *et al.*, 2002; Kull *et al.*, 2005).

There are many studies which show no effect or worsening of the symptoms of allergy. Critical evaluation showed, however, that many of those studies were of low quality (Friedman & Zeiger, 2005). This was also illustrated by meta–analyses of the data (Gdalevich *et al.*, 2001a; Gdalevich *et al.*, 2001b). Exclusive breastfeeding was found to reduce asthma risk and any breastfeeding diminished wheezing for at least the first ten years of life, regardless of the family history of asthma (van Odijk *et al.*, 2003). With breastfeeding longer than four months, the protection improved. Breastfeeding also protected against atopic dermatitis in infancy, but not against atopy later in life.

Exclusive breastfeeding resulted in less wheezing the first two years of life unrelated to the mother's asthma status in a large prospective study in the USA (Wright *et al.*, 2001). But if the mother had asthma, it related to a higher rate of asthma in their atopic children starting from the age of six years. On the other hand, this was not seen in an Australian study (Oddy *et al.*, 2002).

It is possible that withholding solid food during breastfeeding may delay or reduce later risk of allergy (Kull *et al.*, 2002; Oddy *et al.*, 1999). This supports the WHO recommendation of exclusive breastfeeding for six months. In addition, exclusion of allergenic food from the maternal diet resulted in improvement in breastfed infants with colic presentation according to a randomized controlled trial (Hill *et al.*, 2005).

A recent report from a poor area in South Africa suggested that prolonged breastfeeding protected against allergic disease, especially hay fever, but only in children of allergic parents (Obihara *et al.*, 2005). A large Swedish study did not find exclusive breastfeeding to influence the risk of eczema during the first year of life (Ludvigsson *et al.*, 2005).

It is obvious that it is difficult to definitely conclude on the basis of the available data whether or not breastfeeding protects against various forms of allergic diseases. This has many explanations in addition to the fact that it is very difficult to design and run well controlled studies of breastfeeding.

One factor which has not been taken into consideration in previous studies of breastfeeding and risk of allergy in the offspring is the possible presence of subclinical mastitis (Filteau *et al.*, 2003). This condition, which may be very common, was found to increase the risk of atopic dermatitis in the offspring of atopic, but not of non-atopic, mothers (Benn *et al.*, 2004). The same main author showed in another study that current breastfeeding was not associated with atopic dermatitis, but exclusive breastfeeding for at least four months was linked to an increased risk of atopic dermatitis if no parent was allergic (IRR=1.29, 95% CI:1.06-1.55), but not if one or two parents were allergic (Benn *et al.*, 2004). Whether or not the milk can affect the risk of allergy development may relate to its content of components, like CD14 which may help promote the appearance of regulatory T cells which may control and prevent allergy-inducing immune responses. A report from Finland showed a significant association between risk of atopy in the child and low levels of CD14 and SIgA antibodies in the mother's colostrum (Savilahti *et al.*, 2005). Another factor which might increase the risk of allergy in the child is delivery by cesarean section, presumably because it prevents the microbial colonization with the mother's fecal flora that normally takes place at vaginal delivery (Renz-Polster *et al.*, 2005; Laubereau *et al.*, 2005). That microbial flora seems to be important for the induction of regulatory T cells which presumably prevent untoward immune reactivity, such as allergic diseases.

The type of lipids in the mother's diet may also influence the effect of whether or not breastfeeding can protect against allergic diseases in the offspring. A study in rats showed that a low ratio of n-6/n-3 fatty acids of 0.4 in the mother's diet resulted in tolerance to a potential allergen in the breastfed offspring, whereas a ratio close to what is common in food today, around nine, gave an immune response that included potentially allergy-inducing IgE antibodies (Korotkova *et al.*, 2004a; 2004b). Human studies agree with these findings (Reichardt *et al.*, 2004; Hoppu *et al.*, 2005). In addition, supplementation with fish oil during pregnancy increased both levels of CD14 and SIgA in the milk (Dunstan *et al.*, 2004). A recent comment suggests that in discussions of whether or not breastfeeding prevents allergy, it is important to include information as to the mothers' intake of polyunsaturated fatty acids, e.g., by determining the n-6/n-3 ratio (Das, 2004).

In conclusion, it may be said against this background that at this time it is very difficult to clearly say whether or not breastfeeding will protect a baby against allergy. Obviously, it does in many cases, but we do not have easy measures today to tell which they are. The fact is, however, that in most instances the effect of breastfeeding on the appearance of allergy in the offspring, whether positive or negative, is not very strong. Thus, the risk of allergy should not be a strong argument against or for breastfeeding. It should also be noted that there are many other factors which influence whether or not a child will attract allergic disease. For instance, a large Danish study showed that the risk of eczema increased significantly with each infection before the age of six months (Benn *et al.*, 2004). But the risk decreased if there was exposure to siblings, day care, pet ownership, and farm residence. Most likely, these latter conditions work against allergy development via effects on the intestinal microflora as previously discussed.

Breastfeeding, Autoimmune, and Other Inflammatory Diseases

Earlier studies have indicated that breastfeeding may reduce the risk of developing diabetes mellitus type 1 (Hanson, 2004b). In a recent Czeck study, no breastfeeding was associated with an increased risk of diabetes type 1 with OR=1.93 (95% CI:1.33-2.80). The risk decreased with increased duration of breastfeeding; breastfeeding for >12 months reduced the risk with an OR= 0.42 (95% CI: 0.22 - 0.81) (Malcova *et al.*, 2006).

The risk of diabetes type 2, or non-insulin dependent diabetes, may also be reduced by breastfeeding (Young *et al.*, 2002). A systematic review of the literature on breastfeeding and diabetes type 2 indicated that having been breastfed for at least 2 months seems to diminish the risk of diabetes type 2 (Taylor *et al.*, 2005). Another observation was reported from the large Nurse's Health Studies in the USA: the longer these women had breastfed the lower their incidence of type 2 diabetes (Stuebe *et al.*, 2005). This effect lasted up to 15 years after their last lactation period.

Recent studies provide evidence that breastfeeding may protect against rheumatoid arthritis (Jacobsson *et al.*, 2003). There is information that breastfeeding also protects the breastfeeding mother against future rheumatoid arthritis (Karlson *et al.*, 2004).

Children with celiac disease start to have their symptoms when given gluten-containing food. Breastfeeding protects against celiac disease, but it seems they need to start receiving gluten while still breastfeeding (Fålth-Magnusson *et al.*, 1996; Ivarsson *et al.*, 2002; Akobeng *et al.*, 2006). It is not known whether this protection lasts into adulthood.

A recent meta-analysis concluded that the findings support the hypothesis that breastfeeding reduces the risk of inflammatory bowel disease, i.e., ulcerative colitis and Crohn's disease (Klement *et al.*, 2004).

Breastfeeding, Obesity, and Cardiovascular Disease

Numerous studies have investigated whether or not breastfeeding can reduce the risk of obesity. Several studies, some very large, show such an effect (von Kries *et al.*, 1999; Toschke *et al.*, 2002). A dose-dependent protective effect was supported by one meta analysis (Harder *et al.*, 2005) and also by another study (Arenz *et al.*, 2005). The effect remained into adolescence (Gillman *et al.*, 2006).

Other investigations have not confirmed this effect on obesity, suggesting that the noted effects are due to unmeasured confounding variables (Nelson *et al.*, 2005). The protective effect against overweight was not seen in Brazilian children (Araujo *et al.*, 1993), but was noted in Mexican immigrants to the USA (Kersey *et al.*, 2005). In a very large investigation of a US population, a protective effect was found among non-Hispanic whites, but not among Blacks and Hispanics (Grummer-Strawn & Mei, 2004). In another study from the USA, breastfeeding only reduced obesity at age four years among white families, with mothers who were not smoking during pregnancy, and only if breastfeeding had continued without formula for at least 16 weeks or with formula for at least 26 weeks (Bogen *et al.*, 2004). A Norwegian investigation showed an effect of breastfeeding against overweight and obesity in adolescence, but with a weaker effect on adult weight (Kvaavik *et al.*, 2005). In an Australian cohort, breastfeeding reduced overweight at age one, but not at eight years of age (Burke *et al.*, 2005).

It is not easy to summarize this information, but it seems that breastfeeding may protect against overweight and obesity, although at a rather low level with increasing age and with many factors that may impair this effect (Owen *et al.*, 2005).

There is interesting information from one of the few controlled randomized studies of breast versus formula feeding suggesting that breastmilk permanently reduced symptoms of cardiovascular disease into adolescence (Singhal & Lucas, 2004a; Singhal *et al.*, 2004b). This included symptoms like hypertension, dyslipidemia, obesity, and insulin resistance. It is difficult to ascertain the presence of such effects over several years. Further analyses will be required, but some support for effects on blood pressure has been noted at the age of five years (Lawlor *et al.*, 2004) and later according to a meta-study (Martin *et al.*, 2005c). Recent reports indicate that breastfeeding may be linked to a reduced risk for atherosclerosis in adult life (Martin *et al.*, 2005a). It has been considered that breastfeeding affects numerous functional systems in the breastfed offspring via the many signals from the mother to the infant in the milk, such as hormones, cytokines, chemokines, etc. The milk contains or affects the levels in the infant of, for instance, leptin, grehlin, and insulin-like growth factor, IGF-I (Savino *et al.*, 2005). Leptin, which has cytokine structure, has multiple effects on the immune system and on metabolism. Levels of IGF-I in children are related to breastfeeding and have been considered to possibly underlie associations between breastfeeding and adult chronic disease (Martin *et al.*, 2005d).

Breastfeeding and Tumors

Breastfeeding prevents cancers in childhood according to a meta-analysis (Martin *et al.*, 2005b). The protection of having been breastfed included a nine percent lower risk for acute lymphoblastic leukemia, 24% lower risk for Hodgkin's disease, and 41% lower risk for neuroblastoma. It was suggested that increasing breastfeeding from 50% to 100% would prevent at most five percent of the cases of childhood acute leukemia or lymphoma.

Breastfeeding did not result in a reduced risk of cancers in adulthood, such as prostatic, colorectal, or gastric cancers, but did reduce the risk of premenopausal breast cancer (Martin *et al.*, 2005e). Mothers who had breastfed more than three children had a 50% reduced risk of breast cancer (Zheng *et al.*, 2001). A critical review of several studies demonstrated that each pregnancy reduced the risk of breast cancer by seven percent and breastfeeding reduced the risk by an additional 4.3% for each year of breastfeeding. There were no differences in breast cancer rates related to age, menopausal status, ethnic origin, or age of the mother at delivery. A study of Mormon women showed that their many pregnancies and breastfeeding periods related to a lower rate of breast cancer (Daniels *et al.*, 2004).

It is not known how breastfeeding may protect against malignancies, but as has been discussed above, the major human milk protein α-lactalbumin can attain a shape called HAMLET that makes it able to kill malignant human cells (Svanborg *et al.*, 2003).

It seems that exclusive breastfeeding may have a long-term protective effect against chronic infections with *Helicobacter pylori*. Protection against chronic infection with this microorganism might result in a reduced risk of the complication of gastric ulcer (Pearce *et al.*, 2005).

The possible mechanisms behind long-term effects of breastfeeding on infections, inflammatory diseases, and certain tumors are outside the scope of this brief chapter, but have been discussed recently (Hanson, 2004b).

MICROBES THAT MAY BE PRESENT IN HUMAN MILK

Bacteria

When human milk reaches the sucking baby, it is not sterile. It carries a normal microbial flora, including bacteria like *Staphylococcus epidermidis, Streptococcus salivarius* and *mitis,* as predominant strains in 30-60% of milk samples according to a study from Finland (Heikkila & Saris, 2003). Lactobacilli like *L. rhamnosus* and *crispatus, Lactococcus lactis,* and *Leuconostoc mesenteroides* which all produce lactic acid were present together with *Enterococcus faecalis* and Enterococci in 12.5% of the milk samples. *Staph. aureus* were uncommon, possibly due to inhibitory effects by the listed normal flora. A Spanish investigation showed the presence in milk of potentially probiotic bacteria like *Lactobacillus gasseri* and *Enterococcus faecium* (Martin *et al.*, 2003).

Staph. aureus are common on the mother's breast, nose, and skin in recent Swedish studies. This is presumably the origin of the *S. aureus* often found in the gut of Swedish infants (Lindberg *et al.*, 2000). There is no evidence that the presence of these *S. aureus* cause any problems as discussed in the initial section. Milk has also been reported to occasionally contain group B *Streptococci, Campylobacter, Salmonella, Mycobacterium tuberculosis,* and *Borrelia burgdorferi* (Law *et al.*, 1989; Sharp, 1989).

Clinical and Subclinical Mastitis

Clinical mastitis is a very painful condition caused by inflammation. It appears in 24-33% of lactating mothers in Western countries (Fetherston *et al.*, 2001). Mastitis ranges from a relatively short-lasting, painful inflammatory process to an intense, longer lasting process with severe symptoms (Thomsen *et al.*, 1983).

The mammary glands are part of the mucosal immune system, involving all exocrine glands and all mucosal membranes, e.g., in the respiratory and gastrointestinal tract (Hanson, 2004a; Hanson, 2004b). This means that its defense against microbes entering via the glandular mucosa depends on the SIgA antibody system and the SIgA antibodies excreted in the milk (Hanson, 2004b). They act without inducing inflammation. In contrast, the general inflammatory host defense system acting in tissues functions via blood antibodies like IgM and IgG, activating the complement system which brings in phagocytes like neutrophils and macrophages. These cells produce numerous pro-inflammatory cytokines, resulting in even more pro-inflammatory cells. During the course of mastitis, it is likely that such an inflammatory defense has been activated without the presence of microbes and a painful inflammation typical of host defense in tissues, but not of the mucosal immune defense, appears (Prentice *et al.*, 1985).

This form of mastitis has been successfully prevented by induction of the anti-secretory factor in milk. The controlled study was done with mothers either eating an ordinary cereal or a special cereal which induces the protective anti-secretory factor (Svensson *et al.*, 2004). We find that mastitis is much less common in poor regions in rural Pakistan (personal communication, F. Jalil). This is possibly because these mothers presumably had significant levels of the potentially protective anti-secretory factor which is also induced by exposure to bacterial enterotoxins Efficient emptying of the mammary gland may also be helpful against mastitis, as well as anti-inflammatory treatment. It is likely, but not yet proven, that the anti-secretory factor also might be used for treatment, not just prophylaxis.

Subclinical mastitis is defined by an increase of sodium in the milk, best expressed as a ratio to potassium: Na/K. Levels above 1.0 are regarded as indicative of breastfeeding problems that may be severe enough to impair the infant's weight gain (Filteau, 2003). The increased Na/K ratio in milk relates to an elevation of the cytokine IL-8 in milk (Filteau, 1999). This cytokine is strongly chemotactic for neutrophils, presumably bringing additional such cells into the mammary glands. There they would cause a subclinical inflammation by the pro-inflammatory cytokines they produce when they are activated by IL-8 and possibly other cytokines appearing during this process. It seems likely that subclinical mastitis has a similar pathogenesis as clinical mastitis of the inflammatory kind without infection; only that subclinical mastitis is mild enough not to give any apparent local symptoms. Subclinical mastitis is known from the bovine species and relates to decreased milk production (Filteau 2003; Shuster, 1995).

Viruses

HIV-1

About 750,000 children worldwide get infected with HIV-1 every year. This means that 1800 children are infected every day. Most of them obtain the infection from their HIV-positive mothers. This occurs in about 15-20% of HIV-positive pregnancies, but with prolonged breastfeeding, this risk almost doubles to 35-40% (Newell, 2006). In some countries, the risk of HIV transfer from mother to infant has been reduced to less than two percent using anti-retroviral prophylaxis, elective cesarean section, and refraining from breastfeeding. In areas where avoidance of breastfeeding or elective cesarean section are not safe, it has been found that anti-retroviral treatment before and after delivery can half the risk to ten percent at six weeks, but via subsequent breastfeeding the overall risk reaches some 20%.

HIV in the milk is clearly an important factor, but the infective dose is unknown and mothers may have detectable virus in the milk without transmitting the infection. There is a relation between transmission and level of breastmilk virus, but postnatal transmission without detectable virus in the milk has also been noted (Rousseau, 2003; Manigart, 2004; Willumsen, 2003). Most likely, conditions in the infant, such as a healthy intestinal mucosa without inflammation, help to resist infection (Jamieson *et al.*, 2003). The level of HIV in the milk is highly variable and may even differ between breasts (Willumsen *et al.*, 2001).

It has been found that the HIV load in the milk is increased mainly in relation to poor maternal health as reflected by the need for antibiotics, raised inflammatory marker in the form of α_1-acid glycoprotein (AGP), and an increased Na/K ratio in milk signifying the presence of subclinical mastitis (Phiri *et al.*, 2006). This study showed that the plasma viral load was only weakly related to the milk viral load and cracked nipples did not relate to the viral load comparing different breasts. Systemic illness, as measured with AGP, and local breast inflammation, as indicated by increased Na/K ratio in the milk, related to the viral load. The viral load was also related to the need for antibiotics, presumably signifying more severe HIV disease of the mother (Phiri *et al.*, 2006). Poor infant feeding practices were associated with high Na/K ratio in the milk indicating the presence of subclinical mastitis as found in previous work (Flores *et al.*, 2002). There was no change in the viral load if breastfeeding was exclusive or if solids were added to the infant's diet. It seems that consistently supporting maternal health is paramount for decreasing the milk viral load and diminishing the risk of HIV transfer from mother to infant.

WHO recommends avoidance of all breastfeeding when replacement feeding is affordable, feasible, acceptable, sustainable, and safe. Otherwise, exclusive breastfeeding followed by early cessation is recommended (WHO, 2003). A study based on the most recent data on risks of postnatal transfer of HIV when using mixed or exclusive breastfeeding investigated the outcomes of the various forms of feeding using simulation models (Piwoz & Ross, 2005). If the infant mortality rate was <25/1000 live births, replacement feeding gave the highest HIV-free survival. If it was >25/1000, then exclusive breastfeeding up to six months followed by early cessation of breastfeeding gave the best outcome. If infant mortality was put at >/= 101/1000, then replacement feeding gave a better outcome than no postnatal interventions. However, a recent study based on 9424 children and their mothers from Ghana, India, and Peru indicated that the risk of death of not breastfeeding has been underestimated (Bahl *et al.*, 2005). The hazard ratio (HR) was 10.5 (95% CI=5.0-22.0; $p < 0.001$), comparing mortality for non-breastfed with predominantly breastfed. Partially breastfed compared with predominantly breastfed also showed a higher risk (HR=2.46; 95% CI=1.44-4.18; $p < 0.001$). There was no significant difference in protection comparing exclusively and predominantly breastfed. A large investigation from Zimbabwe recently showed that exclusive breastfeeding substantially reduced breastfeeding-associated HIV transmission (Iliff *et al.*, 2005).

A single dose of nevirapine treatment decreased the infectivity of milk in an African study (Chung *et al.*, 2005). It would be desirable that the more effective standardized, long-course, triple anti-retroviral treatment applied in Brazil, Europe, and the USA should also be made available in resource-poor regions for improved safety (Chersich *et al.*, 2005). Each year in the USA, 6-7000 women infected with HIV give birth. The importance of finding these women by testing is stressed so that they can get the recommended treatment to avoid infecting their babies: combination anti-retroviral treatment, elective cesarean section in selected patients, and avoidance of breastfeeding (Chou *et al.*, 2005).

Heating breastmilk as a possible way to avoid transfer of infective HIV was investigated. It seems that flash-heating may be superior to pasteurization for killing the virus (Israel-Ballard *et al.*, 2005). Infectivity of milk may also be decreased or prevented using the microbicide, sodium dodecyl sulfate, which is biodegradable, of little or no toxicity, and inexpensive (Urdaneta *et al.*, 2005). Various practices to prevent HIV transfer via the milk were recently reviewed, discussing their advantages and disadvantages (Urdaneta *et al.*, 2006).

The concentration of α-defensin in the milk was significantly related to a decreased risk of intrapartum and postnatal HIV transmission suggesting that this compound may help prevent HIV transmission to breastfed babies (Kugn *et al.*, 2005). Human milk often contained SIgA and IgG antibodies against the CCR5 co-receptor used by HIV-1 strains to infect human cells. This may signify yet another mode of defense provided by milk against HIV (Gouhlal, 2005). T lymphocytes directed against HIV were also found in human milk and may possibly support in the defense against transfer of HIV to the infant during breastfeeding (Sabbaj, 2005). Human milk commonly contains a blood group-related sugar structure, the Lewis X (Le^x). This was shown to block HIV-1 virus from binding to and infecting $CD4^+$ T lymphocytes (Naarding *et al.*, 2005). This may be important for preventing transfer of HIV infection to breastfed infants.

These recent observations suggest that it might become possible to define which mothers have a lower risk of infecting infants by breastfeeding. It may also become feasible to provide practical modes of destroying HIV in milk. It is to be hoped that with expanding knowledge measures will become available so that breastfeeding by an HIV-infected mother will carry no risk for her infant. Sadly, at this time the potential risk of HIV transfer has contributed to diminishing rates of breastfeeding in some regions (Labbok *et al.*, 2004). This is most unfortunate since breastfeeding offers several substantial advantages as summarized in this chapter.

Breastfeeding by mothers with untreated HIV-infection did not relate to increased maternal mortality (Kugn *et al.*, 2005).

HIV-2

There is no information at this time that HIV-2 can be transferred via milk.

Human T Cell Leukemia virus (HTLV)

This virus causes adult T cell leukemia-lymphoma and can be transferred via breastfeeding as recently briefly reviewed (Hanson, 2004b). This occurs mainly in southwest Japan, but has lately been found in several other parts of the world, like Africa, South America, the Middle East, and the Caribbean. It has not yet been proven that those infected by breastfeeding develop T cell malignancies, but breastfeeding has been discouraged in southern Japan as they are trying to interrupt the epidemic.

Cytomegalovirus (CMV)

A woman who has had a primary CMV infection develops an immune response and the infection becomes latent. During pregnancy, the virus often gets reactivated and may be transferred to the offspring via the placenta, during delivery, and in about 25% of cases via the milk (Numazaki, 1997).

SUMMARY

The sterile newborn is delivered into a world full of microbes. It handles this by expanding and developing its own host defense mechanisms. In the meantime, it is supported by help from the mother via her blood antibodies arriving over the placenta and via multiple defense factors present in her milk.

This chapter describes how being delivered next to the mother's anus provides the best chance for the newborn to pick up the most harmless bacteria around. These microbes quickly expand in the baby during the first year of life, especially in the gut of the infant, competing for space and nutrients with potentially dangerous bacteria also present in the surroundings.

The infant's own defense systems are relatively complete at full term delivery, but small. Several defense functions remain somewhat limited in early life. While the infant's specific immune system expands during the first year of life, it is supported by the mother in two ways:

1. IgG antibodies are transferred via the placenta from the mother to the infant during pregnancy. At delivery, the concentration is relatively similar in the mother and the infant, then decreases rapidly in the infant during the first several months. These antibodies help defend the infant's

tissues via immunological mechanisms which always work by causing an inflammatory response. Besides protection, this causes side effects, such as malaise, tiredness, loss of appetite, and eventually fever, pain, etc.

2. The other mode of protection of the infant is via breastfeeding. Breastfeeding provides numerous defense components and signals to the infant, all of which protect against many different forms of infectious diseases by preventing microbes from reaching the baby's mucosal membranes and deeper tissues so that no inflammatory defense is initiated. Therefore, this kind of defense causes no symptoms and no impairment of appetite and vivacity. Thus breastfeeding, especially exclusive breastfeeding, has been shown to significantly reduce infant mortality, especially in poor regions, but also in well-to-do areas. Protection has been demonstrated against neonatal sepsis, meningitis, and necrotizing enterocolitis. A weak effect has been shown against sudden infant death syndrome. Breastfeeding also gives significant protection against diarrhea, otitis media, lower respiratory tract infections, and, likely, urinary tract infections.

Some, but not all, studies show that breastfeeding may enhance certain vaccine responses. There is some evidence that the enhanced protection resulting from breastfeeding may last for one or several years after the termination of breastfeeding against otitis media, diarrhea, respiratory and urinary tract infections.

Breastfeeding also has effects against certain immunological diseases, which are caused by the same mechanisms which normally protect us against infection. Allergy is such a disease where the special symptoms are caused by the inflammation induced by the immune response erroneously reacting against food, pollen, etc. The effect of breastfeeding on allergic diseases is very complex. It may be preventive in some instances, but have reverse effects in other instances. In either case, the effects are usually moderate, possibly more often protective. There is also evidence that breastfeeding may decrease the risk of certain immunological diseases caused by the immune system reacting with its own tissues. Much more data is needed, but there are suggestions that breastfeeding may decrease the risk of diabetes type 1 and 2, rheumatoid arthritis, celiac disease, ulcerative colitis, Crohn's disease, obesity, and cardiovascular disease. The evidence for such protective effects is good against celiac disease, but needs further proof for many of the other diseases. Furthermore, there are suggestions that breastfeeding may reduce the risk for lymphoblastic leukemia, Hodgkin's disease, and neuroblastoma.

It should be mentioned that studies of protective effects of breastfeeding are difficult to do with optimal techniques: that of randomized, blinded placebo-controlled studies. It is obviously not easy or possible to optimally randomize and blind studies of breastfeeding. This means that one should remain cautious not to over interpret the results presented.

Human milk normally contains bacteria, which with few exceptions are harmless. Mastitis is a very painful inflammatory, not infectious, condition in the mammary gland which can be prevented with the anti-secretory factor. Subclinical mastitis causes no clinical symptoms, but may be common in some populations and is linked to increased risk of transfer of HIV-1 to the breastfed infant.

The transfer of HIV-1 from mother to infant is a very sad and terrible problem. About 1800 children are infected with HIV every day in the world, most of them from their infected mothers. Using antiviral treatment, elective cesarean section, and refraining from breastfeeding, the transfer has been reduced to <2%. But in areas where these measures are not safe or available, the risk of transfer of HIV remains around 20%.

Very active and promising research is trying to find ways to make breastfeeding safer in these situations.

References

Aaby P, Marx C, Trautner S, Rudaa D, Hasselbalch H, Jensen H, *et al.* Thymus size at birth is associated with infant mortality: a community study from Guinea-Bissau. *Acta Paediatr.* 2002; 91:698-703.

Adinolfi M, Glynn AA, Lindsay M, Milne CM. Serological properties of gamma-A antibodies to Escherichia coli present in human colostrum. *Immunology.* 1966; 10:517-26.

Adlerberth I, Carlsson B, de Man P, Jalil F, Khan SR, Larsson P, *et al.* Intestinal colonization with enterobacteriaceae in Pakistani and Swedish hospital-delivered infants. *Acta Paediatr Scand.* 1991; 80:602-10.

Adlerberth I, Hanson LÅ, Wold AE. Ontogeny of the intestinal flora. In: Sanderson IR, Walker WA, editors.

Development of the Gastrointestinal Tract. Hamilton, Ontario: BC Dexter Inc; 1999. p. 279-92.

Adlerberth I, Lindberg E, Åberg N, Hesselmar B, Saalman R, Strannegård IL, *et al.* Reduced enterobacterial and increased staphylococcal colonization of the infantile bowel: an effect of hygienic lifestyle? *Pediatr Res.* 2006; 59:96-101.

Ahrne S, Lonnermark E, Wold AE, Åberg N, Hesselmar B, Saalman R, *et al.* Lactobacilli in the intestinal microbiota of Swedish infants. *Microbes Infect.* 2005; 7:1256-62.

Akobeng AK, Ramanan AV, Buchan I, Heller RF. Effect of breast feeding on risk of coeliac disease: a systematic review and meta-analysis of observational studies. *Arch Dis Child.* 2006; 91:39-43.

Alm B, Wennergren G, Norvenius SG, Skjaerven R, Lagercrantz H, Helweg-Larsen K, *et al.* Breast feeding and the sudden infant death syndrome in Scandinavia, 1992-95. *Arch Dis Child.* 2002; 86:400-2.

Araujo CL, Victora CG, Hallal PC, Gigante DP. Breastfeeding and overweight in childhood: evidence from the Pelotas 1993 birth cohort study. *Int J Obes* (Lond). 2005; 30;500-6.

Arenz S, von Kries R. Protective effect of breastfeeding against obesity in childhood. Can a meta-analysis of observational studies help to validate the hypothesis? *Adv Exp Med Biol.* 2005; 569:40-48.

Armogida SA, Yannaras NM, Melton AL, Srivastava MD. Identification and quantification of innate immune system mediators in human breast milk. *Allergy Asthma Proc.* 2004; 25:297-304.

Arnon SS, Damus K, Thompson B, Midura TF, Chin J. Protective role of human milk against sudden death from infant botulism. *J Pediatr.* 1982; 100:568-73.

Ashraf RN, Jalil F, Aperia A, Lindblad BS. Additional water is not necessary in healthy breastfed babies in a hot climate. *Acta Paediatr.* 1993; 82:1007-11.

Ashraf RN, Jalil F, Zaman S, Karlberg J, Khan SR, Lindblad BS, *et al.* Breastfeeding and protection against neonatal sepsis in a high risk population. *Arch Dis Childh.* 1991; 66:488-90.

Bahl R, Frost C, Kirkwood BR, Edmond K, Martines J, Bbandari N, *et al.* Infant feeding patterns and risks of death and hospitalization in the first half of infancy: multicentre cohort study. *Bull World Health Organ.* 2005; 83:418-26.

Balmer SE, Wharton BA. Diet and faecal flora in the newborn: breast milk and infant formula. *Arch Dis Child.* 1989; 64:1672-77.Bell EF. Preventing necrotizing enterocolitis: what works and how safe? *Pediatrics.* 2005; 115:173-74.

Bendelac A, Medzhitov R. Adjuvants of immunity: harnessing innate immunity to promote adaptive immunity. *J Exp Med.* 2002; 195:F19-23.

Benn CS, Böttcher MF, Pedersen BV, Filteau SM, Duchén K. Mammary epithelial paracellular permeability in atopic and non-atopic mothers versus childhood atopy. *Pediatr Allergy Immunol.* 2004; 15:123-26.

Benn CS, Melbye M, Wohlfahrt J, Björkstén B, Aaby P. Cohort study of sibling effect, infectious diseases, and risk of atopic dermatitis during first 18 months of life. *BMJ.* 2004a; 328:1223.

Benn CS, Wohlfahrt J, Aabye P, Westergaard T, Benfeldt E, Michaelsen KF, et al. Breastfeeding and risk of atopic dermatitis during the first 18 months of life by parental history of allergy. *Am J Epidemiol.* 2004b; 160:217-23.

Benno Y, Sawada K, Mitsuoka T. The intestinal microflora of infants: composition of fecal flora in breast-fed and bottle-fed infants. *Microbiol Immunol.* 1984; 28:975-86.

Bergmann RL, Edenharter G, Bergmann KE, Forster J, Bauer CP, Wahn V, *et al.* Atopic dermatitis in early infancy predicts allergic airway disease at 5 years. *Clin Exp Allergy.* 1998; 28:965-70.

Bhutta ZA, Yusuf K. Neonatal sepsis in Karachi: factors determining outcome and mortality. *J Trop Pediatr.* 1997; 43:65-70.

Bogen DL, Hanusa BH, Whitaker RC. The effect of breast-feeding with and without formula use on the risk of obesity at 4 years of age. *Obes Res.* 2004; 12:1527-35.

Böttcher MF, Jenmalm MC, Björkstén B, Garofalo RP. Chemoattractant factors in breast milk from allergic and nonallergic mothers. *Pediatr Res.* 2000; 47:592-7.

Bouhlal H, Latry V, Requena M, Aubry S, Kaveri SV, Kazatchkine MD, *et al.* Natural antibodies to CCR5 from breast milk block infection of macrophages and dendritic cells with primary R5-tropic HIV-1. *J Immunol.* 2005; 174:7202-9.

Brandtzaeg P. The secretory immunoglobulin system: regulation and biological significance. Focusing on human mammary glands. *Adv Exp Med Biol.* 2001; 503:1-16.

Bullen CL, Tearle PV. Bifidobacteria in the intestinal tract of infants: an in-vitro study. *J Med Microbiol.* 1976; 9:335-44.

Burke V, Beilin LJ, Simmer K, Oddy WH, Blake KV, Doherty D, *et al.* Breastfeeding and overweight: longitudinal analysis in an Australian birth cohort. *J Pediatr.* 2005; 147:56-61.

Butte NF, Goldblum RM, Fehl LM, Loftin K, Smith EO, Garza C, *et al.* Daily ingestion of immunologic components in human milk during the first four months of life. *Acta Paediatr Scand.* 1984; 73:296-301.

Campbell Jr DA, Lorber MI, Sweeton JC, Turcotte JG, Niederhuber JE, Beer AE. Breast feeding and maternal-donor renal allografts. Possibly the original donor-specific transfusion. *Transplantation.* 1984; 37:340-44.

Carbonare CB, Carbonare SB, Carneiro-Sampaio MM. Secretory immunoglobulin A obtained from pooled human colostrum and milk for oral passive immunization. *Pediatr Allergy Immunol.* 2005; 16:574-81.

Cesar JA, Victora CG, Barros FC, Santos IS, Flores JA. Impact of breast feeding on admission for pneumonia during postneonatal period in Brazil: nested case-control study. *BMJ.* 1999; 318:1316-20.

Chantry CJ, Howard CR, Auinger P. Full breastfeeding duration and associated decrease in respiratory tract infection in US children. *Pediatrics.* 2006; 117:425-32.

Chen A, Rogan WJ. Breastfeeding and the risk of postneonatal death in the United States. *Pediatrics.* 2004; 113:e435-9.

Chersich MF, Gray GE. Progress and Emerging Challenges in Preventing Mother-to-Child Transmission. *Curr Infect Dis Rep.* 2005; 7:393-400.

Chien PF, Howie PW. Breast milk and the risk of opportunistic infection in infancy in industrialized and non-industrialized settings. *Adv Nutr Res.* 2001; 10:69-104.

Chong DS, Yip PS, Karlberg J. Maternal smoking: an increasing unique risk factor for sudden infant death syndrome in Sweden. *Acta Paediatr.* 2004; 93:471-78.

Chou R, Smits AK, Huffman LH, Fu R, Korthuis PT. Prenatal screening for HIV: A review of the evidence for the U.S. Preventive Services Task Force. *Ann Intern Med.* 2005; 143:38-54.

Chung MH, Kiarie JN, Richardson BA, Lehman DA, Overbaugh J, John-Stewart GC. Breast milk HIV-1 suppression and decreased transmission: a randomized trial comparing HIVNET 012 nevirapine versus short-course zidovudine. *Aids.* 2005; 19:1415-22.

Clemens J, Rao M, Eng M, Ahmed F, Ward R, Huda S, et al. Breast-feeding and the risk of life-threatening rotavirus diarrhea: Prevention or postponement? *Pediatrics.* 1993; 92:680-5.

Coconnier MH, Bernet MF, Kerneis S, Chauviere G, Fourniat J, Servin AL. Inhibition of adhesion of enteroinvasive pathogens to human intestinal Caco-2 cells by Lactobacillus acidophilus strain LB decreases bacterial invasion. *FEMS Microbiol Lett.* 1993; 110:299-305.

Coconnier MH, Lievin V, Lorrot M, Servin AL. Antagonistic activity of Lactobacillus acidophilus LB against intracellular Salmonella enterica serovar Typhimurium infecting human enterocyte-like Caco-2/TC-7 cells. *Appl Environ Microbiol.* 2000; 66:1152-7.

Cole A. New cases of asthma in children in England and Wales has fallen by two thirds. *BMJ.* 2005; 330:691.

Coppa GV, Zampini L, Galeazzi T, Facinelli B, Ferrante L, Capretti R, *et al.* Human Milk Oligosaccharides Inhibit the Adhesion to Caco-2 Cells of Diarrheal Pathogens: Escherichia coli, Vibrio cholerae, and Salmonella fyris. *Pediatr Res.* 2006; 59:377-82.

Costello A, White H. Reducing global inequalities in child health. *Arch Dis Child.* 2001; 84:98-102.

Cruz JR, Gil L, Cano F, Caceres P, Pareja G. Breast milk anti Escherichia coli heat-labile toxin IgA antibodies protect against toxin-induced infantile diarrhoea. *Acta Paediatr Scand.* 1988; 77:658-62.

Cushing AH, Samet JM, Lambert WE, Skipper BJ, Hunt WC, Young SA, *et al.* Breastfeeding reduces risk of respiratory illness in infants. *Am J Epidemiol.* 1998; 147:863-70.

Daniels M, Merrill RM, Lyon JL, Stanford JB, White GL Jr. Associations between breast cancer risk factors and religious practices in Utah. *Prev Med.* 2004; 38:28-38.

Das UN. Breast-feeding, atopy, and asthma. *J Allergy Clin Immunol.* 2004; 113:1002; author reply -3.

de la Cochetiere MF, Piloquet H, des Robert C, Darmaun D, Galmiche JP, Roze JC. Early intestinal bacterial colonization and necrotizing enterocolitis in premature infants: the putative role of Clostridium. *Pediatr Res.* 2004; 56:366-70.

de Silva A, Jones PW, Spencer SA. Does human milk reduce infection rates in preterm infants? A systematic review. *Arch Dis Child Fetal Neonatal Ed.* 2004; 89:F509-13.

Decker MD, Edwards KM, Bradley R, Palmer P. Comparative trial in infants of four conjugate Haemophilus influenzae type b vaccines. *J Pediatr.* 1992; 120:184-9.

Deubzer HE, Obaro SK, Newman VO, Adegbola RA, Greenwood BM, Henderson DC. Colostrum obtained from women vaccinated with pneumococcal vaccine during pregnancy inhibits epithelial adhesion of Streptococcus pneumoniae. *J Infect Dis.* 2004; 190:1758-61.

Dewey KG, Heinig MJ, Nommsen-Rivers LA. Differences in morbidity between breast-fed and formula-fed infants. *J Pediatr.* 1995; 126:696-702.

Dias S, Silva H Jr, Cumano A, Vieira P. Interleukin-7 is necessary to maintain the B cell potential in common lymphoid progenitors. *J Exp Med.* 2005; 201:971-9.

Duffy LC, Byers TE, Riepenhoff-Talty M, La Scolea LJ, Zielezny M, Ogra PL. The effects of infant feeding on rotavirus-induced gastroenteritis: A prospective study. *Am J Publ Health.* 1986; 76:259-63.

Duncan B, Ey J, Holberg CJ, Wright AL, Martinez FD, Taussig LM. Exclusive breast-feeding for at least 4 months protects against otitis media. *Pediatrics.* 1993; 91:867-72.

Dunstan JA, Roper J, Mitoulas L, Hartmann PE, Simmer K, Prescott SL. The effect of supplementation with fish oil during pregnancy on breast milk immunoglobulin A, soluble CD14, cytokine levels and fatty acid composition. *Clin Exp Allergy.* 2004; 34:1237-42.

Edmond K, Zandioh C, Quigley MA, Amenga-Etego S, Owusu-Agyei S, Kirkwood BR. Delayed breastfeeding initiation increases the risk of neonatal mortality. *Pediatrics.* 2006; 117:380-86.

Ellison RT. The effects of lactoferrin on gram-negative bacteria. In: Hutchens TW, Rumball SV, Lönnerdal B, editors. *Advances in Experimental Medicine and Biology Lactoferrin: Structure and Function.* New York: Plenum Press; 1994. p. 71-90.

Espinoza F, Paniagua M, Hallander H, Svensson L, Strannegård Ö. Rotavirus infections in young Nicaraguan children. *Pediatr Infect Dis J.* 1997; 16:564-71.

Favre L, Spertini F, Corthesy B. Secretory IgA possesses intrinsic modulatory properties stimulating mucosal and systemic immune responses. *J Immunol.* 2005; 175:2793-800.

Fetherston CM, Lee CS, Hartmann PE. Mammary gland defense: the role of colostrum, milk and involution secretion. *Adv Nutr Res.* 2001; 10:167-98.

Field CJ. The immunological components of human milk and their effect on immune development in infants. *J Nutr.* 2005; 135:1-4.

Filteau S. The influence of mastitis on antibody transfer to infants through breast milk. *Vaccine.* 2003; 21:3377-81.

Filteau SM, Rice AL, Ball JJ, Chakraborty J, Stoltzfus R, de Francisco A, *et al.* Breast milk immune factors in Bangladeshi women supplemented postpartum with retinol or beta-carotene. *Am J Clin Nutr.* 1999; 69:953-58.

Fituch CC, Palkowetz KH, Goldman AS, Schanler RJ. Concentrations of IL-10 in preterm human milk and in milk from mothers of infants with necrotizing enterocolitis. *Acta Paediatr.* 2004; 93:1496-500.

Fleming PJ, Blair PS, Ward Platt M, Tripp J, Smith IJ. Sudden infant death syndrome and social deprivation: assessing epidemiological factors after post-matching for deprivation. *Paediatr Perinat Epidemiol.* 2003; 17:272-80.

Flores M, Filteau S. Effect of lactation counselling on subclinical mastitis among Bangladeshi women. *Ann Trop Paediatr.* 2002; 22:85-88.

Ford K, Labbok M. Breast-feeding and child health in the United States. *J Biosoc Sci.* 1993; 25:187-94.

Friedman NJ, Zeiger RS. The role of breast-feeding in the development of allergies and asthma. *J Allergy Clin Immunol.* 2005; 115:1238-48.

Furman L, Taylor G, Minich N, Hack M. The effect of maternal milk on neonatal morbidity of very low-birth-weight infants. *Arch Pediatr Adolesc Med.* 2003; 157:66-71.

Furukawa M, Narahara H, Yasuda K, Johnston JM. Presence of platelet-activating factor-acetylhydrolase in milk. *J Lipid Res.* 1993; 34:1603-9.

Fälth-Magnusson K, Franzén L, Jansson G, Laurin P, Stenhammar L. Infant feeding history shows distinct differences between Swedish celiac and reference children. *Pediatr Allergy Immunol.* 1996; 7:1-5.

Gartner LM, Morton J, Lawrence RA, Naylor AJ, O'Hare D, Schanler RJ, et al. Breastfeeding and the use of human milk. *Pediatrics.* 2005; 115:496-506.

Gdalevich M, Mimouni D, David M, Mimouni M. Breast-feeding and the onset of atopic dermatitis in childhood: a systematic review and meta-analysis of prospective studies. *J Am Acad Dermatol.* 2001a; 45:520-27.

Gdalevich M, Mimouni D, Mimouni M. Breast-feeding and the risk of bronchial asthma in childhood: a systematic review with meta-analysis of prospective studies. *J Pediatr.* 2001b; 139:261-66.

Gianino P, Mastretta E, Longo P, Laccisaglia A, Sartore M, Russo R, *et al.* Incidence of nosocomial rotavirus infections, symptomatic and asymptomatic, in breast-fed and non-breast-fed infants. *J Hosp Infect.* 2002; 50:13-17.

Gilbert JV, Plaut AG, Longmaid B, Lamm ME. Inhibition of bacterial IgA proteases by human secretory IgA and serum. *Ann NY Acad Sci.* 1983; 409:625-36.

Gillman MW, Rifas-Shiman SL, Berkey CS, Frazier AL, Rockett HR, Camargo CA Jr, *et al.* Breast-feeding and overweight in adolescence. *Epidemiology.* 2006; 17:112-14.

Glass RI, Stoll BJ. The protective effect of human milk against diarrhoea: a review of studies from Bangladesh. *Acta Paediatr Scand.* 1989; 351:131-36.

Glass RI, Svennerholm AM, Stoll BJ, Khan SR, Hassain KMB, Huq MI, *et al.* Protection against cholera in breast-fed children by antibodies in breast-milk. *N Engl J Med.* 1983; 308:1389-92.

Goldblum RM, Goldman AS, Garza C, Johnson CA, Nichols BL. Human milk banking. II. Relative stability of immunologic factors in stored colostrum. *Acta Paediatr Scand.* 1982; 71:143-44.

Gordon AE, Saadi AT, MacKenzie DA, Molony N, James VS, Weir DM, *et al.* The protective effect of breast feeding in relation to sudden infant death syndrome (SIDS): III. Detection of IgA antibodies in human milk that bind to bacterial toxins implicated in SIDS. *FEMS Immunol Med Microbiol.* 1999; 25:175-82.

Grummer-Strawn LM, Mei Z. Does breastfeeding protect against pediatric overweight? Analysis of longitudinal data from the Centers for Disease Control and Prevention Pediatric Nutrition Surveillance System. *Pediatrics.* 2004; 113:81-86.

Gustafsson L, Hallgren O, Mossberg AK, Pettersson J, Fischer W, Aronsson A, *et al.* HAMLET kills tumor cells by apoptosis: structure, cellular mechanisms, and therapy. *J Nutr.* 2005; 135:1299-303.

Gustafsson L, Leijonhufvud I, Aronsson A, Mossberg AK, Svanborg C. Treatment of skin papillomas with topical alpha-lactalbumin-oleic acid. *N Engl J Med.* 2004; 350:2663-72.

Hahn-Zoric M, Fulconis F, Minoli I, Moro M, Carlsson B, Böttiger M, *et al.* Antibody responses to parenteral and oral vaccines are impaired by conventional and low protein formulas as compared to breast-feeding. *Acta Paediatr Scand.* 1990; 79:1137-42.

Häkansson A, Zhivotovsky B, Orrenius S, Sabharwal H, Svanborg C. Apoptosis induced by a human milk protein. *Proc Natl Acad Sci USA.* 1995; 92:8064-68.

Halpern MD, Holubec H, Dominguez JA, Williams CS, Meza YG, McWilliam DL, *et al.* Up-regulation of IL-18 and IL-12 in the ileum of neonatal rats with necrotizing enterocolitis. *Pediatr Res.* 2002; 51:733-39.

Hanson LÅ, Ashraf R, Zaman S, Karlberg J, Khan SR, Lindblad B, *et al.* Breastfeeding is a natural contraceptive and prevents disease and death in infants, linking infant mortality and birth rates. *Acta Paediatr.* 1994; 83:3-6.

Hanson LÅ, Korotkova M, Lundin S, Håversen L, Silfverdal S, Mattsby-Baltzer I, *et al.* The transfer of immunity from mother to child. *Ann NY Acad Sci.* 2003; 987:1-8.

Hanson LÅ. *Allergy. Nature Encyclopedia of Life Sciences* (online). London: Nature Publishing Group; 2003. p. Available from www.els.net.

Hanson LÅ, Korotkova M, Telemo E. Human milk, its components and their immunobiological function. In: J Mestecky JB, ME Lamm, L Mayer, J McGhee, W Strober, editor. *Mucosal Immunology.* Third edition ed. San Diego: Academic Press; 2004a. p. 1795-827.

Hanson LÅ. *Immunobiology of Human Milk. How Breastfeeding Protects Babies.* Amarillo, TX, USA: Pharmasoft Publ; 2004b.

Harabuchi Y, Faden H, Yamanaka N, Duffy L, Wolf J, Krystofik D. Human milk secretory IgA antibody to nontypeable Haemophilus influenzae: possible protective effects against nasopharyngeal colonization. *J Pediatric.* 1994; 124:193-98.

Harder T, Bergmann R, Kallischnigg G, Plagemann A. Duration of breastfeeding and risk of overweight: a meta-analysis. *Am J Epidemiol.* 2005; 162:397-403.

Håversen L, Ohlsson BG, Hahn-Zoric M, Hanson LÅ, Mattsby-Baltzer I. Lactoferrin down-regulates the LPS-induced cytokine production in monocytic cells via NF-kappaB. *Cell Immunol.* 2002; 220:83-95.

Håversen LÅ, Baltzer L, Dolphin G, Hanson LÅ, Mattsby-Baltzer I. Anti-inflammatory activities of human lactoferrin in acute dextran sulphate-induced colitis in mice. *Scand J Immunol.* 2003; 57:2-10.

Håversen LÅ, Engberg I, Baltzer L, Dolphin G, Hanson LÅ, Mattsby-Baltzer I. Human lactoferrin and peptides derived from a surface-exposed helical region reduce experimental Escherichia coli urinary tract infection in mice. *Infect Immun.* 2000; 68:5816-23.

Hawkes JS, Neumann MA, Gibson RA. The effect of breast feeding on lymphocyte subpopulations in healthy term infants at 6 months of age. *Pediatr Res.* 1999; 45:648-51.

Hayani KC, Guerrero ML, Morrow AL, Gomez HF, Winsor DK, Ruiz-Palacios GM, *et al.* Concentration of milk secretory immunoglobulin A against Shigella virulence plasmid-associated antigens as a predictor of symptom status in Shigella-infected breast-fed infants. *J Pediatr.* 1992; 121:852-6.

Heikkila MP, Saris PE. Inhibition of Staphylococcus aureus by the commensal bacteria of human milk. *J Appl Microbiol.* 2003; 95:471-8.

Hernell O, Ward H, Blackberg L, Pereira ME. Killing of Giardia lamblia by human milk lipases: an effect mediated by lipolysis of milk lipids. *J Infect Dis.* 1986; 153:715-20.

Herrera-Insua I, Gomez HF, Diaz-Gonzalez VA, Chaturvedi P, Newburg DS, Cleary TG. Human milk lipids bind Shiga toxin. *Adv Exp Med Biol.* 2001; 501:333-39.

Hill DJ, Roy N, Heine RG, Hosking CS, Francis DE, Brown J, *et al.* Effect of a low-allergen maternal diet on colic among breastfed infants: a randomized, controlled trial. *Pediatrics.* 2005; 116:709-15.

Hobcraft JN, McDonald JW, Rutstein SO. Demographic determinants of infant and early child mortality: A comparative analysis. *Population Studies.* 1985; 39:363-85.

Hogquist KA, Baldwin TA, Jameson SC. Central tolerance: learning self-control in the thymus. *Nat Rev Immunol.* 2005; 5:772-82.

Hoppu U, Rinne M, Lampi AM, Isolauri E. Breast milk fatty acid composition is associated with development of atopic dermatitis in the infant. *J Pediatr Gastroenterol Nutr.* 2005; 41:335-38.

Howie PW, Forsyth JS, Ogston SA, Clark A, Florey CV. Protective effect of breast feeding against infection. *BMJ.* 1990; 300:11-16.

Huffman SL, Zehner ER, Victora C. Can improvements in breast-feeding practices reduce neonatal mortality in developing countries? *Midwifery.* 2001; 17:80-92.

Hylander MA, Strobino DM, Dhanireddy R. Human milk feedings and infection among very low birth weight infants. *Pediatrics.* 1998; 102:E38.

Iliff PJ, Piwoz EG, Tavengwa NV, Zunguza CD, Marinda ET, Nathoo KJ, *et al.* Early exclusive breastfeeding reduces the risk of postnatal HIV-1 transmission and increases HIV-free survival. *Aids.* 2005; 19:699-708.

Isaacs CE. Human milk inactivates pathogens individually, additively, and synergistically. *J Nutr.* 2005; 135:1286-88.

Israel-Ballard K, Chantry C, Dewey K, Lönnerdal B, Sheppard H, Donovan R, *et al.* Viral, nutritional, and bacterial safety of flash-heated and pretoria-pasteurized breast milk to prevent mother-to-child transmission of HIV in resource-poor countries: a pilot study. *J Acquir Immune Defic Syndr.* 2005; 40:175-81.

Ivarsson A, Hernell O, Stenlund H, Persson LÅ. Breast-feeding protects against celiac disease. *Am J Clin Nutr.* 2002; 75:914-21.

Jacobsson LT, Jacobsson ME, Askling J, Knowler WC. Perinatal characteristics and risk of rheumatoid arthritis. *BMJ.* 2003; 326:1068-69.

Jamieson DJ, Sibailly TS, Sadek R, Roels TH, Ekpini ER, Boni-Ouattara E, *et al.* HIV-1 viral load and other risk factors for mother-to-child transmission of HIV-1 in a breast-feeding population in Cote d'Ivoire. *J Acquir Immune Defic Syndr.* 2003; 34:430-36.

Janeway CA, Travers P, Walport M, Schlomchik M. *Immunobiology. The immune system in health and disease.* 5 ed. New York: Garland Science Publishing; 2005.

Jia HP, Starner T, Ackermann M, Kirby P, Tack BF, McCray PB Jr. Abundant human beta-defensin-1 expression in milk and mammary gland epithelium. *J Pediatr.* 2001; 138:109-12.

Karlson EW, Mandl LA, Hankinson SE, Grodstein F. Do breast-feeding and other reproductive factors influence future risk of rheumatoid arthritis? Results from the Nurses' Health Study. *Arthritis Rheum.* 2004; 50:3458-67.

Karlsson H, Hessle C, Rudin A. Innate immune response of human neonatal cells to bacteria from the normal gastrointestinal flora. *Infect Immun.* 2002; 70:6688-96.

Karlsson MR, Rugtveit J, Brandtzaeg P. Allergen-responsive CD4+CD25+ regulatory T cells in children who have outgrown cow's milk allergy. *J Exp Med.* 2004; 199:1679-88.

Kelly D, Campbell JI, King TP, Grant G, Jansson EA, Coutts AGP, Pettersson S, Conway S. Commensal anarobic gut bacteria attenuate inflammation by regulating nuclear-cytoplasmic shuttling of PPAR-g and RelA. *Nature Immunology.* 2004; 5:104-12.

Kero P, Piekkala P. Factors affecting the occurrence of acute otitis media during the first year of life. *Acta Paediatr Scand.* 1987; 76:618-23.

Kersey M, Lipton R, Sanchez-Rosado M, Kumar J, Thisted R, Lantos JD. Breast-feeding history and overweight in Latino preschoolers. *Ambul Pediatr.* 2005; 5:355-58.

Kleessen B, Bunke H, Tovar K, Noack J, Sawatzki G. Influence of two infant formulas and human milk on the development of the faecal flora in newborn infants. *Acta Paediatr.* 1995; 84:1347-56.

Klement E, Cohen RV, Boxman J, Joseph A, Reif S. Breastfeeding and risk of inflammatory bowel disease: a systematic review with meta-analysis. *Am J Clin Nutr.* 2004; 80:1342-52.

Korotkova M, Telemo E, Hanson LÅ, Strandvik B. The ratio of n-6 and n-3 essential fatty acids in maternal milk influences the induction of neonatal immunological tolerance to ovalbumin. *Clin Exp Immunol.* 2004a; 137:237-44.

Korotkova M, Telemo E, Hanson LÅ, Strandvik B. Modulation of neonatal immunological tolerance to ovalbumin by maternal essential fatty acid intake. *Pediatr Allergy Immunol.* 2004b; 15:112-22.

Kramer MS, Chalmers B, Hodnett ED, Sevkovskaya Z, Dzikovich I, Shapiro S, *et al.* Promotion of Breastfeeding Intervention Trial (PROBIT): a randomized trial in the Republic of Belarus. *JAMA.* 2001; 285:413-20.

Kramer MS, Guo T, Platt RW, Sevkovskaya Z, Dzikovich I, Collet JP, *et al.* Infant growth and health outcomes associated with 3 compared with 6 mo of exclusive breastfeeding. *Am J Clin Nutr.* 2003; 78:291-95.

Kuhn L, Kasonde P, Sinkala M, Kankasa C, Semrau K, Vwalika C, *et al.* Prolonged breast-feeding and mortality up to two years post-partum among HIV-positive women in Zambia. *Aids.* 2005; 19:1677-81.

Kuhn L, Trabattoni D, Kankasa C, Semrau K, Kasonde P, Lissoni F, *et al.* Alpha-defensins in the prevention of HIV transmission among breastfed infants. *J Acquir Immune Defic Syndr.* 2005; 39:138-42.

Kull I, Almqvist C, Lilja G, Pershagen G, Wickman M. Breastfeeding reduces the risk of asthma during the first 4 years of life. *J Allergy Clin Immunol.* 2005; 114:657-61.

Kull I, Wickman M, Lilja G, Nordvall SL, Pershagen G. Breast feeding and allergic diseases in infants - a prospective birth cohort study. *Arch Dis Child.* 2002; 87:478-81.

Kvaavik E, Tell GS, Klepp KI. Surveys of Norwegian youth indicated that breast feeding reduced subsequent risk of obesity. *J Clin Epidemiol.* 2005; 58:849-55.

Kvistgaard AS, Pallesen LT, Arias CF, Lopez S, Petersen TE, Heegaard CW, *et al.* Inhibitory effects of human and bovine milk constituents on rotavirus infections. *J Dairy Sci.* 2004; 87:4088-96.

Labbok MH, Clark D, Goldman AS. Breastfeeding: maintaining an irreplaceable immunological resource. *Nat Rev Immunol.* 2004; 4:565-72.

Labbok MH, Hight-Laukaran V, Peterson AE, Fletcher V, von Hertzen H, Van Look PF. Multicenter study of the Lactational Amenorrhea Method (LAM): I. Efficacy, duration, and implications for clinical application. *Contraception.* 1997; 55:327-36.

Lange S, Lönnroth I. The antisecretory factor: synthesis, anatomical and cellular distribution, and biological action in experimental and clinical studies. *Int Rev Cytol.* 2001; 210:39-75.

Langrish CL, Buddle JC, Thrasher AJ, Goldblatt D. Neonatal dendritic cells are intrinsically biased against Th-1 immune responses. *Clin Exp Immunol.* 2002; 128:118-23.

Laubereau B, Brockow I, Zirngibl A, Koletzko S, Gruebl A, von Berg A, *et al.* Effect of breast-feeding on the development of atopic dermatitis during the first 3 years of life--results from the GINI-birth cohort study. *J Pediatr.* 2004; 144:602-7.

Laubereau B, Filipiak-Pittroff B, von Berg A, Grubl A, Reinhart D, Wichmann HE, Koletzko S, Reading R. Caecarean section and gastrointestinal symptoms, atopic dermatitis, and sensitization during the first year of life. *Child Care Health Dev.* 2005; 1:124-25.

Law BJ, Urias BA, Lertzman J, Robson D, Romane L. Is ingestion of milk-associated bacteria by premature infants fed raw human milk controlled by routine bacteriologic screening? *J Clin Microbiol.* 1989; 7:1560-66.

Lawlor DA, Najman JM, Sterne J, Williams GM, Ebrahim S, Davey-Smith G. Associations of parental, birth, and early life characteristics with systolic blood pressure at 5 years of age: findings from the Mater-University study of pregnancy and its outcomes. *Circulation.* 2004; 110:2417-23.

Levy O. Innate immunity of the human newborn: distinct cytokine responses to LPS and other Toll-like receptor agonists. *J Endotoxin Res.* 2005; 11:113-16.

Lievin V, Peiffer I, Hudault S, Rochat F, Brassart D, Neeser JR, *et al.* Bifidobacterium strains from resident infant human gastrointestinal microflora exert antimicrobial activity. *Gut.* 2000; 47:646-52.

Lindberg E, Adlerberth I, Hesselmar B, Saalman R, Strannegård IL, *et al.* High rate of transfer of Staphylococcus aureus from parental skin to infant gut flora. *J Clin Microbiol.* 2004; 42:530-34.

Lindberg E, Nowrouzian F, Adlerberth I, Wold AE. Long-time persistence of superantigen-producing Staphylococcus aureus strains in the intestinal microflora of healthy infants. *Pediatr Res.* 2000; 48:741-47.

Lindstrand A, Smedman L, Gunnlaugsson G, Troye-Blomberg M. Selective compartmentalization of gammadelta-T lymphocytes in human breastmilk. *Acta Paediatr.* 1997; 86:890-91.

Liu E, Tu W, Law HK, Lau YL. Decreased yield, phenotypic expression and function of immature monocyte-derived dendritic cells in cord blood. *Br J Haematol.* 2001; 113:240-46.

Long K, Vasquez-Garibay E, Mathewson J, de la Cabada J, DuPont H. The impact of infant feeding patterns on infection and diarrheal disease due to enterotoxigenic Escherichia coli. *Salud Publica Mex.* 1999; 41:263-70.

Lord G. Role of leptin in immunology. *Nutr Rev.* 2002; 60:S35-8; discussion S68-84.

Lucas A, Cole TJ. Breast milk and neonatal necrotising enterocolitis. *Lancet.* 1990; 336:1519-23.

Ludvigsson JF, Moström M, Ludvigsson J, Duchén K. Exclusive breastfeeding and risk of atopic dermatitis in some 8300 infants. *Pediatr Allergy Immunol.* 2005; 16:201-8.

Lundequist B, Nord CE, Winberg J. The composition of the faecal microflora in breastfed and bottle fed infants from birth to eight weeks. *Acta Paediatr Scand.* 1985; 74:45-51.

Malcova H, Sumnik Z, Drevinek P, Venhacova J, Lebl J, Cinek O. Absence of breast-feeding is associated with the risk of type 1 diabetes: a case-control study in a population with rapidly increasing incidence. *Eur J Pediatr.* 2006; 165:114-19.

Manigart O, Crepin M, Leroy V, Meda N, Valea D, Janoff EN, *et al.* Effect of perinatal zidovudine prophylaxis on the evolution of cell-free HIV-1 RNA in breast milk and on postnatal transmission. *J Infect Dis.* 2004; 190:1422-28.

Mårild S, Hansson S, Jodal U, Oden A, Svedberg K. Protective effect of breastfeeding against urinary tract infections. *Acta Paediatri.* 2004; 93:164-68.

Mårild S, Jodal U, Hanson LÅ. Breastfeeding and urinary-tract infection. *Lancet.* 1990; 336:942.

Marodi L. Deficient interferon-gamma receptor-mediated signaling in neonatal macrophages. *Acta Paediatr.* 2002; 91 (Suppl 438): 117-19.

Marshall-Clarke S, Reen D, Tasker L, Hassan J. Neonatal immunity: how well has it grown up? *Immunol Today.* 2000; 21:35-41.

Martin R, Langa S, Reviriego C, Jiminez E, Marin ML, Xaus J, *et al.* Human milk is a source of lactic acid bacteria for the infant gut. *J Pediatr.* 2003; 143:754-58.

Martin RM, Ebrahim S, Griffin M, Davey-Smith G, Nicolaides AN, Georgiou N, et al. Breastfeeding and atherosclerosis: intima-media thickness and plaques at 65-year follow-up of the Boyd Orr cohort. *Arterioscler Thromb Vasc Biol.* 2005a; 25:1482 88.

Martin RM, Gunnell D, Owen CG, Smith GD. Breast-feeding and childhood cancer: A systematic review with meta analysis. *Int J Cancer.* 2005b; 117:1020-31.

Martin RM, Gunnell D, Smith GD. Breastfeeding in infancy and blood pressure in later life: systematic review and meta-analysis. *Am J Epidemiol.* 2005c; 161:15-26.

Martin RM, Holly JM, Smith GD, Ness AR, Emmett P, Rogers I, *et al.* Could associations between breastfeeding and insulin-like growth factors underlie associations of breastfeeding with adult chronic disease? The Avon Longitudinal Study of Parents and Children. *Clin Endocrinol* (Oxf). 2005d; 62:728-37.

Martin RM, Middleton N, Gunnell D, Owen CG, Smith GD. Breast-feeding and cancer: the Boyd Orr cohort and a systematic review with meta-analysis. *J Natl Cancer Inst.* 2005e; 97:1446-57.

Mata LJ, Urrutia JJ, García RF, Béhar M. Shigella infection in breast-fed Guatemalan Indian neonates. *Amer J Dis Child.* 1969; 117:142-6.

McGuire W, Anthony MY. Donor human milk versus formula for preventing necrotising enterocolitis in preterm infants: systematic review. *Arch Dis Child Fetal Neonatal Ed.* 2003; 88:F11-14.

Morrow AL, Reves RR, West MS, Guerrero ML, Ruiz-Palacios GM, Pickering LK. Protection against infection with Giardia lamblia by breast-feeding in a cohort of Mexican infants. *J Pediatr.* 1992; 121:363-70.

Morrow AL, Ruiz-Palacios GM, Altaye M, Jiang X, Guerrero ML, Meinzen-Derr JK, *et al.* Human milk oligosaccharides are associated with protection against diarrhea in breast-fed infants. *J Pediatr.* 2004; 145:297-303.

Murakami M, Dorschner RA, Stern LJ, Lin KH, Gallo RL. Expression and secretion of cathelicidin antimicrobial peptides in murine mammary glands and human milk. *Pediatr Res.* 2005; 57:10-15.

Naarding MA, Ludwig IS, Groot F, Berkhout B, Geijtenbeek TB, Pollakis G, *et al.* Lewis X component in human milk binds DC-SIGN and inhibits HIV-1 transfer to CD4+ T lymphocytes. *J Clin Invest.* 2005; 115:3256-64.

Nafstad P, Jaakkola JJ, Hagen JA, Botten G, Kongerud J. Breastfeeding, maternal smoking and lower respiratory tract infections. *Eur Respir J.* 1996; 9:2623-29.

Narayanan I, Prakash K, Prabhakar AK, Gujral VV. A planned prospective evaluation of the anti-infective property of varying quantities of expressed human milk. *Acta Paediatr Scand.* 1982; 71:441-45.

Nelson EA, Yu LM, Williams S. International Child Care Practices study: breastfeeding and pacifier use. *J Hum Lact.* 2005; 21:289-95.

Nelson MC, Gordon-Larsen P, Adair LS. Are adolescents who were breast-fed less likely to be overweight? Analyses of sibling pairs to reduce confounding. *Epidemiology.* 2005; 16:247-53.

Newburg DS, Peterson JA, Ruiz-Palacios GM, Matson DO, Morrow AL, Shults J, *et al.* Role of human-milk lactadherin in protection against symptomatic rotavirus infection. *Lancet.* 1998; 351:1160-64.

Newburg DS, Ruiz-Palacios GM, Morrow AL. Human milk glycans protect infants against enteric pathogens. *Annu Rev Nutr.* 2005; 25:37-58.

Newell ML. Current issues in the prevention of mother-to-child transmission of HIV-1 infection. *Trans R Soc Trop Med Hyg.* 2006; 100:1-5.

Ngom PT, Collinson A, Pido-Lopez J, Henson S, Prentice A, Aspinall R. Improved thymic function in exclusively breast-fed babies is associated with higher breast milk IL-7. *Am J Clin Nutr.* 2004; 80:722-28.

Nikawa H, Samaranayake LP, Tenovuo J, Hamada T. The effect of antifungal agents on the in vitro susceptibility of Candida albicans to apo-lactoferrin. *Arch Oral Biol.* 1994; 39:921-23.

Noverr MC, Huffnagle GB. The 'microflora hypothesis' of allergic diseases. *Clin Exp Allergy.* 2005; 35:1511-20.

Nowrouzian FL, Monstein HJ, Wold AE, Adlerberth I. Effect of human milk on type 1 and P-fimbrial mRNA expression in intestinal Escherichia coli strains. *Lett Appl Microbiol.* 2005; 40:74-80.

Numazaki K. Human cytomegalovirus infection of breast milk. *FEMS Immunol Med Microbiol.* 1997; 18:91-98.

Obaro SK, Deubzer HE, Newman VO, Adegbola RA, Greenwood BM, Henderson DC. Serotype-specific pneumococcal antibodies in breast milk of Gambian women immunized with a pneumococcal polysaccharide vaccine during pregnancy. *Pediatr Infect Dis J.* 2004; 23:1023-29.

Obihara CC, Marais BJ, Gie RP, Potter P, Bateman ED, Lombard CJ, *et al.* The association of prolonged breastfeeding and allergic disease in poor urban children. *Eur Respir J.* 2005; 25:970-77.

Oddy WH, Holt PG, Sly PD, Read AW, Landau LI, Stanley FJ, *et al.* Association between breast feeding and asthma in 6 year old children: findings of a prospective birth cohort study. *BMJ.* 1999; 319:815-19.

Oddy WH, Peat JK, de Klerk NH. Maternal asthma, infant feeding, and the risk of asthma in childhood. *J Allergy Clin Immunol.* 2002; 110:65-67.

Oddy WH, Sly PD, de Klerk NH, Landau LI, Kendall GE, Holt PG, *et al.* Breast feeding and respiratory morbidity in infancy: a birth cohort study. *Arch Dis Child.* 2003; 88:224-28.

Owen CG, Martin RM, Whincup PH, Davey-Smith G, Gillman MW, Cook DG. The effect of breastfeeding on mean body mass index throughout life: a quantitative review of published and unpublished observational evidence. *Am J Clin Nutr.* 2005; 82:1298-307.

Pabst HF, Spady DW. Effect of breast-feeding on antibody response to conjugate vaccine. *Lancet.* 1990; 336:269-70.

Pearce MS, Thomas JE, Campbell DI, Parker L. Does increased duration of exclusive breastfeeding protect against Helicobacter pylori infection? The Newcastle Thousand Families Cohort Study at age 49-51 years. *J Pediatr Gastroenterol Nutr.* 2005; 41:617-20.

Penders J, Vink C, Driessen C, London N, Thijs C, Stobberingh EE. Quantification of Bifidobacterium spp., Escherichia coli and Clostridium difficile in faecal samples of breast-fed and formula-fed infants by real-time PCR. *FEMS Microbiol Lett.* 2005; 243:141-47.

Phiri W, Kasonka L, Collin S, Makasa M, Sinkala M, Chintu C, *et al.* Factors influencing breast milk HIV RNA viral load among Zambian women. *AIDS Res Hum Retrov.* 2006; 22:607-14.

Pisacane A, de Luca U, Criscuolo L, Vaccaro F, Valiante A, Inglese A, *et al.* Breast feeding and hypertrophic pyloric stenosis: population based case-control study. *BMJ.* 1996; 312:745-46.

Pisacane A, de Luca U, Impagliazzo N, Russo M, de Caprio C, Caracciolo G. Breast feeding and acute appendicitis. *BMJ.* 1995; 310:836-37.

Pisacane A, Graziano L, Mazzarella G, Scarpellino B, Zona G. Breastfeeding and urinary tract infection. *J Pediatr.* 1992; 120:87-89.

Pisacane A, Impagliazzo N, de Caprio C, Criscuolo L, Inglese A, Mendes Pereira da Silva MC. Breast feeding and tonsillectomy. *BMJ.* 1996; 312:746-47.

Piwoz EG, Ross JS. Use of population-specific infant mortality rates to inform policy decisions regarding HIV and infant feeding. *J Nutr.* 2005; 135:1113-19.

Porro E, Indinnimeo L, Antognoni G, Midulla F, Criscione S. Early wheezing and breast feeding. *Asthma.* 1993; 30:23-28.

Prentice A, Prentice AM, Lamb WH. Mastitis in rural Gambian mothers and the protection of the breast by milk antimicrobial factors. *Trans R Soc Trop Med Hyg.* 1985; 79:90-95.

Rask C, Evertsson S, Telemo E, Wold AE. A full flora, but not monocolonization by Escherichia coli or lactobacilli, supports tolerogenic processing of a fed antigen. *Scand J Immunol.* 2005; 61:529-35.

Reichardt P, Muller D, Posselt U, Vorberg B, Diez U, Schlink U, *et al.* Fatty acids in colostrum from mothers of children at high risk of atopy in relation to clinical and laboratory signs of allergy in the first year of life. *Allergy.* 2004; 59:394-400.

Renz-Polster H, David MR, Buist AS, Vollmer WM, O'Connor EA, Frazier EA, *et al.* Caesarean section delivery and the risk of allergic disorders in childhood. *Clin Exp Allergy.* 2005; 35:1466-72.

Ribeiro-do-Couto LM, Boeije LC, Kroon JS, Hooibrink B, Breur-Vriesendorp BS, Aarden LA, *et al.* High IL-13 production by human neonatal T cells: neonate immune system regulator? *Eur J Immunol.* 2001; 31:3394-402.

Roine I, Fernandez JA, Vasquez A, Caneo M. Breastfeeding reduces immune activation in primary respiratory syncytial virus infection. *Eur Cytokine Netw.* 2005; 16:206-10.

Ronnestad A, Abrahamsen TG, Medbo S, Reigstad H, Lossius K, Kaaresen PI, *et al.* Septicemia in the first week of life in a Norwegian national cohort of extremely premature infants. *Pediatrics.* 2005; 115:262-68.

Rosen IA, Håkansson A, Aniansson G, Hansson C, Andersson B, *et al.* Antibodies to pneumococcal polysaccharides in human milk: lack of relationship to colonization and acute otitis media. *Pediatr Infect Dis J.* 1996; 15:498-507.

Rousseau CM, Nduati RW, Richardson BA, Steele MS, John-Stewart GC, Mbori-Ngacha DA, *et al.* Longitudinal analysis of human immunodeficiency virus type 1 RNA in breast milk and of its relationship to infant infection and maternal disease. *J Infect Dis.* 2003; 187:741-47.

Ruiz-Palacios GM, Calva JJ, Pickering LK, Lopez-Vidal Y, Volkow P, Pezzarossi H, *et al.* Protection of breast-fed infants against Campylobacter diarrhea by antibodies in human milk. *J Pediatr.* 1990; 116:707-13.

Saarinen UM. Prolonged breast feeding as prophylaxis for recurrent otitis media. *Acta Paediatr Scand.* 1982; 71:567-71.

Sabbaj S, Ghosh MK, Edwards BH, Leeth R, Decker WD, Goepfert PA, *et al.* Breast milk-derived antigen-specific CD8+ T cells: an extralymphoid effector memory cell population in humans. *J Immunol.* 2005; 174:2951-56.

Salminen SJ, Gueimonde M, Isolauri E. Probiotics that modify disease risk. *J Nutr.* 2005; 135:1294-98.

Salzman NH, Polin RA, Harris MC, Ruchelli E, Hebra A, Zirin-Butler S, *et al.* Enteric defensin expression in necrotizing enterocolitis. *Pediatr Res.* 1998; 44:20-26.

Savilahti E, Siltanen M, Kajosaari M, Vaarala O, Saarinen KM. IgA antibodies, TGF-beta1 and -beta2, and soluble CD14 in the colostrum and development of atopy by age 4. *Pediatr Res.* 2005; 58:1300-5.

Savino F, Fissore MF, Grassino EC, Nanni GE, Oggero R, Silvestro L. Ghrelin, leptin and IGF-I levels in breast-fed and formula-fed infants in the first years of life. *Acta Paediatr.* 2005; 94:531-37.

Schanler RJ, Shulman RJ, Lau C, Smith EO, Heitkemper MM. Feeding strategies for premature infants: randomized trial of gastrointestinal priming and tube-feeding method. *Pediatrics.* 1999; 103:434-39.

Schelonka RL, Infante AJ. Neonatal immunology. *Seminars in perinatology.* 1998; 22:2-14.

Schultz C, Temming P, Bucsky P, Gopel W, Strunk T, Hartel C. Immature anti-inflammatory response in neonates. *Clin Exp Immunol.* 2004; 135:130-36.

Sharp JCM. Milk-born infection. *J Med Microbiol.* 1989; 29.

Shuster DE, Kehrli ME Jr, Baumrucker CR. Relationship of inflammatory cytokines, growth hormone, and insulin-like growth factor-I to reduced performance during infectious disease. *Proc Soc Exp Biol Med.* 1995; 210:140-49.

Siegrist CA. Mechanisms by which maternal antibodies influence infant vaccine responses: review of hypotheses and definition of main determinants. *Vaccine.* 2003; 21:3406-12.

Silfverdal SA, Bodin L, Hugosson S, Garpenholt Ö, Werner B, Esbjörner E, *et al.* Protective effect of breastfeeding on invasive Haemophilus influenzae infection: A case-control study in Swedish preschool children. *Int J Epidemiol.* 1997; 26:443-50.

Silfverdal SA, Bodin L, Olcen P. Protective effect of breastfeeding: an ecologic study of Haemophilus influenzae meningitis and breastfeeding in a Swedish population. *Int J Epidemiol.* 1999; 28:152-56.

Silfverdal SA, Bodin L, Ulanova M, Hahn-Zoric M, Hanson LÅ, *et al.* Long term enhancement of the IgG2 antibody response to Haemophilus influenzae type b by breast-feeding. *Pediatr Infect Dis J.* 2002; 21:816-21.

Silfverdal SA, Ekholm L. Influence of breastfeeding on the antibody response to Hib and pneumococcal conjugate vaccines given at 3, 5, and 12 months of age. *Adv Exp Med Biol.* 2007a; in press.

Silfverdal SA, Montgomery SM. Breastfeeding protects against more severe manifestations of clinical measles infection. 2007b; submitted.

Singhal A, Cole TJ, Fewtrell M, Lucas A. Breastmilk feeding and lipoprotein profile in adolescents born preterm: follow-up of a prospective randomised study. *Lancet.* 2004a; 363:1571-78.

Singhal A, Lucas A. Early origins of cardiovascular disease: is there a unifying hypothesis? *Lancet.* 2004b; 363:1642-45.

Sinha A, Madden J, Ross-Degnan D, Soumerai S, Platt R. Reduced risk of neonatal respiratory infections among breastfed girls but not boys. *Pediatrics.* 2003; 112:e303.

Sipilä M, Karma P, Pukander J, Timonen M, Kataja M. The Bayesian approach to the evaluation of risk factors in acute and recurrent acute otitis media. *Acta Otolaryngol.* 1988; 106:94-101.

Stark PL, Lee A. The microbial ecology of the large bowel of breast-fed and formula-fed infants during the first year of life. *J Med Microbiol.* 1982; 15:189-203.

Stephens S, Kennedy CR, Lakhani PK, Brenner MK. In vivo immune responses of breast- and bottle-fed infants to tetanus toxoid antigen and to normal gut flora. *Acta Paediatr Scand.* 1984; 73:426-32.

Stuebe AM, Rich-Edwards JW, Willett WC, Manson JE, Michels KB. Duration of lactation and incidence of type 2 diabetes. *JAMA.* 2005; 294:2601-10.

Svanborg C, Ågerstam H, Aronson A, Zjerkvist R, Duringer C, Fischer W, *et al.* HAMLET kills tumor cells by an apoptosis-like mechanism - cellular, molecular and therapeutic aspects. *Adv Cancer Res.* 2003; 88:1-29.

Svensson K, Lange S, Lönnroth I, Widström AM, Hanson L Å. Induction of anti-secretory factor in human milk may prevent mastitis. *Acta Paediatr.* 2004; 93:1228-31.

Taylor JS, Kacmar JE, Nothnagle M, Lawrence RA. A systematic review of the literature associating breastfeeding with type 2 diabetes and gestational diabetes. *J Am Coll Nutr.* 2005; 24:320-26.

Tellez A, Palm D, Weiland M, Aleman J, Winiecka-Krusnell J, Linder E, *et al.* Secretory antibodies against Giardia intestinalis in lactating Nicaraguan women. *Parasite Immunol.* 2005; 27:163-69.

Thomsen AC, Hansen KB, Möller BR. Leukocyte counts and microbiologic cultivation in the diagnosis of puerperal mastitis. *Am J Obstet Gynecol.* 1983; 146:938-41.

Toschke AM, Vignerova J, Lhotska L, Osancova K, Koletzko B, *et al.* Overweight and obesity in 6- to 14-year-old Czech children in 1991: protective effect of breast-feeding. *J Pediatr.* 2002; 141:764-69.

Uauy R, Araya M. Novel oligosaccharides in human milk: understanding mechanisms may lead to better prevention of enteric and other infections. *J Pediatr.* 2004; 145:283-85.

Urdaneta S, Berlin CM, Howett MK. Alternative modified infant-feeding practices to prevent postnatal transmission of human immunodeficiency virus type 1 through breast milk: past, present and future. *J Human Lact.* 2006; 22:75-88.

Urdaneta S, Wigdahl B, Neely EB, Berlin CM Jr, Schengrund CL, Lin HM, *et al.* Inactivation of HIV-1 in breast milk by treatment with the alkyl sulfate microbicide sodium dodecyl sulfate (SDS). *Retrovirology.* 2005; 2:28.

van den Bogaard C, van den Hoogen HJM, Huygen FJA, van Weel C. The relationship between breast-feeding and early childhood morbidity in a general population. *Fam Med.* 1991; 23:510-15.

van Odijk J, Kull I, Borres MP, Brandtzaeg P, Edberg U, Hanson LÅ, *et al.* Breastfeeding and allergic disease: a multidisciplinary review of the literature (1966-2001) on the mode of early feeding in infancy and its impact on later atopic manifestations. *Allergy.* 2003; 58:833-43.

Victora CG, Smith PG, Vaughan JP, Nobre LC, Lombardi C, Teixeira AM, *et al.* Evidence for protection by breast-feeding against infant deaths from infectious diseases in Brazil. *Lancet.* 1987; 2:319-22.

Victora CG. Case-control studies of the influence of breast-feeding on child morbidity and mortality: methodological issues. In: Atkinson S, Hanson L, Chandra R, editors.

Human Lactation 4, Breastfeeding, Nutrition, Infection and Infant Growth in Developed and Emerging Countries. St John's, Newfoundland, Canada: ARTS Biomedical Publisher; 1990. p. 405-18.

von Kries R, Koletzko B, Sauerwald T, von Mutius E, Barnert D, Grunert V, *et al.* Breast feeding and obesity: cross sectional study. *BMJ.* 1999; 319:147-50.

Walterspiel JN, Morrow AL, Guerrero ML, Ruiz-Palacios GM, Pickering LK. Secretory anti-Giardia lamblia antibodies in human milk: protective effect against diarrhea. *Pediatrics.* 1994; 93:28-31.

Watemberg N, Dagan R, Arbelli Y, Belmaker I, Morag A, Hessel L, *et al.* Safety and immunogenicity of Haemophilus type b-tetanus protein conjugate vaccine, mixed in the same syringe with diphtheria-tetanus-pertussis vaccine in young infants. *Pediatr Infect Dis.* 1991; 10:758-61.

Weisz-Carrington P, Roux ME, McWilliams M, Phillips-Quagliata JM, Lamm ME. Hormonal induction of the secretory immune system in the mammary gland. *Proc Natl Acad Sci USA.* 1978; 75:2928-32.

WHO, UNFPA, UNAIDS. *HIV and infant feeding: guidelines for decision-makers.* WHO document WHO/FRH/NUT/CHD/. 2003; 98:1.

WHO. Effect of breastfeeding on infant and child mortality due to infectious diseases in less developed countries: a pooled analysis. WHO Collaborative Study Team on the Role of Breastfeeding on the Prevention of infant Mortality. *Lancet.* 2000; 355:451-55.

WHO. Factors affecting the immunogenicity of oral poliovirus vaccine: a prospective evaluation in Brazil and the Gambia. WHO Collaborative Study Group On Oral Poliovirus Vaccination. *J Infect Dis.* 1995; 95:1097-106.

Willumsen JF, Filteau SM, Coutsoudis A, Newell ML, Rollins NC, Coovadia HM, *et al.* Breastmilk RNA viral load in HIV-infected South African women: effects of subclinical mastitis and infant feeding. *Aids.* 2003; 17:407-14.

Willumsen JF, Newell ML, Filteau SM, Coutsoudis A, Dwarika S, York D, *et al.* Variation in breastmilk HIV-1 viral load in left and right breasts during the first 3 months of lactation. *Aids.* 2001; 15:1896-98.

Winberg J, Wessner G. Does breast milk protect against septicaemia in the newborn? *Lancet.* 1971; 1:1091-94.

Wright AL, Holberg CJ, Martinez FD, Morgan WJ, Taussig LM. Breast-feeding and lower respiratory tract illness in the first year of life. *BMJ.* 1989; 299:946-49.

Wright AL, Holberg CJ, Taussig LM, Martinez FD. Factors influencing the relation of infant feeding to asthma and recurrent wheeze in childhood. *Thorax.* 2001; 56:192-97.

Young TK, Martens PJ, Taback SP, Sellers EA, Dean HJ, Cheang M, *et al.* Type 2 diabetes mellitus in children: prenatal and early infancy risk factors among native Canadians. *Arch Pediatr Adolesc Med.* 2002; 156:651-55.

Zaman S, Mannan J, Lange S, Lönnroth I, Hanson LÅ. Efficacy of anti-secretory factor in reducing severity and duration of acute and prolonged diarrhoeal illness in children 6-24 months of age - a placebo controlled trial. 2007; submitted.

Zheng T, Holford TR, Mayne ST, Owens PH, Zhang Y, Zhang B, *et al.* Lactation and breast cancer risk: a case-control study in Connecticut. *Br J Cancer.* 2001; 84:1472-76.

Chapter 11

Human Milk and Infectious Diseases

E. Stephen Buescher

INTRODUCTION

Human milk is a complex and sophisticated biomaterial that provides the infant protection, nourishment, and information. Its transfer from mother to infant usually occurs in an environment of intimate contact, the process called breastfeeding, which provides the infant the additional benefits of warmth and attention. As a biological fluid, milk has the potential to transmit disease directly from the mother to the recipient infant. The intimate contact necessary for breastfeeding presents further opportunities for transmission of infectious agents from either mother-to-infant or infant-to-mother.

When modern life precludes the process of breastfeeding, human milk that has first been expressed from the breast is often substituted. Milk expression by hand or by breast pump introduces an additional set of factors related to the collection, storage/preservation, and re-administration methods used that can alter the infectious risks associated with human milk feeding.

The intent of this chapter is to address the aspects of human milk feeding that relate to infectious diseases, including the agents to consider, the infectious conditions they can cause in the mother-infant dyad, and the general approaches to prevention and/or treatment of these conditions.

The Microbial Flora of the Breast

The microbial flora of the breast, breastmilk, and the infant's mouth all appear to be related. Studies done at the time of breast surgery have demonstrated that the breast has a cutaneous flora, and that about 60-90% of deep cultures are positive for similar organisms (Thornton *et al.*, 1988; Ransjo *et al.*, 1985). Classical skin flora organisms (coagulase negative staphylococci, diphtheroids, *Propionibacteria*) predominate in all sites and are thought to protect the breast in the same ways as normal floras in other tissues do. One study of nipple secretion flora in non-lactating breasts found coagulase negative staphylococci most frequently (67%), with Bacillus and diphtheroids also recovered in a few breast samples (Courtiss *et al.*, 1979). Studies of the oral flora of infants following vaginal delivery indicate this flora is initially similar to that of the maternal vagina. By seven days of age, it changes to include enteric Gram-negative rods, various species of anaerobes (Kononen *et al.*, 1992), α-hemolytic streptococci (Rotimi & Duerden, 1981), and coagulase negative staphylococci (Hegde & Munshi, 1998).

Studies of the microbial flora of expressed breastmilk have shown that nearly 80% of samples contain coagulase negative staphylococci, five percent contain *Staphylococcus aureus*, five percent contain streptococci, and five percent contain Gram-negative bacilli (Law *et al.*, 1989). Considering these studies, coagulase negative staphylococci appear to be the most prominent routine flora of the breast and infant mouth, with other typical "skin flora" significantly less prominent as flora. Presence of Gram-negative bacilli, α-hemolytic streptococci, and other skin flora are significantly less frequent. True pathogens, such as *Staphylococcus aureus* and *Staphylococcus agalactiae*, are only infrequently isolated in the large studies examining flora; however, their recovery from milk in instances where infants develop severe disease (Arias-Camison, 2003; Bejaro *et al.*, 2004) suggest their presence in milk may indicate some increased degree of risk for disease development in the breastfed infant. Similarly, Gram-negative bacilli are low-frequency contaminants of normal milk; however, in instances where human milk collecting or processing equipment has become contaminated, outbreaks of disease caused by these organisms have been described (Donowitz *et al.*, 1981; Gras-Le Gruen *et al.*, 2003). This is not to say that microbial contamination in general should be considered a risk. In a study examining the feeding of 10,000+ expressed milk samples to premature infants in which over 80% contained contaminating microorganisms (Law *et al.*, 1989), the authors note "... surprisingly few, if any, adverse events that could be directly related to ingestion of bacteria in raw breastmilk." In fact, a recent study suggests that human milk is the source for the lactic acid bacteria that colonize the nursing infant's GI tract (Martin *et al.*, 2003), providing the unique and protective intestinal flora of the breastfed infant.

Mastitis

Lactational mastitis, the development of redness, warmth, swelling, and pain in the lactating breast with associated fever, is common in breastfeeding mothers. Estimates of its frequency vary from 4-33% depending on the data collection method used (Amir *et al.*, 2004; Jonsson & Pulkkinen, 1994; Fetherston, 1997). Recent prospectively collected data suggest a rate of about 27% (Fetherston, 1997).

Development of mastitis results from milk stasis and duct distention, pressure related milk flow obstruction, and subsequent development of bacterial infection of the pooled milk. This pathogenesis explains why it is a condition most frequently seen in the first four weeks postpartum (Fetherston, 1997); why its risk factors include breast engorgement, poorly fitting/ constricting breast support garments, nipple pain during a feed, cracked nipples, and nipple dissymmetry after a feeding; and why more frequent feeding is a protective factor (Fetherston, 1998). Progression from mastitis to breast abscess is the last phase of pathogenesis and occurs in about 3 to 5% of mastitis cases (Amir *et al.*, 2004; Marshall *et al.*, 1975). Both retrograde flow of milk within the ducts following the milk ejection reflex (Ramsay *et al.*, 2004) and nipple manipulation by the nursing infant's tongue potentially explain how surface flora gain access to the intramammary ducts. Not surprisingly, studies of infectious agents isolated from women with mastitis have shown pathogen distributions largely consistent with the flora found on the nipple, breast surface, and infant oral cavity (Osterman & Rahm, 2000) with one exception, *Staphylococcus aureus*, (Matheson *et al.*, 1988) which is not prominent in any of the normal floras.

Management of the milk stasis-mastitis continuum centers around rest and achieving effective milk removal from the distended breast (Academy of Breastfeeding Medicine 2006). Often, the nursing infant is the most effective device for achieving the latter, so more frequent nursing at the affected breast is a long-standing recommendation for treatment along with local heat and massage/milk expression. Delay in administration of antibiotics that treat *S. aureus* is associated with breast abscess development (Devereux, 1970). Most physicians consider presence of a breast abscess a contraindication to nursing because of the risk of abscess rupture during nursing with resultant consumption of large numbers of organisms by the infant (American Academy of Pediatrics, 2006a).

MICROBIAL CONTAMINATION OF HUMAN MILK

Because the human breast has a microbial flora both on its surface and in the interior milk collecting system, human milk is expected to contain microbial contaminants. In the term infant who is breastfeeding, this flora is of little concern because the numbers of organisms vary, but are usually low, most are non-pathogenic, they are similar to the flora found in the mouth of the infant, and the milk is being consumed immediately. When milk is expressed, however, consideration must be given to the environment where collection is taking place, the method used for collection, the container used for storage, the duration and temperature of storage, the method and duration of feeding, and the developmental maturity of the infant receiving the milk.

Prior to expression of milk by hand or by device, the surface of the breast and the hands should be cleaned. Hands should be washed with soap, but breast surface cleansing with either water or soap and water appears to be equally efficient (Thompson *et al.*, 1997). Because collection of manually expressed milk into sterile containers may not be practical in all instances, containers that have been rinsed with dilute bleach solution (1% hypochlorite) then drained can be substituted with good effect (Jones *et al.*, 1979). If a breast pump is used for milk collection, it is crucial that the device be cleaned regularly and maintained in good condition, as outbreaks of illness in neonatal nurseries have been associated with contaminated breast pump fixtures (Donowitz *et al.*, 1981; Gransden *et al.*, 1986). When microbial contamination of expressed milk collected in different environments has been examined, microbial load is greater when the milk is collected in less controlled environments: greater when collected at home versus in the hospital (Boo *et al.*, 2001). Storage of expressed human milk for up to six hours at room temperature (Hamosh *et al.*, 1996) and up to 72 hours when refrigerated is considered safe (Ogundele, 2000), but the shortest storage duration under any condition should be the goal. Most human milk collected for use in hospitalized premature infants is collected/used immediately or collected and promptly frozen. A large study examining contamination of expressed milk fed to premature infants showed no attributable adverse events after feeding specimens with microbial loads from 10^4-10^8/mL (specimens cultured at the time of feeding) (Law *et al.*, 1989). If feeding is prolonged (e.g., slow drip feeds via gastric tube), the "hang time" of the milk can become an issue because of microbial growth. At present, hang times of greater than four hours are recommended (Lemons, 1983).

Because microbial contamination of expressed human milk is the rule, processing expressed raw milk to decrease its microbial content has been examined. Pasteurization is effective at eliminating bacteria (Jeffery *et al.*, 2003), HIV (Israel-Ballard *et al.*, 2005), and CMV (Welsh *et al.*, 1979), but results in diminution of some components thought to be beneficial to the breastfed infant (Raptopoulou-Gigi *et al.*, 1977; Hernandez *et al.*, 1979). When less aggressive heating is used, preservation of milk components is improved at the cost of incomplete elimination of contaminating organisms. When it has been examined, feeding of pasteurized human milk results in less protection against infection (Narayanan *et al.*, 1984). Freeze/thaw of milk eliminates HTLV-1 (Ando *et al.*, 2004) and decreases (but does not eliminate) the infectivity of CMV in human milk (Forsgren, 2004).

MYCOBACTERIAL DISEASES

Tuberculosis

Tuberculosis continues to be a threat in both the under-developed and developed worlds. The myriad presentations, confounding factors, host immunocompetence, and often silent progression of this disease make its recognition and management both diagnostic and clinical challenges. Differentiation between *Mycobacterium tuberculosis* infection and disease is an important concept because tuberculosis infection in the lactating mother is of little concern, while tuberculosis disease is a serious risk to the breastfed infant. Aerosolization of organisms from untreated cavitary tuberculosis lung disease via coughing is the primary mechanism for spreading infection. Therefore, the close contact of the nursing infant with the mother, the mother's respiratory secretion droplets, and the marked susceptibility of small infants to development of *M. tuberculosis* disease create a dangerous situation for the infant. The danger of the situation is reflected in the recommendation of the American Academy of Pediatrics that mothers with active pulmonary tuberculosis (positive tuberculin skin test and chest X-ray consistent with tuberculosis disease) be separated from their infants until they are receiving appropriate anti-tuberculosis therapy (American Academy of Pediatrics, 2006b). In contrast, if tuberculosis infection but not disease is present, i.e., the skin test is positive and the chest x-ray is either normal or abnormal without any evidence of tuberculosis disease, separation of mother and infant is not recommended. In the "between" situation where the skin test is positive and the chest x-ray is interpreted as showing "possibly contagious tuberculosis," the recommendation remains to separate mother and infant, but it is modified by factors such as the likelihood of multi-drug resistant *M. tuberculosis* being involved and whether the infant is being treated with anti-tuberculous medications.

The World Health Organization does not recommend separation of the mother and infant in the case of active tuberculosis disease in the mother; rather, it recommends treatment of the mother and simultaneous preventative chemotherapy for the infant, followed by BCG vaccination (Division of Child Health and Development Update, 1998).

While it is clearly possible for *M. tuberculosis* to be present and transmissible in the mother's milk, this is decidedly uncommon unless tuberculous mastitis is present. Therefore, in maternal tuberculosis disease where the infant and mother are separated, continued infant feeding with expressed human milk is considered appropriate.

The medications used to treat tuberculosis infection and disease are likely to be passed to the infant in small amounts via the mother's milk and are not considered to pose a threat to the nursing infant. Nor are the amounts passed considered adequate to treat tuberculosis in the infant.

Hansen's Disease

Hansen's disease is a chronic progressive condition caused by *Mycobacterium leprae* that most commonly involves the skin, peripheral nerves, and upper respiratory mucosa. It occurs most commonly in the under-developed world. Approximately 90% of cases in the USA occur in immigrants/refugees from areas with endemic disease. The incubation period is usually less than one year and presentation during pregnancy or the puerperium is common (Dundan *et al.*, 1981). Organisms likely to be *M. leprae* have been visualized in the mammary secretions and milk (Pedly, 1967; Girdhar *et al.*, 1981) of non-lactating women and lactating women, respectively, with the infection. However, the World Health Organization does not consider Hansen's Disease a contraindication to breastfeeding.

Mycobacterium Avium Subsp Paratuberculosis

Mycobacterium avium subsp *paratuberculosis* is the cause of a chronic gastrointestinal granulomatous disease in cattle, Johne's Disease. It can be transmitted through the milk of infected cows to their young. Significant debate is ongoing as to role of this organism in Crohn's disease in humans, as it has been isolated from the GI tract and blood of a subset of these patients. It has also been isolated from the breastmilk of patients with Crohn's disease (Naser *et al.*, 2000). At present, there are no recommendations regarding breastfeeding by patients with Crohn's disease regarding transmission of this organism.

VIRAL DISEASES

Mumps

Mumps is an enveloped, negatively stranded RNA virus of the *Paramyxoviridae* family. It causes a common childhood infectious disease (fever, parotitis) that is transmitted through contact with infected respiratory secretions. Mumps virus can be isolated from saliva seven days before and up to nine days after onset of parotid swelling, but patients are most infectious for the one to two days preceding and approximately five days following symptom onset. Since introduction of an attenuated live virus vaccine in the late 1960's, fewer than 500 cases/year occur in the USA. Current recommendations are for two doses of vaccine in childhood, at 12 months and at 4-6 years of age. Transmission from a mother to her infant could occur via respiratory droplets or via breastmilk (Kilham, 1951). Vaccinated persons do not transmit the attenuated virus. Neither mumps disease nor mumps vaccination is a contraindication to breastfeeding.

Measles

Rubeola (measles) virus is an enveloped, single-stranded, negative sense RNA virus of the *Paramyxoviridae* family that causes a common childhood infectious disease called measles. It is spread via aerosolized droplets from the respiratory tract of infected individuals. Symptoms (fever, rash, upper respiratory tract symptoms) occur eight to twelve days after exposure. Contagiousness is greatest during the prodromal period (seven to ten days after exposure), persisting through the fourth day after onset of the rash, and symptomatic infection occurs in essentially all susceptible persons who are exposed. A live, attenuated vaccine was introduced in the early 1960's which is 95% effective at producing immunity. Currently, two doses of vaccine are recommended during childhood: the first at 12 to 15 months of age, the second at either 4 to 6 or 11 to 12 years of age. The attenuated vaccine virus is not transmitted from human to human, and neither the rubeola virus nor the attenuated vaccine virus has been documented to be shed in human milk. Thus, there is no specific contraindication to breastfeeding.

Rubella

Rubella (German Measles) was in the past a common childhood exanthem that caused mild illness in children, but could cause congenital ophthalmologic, cardiac, and/or neurologic anomalies when infection occurred in pregnant females. Attenuated rubella vaccine was introduced in 1960, which has subsequently decreased the incidence of rubella in the USA by approximately 99% compared to the pre-vaccine era.

Both wild and vaccine strains of rubella virus have been isolated from breastmilk, but significant resulting illness has not been observed in nursing infants (Losonsky *et al.*, 1982). Rubella vaccination is contraindicated in pregnancy, but post-partum vaccination of women not previously immunized is recommended and such immunization does not alter breastfeeding (Atkinson *et al.*, 2002).

Varicella

Varicella-Zoster virus (VZV) is the herpesvirus that causes chickenpox and zoster. Once primary infection (chickenpox) occurs, VZV is carried by the host for the rest of their life, and should reactivation and clinical manifestations occur, it is called zoster (shingles). In immunocompromised individuals, reactivation may occur as disseminated zoster which is clinically indistinguishable from chickenpox. Development of chickenpox in a mother during the first 20 weeks of gestation results in varicella embryopathy in about 2% of infants, with manifestations of limb atrophy, skin scarring, and sometimes CNS and eye findings. Infection in the second 20 weeks can result in inapparent varicella in the fetus. Development of zoster in a child without preceding varicella may suggest this type of intrauterine infection. Maternal chickenpox from five days before birth through two days after birth is associated with development of severe illness in the newborn (American Academy of Pediatrics, 2006c), presumably because of intensive transplacental exposure without passage of maternal antibody against VZV.

Chickenpox is considered highly contagious, and contagiousness starts one to two days before the rash appears. Chickenpox in the lactating mother almost assuredly results in exposure of the nursing infant, but beyond the 48 hours following birth, development of chickenpox in the mother is not an indication for treatment of the infant with Varicella-Zoster immune globulin. Several reports indicate that VZV DNA can be detected in the breastmilk of mothers with chickenpox (Yoshida *et al.*, 1992) or zoster (Yoshida *et al.*, 1995), but this is not considered a contraindication to breastfeeding because exposure of the breastfeeding infant to VZV has likely already occurred. It could be argued, however, that raw expressed milk from a mother donating her milk to other infants should not be used if the donor mother develops chickenpox or zoster.

An attenuated VZV vaccine is now used to prevent chickenpox, and universal immunization of infants (less than 12 months old) and immunization of susceptible older children and adolescents without contraindications are recommended. Person-to-person transmission of the vaccine virus is rare and has only occurred when a rash develops in the immunized individual. Neither vaccine virus nor vaccine virus DNA appears to be excreted in human milk (Bohlke *et al.*, 2003).

Treatment of VZV infection with acyclovir is well accepted. Because VZV is less sensitive to acyclovir than HSV-1 or -2 and oral bioavailability is only about 10% of the administered dose, intravenous therapy is usually used to treat non-Zoster VZV infection. Valacyclovir is an oral agent that is converted to acyclovir, and both acyclovir and Valacyclovir treatment results in breastmilk acyclovir levels several times higher than average plasma levels, but the resulting dose to the infant is not therapeutically significant.

Epstein-Barr Virus

EBV is the herpesvirus associated with infectious mononucleosis, and much more infrequently, certain lymphoproliferative disorders in immunocompromised individuals, Burkitt's lymphoma, and nasopharyngeal carcinoma. EBV infection is usually acquired in childhood, and then becomes a life-long latent infection controlled by cell-mediated immunity. EBV DNA has been detected in 46% of solicited donor milk specimens (Junker *et al.*, 1991). However, based on sero-epidemiologic examination of breastfed or bottle-fed infants 12-23 months of age in Japan, breastmilk is not a significant source for early EBV infection (Kusuhara *et al.*, 1997).

Human Herpesvirus 6

HHV6 is the herpesvirus that causes roseola (exanthem subitum), an undifferentiated febrile illness common in childhood. One seroepidemiologic study has observed that breastmilk was not a significant source for HHV6 infections in infants (Kusuhara *et al.*, 1997).

Herpes SimplexVirus

Herpes simplex virus commonly causes oropharyngeal (HSV-1) and genital (HSV-2) infections in humans. It can cause intrauterine infection of the fetus, or encephalitis, disseminated, or superficial skin/mucosal infections in infants due to acquisition of the virus at the time of birth. Encephalitic infections are infrequent in older children and adults, but disseminated infections can occur in the face of immunocompromise. As with the other herpesviruses, once acquired it is carried for life, typically as latent infection with recurrent episodes of clinical disease. The newborn infant is considered particularly vulnerable to infection when primary maternal genital infection is present at the time of birth (approximately 50% attack rate). Recurrent genital infection at birth has significantly lower risk - less than five percent.

Transmission from mother to infant beyond the puerperium can occur, but is uncommon. The usual mechanism is contact with a cutaneous vesicle, such as a finger whitlow or lip fever blister. Several reports describe development of HSV infections, one fatal, associated with either a cutaneous breast lesion or HSV isolation from the mother's milk, but in at least one instance, it could not be definitively determined whether transmission was mother-to-infant or infant-to-mother (Sullivan-Bolyai *et al.*, 1983; Kibrick, 1979; Dunkle *et al.*, 1979; Quin & Lofberg, 1978; Sealander & Kerr, 1989). Genital or oral HSV infections in a lactating mother are not considered contraindications to breastfeeding as long as good handwashing and avoidance of contact with cutaneous lesions are maintained. Presence of an HSV lesion on the breast is considered a strong indication to avoid breastfeeding and collection/feeding of expressed milk until the lesion is dried and crusted. In any situation involving HSV exposure, the infant must be observed closely for development of symptoms suggestive of HSV infection.

Acyclovir is used for treatment of HSV infections, and this agent appears in the breastmilk of women as described above for VZV.

Cytomegalovirus

Cytomegalic Inclusion Disease is the condition caused by Cytomegalovirus (CMV). CMV is a DNA virus in the herpesvirus family, and as with other herpesviruses, it causes lifelong infection. For normal hosts, acquisition of CMV typically occurs in early childhood with asymptomatic infection most common. Less commonly, a self-limited syndrome of fever and adenopathy can occur. In compromised hosts, syndromes of pneumonitis, colitis, hepatitis, and retinitis can occur. Delayed acquisition of primary CMV infection until pregnancy frequently results in intrauterine infection, which has no manifestations at birth in the majority (90%) of infected infants. Subsequently, however, development of deafness and learning disability can occur. Approximately 10% of congenitally infected infants have severe disease, which can include intrauterine growth retardation, hepatosplenomegaly, purpura, hepatitis, microcephaly, intracerebral calcifications, or retinitis. Vertical transmission can also result from passage through an infected birth canal and/or by ingestion of breastmilk. Term infants infected by either of these routes usually do not develop clinical illness. However, premature infants acquiring infection by these routes are at risk of developing symptomatic illness, and there-in lies the area of concern about feeding infants milk from mothers shedding CMV (Bryant *et al.*, 2002). Between 60-95% of CMV seropositive mothers excrete CMV DNA in their milk (Meier *et al.*, 2005; Jim *et al.*, 2004). Approximately 38% of premature infants breastfed by mothers excreting CMV became infected (Hamprecht *et al.*, 2001). The more premature the infant, the more likely illness is to result from infection: about 30% of infants with birth weights <1500 g (Yeager *et al.*, 1983) and up to 80% in infants under 26 weeks gestation (Vochem *et al.*, 1998). Long-term effects of postnatally acquired CMV infection on neurodevelopment and hearing in premature infants appear to be minimal (Vollmer *et al.*, 2004), but instances of severe acute CMV illness in these groups are well documented (Meier *et al.*, 2005; Gessler *et al.*, 2004). In light of this, caution must be exercised in the use of human milk from CMV-positive mothers for feeding of premature infants, with careful consideration of its risks and benefits.

Enteroviruses

The genus Enterovirus is comprised of small RNA viruses that include the Coxsackieviruses, Echoviruses, Polioviruses, and Enteroviruses. These agents reproduce in the upper respiratory and GI tracts and are spread either by respiratory secretion droplets or fecal-oral contamination. There is currently no evidence for their transmission through breastmilk, but there is likely a risk associated with breastfeeding because of its close mother-infant contact. Infants younger than one year of age are infected at rates several times higher than observed in older children and adults, and infections are recognized most frequently in infants less than three months of age. A large variety of clinical syndromes, including febrile rash illness, aseptic meningitis, myositis, pericarditis, and neonatal infection syndromes have been ascribed to these agents. Intensive examination of breastfeeding effects on infant responses to polio vaccination has documented that breastfeeding does not interfere with polio vaccination (John *et al.*, 1976). Antibody responses in human milk following poliovirus (wild or vaccine) exposures vary with the type of exposure: natural exposure being better than inactivated vaccine exposure, and inactivated vaccine exposure better than attenuated vaccine exposure (Zaman *et al.*, 1993).

Hepatitis A

The hepatitis A virus, an RNA virus in the picornavirus group, causes a self-limited hepatitis syndrome without a chronic phase. Close personal contact that facilitates fecal-oral contamination is the usual mechanism for spread. Perinatal transmission is rare; transmission via breastmilk is not described. However, the intimate contact of breastfeeding may facilitate transmission if fecal-oral contamination occurs. Potential for transmission is greatest when fecal excretion of virus is highest during the one to two weeks preceding onset of clinical symptoms (jaundice, fever, malaise, nausea, anorexia). Transmission is minimal by one week after onset of jaundice. Asymptomatic illness is common in small children, its presence being recognized only after development of symptomatic (icteric) illness in adult contacts of an infected child.

No treatment is available for Hepatitis A. Prevention can be achieved through passive immunization using pooled human immunoglobulin within two weeks of exposure. More recently, vaccination using formalin-inactivated virus has been approved for children greater than two years old and adults given in a two dose schedule (six months between doses). If maternal disease develops between two weeks before and one week after birth, some experts recommend treatment of the newborn with pooled immunoglobulin (0. 02 mL/kg). Development of severe disease in healthy infants occurs very infrequently. Regardless of the approach taken, it is prudent for breastfeeding mothers with Hepatitis A to assure good handwashing before and after all breastfeeding activities.

Hepatitis B

Hepatitis B is a DNA virus transmitted by blood and body fluids. It causes an acute hepatitis syndrome that may develop into a chronic and/or progressive infection. Asymptomatic infections can occur. When acquired perinatally (usually via blood exposures during labor and delivery), Hepatitis B very frequently becomes a chronic infection, and up to 25% of these chronic infections will develop hepatocellular carcinoma in mid-life.

Diagnosis of Hepatitis B is based on detection of Hepatitis B surface antigen (HBsAg) in the blood, and any person who is HBsAg-positive is considered potentially infectious. HBsAg is present in the blood of individuals with either acute or chronic infection. In reality, the individuals with the highest potential for disease transmission are those with Hepatitis Be Antigen (HBeAg) in their blood as this indicates active replication of Hepatitis B virus. The blood and body fluids of these individuals are considered exquisitely infectious.

Current recommendations for management of infants born to women with active or chronic hepatitis B infection (i.e., HBsAg-positive) are for administration of Hepatitis B immune globulin (HBIg) and Hepatitis B vaccine at different sites within twelve hours of birth, and two subsequent vaccine doses are to be given at one to two months and six months after birth (American Academy of Pediatrics, 2006). For infants of HBsAg-positive mothers weighing less than 2 kg, both HBIg and vaccine should be administered within twelve hours of birth, but three subsequent doses of vaccine should be administered at one, two to three, and six to seven months of age.

Although Hepatitis B virus DNA can be detected in the milk of lactating women with either chronic carriage or acute infection, epidemiologic studies suggest that the rate of Hepatitis B transmission via breastfeeding is quite low (Beasley *et al.*, 1975). Hence, neither the World Health Organization nor the American Academy of Pediatrics considers maternal Hepatitis B infection a contraindication to either breastfeeding or human milk feeding. When recommended immunoprophylaxis of the infant is performed after birth, the rate of transmission of Hepatitis B to infants from mothers with chronic infection is not different for breastfed versus formula-fed infants (Hill *et al.*, 2005). If nipple cracking/bleeding is present in a mother with Hepatitis B, it is considered prudent for the mother to refrain from breastfeeding her infant or expressing milk for feeding until the wound is healed.

Hepatitis C

Hepatitis C virus causes illness with or without an acute hepatitis syndrome that frequently (60-70% of infected adults) develops into chronic hepatitis. The causative agent is an RNA virus that is transmitted most effectively by percutaneous exposures to infected blood. All individuals with antibody against Hepatitis C virus are considered to be infectious. The risk of perinatal transmission from mother to infant averages about 5 to 6% and occurs in women who have Hepatitis C RNA in their blood at the time of birth. Approximately $^1/_3$ - ½ of mother-to-child transmission appears to occur in utero (Mok *et al.*, 2005). Hepatitis C RNA is not present in breastmilk (Polywka *et al.*, 1999) and the risk of transmission via breastfeeding appears to be low (Mast, 2004). However, as with mothers acutely infected with or carriers of Hepatitis B, it is considered prudent for the mother with Hepatitis C who has nipple cracking or bleeding to refrain from breastfeeding her infant or expressing milk for feeding until the wound is healed.

Hepatitis E

Hepatitis E virus causes an acute hepatitis syndrome similar to that caused by Hepatitis A virus that is transmitted by fecal-oral contamination. It is an RNA virus. In one study, about 5% of infants born to mothers with Hepatitis E developed acute hepatic disease within two weeks of birth, and all of these infants had been formula-fed because of acute maternal disease (Chibber *et al.*, 2004). No breastfed infants of mothers with Hepatitis E developed acute disease, leading the authors to conclude that it appears breastfeeding is safe in this disease. It would appear prudent, however, for mothers with Hepatitis E to exercise caution with their infants, taking care to perform good handwashing before and after breastfeeding.

Hepatitis G

Hepatitis G is an RNA virus frequently detected in persons exposed to human blood or with liver disease. Mother-to-infant transmission occurs, but what mechanisms other than pure vertical transmission occur are presently unknown (Menendez *et al.*, 1999). No data currently exist about transmission via breastmilk. As with Hepatitis B and C, it would seem prudent for lactating women with Hepatitis G to avoid breastfeeding if they develop cracked/bleeding nipples because it appears exposure to infected human blood is a risk factor.

Transfusion Transmitted Virus

In 1977, a new hepatitis-associated DNA virus was isolated from the serum of a patient with post-transfusion hepatitis. It is argued whether this new agent, Transfusion-Transmitted Virus (TTV), can be transplacentally passed (Gerner *et al.*, 2000; Iso *et al.*, 2001), but there is agreement that viral DNA can be detected in human milk (Gerner *et al.*, 2000; Iso *et al.*, 2001; Bagaglio *et al.*, 2002). However, no disease activity could be identified due to mother-to-infant transmission.

Human T-cell LymphotrophicVirus Type One

HTLV-1 causes endemic infection in selected parts of the world, including Japan, the Caribbean, and parts of South America. Long-term infection is associated with development of a tropical spastic paraparesis in adults. HTLV-1 is transmitted by body fluids from an infected individual. Human milk has been implicated as mediating mother-to-infant transmission (Wiktor *et al.*, 1997), with longer duration feeding increasing the risks. Overnight freezing of expressed human milk eliminates its infectivity (Ando *et al.*, 2004).

Human Immunodeficiency Virus

HIV causes a chronic infection that results in progressive loss of T-cells with subsequent development of opportunistic infections which define the Acquired Immunodeficiency Syndrome (AIDS). Acquisition of HIV by children or adults occurs via sexual activity, blood product administration, intravenous drug use, or intrauterine infection. Two types of HIV are recognized, HIV-1 and HIV-2: the former is the cause of the large majority of HIV infections worldwide, the latter is rare outside of west Africa. The major routes of mother-to-infant transmission of HIV are intrauterine (5-10%), peripartum (10-15%), and through breastfeeding (5-20%) (Public Health Service Task Force, 2005). Factors such as maternal treatment with highly active anti-retroviral therapy; prepartum/intrapartum azidothymidine (AZT, zidovudine), AZT + lamivudine, or nevirapine treatment of the mother (Public Health Service Task Force, 2005; Taha *et al.*, 2004); cesarean section delivery; and post-partum treatment of the exposed infant with AZT or neviripine all decrease the rate of peripartum mother-to-infant transmission (Public Health Service Task Force, 2005; European Collaborative Study, 2005). HIV transmission from mother-to-infant can occur via human milk (Nduati *et al.*, 2000). Because of this, counseling the HIV-infected mother about the risks and benefits of the different feeding options available is crucial. In regions where affordable, acceptable, feasible, sustainable, and safe alternatives to breastfeeding are available, complete avoidance of breastfeeding is recommended because it is presently the only approach that absolutely prevents transmission by breastfeeding (Read, 2003). In environments where alternatives are not appropriate, the WHO currently recommends counseling the HIV-infected mother about the risks and benefits of the different feeding options available and to consider breastfeeding as the feeding method with the fewest associated risks (HIV and Infant Feeding, 2003). If breastfeeding by the HIV-positive mother is chosen, she should be encouraged to breastfeed exclusively, as existing data indicate higher rates of mother to infant transmission when mixed feedings are given (Coutsoudis, 2000). In addition, breastfeeding should be discontinued as soon as feasible taking into consideration the local circumstances, the mother's situation, and the risks of replacement feeding, including malnutrition and acquisition of other non-HIV infections (Global Strategy for Infant and Young Child Feeding, 2001).

Expressed milk from HIV infected women can be heat treated ("Pretoria pasteurization") to inactivate HIV (Jeffery *et al.*, 2001; Israel-Ballard *et al.*, 2005). In this method intended to be applicable in the home environment, heat is transferred from 450 mL of water (heated to the boiling point) to 50 mL of milk by pouring the hot water into a one quart aluminum pot and placing a glass jar (16 oz peanut butter jar) containing the milk into this water. This results in milk temperatures of 56 to 62.5 degrees Celsius for approximately fifteen minutes, with inactivation of HIV and the bulk of bacterial contaminants (Jeffery *et al.*, 2003). A second method, also applicable at home, called "flash heating" uses the same glass peanut butter jar containing 50 mL of milk, but places the jar in water and both are heated until the water achieves a rolling boil. At this point, the milk is removed and allowed to cool to body temperature before feeding (Israel-Ballard *et al.*, 2005). This method inactivates HIV slightly better than Pretoria pasteurization and is also effective at destroying bacterial contaminants in the milk.

West Nile Virus

Illnesses caused by this mosquito-borne virus include asymptomatic infection (80%), West Nile Fever (20%), and West Nile encephalitis (<1%) (Huhn *et al.*, 2003). Intrauterine transmission (Hayes & O'Leary, 2004) and likely breastmilk transmission have occurred (MMWR, West Nile Transmission, 2002). Treatment for West Nile encephalitis is supportive, but administration of human intravenous immunoglobulins containing high titers of antibody against West Nile Virus are currently being studied (Halry *et al.*, 2003).

Vaccinia

World-wide eradication of smallpox was achieved in 1980. Unfortunately, increasing concern that variola, the virus that causes smallpox, could be used as an agent of bioterrorism has resurrected the use of vaccinia virus to vaccinate against smallpox in some populations. Vaccination produces a pustule at the needle scarification site that heals and scars over 28 days. As long as this process remains localized at the site of vaccine administration, there is little concern for complications. However, the vaccination site pustule contains infectious vaccinia virus, and rupture of the pustule by scratching, trauma, etc. can lead to spread of the vaccination process locally or to distant sites (inadvertent inoculation) on the vaccinee, or spread to other individuals (Cono *et al.*, 2003). In small percentages of vaccinees, generalized vaccinia, progressive vaccinia, post-vaccinial encephalopathy, or encephalomyelitis can occur. Because fetal vaccinia can occur when pregnant women are vaccinated, vaccination is currently contraindicated in pregnancy. Vaccinated women are advised to avoid pregnancy for at least a month after vaccination, and pregnant women are advised to avoid close contact with anyone who has received smallpox vaccination until the vaccination scab falls away (Smallpox Vaccination Information). For breastfeeding women, vaccination is also contraindicated because of the risk of spread to the infant by contact. Tertiary spread of vaccinia to a breastfeeding infant has been reported, demonstrating the potential risk to the infant from even indirect familial contact with a vaccinee (Garde *et al.*, 2004). If a breastfeeding mother is vaccinated, she should cease breastfeeding (but can maintain her milk production by expressing and discarding her milk) until the scab fully separates from the vaccination site. It is unknown whether the vaccinia virus or antibodies against it are transmitted by breastmilk. These recommendations will undoubtedly be revised should a case of smallpox occur.

BACTERIAL DISEASES

Group B ß-Hemolytic Streptococcus

At least thirteen reports and case series starting in the late 1970's describe transmission of *Streptococcus agalactiae* to infants via mother's milk (Kenny, 1977; Rench & Baker, 1987; Bingen *et al.*, 1992; Godambe *et al.*, 2005). In some mothers, clinical mastitis was present, while in others, there was no evidence of mammary inflammation/infection despite positive milk cultures. Disease in the infant was typically late onset (6 to 68 days post-partum), and sibling or recurrent infections have occurred in some instances before the association with human milk feedings was made (Olver *et al.*, 2000).

Staphylococcus Aureus

As a "true pathogen," *Staphylococcus aureus* is capable of causing a wide spectrum of disease. In the lactating mother, this may be mastitis, breast abscess, sore nipples, boils, and/or skin infection (Amir, 1996). In the infant, this may be sepsis, pneumonia (Thomas *et al.*, 2001), scalded skin syndrome (Katzman & Wald, 1987), or superficial colonization. Colonization and sharing of *S. aureus* as a flora between mother and infant outside of breastfeeding has been demonstrated (Peacock *et al.*, 2003; Kawada *et al.*, 2003), and transmission from mother to infant via breastmilk has been rigorously documented in some cases (Behari *et al.*, 2004). Both methicillin-resistant and methicillin-susceptible strains of *S. aureus* have been described in the latter situations, and maternal signs and symptoms of mastitis may or may not be present.

Gram-Negative Rods

In almost all series examining the flora of expressed human milk, 3-28% of specimens contain enteric or non-enteric Gram-negative rods (Law *et al.*, 1989; Olowe *et al.*, 1987) in amounts ranging from 10^4-10^8/mL (Law *et al.*, 1989). Although these numbers may sound large, studies examining home-prepared infant formula contamination in developing countries have shown similar or greater contamination of home-prepared milk feeds (Suthienkul *et al.*, 1999; Morais *et al.*, 2005), i.e., a geometric mean of 2.9×10^6 Gram-negative rod CFU/mL of milk (Botsford, 1986). Reports of clinical illness/feeding intolerance resulting from breastfeeding of human milk contaminated with Gram-negative rods are rare. However, feeding of contaminated expressed human milk, usually to preterm infants, may have: 1) no effect (Law *et al.*, 1989); 2) result in feeding intolerance (Thomas *et al.*, 2001); or 3) result in severe infection in the infant (Donowitz *et al.*, 1981; Youssef *et al.*, 2002). In most reports where severe infections have occurred, a contaminated breast pump is the culprit, emphasizing the need to clean and maintain both electric and manual breast pump devices (Liebhaber *et al.*, 1978), whether they are in a healthcare institution or at home (Boo *et al.*, 2001). Ironically, the same applies to devices used to sterilize and prepare expressed human milk (Gras-Le Gruen, 2003).

Brucellosis

In most instances, infections caused by *Brucella* sp. are the result of contact with infected animals, their products of conception, or through ingestion of infected meat, milk, or milk products. Transmission from human-to-human is uncommon, but has been reported with blood transfusion or bone marrow transplanted from infected donors. Neonatal infection can occur transplacentally or during delivery. Two case reports suggest that transmission may also be possible through breastmilk (al-Eissa, 1990; Palanduz, 2000). Brucellosis is typically difficult to recognize and diagnose: it is often a systemic illness with non-specific patient complaints and few physical findings. Definitive diagnosis requires isolation of the *Brucella* sp. from blood, bone marrow, or other tissue: more typically, presumptive diagnosis is made based on serologic testing.

Melioidosis

In Southeast Asia and many tropical areas of the world, infection with *Burkholderia pseudomallei* results in melioidosis. This organism is present in the soil and surface water and is typically acquired by inoculation to produce localized disease. Septicemic disease can result from subsequent hematogenous spread, as can disease in almost any organ system. Transmission by inhalation and ingestion can also occur, with both transplacental and transmammary transmission documented in goats. One report of two cases from northern Australia strongly suggests that transmission via human milk can also occur (Ralph *et al.*, 2004). In both instances, the mothers had mastitis.

Anthrax

The disease caused by *Bacillus anthracis*, anthrax, is not considered to be transmissible from human to human. It is acquired by inhalation or inoculation of *B. anthracis* spores, and spores are not formed by this organism under conditions of acute infection. Based on the bioterrorism attacks in the United States in the fall of 2001 in which spores were disseminated in several environments with subsequent development of acute infections, recommendations for antimicrobial prophylaxis in breastfeeding mothers and children were made (MMWR Anthrax Rec, 2001). Ciprofloxacin or doxycycline are the preferred agents for chemoprophylaxis in adults, including breastfeeding women. Both agents are considered safe in breastfeeding because the amounts of either drug transferred to the infant in the milk are very small. However, prophylaxis is usually prescribed for 60 days, and data on the safety of long term use for the infant do not exist. Therefore, in situations where the *B. anthracis* strain is known to be penicillin susceptible and there is no other contraindication for its use in the mother, amoxicillin is considered an appropriate alternative to ciprofloxacin or doxycycline for prophylaxis in the mother. Mothers who are concerned about long-term exposure of their infants to ciprofloxacin or doxycycline in their milk can consider expressing and then discarding their milk so that breastfeeding can be resumed at the completion of their prophylaxis. For prophylaxis in children, either ciprofloxacin or doxycycline should be used until it is known whether the anthrax isolate is penicillin susceptible. Because of the potential for adverse effects with prolonged use of these agents, amoxicillin is considered an option for completion of the 60 days of prophylaxis in penicillin susceptible isolates.

Salmonellosis

Three reports describe transmission of *Salmonella* sp. to the infant via breastmilk (Chen *et al.*, 2005; Fleischrocker *et al.*, 1972; Qutaishat *et al.*, 2003). Although Salmonellosis is usually an enteric infection that is spread by fecal-oral contamination, bacteremia is common during enteritis and would provide a potential mechanism by which breastmilk could become contaminated. *Salmonella* sp. enteritis in infants less than six months of age carries greater risks of developing invasive disease than in older children - meningitis being the greatest concern. To prevent transmission, good hand washing before and after breastfeeding is appropriate to prevent fecal-oral transmission. Salmonella gastroenteritis in older children and adults is usually a self-limited illness, and it is not usual practice to treat it with antibiotics unless infection is severe, because antibiotic treatment tends to prolong Salmonella fecal carriage. Therefore, it may be advisable to cease breastfeeding for a day or two until the acute illness passes, maintaining lactation and milk production by milk expression, and discarding the expressed milk.

Infant Botulism

Intoxication by toxins produced by *Clostridium botulinum* produces the clinical condition called botulism. Clostridia are spore-forming anaerobic organisms typically associated with putrefaction, which usually makes their presence quite notable. Botulinal toxin is produced by actively growing *C. botulinum* and is renowned for its extreme potency: the dose needed to cause botulism can be less than a billionth of a gram. In adults, most cases of botulism result from either wounds contaminated with *C. botulinum* spores that germinate or from ingestion and absorption of the toxin. Of note, the toxin does not appear to be passed to the infant in mother's milk (Middaugh, 1978). In contrast, "infant botulism" is a "toxicoinfection" that results from ingestion of *C. botulinum* spores (which are both ubiquitous in the environment and often present in commercial honey) (Arnon *et al.*, 1979), germination of the spores in a permissive GI environment, toxin production by the intraluminally growing *C. botulinum*, and absorption of the toxin to produce symptoms and signs. The permissive GI environment is thought to be crucial for development of infant botulism, with both the putrefactive flora of formula-fed and the fermentative flora of human milk-fed infants thought to limit permissiveness of the GI tract. At the time of weaning from either formula or human milk, perturbation of the non-permissive flora likely allows germination of ingested *C. botulinum* spores in the GI tract with subsequent development of infant botulism (Arnon *et al.*, 1979). Perhaps not surprisingly, the average age of hospitalized formula-fed infants with infant botulism is about half that of hospitalized breastfed infants with the condition (7.6 vs. 13.8 weeks) (Arnon *et al.*, 1982). It has also been suggested that human milk or other factors associated with breastfeeding may moderate the severity of infant botulism because of differences in the frequency of Sudden Infant Death Syndrome related to infant botulism in formula-fed vs. breastfed infants (Arnon *et al.*, 1982).

Syphilis

This condition, caused by the spirochete *Treponema pallidum*, is a disseminated, slowly progressive infection that can produce devastating cardiovascular and central nervous system effects in its late phase. Most commonly, it is acquired as a sexually transmitted disease, although acquisition by blood transfusion, transplantation, and congenital infection occur. A broad range of clinical manifestations is a hallmark of this condition, but the usual presentation of primary infection is a small painless ulceration, the chancre, which appears at the site of initial infection. Primary infection leads to dissemination, which then produces the secondary and tertiary phases of syphilis over months to years. Congenital infection can vary from asymptomatic to stillbirth: determination whether the central nervous system is involved in congenital syphilis is crucial for management.

Whether human milk transmission of *T. pallidum* can occur is unknown. Because the organism cannot be cultured, congenital transmission occurs and diagnosis of symptomatic cases is based on serology, it is difficult to be definitive about this. One report describes transmission of syphilis from infant-to-breast where a congenitally infected infant with a mouth lesion was nursed by a woman other than its mother (Hamel, 1950). In the situation where a lactating mother is found to have syphilis, she should be evaluated and treated as appropriate for her stage of disease. Her infant should also be tested for syphilis, with a low threshold for treatment because of the subtleties of syphilis diagnosis and its long-term effects when left untreated.

Q-fever

Coxiella burnetii is the causative agent of an uncommon systemic illness in humans called Q-fever. This agent is an intracellular rickettsial pathogen whose reservoir in nature is primarily farm animals, such as goats, sheep, and cattle, but domestic dogs, cats, and other mammals can transmit infection to humans. Fine particle aerosols of infected birth fluids or dust contaminated with these fluids are inhaled by humans resulting in pulmonary infection which can disseminate. Breastfeeding has not been proven to transmit the infection, but through both transmission and serologic testing in animals, about five percent of milk samples obtained from Indian women had either anti-*C. burnetii* antibody or infectious *Coxiella* in their milk (Kumar *et al.*, 1981). Thus it would appear than human milk transmission is possible.

PARASITIC INFECTIONS

Strongyloidiasis

Strongyloidiasis is the endoparasitic worm infestation that is caused by *Strongyloides* species. In humans, the large majority of cases are caused by *Strongyloides stercoralis*. In Papua/New Guinea and Africa, *Strongyloides fulleborni*, a common cause of strongyloidiasis in non-human primates, can also cause human infection. Strongyloidiasis is endemic in tropical and subtropical regions and is acquired via penetration of the skin by infective (filariform) larvae, usually through barefoot contact with infected soil. After skin penetration, the larvae enter the circulation and are transported to the lungs where they emerge, move to and up the trachea, are swallowed, and then mature to adult females in the intestine. The adults lay eggs in the duodenum and proximal jejunum, which hatch and mature into non-infectious (rhabditiform) larvae that are either passed in the stool, or less frequently, undergo a molt in the host's bowel to become filariform and re-enter the hosts tissues (auto-infection) to repeat the cycle. In immunocompromised hosts, auto-infection is more common and can result in disseminated strongyloidiasis.

In rural Africa, acquisition of strongyloidiasis was documented in 34% of infants less than 200 days old: *S. fulleborni* larvae were found in the breastmilk of one of 25 mothers examined, indicating transmammary passage and the possibility of breastmilk transmission (Brown & Girardeau, 1977). Transmammary passage of *Strongyloides* sp. has been documented in other species, including horses, buffalo, rats, sheep, and dogs, supporting the likelihood it can occur in man.

Hookworm

Hookworm infestation in humans can be caused by either *Ancylostoma duodenale* or *Necator americanus*. Infection is usually acquired though barefoot skin contact with contaminated soil. Alternatively, ingestion of contaminated food can result in oral acquisition of infection by *A. duodenale*. Filariform larvae penetrate the skin/oral mucosa and via the circulation or lymphatics, make their way to the lungs. After entry into the alveoli, the larvae move to and up the trachea, are swallowed, and pass to the small intestine. There, the larvae mature to adults, attach to the bowel wall by their mouths and feed on the host's blood. Adult males and females mate in the bowel, resulting in release of eggs into the feces. The eggs pass with the stool and require time to hatch and develop into filariform larvae outside the host in order to repeat the cycle.

One report documents the presence of *N. Americanus* larvae in human milk (Setasuban *et al.*, 1980), indicating transmammary passage of this agent. Reports of neonatal/infantile hookworm infection in Africa and China (Yu *et al.*, 1995; Griffin, 1981; Nwosu, 1981), usually involving *A. duodenale*, strongly imply this parasite can also be passed by the transmammary route.

Chagas Disease

Trypanosoma cruzi infection can result from the bite of an infected reduviid bug, blood transfusion, transplantation, or oral ingestion. It can also be acquired transplacentally or by laboratory infection. The resulting condition is called Chagas Disease. Following acute infection, parasites distribute widely into the tissues, but with preference for reticuloendothelial, neural, skeletal, smooth, and cardiac muscle tissues. Resulting interstitial inflammation, necrosis, and scarring ultimately alter tissue function. The acute phase is followed by a period of disease quiescence, the indeterminate stage, during which low-level parasitemia persists and may last for years. Over time, however, continuing infection causes chronic cardiac, neurologic, and digestive tract damage which can result in heart failure, central nervous system dysfunction, megaesophagus, and megacolon during the chronic stage.

Intrauterine infection can occur when mothers are in the indeterminate or chronic stages and is usually associated with hepatosplenomegaly, fever, seizures, hypotonia, and hyporeflexia in the infected infant. Prognosis is poor. Transmission through human milk has been reported, but this could have resulted from cracked/bleeding nipples rather than the presence of *T. cruzii* in the milk. Several attempts to identify the organism in milk have failed (Bittencourt, 1988; Amato *et al.*, 1992). At present, the World Health Organization does not consider chronic Chagas disease to be a contraindication to breastfeeding.

Several studies have examined treatment methods for expressed milk containing *T. cruzi*. Pasteurization (Ferreira, 2001) and microwave heating to 63° C (Santos Ferreira *et al.*, 2003) have both been demonstrated to inactivate *T. cruzi* seeded into human milk.

Scabies

Ectoparasitic skin infestation by the mite *Sarcoptes scabiei* var *hominis* is the cause of scabies. Intense pruritus is the most common clinical manifestation, usually in association with a variety of different dermatoses. In normal adults, sites of involvement include the finger webs, wrists, abdomen, buttock, axillary folds, inframammary folds, and male external genitalia. Involvement of breast areola can occur. Scabies is highly contagious and development of infantile scabies has been associated with nipple scabies (Hass & Stuttgen, 1987), implying that transmission during breastfeeding can occur. Infantile scabies is notorious for its more difficult diagnosis, often presenting as a generalized eruption with involvement of face, scalp, soles, and palms. Development of papules, vesiculopustules, or nodules with secondary eczematous or impetiginous changes is common (Paller, 1993). Misdiagnosis as other conditions or progression to crusted ("Norwegian") scabies (both often associated with topical steroid treatments) are common in infants (Janik-Moszant *et al.*, 2003; Kim *et al.*, 2002; Camassa *et al.*, 1995). Treatment of small infants with permethrin 5% cream is effective (Quarterman & Lesher, 1994) and avoids the potential toxicity associated with topical lindane use (Bhalla & Thami, 2004). Simultaneous treatment of other infested family members is usually indicated when an infant with scabies is identified (Paller, 1993).

FUNGAL INFECTIONS

Candidosis

Mammary Candidosis is a confusing and contentious clinical entity because rigorous data documenting its clinical parameters, diagnostic criteria, and treatment

Table 1. Breastmilk Provides Protection From:

Infectious Disease	References
All infections	*J Pediatr.* 1995; 126:191-197. *J Hum Lact.* 1996; 12:27-30.
Infections requiring hospitalization	*Pediatrics.* 1980; 65:1121-1124.
Death from infection	*Lancet.* 1987; 2:319-321.
Otitis media	*J Pediatr.* 1995; 126:696-702. *Clin Infect Dis.* 1996; 22:1079-1083. *J Infect Dis.* 1989; 160:83-94.
Infant respiratory illness	*Am J Epidemiol.* 1998; 147:863-870.
Upper respiratory infection (h/o prematurity)	*J Perinatol.* 2002; 22:354-359.
Acute respiratory infection	*Saudi Med J.* 2 2001; 2:347-350. *J Nutr.* 1997; 127:436-443.
Respiratory infection	*Int J Epidemiol.* 1984; 13:447-453. *J Pediatr.* 1995; 126:191-197.
Wheezing lower respiratory illness	*Arch Dis Child.* 2003; 88:224-228.
Pneumonia	*Pediatrics.* 1998; 101:837-844.
	Pediatrics. 1994; 93:977-985.
Pneumonia/bronchiolitis	*Acta Paediatr.* 1994; 83:714-718.
Parainfluenza bronchiolitis	*Am J Dis Child.* 1986; 140:34-40.
Invasive *Hemophilus influenzae*	*Int J Epidemiol.* 1997; 26:443-450.
Death from respiratory infection	*BMJ.* 2001; 323:1-5.
	Int J Epidemiol. 1989; 18:918-925.
Diarrheal illness	*J Pediatr.* 1995; 126:696-702.
Diarrhea	*J Nutr.* 1997; 127:436-443.
	Pediatrics. 1990; 86:874-882.
Persistent diarrhea	*Int J Epidemiol.* 1991; 20:1064-1072.
Gastrointestinal infection	*Am J Clin Nutr.* 2003; 78:291-295.
	J Pediatr. 1995; 126:191-197.
Gastroenteritis	*Pediatrics.* 1998; 101:837-844.
Gastrointestinal illness	*Am J Dis Child.* 1984; 138:629-632.
Rotavirus	*J Hosp Infect.* 2002; 50:13-17.
	Am J Epidemiol. 1999; 150:770-777.
Severe rotavirus infection	*Pediatrics.* 1993; 92:680-685.
Giardia	*Scand J Infect Dis.* 2003; 35:322-325. *Am J Trop Med Hyg.* 2001; 65:257-260. *Pediatrics.* 1994; 93:28-31. *J Pediatr.* 1992; 121:363-370.
Campylobacter diarrhea	*J Pediatr.* 1990; 116:707-713.
Cholera	*N Engl J Med.* 1983; 308:1389-1392.
Severe shigellosis	*Am J Epidemiol.* 1986; 123:710-720. *Pediatrics.* 1992; 90:406-411.
Salmonella	*Am J Dis Child.* 1980; 134:147-152. *Clin Infect Dis.* 2004; 38 Suppl 3:S262-S270. *Acta Paediatr.* 1996; 85:804-808.
Death from diarrhea	*BMJ.* 2001; 323:1-5. *Am J Epidemiol.* 1989; 129:1032-1041.
UTI	*Acta Paediatr.* 2004; 93:164-168. *J Pediatr.* 1992; 120:87-89.

VLBW infant infections	*Pediatrics.* 1998; 102:E38.
VLBW sepsis	*Arch Pediatr Adolesc Med.* 2003; 157:66-71.
Necrotizing Enterocolitis	*Arch Dis Child Fetal Neonatal Ed.* 2003; 88:F11-F14.
Ascaris infection	*Indian J Pediatr.* 1983; 50:493-495.
Breastmilk Provides No Protection From:	
Infections (industrialized countries)	*JAMA.* 1986; 256:887-892.
Otitis media	*Pediatrics.* 1990; 85:464-471.
Upper respiratory infections	*Singapore Med J.* 1998; 39:551-556. *Am J Dis Child.* 1984; 138:629-632.
Respiratory infections	*Pediatrics.* 1982; 70:239-245.
Upper respiratory infection	*Pediatrics.* 1990; 85:464-471.
Lower respiratory illness	*Pediatrics.* 1990; 85:464-471.
NP colonization by bacterial respiratory pathogens	*J Clin Microbiol.* 1993; 31:2674-2678.
Pertussis-like illness	*Acta Paediatr.* 1994; 83:714-718.
Gastrointestinal infections	*Singapore Med J.* 1998; 39:551-556.
Gastroenteritis	*Pediatrics.* 1990; 85:464-471.
Rotavirus infection	*Pediatrics.* 1993; 92:680-685.
VLBW infant infections	*Arch Dis Child Fetal Neonatal Ed.* 2004; 89:F509-F513.
Hookworm infection	*Indian J Pediatr.* 1983; 50:493-495.

options are not available. While there is little doubt that Candida species are common causes of oral infection (thrush) in infants, can cause vulvo-vaginal infection in women (particularly following disruption of normal flora by antibiotic therapy), and cause superficial infection of macerated skin (e.g., candidal diaper rashes), their abilities to cause invasive infections are usually limited without a foreign body present (e.g., a vascular catheter), an underlying disease (diabetes), or an immunosuppressive condition. In the breastfeeding woman, chronic nipple and breast pain, particularly lancinating deep breast pain (Amir & Pakula, 1991), is frequently ascribed to "mammary candidosis" and topical/enteral treatment with anti-candidal agents for both mother and infant is given (Brent, 2001). The difficulty is that directed study of women with the pain thought to be characteristic of "candidosis" has produced unimpressive results: while *Candida albicans* was recovered from the nipple/milk of 12/61 (nineteen percent) women with nipple pain (Amir *et al.*, 1996) compared to 3% of controls, *Staphylococcus aureus* was isolated from 42% and 5% of the same groups: curiously, the authors implicated *C. albicans* rather than *S. aureus* as being causative. In a second smaller study, *C. albicans* was present in the milk of 25% of women with "characteristic" deep pain compared to 15% of controls, while skin flora bacteria were recovered in 95% and 20% of the same groups (Thomassen *et al.*, 1998). In this study, the authors concluded "deep pain" clearly did not identify the women from whom *Candida* sp. would likely be isolated from their milk, and implied bacteria could not be excluded as causative in either nipple or "deep pain" syndromes. One study suggests recovery of *Candida* sp. from human milk may be limited by the large quantities of iron unsaturated lactoferrin present in breastmilk (which appears to suppress candidal growth) and that iron supplementation to saturate the lactoferrin present before culture will increase culture yields by about three-fold (Morrill *et al.*, 2003). Recently, the signs and symptoms associated with mammary candidosis were examined for their relationship with recovery of *Candida* sp. from the nipple or expressed milk at two weeks post-partum (Francis-Mirrill *et al.*, 2004). In this part of the study, nipple soreness, nipple burning, breast pain, stabbing breast pain, shiny skin, or skin flaking of the nipple/areola had poor sensitivity (0-44%) for predicting recovery of *Candida* species from the iron-supplemented breastmilk. The authors then re-interviewed participants seven weeks later (without reculturing) and found that subsequent development of the signs/symptoms of interest was common. This resulted in improvement of sensitivity (39-83%) and specificity (51-91%). However, the positive predictive value of the best indicators (shiny or flaky nipple/areola skin) was modest (50% and 45%) and because other causes (i.e., bacteria) for the signs and symptoms of interest were not considered, the questions regarding diagnosis and clinical significance of "mammary candidosis" remain largely unanswered.

PROTECTION AGAINST INFECTION MEDIATED BY BREASTFEEDING OR HUMAN MILK FEEDING

This characteristic of human milk is one of its most striking effects on infants. Two explanations for these broad effects exist: the anti-infectious/anti-inflammatory components contained in human milk and human milk's minimal microbial contamination, relative to other infant foods and water. The former includes multiple milk components - immunoglobulins, soluble receptors, binding activities, oligosaccharides, glycoconjugates, specialized fecal flora, and biologic activities, while the latter is the basis for the "weanling's dilemma" - the trade-off between increased risk of infectious disease versus increased caloric density of other foods - that must be addressed when exclusive human milk feeding ceases. **Table 1** illustrates the broad range of infectious agents and infectious conditions that breastfeeding/ human milk feeding protect against in the human infant.

References

Academy of Breastfeeding Medicine. Protocol #4: *Mastitis.* [protocol page on Internet]. New Rochelle, NY: ABM; [no date listed; cited 2006 August 30]. Available from: http://www.bfmed.org/index.asp.

al-Eissa YA. Probable breast-milk borne brucellosis in a young infant. *Ann Trop Pediatr.* 1990; 10:305-307.

Amato Neto V, Matsubara L, Campos R, Moreira AA, Pinto PL, *et al.* Trypanosoma cruzi in the milk of women with chronic Chagas disease. *Rev Hosp Clin Fac Med Sao Paulo.* 1992; 47:10-11.

American Academy of Pediatics. Varicella-zoster infections. In: Pickering LK (ed.). *Red book: 2006 report of the committee on infectious diseases.* 27th ed. Elk Grove Village, IL: American Academy of Pediatrics; 2006. p. 711.

American Academy of Pediatrics. Human milk. In: Pickering LK (ed.). *Red book: 2006 report of the committee on infectious diseases.* 27th ed. Elk Grove Village, IL: American Academy of Pediatrics; 2006. p. 124-25.

American Academy of Pediatrics. Tuberculosis. In: Pickering LK (ed.). *Red book: 2006 report of the committee on infectious diseases.* 27th ed. Elk Grove Village, IL: American Academy of Pediatrics; 2006. p. 695.

American Academy of Pediatrics. Hepatitis B. In Pickering LK (ed.). *Red book: 2006 report of the committee on infectious diseases.* 27th ed. Elk Grove Village, IL; American Academy of Pediatrics; 2006. p. 345-47.

Amir L. Breastfeeding and staphylococcus aureus: three case reports. *Breastfeed Rev.* 2002; 10:15-18.

Amir LH, Forster D, McLachlan H, Lumley J. Incidence of breast abscess in lactating women: report from an Australian cohort. *BJOG.* 2004; 111:1378-81.

Amir LH, Garland SM, Dennerstein L, Farish SJ. Candida albicans: is it associated with nipple pain in lactating women? *Gynecol Obstet Invest.* 1996; 41:30-34.

Amir LH, Pakula S. Nipple pain, mastalgia and candidiasis in the lactating breast. *Aust N Z J Obstet Gynaecol.* 1991; 31:378-80.

Ando Y, Ekuni Y, Matsumoto Y, Nakano S, Saito K, *et al.* Long-term serological outcome of infants who received frozen-thawed milk from human T-lymphotropic virus type-I positive mothers. *J Obstet Gynaecol Res.* 2004; 30:436-38.

Arias-Camison JM. Late onset group B streptococcal infection from maternal expressed milk in a very low birth weight infant. *J Perinatol.* 2003; 23:691-92.

Arnon SS, Damus K, Thompson B, Midura TF, Chin J. Protective role of human milk against sudden death in infant botulism. *J Pediatr.* 1982; 100:568-73.

Arnon SS, Midura TF, Damus K, Thompson B, Wood RM, *et al.* Honey and other environmental risk factors for infant botulism. *J Pediatr.* 1979; 94:331-336.

Atkinson WL, Pickering LK, Schwartz B, Weniger BG, Iskander JK, *et al.* General recommendations on immunization. *MMWR.* 2002; 51(RR02):1-36.

Bagaglio S, Sitia G, Prati D, Cella D, Hasson H, *et al.* Mother-to-child transmission of TT virus: sequence analysis of non-coding region of TT virus in infected mother-infant pairs. *Arch Virol.* 2002; 147:803-12.

Beasley RP, Stevens CE, Shiao IS, Meng HC. Evidence against breast-feeding as a mechanism for vertical transmission of hepatitis B. *Lancet.* 1975; 2:740-41.

Behari P, Englund J, Alcasid G, Garcia-Houchins S, Weber SG. Transmission of methicillin-resistant Stapylococcus aureus to preterm infants through breast milk. *Infect Control Hosp Epdemiol.* 2004; 25:778-80.

Bhalla M, Thami GP. Reversible neurotoxicity after an overdose of topical lindane in an infant. *Pediatr Dermatol.* 2004; 21:597-99.

Bingen E, Denamur E, Lambert-Zechovsky N, Aujard Y, Brahimi N, *et al.* Analysis of DNA restriction fragment length polymorphism extends the evidence for breast milk transmission of Streptococcus agalactiae late onset neonatal infection. *J Infect Dis.* 1992; 165:569-73.

Bittencourt AL, Sadigursky M, Da Silva AA, Menezes CA, Marianetti MM, *et al.* Evaluation of Chagas' disease transmission through breast-feeding. *Mem Inst Oswaldo Cruz.* 1988; 83:37-39.

Bohlke K, Gail K, Jackson LA, Schmid DS, Starkovich P, *et al.* Post-partum varicella vaccination: is the vaccine virus excreted in breast milk? *Obstet Gynecol.* 2003; 102:970-77.

Boo NY, Nordiah AJ, Alfizah H, Nor-Rohaini AH, Lim VK. Contamination of breast milk obtained by manual expression and breast pumps in mothers of very low birth weight infants. *J Hosp Infect.* 2001; 49:274-81.

Boo NY, Nordiah AJ, Alfizah H, Nor-Rohaini AH, Lim VK. Contamination of breast milk obtained by manual expression and breast pumps in mothers of very low birthweight infants. *J Hosp Infect.* 2001; 49:274-81.

Botsford KB, Weinstein RA, Boyer KM, Nathan C, Carman M, *et al.* Gram negative bacilli in human milk feedings: quantitation and clinical consequences for premature infants. *J Pediatr.* 1986; 109:707-10.

Brent NB. Thrush in the breastfeeding dyad: results of a survey on diagnosis and treatment. *Clin Pediatr.* 2001; 40:503-06.

Brown RC, Girardeau HF. Transmammary passage of Strongyloides sp. larvae in the human host. *Am J Trop Med Hyg.* 1977; 26:215-19.

Bryant P, Morley C, Garland S, Curtis N. Cytomegalovirus transmission from breast milk in premature babies: does it matter? *Arch Dis Child Fetal Neonatal Ed.* 2002; 87:F75-F77.

Camassa F, Fania M, Ditano G, Silvestris AM, Lomuto M. Neonatal scabies. *Cutis.* 1995; 56:210-12.

Centers for Disease Control. *Smallpox vaccination information for women who are pregnant or breastfeeding.* [page on Internet]. Atlanta, GA: CDC; [last reviewed 2004 July 30; last updated 2003 May 6]. Available from: http://www.bt.cdc.gov/agent/smallpox/vaccination/preg-factsheet.asp.

Chen TL, Thien PF, Liaw SC, Fung CP, Siu LK. First report of Salmonella enterica serotype panama meningitis associated with consumption of contaminated breast milk by a neonate. *J Clin Microbiol.* 2005; 43:5400-2.

Chibber RM, Usmani MA, Al-Sibai MH. Should HEV infected mothers breast feed? *Arch Gynecol Obstet.* 2004; 270:15-20.

Cono J, Casey CG, Bell DM. Smallpox vaccination and adverse reactions. *MMWR.* 2003; 52(RR04):1-28.

Courtiss EH, Goldwyn RM, Anastasi GW. The fate of breast implants with infections around them. *Plas Reconstruct Surg.* 1979; 63:812-16.

Coutsoudis A. Influence of infant feeding patterns on early mother-to-child transmission of HIV-1 in Durban, South Africa. *Ann NY Acad Sci.* 2000; 918:136-44.

Devereux WP. Acute puerperal mastitis. *Am J Obstet Gynecol.* 1970; 108:78-81.

Division of Child Health and Development Update. Breastfeeding and maternal tuberculosis. *WHO.* 1998; 23.

Donowitz LG, Marsik FJ, Fisher KA, Wenzel RP. Contaminated breast milk: a source of Klebsiella bacteremia in a newborn intensive care unit. *Rev Infect Dis.* 1981; 3:716-20.

Duncan ME, Melsom R, Pearson JMH, Ridley DS. The association of pregnancy and leprosy. *Lepr Rev.* 1981; 52:245-62.

Dunkle LM, Schmidt RR, O'Connor DM. Neonatal herpes simplex infection possibly acquired via maternal breast milk. *Pediatrics.* 1979; 63:250-51.

European Collaborative Study. Mother-to-child transmission of HIV infection in the era of highly active anti-retroviral therapy. *Clin Infect Dis.* 2005; 40:458-65.

Ferreira CS, Martinho PC, Amato Neto V, Cruz RR. Pasteurization of human milk to prevent transmission of Chagas disease. *Rev Inst Med Trop Sao Paulo.* 2001; 43:161-62.

Fetherston C. Characteristics of lactation mastitis in a western Australian cohort. *Breastfeed Rev.* 1997; 5:5-11.

Fetherston C. Risk factors for lactation mastitis. *J Hum Lact.* 1998; 14:101-9.

Fleischrocker G, Vutuc C, Werner HP. Infection of a newborn infant by breast milk containing Salmonella typhimurium. *Wein Klin Wochenschr.* 1972; 84:394-95.

Forsgren M. Cytomegalovirus in breast milk: reassessment of pasteurization and freeze-thawing. *Pediatr Res.* 2004; 56:526-28.

Francis-Morrill J, Heinig MJ, Pappagianis D, Dewey KG. Diagnostic value of signs and symptoms of mammary candidosis among lactating women. *J Hum Lact.* 2004; 20:288-95.

Garde V, Harper D, Fairchok MP. Tertiary contact vaccinia in a breastfeeding infant. *JAMA.* 2004; 291:725-27.

Gerner P, Oettinger R, Gerner W, Falbrede J, Wirth S. Mother to infant transmission of TT virus: prevalence, extent and mechanism of vertical transmission. *Pediatr Infect Dis J.* 2000; 19:1074-77.

Gessler P, Bischoff GA, Wiegand D, Essers B, Bossart W. Cytomegalovirus-associated necrotizing enterocolitis in a preterm twin after breastfeeding. *J Perinatol.* 2004; 24:124-26.

Girdhar A, Girdhar BK, Ramu G, Desikan KV. Discharge of M. leprae in milk of leprosy patients. *Lepr India.* 1981; 53:390-94.

Global strategy for infant and young child feeding. Document A54/7, World Health Organization, 54th World Health Assembly, Provisional Agenda Item 13.1, April 9, 2001.

Godambe S, Shah PS, Shah V. Breast milk as a source of late onset neonatal sepsis. *Pediatr Infect Dis J.* 2005; 214:381-82.

Gransden WR, Webster M, French GL, Phillips I. An outbreak of Serratia marcescens transmitted by contaminated breast pumps in a special care baby unit. *J Hosp Infect.* 1986; 7:149-54.

Gras-Le Gruen C, Lepelletier D, Debillon T, Gournay V, Espaze E, *et al.* Contamination of a milk bank pasteuriser causing a pseudomonas aeruginosa outbreak in a neonatal intensive care unit. *Arch Dis Child Fetal Neonatal Ed.* 2003; 88:F434-35.

Griffin L. Studies on the incidence and seasonal pattern of hookworm infection in lactating mothers and the possible transmission to infants via the breastmilk, in Mombasa and Machakos, Kenya. *Cent Afr J Med.* 1981; 27:214-19.

Haas N, Stuttgen G. Facial involvement in scabies of infancy. *Hautarzt.* 1987; 39:622-23.

Halry M, Retter AS, Fowler D, Gea-Banacloche J, O'Grady NP. The role of intravenous immunoglobulin in the treatment of West Nile virus encephalitis. *Clin Infect Dis.* 2003; 37: e88-e90.

Hamel J. Primary chancre of the left breast after multiple suckling of an unrelated syphilitic infant. *Dermatol Wochenschr.* 1950; 121:303.

Hamosh M, Ellis LA, Pollock DR, Henderson TR, Hamosh P. Breastfeeding and the working mother: effect of time and temperature of short-term storage on proteolysis, lipolysis and bacterial growth in milk. *Pediatrics.* 1996; 97:492-98.

Hamprecht K, Maschmann J, Vochem M, Dietz K, Speer CP, *et al.* Epidemiology of transmission of cytomegalovirus from mother to preterm infant by breastfeeding. *Lancet.* 2001; 357:513-18.

Hayes EB, O'Leary DR. West Nile Virus infection: a pediatric perspective. *Pediatrics.* 2004; 11:1375-81.

Hegde S, Munshi AK. Influence of the maternal vaginal microbiota on the oral microbiota of the newborn. *Clin Pediatr Dent.* 1998; 22:317-21.

Hernandez J, Lemons P, Lemons J, Todd J. Effect of storage processes on the bacterial growth inhibiting activity of human breast milk. *Pediatrics.* 1979; 63:597-601.

Hill JB, Sheffield JS, Kim MJ, Alexander JM, Sercely B, *et al.* Risk of hepatitis B transmission in breast-fed infants of chronic hepatitis B carriers. *Obstet Gynecol.* 2002; 99:1049-52.

Huhn GD, Sejvar JJ, Montgomery SP, Dworkin MS. West Nile Virus in the United States: an update on an emerging infectious disease. *Am Fam Physician.* 2003; 68:653-60.

Iso K, Suzuki Y, Takayama M. Mother-to-infant transmission of TT-virus in Japan. *Int J Gynecol Obstet.* 2001; 75:11-19.

Israel-Ballard K, Chantry C, Dewey K, Lonnerdal B, Sheppard H, *et al.* Viral, bacterial and nutritional safety of flash-heated and pretoria-pasteurized breast milk to prevent mother-to-child transmission of HIV in resource-poor countries: a pilot study. *J Acquir Immune Defic Sydr.* 2005; 40:175-81.

Janik-Moszant A, Tomaszewska R, Szczepanski T, Sonta-Jakimczyk D, Pobudejska A. Infantile scabies or Langerhans cell histiocytosis? *Med Pediatr Oncol.* 2003; 40:111-12.

Jeffery BS, Soma-Pillay P, Makin J, Moolman G. The effect of Praetoria pasteurization on bacterial contamination of hand-expressed human breastmilk. *J Trop Pediatr.* 2003; 49:240-44.

Jeffery BS, Webber L, Mokhondo KR, Erasmus D. Determination of the effectiveness of inactivation of human immunodeficiency virus by Pretoria pasteurization. *J Trop Pediatr.* 2001; 47:345-49.

Jim WT, Shu CH, Chiu NC, Kao HA, Hung HY, *et al.* Transmission of cytomegalovirus from mothers to preterm infants by breast milk. *Pediatr Infect Dis J.* 2004; 23:848-51.

John TJ, Devarajan LV, Luther L, Vijayarathnam P. Effect of breastfeeding on seroresponse of infants to oral polio vaccination. *Pediatrics.* 1976; 57:47-53.

Jones CL, Jennison RF, D'Souza SW. Bacterial contamination of expressed breast milk. *Br Med J.* 1979; 2:1320-22.

Jonsson S, Pulkkinen MO. Mastitis today: incidence, prevention and treatment. *Ann Chir Gynaecol Suppl.* 1994; 208:84-87.

Junker AK, Thomas EE, Radcliffe A, Forsyth RB, Davidson AG, *et al.* Epstein-Barr virus shedding in breast milk. *Am J Med Sci.* 1991; 302:220-23.

Katzman DK, Wald ER. Staphylococcal scalded skin syndrome in a breast-fed infant. *Pediatr Infect Dis J.* 1987; 6:295-96.

Kawada M, Okuzumi K, Hitomi S, Sugishita C. Transmission of Staphylococcus aureus between healthy, lactating mothers and their infants by breastfeeding. *J Hum Lact.* 2003; 19:411-17.

Kenny JF. Recurrent group B streptococcal disease in an infant associated with the ingestion of infected mother's milk. *J Pediatr.* 1977; 91:158-59.

Kibrick S. Herpes simplex virus in breast milk. *Pediatrics.* 1979; 64:390.

Kilham L. Mumps virus in human milk and in milk of infected monkey. *JAMA.* 1951; 146:1231-32.

Kim KJ, Roh KH, Choi JH, Sung KJ, Moon KC, *et al.* Scabies incognito presenting as urticaria pigmentosa in an infant. *Pediatr Dermatol.* 2002; 19:409-11.

Kononen E, Asikainen S, Jousimies-Somer H. The early colonization of Gram negative bacteria in edentulous infants. *Oral Microbiol Immunol.* 1992; 7:28-31.

Kumar A, Yadav MP, Kakkar S. Human milk as a source of Q-fever infection in breast-fed babies. *Indian J Med Res.* 1981; 73:510-12.

Kusuhara K, Takabayashi A, Ueda K, Hidaka Y, Minamishima I, *et al.* Breast milk is not a significant source for early Epstein-Barr or human herpesvirus 6 infection in infants. A seroepidemiologic study in 2 endemic areas of human T-cell lymphotropic virus type I in Japan. *Microbiol Immunol.* 1997; 41:309-12.

Law BJ, Urias BA, Lertzman J, Robson D, Romance L. Is ingestion of milk-associated bacteria by premature infants fed raw human milk controlled by routine bacteriologic screening? *J Clin Microbiol.* 1989; 27:1560-66.

Lemons PM, Miller K, Eitzen H, Strodtbeck F, Lemons JA. Bacterial growth in human milk during continuous feeding. *Am J Perinatol.* 1983; 1:76-80.

Liebhaber M, Lewiston NJ, Asquith MT, Sunshine P. Comparison of bacterial contamination with two methods of human milk collection. *J Pediatr.* 1978; 92:236-37.

Livingstone VH, Willis CE, Berkowitz J. Staphylococcus aureus and sore nipples. *Can Fam Physician.* 1996. 42:654-59.

Long SS, Gajewski JL, Brown LW, Gilligan PH. Clinical, laboratory and environmental features of infant botulism in southeastern Pennsylvania. *Pediatrics.* 1985; 75:935-41.

Losonsky GA, Fishaut JM, Strussenberg J, Ogra PL. Effect of immunization against rubella on lactation products. II. Maternal-neonatal interactions. *J Infect Dis.* 1982; 145:661-66.

Marshall BR, Hepper JK, Zirbel CC. Sporadic puerperal mastitis. An infection that need not interrupt lactation. *JAMA*. 1975; 233:1377-79.

Martin R, Langa S, Reviriego C, Jiminez E, Martin ML, *et al.* Human milk is a source of lactic acid bacteria for the infant gut. *J Pediatr.* 2003; 143:754-58.

Mast EE. Mother-to-infant hepatitis C virus transmission and breastfeeding. *Adv Exp Med Biol.* 2004; 554:211-16.

Matheson I, Aursnes I, Horgen M, Aabo O, Melby K. Bacteriological findings and clinical symptoms in relation to clinical outcome in pueroperal mastitis. *Acta Obstet Gynecol Scand.* 1988; 67:723-26.

Meier J, Lienicke U, Tschirch E, Kruger DH, Wauer RR, *et al.* Human cytomegalovirus reactivation during lactation and mother-to-child transmission in preterm infants. *J Clin Microbiol.* 2005; 43:1318-24.

Menendez C, Sanchez-Tapias JM, Alonso PL, Gimenez-Barcons M, Kahigwa E, *et al.* Molecular evidence of mother-to-infant transmission of hepatitis G among women without known risk factors for parenteral infections. *J Clin Microbiol.* 1999; 37:2333-36.

Middaugh J. Botulism and breast milk. *N Engl J Med.* 1978; 298:343.

Mok J, Pembrey L, Tovo PA, Newell ML: European Pediatric Hepatitis C Network. When does mother to child transmission of hepatitis C virus occur? *Arch Dis Child Fetal Neonatal Ed.* 2005; 90:F156-60.

Morais TB, Sigulem DM, de Sousa Maranhao H, de Morais MB. Bacterial contamination and nutrient content of home-prepared milk feeding bottles of infants attending a public outpatient clinic. *J Trop Pediatr.* 2005; 51:87-92.

Morrill JF, Pappagianis D, Heinig MJ, Lonnerdal B, Dewey KG. Detecting *Candida albicans* in human milk. *J Clin Microbiol.* 2003; 41:475-78.

Narayanan I, Prakash K, Murthy NS, Gujral VV. Randomized controlled trial of effect of raw and holder pasteurized human milk and of formula supplements on incidence of neonatal infection. *Lancet.* 1984; 2:1111-13.

Naser SA, Schwartz D, Shafran I. Isolation of Mycobacterium avium subsp paratuberculosis from breast milk of Crohn's disease patients. *Am J Gastroenterol.* 2000; 95: 1094-95.

Nduati R, John G, Mbori-Ngacha D, Richardson B, Overbaugh J, *et al.* Effect of breastfeeding and formula feeding on transmission of HIV-1. A randomized clinical trial. *JAMA*. 2000; 283:1167-74.

Nwosu AB. Human neonatal infections with hookworms in an endemic area of southern Nigeria. A possible transmammary route. *Trop Geogr Med.* 1981; 33:105-11.

Ogundele MO. Techniques for the storage of human breast milk: implications for anti-microbial functions and safety of stored milk. *Eur J Pediatr.* 2000; 159:793-97.

Olowe SA, Ahmed I, Lawal SF, Ransome-Kuti S. Bacteriological quality of raw human milk: effect of storage in a refrigerator. *Ann Trop Paediatr.* 1987; 7:233-37.

Olver WJ, Bond DW, Boswell TC, Watkin SL. Neonatal group B streptococcal disease associated with infected breast milk. *Arch Dis Child Neonatal Ed.* 2000; 83:F48-49.

Osterman KL, Rahm VA. Lactation mastitis: bacterial cultivation of breast milk, symptoms, treatment and outcome. *J Hum Lact.* 2000; 16:297-302.

Palanduz A, Palanduz S, Guler K, Guler N. Brucellosis in a mother and her young infant: possible transmission by breast milk. *Int J Infect Dis.* 2000; 4:55-56.

Paller AS. Scabies in infants and children. *Semin Dermatol.* 1993; 12:3-8.

Peacock SJ, Justice A, Griffiths D, de Silva GDI, Kantzanou MN, *et al.* Determinants of acquisition and carriage of Staphylococcus aureus in infancy. *J Clin Microbiol.* 2003; 41:5718-25.

Pedley JC. The presence of M. leprae in human milk. *Pepr Rev.* 1967; 38:239-42.

Polywka S, Schroter M, Feucht HH, Zollner B, Laufs R. Low risk of vertical transmission of hepatitis C virus by breast milk. *Clin Infect Dis.* 1999; 29:1327-29.

Possible West Nile Virus transmission to an infant through breastfeeding. *MMWR.* 2002; 51(39):877-78.

Public Health Service Task Force. Recommendations for use of antiretroviral drugs in pregnant HIV-1 infected women for maternal health and interventions to reduce perinatal HIV-1 transmission in the United States. From: DHHS. *AIDS info* [homepage on the Internet]. Rockville, MD: NIH; [cited 2005 Nov 17]. Available from: http://AIDSinfo.nih.gov.

Quarterman MJ, Lesher JL. Neonatal scabies treated with permethrin 5% cream. *Pediatr Dermatol.* 1994; 11:264-66.

Quin PT, Lofberg JV. Maternal herpetic breast infection: another hazard of neonatal herpes simplex. *Med J Aust.* 1978; 2:411-12.

Qutaishat SS, Stemper ME, Spencer SK, Borchardt MA, *et al.* Transmission of Salmonella enterica serotype typhimurium DT104 to infants through mother's milk. *Pediatrics.* 2003; 111:1442-46.

Ralph A, McBride J, Currie BJ. Transmission of Burkholderia pseudomallei via breast milk in northern Australia. *Pediatr Infect Dis J.* 2004; 23:1169-71.

Ramsay DT, Kent JC, Owens RA, Hartmann PE. Ultrasound imaging of milk ejection in the breast of lactating women. *Pediatrcs.* 2004; 113:361-67.

Ransjo U, Asplund OA, Gylbert L, Jurell G. Bacteria in the female breast. *Scand J Plast Reconstr Surg.* 1985; 19:87-89.

Raptopoulou-Gigi M, Marwick K, McClelland DB. Antimicrobial proteins in sterilized human milk. *Br Med J.* 1977; 1:12-14.

Read JS, Committee on Pediatric AIDS. Human milk, breastfeeding and transmission of human immunodeficiency virus type 1 in the United States. *Pediatrics.* 2003; 112:1196-1205.

Recommendations for antimicrobial prophylaxis for children and breastfeeding mothers and treatment of children with anthrax. *MMWR.* 2001; 50:1014-16.

Rench MA, Baker CJ. Group B streptococcal breast abscess in a mother and mastitis in her infant. *Obstet Gynecol.* 1987; 73:875-77.

Rotimi VO, Duerden BI. The development of the bacterial flora in normal neonates. *J Med Microbiol.* 1981; 14:51-62.

Santos Ferreira C, Amato Neto V, Gakiya E, Bezerra RC, Alarcon RS. Microwave treatment of human milk to prevent transmission of Chagas disease. *Rev Inst Med Trop Sao Paulo.* 2003; 45:41-42.

Sealander JY, Kerr CP. Herpes simplex of the nipple: infant-to-mother transmission. *Am Fam Physician.* 1989; 39:111-13.

Setasuban P, Punsri W, Meunnoo C. Transmammary transmission of Necator americanus larva in the human host. *Southeast Asian J Trop Med Public Health.* 1980; 11:535-38.

Sullivan-Bolyai JZ, Fife KH, Jacobs RF, Miller Z, Corey L. Disseminated neonatal herpes simplex type 1 from a maternal breast lesion. *Pediatrics.* 1983; 71:455-57.

Suthienkul O, Siripanichgon K, Promachat P, Echeverria P, Lexsomboon U, *et al.* Bacterial contamination of bottle milk in infants under 6 months in Children's Hospital, Bangkok, Thailand. *Southeast Asian J Trop Med Public Health.* 1999; 30:770-75.

Taha TE, Kumwenda NI, Hoover DR, Fiscus SA, Kafulafula G, *et al.* Neviripine and zidovudine at birth to reduce perinatal transmission of HIV in an African setting: a randomized controlled trial. *JAMA.* 2004; 292:202-9.

Thomas IL, Marianai-Kurkdjian P, Collignon A, Gravet A, Clermont O, *et al.* Breast milk transmission of a Panton-Valentine leukocudin-producing Staphylococcus aureus strain causing infantile pneumonia. *J Clin Microbiol.* 2001; 39:728-29.

Thomassen P, Johansson VA, Wassberg C, Petrini B. Breast-feeding, pain and infection. *Gynecol Obstet Invest.* 1998; 46:73-74.

Thompson N, Pickler RH, Munro C, Shotwell J. Contamination in expressed breast milk following breast cleansing. *J Hum Lact.* 1997; 13:127-30.

Thornton JW, Argenta LC, McClatchey KD, Marks MW. Studies of the endogenous flora of the breast. *Ann Plastic Surg.* 1988; 20:39-42.

Vochem M, Hamprecht K, Jahn G, Speer CP. Transmission of cytomegalovirus to preterm infants through breast milk. *Pediatr Infect Dis J.* 1998; 17:53-58.

Vollmer B, Seibold-Weiger K, Schmitz-Salue C, Hamprecht K, Goelz R, *et al.* Postnatally acquired cytomegalovirus infection via breast milk: effects on hearing and development in preterm infants. *Pediatr Infect Dis J.* 2004; 23:322-27.

Welsh JK, Arsenakis M, Coelen RJ, May JT. Effect of antiviral lipids, heat, and freezing on the activity of viruses in human milk. *J Infect Dis.* 1979; 140:322-28.

Wiktor SZ, Pate EJ, Rosenberg PS, Barnett M, Palmer P, *et al.* Mother-to-child transmission of human T-cell lymphotropic virus type I associated with prolonged breast-feeding. *J Hum Virol.* 1997; 1:37-44.

World Health Organization. *HIV and infant feeding: guidelines for decision makers.* Geneva: World Health Organization; 2003.

Yeager AS, Palumbo PE, Malachowski N, Ariagno RL, Stevenson DK. Sequellae of maternally derived cytomegalovirus infections in premature infants. *J Pediatr.* 1983; 102:918-22.

Yoshida M, Tezuka T, Hiruma M. Detection of varicella-zoster virus DNA in maternal breast milk from a mother with herpes zoster. *Clin Diagn Virol.* 1995; 4:61-65.

Yoshida M, Yamagami N, Tezuka T, Hondo R. Case report: detection of varicella-zoster virus DNA in maternal breast milk. *J Med Virol.* 1992; 38:108-10.

Youssef RF, Darcy E, Barone A, Borja MT, Leggiadro RJ. Expressed breast milk as a source of neonatal sepsis. *Pediatr Infect Dis J.* 2002; 21:888-89.

Yu SH, Jiang ZX, Xu LQ. Infantile hookworm disease in China. *A review. Acta Trop.* 1995; 59:265-70.

Zaman S, Carlsson B, Morikawa S, Jeansson S, Narayanan I, *et al.* Poliovirus antibody titres, relative affinity, and neutralising capacity in maternal milk. *Arch Dis Child.* 1993; 68:198-201.

SECTION III

MANAGEMENT - INFANT

Chapter 12

Human Milk, Breastfeeding, and the Preterm Infant

Nancy E. Wight and Jane A. Morton

INTRODUCTION

Although advancements in neonatal intensive care have improved survival for premature infants dramatically in the last 35 years, the percent of premature and low birth weight infants continues to rise, 12.7% and 8.2%, respectively (Hamilton *et al.*, 2007; Child Trends Data Bank, 2005). The benefits of human milk for term infants are well recognized (American Academy of Pediatrics Section on Breastfeeding, 2005; Cunningham, 1995). Human milk is species-specific and has been adapted through evolution to meet the needs of the human infant, supporting growth, development, and survival (Goldman *et al.*, 1998). It has only been in the very recent past that significantly preterm infants have survived and that attention has been paid to the crucial role of nutrition in the long-term outcomes for these infants.

Current research confirms that human milk especially benefits the preterm infant through: host defense, gastrointestinal development, special nutrition, neurodevelopmental outcome, (indirectly) a physically and psychologically healthier mother, and ultimately, economic and environmental benefits (California Perinatal Quality Care Collaborative, 2004; Weimer, 2001; Wight, 2001a). Human milk has been rediscovered as one of the key factors in improving overall infant outcomes and is now the standard of care in the NICU (American Academy of Pediatrics Section on Breastfeeding, 2005; California Perinatal Quality Care Collaborative, 2004; California Perinatal Quality Care Collaborative, 2005; Schanler *et al.*, 2005).

All premature infants are not the same (Lawrence & Lawrence, 2005b). Infants who are born weighing less than 2500 grams (<5lb8oz) are classified as low birth weight (LBW); infants born weighing less than 1500 grams (<3lb5oz) are termed very low birth weight (VLBW); and infants born at less than 1000 grams (<2lb3oz) are termed extremely low birth weight (ELBW). Infants born at less than 37 completed weeks are considered premature (American Academy of Pediatrics & American College of Obstetricians and Gynecologists, 2002). Infants who are less than the tenth percentile for weight at any gestation are classified as small for gestational age (SGA). Given advances in medical technology and therapies, predominantly in the area of respiratory support, survival of preterm infants has improved significantly for all but the tiniest, most immature infants (**Table 1**).

Nutrition appropriate for a 2000 gram preterm infant is considerably different from that needed by a 500 gram, 24 week premature infant. Optimal nutritional management, adjusted for gestational age and nutritional status at birth, is a key factor in improving the quality of survival, as well as survival itself.

HISTORICAL PERSPECTIVE

Throughout history, all civilizations have found alternatives when mothers either could not or would

Table 1. Preterm Births and Survival

Preterm Births: 2003		Weight at 50 % Survival (in USA)	
US (4.1 million)	LBW (7.9%) ~ 324,000/yr	1970	1500 g
	VLBW (1.4%) ~ 58,000	1980	1000 g
	ELBW (0.7%) ~ 29,000	1990	750 g
World (200 million)	LBW (15%) ~ 30,000,000	1995	600 g
	VLBW (3%) ~ 6,000,000	2000	500 g
	ELBW (1.5%) ~ 3,000,000	2005	500 g

Source: NCHS, 2003: www.cdc.gov/nchs/fastats/birthwt.htm

not breastfeed their infants (Fildes, 1986). Wet nursing provided better infant survival than dry nursing (animal milks or other adult foods) (Baumslag & Michels, 1995). However, up until the late 19th century, most preterm infants died, regardless of type of feeding. The tiny infants that survived were usually close to term and small for gestational age.

Obstetricians Pierre Budin (1846-1907) and his mentor, Stephane Tarnier (1828-1897), are usually credited with the creation of perinatal medicine through their care of preterm infants ("weaklings" as they were called at the time) at L'Hôpital Maternité in Paris. Their key principles of care were: warmth, protection from infection, and nutrition, preferably breastmilk.

After visiting European premature centers, Dr. Julius H. Hess (1876-1955) started the first center for preterm infants in the United States at Michael Reese Hospital in Chicago and published the first book on the premature infant. Hess advocated human milk as the feeding of choice, starting in the second 12 hours of life with milk provided by a wet nurse (Hess, 1922). In the second version of his textbook 20 years later, he still advocated the use of breastmilk, but recommended delaying feedings for as long as four days in fear of aspiration and renal intolerance (Hess & Lundeen, 1941). During this time, the infant was to receive a physiologic salt solution subcutaneously.

Research in the 1940s noted that infants fed a diluted "half-skimmed cow's milk formula" gained weight more rapidly than those fed breastmilk, presumably due to the higher protein content of cow's milk (Gordon *et al.*, 1947). Other studies suggested that human milk required supplementation with calcium and phosphorus for optimum bone mineralization (Greer, 2001). As a result, the 1958 revision of Hess's textbook downplayed the promotion of breastmilk for preterm infants and included an expanded section on "artificial feeding" (Lundeen & Kunstadter, 1958).

In the 1970s, research suggested that the quality, as well as the quantity, of proteins were important in preterm nutrition and that feeding too much protein (4.5 g/kg/d) could lead to azotemia, hyperammonemia, and metabolic acidosis in some infants (Greer, 2001) and lactobezoars (Erenberg *et al.*, 1979). Mothers' own milk was noted to provide better growth than pooled mature donor milk (Gross, 1983), but no milk or formula achieved the intrauterine rate of growth. Lacking evidence that the intrauterine rate of growth was the appropriate standard for preterm infants ex-utero, the American Academy of Pediatrics, in its first statement on the nutritional needs of low birth weight infants, concluded that "the optimal diet for the low birth weight infant may be defined as the one that supports a rate of growth approximating that of the third trimester intrauterine life, without imposing stress on the developing metabolic or excretory systems" (American Academy of Pediatrics, 1977).

By the 1980s, human milk was found in almost every hospital with an NICU. At that time, a crisis arose due to inconsistent practices regarding pasteurization and usage. Occasional NICU epidemics of sepsis and necrotizing enterocolitis from contaminated milk of one mother used for several NICU infants and the recognition that human immunodeficiency virus (HIV) and other viral pathogens could be transmitted through the use of fresh donor milk, caused all but a handful of milk banks in the U.S. to close (Arnold & Erickson, 1988; Jones, 2003). The 1980s also saw the commercial development of preterm formulas with higher protein, calcium, phosphorus, and vitamins than term formulas (Greer, 2001), resulting in more rapid growth without the metabolic complications seen in the 1970s (Cooper *et al.*,

1984; Schanler & Oh, 1985; Tyson, 1983). Human milk alone was generally perceived to be inadequate to meet the needs of the preterm infant, although an increasing number of studies reported evidence for the benefits of human milk.

With the development of commercially available human milk fortifiers in the 1980s and 1990s, human milk with fortification became the standard of care for the low birth weight infant in the U.S. (Greer, 2001). Although comparative studies continued to show that infants fed special preterm formulas grew faster than those fed fortified human milk (Atkinson *et al.*, 1981b; Schanler & Garza, 1987; Schanler *et al.*, 1999c), many other countries either could not afford or preferred not to use commercial multi-component human milk fortifiers, preferring instead to increase feeding volume and/or add specific nutrients, such as protein, calcium, and phosphorus. NICUs in the U.S. did not use these higher volumes due to concerns regarding fluid overload aggravating pulmonary and cardiovascular status. Although "extrauterine growth restriction" has been associated with both short-term and long-term morbidities (Clark *et al.*, 2003), optimal extrauterine growth rate(s) are yet to be determined. Too rapid growth in infancy, especially "catch-up" growth for in-utero growth-restricted infants, is also associated with later morbidities (Griffin, 2002; Singhal, 2006; Lucas, 2005c).

Having established the superiority of human milk feedings with benefits especially magnified in VLBW infants, a current barrier is the shortage of supply of mothers' own milk. Increasingly, research is focusing on the potential to improve milk production in the pump-dependent mother (Mitoulas *et al.*, 2002) and the use of donor human milk (Schanler *et al.*, 2005; Wight, 2001a).

In the 21st century, human milk is the standard of care for all infants, including preterm infants:

"Human milk is species-specific, and all substitute feeding preparations differ markedly from it, making human milk uniquely superior for infant feeding... In addition, human milk-fed premature infants receive significant benefits with respect to host protection and improved developmental outcomes compared with formula-fed premature infants... Hospitals and physicians should recommend human milk for premature and other high risk infants either by direct breastfeeding and/or using the mother's own expressed milk" (American Academy of Pediatrics Section on Breastfeeding, 2005).

PRETERM DEVELOPMENTAL PHYSIOLOGY

Healthy, full-term infants are programmed to make the transition from their intrauterine continuous parenteral nutrition via the umbilical cord to extrauterine intermittent enteral support via breastmilk. Human milk is a complex fluid that simultaneously provides nutrients and bioactive components that facilitate the adaptive, functional changes required for the optimal transition from intrauterine to extrauterine life (Donovan, 2006). Although still immature compared to adults and undergoing significant postnatal growth and functional adaptation, term infants usually make the transition without much difficulty. Preterm infants, however, suffer not only from gastrointestinal immaturity, but also from functional immaturity of all organs and physiologic systems, as well as specific illnesses and complications, which further confound their transition from fetus to newborn.

Gastrointestinal Tract

Amniotic fluid provides the first luminal stimulus to the developing fetus with the third trimester fetus receiving 10-14% of energy and protein requirements from ingested amniotic fluid (Underwood & Sherman, 2006). Postnatally, breastmilk provides the continuum of luminal stimulation for the neonate. Human milk components actively protect the infant from pathogenic infection and facilitate the establishment of the microbiota, which is necessary to activate the mucosal immune system (Donovan, 2006; Goldman, 2000). As such, human milk constitutes a "communication vehicle" or link between the mother and the infant that reduces the infant's disease risk (Donovan, 2006; Walker, 2004).

The gut is the largest immune organ of the body. Instead of protecting the baby, the dysfunctional gut of the preterm infant can become a risk factor. The intestinal ecosystem is composed of three closely interacting components: host cells, nutrients, and microflora (Caicedo *et al.*, 2005). Caicedo *et al.* describe how the developing intestinal ecosystem and the immune system work in concert. The first component, the highly immunoreactive intestinal submucosa, underlies only a fragile, single layer of epithelial cells. The second component is the intestinal flora. At birth, the intestine is sterile, but rapidly becomes colonized. In one study of infants greater than 34 weeks gestation, the most important determinants of the gut microbiotic composition in these infants were the mode of delivery, type of feeding, gestational age, hospitalization, and antibiotic use (Penders *et al.*, 2006). In the preterm infant, delayed feeding, antibiotics, formula feeding, total parenteral nutrition, or nursing in incubators may delay or impair the intestinal colonization process.

So-called "cross-talk" between the epithelium and commensal bacteria modulates proinflammatory mediators, preventing propagation of inflammation locally and at distal sites (lung and brain). The third component, the nutrients, not only supports the prevalence of beneficial microflora (*Bifidobacterium* and *Lactobacilli*), but additionally inhibits the growth of pathogenic microbes with factors such as lactoferrin and secretory IgA. As human milk contains a wide variety of biologically active components, it can be considered a "symbiotic;" a substance that has the properties of both a probiotic ("good" bacteria) and a prebiotic (nutritional substrates that promote the growth of probiotic bacteria). The feeding of human milk is an immediate way to promote the development of the intestinal ecosystem in both the term and preterm neonate (Caicedo *et al.*, 2005).

Digestive Development

Not only is human milk the appropriate "prebiotic" nutrient required to support the immune system, it is needed urgently and in high volume. The longer the delay in establishing full human milk feeds, the greater the risk (Ronnestad *et al.*, 2005). Yet, the capacity to tolerate rapid advancement to feedings is severely compromised in this population.

The gastrointestinal (GI) tract is one of the first structures visible in the developing embryo. The intestine grows very rapidly during the second trimester, slows down, then continues to increase more rapidly than body length for three to four years of life (Newell, 2000). The ontogenic timetable is complex (**Figure 1**). The stomach proton pump is active from 13 weeks gestation with intrinsic factor and pepsin secreted a few weeks later (Newell, 2000). Gastric acid secretion is present and can lower stomach pH to less than 4.0, even in extremely preterm infants. Very preterm infants also demonstrate pancreatic exocrine secretion and can digest fat, protein, and carbohydrate (Newell, 2000). Although pancreatic lipase and bile salts are minimal in ELBW infants, human milk provides lipases and other digestive enzymes (Lawrence & Lawrence, 2005b). In the intestinal mucosa, villus development and cellular differentiation occur early in the second trimester (Newell, 2000). At the beginning of the third trimester, lactase activity is around 5% of adult levels, but feeding human milk increases the levels (Shulman *et al.*, 1998).

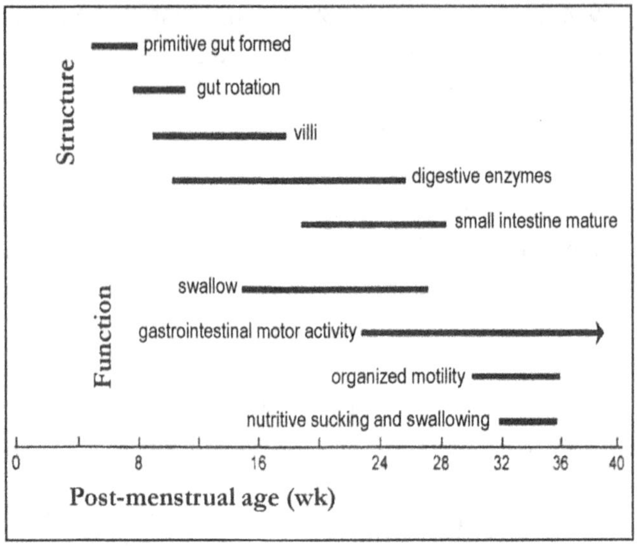

Figure 1. The ontogenic timetable of GI development Source: Newell, 2000. Figure reprinted with permission, copyright Elsevier.

Table 2. Factors Affecting Gastric Emptying

Faster Gastric Emptying	No Effect	Slower Gastric Emptying
Breast milk	Phototherapy	Prematurity
Glucose polymers	Feed temperature	Formula milk
Starch	Nonnutritive sucking	Caloric density
Medium-chain triglycerides		Fatty acids
Prone position		Dextrose concentration
		Long-chain triglycerides
		Osmolality
		Illness

Source: Newell, 2000. Table reprinted with permission, copyright Elsevier.

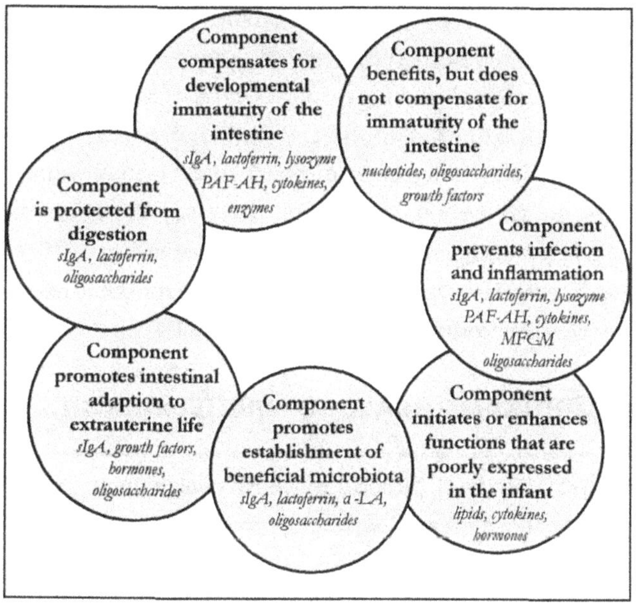

Figure 2. Strategies for beneficial effects of bioactive agents in Human Milk (HM). HM contains bioactive agents with overlapping and synergistic effects on intestinal development of neonates. Source: Donovan, 2006. Figure reprinted with permission, copyright Elsevier.

Slow gastric emptying is common in the preterm infant and presents as failure to tolerate milk feeds. Gastric emptying is faster with human milk and is retarded by formula and increased osmolality (**Table 2**) (Newell, 2000). Fortifying human milk delays gastric emptying significantly (Ewer & Yu, 1996; McClure & Newell, 1996).

Maturation of small intestinal motility and tolerance to feeds is enhanced by previous exposure to enteral nutrition (Berseth, 1996; Bisset *et al.*, 1989; McClure & Newell, 1999). Small volumes of undiluted milk lead most rapidly to a more mature feed response (Newell, 2000). Gastro-anal transit time is slower in preterm infants than their term counterparts. Stools are more varied and frequent in infants who receive human milk (Newell, 2000). An overall schema for the bioactive factors in human milk is seen in **Figure 2**.

Development of the Immune System

Reciprocal relationships between the production of immune factors by the lactating mammary gland and the production of those defense agents during early infancy are found in all mammalian species (Goldman *et al.*, 1994; Goldman *et al.*, 1998). Defense factors in human milk include direct antimicrobial agents, anti-inflammatory factors, immunomodulators, and leukocytes. Protective immune factors in breastmilk coat the GI and upper respiratory tracts via mucosa-associated lymphoid tissue and prevent invasion of mucous membranes by respiratory and enteric pathogens. Inadequacies in the newborn's mucosal defenses are passively provided by protective substances in human milk or by an active, accelerated stimulation of the infants' immune system by trophic factors and cytokines secreted into human milk (Goldman *et al.*, 2003; Walker, 2004). Since the premature infant's immune system is even more immature and his survival more precarious than that of a full-term newborn, the importance of ingesting his mother's own milk is even more apparent (Schanler *et al.*, 1986; Walker, 2004).

In addition, milk of mothers who deliver prematurely differs in composition from milk of mothers who deliver at term, both in terms of nutrients and bioactive factors (Groer & Walker, 1996; Schanler & Atkinson, 1999). Preterm milk appears to have a higher concentration of growth factors, hormones, anti-inflammatory factors, immunomodulators, immunoglobulins, and live infection-fighting cells than term milk (Groer & Walker, 1996; Gross *et al.*, 1981a), thus meeting the needs of these extremely immature infants (**Table 3**).

Other Organs/Systems Development

Although the respiratory system is clearly the most important organ system in establishing early survival,

Table 3. Comparison of Anti-infective Properties in Colostrum of Preterm vs. Term Mothers

Factor	Preterm Colostrum	Term Colostrum
Total protein (g/L)	0.43 ± 1.3	0.31 ± 0.05
IgA (mg/g protein)	310.5 ± 70	168.2 ± 21
IgG (mg/g protein)	7.6 ± 3.9	8.4 ± 1
IgM (mg/g protein)	39.6 ± 23	36.1 ± 16
Lysozyme (mg/g protein)	1.5 ± 0.5	1.1 ± 0.3
Lactoferrin (mg/g protein)	165 ± 37	102 ± 25
Total cells/ ml^3	6794 ± 1946	3064 ± 424
Macrophages	4041 ± 1420	1597 ± 303
Lymphocytes	1850 ± 543	954 ± 143
Neutrophils	842 ± 404	512 ± 178

Source: Lawrence & Lawrence, 2005b. Table reprinted with permission, copyright Elsevier/Mosby.

all preterm infants experience the effects of multiple organ and system immaturities. As noted above, human milk provides some degree of mucosal immunity for the respiratory and GI systems. In addition, immunoglobulins and other antimicrobial factors can be absorbed through the immature gut mucosa to protect other organs, such as the immature urinary tract (Goldblum *et al.*, 1989; Pisacane *et al.*, 1992).

In utero, red blood cell (RBC) production is controlled exclusively by fetal erythropoietin produced in the liver. At birth, the site of erythropoietin production changes from the liver to the kidney by an unknown mechanism. An abrupt increase in PaO2 causes serum erythropoietin to fall, shutting down RBC production for six to eight weeks, contributing to physiologic anemia and anemia of prematurity (Stockman & deAlarcon, 1992). Human milk contains significant concentrations of erythropoietin which tend to resist proteolytic degradation (Kling, 2002; Semba & Juul, 2002; Kling *et al.*, 1998). Erythropoietin receptors are widely distributed in human tissues, including the GI tract, endothelial cells, spinal cord, and brain, suggesting that erythropoietin plays a wider role in infant development (Kling, 2002; Semba & Juul, 2002).

Preterm infants fed maternal or banked breastmilk have significantly higher peak bilirubin concentrations and more prolonged jaundice than infants fed artificial preterm formula (Lucas & Baker, 1986; Kumar *et al.*, 2006; Mancuso *et al.*, 2006). However, bilirubin has been shown to be a potent anti-oxidant (Kumar *et al.*, 2006; Mancuso *et al.*, 2006), and a randomized controlled trial of allowing higher bilirubin levels in preterm infants is currently in the data analysis phase.

Environmental Issues

Preterm infants are likely to experience prolonged hospitalization, invasive procedures, and separation from their mothers. The NICU environment is a source of nosocomial infections with resistant organisms and nonphysiologic treatments as compared to the in utero environment. Endotracheal tubes sustain life, but bypass upper airway defenses, leading to respiratory infections. Umbilical catheters and other vascular lines provide portals for bacterial entry. Hospital equipment, staff, and even the infant's family are carriers of bacterial, viral, and fungal pathogens, despite careful attention to infection control procedures.

The "enteromammary system" (Groer & Walker, 1996; Kleinman & Walker, 1979) produces specific IgA antibodies against antigens in the mother's environment. Through skin-to-skin contact with her preterm infant in the NICU, a lactating mother's more mature immune system can be exposed to and make specific antibodies against pathogens in the infant's environment. These antibodies are transferred rapidly to the mother's milk to protect her immature infant (Walker, 2004).

NUTRITIONAL GOALS FOR PRETERM INFANTS

In the neonatal period, low birth weight and preterm infants have greater nutritional needs than at any time in their lives (Schanler, 2003). For example, the accretion of neuronal mass is greater in the last trimester than in the first three months of a term infant's life. Without the last trimester, when many constituents, such as iron, are actively transported across the placenta to meet growth demands and fill storage organs, the preterm infant faces the most demanding growth period with a nutritional deficit. In addition, their medical condition may contribute to increased nutrient needs. The stress of common pathophysiologic events (hypotension, hypoxia, acidosis, infection, surgical intervention), and their therapies (antibiotics, corticosteroids), as well as physiologic immaturity of all organ systems are significant impediments to growth, even if full nutrition can be achieved rapidly (Schanler, 2003).

The goals of nutrition for the preterm infant are to:

- define and achieve a standard of short-term growth;
- meet the unique nutritional needs of prematurity;
- prevent feeding-related morbidities; and
- optimize long-term outcome (California Perinatal Quality Care Collaborative, 2004).

Define and Achieve Growth Standards

The nutritional reference standard for the term newborn is the exclusively breastfed infant. The World Health Organization (WHO) recently published growth reference standards based on optimal infant feeding (including breastfeeding), optimal health care, and optimal environmental conditions (World Health Organization, 2006). These growth charts describe how all the world's children should grow from birth to five years of age. Although normative data exist for longitudinal growth of infants born at various gestational

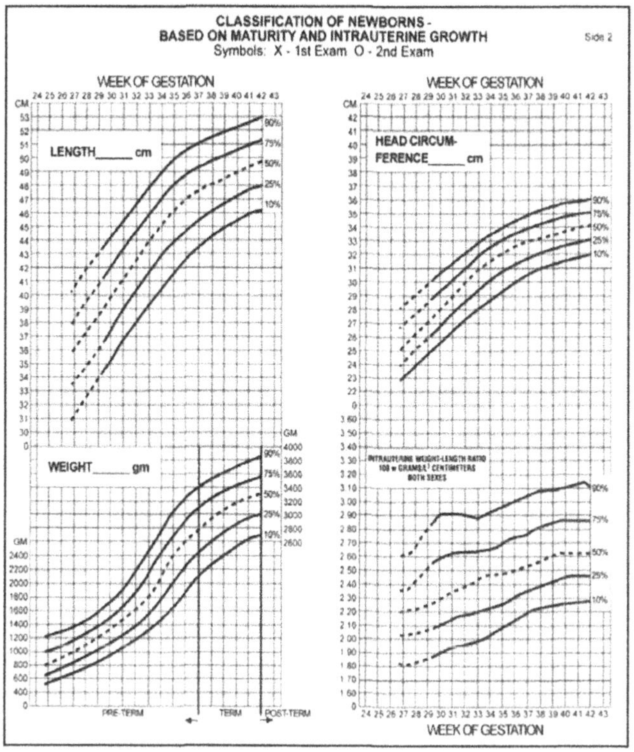

Figure 3. In utero growth curves

Source: Developed by Jacob L. Kay, MD, in conjunction with Mead Johnson Nutritionals. Reprinted with permission of Mead Johnson & Company.

ages (Ehrenkranz *et al.*, 1999), an optimal growth standard comparable to the WHO data for term infants does not exist for preterm infants. Instead, the current growth standard used is the estimated intrauterine nutrient accretion rate at corresponding stages during the last trimester of pregnancy (Schanler, 2003). The currently accepted goal is to approximate the in utero growth of a normal fetus of the same postmenstrual age in both body weight and body composition, while maintaining normal concentrations of blood and tissue nutrients (American Academy of Pediatrics Committee on Nutrition, 2004). The optimal reference standard may be different given the significant differences in the in utero and extrauterine environments, the extreme differences in condition at birth, and the degrees of illness for the wide range of premature infants (**Figure 3**).

Growth is an important health outcome for preterm infants with in-hospital growth velocity affecting both neurodevelopmental and growth outcomes at 18-22 months of age (Ehrenkranz *et al.*, 2006). Despite this, National Institute of Child and Human Development (NICHD) data reveal that over 90% of infants who are less than 1000 grams at birth are discharged weighing less than the tenth percentile for corrected gestational age (Dusick *et al.*, 2003). The term "extrauterine growth restriction" has been used to describe this phenomenon of turning appropriate for gestational age infants at birth into small for gestational age infants at discharge (Clark *et al.*, 2003).

Meet the Unique Nutritional Needs of Prematurity

An infant born at term will increase his brain weight by 40% over the first eight weeks of life. A preterm infant born at 28 weeks gestation must double the weight of his brain (100% increase) in the first eight weeks to match in utero growth rates. This difference in growth rate explains why a nutritional deficiency early on can be more damaging in the preterm infant compared to the term infant. The energy and nutrient requirements of preterm and LBW infants vary enormously, depending on birth weight, gestational age, degree of intrauterine growth restriction, medical complications, nutritional status, clinical management, and the model and assumptions used to establish the "requirements." In addition, the VLBW infant (less than 1500 grams) has several unique aspects of nutrition that must be considered (**Table 4**). Human milk alone may not meet all these special needs.

Table 4. Special Nutritional Conditions of VLBW Infants

Less Energy Reserves (carbohydrate and fat)	Greater Oxygen Consumption during Growth
Higher organ : muscle mass ratio (resulting in higher metabolic rate)	Higher rate of protein synthesis and turnover (inversely proportional to gestational age)
Higher energy cost due to transepidermal water loss	Higher total body water content
More prone to hyperglycemia (despite higher energy needs for energy and brain metabolism)	Higher rate of fat deposition (despite higher EFA needs for brain and vascular development)
Immature gastrointestinal peristalsis	Limited production of gut digestive enzymes and growth factors
High incidence of stressful events	Excess urinary water and solute losses

Table 5. Comparison of Enteral Intake Recommendations for Growing Preterm Infants in Stable Clinical Condition

Nutrients per 100 Kcal †	Consensus Recommendations*		AAPCON‡	ESPGAN-CON‡
	<1000 g	>1000 g		
Water, mL	125-167	125-167	...	115-154
Energy, kcal	100	100	100	100
Protein, g	3.0-3.16	2.5-3.0	2.9-3.3	2.25-3.1
Carbohydrate, g			9.13	7-14
Lactose, g	3.16-9.5	3.16-9.8	..	...
Oligomers, g	0-7.0	0-7.0	...	...
Fat, g			4.5-6.0	3.6-7
Linoleic acid, g	0.44-1.7	0.44-1.7	0.4+	0.5-1.4
Linolenic acid, g	0.11-0.44	0.11-0.44	..	>0.055
C18:2/C18:3	>5	>5		5-15
Vitamin A, USP units	583-1250	583-1250	75-225	270-450
With lung disease	2250-2333	2250-2333	...	...
Vitamin D, USP units	125-333	125-333	270	800-1600/d
Vitamin E, USP units			>1.1	0.6-10
Supplement, HM§	2.9	2.9	...	...
Vitamin K_1, µg	6.66-8.33	6.66-8.33	4	4-15
Ascorbate, mg	15-20	15-20	35	7-40
Thiamin, µg	150-200	150-200	>40	20-250
Riboflavin, µg	200-300	200-300	>60	60-600
Pyridoxine, µg	125-175	125-175	>35	35-250
Niacin, mg	3-4	3-4	>0.25	0.8-5.0
Pantothenate, mg	1-15	1-15	>0.30	>0.3
Biotin, µg	3-5	3-5	>1.5	>1.5
Folate, µg	21-42	21-42	33	>60
Vitamin B_{12}, µg	0.25	0.25	>0.15	>0.15
Sodium, mg	38-58	38-58	48-67	23-53
Potassium, mg	65-100	65-100	66-98	90-152
Chloride, mg	59-89	59-89	...	57-89
Calcium, mg	100-192	100-192	175	70-140
Phosphorus, mg	50-117	50-117	91.5	50-87
Magnesium, mg	6.6-12.5	6.6-12.5	...	6-12
Iron, mg	1.67	1.67	1.7-2.5	1.5
Zinc, µg	833	833	>500	550-1100
Copper, µg	100-125	100-125	90	90-120
Selenium, µg	1.08-2.5	1.08-2.5	...	.
Chromium, µg	0.083-0.42	0.083-0.42	...	..
Manganese, µg	6.3	6.3	>5	1.5-7.5
Molybdenum, µg	0.25	.25	..	...
Iodine, µg	25-50	25-50	5	10-45
Taurine, mg	3.75-7.5	3.75-7.5	.	..
Carnitine, mg	2.4	2.4	...	>1.2
Inositol, mg	27-67.5	27-67.5	...	...
Choline, mg	12-23.4	12-23.4	...	...

*Source: AAP Committee on Nutrition, 2004. Used with permission of the American Academy of Pediatrics.
† 120 kcal/kg/d was used where a conversion was made from per kg recommendations.
‡ AAPCON indicates American Academy of Pediatrics, Committee on Nutrition; ESPGAN-CON, European Society of Pediatric Gastroenterology and Nutrition, Committee on Nutrition of the Preterm Infant.
§HM = human milk.

The recommended parenteral and enteral intakes of preterm infants for each nutrient at various weights and gestational ages are usually calculated using the factorial approach: deposition plus losses (absorption, urinary, stool, cutaneous), and are found in many neonatal nutrition references (American Academy of Pediatrics Committee on Nutrition, 1985; American Academy of Pediatrics Committee on Nutrition, 2004; Committee on Nutrition of the Preterm Infant - European Society of Paediatric Gastroenterology and Nutrition (ESPGAN), 1987; Schanler, 2003; Tsang *et al.*, 1993; Hay, 1991) (**Table 5**). Even though human milk produced by mothers who deliver prematurely is somewhat different from the milk of mothers who deliver at term (see below), nutrient intake may be limited by milk composition, availability, and fluid volume realities or restrictions. One of the most important nutritional discoveries in the last ten years has been the recognition that protein intake (both quantity and quality) and protein-energy ratio are more important in developing healthy lean body mass than just increasing caloric intake (Anderson & Aziz, 2006; Rigo & Senterre, 2006). The smaller and more immature the infant, the higher the protein turnover and protein requirement (Tsang *et al.*, 1993).

Prevent Feeding-Related Morbidities

Preterm infants are vulnerable to both under and over-nutrition. Immaturity of the liver, kidneys, and intestine, as noted above, can predispose to significant morbidity in this area. Necrotizing enterocolitis, feeding intolerance, and prolonged hospitalization are all more common in artificially fed infants (Lucas & Cole, 1990; Schanler *et al.*, 1999b), but can occur in any infant. Prolonged fasting and parenteral nutrition due to severe illness causes gut atrophy and can lead to infection and liver compromise. Restriction of calcium and phosphorous intake because of fluid restriction or inappropriate supplementation can lead to osteoporosis and fractures. Most importantly, inappropriate nutrition can prevent a preterm infant from reaching his full physical and intellectual potential (Martinez & Desai, 1995).

Optimize Long-Term Outcomes

Whether considering in utero nutrition (Barker, 1992b; Barker, 2004a; Barker *et al.*, 2002; Godfrey & Barker, 2000) or early newborn nutrition (Lucas, 1990; Lucas, 2005a; Lucas, 2005b), it is now clear that early nutrition can permanently affect long term outcomes, such as growth, glucose tolerance, insulin sensitivity, blood pressure, cardiovascular disease, allergic response, and neurocognitive development (Barker, 1992c; Barker, 1992d; Barker, 1992a; Barker, 2002; Barker, 2003; Barker, 2004b; Barker, 2005; Barker & Bagby, 2005; Barker *et al.*, 2005a; Barker *et al.*, 2005b; Bhargava *et al.*, 2004; Day *et al.*, 2004; Eriksson *et al.*, 2003; Kajantie *et al.*, 2002; Lucas, 2005a; Lucas, 2005b; Lucas *et al.*, 1990; Lucas *et al.*, 1998; Lucas *et al.*, 1992b; Osmond & Barker, 2000). (See below). The term proposed for early nutritional effects on long term health is "nutritional programming" (Lucas, 1990). New evidence suggests that early nutrition affects gene expression (epigenetics) (Feil, 2006; James, 2006; Waterland, 2006).

NUTRITIONAL "BEST PRACTICES" FOR THE PRETERM INFANT

Early Parenteral Nutrition

At birth, a preterm infant is abruptly disconnected from the ideal source of parenteral nutrition – the placenta (California Perinatal Quality Care Collaborative, 2005). Although intravenous (IV) fluids are standard for preterm or ill infants upon admission to the NICU, parenteral nutrition (protein, lipid, vitamins) used to be delayed for several days. Since the late 1980's, it has been clear that earlier institution of parenteral nutrition was associated with improved growth and outcome (Georgieff *et al.*, 1989), and there has been a gradual shift in favor of starting parenteral nutrition in the first day or two (Pauls *et al.*, 1998; Wilson *et al.*, 1997; Saini *et al.*, 1989; Thureen *et al.*, 2003; Porcelli & Sisk, 2002; Ziegler *et al.*, 2002; Kerner, 2003). Very low birth weight infants (VLBW) lose large amounts of body protein over the first few days of life if protein is not provided immediately. This early protein loss, when added to the normal daily in utero protein accretion, produces a protein debt (Dusick *et al.*, 2003; Embleton *et al.*, 2001) which may never be recovered.

Early parenteral nutrition, providing a minimum of sixty-eighty non-protein kcal/kg/day and two gm/kg/day protein has been shown to improve nitrogen balance, energy intake, and protein synthesis, and affect better weight gain without adverse effects (Ibrahim *et al.*, 2004; Porcelli & Sisk, 2002; Saini *et al.*, 1989; Thureen *et al.*, 2003). Similarly, early lipid intake improves nutrition

Table 6. Effects of Gut Lumenal Starvation

Nutritional
- Steatorrhea
- Protein-losing enteropathy
- Decreased circulating gut peptides
- Decreased enzyme levels
- Decreased nutrient transport

Morphology/Development
- Decreased synthesis of new epithelial cells
- Fusion/flattening of cells
- Edema

Host Resistance
- Decreased secretion of IgA, Mucin
- Increased uptake of macromolecules
- Bacterial overgrowth
- Direct damage to mucosal barrier

Source: La Gamma &Browne, 1994. Table reprinted with permission, copyright Elsevier.

Table 7. Effects of Early Enteral Intake on Infants Weighing Less Than 1500 Grams

- No change or decrease in NEC incidence
- Less cholestatic jaundice
- Less osteopenia
- Less physiologic jaundice
- Increased glucose tolerance
- Better weight gain
- Earlier tolerance of full enteral intake
- Increased gut hormones
- Induction of digestive enzymes
- Improved antral-duodenal coordination
- Allows gut colonization (Vit K production)
- Earlier maturation of brush border
- Prevents atrophy and starvation effects

Source: La Gamma & Browne, 1994. Table reprinted with permission, copyright Elsevier.

by preventing essential fatty acid deficiency, acting as an energy source, a precursor for eicosanoids, and a substitute for cerebral arachadonic and docosahexaenoic acid synthesis. Early animal studies and theoretical concerns regarding slow infusion of lipids causing pulmonary hypertension and leading to chronic lung disease have not been confirmed by recent clinical trials (Ibrahim *et al.*, 2004; Thureen *et al.*, 2003).

Minimal Enteral Nutrition (MEN) (AKA "trophic feeds" or "GI priming")

In utero, the fetal gastrointestinal tract is constantly active, swallowing amniotic fluid, absorbing fluid and some nutrition, performing rudimentary peristalsis, and forming meconium. The objective of feeding during the early days of life is to stimulate gut maturation, hormone release, and motility, and to support the immune system, *not* to provide full enteral nutrition. Although it was never shown that prolonged withholding of feedings actually prevented necrotizing enterocolitis (NEC), some form of this strategy was widely adopted in the 1970s and 1980s (California Perinatal Quality Care Collaborative, 2005). Artificially starving the gut at birth leads to atrophy of the gut with multiple nutritional, morphologic, and host resistance pathologies (La Gamma & Browne, 1994) (**Table 6**), so that withholding feedings may actually render subsequently introduced feedings less safe (Ziegler *et al.*, 2002). A recent pilot trial found that feeding a sterile, isotonic, noncaloric enteral solution patterned after human amniotic fluid improved tolerance of milk feedings in infants with a history of feeding intolerance (Barney *et al.*, 2006).

Withholding of feedings was eventually re-evaluated with a number of trials of early introduction of feedings (Heicher, 1976; La Gamma, 1985; Lucas, 1986; Ostertag, 1986; Dunn, 1988; Slagle, 1988; Berseth, 1992b; Meetz, 1992; Thureen, 1999; Schanler, 2003). A systematic review of the results of published trials (Tyson & Kennedy, 2000) concluded that early introduction of feedings shortens the time to full feeds and to discharge and does not increase the incidence of NEC, although they noted some problems with individual studies. A controlled study involving 100 LBW infants (McClure, 2000) confirmed these findings and found, in addition, a significant reduction in serious infections with "early" introduction of feedings. Early enteral intake appears both safe and physiologically advantageous for VLBW infants (Ronnestad *et al.*, 2005) (**Table 7**).

Most infants in the GI priming studies were fed with umbilical artery catheters in place, yet the studies still noted a decreased incidence of necrotizing enterocolitis (Davey *et al.*, 1994; Dunn *et al.*, 1988; Schanler *et al.*, 1999b). Although feeding an infant with a patent ductus arteriosus (PDA) is thought to be risky, a recent study of feedings during indomethacin therapy for a persistent ductus arteriosus found otherwise (Bellander *et al.*, 2003). Further research is needed to ascertain just how "unstable" an infant needs to be before feedings are withheld. Unquestionably, human milk is the safest choice for early enteral feedings, with few exceptions.

Standards/Measurement/Protocols. In light of the current variations in feeding practice, paying close attention to feeding parameters with a standardized feeding regimen appears to significantly decrease NEC and improve nutrition (Kamitsuka *et al.*, 2000; Patole *et al.*, 2003). Infant weight, length, head circumference, and biochemical parameters should be followed at appropriate intervals (California Perinatal Quality Care Collaborative, 2005). Mother's milk volume should also be monitored. Every NICU that cares for VLBW infants should have a neonatal nutritionist as part of the team to measure infant growth and outcomes, calculate and relate parenteral nutrition and enteral intakes to current growth and medical conditions, suggest improvements in nutritional management, manage the formulary of premature infant supplements, and make nutritional plans with goals and resource referral information at discharge (Kuzma-O'Reilly *et al.*, 2003; Olsen *et al.*, 2005; Rubin *et al.*, 1997; Valentine & Schanler, 1993; Anderson, 2002).

Use of Human Milk

Research to date supports, and the consensus is growing, that human milk (with appropriate fortification for the very low birth weight infant) is the standard of care for preterm, as well as term infants (American Academy of Pediatrics Section on Breastfeeding, 2005; Schanler, 1998; Schanler, 2001; Schanler *et al.*, 1999a; Schanler *et al.*, 1999b; Schanler & Atkinson, 1999).

As the objective of feeding during the early days of life is to stimulate gut hormone maturation, stimulate gut hormone release, induce gut motility, and enable the growth of beneficial microflora to support the immune system, the preferred feeding is breastmilk, preferably started on day one (American Academy of Pediatrics Section on Breastfeeding, 2005; Schanler, 2003; Ziegler *et al.*, 2002). Colostrum contains high concentrations of antimicrobial, anti-inflammatory, and immunomodulating factors, and prepares the gut for mature milk (Goldman *et al.*, 1994; Caicedo *et al.*, 2005). Feedings should be started with full strength, unfortified milk (Berseth *et al.*, 1992; Koenig *et al.*, 1995).

SHORT TERM BENEFITS OF HUMAN MILK FOR PRETERM INFANTS

Host Defense

Human milk has multiple interactive factors, each of which may have multiple functions, thought to protect the preterm infant from infection (Ogra & Rassin, 1995; Lawrence, 2005; Buescher, 1994). After controlling for confounders, receiving expressed breastmilk was one of three factors significantly associated with survival in extremely low birth weight (ELBW) infants (odds ratio 57.5, 95% confidence interval 7-474, $p=0.0002$) (Boo *et al.*, 2000).

Human milk reduces the incidence and severity of necrotizing enterocolitis (NEC), an acute inflammatory bowel disease which may lead to perforation and peritonitis in preterm infants (Beeby & Jeffery, 1992; Santulli *et al.*, 1975; Kliegman *et al.*, 1979; Gross, 1983; Guthrie *et al.*, 2003; Boo & Goh, 1999; Schanler *et al.*, 2005; Schanler *et al.*, 1999b; Lucas & Cole, 1990; Schanler *et al.*, 1985; Pitt *et al.*, 1977; Buescher, 1994; Yu *et al.*, 1981; Narayanan *et al.*, 1980; Narayanan *et al.*, 1984a; Narayanan *et al.*, 1981; McGuire & Anthony, 2003). Even partial feeding of human milk can reduce the incidence of NEC (Narayanan *et al.*, 1980; Lucas & Cole, 1990). Many human milk factors have been associated with the decrease in NEC, including immunoglobulins A and G (Eibl *et al.*, 1988), epidermal growth factor (Dvorak *et al.*, 2004; Dvorak, 2004; Dvorak *et al.*, 2003a), platelet activating factor acetylhydrolase (Reber & Nankervis, 2004; Moya *et al.*, 1994; Furukawa *et al.*, 1993), lactoferrin (Schanler *et al.*, 1986) and the cytokine interleukin-10 (Dvorak *et al.*, 2003b).

Human milk is also associated with protection from sepsis and other infections (el-Mohandes *et al.*, 1997; Furman *et al.*, 2003; Narayanan *et al.*, 1980; Narayanan *et al.*, 1981; Narayanan *et al.*, 1984a; Narayanan *et al.*, 1982; Ronnestad *et al.*, 2005; Schanler *et al.*, 2005; Schanler *et al.*, 1999b; Uraizee & Gross, 1989). A systematic review (de Silva *et al.*, 2004) of six cohort and three randomized controlled trials concluded that existing studies did not prove that human milk prevented infection in preterm VLBW infants because of methodological problems, including small sample size, failure to adjust for confounding variables, and inadequate definitions of human milk feedings and outcomes. Countering these criticisms in a letter to the editor (Furman, 2006) referring to her 2003 study (Furman *et al.*, 2003), Dr. Furman clearly demonstrated that a threshold amount of at least 50 ml/kg/d of maternal milk through week four of life reduced the rate of sepsis in preterm infants (Furman *et al.*, 2003). No study has demonstrated an increased rate of infection in preterm infants fed maternal milk. Two more recent studies confirmed that maternal milk (Schanler *et al.*, 2005) and a combination of maternal milk and donor milk used for early initiation of feedings (Ronnestad *et al.*, 2005) clearly reduced late onset sepsis in preterm infants.

One of the major protective effects of human milk on the recipient infant operates through the "enteromammary system" (Groer & Walker, 1996; Kleinman & Walker, 1979). Exposure of mothers to the NICU environment through skin-to-skin contact with their preterm infants can "induce" mothers to make specific antibodies against the nosocomial pathogens in their infants' environment (Walker, 2004; Schanler, 2001).

Gastrointestinal Development

Human milk has multiple factors that stimulate growth, motility, and maturation of the intestine (Donovan, 2006; Groer & Walker, 1996; Walker, 2004; Martin & Walker, 2006). Human milk is associated with a faster decrease in intestinal permeability than artificial milks (Catassi *et al.*, 1995) and an increase in intestinal lactase activity at ten days if human milk, rather than artificial milks, are fed from day four (Shulman *et al.*, 1998). Human milk promotes more rapid gastric emptying than formulas (Ewer & Yu, 1996; Cavell, 1981), resulting in less residuals and faster realization of full enteral feedings (Schanler *et al.*, 1999b; Lucas & Cole, 1990; Uraizee & Gross, 1989; Boo & Goh, 1999). Reaching full feedings faster means fewer days of IV's, less side effects from TPN, less infections and infiltrations from IV's, and less costly and fewer hospital days (Schanler *et al.*, 2005; Schanler *et al.*, 1999b).

Special Nutrition

Milk from mothers who deliver prematurely (preterm milk) has been shown to be somewhat different from milk of mothers who deliver at term (term milk). Since the first report of higher concentrations of nitrogen in preterm milk (Atkinson *et al.*, 1978), many publications have described differences in milk composition relative to gestational age at birth. Preterm milk has been noted to have increased amounts of nitrogen, total protein, immune proteins, total lipids, medium-chain fatty acids, total energy, and some vitamins and minerals, as well as trace elements (Atkinson, 1995; Barros & Carneiro-Sampaeio, 1983; Bitmar *et al.* 1983; Lepage *et al.*, 1984; Anderson *et al.*, 1981; Butte *et al.*, 1984; Gross *et al.*, 1981b; Gross *et al.*, 1980; Schanler & Oh, 1980). The degree of prematurity and whether infants are born appropriate or small for gestational age may also play a role in milk composition (Barros & Carneiro-Sampaeio, 1983; Lepage *et al.*, 1984). Some studies did not find a difference between term and preterm milk (Sann *et al.*, 1981; Udipi *et al.*, 1985), but no studies have found lesser concentrations of nutrients in preterm milk at similar stages of lactation (Schanler & Atkinson, 1999). The lack of agreement between studies may reflect not only small sample size because of the greater inter-individual variability of milk composition in preterm milk, but also milk sample collection methods and inclusion of wide ranges of gestational age (Atkinson, 2000).

In addition, preterm milk seems to have a higher concentration of growth factors and hormones to aid in the development of the gut and other organs. Preterm milk has more live infection fighting cells, immunoglobulins, like secretory IgA, epidermal growth factor (Dvorak *et al.*, 2003a), anti-inflammatory factors, and immunomodulators than term milk (Groer & Walker, 1996; Gross *et al.*, 1981a). There is a trend for nutrient and immunologic factor concentrations in preterm milk to decrease as lactation progresses, a pattern also observed in term milk (Schanler & Atkinson, 1999). The physiological basis of reported differences between preterm and term milk theoretically may be due to the immaturity of the mammary gland with increased paracellular leakage of serum proteins (e.g., immune proteins) and ions (e.g., sodium and chloride) (Schanler & Atkinson, 1999).

Given the innumerable protective properties of bioactive human milk concentrated in colostrum, the first feedings can be called the infant's "first immunization." The urgency and importance of reducing morbidity and mortality by providing the first small volume in the early hours of life is under investigation (Edmond *et al.*, 2006; Rodriguez & Caplan, 2006).

LONG TERM BENEFITS OF HUMAN MILK FOR PRETERM INFANTS

Neurodevelopmental Outcome

A meta-analysis of 20 studies comparing cognitive development in breastfed and artificially-fed infants concluded that breastfeeding was associated with higher scores in all measured parameters, that developmental achievements persisted at least through adolescence, and that the benefit of human milk was strongest for children of low birth weight (Anderson *et al.*, 1999). There is significant evidence that human milk confers neurodevelopmental advantages (Lucas *et al.*, 1992a; Lucas *et al.*, 1998; Lucas *et al.*, 1992b; Morley, 2002; Morley *et al.*, 1988; Morley & Lucas, 2000; Vohr *et al.*, 2006; Feldman & Eidelman, 2003; Amin *et al.*, 2000; Bier *et al.*, 2002; Elwood *et al.*, 2005; Smith *et al.*, 2003a; Lucas *et al.*, 1994; Gale & Martyn, 1996; Pollock, 1989; Jacobson & Jacobson, 1992; Hart *et al.*, 2003; Horne *et al.*, 2004; Hagan *et al.*, 1996; Sacker *et al.*, 2006; O'Connor *et al.*, 2003); however, the direct relationship between human milk feeding and IQ has been challenged (Der *et al.*, 2006; Jacobson *et al.*, 1999; Furman *et al.*, 2004) because of the complexity of the many factors which contribute to an infant's neurodevelopmental outcome (Burgard, 2003; Rey, 2003).

The Der *et al.* study (Der *et al.*, 2006) itself was challenged by no less than 14 letters to the editor (BMJ, 2006) criticizing the age of the data, methodologies, definitions, and statistics. All researchers have made some adjustments for confounding variables between groups, especially socioeconomic status and maternal education, but parenting variables are difficult to quantify (King & Jones, 2005). Due to the ethical constraints of randomizing infants to their own mother's milk or formula, the majority of the studies have been observational (King & Jones, 2005).

Randomized allocation of infants to human milk in the form of donated milk has rarely been done (Lucas *et al.*, 1994; Schanler *et al.*, 2005), and only Lucas *et al.* followed long term neurodevelopment. In this study, infants were randomized to donor human milk or an early form of preterm formula, either as the sole source of nutrition or as a supplement to mother's own expressed breastmilk. At eighteen months, there was no difference in development despite the lower nutritional content of the donor milk (Lucas *et al.*, 1994). Further follow up of this cohort of preterm infants revealed higher IQ scores (eight points) in those infants fed their own mother's milk (Lucas *et al.*, 1998; Lucas *et al.*, 1992b; Lucas *et al.*, 1996).

The long-chain polyunsaturated fatty acids (especially docosahexaenoic acid and arachidonic acid) found in both term and preterm milk have been implicated in optimal brain development and retinal maturation (Anderson *et al.*, 1999; Uauy *et al.*, 1990; Carlson *et al.*, 1993; Faldella *et al.*, 1996). A reduction in the incidence and severity of retinopathy of prematurity (ROP), a disease of premature infants that can cause visual impairment and blindness, has also been demonstrated (Schanler *et al.*, 2005; DiBiasie, 2006; Hylander *et al.*, 2001; Hallman *et al.*, 1992; Furman *et al.*, 2003) with the use of human milk.

Immunomodulation

Preterm infants fed human milk continue to benefit even after discharge. They have fewer hospital admissions in the first year of life (Elder *et al.*, 1999) and less respiratory infections (Blaymore Bier *et al.*, 2002). In addition, ulcerative colitis, Crohn's disease, diabetes, and allergic diseases may be reduced in breastfed preterm infants as in full-term infants (American Academy of Pediatrics Section on Breastfeeding, 2005).

Other Potential Benefits

Evidence is accumulating that early nutrition has long term effects on health into adulthood, including cardiovascular disease risk and bone health (Lucas, 2005a). Adolescent blood pressure, lipid ratios, and C-reactive protein levels have been positively affected by mother's own and donor human milk given to preterm infants (Lucas, 2005a; Singhal, 2006; Singhal *et al.*, 2004; Singhal *et al.*, 2001). Human milk contains many antioxidants and may prevent diseases mediated by oxygen free radicals in VLBW infants (Shoji *et al.*, 2004; Friel *et al.*, 2002).

A definite benefit for the preterm infant is a physically and psychologically healthier mother. Mothers of preterm infants, like mothers of full-term infants, can

Table 8. Preterm Milk Over Time

Milk Component	Preterm Mother's Milk: Colostrum	Transit.	Mature	Term Mature
Total Protein g/dL	30	24	15	12
IgA, mg/g protein	109	92	64	83
NPN % total N	15	18	17	24
Na, mmol/L	22.2	11.6	8.8	9.0
Ca, mmol/L	6.8	8	7.2	6.5

Source: Adapted from Schanler & Atkinson, 1999. Reprinted with permission of Springer Science and Business Media.
Transit. = transitional milk

be expected to have a decreased risk of pre-menopausal breast cancer, ovarian cancer, and osteoporosis, reduced life-time blood loss (improved iron status), and a delay in fertility post-partum (Labbok, 2001). By providing an alternate focus for the mother, expressing milk for a preterm infant can relieve the guilt of delivering an ill, preterm infant. It can also increase a mother's sense of self-competency (Labbok, 2001), her sense of control in a stressful situation, and her claim on her infant (Meier, 2003; Miracle *et al.*, 2004; Kavanaugh *et al.*, 1997).

The economic impact of NOT breastfeeding is significant with increased health care costs for both acute (Ball & Wright, 1999; Weimer, 2001) and chronic diseases, losses for both employees and employers, and unnecessary excess use of natural resources to make and dispose of the waste products of artificial milks (Ball & Bennett, 2001). If the prevalence of breastfeeding in the hospital were increased from 64% to 75%, it is estimated that over $90 million would be saved each year in excess costs for treating NEC, and many premature infant lives would be saved (Weimer, 2001).

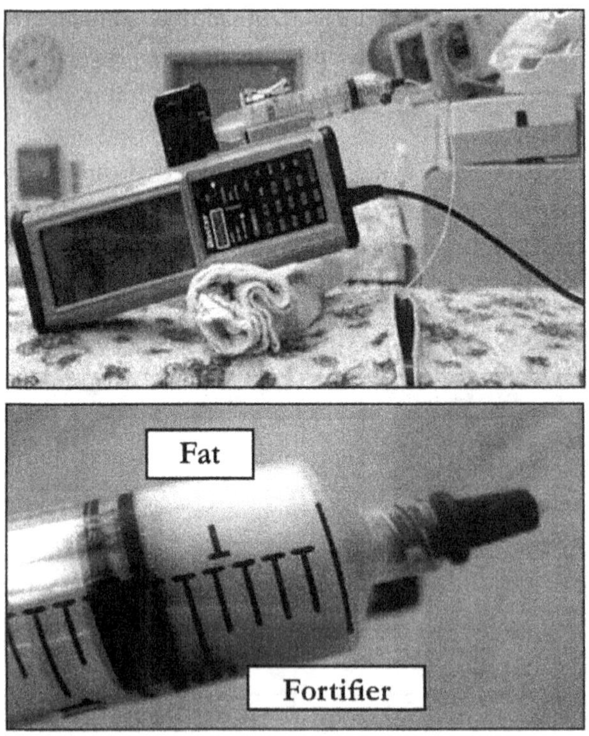

(photos courtesy of N Wight)

Figure 4. Loss of fat and fortifier by poor orientation of feeding syringe

NUTRITIONAL CHALLENGES OF HUMAN MILK FOR PRETERM INFANTS

Exclusive feeding of unfortified human milk in preterm infants (especially those less than 1500 grams) is associated with poorer growth rates and nutritional deficits both during and after hospitalization (Atkinson *et al.*, 1981a; Atkinson *et al.*, 1983; Cooper *et al.*, 1984; Kashyap *et al.*, 1990; Gross, 1983). Protein nutritional status indicators are lower than with preterm formula or fortified human milk and decline over time in preterm infants fed unfortified human milk (Atkinson *et al.*, 1981a; Kashyap *et al.*, 1990; Polberger *et al.*, 1990). Low intakes of calcium and phosphorus in unfortified human milk result in elevated calcium and alkaline phosphatase levels and low serum phosphorous (Pettifor *et al.*, 1989; Atkinson *et al.*, 1983), and eventually a reduction in height (Fewtrell *et al.*, 2000; Lucas *et al.*, 1989). Low milk sodium intake may contribute to late hyponatremia (Roy *et al.*, 1976).

The nutritional adequacy of human milk for preterm infants may be limited for several reasons. Premature infants are often restricted as to volume of milk given due to concerns regarding chronic lung disease, the ductus arteriosus, and necrotizing enterocolitis. Variability of composition, although perfect for a full term infant feeding ad libitum, is not ideal for the preterm infant with increased nutrient needs. While the milk of mothers who deliver preterm has increased protein, IgA, and sodium, the milk changes over the first few weeks to a composition similar to term human milk (**Table 8**). Unfortunately, the nutrient needs of the preterm infant, especially those less than 1500 grams, do not change nearly as fast. The content of other nutrients in preterm milk (e.g., calcium and phosphorus) do not change notably through lactation, but are too low to meet the needs of many preterm infants.

In addition, loss of nutrients and other components of the milk may occur with expression, storage, and feeding methods (**Figure** 4) (Ogundele, 2002; Fidler *et al.*, 2001; Stocks *et al.*, 1985; Narayanan *et al.*, 1984b; Mehta *et al.*, 1988; Greer *et al.*, 1984). As much of the variation in energy content is due to the fat content of the milk (Schanler, 2001), adherence of fat to the tubing may decrease the infant's main source of energy. Three hours of light exposure can decrease the breastmilk riboflavin by 50% and Vitamin A by 70% (Bates *et al.*, 1985).

OVERCOMING NUTRITIONAL CHALLENGES OF HUMAN MILK FOR PRETERM INFANTS

Volume

Increasing the volume of human milk is one way of increasing nutrient intake. The historic target for premature infants of 150 mL/kg/day of enteral feedings may be inadequate to overcome prior nitrogen deficits and establish optimal growth. A randomized trial of enteral feeding volumes (150 and 200 mL/kg/d) of infants born less than 30 weeks gestation, once they reached full enteral feeds, found that individual milk volume requirements for adequate weight gain without significant adverse effects varied between 150-200 mL/kg/d (Kuschel *et al.*, 2000). Increased milk intakes were associated with increased daily weight gains and a greater weight at 35 weeks, but there was no difference in any growth parameter at one year or in morbidity. Ziegler suggests that feeding volume should be increased until the infant shows signs that GI capacity has been reached, then kept at that volume through daily adjustment of the feeding volume (Ziegler *et al.*, 2002). Restricting feeding volume until a weight plateau has been identified is the most common cause of growth delay (Hay *et al.*, 1999). It has been suggested that fortified human milk must be fed at approximately 180 mL/kg/d if ELBW infants are to achieve adequate growth, nutrient retention, and biochemical indices of nutritional status (Hay *et al.*, 1999).

Hindmilk "Fortification"

As hindmilk may have a two to three-fold greater fat content than foremilk, hindmilk can be used to increase caloric intake if the mother's milk production is in excess of the infant's needs (Schanler, 2005b). Although one study demonstrated increased weight gain with short-term hindmilk fortification (Valentine *et al.*, 1994), a subsequent study showed no difference in weight, length, head circumference, mid-arm circumference, or skin fold thickness after twenty-eight days of hindmilk feeding (Payanikli *et al.*, 2004). There were no adverse effects on serum chemistries. It is important to note that the protein content of foremilk and hindmilk are the same (Valentine *et al.*, 1994).

MULTI-NUTRIENT FORTIFICATION

Studies have repeatedly demonstrated that protein and multinutrient fortification of human milk is associated with short-term growth advantages (weight, length, and head circumference) for infants less than 34 weeks gestation or birthweight less than 1800 grams when fortified human milk is given both during and after the infant's initial hospitalization (Kuschel & Harding, 2004; Schanler, 1998; Schanler, 2003). In addition, VLBW (less than 1500 grams) infants grow faster and have higher bone mineral content up to one year of age if provided with additional nutrients, especially protein, calcium, and phosphorus (Friel *et al.*, 1993; Worrell *et al.*, 2002). However, exclusively breastfed former preterm infants tend to "catch-up" if given sufficient time (two to eight years) (Backstrom *et al.*, 1999; Morley & Lucas, 2000; Schanler *et al.*, 1992).

Although a weight gain of greater than 15 grams per day is recommended, the optimal growth rate (reference target) has not yet been established. It is unclear whether the rapid catch-up growth seen with aggressive supplementation is of benefit or harm for long-term overall health, growth, and neurodevelopment (Griffin, 2002; Hall, 2001; Singhal *et al.*, 2007).

Current guidelines recommend fortification of breastmilk be initiated well before a full feeding volume is reached in VLBW (less than 1500 grams) infants (Ziegler *et al.*, 2002) and may need to be continued post-discharge. Some infants between 1500-2000 grams, and those infants with special nutrient needs (e.g., chronic lung disease or cardiac problems) may also require fortification. Studies of feeding types and their advancement have usually started fortifiers at enteral feeds of 100 mL/kg/d, but there is no research to suggest that starting earlier (50-75 mL/kg/day) is harmful. Also, many studies do not specify whether "full" fortification (1 packet powder per 25 mL EBM) or "half" fortification is used to start.

There is no research as to how fast to "advance" fortification, but multiple studies demonstrate no increase in feeding intolerance or NEC with multinutrient fortifiers (Kuschel & Harding, 2004; Lucas *et al.*, 1996; Schanler *et al.*, 1999b; Moody *et al.*, 2000). Care must be taken that large doses of multiple additives do not raise the osmolality of breastmilk (or formula) to unacceptable levels (Srinivasan *et al.*, 2004). There is no general agreement as to when fortifiers should be discontinued.

VLBW infants fed human milk can benefit from vitamin supplementation, most specifically vitamins A,

C, and D. Patients with or recovering from cholestasis may also require additional fat-soluble vitamins (A, D, E, K). The AAP currently recommends that preterm infants (<1000 grams birthweight) receive 6 - 12 IU/kg/day Vitamin E enterally, which maybe supplied either by preterm formula or by fortification of human milk (American Academy of Pediatrics Committee on Nutrition, 2004). When powdered commercial fortifier is used, no additional vitamin supplements are needed. Iron supplementation should be given to VLBW infants fed human milk at a dose of two mg/kg/d starting at one month until 12 months of age.

VLBW infants are at significant risk for chemical and clinical osteopenia due to inadequate calcium and phosphorous intake, dysfunctional vitamin D metabolism, and/or excessive renal losses of these minerals (which may be exacerbated by diuretics, especially furosemide). In one series, over half of the infants with a birthweight less than 1000 grams and nearly 25% of those with a birthweight less than 1500 grams had radiographic evidence of rickets (Backstrom *et al.*, 1996). VLBW infants receiving breastmilk that is fortified with commercially available products receive additional calcium and phosphorus in a quantity associated with improved growth (Wauben *et al.*, 1998; Kuschel & Harding, 2004). Supplementation of a premature's diet with vitamin D beyond 200-400 IU/day has not been found to increase later bone density (Backstrom *et al.*, 1999).

Fortification Concerns

Gastric emptying is prolonged to times equal with formulas when fortifiers are added to human milk (Ewer & Yu, 1996). As noted above, clinical concerns regarding feeding tolerance with fortifiers have not been verified in research. Concerns remain regarding changing the milk (altered immune function, contamination and increased bacterial growth, bioavailability of nutrients), introduction of bovine proteins and plant oils, and an overall change in GI flora.

Fortification does not appear to significantly alter bacterial counts if the fortified milk is used within 24 hours (Jocson *et al.*, 1997). This study also found that IgA content was not affected by fortification, storage temperature, or storage duration. Another study found that fortification did not decrease the total IgA content, but did decrease E. coli-specific IgA and also decreased lysozyme activity (Quan *et al.*, 1994). One study suggested that the fortifier with more iron and MCT (medium chain triglycerides) oil increased bacterial counts in human milk more than another brand (Chan, 2003). Subsequent studies demonstrated equal bacterial growth in milk fortified with the two brands up to six hours (Telang *et al.*, 2005) and up to 72 hours (Santiago *et al.*, 2005) with total bacterial colony counts declining from zero to 72 hours in both fortified milks. Although the fortifier did not affect the bacterial inhibition in another study, the addition of iron alone reduced the antimicrobial effect of human milk against E. coli, S. aureus, P. aeruginosa, and Candida (Ovali *et al.*, 2006).

Askin and Diehl-Jones (Askin & Diehl-Jones, 2002) studied paired samples of fortified and unfortified preterm milk and found that bacterial counts were significantly increased in the fortified samples after four hours at room temperature. They also noted a 20% decrease in epidermal growth factor titers (EGF) in the same time period. EGF is believed to play a role in reducing NEC in preterm infants.

Any formula or fortifier intake will change the GI flora significantly, and for a considerable time (Rubaltelli *et al.*, 1998), affecting the "cross-talk" between the commensal bacteria and the intestinal epithelium. At present, it does not appear that fortification of human milk increases necrotizing enterocolitis (Schanler *et al.*, 1999b; Schanler *et al.*, 2005).

At present, there are both liquid fortifiers and powdered fortifiers; both essentially preterm formulas

AAP 2006 RED BOOK

1. Outbreaks from gram negative bacterial infections in NICUs occasionally have been attributed to contaminated human milk specimens that have been collected or stored improperly.
2. Milk from other than the biologic mother should be treated according to Human Milk Banking Association of North America (HMBANA) guidelines.
3. Routine culturing or heat treatment of mother's milk fed to her infant has not been demonstrated to be necessary or cost-effective.

(American Academy of Pediatrics, 2006, p. 125.)

to be added to human milk. The powdered products have the advantage of not diluting the human milk and appear to be preferred by parents (Fenton *et al.*, 2000). A comparison of the two products suggests the liquid preparation results in lower protein, calcium, phosphorus, and zinc intakes (Schanler *et al.*, 1999b).

New Directions in Fortification

Ideally, each sample of human milk should be analyzed for macro and micro-nutrient content and fortified with only the nutrients required by that infant. Such individualized lactoengineering is not practical or cost-effective at this time. However, commercial efforts are underway to tailor donated human milk to more closely meet the needs of preterm infants and to produce a human milk fortifier made from donated human milk. Although a good idea in theory, there is no research available at the present time to demonstrate the effectiveness of these products.

Probiotics are live, non-pathogenic microbial preparations that colonize the intestine and provide benefit to the host (Schanler, 2006). "They normalize intestinal microflora, increase mucosal barrier function, reduce intestinal permeability, enhance immune defenses, and improve enteral nutrition" (Schanler, 2006). Probiotics appear to enhance feeding tolerance in preterm infants (Kitajima *et al.*, 1997) and may have an additive effect with breastfeeding on gut immunity (Rinne *et al.*, 2005). Because of the immunocompromised status of preterm infants, systemic infection as a result of probiotic treatment is a possibility (Land *et al.*, 2005). More research as to the safety and efficacy of each strain is necessary before probiotics are widely used in preterm infants.

INFECTION CONCERNS REGARDING HUMAN MILK FOR PRETERM INFANTS

While human milk has considerable host defense properties, it can still be contaminated with pathogenic microorganisms during expression, storage, and feeding. Human milk can also transmit many different maternal bacterial and viral illnesses (American Academy of Pediatrics, 2006). Group B streptococcal disease and methicillin-resistant staphylococcus aureus have been implicated in morbidity and mortality in preterm infants fed contaminated milk (Arias-Camison, 2003; Godambe *et al.*, 2005; Olver *et al.*, 2000; Gastelum *et al.*, 2005). Infectious mastitis does not pose a risk for the full-term healthy infant, but may increase risk to the VLBW infant. The risk of using breastmilk from a mother with a potentially transmittable illness or medication must be weighed against both the short-term and long-term risks of withholding human milk from the preterm infant.

Current infectious contraindications to using mother's milk in developed countries include human immunodeficiency virus (HIV/AIDS), Human T-Lymphotrophic virus types 1 and 2 (HTLV 1 & 2), and active tuberculosis prior to treatment. Other maternal illnesses may require temporary "pump and dump" until the mother is no longer infectious (varicella-zoster, measles, herpes on the breast). Although infants of women with Hepatitis B virus (HBV) may breastfeed, the infant should receive hepatitis B vaccine and immunoglobulin. Transmission of Hepatitis C is theoretically possible, but transmission through breastfeeding has not been documented (American Academy of Pediatrics, 2006).

The most common source of angst for neonatologists is a very preterm infant of a mother who is positive for cytomegalovirus (CMV) or whose CMV status is unknown (Schanler, 2005a). CMV is shed intermittently in human milk (along with the antibody), and transmission is common; although active disease is rare, except in VLBW infants in some studies (Ekema *et al.*, 2006; Kerrey *et al.*, 2006; Hamprecht *et al.*, 2005; Doctor *et al.*, 2005; Morgan *et al.*, 2003; Mussi-Pinhata *et al.*, 2004; Cheong *et al.*, 2004; Vollmer *et al.*, 2004; Iwanaga *et al.*, 2004; Bradshaw & Moore, 2003; Bryant *et al.*, 2002; Sharland *et al.*, 2002; Maschmann *et al.*, 2001; Vochem *et al.*, 1998; Neuberger *et al.*, 2006; Schleiss, 2006b; Schleiss, 2006a; Meier *et al.*, 2005; Miron *et al.*, 2005; Jim *et al.*, 2004; Willeitner, 2004; Gessler *et al.*, 2004; Yasuda *et al.*, 2003; Hamprecht *et al.*, 2001). The use of fresh colostrum may pose less of a concern than milk pumped after the first week (Yasuda *et al.*, 2003). Decisions about using breastmilk from CMV positive mothers should balance the risk of active CMV disease and the risks of not receiving human milk. Freezing may decrease CMV infectivity, but does not reliably eliminate it (American Academy of Pediatrics Committee on Infectious Diseases, 2006). Interventions to screen breastmilk or render it non-infectious have met with variable success (Maschmann *et al.*, 2006; Curtis *et al.*, 2005; Forsgren, 2004).

WHO/UNICEF Joint Statement

"Where it is not possible for the biologic mother to breastfeed, the first alternative, if available, should be the use of human milk from other sources. Human milk banks should be made available in appropriate situations."

(WHO/UNICEF, 1980)

AAP: Breastfeeding and the Use of Human Milk

"Banked human milk may be a suitable feeding alternative for infants whose mothers are unable or unwilling to provide their own milk."

"Fresh human milk from unscreened donors is not recommended because of the risk of transmission of infectious agents."

(American Academy of Pediatrics Section on Breastfeeding, 2005)

DONOR HUMAN MILK FOR PRETERM INFANTS

Although mothers' own milk is clearly best, human milk banking has a long tradition in many countries and a recognized role in the care of preterm and ill infants (Williamson *et al.*, 1978b; Lawrence & Lawrence, 2005a; Arnold, 2005). The American Academy of Pediatrics established its first formal guidelines for human milk banks in 1943 (American Academy of Pediatrics Committee on Mother's Milk, 1943). Initially, milk was dispensed unprocessed from approximately 50 U.S. milk banks, but with the threat of HIV, the return of tuberculosis, and drug abuse, by 2000, all but five of the milk banks had closed. Those that remained formed the Human Milk Banking Association of North America (HMBANA) in 1985 and adopted strict procedures for donor screening, milk processing (pasteurization), milk storage, and shipping (Human Milk Banking Association of North America, 2005).

With the explosion of research on the possible medical uses of human milk components and the recognition of the benefits of human milk for preterm infants, more attention has been focused on donor human milk and the number of U.S. non-profit milk banks has increased to ten, with one for-profit milk bank, as of the end of 2006. During 2003, North American milk banks processed more than 500,000 ounces of donated human milk that was used for individuals with a variety of diagnoses (Updegrove, 2005). Brazil leads the world with over 180 milk banks processing more than 215,000 liters of donated milk for over 300,000 premature and low birth weight infants, saving the country's Ministry of Health more than $540 million per year (Arnold, 2005; IBFAN, 2001). In 2002, the World Health Assembly unanimously endorsed the Global Strategy for Infant and Young Child Feeding, which recommends banked donor milk as an option when an infant cannot breastfeed or mother's expressed breastmilk is unavailable (World Health Organization & UNICEF, 2003).

Donor Milk Recipients

While the largest numbers of recipients of heat-treated donor human milk are preterm infants, the largest volume of milk is used by older infants and adults. The usual recipients of banked donor milk are the VLBW (less than 1500 grams) infants whose mothers cannot provide breastmilk for various reasons: maternal illness, medications, substance abuse, or poor social support and resources (Wight, 2001a). Other potential recipients are infants with severe allergies, feeding intolerance, short gut syndrome, malabsorption, and other GI problems who cannot tolerate artificial milks. Post-surgical infants may have feedings advanced more quickly when human milk is used as the initial feeding (Rangecroft *et al.*, 1978; Riddell, 1989). As pasteurized milk is devoid of any functional cells, infants with immune deficiencies may benefit from the immunoglobulins and other immune factors without the fear of graft versus host disease (Wight, 2001a; Tully, 1990).

Donor milk has been used to supply IgA to adult liver transplant patients who were IgA deficient (Merhav *et al.*, 1995), in patients in immune suppression because of chemotherapy or bone marrow transplant (Asquith *et al.*, 1987) and in a young adult male with severe gastro-esophageal reflux (Wiggins & Arnold, 1998). Human milk components are under active investigation regarding their ability to induce apoptosis in cancer cells and decrease viral replication (papilloma virus). Human milk has been used for centuries in the treatment of conjunctivitis, otitis externa, and wound healing.

Donor Milk Banking

Human milk donors are usually mothers of healthy term infants between the ages of two and six months (Lindemann *et al.*, 2004), but mothers of preterm infants (less than 32 weeks) also donate excess milk. The donors receive a full health and lifestyle risk screening as well as serologic screening for HIV 1 and 2, HTLV

Table 9. Effects of Heat Treatment on Human Milk Components

	Remaining Activity	
Component	56°C X 30 min	62.5°C X 30 min
S. Aureus	100% killed	100% killed
E. Coli	100% killed	100% killed
Lactoferrin	72%	22%
IgA	84%	51%
Folic acid	72%	57%
Lysozyme	132%	100%
Phosphatase	23%	1.4%

Source: Adapted from Arnold & Larson, 1993. Table reprinted with permission, copyright Elsevier.

1 and 2, hepatitis B and C, syphilis, and tuberculosis. Medical release forms are obtained to allow the milk bank to contact the prenatal and infant's care providers (Updegrove, 2005). The mother is given a unique donor identification number and delivers her frozen expressed milk to the milk bank or a collection depot.

In the milk bank, the milk is carefully logged in, thawed to slurry, and cultured for pathogens. Milk testing positive for staphylococcus aureus, methicillin-resistant S. aureus, pseudomonas, bacillus species, or an excess of normal stool flora is discarded without further processing. HMBANA milk banks then pasteurize the milk (62.5°C for 30 minutes) while other milk banks may use a variant of the high-temperature short time (HTST) process (72°C for 5-15 seconds). A second culture is obtained after the heating process for quality control, and milk with any bacterial growth is discarded. The milk is then given lot numbers and expiration dates, stored, and shipped frozen upon prescription to the hospital or patient.

Table 10. Impact of Processing on Immunologic Properties

Factor (NC = No Change)	Storage 0-4°C	Storage -20°C	Heat-Treatment 56°C X 30 min
IgA	NC	NC	Stable (↓@ 62.5°C)
SIgA	NC	NC	Stable (↓@ 62.5°C)
Lactoferrin	NC	NC	NC (↓@ 62.5°C)
Lysozyme	NC	NC	NC (↓@ 62.5°C)
C3 Complement	NC	NC	NC
Bifidum Factor	NC	NC	Stable

Source: Adapted from Lawrence, 1999.

Changes in Human Milk with Processing

The effects of freezing, heating, and handling of human milk are cumulative and affect both the immunologic and nutritional qualities of the milk, as well as the bacterial and viral content. Heat treatment at 56°C (133°F) or greater for 30 minutes reliably eliminates all functional white blood cells and bacteria, inactivates human immunodeficiency virus (HIV) (Orloff *et al.*, 1993) and human T-lymphotrophic virus (Yamato *et al.*, 1986), and decreases the titers of other viruses. Holder pasteurization (62.5°C [144.5°F] for 30 minutes) reliably inactivates HIV and CMV, and will eliminate or significantly decrease titers of most other viruses (American Academy of Pediatrics Committee on Infectious Diseases, 2006; Lawrence & Lawrence, 2005a). HTST heat treatment for five seconds destroys all bacteria and for 15 seconds makes CMV activity undetectable (Goldblum *et al.*, 1984).

Immunologic factors are variously affected by heat treatment and many studies have found different values for different milk components based on differing milk specimens, handling techniques, and assays. With Holder pasteurization, a significant amount of the IgA, bifid growth factor, and lysozyme remain, lipids are unaffected, but 57% of the lactoferrin and most of the IgG are destroyed (Evans *et al.*, 1978; Ford *et al.*, 1977; Lawrence, 1999; Lawrence & Lawrence, 2005a; Welsh & May, 1979).

Transforming growth factors α and β2, present in human milk, are involved in growth, differentiation, and repair of human intestinal epithelial cells, and are unchanged after pasteurization (McPherson & Wagner, 2001) (**Table 9**).

In general, nutritional components may be altered somewhat, but Holder pasteurization does not appear to influence nitrogen retention in LBW infants (Schmidt, 1982). Vitamins A, D, E, B_2, and B_6, choline, niacin, and pantothenic acid are only slightly affected by pasteurization, while thiamine was reduced up to 25%, biotin up to 10%, and vitamin C up to 35% (Van Zoeren-Grobben *et al.*, 1987). The essential fatty acids found naturally in human milk, arachadonic acid and docosahexaenoic acid, are not affected by pasteurization (Fidler *et al.*, 2001; Fidler *et al.*, 1998; Luukkainen *et al.*, 1995) (**Table 10**).

Freezing affects lipids in human milk by breaking down fat globules, thereby increasing the surface available for lipase activity (Garza *et al.*, 1986), and lessening the palatability of the milk to the infant. Microwaving clearly decreases the anti-infective properties of human milk; the higher the temperature, the greater the effect (Quan *et al.*, 1992). Readers are referred to a helpful review article with many further references regarding the contents of processed donor human milk (Tully *et al.*, 2001). To better preserve the immunologic and nutrient components of human milk, yet preclude transmission of pathogens, experiments are underway using varying heating techniques, lyophilization, and irradiation (Arnold, 2005).

DONOR HUMAN MILK FOR PRETERM INFANTS: BENEFITS

Donor human milk is species-specific and as noted above, even when processed, retains much of its nutritional and immunologic value (Goes *et al.*, 2002), while preterm formulas provide only basic nutrition. Protective effects of human milk on infection rates have been observed with the use of *both* fresh and pasteurized milk (Lucas & Cole, 1990; Narayanan *et al.*, 1980; Narayanan *et al.*, 1984a). Lucas and Cole (Lucas & Cole, 1990) found a dose-response decrease in NEC with both mother's own and pasteurized donor human milk. In a randomized, controlled trial of 226 high-risk neonates, Narayanan *et al.* (Narayanan *et al.*, 1984a) demonstrated that infants given only raw human milk or pasteurized human milk had similar (10.5% vs 14.3%) infection rates. However, when formula was added to each, the heat-treated milk had less protective effect than the raw human milk on infection rates (33% vs 16%) (see below). In Norway, where fresh and pasteurized donor human milk are used routinely for VLBW infants, late-onset sepsis was reduced by early feeding of both mothers' own and donor milk (Ronnestad *et al.*, 2005). Two meta-analyses of the limited available literature prior to 2005 (McGuire & Anthony, 2003; Boyd *et al.*, 2006) found significant reductions in NEC with pasteurized donor human milk.

DONOR HUMAN MILK FOR PRETERM INFANTS: CONCERNS

Nutritional Concerns

As donor human milk is usually milk from mothers of term infants, the nutritional content may be of more concern than mothers' own milk, with insufficient protein, calcium, phosphorus, and sodium for optimal growth. Variability of composition, alteration of nutrients with processing, and loss of nutrients during storage and feeding are also concerns. Although caloric content is not significantly different, lower protein levels in term donor milk result in slower growth (**Figure 5**) (Schanler *et al.*, 2005; Stein *et al.*, 1986; Schmidt, 1982; Williamson *et al.*, 1978a; Williamson *et al.*, 1978b). This can be overcome with fortification, just as with mothers' own milk.

	MOM	Pooled Term	pValue
Days to regain birth weight	11.5	17.2	< 0.0001
Days from regained birth weight to 1800 gm	32	44	< 0.0001
Growth (gm/d)	16	12	< 0.0001
Increase in head circ (cm/wk)	0.77	0.74	0.8
Increase in length (cm/wk)	0.77	0.76	0.5
Adapted from: Stein *et al.*, 1986 MOM = Mothers' Own Milk			

Figure 5. Pooled pasteurized breastmilk and untreated own mother's milk in the feeding of VLBW babies: a RCT. Adapted from: Stein *et al.*, 1986.

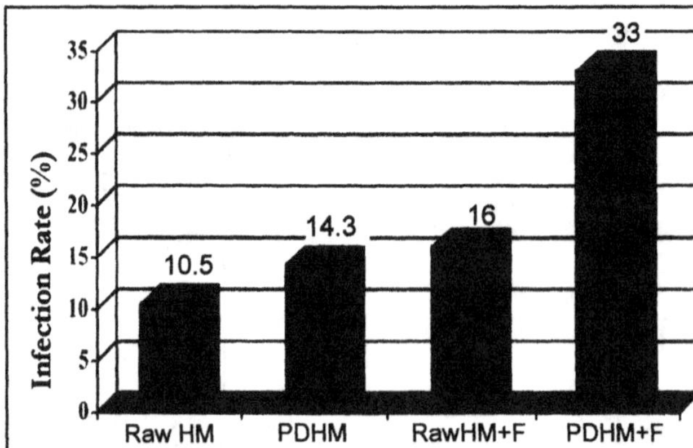

HM = human milk; PDHM = pasteurized donor human milk; F = formula
Adapted from Narayanan *et al.*, 1984a. Figure reprinted with permission from Elsevier.

Figure 6. Infection Rates in High Risk Infants

	2004	2005
▪ Prematurity	77%	71%
▪ Feeding intolerance	19%	14%
▪ IUGR	-	6.5%
▪ Post-NEC	3%	3.3%
▪ Post GI surgery	3%	4.3%
▪ Surrogate pregnancy	3 %	1.1%
▪ ISAM	1.5%	-
▪ Parent request (no medical indication)	1.5%	-
▪ Interval delivery	0.7%	-

Total > 100% as some with > 1 indication
IUGR = intrauterine growth restriction
ISAM = infant of substance-abusing mother

Figure 7. Indication for Donor Milk

In a randomized, blinded trial of pasteurized donor human milk used as a supplement to mother's own milk when not enough mother's own milk was available for 23-29 week infants, Schanler *et al.* (Schanler *et al.*, 2005) found that donor milk offered little short-term advantage over preterm formula for feeding extremely preterm infants. Weight gain was less with donor milk supplementation, and length of stay and retinopathy of prematurity were similar to the preterm formula supplemented group. There was a decrease in NEC and a small decrease in late onset sepsis in the donor milk supplemented group which were not statistically significantly different from the preterm formula group, possibly due to lower than expected rates of these illnesses in all groups. There was a significant decrease in chronic lung disease with both mothers' own and donor human milk. Importantly, use of mothers' own milk was associated with a significant decrease in length of stay, NEC, late-onset sepsis, chronic lung disease, and retinopathy of prematurity (Schanler *et al.*, 2005). In this study, only 27% of the mothers who intended to breastfeed had enough milk to meet their infant's needs, and all infants in the study received at least 50% of their intake as mothers' own milk. An interesting finding was that mothers who did the most kangaroo care had the best milk supply, and there was no increase in infant infection with kangaroo care.

Infection Concerns

As noted above, adding fortifier or formula may change the immune competence of the milk. Narayanan (Narayanan *et al.*, 1984a) found a significant increase in infection when formula was added to pasteurized donor milk, but not when it was added to the raw milk (**Figure 6**).

Pasteurized donor human milk is sterile when shipped from the milk bank. Although bacterial contamination during storage and feeding is a possibility, bacterial contamination with processing has not been reported in the U.S.

Neonatologists' Concerns

A survey study of California neonatologists' attitudes and knowledge base of human milk and donor human milk for preterm infants (Wight, 2003b) found strong support for mothers' own milk use in the NICU, but a significant lack of basic knowledge about human milk and donor milk. Few neonatologists were aware that breastmilk is not normally sterile or that pasteurized donor milk is. Most neonatologists had no experience with donor milk in their training or clinical practice. Key concerns identified were: accessibility and logistics of obtaining milk; safety and infection control issues; social acceptability and legal issues; and nutritional adequacy and efficacy issues. Obviously more research and education are needed in this area.

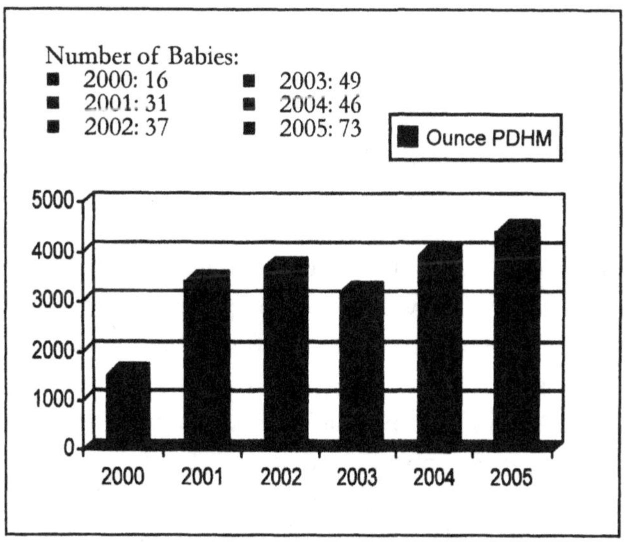

Figure 8. Amount of donor milk used by year

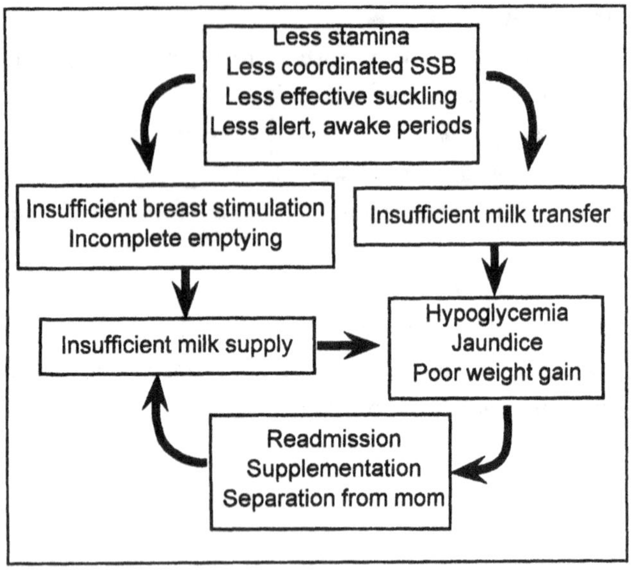

Figure 9. Near-Term Infant Breastfeeding Cascade
Source: Wight, 2003. Figure reprinted with permission from SLACK Inc.

USE OF PASTEURIZED DONOR HUMAN MILK IN THE NICU

The use of heat-treated donor human milk is increasing in U.S. NICUs. Indications for pasteurized donor human milk were tracked in one NICU (**Figure** 7) (Wight, 2006). Amounts used were also tallied (**Figure 8**). The most common indication was prematurity, and the most common uses were for trophic feedings before mother's own colostrum was available and when a mother's milk supply was insufficient to meet her VLBW infant's needs.

Logistics

As with any medication or procedure in the hospital, the use of donor human milk should be regulated with appropriate policies, procedures, and quality control. Surrogate mothers' milk is used routinely, but it is recommended that fresh milk from a relative or friend be screened the same as a donor to a milk bank (California Perinatal Quality Care Collaborative, 2005). Just as with mothers' own milk, appropriate procedures for monitoring freezer temperature and handling donor milk are essential.

Donor milk can be ordered as needed for individual infants, or a supply can be kept on hand in the NICU for immediate use when ordered by the physician. Lot numbers of the milk are recorded when the infant is fed. Some NICUs use informed consent forms, others use information sheets, and, in others, it is simply the standard of care.

Commercial Development of Donor Human Milk Products

Commercial milk banking can be compared to commercial blood banking, with individuals donating their milk, the milk bank processing the milk into various components or products, then selling the products back to the hospital. Benefits of this approach are the possibility of decreased cost of the donor milk with economies of scale (not yet realized), lactoengineering of components or mixtures for special populations (e.g., the premature infant or cancer therapy), and most importantly, the recognition of the economic value of human milk. Possible concerns include mothers or collection depots selling milk with potential falsification of screening or harm to the mother's own infant, and a competing system for milk donation, with no guarantee that those who need the milk will receive it. Processes for producing many components of human milk are already patented.

BREASTFEEDING THE LATE PRETERM INFANT

Preterm infants of 34-36 weeks comprise almost 75% of all preterm singleton births (Davidoff *et al.*, 2006). In addition, deliveries from 37-39 weeks gestation have increased 11% from 1993-2003 in the U.S. (Martin, 2005). Born only a few weeks early, and often only slightly smaller than a full-term infant, "near-term", "borderline premature", or, the now preferred term, "late preterm", infants are all too frequently treated as

Table 11. Post-Discharge Nutritional Monitoring

Nutritional Assessment	Action Values
Growth	
Weight gain	< 20-25 gm/day
Linear growth	< 0.5-1 cm/wk
Head circumference	< 0.5 cm/wk
Biochemical Assessment	
Phosphorus	< 4.5 mg/dL
Alkaline phosphatase	> 450 IU/L
BUN	< 5 mg/ml
Pre-albumin/transthyretin	< 10 mg/dL

Source: Modified from Hall, 2000; 2001.

full-term, although they are at significantly greater risk for health and developmental problems (Institute of Medicine, 2006; Wang *et al.*, 2004) and complications of feeding. Lacking the last few weeks of in utero growth and development, these infants may demonstrate a more subtle immaturity requiring a trained eye and proactive management to prevent subsequent problems. The recommended definition for the late preterm is 34 $^{0/7}$ to 36 $^{6/7}$ weeks (Engle, 2006).

Neither size nor gestational age can reliably predict maturity of all organ systems. All problems of the term infant are magnified in the late preterm infant with higher risks for hypothermia, hypoglycemia, jaundice and kernicterus, excessive weight loss and dehydration, fever secondary to dehydration, slow weight gain, failure to thrive, prolonged artificial milk supplementation, hospital readmission, and breastfeeding failure (**Figure 9**) (Edmonson *et al.*, 1997; Neifert, 2001; Soskolne *et al.*, 1996; Tomashek *et al.*, 2006; Wang *et al.*, 2004; Moritz *et al.*, 2005; Tarcan *et al.*, 2005, Hall *et al.*, 2000). There is a huge variability in breastfeeding ability in this group with many infants and mothers having significant problems initiating and maintaining breastfeeding. Late preterm infants may have special needs. Close follow-up is essential to prevent unnecessary morbidity and the loss of a successful breastfeeding relationship (Academy of Breastfeeding Medicine, 2004a; Wight, 2003a).

There are two basic principles involved in breastfeeding the late preterm infant:

- Feed the baby, and
- Establish and maintain the mother's milk supply.

At delivery, all infants should be quickly dried, assessed, and if stable, placed immediately in uninterrupted skin-to-skin contact with their mother until the first breastfeed is accomplished. After the initial few hours of skin-to-skin contact, the infant should have a complete physical exam, including a gestational age assessment, and necessary procedures should be performed in the mother's room if possible.

Mothers of late preterm infants should be instructed to express milk after every feeding attempt, or approximately every three hours. Using a combination of frequent hand expression (>5 times per day in the first three days) in addition to pumping has been shown to increase production more effectively than reliance on electric pumping alone (Jones *et al.*, 2001; Morton *et al.*, 2007a). An instructional video on the technique can be found at http://newborns.stanford.edu/Breastfeeding/HandExpression.html.

A lactation consultant or other breastfeeding knowledgeable professional should evaluate the dyad within 24 hours of delivery and daily. Many late preterm infants will require at least some supplementation, and most are not discharged exclusively feeding at the breast.

A multidisciplinary post-discharge feeding plan should be developed before discharge and approved by all involved: parents, lactation consultant, current and follow-up physician. Equipment needs, such as an electric breast pump with a "double-pump" kit (to enable pumping both breasts at the same time), home scale, nipple shields, milk storage bottles, etc., should be arranged (Wight, 2003a). A follow-up visit with the physician is recommended 24-48 hours after discharge, then weekly until the infant is fully, exclusively breastfeeding or at least 40 weeks corrected age. To provide consistency, written policies and procedures should be evidence-based and delineate a pathway for care for late preterm infants, as well as procedures for alternate feeding methods, supplementation, and assessments.

BREASTFEEDING THE NICU GRADUATE

The multiple benefits of breastmilk and breastfeeding should not terminate at hospital discharge. Adequate support should be arranged to allow each mother to reach her breastfeeding goal while ensuring appropriate growth and nutrition for the infant. The optimal growth rate (reference target) has not yet been established for post-discharge preterm infants (Schanler, 2005c). Although preterm infants fed "follow-up" formulas tend to gain weight and bone mineral content faster than exclusively breastfed infants, it is unclear whether the rapid catch-up growth seen with supplementation is of benefit or harm for long term overall health, growth and neurodevelopment, cardiovascular health, or insulin resistance (Griffin, 2002; Hall, 2001; Regan *et al.*, 2006).

All infants less than 34 weeks or less than 1800 grams at birth, and other larger infants with nutritional risk factors (chronic lung disease, short gut, neurologic impairment, etc.), should have a complete nutritional assessment prior to discharge which should include both growth parameters (weight, length, head circumference) and biochemical measurements (phosphorus, alkaline phosphatase, urea nitrogen, transthyretin/prealbumin)

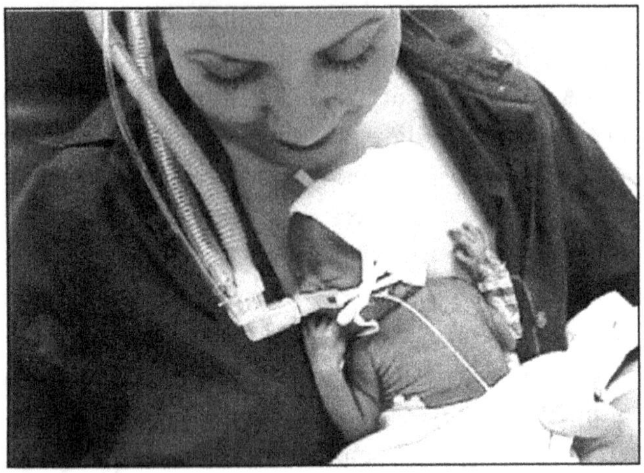

Figure 10. Kangaroo care. Photo courtesy of N. Wight.

(Academy of Breastfeeding Medicine, 2004b; Griffin, 2002; Hall, 2001). If the infant is taking ≥ 160-180 cc/kg/day and growth parameters are normal (**Table 11**) or improving on human milk alone for a week or more prior to discharge, human milk alone should be adequate post-discharge.

If supplementation is deemed necessary, breastfeeding can be supported by having the mother directly breastfeed, then substitute from one to four feedings (as calculated for nutritional needs) per 24 hours of preterm or post-discharge enhanced formula to reach growth and biochemical goals (Academy of Breastfeeding Medicine, 2004b). Alternately, powdered follow-up formula can be added to expressed breastmilk as a fortifier. Multivitamins and iron are also usually needed post-discharge. Repeat biochemical assessments help to adjust the diet over time.

In the week prior to discharge, an individualized nutritional plan should be prepared in coordination with the neonatologist, lactation consultant, dietitian, post-discharge primary physician, and family. For VLBW infants, the in-hospital growth chart as well as a discharge summary should sent home with the patient. Most infants born at <1500 grams will receive some supplementation at discharge (often 35-36 weeks corrected gestational age in the U.S.) and will transition over the next four to eight weeks to full exclusive breastfeeding (Hurst *et al.*, 2000). A full milk supply at discharge is one of the best predictors of successful breastfeeding post-discharge (Furman *et al.*, 2002; Wooldridge & Hall, 2003).

Mothers should continue to pump to maintain milk supply for at least one to two months post-discharge. Kangaroo care should also be continued after discharge home. Although preterm birth may not limit milk production capacity, preterm infants are vulnerable to under consumption until term corrected age or beyond (Meier, 2003), so close monitoring is critical. Breastfeeding educational and promotional efforts, as well as support groups, have been shown to improve breastfeeding rates in the hospital and at discharge (Meier *et al.*, 2004; Merewood *et al.*, 2006b; Sisk *et al.*, 2004; Sisk *et al.*, 2006). "Graduate" mothers should be encouraged to continue to attend these support groups as they can both give and receive support and information.

MANAGING BREASTFEEDING IN THE NICU

For a mother, the decision to provide milk for a VLBW infant is quite distinct from the decision to breastfeed a healthy, term infant (California Perinatal Quality Care Collaborative, 2004). First, the decision is usually made based on health-related issues (i.e., the vulnerability of the infant puts him at greater risk of diseases from which breastmilk may protect him). Second, mothers who did not intend to breastfeed, often decide to pump, while not planning to feed at the breast (Meier *et al.*, 2000a). Third, mothers are highly influenced by the advice of professionals who care for the infant, feeling thankful for (not coerced by) their guidance and even resentful if misinformed about formula being equally acceptable (Miracle *et al.*, 2004).

The volume of milk produced by a pump-dependent mother is the strongest determinant of the duration and exclusivity of breastfeeding the very low birth weight (VLBW, less than 1500 grams) infant. Early, frequent, and effective breastfeeding or milk expression, usually using a hospital grade, automatic-cycling electric "double" pump, has been shown to be the most important factor in establishing normal lactation (Furman *et al.*, 2002; Smith *et al.*, 2003b; Wooldridge & Hall, 2003). Ongoing monitoring of a mother's milk supply via a pumping log can provide opportunity for intervention before the milk supply is irretrievably low.

Breast massage has been shown to improve milk production both in mothers who double pump (both breasts simultaneously) as well as those who pump sequentially (Jones *et al.*, 2001). Manual expression, used in conjunction with electric pumping, may facilitate the collection of small volumes of colostrum and help initiate milk flow when the breasts are engorged. It is very common for a mother of a preterm infant to have her milk supply decrease after four to six weeks of pumping, as she resumes her normal daily routine or returns to work (Ehrenkranz & Ackerman, 1986; Hill *et al.*, 1999). As milk production is positively related to feeding frequency and degree of emptying (Daly & Hartmann, 1995b; Daly & Hartmann, 1995a; Daly *et al.*, 1996), treatment of insufficient milk is centered on increasing the frequency and thoroughness of milk removal. A recent study suggests that combining breast expression and massage with electric pumping may increase milk output. Mothers pumped while applying manual pressure over areas of firmness in the breast (manually assisted pumping = MAP). Without increasing frequency or duration of pumping, milk output increased over several weeks from an average of 591 mL/day to a post-instruction output of 862 mL/day (Morton *et al.*, 2007b).

Many medications and herbal therapies have been recommended as galactogogues (a material that stimulates the production of milk) (Wight & Montgomery, 2004; Wight, 2001b). Detailed, evidence-based recommendations for all phases of breastmilk collection, storage, thawing, and feeding are available (Human Milk Banking Association of North America, 2005). Appropriate steps should be taken to ensure an individual mother's milk is given only to her own child, unless the milk has been heat-treated under standardized conditions (American Academy of Pediatrics Committee on Infectious Diseases, 2006).

Skin-to-skin care (**Figure 10**) has been shown safe and effective in promoting physiologic stability and breastfeeding in preterm infants (DiMenna, 2006). Clinical trials of non-nutritive sucking on a pacifier have been shown to decrease length of stay and facilitate transition to oral feeding for preterm infants (Pinelli & Symington, 2005). A natural extension of kangaroo care, non-nutritive breastfeeding ("dry" breastfeeding or "tasting") offers the mother and infant the chance to practice positioning for breastfeeding and infant suckling before the infant is ready to fully coordinate suck, swallow, and breathing (Narayanan *et al.*, 1991). Infants should be transitioned to oral feedings when physiologically capable, not based on arbitrary weight or gestational age criteria (Lau & Hurst, 1999; Medoff-Cooper, 2000; Nyqvist *et al.*, 1999; Lau, 2006; Siddell & Froman, 1994).

Test weighing, done by standard protocol, appears to be a valid measure of intake at the breast and can be used to determine need for supplementation (Meier *et al.*, 1994; Scanlon *et al.*, 2002). Alternative feeding methods have been sought for both term and preterm infants with the presumption that bottle-feeding would interfere with the establishment of breastfeeding. In the absence of additional research, every effort should be made to accommodate mothers' preferences as to feeding methods as long as appropriate weight gain is maintained. Weak sucking pressures found in preterm infants may result in difficulty maintaining attachment to the breast and, therefore, ineffective milk transfer (Lau *et al.*, 1997). Nipple shields can be used, when appropriate, to maximize milk transfer at the breast (Clum & Primomo, 1996; Meier *et al.*, 2000b).

THE BREASTFEEDING SUPPORTIVE NICU

There are multiple barriers to breastfeeding the preterm infant: the intimidating physical environment of the NICU; individual infant medical factors; ill, stressed or medicated mothers; the family environment and experience with breastfeeding; and financial constraints (e.g., breast pump rental). The most significant barrier is often the healthcare system and well-meaning but misinformed health care providers. Inconsistent, inaccurate information and lack of support by health care professionals have been cited as reasons for breastfeeding failure among many groups of mothers (Ellis & Hewat, 1983; Humenick *et al.*, 1998; Raisler, 1993; Winikoff *et al.*, 1986; Winikoff *et al.*, 1987).

Antepartum hospital stays are opportunities for dispelling myths (e.g., "*I can't breastfeed because I have a premature infant.*") and for providing anticipatory guidance regarding procedures to ensure a full milk supply and safe storage and use of pumped milk. Although all healthcare professionals who care for mothers and infants should have a general knowledge of lactation physiology and breastfeeding management, supporting the mother of a NICU infant often requires special knowledge, skill, and experience. Several models of support have been developed (Hurst *et al.*, 1998; Jones, 1995; Meier *et al.*, 1993).

> *"An obstetrician's advice is critical to the mother's decision-making. It takes very little time and effort. It's your gift to the mother, and it's her gift to her baby."*
>
> John T. Queenan MD, Deputy Editor
> *Obstetrics & Gynecology*
> July 2003; 102(1):3-4

Having International Board Certified Lactation Consultants (IBCLC) on staff is one method to assist in increasing breastfeeding rates in the NICU through staff and mother education, clinical consultation, and support (Baker & Rasmussen, 1997; Gonzalez *et al.*, 2003; Hurst *et al.*, 1998; Kuzma-O'Reilly *et al.*, 2003; Merewood *et al.*, 2003; Castrucci *et al.*, 2006). In some units, well-trained NICU RNs and peer counselors may have the knowledge and experience to counsel and manage complicated NICU breastfeeding issues (Meier, 2003; Meier, 2001). NICU peer counselors have been shown to significantly increase the odds of breastfeeding at two, four, eight, and 12 weeks after birth (Merewood *et al.*, 2006b). Postnatal peer counseling was also found to increase both exclusive and any breastfeeding of term LBW infants at six months (Agrasda *et al.*, 2005).

In addition to a basic breastfeeding policy for birthing hospitals, the NICU should have its own NICU breastmilk/breastfeeding policy or policies to cover, at a minimum:

- basic principles
- collection, storage, and handling of a mother's own milk for her infant
- misadministration of one mother's milk to another mother's infant.

NICUs using fresh and/or heat-treated donor human milk should also have policies and procedures covering this area (California Perinatal Quality Care Collaborative, 2004; California Perinatal Quality Care Collaborative, 2005).

The use of human milk and breastfeeding in preterm, vulnerable infants requires staff educated on the science of human milk, the physiology of milk production, and the best practices to facilitate transition to direct breastfeeding. "Providing this care and support to families in the intensive care nursery requires time, positive attitudes, and encouragement by all members of the healthcare team. In order to improve outcomes of vulnerable infants, the provision of human milk must be viewed not as a choice but a necessity of care" (Spatz, 2006).

CONCLUSIONS

Mothers of premature infants are less likely to breastfeed than mothers of healthy, term infants (Bell & McGrath, 1996; Ehrenkranz *et al.*, 1985; Furman *et al.*, 1998; Hill *et al.*, 1997; Lefebvre & Ducharme, 1989; Meier *et al.*, 1993; Merewood *et al.*, 2006a). While an average of 69-71% of term infants in the U.S. does any breastfeeding in the hospital before discharge (Li *et al.*, 2005; Ryan *et al.*, 2002), the average rate of preterm infants receiving *any* breastmilk at hospital discharge is approximately 50% (Furman *et al.*, 1998; Hill *et al.*, 1997). This is especially concerning because the evidence suggests that human milk may especially benefit premature and high-risk infants (Schanler, 2001).

Other countries seem to have more success with breastfeeding in the NICU and at discharge (Flacking *et al.*, 2003; Nyqvist, 2005; Reinert do Nascimento & Issler, 2005). In the U.S., the average corrected age of preterm infants at discharge is 35-36 weeks and the average weight is 1800-2000 grams, but infants vary enormously in age, weight, medical condition, and nutritional needs. In many parts of the world, preterm infants are discharged much heavier and older than in the U.S. and have, therefore, had much more opportunity to mature and learn to breastfeed.

Providing lactation support in the NICU is not without cost. Lactation consultants, staff education, pump kits and other supplies, non-commercial patient education materials, breastmilk storage bottles and caps, and dedicated space and equipment for pumping are expenses to the NICU. However, when both the general cost savings from breastfeeding (Ball & Wright, 1999; Weimer, 2001) and the specific cost savings to the NICU through reduced NEC, late-onset sepsis, shorter hospital stays, and less use of hospital resources, such as total parenteral nutrition (Schanler *et al.*, 2005; Schanler *et al.*, 1999c; Wight, 2001a) are considered, the investment gives dramatic returns.

Of course, the most important benefit of lactation support in the NICU is the decreased morbidity and mortality and improved long-term outcomes associated with the provision of human milk for preterm and ill newborns. Animal data and a few recent human studies suggest that the neuroendocrinology of the lactating mother may down-regulate the magnitude of the maternal postpartum stress response (Groer *et al.*, 2002). Several studies indicate that providing milk for their infants helps mothers cope with the emotional stresses surrounding the NICU experience and gives them a tangible claim on their infants (Kavanaugh, 1997; Spanier-Mingolelli, 1998).

In summary, human milk is much more than nutrition and is an important factor in the transition from fetus to infant. With attention to the special needs of preterm infants and support for their mothers, more infants will benefit from breastmilk in the NICU and after discharge.

References

Academy of Breastfeeding Medicine. ABM protocol # 10: Breastfeeding the near-term infant (35-37 weeks gestation). 2004a. Available from: http://www.bfmed.org/ace-files/protocol/near_term.pdf.

Academy of Breastfeeding Medicine. Clinical protocol #12: Transitioning the breastfeeding/breastmilk-fed premature infant from the neonatal intensive care unit to home. 2004b. Available from: www.bfmed.org.

Agrasda G, Gustafsson J, Kylberg E, Ewald U. Postnatal peer counselling on exclusive breastfeeding of low-birthweight infants: A randomized, controlled trial. *Acta Paediatr.* 2005; 94:1109-15.

American Academy of Pediatrics Committee on Nutrition. Nutritional needs of low-birth-weight infants. *Pediatrics.* 1985; 75:976-86.

American Academy of Pediatrics. Human milk. In: Pickering LK, Baker CJ, Long SS, McMillan JA (eds.). *Red book: 2006 Report of the Committee on Infectious Diseases.* 27th Ed. Elk Grove Village, IL: American Academy of Pediatrics; 2006. p. 123-30.

American Academy of Pediatrics and the American College of Obstetricians and Gynecologists. Appendix E: Standard terminology for reporting of reproductive health statistics in the United States. *Guidelines for perinatal care.* 5th Ed. Elk Grove Village, IL: American Academy of Pediatrics; 2002.

American Academy of Pediatrics Committee on Infectious Diseases. *2006 Red book: Report of the Committee on Infectious Diseases.* Elk Grove Village, IL: American Academy of Pediatrics; 2006.

American Academy of Pediatrics Committee on Mother's Milk. Operation of mother's milk bureaus. *J Pediatr.* 1943; 23:112.

American Academy of Pediatrics Committee on Nutrition. Chapter 2: Nutritional needs of the preterm infant. In: Kleinman RE (ed). *Pediatric nutrition handbook.* 5th Ed. Elk Grove Village, IL: American Academy of Pediatrics; 2004. p. 23.

American Academy of Pediatrics Committee on Nutrition. Nutritional needs of low-birth-weight infants. *Pediatrics.* 1977; 60:519-30.

American Academy of Pediatrics Section on Breastfeeding. Policy Statement. Breastfeeding and the use of human milk. *Pediatrics.* 2005; 115(2):496-506.

Amin SB, Merle KS, Orlando MS, Dalzell LE, Guillet R. Brainstem maturation in premature infants as a function of enteral feeding type. *Pediatrics.* 2000; 106(2 Pt 1):318-22.

Anderson DM. Nutritional assessment and therapeutic interventions for the preterm infant. *Clin Perinatol.* 2002; 29(2):313-26.

Anderson G, Aziz A. Multifunctional roles of dietary proteins in the regulation of metabolism and food intake: Application to feeding infants. *J Pediatr.* 2006; 149(5):S74-79.

Anderson GH, Atkinson SA, Bryan MH. Energy and macronutrient content of human milk during early lactation from mothers giving birth prematurely and at term. *Am J Clin Nutr.* 1981; 34(2):258-65.

Anderson JW, Johnstone BM, Remley DT. Breast-feeding and cognitive development: a meta-analysis. *Am J Clin Nutr.* 1999; 70(4):525-35.

Arias-Camison JM. Late onset group B streptococcal infection from maternal expressed breast milk in a very low birth weight infant. *J Perinatol.* 2003; 23(8):691-92.

Arnold L, Erickson M. The early history of milk banking in the USA. *J Hum Lact.* 1988; 4(3):112-13.

Arnold LD, Larson E. Immunologic benefits of breast milk in relation to human milk banking. *Am J Infect Control.* 1993; 21(5):235-42.

Arnold LDW. Chapter 14: Donor human milk banking. In: Riordan J (ed). *Breastfeeding and human lactation.* 3rd Ed. Boston: Jones and Bartlett; 2005. p. 409-34.

Askin DF, Diehl-Jones W. Effects of human milk fortifier on bacterial growth and cytokines in breast milk. In: *Proceedings of the annual meeting.* San Francisco, CA: American Society for Cell Biology; 2002.

Asquith MT, Pedrotti PW, Stevenson DK, Sunshine P. Clinical uses, collection, and banking of human milk. *Clin Perinatol.* 1987; 14(1):173-85.

Atkinson SA. The effects of gestational age at delivery on human milk components. In: Jensen RG (ed). *Handbook of milk composition.* San Diego: Academic Press; 1995. p. 222-37.

Atkinson SA. Human milk feeding of the micropremie. *Clin Perinatol.* 2000; 27(1): 235-47.

Atkinson SA, Bryan MH, Anderson GH. Human milk: difference in nitrogen concentration in milk for mothers of term and premature infants. *J Pediatr.* 1978; 93:67-69.

Atkinson SA, Bryan MH, Anderson GH. Human milk feeding in premature infants: protein, fat, and carbohydrate balances in the first two weeks of life. *J Pediatr.* 1981a; 99(4):617-24.

Atkinson SA, Radde IC, Anderson GH. Macromineral balances in premature infants fed their own mothers' milk or formula. *J Pediatr.* 1983; 102(1):99-106.

Backstrom M, Maki R, Kuusela A, *et al.* The long-term effect of early mineral, vit D, and breast milk intake on bone mineral status in 9-to 11-year-old children born prematurely. *J Pediatr Gastroenterol Nutr.* 1999; 29:575-82.

Backstrom MC, Kuusela AL, Maki R. Metabolic bone disease of prematurity. *Ann Med.* 1996; 28(4):275-82.

Baker BJ, Rasmussen TW. Organizing and documenting lactation support of NICU families. *J Obstet Gynecol Neonatal Nurs.* 1997; 26(5):515-21.

Ball TM, Bennett DM. The economic impact of breastfeeding. *Pediatr Clin NA.* 2001; 48(1):253-62.

Ball TM, Wright AL. Health care costs of formula-feeding in the first year of life. *Pediatrics.* 1999; 103(4 Part 2):870-76.

Barker DJ. The effect of nutrition of the fetus and neonate on cardiovascular disease in adult life. *Proc Nutr Soc.* 1992a; 51(2):135-44.

Barker DJ. Fetal growth and adult disease. *Br J Obstet Gynaecol.* 1992b; 99(4): 275-76.

Barker DJ. The fetal origins of adult hypertension. *J Hypertens Suppl.* 1992c; 10(7):S39-44.

Barker DJ. The fetal origins of diseases of old age. *Eur J Clin Nutr.* 1992d; 46 Suppl 3:S3-9.

Barker DJ. Fetal programming of coronary heart disease. *Trends Endocrinol Metab.* 2002; 13(9):364-68.

Barker DJ. Commentary: Developmental origins of raised serum cholesterol. *Int J Epidemiol.* 2003; 32(5):876-77.

Barker DJ. The developmental origins of adult disease. *J Am Coll Nutr.* 2004a; 23(6 Suppl):588S-95S.

Barker DJ. The developmental origins of chronic adult disease. *Acta Paediatr Supp.*,2004b; 93(446):26-33.

Barker DJ. The developmental origins of insulin resistance. *Horm Res.* 2005; 64 Suppl 3:2-7.

Barker DJ, Bagby SP. Developmental antecedents of cardiovascular disease: a historical perspective. *J Am Soc Nephrol.* 2005; 16(9):2537-44.

Barker DJ, Eriksson JG, Forsen T, Osmond C. Fetal origins of adult disease: strength of effects and biological basis. *Int J Epidemiol.* 2002; 31(6):1235-39.

Barker DJ, Eriksson JG, Forsen T, Osmond C. Infant growth and income 50 years later. *Arch Dis Child.* 2005a; 90(3):272-73.

Barker DJ, Osmond C, Forsen TJ, Kajantie E, Eriksson JG. Trajectories of growth among children who have coronary events as adults. *N Engl J Med.* 2005b; 353(17):1802-09.

Barney CK, Purser N, Christensen RD. A phase 1 trial testing an enteral solution patterned after human amniotic fluid to treat feeding intolerance. *Adv Neonatal Care.* 2006; 6(2):89-95.

Barros MD, Carneiro-Sampaeio MMS. Milk composition in low birth weight infants' mothers. *Acta Paediatr Scand.* 1983; 73:693-94.

Bates CJ, Liu DS, Fuller NJ, Lucas A. Susceptibility of riboflavin and vitamin A in breast milk to photodegradation and its implications for the use of banked breast milk in infant feeding. *Acta Paediatr Scand.* 1985; 74(1):40-44.

Baumslag N, Michels D. *Milk, money and madness.* Westport: Bergin & Garvey; 1995.

Beeby PJ, Jeffery H. Risk factors for necrotising enterocolitis: the influence of gestational age. *Arch Dis Child.* 1992; 67(4 Spec No):432-35.

Bell RP, McGrath JM. Implementing a research-based kangaroo care program in the NICU. *Nurs Clin North Am.* 1996; 31(2):387-403.

Bellander M, Ley D, Polberger S, Hellstrom-Westas L. Tolerance to early human milk feeding is not compromised by indomethacin in preterm infants with persistent ductus arteriosus. *Acta Paediatr.* 2003; 92(9):1074-78.

Berseth CL. Gastrointestinal motility in the neonate. *Clin Perinatol.* 1996; 23: 179-90.

Berseth CL, Nordyke CK, Valdes MG, Furlow Bl, Go VL. Responses of gastrointestinal peptides and motor activity to milk and water feedings in preterm and term infants. *Pediatr Res.* 1992; 31: 587-90.

Bhargava SK, Sachdev HS, Fall CH, Osmond C, Lakshmy R, Barker DJ, *et al.* Relation of serial changes in childhood body-mass index to impaired glucose tolerance in young adulthood. *N Engl J Med.* 2004; 350(9):865-75.

Bier JA, Oliver T, Ferguson AE, Vohr BR. Human milk improves cognitive and motor development of premature infants during infancy. *J Hum Lact.* 2002; 18(4): 361-67.

Bisset WM, Watt JB, Rivers JPA, Milla PJ. Postprandial motor response of the small intestine to enteral feeds in preterm infants. *Arch Dis Child.* 1989; 64:1356-61.

Bitmar J, Wood DL, Hamosh M, Hamosh P, Mehta NR. Comparison of the lipid composition of breast milk from mothers of term and preterm infants. *Am J Clin Nutr.* 1983; 38:300-12.

Blaymore Bier JA, Oliver T, Ferguson A, Vohr BR. Human milk reduces outpatient upper respiratory symptoms in premature infants during their first year of life. *J Perinatol.* 2002; 22(5):354-59.

BMJ. Rapid responses to: Effect of breast feeding on intelligence in children: prospective study, sibling pairs analysis, and meta-analysis. 2006. Available **from:** www.bmj.com/cgi/eletters/333/7575/945.

Boo NY, Goh ES. Predictors of breastfeeding in very low birthweight infants at the time of discharge from hospital. *J Trop Pediatr.* 1999; 45(4):195-201.

Boo NY, Puah CH, Lye MS. The role of expressed breastmilk and continuous positive airway pressure as survival in extremely low birthweight infants. *J Trop Pediatr.* 2000; 46:15-20.

Boyd CA, Quigley MA, Brocklehurst P. Donor breast milk versus infant formula for preterm infants: a systematic review and meta-analysis. *Arch Dis Child Fetal Neonatal Ed.* 2007; 92(3):F169-75.

Bradshaw JH, Moore PP. Perinatal cytomegalovirus infection associated with lung cysts. *J Paediatr Child Health.* 2003; 39(7):563-66.

Bryant P, Morley C, Garland S, Curtis N. Cytomegalovirus transmission from breast milk in premature babies: does it matter? *Arch Dis Child Fetal Neonatal Ed.* 2002; 87(2): F75-77.

Buescher ES. Host defense mechanisms of human milk and their relations to enteric infections and necrotizing enterocolitis. *Clin Perinatol.* 1994; 21(2): 247-62.

Burgard P. Critical evaluation of the methodology employed in cognitive development trials. *Acta Paediatr.* 2003; 92 (suppl.):6-10.

Butte NF, Garza C, Johnson CA, Smith EO, Nichols BL. Longitudinal changes in milk composition of mothers delivering preterm and term infants. *Early Hum Dev.* 1984; 9(2):153-62.

Caicedo RA, Schanler RJ, Li N, Neu J. The developing intestinal ecosystem: Implications for the neonate. *Pediatr Res.* 2005. 58(4):625-28.

California Perinatal Quality Care Collaborative. P. Q. I. P. Toolkit: Nutritional support of the VLBW infant, part 1. California Perinatal Quality Care Collaborative. Perinatal Quality Improvement Panel; 2004. Available from: www.cpqcc.org.

California Perinatal Quality Care Collaborative. P. Q. I. P. Toolkit: Nutritional support of the VLBW infant, part 2. California Perinatal Quality Care Collaborative. Perinatal Quality Improvement Panel; 2005. Available from: www.cpqcc.org.

Carlson SE, Werkman SH, Rhodes PG, Tolley EA. Visual-acuity development in healthy preterm infants: effect of marine-oil supplementation. *Am J Clin Nutr.* 1993; 58(1):35-42.

Castrucci B, Hoover K, Lim S, Maus K. A comparison of breastfeeding rates in an urban birth cohort among women delivering infants at hospitals that employ and do not employ lactation consultants. *J Public Health Manag Pract.* 2006; 12(6): 578-85.

Catassi C, Bonucci A, Coppa GV, Carlucci A, Giorgi PL. Intestinal permeability changes during the first month: effect of natural versus artificial feeding. *J Pediatr Gastroenterol Nutr.* 1995; 21(4):383-86.

Cavell B. Gastric emptying in infants fed human milk or infant formula. *Acta Paediatr Scand.* 1981; 70:639-41.

Chan GM. Effects of powdered human milk fortifiers on the antibacterial actions of human milk. *J Perinatol.* 2003; 23(8):620-23.

Cheong JL, Cowan FM, Modi N. Gastrointestinal manifestations of postnatal cytomegalovirus infection in infants admitted to a neonatal intensive care unit over a five year period. *Arch Dis Child Fetal Neonatal Ed.* 2004; 89(4): F367-69.

Child Trends DataBank. Child Trends DataBank. Vol. 2006. Available from: http://www.childtrendsdatabank.org/.

Clark RH, Wagner CL, Merritt RJ, Bloom BT, Neu J, Young TE, Clark DA. Nutrition in the neonatal intensive care unit: How do we reduce the incidence of extrauterine growth restriction? *J Perinatol.* 2003; 23:337-44.

Clum D, Primomo J. Use of a silicone nipple shield with premature infants. *J Hum Lact.* 1996; 12(4):287-90.

Committee on Nutrition of the Preterm Infant - European Society of Paediatric Gastroenterology and Nutrition (ESPGAN). *Nutrition and feeding of preterm infants.* Oxford, England: Blackwell Scientific Publications; 1987.

Cooper PA, Rothberg AD, Pettifor JM, Bolton KD, Davenhuis S. Growth and biochemical response of premature infants fed pooled preterm mik or special formula. *J Pediatr Gastroenterol Nutr.* 1984; 3:749-54.

Cunningham AS. Chapt 9: Breastfeeding: Adaptive behavior for child health and longevity. In: Stewart-Macadam P, Dettwyler KA (eds.). *Breastfeeding: Biocultural perspectives.* New York: Aldine de Gruyter; 1995.

Curtis N, Chau L, Garland S, Tabrizi S, Alexander R, Morley CJ. Cytomegalovirus remains viable in naturally infected breast milk despite being frozen for 10 days. *Arch Dis Child Fetal Neonatal Ed.* 2005; 90(6): F529-30.

Daly SE, Hartmann PE. Infant demand and milk supply. Part 1: Infant demand and milk production in lactating women. *J Hum Lact.* 1995a; 11(1):21-26.

Daly SE, Hartmann PE. Infant demand and milk supply. Part 2: The short-term control of milk synthesis in lactating women. *J Hum Lact.* 1995b;11(1):27-37.

Daly SE, Kent JC, Owens RA, Hartmann PE. Frequency and degree of milk removal and the short-term control of human milk synthesis. *Exp Physiol.* 1996; 81(5):861-75.

Davey AM, Wagner CL, Cox C, Kendig JW. Feeding premature infants while low umbilical artery catheters are in place: a prospective, randomized trial. *J Pediatr.* 1994; 124(5 Pt 1):795-99.

Davidoff MJ, Dias T, Damus K, Russell R, Bettegowda VR, Dolan S, *et al.* Changes in the gestational age distribution among U.S. singleton births: impact on rates of late preterm birth, 1992 to 2002. *Semin Perinatol.* 2006; 30(1):8-15.

Day IN, Chen XH, Gaunt TR, King TH, Voropanov A, Ye S, *et al.* Late life metabolic syndrome, early growth, and common polymorphism in the growth hormone and placental lactogen gene cluster. *J Clin Endocrinol Metab.* 2004; 89(11):5569-76.

de Silva A, Jones PW, Spencer SA. Does human milk reduce infection rates in preterm infants? A systematic review. *Arch Dis Child Fetal Neonatal Ed.* 2004; 89:F509-13.

Der G, Batty GD, Deary IJ. Effect of breast feeding on intelligence in children: prospective study, sibling pairs analysis, and meta-analysis. *BMJ.* 2006; 333(7575):945. Epub 2006 Oct 4.

DiBiasie A. Evidence-based review of retinopathy of prematurity prevention in VLBW and ELBW infants. *Neonatal Netw.* 2006; 25(6):393-403.

DiMenna L. Considerations for implementation of a neonatal kangaroo care protocol. *Neonatal Network.* 2006; 25(6):405-12.

Doctor S, Friedman S, Dunn MS, Asztalos EV, Wylie L, Mazzulli T, *et al.* Cytomegalovirus transmission to extremely low-birthweight infants through breast milk. *Acta Paediatr.* 2005; 94(1):53-58.

Donovan S. Role of human milk components in gastrointestinal development: Current knowledge and future needs. *J Pediatr.* 2006; 149(5):S49-61.

Dunn L, Hulman S, Weiner J, Kliegman R. Beneficial effects of early hypocaloric enteral feeding on neonatal gastrointestinal function: preliminary report of a randomized trial. *J Pediatr.* 1988; 112(4):622-29.

Dusick AM, Poindexter BB, Ehrenkranz RA, Lemons JA. Growth failure in the preterm infant: can we catch up? *Semin Perinatol.* 2003; 27(4):302-10.

Dvorak B. Epidermal growth factor and necrotizing enterocolitis. *Clin Perinatol.* 2004; 31(1):183-92.

Dvorak B, Fituch CC, Williams CS, Hurst NM, Schanler RJ. Increased epidermal growth factor levels in human milk of mothers with extremely premature infants. *Pediatr Res.* 2003a; 54(1):15-19.

Dvorak B, Fituch CC, Williams CS, Hurst NM, Schanler RJ. Concentrations of epidermal growth factor and transforming growth factor-alpha in preterm milk. *Adv Exp Med Biol.* 2004; 554:407-9.

Dvorak B, Halpern MD, Holubec H, Dvorakova K, Dominguez JA, Williams CS, *et al.* Maternal milk reduces severity of necrotizing enterocolitis and increases intestinal IL-10 in a neonatal rat model. *Pediatr Res.* 2003b; 53(3):426-33.

Edmond KM, Zandoh C, Quigley MA, Amenga-Etego S, Owusu-Agyei S, Kirkwood BR. Delayed breastfeeding initiation increases risk of neonatal mortality. *Pediatrics.* 2006; 117(3):e380-86.

Edmonson M, Stoddard J, Owens L. Hospital readmission with feeding related problems after early postpartum discharge of normal newborns. *JAMA.* 1997; 278:299-303.

Ehrenkranz R, Ackerman B, Mezger J, Bracken M. Breastfeeding premature infants: incidence and success. *Pediatr Res.* 1985; 19:199A (abstract # 530).

Ehrenkranz RA, Ackerman BA. Metoclopramide effect on faltering milk production by mothers of premature infants. *Pediatrics.* 1986; 78(4):614-20.

Ehrenkranz RA, Dusick AM, Vohr BR, Wright LL, Wrage LA, Poole WK. Growth in the neonatal intensive care unit influences neurodevelopmental and growth outcomes of extremely low birth weight infants. *Pediatrics.* 2006; 117(4):1253-61.

Ehrenkranz RA, Younes N, Lemons JA, Fanaroff AA, Donovan EF, Wright LL, *et al.* Longitudinal growth of hospitalized very low birth weight infants. *Pediatrics.* 1999; 104(2 Pt 1):280-89.

Eibl MM, Wolf HM, Furnkranz H, Rosenkranz A. Prevention of necrotizing enterocolitis in low-birth-weight infants by IgA-IgG feeding. *N Engl J Med.* 1988; 319(1):1-7.

Ekema G, Pedersini P, Milianti S, Ubertazzi M, Minoli D, Manciana A. Colonic stricture mimicking Hirschsprung's disease: a localized cytomegalovirus infection. *J Pediatr Surg.* 2006; 41(4):850-52.

el-Mohandes AE, Picard MB, Simmens SJ, Keiser JF. Use of human milk in the intensive care nursery decreases the incidence of nosocomial sepsis. *J Perinatol.* 1997; 17(2):130-34.

Elder DE, Hagan R, Evans SF, Benninger HR, French NP. Hospital admissions in the first year of life in very preterm infants. *J Paediatr Child Health.* 1999: 35(2):145-50.

Ellis DJ, Hewat RJ. Do nurses help or hinder mothers who breastfeed? *J Adv Nurs.* 1983; 8(4):281-88.

Elwood PC, Pickering J, Gallacher JE, Hughes J, Davies D. Long term effect of breast feeding: cognitive function in the Caerphilly cohort. *J Epidemiol Community Health.* 2005; 59(2):130-33.

Embleton NE, Pang N, Cooke RJ. Postnatal malnutrition and growth retardation: an inevitable consequence of current recommendations in preterm infants? *Pediatrics.* 2001; 107(2):270-73.

Engle WA. A recommendation for the definition of "late preterm" (near-term) and the birth weight-gestational age classification system. *Semin Perinatol.* 2006; 30(1): 2-7.

Erenberg A, Shaw RD, Yousefzadeh D. Lactobezoar in the low-birth-weight infant. *Pediatrics.* 1979; 63(4): 642-46.

Eriksson JG, Forsen TJ, Osmond C, Barker DJ. Pathways of infant and childhood growth that lead to type 2 diabetes. *Diabetes Care.* 2003; 26(11): 3006-10.

Evans TJ, Ryley HC, Neale LM, Dodge JA, Lewarne VM. Effect of storage and heat on antimicrobial proteins in human milk. *Arch Dis Child.* 1978; 53(3): 239-41.

Ewer AK, Yu VY. Gastric emptying in pre-term infants: the effect of breast milk fortifier. *Acta Paediatr.* 1996; 85(9):1112-15.

Faldella G, Govoni M, Alessandroni R, Marchiani E, Salvioli GP, Biagi PL, *et al.* Visual evoked potentials and dietary long chain polyunsaturated fatty acids in preterm infants. *Arch Dis Child Fetal Neonatal Ed.* 1996; 75(2):F108-12.

Feil R. Environmental and nutritional effects on the epigenetic regulation of genes. *Mutat Res.* 2006; 600(1-2):46-57.

Feldman R, Eidelman AI. Direct and indirect effects of breast milk on the neurobehavioral and cognitive development of premature infants. *Dev Psychobiol.* 2003; 43(2):109-19.

Fenton TR, Tough SC, Belik J. Breast milk supplementation for preterm infants: parental preferences and postdischarge lactation duration. *Am J Perinatol.* 2000; 17(6): 329-33.

Fewtrell MS, Cole TJ, Bishop NJ, Lucas A. Neonatal factors predicting childhood height in preterm infants: evidence for a persisting effect of early metabolic bone disease? *J Pediatr.* 2000; 137(5):668-73.

Fidler N, Sauerwald TU, Demmelmair H, Koletzko B. Fat content and fatty acid composition of fresh, pasteurized, or sterilized human milk. *Adv Exp Med Biol.* 2001; 501:485-95.

Fidler N, Sauerwald TU, Koletzko B, Demmelmair H. Effects of human milk pasteurization and sterilization on available fat content and fatty acid composition. *J Pediatr Gastroenterol Nutr.* 1998; 27(3):317-22.

Fildes V. *Breast, bottles, and babies.*, Edinburgh: Edinburgh University Press; 1986.

Flacking R, Nyqvist KH, Ewald U, Wallin L. Long-term duration of breastfeeding in Swedish low birth weight infants. *J Hum Lact.* 2003; 19(2):157-65.

Ford JE, Law BA, Marshall VM, Reiter B. Influence of the heat treatment of human milk on some of its protective constituents. *J Pediatr.* 1977; 90(1): 29-35.

Forsgren M. Cytomegalovirus in breast milk: reassessment of pasteurization and freeze-thawing. *Pediatr Res.* 2004; 56(4):526-28.

Friel J, Andrews W, Matthew JEA. Improved growth of very low birthweight infants. *Nutr Res.* 1993; 13:611-20.

Friel JK, Martin SM, Langdon M, Herzberg GR, Buettner GR. Milk from mothers of both premature and full-term infants provides better antioxidant protection than does infant formula. *Pediatr Res.* 2002; 51(5):612-18.

Furman L. Yes, human milk does reduce infection rates in very low birthweight infants. *Arch Dis Child Fetal Neonatal Ed.* 2006; 91:F78.

Furman L, Minich N, Hack M. Correlates of lactation in mothers of very low birth weight infants. *Pediatrics.* 2002; 109(4):e57. Available from: www.pediatrics.org/cgi/content/full/109/4/e57.

Furman L, Minich NM, Hack M. Breastfeeding of very low birth weight infants. *J Hum Lact.* 1998; 14(1):29-34.

Furman L, Taylor G, Minich N, Hack M. The effect of maternal milk on neonatal morbidity of very low-birth-weight infants. *Arch Pediatr Adolesc Med.* 2003; 157(1):66-67.

Furman L, Wilson-Costello D, Friedman H, Taylor HG, Minich N, Hack M. The effect of neonatal maternal milk feeding on the neurodevelopmental outcome of very low birth weight infants. *J Dev Behav Pediatr.* 2004; 25(4):247-53.

Furukawa M, Lee EL, Johnston JM. Platelet-activating factor-induced ischemic bowel necrosis: the effect of platelet-activating factor acetylhydrolase. *Pediatr Res.* 1993; 34(2):237-41.

Gale CR, Martyn CN. Breastfeeding, dummy use, and adult intelligence. *Lancet.* 1996; 347(9008):1072-75.

Garza C, Hopkinson JM, Schanler RJ. Human Milk Banking. In: Howell RR, Morriss RH, Pickering LK (eds.). *Human milk in infant nutrition and health.* Springfield, IL: Charles C. Thomas; 1986. p. 225-55.

Gastelum DT, Dassey D, Mascola L, Yasuda LM. Transmission of community-associated methicillin-resistant Staphylococcus aureus from breast milk in the neonatal intensive care unit. *Pediatr Infect Dis J.* 2005; 24(12):1122-24.

Georgieff M, Mills M, Lindeke L, Iverson S, Johnson D, Thompson T. Changes in nutritional management and outcome of very-low-birth-weight infants. *Am J Dis Child.* 1989; 143(1):82-85.

Gessler P, Bischoff GA, Wiegand D, Essers B, Bossart W. Cytomegalovirus-associated necrotizing enterocolitis in a preterm twin after breastfeeding. *J Perinatol.* 2004; 24(2):124-26.

Godambe S, Shah PS, Shah V. Breast milk as a source of late onset neonatal sepsis. *Pediatr Infect Dis J.* 2005; 24(4):381-82.

Godfrey KM, Barker DJ. Fetal nutrition and adult disease. *Am J Clin Nutr.* 2000; 71(Suppl 5):1344S-52S.

Goes HC, Torres AG, Donangelo CM, Trugo NM. Nutrient composition of banked human milk in Brazil and influence of processing on zinc distribution in milk fractions. *Nutrition.* 2002; 18(7-8):590-94.

Goldblum RM, Dill CW, Albrecht TB, Alford ES, Garza C, Goldman AS. Rapid high-temperature treatment of human milk. *J Pediatr.* 1984; 104(3):380-85.

Goldblum RM, Schanler RJ, Garza C, Goldman AS. Human milk feeding enhances the urinary excretion of immunologic factors in low birth weight infants. *Pediatr Res.* 1989; 25(2):184-88.

Goldman A, Cheda S, Keeney S, Schmalstieg F, Schanler R. Immunologic protection of the preterm newborn by human milk. *Sem Perinatol.* 1994; 18(6):495-501.

Goldman AS. Modulation of the gastrointestinal tract of infants by human milk. interfaces and interactions. An evolutionary perspective. *J Nutr.* 2000; 130, 426S-31S.

Goldman AS, Chheda S, Garofalo R. Evolution of immunologic functions of the mammary gland and the postnatal development of immunity. *Pediatr Res.* 1998; 43(2):155-62.

Goldman AS, Goldblum RM, Schmalsteig Jr FC. Chapter 32: Protective properties of human milk. In: Walker DJ, Watkins J, Duggan C, editors. *Nutrition in pediatrics: Basic science and clinical applications.* 3rd Ed. Hamilton Ontario: BC Decker Inc; 2003.

Gonzalez KA, Meinzen-Derr J, Burke BL, Hibler AJ, Kavinsky B, Hess S, *et al.* Evaluation of a lactation support service in a children's hospital neonatal intensive care unit. *J Hum Lact.* 2003; 19(3):286-92.

Gordon H, Levine S, Deamer W, McNamara H. Feeding of premature infants. A comparison of human and cow's milk. *Am J Dis Child.* 1947; 73:442-52.

Greer FR. Feeding the premature infant in the 20th century. *J Nutr.* 2001; 131(2): 426S-30S.

Greer FR, McCormick A, Loker J. Changes in fat concentration of human milk during delivery by intermittent bolus and continuous mechanical pump infusion. *J Pediatr.* 1984; 105(5):745-49.

Griffin IJ. Postdischarge nutrition for high risk neonates. *Clin Perinatol.* 2002; 29(2):327-44.

Groer MW, Walker WA. What is the role of preterm human milk supplement in the host defenses of the preterm infant? Science vs. fiction. *Adv Pediatr.* 1996; 43:335-58.

Gross SJ. Growth and biochemical response of preterm infants fed human milk or modified infant formula. *N Engl J Med.* 1983; 308(5):237-41.

Gross SJ, Buckley RH, Wakil SS, McAllister DC, David RJ, Faix RG. Elevated IgA concentration in milk produced by mothers delivered of preterm infants. *J Pediatr.* 1981a; 99(3):389-93.

Gross SJ, David RJ, Bauman L, Tomarelli RM. Nutritional composition of milk produced by mothers delivering preterm. *J Pediatr.* 1980; 96(4):641-44.

Gross SJ, Geller J, Tomarelli RM. Composition of breast milk from mothers of preterm infants. *Pediatrics.* 1981b; 68(4):490-93.

Guthrie SO, Gordon PV, Thomas V, Thorp JA, Peabody J, Clark RH. Necrotizing enterocolitis among neonates in the United States. *J Perinatol,* 2003; 23(4):278-85.

Hagan R, French N, Evans S, Al E. Breast feeding, distractibility and IQ in very preterm infants. *Pediatr Res.* 1996; 39:266A.

Hall RT. Nutritional follow-up of the breastfeeding premature infant after hospital discharge. *Pediatr Clin North Am.* 2001; 48(2):453-60.

Hall RT, Simon S, Smith MT. Readmission of breastfed infants in the first 2 weeks of life. *J Perinatol.* 2000; 20(7):432-37.

Hallman M, Bry K, Hoppu K, Lappi M, Pohjavuori M. Inositol supplementation in premature infants with respiratory distress syndrome. *N Engl J Med.* 1992; 326(19):1233-39.

Hamilton BE, Minino AM, Martin JA, Kochanek KD, Strobino DM, Guyer B. Annual summary of vital statistics: 2005. *Pediatrics.* 2007; 119(2):345-60.

Hamprecht K, Goelz R, Maschmann J. Breast milk and cytomegalovirus infection in preterm infants. *Early Hum Dev.* 2005; 81(12):989-96.

Hamprecht K, Maschmann J, Vochem M, Dietz K, Speer CP, Jahn G. Epidemiology of transmission of cytomegalovirus from mother to preterm infant by breastfeeding. *Lancet.* 2001; 357(9255):513-18.

Hart S, Boylan LM, Carroll S, Musick YA, Lampe RM. Brief report: breast-fed one-week-olds demonstrate superior neurobehavioral organization. *J Pediatr Psychol.* 2003; 28(8):529-34.

Hay WW. *Neonatal Nutrition and Metabolism.* St Louis: Mosby Year Book; 1991.

Hay WW, Lucas A, Heird WC, Ziegler EE, Levin E, Grave GD, *et al.* Workshop summary: Nutrition of the extremely low birth weight infant. *Pediatrics.* 1999; 104(6):1360-68.

Hess J. *Premature and congenitally diseased infants.* Philadelphia: Lea & Febiger; 1922.

Hess J, Lundeen E. *The premature infant. Its medical and nursing care.* Philadelphia: JB Lippincott; 1941.

Hill PD, Aldag JC, Chatterton RT, Jr. Breastfeeding experience and milk weight in lactating mothers pumping for preterm infants. *Birth,* 1999; 26(4):233-38.

Hill PD, Ledbetter RJ, Kavanaugh KL. Breastfeeding patterns of low-birth-weight infants after hospital discharge. *J Obstet Gynecol Neonatal Nurs.* 1997; 26(2):189-97.

Horne RS, Parslow PM, Ferens D, Watts AM, Adamson TM. Comparison of evoked arousability in breast and formula fed infants. *Arch Dis Child.* 2004; 89(1):22-25.

Human Milk Banking Association of North America. *Best practice for expressing, storing and handling human milk in hospitals, homes and child care settings.* Raleigh: Human Milk Banking Association of North America; 2005.

Humenick SS, Hill PD, Spiegelberg PL. Breastfeeding and health professional encouragement. *J Hum Lact.* 1998; 14(4):305-10.

Hurst N, Meier P, Engstrom J. Milk volume consumed at breast during the first month post-discharge (PDC) for preterm infants (PT): Implications for management of breastfeeding and infant growth. *Pediatr Res.* 2000; 47:197A.

Hurst NM, Myatt A, Schanler RJ. Growth and development of a hospital-based lactation program and mother's own milk bank. *J Obstet Gynecol Neonatal Nurs.* 1998; 27(5):503-10.

Hylander MA, Strobino DM, Pezzullo JC, Dhanireddy R. Association of human milk feedings with a reduction in retinopathy of prematurity among very low birthweight infants. *J Perinatol.* 2001; 21(6):356-62.

IBFAN. Brazil leads the world in human milk banks. *IBFAN INFO.* 2001; 3(4):5.

Ibrahim HM, Jeroudi MA, Baier RJ, Dhanireddy R, Krouskop RW. Aggressive early total parental nutrition in low-birth-weight infants. *J Perinatol.* 2004; 24(8):482-86.

Institute of Medicine. *Preterm birth: causes, consequences, and prevention.* Washington, DC: Institute of Medicine; 2006.

Iwanaga M, Zaitsu M, Ishii E, Nishimura Y, Inada S, Yoshiki H, Okinami S, *et al.* Protein-losing gastroenteropathy and retinitis associated with cytomegalovirus infection in an immunocompetent infant: a case report. *Eur J Pediatr.* 2004; 163(2):81-84.

Jacobson SW, Chiodo LM, Jacobson JL. Breastfeeding effects on intelligence quotient in 4- and 11-year-old children. *Pediatrics.* 1999; 103(5):e71.

Jacobson SW, Jacobson JL. Breastfeeding and intelligence. *Lancet.* 1992; 339(8798):926.

James P. Marabou 2005: Nutrition and human development. *Nutr Rev.* 2006; 64(5 Pt 2):S1-11; discussion S72-91.

Jim WT, Shu CH, Chiu NC, Kao HA, Hung HY, Chang JH, *et al.* Transmission of cytomegalovirus from mothers to preterm infants by breast milk. *Pediatr Infect Dis J.* 2004; 23(9):848-51.

Jocson MAL, Mason EO, Schanler RJ. The effects of nutrient fortification and varying storage conditions on host defense properties of human milk. *Pediatrics.* 1997; 100:240-43.

Jones E. Strategies to promote preterm breastfeeding. *Mod Midwife.* 1995; 5(3):8-11.

Jones E, Dimmock PW, Spencer SA. A randomised controlled trial to compare methods of milk expression after preterm delivery. *Arch Dis Child Fetal Neonatal Ed.* 2001; 85(2):F91-95.

Jones F. History of North American donor milk banking: one hundred years of progress. *J Hum Lact.* 2003; 19(3):313-18.

Kajantie E, Phillips DI, Andersson S, Barker DJ, Dunkel L, Forsen T, *et al.* Size at birth, gestational age and cortisol secretion in adult life: foetal programming of both hyper- and hypocortisolism? *Clin Endocrinol (Oxf).* 2002; 57(5):635-41.

Kamitsuka MD, Horton MK, Williams MA. The incidence of necrotizing enterocolitis after introducing standardized feeding schedules for infants between 1250 and 2500 grams and less than 35 weeks of gestation. *Pediatrics.* 2000; 105(2):379-84.

Kashyap S, Schulze KF, Forsyth M, Dell RB, Ramakrishnan R, Heird WC. Growth, nutrient retention, and metabolic response of low-birth-weight infants fed supplemented and unsupplemented preterm human milk. *Am J Clin Nutr.* 1990; 52(2):254-62.

Kavanaugh K, Meier P, Zimmermann B, Mead L. The rewards outweigh the efforts: breastfeeding outcomes for mothers of preterm infants. *J Hum Lact.* 1997; 13(1):15-21.

Kay JL. Classification of newborns - based on maturity and intrauterine growth LB 146 REV 1/07. Evansville, IN: Mead Johnson Nutritionals; 1999. Available from: http://www.meadjohnson.com/professional/pdf/LB146REV_11_99.pdf.. Accessed 6/1/07.

Kerner Jr JA. Chapter 57: Parenteral nutrition. In: Walker W, Watkins J, Duggan C (eds.). *Nutirion in pediatrics: Basic science and clinical applications.* 3rd Ed. Hamilton,Ontario: BC Decker Inc.; 2003. p. 957-85.

Kerrey BT, Morrow A, Geraghty S, Huey N, Sapsford A, Schleiss MR. Breast milk as a source for acquisition of cytomegalovirus (HCMV) in a premature infant with sepsis syndrome: detection by real-time PCR. *J Clin Virol.* 2006; 35(3):313-16.

King C, Jones E. The benefits of human milk for the preterm baby. In: King C, Jones E (eds.). *Feeding and nutrition in the preterm infant.* Edinburgh: Elsevier; 2005. p. 1-13.

Kitajima H, Sumida Y, Tanaka R, *et al.* Early administration of Bifidobacterium breve to preterm infants: randomised controlled trial. *Arch Dis Child.* 1997; 76: F101-7.

Kleinman RE, Walker WA. The enteromammary immune system: an important new concept in breast milk host defense. *Dig Dis Sci.* 1979; 24(11):876-82.

Kliegman RM, Pittard WB, Fanaroff AA. Necrotizing enterocolitis in neonates fed human milk. *J Pediatr.* 1979; 95(3):450 53.

Kling PJ. Roles of erythropoietin in human milk. *Acta Paediatr Suppl.* 2002; 91(438):31-35.

Kling PJ, Sullivan TM, Roberts RA, Philipps AF, Koldovsky O. Human milk as a potential enteral source of erythropoietin. *Pediatr Res.* 1998; 43(2):216-21.

Koenig WJ, Amarnath RP, Hench V, Berseth CL. Manometrics for preterm and term infants: a new tool for old questions. *Pediatrics.* 1995; 95:203-6.

Kumar A, Pant P, Basu S, Rao GR, Khanna HD. Oxidative stress in neonatal hyperbilirubinemia. *J Trop Pediatr.* 2007; 53(1):69-71.

Kuschel CA, Evans N, Askie L, Bredemeyer S, Nash J, Polverino J. A randomized trial of enteral feeding volumes in infants born before 30 weeks' gestation. *J Paediatr Child Health.* 2000; 36(6):581-86.

Kuschel CA, Harding JE. Multicomponent fortified human milk for promoting growth in preterm infants. *Cochrane Database Syst Rev.* 2004; (1): CD000343.

Kuzma-O'Reilly B, Duenas ML, Greecher C, Kimberlin L, Mujsce D, Miller D, *et al.* Evaluation, development, and implementation of potentially better practices in neonatal intensive care nutrition. *Pediatrics.* 2003; 111(4 Pt 2): e461-70.

La Gamma EF, Browne LE. Feeding practices for infants weighing less than 1500 G at birth and the pathogenesis of necrotizing enterocolitis. *Clin Perinatol.* 1994; 21(2):271-306.

Labbok MH. Effects of breastfeeding on the mother. *Pediatr Clin NA.* 2001; 48(1):143-58.

Land HM, Rouster-Stevens K, Woods CR, *et al.* Lactobacillus sepsis associated with probiotic therapy. *Pediatrics.* 2005; 116:517-18.

Lau C. Oral feeding in the preterm infant. *NeoReviews.* 2006; 7(1): e19-e27. Accessed September 2, 2006.

Lau C, Hurst N. Oral feeding in infants. *Curr Probl Pediatr.* 1999; 29(4):105-24.

Lau C, Sheena HR, Shulman RJ, Schanler RJ. Oral feeding in low birth weight infants. *J Pediatr.* 1997; 130(4):561-69.

Lawrence RA. Storage of human milk and the influence of procedures on immunological components of human milk. *Acta Paediatr Suppl.* 1999; 88(430):14-18.

Lawrence RA, Lawrence RM. *Breastfeeding: A guide for the medical profession.* 6th Ed. St. Louis, MO: Elsevier/Mosby; 2005a.

Lawrence RA, Lawrence RM. Chapt 14: Breastfeeding the premature infant. In: Lawrence RA, Lawrence RM (eds.). *Breastfeeding: A guide for the medical profession.* 6th Ed. St. Louis, MO: Elsevier/Mosby; 2005b.

Lawrence RM. Chapter 5: Host-resistance factors and immunologic significance of human milk. In: Lawrence RA, Lawrence RM (eds.). *Breastfeeding: A guide for the medical profession.* Philadelphia: Elsevier-Mosby; 2005. p. 171-214.

Lefebvre F, Ducharme M. Incidence and duration of lactation and lactational performance among mothers of low-birth-weight and term infants. *Can Med Assoc J.* 1989; 140(10):1159-64.

Lepage G, Collet S, Bougle D, Kien LC, Lepage D, Dallaire L, *et al.* The composition of preterm milk in relation to the degree of prematurity. *Am J Clin Nutr.* 1984; 40(5):1042-49.

Li R, Darling N, Maurice E, Barler L, Grummer-Strawn L. Breastfeeding rates in the United States by characteristics of the child, mother, or family: the 2002 National Immunization Survey. *Pediatrics.* 2005; 115(1):e31-37.

Lindemann PC, Foshaugen I, Lindemann R. Characteristics of breast milk and serology of women donating breast milk to a milk bank. *Arch Dis Child Fetal Neonatal Ed.* 2004; 89: F440-41.

Lucas A. Does early diet program future outcome? *Acta Paediatr Scand Suppl.* 1990; 365:58-67.

Lucas A. The developmental origins of adult health and well-being. *Adv Exp Med Biol.* 2005a; 569:13-15.

Lucas A. Long-term programming effects of early nutrition -- implications for the preterm infant. *J Perinatol.* 2005b; 25 Suppl 2:S2-6.

Lucas A, Baker B. Breast milk jaundice in premature infants. *Arch Dis Child.* 1986; 61:1063-67.

Lucas A, Bishop N, King F, Cole T. Randomized trial of nutrition for preterm infants after discharge. *Arch Dis Child.* 1992a; 67:324-27.

Lucas A, Brooke OG, Baker BA, Bishop N, Morley R. High alkaline phosphatase activity and growth in preterm neonates. *Arch Dis Child.* 1989; 64(7 Spec No):902-9.

Lucas A, Brooke OG, Morley R, Cole TJ, Bamford MF. Early diet of preterm infants and development of allergic or atopic disease: randomised prospective study. *BMJ.* 1990; 300(6728):837-40.

Lucas A, Cole TJ. Breast milk and neonatal necrotising enterocolitis. *Lancet.* 1990; 336:1519-23.

Lucas A, Fewtrell MS, Morley R, Lucas PJ, Baker BA, Lister G, *et al.* Randomized outcome trial of human milk fortification and developmental outcome in preterm infants. *Am J Clin Nutr.* 1996; 64(2):142-51.

Lucas A, Morley R, Cole TJ. Randomised trial of early diet in preterm babies and later intelligence quotient. *BMJ.* 1998; 317(7171):1481-87.

Lucas A, Morley R, Cole TJ, Gore SM. A randomised multicentre study of human milk versus formula and later development in preterm infants. *Arch Dis Child Fetal Neonatal Ed.* 1994; 70(2):F141-46.

Lucas A, Morley R, Cole TJ, Lister G, Leeson-Payne C. Breast milk and subsequent intelligence quotient in children born preterm. *Lancet.* 1992b; 339(8788):261-64.

Lundeen E, Kunstadter R. *Care of the premature infant.* Philadelphia: JB Lippincott; 1958.

Luukkainen P, Salo MK, Nikkari T. The fatty acid composition of banked human milk and infant formulas: the choices of milk for feeding preterm infants. *Eur J Pediatr.* 1995; 154(4):316-19.

Mancuso C, Pani G, Calabrese V. Bilirubin: an endogenous scavenger of nitric oxide and reactive nitrogen species. *Redox Rep.* 2006; 11(5):207-13.

Martin CR, Walker WA. Intestinal immune defences and the inflammatory response in necrotising enterocolitis. *Semin Fetal Neonatal Med.* 2006; 11(5):369-77.

Martin J, Hamilton BE, Sutton PD, Ventura SJ, Menacker F, Munson ML. Births: Final data for 2003. In: Centers for Disease Control and Prevention. *National vital statistics reports.* Vol. 54. Atlanta: Centers for Disease Control and Prevention; 2005. p. 17.

Martinez FE, Desai ID. Human milk and premature infants. *World Rev Nutr Diet.* 1995; 78:55-73.

Maschmann J, Hamprecht K, Dietz K, Jahn G, Speer CP. Cytomegalovirus infection of extremely low-birth weight infants via breast milk. *Clin Infect Dis.* 2001; 33(12):1998-2003.

Maschmann J, Hamprecht K, Weissbrich B, Dietz, K, Jahn G, Speer CP. Freeze-thawing of breast milk does not prevent cytomegalovirus transmission to a preterm infant. *Arch Dis Child Fetal Neonatal Ed.* 2006; 91(4):F288-90.

McClure RJ, Newell SJ. Effect of fortifying breast milk on gastric emptying. *Arch Dis Child.* 1996; 74:F60-62.

McClure RJ, Newell SJ. Randomised controlled trial of trophic feeding and gut motility. *Arch Dis Child.* 1999; 80:F54-58.

McGuire W, Anthony MY. Donor human milk versus formula for preventing necrotising enterocolitis in preterm infants: systematic review. *Arch Dis Child Fetal Neonatal Ed.* 2003; 88(1):F11-14.

McPherson RJ, Wagner CL. The effect of pasteurization on transforming growth factor alpha and transforming growth factor beta 2 concentrations in human milk. *Adv Exp Med Biol.* 2001; 501:559-66.

Medoff-Cooper B. Multi-system approach to the assessment of successful feeding. *Acta Paediatr.* 2000; 89(4):393-94.

Mehta NR, Hamosh M, Bitman J, Wood DL. Adherence of medium-chain fatty acids to feeding tubes during gavage feeding of human milk fortified with medium-chain triglycerides. *J Pediatr.* 1988; 112(3):474-76.

Meier J, Lienicke U, Tschirch E, Kruger DH, Wauer RR, Prosch S. Human cytomegalovirus reactivation during lactation and mother-to-child transmission in preterm infants. *J Clin Microbiol.* 2005; 43(3):1318-24.

Meier P. Supporting lactation in mothers with very low birth weight infants. *Pediatric Annals.* 2003; 32(5):317-25.

Meier P, Engstrom J, Spanier-Mingolelli S, *et al.* Dose of own mothers' milk provided by low-income and non-low income mothers of very low birthweight infants (abstract). *Pediatr Res.* 2000a; 47:292A.

Meier PP. Breastfeeding in the special care nursery. Prematures and infants with medical problems. *Pediatr Clin North Am.* 2001; 48(2):425-42.

Meier PP, Brown LP, Hurst NM, Spatz DL, Engstrom JL, Borucki LC, *et al.* Nipple shields for preterm infants: effect on milk transfer and duration of breastfeeding. *J Hum Lact.* 2000b; 16(2):106-14.

Meier PP, Engstrom JL, Crichton CL, Clark DR, Williams MM, Mangurten HH. A new scale for in-home test-weighing for mothers of preterm and high risk infants. *J Hum Lact.* 1994; 10(3):163-68.

Meier PP, Engstrom JL, Mangurten HH, Estrada E, Zimmerman B, Kopparthi R. Breastfeeding support services in the neonatal intensive-care unit. *J Obstet Gynecol Neonatal Nurs.* 1993; 22(4):338-47.

Meier PP, Engstrom JL, Mingolelli SS, Miracle DJ, Kiesling S. The Rush Mothers' Milk Club: breastfeeding interventions for mothers with very-low-birth-weight infants. *J Obstet Gynecol Neonatal Nurs.* 2004; 33(2):164-74.

Merewood A, Brooks D, Bauchner H, MacAuley L, Mehta S. Maternal birthplace and breastfeeding initiation among term and preterm infants: a statewide assessment for Massachusetts. *Pediatrics.* 2006a; 118(4): e1048-54.

Merewood A, Chamberlain LB, Cook JT, Philipp BL, Malone K, Bauchner H. The effect of peer counselors on breastfeeding rates in the neonatal intensive care unit: results of a randomized controlled trial. *Arch Pediatr Adolesc Med.* 2006b; 160(7):681-85.

Merewood A, Philipp BL, Chawla N, Cimo S. The baby-friendly hospital initiative increases breastfeeding rates in a US neonatal intensive care unit. *J Hum Lact.* 2003; 19(2):166-71.

Merhav HJ, Wright HI, Mieles LA, Van Thiel DH. Treatment of IgA deficiency in liver transplant recipients with human breast milk. *Transpl Int,* 1995; 8(4): 327-29.

Miracle DJ, Meier PP, Bennett PA. Mothers' decisions to change from formula to mothers' milk for very-low-birth-weight infants. *J Obstet Gynecol Neonatal Nurs.* 2004; 33(6):692-703.

Miron D, Brosilow S, Felszer K, Reich D, Halle D, Wachtel D, *et al.* Incidence and clinical manifestations of breast milk-acquired Cytomegalovirus infection in low birth weight infants. *J Perinatol.* 2005; 25(5):299-303.

Mitoulas LR, Lai CT, Gurrin LC, Larsson M, Hartmann PE. Effect of vacuum profile on breast milk expression using an electric breast pump. *J Hum Lact.* 2002; 18(4):353-60.

Moody GJ, Schanler RJ, Lau C, Shulman RJ. Feeding tolerance in premature infants fed fortified human milk. *J Pediatr Gastroenterol Nutr.* 2000; 30(4): 408-12.

Morgan MA, el-Ghany el-SM, Khalifa NA, Sherif A, Rasslan LR. Prevalence of cytomegalovirus (CMV) infection among neonatal intensive care unit (NICU) and healthcare workers. *Egypt J Immunol.* 2003; 10(2):1-8.

Moritz ML, Manole MD, Bogen DL, Ayus JC. Breastfeeding-associated hypernatremia: are we missing the diagnosis? *Pediatrics.* 2005; 116(3):e343-47.

Morley R. Breast feeding and cognitive outcome in children born prematurely. *Adv Exp Med Biol.* 2002; 503:77-82.

Morley R, Cole TJ, Powell R, Lucas A. Mother's choice to provide breast milk and developmental outcome. *Arch Dis Child.* 1988; 63(11):1382-85.

Morley R, Lucas A. Randomized diet in the neonatal period and growth performance until 7.5-8 yr of age in preterm children. *Am J Clin Nutr.* 2000; 71(3):822-28.

Morton J, Hall JY, Thairu L Nomanbhoy S, Bhutani R, Carlson S, *et al.* Breast massage maximizes milk volumes of pump-dependent mothers. Abstr#444. Pediatric Academic Societies Meeting. Toronto, CA. May 5-8, 2007b.

Morton J, Hall JY, Thairu L, Nomanbhoy S, Carlson S, Wong RJ, Rhine WD. Early hand expression affects breastmilk production in pump-dependent mothers of preterm infants. Abstr # 7720.9. Pediatric Academic Societies Meeting. Toronto, Canada. May 5-8, 2007.

Moya FR, Eguchi H, Zhao B, Furukawa M, Sfeir J, Osorio M, *et al.* Platelet-activating factor acetylhydrolase in term and preterm human milk: a preliminary report. *J Pediatr Gastroenterol Nutr.* 1994; 19(2):236-39.

Mussi-Pinhata MM, Yamamoto AY, do Carmo Rego MA, Pinto PC, da Motta MS, Calixto C. Perinatal or early-postnatal cytomegalovirus infection in preterm infants under 34 weeks gestation born to CMV-seropositive mothers within a high-seroprevalence population. *J Pediatr.* 2004; 145(5):685-88.

Narayanan I, Mehta R, Choudhury DK, Jain BK. Sucking on the 'emptied' breast: non-nutritive sucking with a difference. *Arch Dis Child.* 1991;66(2):241-4.

Narayanan I, Prakash K, Bala S, Verma RK, Gujral VV. Partial supplementation with expressed breast-milk for prevention of infection in low-birth-weight infants. *Lancet.* 1980; 2(8194):561-63.

Narayanan I, Prakash K, Gujral VV. The value of human milk in the prevention of infection in the high-risk low-birth-weight infant. *J Pediatr.* 1981; 99(3):496-98.

Narayanan I, Prakash K, Murthy NS, Gujral VV. Randomised controlled trial of effect of raw and holder pasteurised human milk and of formula supplements on incidence of neonatal infection. *Lancet.* 1984a; 2(8412):1111-13.

Narayanan I, Prakash K, Prabhakar AK, Gujral VV. A planned prospective evaluation of the anti-infective property of varying quantities of expressed human milk. *Acta Paediatr Scand.* 1982; 71(3):441-45.

Narayanan I, Singh B, Harvey D. Fat loss during feeding of human milk. *Arch Dis Child.* 1984b; 59(5):475-77.

Neifert M. Prevention of breastfeeding tragedies. *Pediatr Clin NA.* 2001; 48(2):273-97.

Neuberger P, Hamprecht K, Vochem M, Maschmann J, Speer CP, Jahn G, *et al.* Case-control study of symptoms and neonatal outcome of human milk-transmitted cytomegalovirus infection in premature infants. *J Pediatr.* 2006; 148(3):326-31.

Newell SJ. Enteral feeding of the micropremie. *Clin Perinato.* 2000; 27(1):221-34.

Nyqvist K. Breastfeeding support in neonatal care: An example of the integration of international evidence and experience. *Newborn & Infant Nursing Reviews.* 2005; 5(1):34-48.

Nyqvist KH, Sjoden PO, Ewald U. The development of preterm infants' breastfeeding behavior. *Early Hum Dev.* 1999; 55(3):247-64.

O'Connor DL, Jacobs J, Hall R, Adamkin D, Auestad N, Castillo M, *et al.* Growth and development of premature infants fed predominantly human milk, predominantly premature infant formula, or a combination of human milk and premature formula. *J Pediatr Gastroenterol Nutr.* 2003; 37(4):437-46.

Ogra PL, Rassin DK. Chapter 4: Human breast milk. In: Remington JS. *Infectious diseases of the fetus and newborn infant.* 4th Ed. Philadelphia: WB Saunders; 1995.

Ogundele MO. Effects of storage on the physicochemical and antibacterial properties of human milk. *Br J Biomed Sci.* 2002; 59(4):205-11.

Olsen IE, Richardson DK, Schmid CH, Ausman LM, Dwyer JT. Dietitian involvement in the neonatal intensive care unit: More is better. *J Am Diet Assoc.* 2005; 105(8):1224-30.

Olver WJ, Bond DW, Boswell TC, Watkin SL. Neonatal group B streptococcal disease associated with infected breast milk. *Arch Dis Child Fetal Neonatal Ed.* 2000; 83(1):F48-49.

Orloff SL, Wallingford JC, McDougal JS. Inactivation of human immunodeficiency virus type I in human milk: effects of intrinsic factors in human milk and of pasteurization. *J Hum Lact.* 1993; 9(1):13-17.

Osmond C, Barker DJ. Fetal, infant, and childhood growth are predictors of coronary heart disease, diabetes, and hypertension in adult men and women. *Environ Health Perspect.* 2000; 108(Suppl 3): 545-53.

Ovali F, Ciftci I, Cetinkaya Z, Bukulmez A. Effects of human milk fortifier on the antimicrobial properties of human milk. *J Perinatol.* 2006; 26(12):761-63.

Patole S, McGlone L, Muller R. Virtual elimination of necrotising enterocolitis for 5 years - reasons? *Med*

Hypotheses. 2003; 61(5-6):617-22.

Pauls J, Bauer K, Versmold H. Postnatal body weight curves for infants below 1000 g birth weight receiving early enteral and parenteral nutrition. *Eur J Pediatr.* 1998; 157(5):416-21.

Payanikli P, *et al.* Hindmilk feeding in VLBW infants. *Pediatric Academic Societies.* Abstract # 2526 & # 2194. 2004.

Penders J, Thijs C, Vink C, Stelma FF, Snijders B, Kummeling I, *et al.* Factors influencing the composition of the intestinal microbiota in early infancy. *Pediatrics.* 2006; 118(2):511-21.

Pettifor JM, Rajah R, Venter A, Moodley GP, Opperman L, Cavaleros M, *et al.* Bone mineralization and mineral homeostasis in very low-birth-weight infants fed either human milk or fortified human milk. *J Pediatr Gastroenterol Nutr.* 1989; 8(2):217-24.

Pinelli J, Symington A. Non-nutritive sucking for promoting physiologic stability and nutrition in preterm infants. *Cochrane Database Syst Rev.* 2005; (4): CD001071.

Pisacane A, Graziano L, Mazzarella G, Scarpellino B, Zona G. Breast-feeding and urinary tract infection. *J Pediatr.* 1992; 120(1): 87-89.

Pitt J, Barlow B, Heird WC. Protection against experimental necrotizing enterocolitis by maternal milk. I. Role of milk leukocytes. *Pediatr Res.* 1977; 11(8):906-9.

Polberger SK, Axelsson IE, Raiha NC. Urinary and serum urea as indicators of protein metabolism in very low birthweight infants fed varying human milk protein intakes. *Acta Paediatr Scand.* 1990; 79(8-9):737-42.

Pollock JI. Mother's choice to provide breast milk and developmental outcome. *Arch Dis Child.* 1989; 64(5):763-64.

Porcelli Jr PJ, Sisk PM. Increased parenteral amino acid administration to extremely low-birth-weight infants during early postnatal life. *J Pediatr Gastroenterol Nutr.* 2002; 34(2):174-79.

Quan R, Yang C, Rubinstein S, Lewiston NJ, Stevenson DK, Kerner Jr A. The effect of nutritional additives on anti-infective factors in human milk. *Clin Pediatr (Phila).* 1994; 33(6):325-28.

Quan R, Yang C, Rubinstein S, Lewiston NJ, Sunshine P, Stevenson DK, *et al.* Effects of microwave radiation on anti-infective factors in human milk. *Pediatrics.* 1992; 89(4 Pt 1):667-69.

Raisler J. Promoting breast-feeding among vulnerable women. *J Nurse Midwifery.* 1993; 38(1):1-4.

Rangecroft L, de San Lazaro C, Scott J. A comparison of the feeding of the post-operative newborn with banked breastmilk or cow's milk feeds. *J Pediatr Surg.* 1978; 13:11-12.

Reber KM, Nankervis CA. Necrotizing enterocolitis: preventative strategies. *Clin Perinatol.* 2004; 31(1):157-67.

Regan F, Cutfield W, Jefferies C, Robinson E, Hofman P. The impact of early nutrition in premature infants on later childhood insulin sensitivity and growth. *Pediatrics.* 2006; 118(5):1943-49.

Reinert do Nascimento M, Issler H. Breastfeeding the premature infant: Experience of a baby-friendly hospital in Brazil. *J Hum Lact.* 2005; 21(1):47-52.

Rey J. Breastfeeding and cognitive development. *Acta Paediatr.* 2003; 92 (suppl.):11-18.

Riddell D. Use of banked human milk for feeding infants with abdominal wall defects. In: *Annual Meeting of the Human Milk Banking Association of North America.* Vancouver, BC, Canada; Oct 15. 1989.

Rigo J, Senterre J. Nutritional needs of premature infants: Current issues. *J Pediatr.* 2006; 149(5):S80-88.

Rinne M, Kalliomaki M, Arvilommi H, Salminen S, Isolauri E. Effect of probiotics and breastfeeding on the Bifidobacterium and Lactobacillus/Enterococcus microbiota and humoral immune responses. *J Pediatr.* 2005; 147:186-91.

Rodriguez NA, Caplan MS. Oropharyngeal administration of own mother's colostrum (OMC) during the first days of life: Effects on immune function of extremely low birth weight (ELBW; BW < 100g) infants - A pilot study. In: *APS/SPR/PAS.* Abstract # 3850.10; April 29-May 2, 2006.

Ronnestad A, Abrahamsen TG, Medbo S, Reigstad H, Lossius K, Kaaresen PI, *et al.* Late-onset septicemia in a Norwegian national cohort of extremely premature infants receiving very early full human milk feeding. *Pediatrics.* 2005; 115(3):e269-76.

Roy RN, Chance GW, Radde IC, Hill DE, Willis DM, Sheepers J. Late hyponatremia in very low birthweight infants (less than 1.3 kilograms). *Pediatr Res.* 1976; 10(5):526-31.

Rubaltelli FF, Biadaioli R, Pecile P, Nicoletti P. Intestinal flora in breast- and bottle-fed infants. *J Perinat Med.* 1998; 26(3):186-91.

Rubin L, Richardson D, Bodarek F, McCormick M. Growth in hospital of VLBW infants. Identification of patient characteristics and inter-NICU differences. *Pediatr Res.* 1997; 41:Abstract 239A.

Ryan A, Wenjun Z, Acosta A. Breastfeeding continues to increase into the new millenium. *Pediatrics.* 2002; 110:1103-9.

Sacker A, Quigley MA, Kelley YJ. Breastfeeding and developmental delay: Findings from the Millennium Cohort Study. *Pediatrics.* 2006; 118(3): e682-89.

Saini J, MacMahon P, Morgan JB, Kovar IZ. Early parenteral feeding of amino acids. *Arch Dis Child.* 1989; 64(10 Spec No):1362-66.

Sann L, Bienvenu F, Lahet C, Bienvenu J, Bethenod M. Comparison of the composition of breast milk from mothers of term and preterm infants. *Acta Paediatr Scand.* 1981; 70(1):115-16.

Santiago MS, Codipilly CN, Potak DC, Schanler RJ. Effect of human milk fortifiers on bacterial growth in human milk. *J Perinatol.* 2005; 25(10):647-49.

Santulli TV, Schullinger JN, Heird WC, Gongaware RD, Wigger J, Barlow B, *et al.* Acute necrotizing enterocolitis in infancy: a review of 64 cases. *Pediatrics.* 1975; 55(3):376-87.

Scanlon K, Alexander M, Serdula M, Davis MK, Bowman BA. Assessment of infant feeding: the validity of measuring milk intake. *Nutr Rev.* 2002; 60(8):235-51.

Schanler R, Burns P, Abrams S, Garza C. Bone mineralization outcomes in human milk-fed preterm infants. *Pediatr Res.* 1992; 31(6):583-86.

Schanler RJ. Fortified human milk: nature's way to feed premature infants. *J Hum Lact.* 1998; 14(1):5-11.

Schanler RJ. The use of human milk for premature infants. *Pediatr Clin North Am.* 2001; 48(1):207-19.

Schanler RJ. Chapter 28: The low birth weight infant. In: Walker W, Watkins J, Duggan C (eds.). *Nutrition in pediatrics: Basic science and clinical applications.* 3rd Ed. Hamilton, Ontario: BC Decker, Inc; 2003. p. 491-514.

Schanler RJ. CMV acquisition in premature infants fed human milk: reason to worry? *J Perinatol.* 2005a; 25(5):297-98.

Schanler RJ. Human milk supplementation for preterm infants. *Acta Paediatr.* 2005b; 94(Suppl 449):64-67.

Schanler RJ. Post-discharge nutrition for the preterm infant. *Acta Paediatr.* 2005c; 94(*Suppl* 449):68-73.

Schanler RJ. Probiotics and necrotising enterocolitis in premature infants. *Arch Dis Child Fetal Neonatal Ed.* 2006; 91:F395-97.

Schanler RJ, Atkinson SA. Effects of nutrients in human milk on the recipient premature infant. *J Mammary Gland Biol Neoplasia.* 1999; 4(3):297-307.

Schanler RJ, Garza C. Improved mineral balance in very low birth weight infants fed fortified human milk. *J. Pediatr.* 1987; 112:452-56.

Schanler RJ, Garza C, Nichols BL. Fortified mothers' milk for very low birth weight infants: results of growth and nutrient balance studies. *J Pediatr,* 1985; 107(3):437-45.

Schanler RJ, Goldblum RM, Garza C, Goldman AS. Enhanced fecal excretion of selected immune factors in very low birth weight infants fed fortified human milk. *Pediatr Res.* 1986; 20(8):711-15.

Schanler RJ, Hurst NM, Lau C. The use of human milk and breastfeeding in premature infants. *Clin Perinatol.* 1999a; 26(2):379-98.

Schanler RJ, Lau C, Hurst NM, Smith EO. Randomized trial of donor human milk versus preterm formula as substitutes for mothers' own milk in the feeding of extremely premature infants. *Pediatrics.* 2005; 116(2):400-6.

Schanler RJ, Oh W. Composition of breast milk obtained from mothers of premature infants as compared to breast milk obtained from donors. *J Pediatr.* 1980; 96(4):679-81.

Schanler RJ, Oh W. Nitrogen and mineral balance in preterm infants fed human milk or formula. *J Pediatr. Gastroenterol Nutr.* 1985; 4:214-19.

Schanler RJ, Shulman RJ, Lau C. Feeding strategies for premature infants: beneficial outcomes of feeding fortified human milk versus preterm formula. *Pediatrics.* 1999b; 103(6 Pt 1):1150-57.

Schleiss MR. Acquisition of human cytomegalovirus infection in infants via breast milk: natural immunization or cause for concern? *Rev Med Virol.* 2006a; 16(2):73-82.

Schleiss MR. Role of breast milk in acquisition of cytomegalovirus infection: recent advances. *Curr Opin Pediatr.* 2006b; 18(1):48-52.

Schmidt E. Effects of varying degrees of heat treatment on milk protein and its nutritional consequences. *Acta Paediatr Scand Suppl.* 1982; 296:41-43.

Semba RD, Juul SE. Erythropoietin in human milk: physiology and role in infant health. *J Hum Lact.* 2002; 18(3):252-61.

Sharland M, Khare M, Bedford-Russell A. Prevention of postnatal cytomegalovirus infection in preterm infants. *Arch Dis Child Fetal Neonatal Ed.* 2002; 86(2):F140.

Shoji H, Shimizu T, Shinohara K, Oguchi S, Shiga S, Yamashiro Y. Suppressive effects of breast milk on oxidative DNA damage in very low birthweight infants. *Arch Dis Child Fetal Neonatal Ed.* 2004; 89:F136-38.

Shulman RJ, Schanler RJ, Lau C, Heitkemper M, Ou CN, Smith EO. Early feeding, feeding tolerance, and lactase activity in preterm infants. *J Pediatr.* 1998; 133(5):645-49.

Siddell EP, Froman RD. A national survey of neonatal intensive-care units: criteria used to determine readiness for oral feedings. *J Obstet Gynecol Neonatal Nurs.* 1994; 23(9):783-89.

Singhal A. Early nutrition and long-term cardiovascular health. *Nutr Rev.* 2006; 64(5 Pt 2):S44-9; discussion S72-91.

Singhal A, Cole TJ, Fewtrell M, Kennedy K, Stephenson T, Elias-Jones A, *et al.* Promotion of faster weight gain in infants born small for gestational age: is there an adverse effect on later blood pressure? *Circulation.* 2007; 115(2):213-20.

Singhal A, Cole TJ, Fewtrell M, Lucas A. Breastmilk feeding and lipoprotein profile in adolescents born preterm: follow-up of a prospective randomised study. *Lancet.* 2004; 363(9421):1571-78.

Singhal A, Cole TJ, Lucas A. Early nutrition in preterm infants and later blood pressure: two cohorts after randomised trials. *Lancet,* 2001; 357(9254): 413-19.

Sisk PM, Lovelady CA, Dillard RG. Effect of education and lactation support on maternal decision to provide human milk for very-low-birth-weight infants. *Adv Exp Med Biol.* 2004; 554:307-11.

Sisk PM, Lovelady CA, Dillard RG, Gruber KJ. Lactation counseling for mothers of very low birth weight infants: effect on maternal anxiety and infant intake of human milk. *Pediatrics.* 2006; 117(1):e67-75.

Smith MM, Durkin M, Hinton VJ, Bellinger D, Kuhn L. Influence of breastfeeding on cognitive outcomes at age 6-8 years: follow-up of very low birth weight infants. *Am J Epidemiol.* 2003a; 158(11):1075-82.

Smith MM, Durkin M, Hinton VJ, Bellinger D, Kuhn L. Initiation of breastfeeding among mothers of very low birth weight infants. *Pediatrics.* 2003b; 111(6 Pt 1):1337-42.

Soskolne E, Schumacher R, Fyock C, Young ML, Schork A. The effect of early discharge and other factors on readmission rates of newborns. *Arch Pediatr Adolesc Med.* 1996; 150:373-79.

Spatz DL. State of the science: use of human milk and breastfeeding for vulnerable infants. *J Perinat Neonatal Nurs.* 2006; 20(1):51-55.

Srinivasan L, Bokiniec R, King C, Weaver G, Edwards AD. Increased osmolality of breast milk with therapeutic additives. *Arch Dis Child Fetal Neonatal Ed.* 2004; 89(6): F514-17.

Stein H, Cohen D, Herman AA, Rissik J, Ellis U, Bolton K, *et al.* Pooled pasteurized breast milk and untreated own mother's milk in the feeding of very low birth weight babies: a randomized controlled trial. *J Pediatr Gastroenterol Nutr.* 1986; 5(2):242-47.

Stockman III JA, deAlarcon PA. Chapter 134: Hematopoiesis and granulopoiesis. In: Polin RA, Fox WW (eds.). *Fetal and neonatal physiology.* Philadelphia: WB Saunders; 1992.

Stocks RJ, Davies DP, Allen F, Sewell D. Loss of breast milk nutrients during tube feeding. *Arch Dis Child.* 1985; 60(2):164-66.

Tarcan A, Tiker F, Vatandas NS, Haberal A, Gurakan B. Weight loss and hypernatremia in breast-fed babies: frequency in neonates with non-hemolytic jaundice. *J Paediatr Child Health.* 2005; 41(9-10):484-87.

Telang S, Berseth CL, Ferguson PW, Kinder JM, DeRoin M, Petschow BW. Fortifying fresh human milk with commercial powdered human milk fortifiers does not affect bacterial growth during 6 hours at room temperature. *J Am Diet Assoc.* 2005; 105(10):1567-72.

Thureen PJ, Melara D, Fennessey PV, Hay Jr WW. Effect of low versus high intravenous amino acid intake on very low birth weight infants in the early neonatal period. *Pediatr Res.* 2003; 53(1):24-32.

Tomashek KM, Shapiro-Mendoza CK, Weiss J, Kotelchuck M, Barfield W, Evans S, *et al.* Early discharge among late preterm and term newborns and risk of neonatal morbidity. *Semin Perinatol.* 2006; 30(2):61-68.

Tsang RC, Lucas A, Uauy R, Zlotkin S (eds.). *Nutritional needs of the preterm infant: Scientific basis and practical guidelines.* Baltimore: Williams & Wilkins; 1993.

Tully DB, Jones F, Tully MR. Donor milk: what's in it and what's not. *J Hum Lact.* 2001; 17(2):152-55.

Tully MR. Banked human milk and the treatment of IgA deficiency and allergy symptoms. *J Hum Lact.* 1990; 6(2):75.

Tyson JE, Kennedy KA. Minimal enteral nutrition for promoting feeding tolerance and preventing morbidity in parenterally fed infants. *Cochrane Database Syst Rev.* 2000; (2):CD000504.

Tyson JE, Lasky RE, Mize CE, Richards CJ, Blair-Smith N, Whyte R, *et al.* Growth, metabolic response and development in very low birth weight infants fed banked human milk or enriched formula: 1. Neonatal findings. *J. Pediatr.* 1983; 103:95-104.

Uauy RD, Birch DG, Birch EE, Tyson JE, Hoffman DR. Effect of dietary omega-3 fatty acids on retinal function of very-low-birth-weight neonates. *Pediatr Res,* 1990; 28(5):485-92.

Udipi SA, Kirksey A, West K, Giacoia G. Vitamin B6, vitamin C and folacin levels in milk from mothers of term and preterm infants during the neonatal period. *Am J Clin Nutr.* 1985; 42(3):522-30.

Underwood MA, Sherman MP. Nutritional characteristics of amniotic fluid. *NeoReviews.* 2006; 7(6):e310-16.

Updegrove K. Human milk banking in the United States. *Newborn Infant Nurs Rev.* 2005; 5(1):27-33.

Uraizee F, Gross SJ. Improved feeding tolerance and reduced incidence of sepsis in sick very low birth weight (VLBW) infants fed maternal milk. *Pediatr Res.* 1989; 25:298A.

Valentine C, Hurst N, Schanler R. Hindmilk improves weight gain in low-birth-weight infants fed human milk. *J Pediatr Gastroenterol Nutr.* 1994; 18(4): 474-77.

Valentine C, Schanler R. Neonatal nutritionist intervention improves nutrition support and promotes cost containment in the management of LBW infants. *J Parenter Enteral Nutr.* 1993; Suppl 46:466.

Van Zoeren-Grobben D, Schrijver J, Van den Berg H, Berger HM. Human milk vitamin content after pasteurisation, storage, or tube feeding. *Arch Dis Child.* 1987; 62(2):161-65.

Vochem M, Hamprecht K, Jahn G, Speer CP. Transmission of cytomegalovirus to preterm infants through breast milk. *Pediatr Infect Dis J.* 1998; 17(1): 53-58.

Vohr BR, Poindexter BB, Dusick AM, McKinley LT, Wright LL, Langer JC, *et al.* Beneficial effects of breast milk in the neonatal intensive care unit on the developmental outcome of extremely low birth weight infants at 18 months of age. *Pediatrics.* 2006; 118(1): e115-23.

Vollmer B, Seibold-Weiger K, Schmitz-Salue C, Hamprecht K, Goelz R., Krageloh-Mann I, *et al.* Postnatally acquired cytomegalovirus infection via breast milk: effects on hearing and development in preterm infants. *Pediatr Infect Dis J.* 2004; 23(4):322-27.

Walker WA. The dynamic effects of breastfeeding on intestinal development and host defense. *Adv Exp Med Biol.* 2004; 554:155-70.

Wang M, Dorer D, Flemming M, Catlin E. Clinical outcomes of near-term infants. *Pediatrics.* 2004; 114(2):372-76.

Waterland RA. Epigenetic mechanisms and gastrointestinal development. *J Pediatr.* 2006; 149(5):S137-42.

Wauben IP, Atkinson SA, Grad TL, Shah JK, Paes B. Moderate nutrient supplementation of mother's milk for preterm infants supports adequate bone mass and short-term growth: a randomized, controlled trial. *Am J Clin Nutr.* 1998; 67(3):465-72.

Weimer J. *The economic benefits of breastfeeding: A review and analysis.* Food and Rural Economics Division, Economic Research Service, US Dept. of Agriculture. Food Assistance and Nutrition Research Report No. 13. 2001. Available from: www.ers.usda.gov/publications/fanrr13/.

Welsh JK, May JT. Anti-infective properties of breast milk. *J Pediatr.* 1979; 94(1): 1-9.

WHO/UNICEF. WHO/UNICEF joint statement, meeting on infant and young child feeding. *J Nurse-Midwifery.* 1980; 25:31-38.

Wiggins PK, Arnold LD. Clinical case history: donor milk use for severe gastroesophageal reflux in an adult. *J Hum Lact.* 1998; 14(2):157-59.

Wight N, Montgomery A.) Use of galactogogues in initiating or maintaining maternal milk supply (protocol #9). *Academy of Breastfeeding Medicine*; 2004.

Wight NE. Commentary: Donor human milk for preterm infants. *J. Perinatol*, 2001a; 21:249-54.

Wight NE. Management of common breastfeeding issues. *Pediatr Clin North Am.* 2001b; 48(2):321-44.

Wight NE. Breastfeeding the borderline (near-term) preterm infant. *Pediatr Ann.* 2003a; 32(5):329-36.

Wight NE. Neonatologists' attitudes and practice on the use of mother's own and pasteurized donor human milk in the NICU. *Academy of Breastfeeding Medicine News and Views.* 2003b; 9(4):32-33; Abstract P21.

Wight NE. NICU donor milk statistics 2004-2005. Personal communication: 2006.

Willeitner A. Transmission of cytomegalovirus (CMV) through human milk: are new breastfeeding policies required for preterm infants? *Adv Exp Med Biol.* 2004; 554:489-94.

Williamson S, Finucane E, Ellis H, Gamsu HR. Effect of heat treatment of human milk on absorption of nitrogen, fat, sodium, calcium, and phosphorus by preterm infants. *Arch Dis Child.* 1978a; 53(7):555-63.

Williamson S, Hewitt JH, Finucane E, Gamsu HR. Organisation of bank of raw and pasteurised human milk for neonatal intensive care. *Br Med J.* 1978b; 1(6110):393-96.

Wilson DC, Cairns P, Halliday HL, Reid M, McClure G, Dodge JA. Randomised controlled trial of an aggressive nutritional regimen in sick very low birthweight infants. *Arch Dis Child Fetal Neonatal Ed.* 1997; 77(1):F4-11.

Winikoff B, Laukaran VH, Myers D, Stone R. Dynamics of infant feeding: mothers, professionals, and the institutional context in a large urban hospital. *Pediatrics.* 1986; 77(3):357-65.

Winikoff B, Myers D, Laukaran VH, Stone R. Overcoming obstacles to breast-feeding in a large municipal hospital: applications of lessons learned. *Pediatrics.* 1987; 80(3):423-33.

Wooldridge J, Hall W. Posthospitalization breastfeeding patterns of moderately preterm infants. *J Perinat Neonat Nurs.* 2003; 17(1):50-64.

World Health Organization. *WHO child growth standards: methods & development.* Geneva: World Health Organization; 2006. Available from: http://www.who.int/childgrowth/en/.

World Health Organization and UNICEF. *global strategy for infant and young child feeding.* Geneva: World Health Organization; 2003. Available from: http://whqlibdoc.who.int/publications/2003/9241562218.pdf.

Worrell L, Thorp J, Tucker R, McKinley LT, Chen J, Chng YM, *et al.* The effects of the introduction of a high-nutrient transitional formula on growth and development of very-low-birth-weight infants. *J Perinatol.* 2002; 22:112-19.

Yamato K, Taguchi H, Yoshimoto S, Fujishita M, Yamashita M, Ohtsuki Y, *et al.* Inactivation of lymphocyte-transforming activity of human T-cell leukemia virus type I by heat. *Jpn J Cancer Res.* 1986; 77(1):13-15.

Yasuda A, Kimura H, Hayakawa M, Ohshiro M, Kato Y, Matsuura O, *et al.* Evaluation of cytomegalovirus infections transmitted via breast milk in preterm infants with a real-time polymerase chain reaction assay. *Pediatrics.* 2003; 111(6 Pt 1):1333-36.

Yu VY, Jamieson J, Bajuk B. Breast milk feeding in very low birthweight infants. *Aust Paediatr J.* 1981; 17(3):186-90.

Ziegler EE, Thureen PJ, Carlson SJ. Aggressive nutrition of the very low birthweight infant. *Clin Perinatol.* 2002; 29(2):225-44.

Chapter 13

Hyperbilirubinemia and Breastfeeding

Lawrence M. Gartner

INTRODUCTION

Increased serum bilirubin (hyperbilirubinemia) in excess of the adult upper range of normal of 1.5 mg/dl is a normal and regular phenomenon in nearly all infants during the early weeks of life and is usually identified as physiologic jaundice of the newborn (Clarkson *et al.*, 1984; Gartner *et al.*, 1977). In most healthy *breastfed* infants, this phenomenon is prolonged for two to 15 weeks of life and is known as *breastmilk jaundice* (Gartner & Arias, 1966; Gartner & Herschel, 2001). This prolongation of unconjugated hyperbilirubinemia (indirect-reacting bilirubin) in the breastfed infant is believed to be of benefit to the young infant by providing a potent antioxidant (bilirubin) at a time of life when other antioxidants are deficient. The phenomenon of *breastmilk jaundice* must be distinguished from abnormal exaggeration of unconjugated hyperbilirubinemia seen occasionally in breastfed infants who have inadequate intake of milk, known as *starvation jaundice of the newborn* (DeCarvalho *et al.*, 1982; Kuhr & Paneth, 1982; Yamauchi & Yamanouchi, 1990; Barrett, 1971; Gronwall & Cornelius, 1970; Gartner *et al.*, 1983). Starvation jaundice may occur as an isolated phenomenon or may be secondary to a pathologic condition, such as sepsis, or any other pathology which reduces caloric intake, including breastfeeding management problems. These two breastfeeding-related conditions must be distinguished from pathologic conditions which cause *increased bilirubin production* (hemolytic syndromes) and inherited disorders of hepatic bilirubin metabolism which prevent clearance of bilirubin from the circulation. In addition, some forms of hyperbilirubinemia are characterized by increased serum concentrations of *conjugated* bilirubin (direct-reacting bilirubin) which usually result from obstruction to biliary drainage or significant disease of the liver parenchyma.

Clinically, all of these disorders are marked by the presence of jaundice or icterus, a yellow discoloration of the skin, mucous membranes, and optic sclerae. It is the appearance of jaundice which usually alerts the clinician to the presence of a potential problem and necessitates clinical and laboratory analyses to determine the cause of the problem and to establish the seriousness of the condition. The time of onset of the jaundice and the level of serum bilirubin will dictate the therapy required, if any.

Concern about the presence of jaundice and hyperbilirubinemia in the newborn is based on the potential for unconjugated bilirubin to enter specific areas of the brain (basal ganglia and cerebellum) and produce permanent loss of critical neurons with moderate to severe life-long neurologic sequelae, known as kernicterus (Hansen & Bratlid, 1986; Volpe, 2001; Van Praagh, 1961; Maisels & Newman, 1995; Ebbesen, 2000). It is the prevention of kernicterus which is paramount in the management of the jaundiced newborn. However, the great majority of jaundiced newborns are not at risk for development of kernicterus. In the case of the breastfed infant with prolonged jaundice, it is essential that states of real risk be distinguished from those of little or no risk, so as not to jeopardize successful breastfeeding (Gartner & Herschel, 2001). The challenge to the clinician is to distinguish levels of risk and to achieve optimal outcomes of both jaundice and breastfeeding.

This chapter will explore the mechanisms of bilirubin metabolism and transport as it occurs in all mammals and the variations which occur in the newborn period without and with breastfeeding. Differential diagnosis, laboratory evaluation, management to prevent brain damage while preserving breastfeeding, and treatment of severe hyperbilirubinemia will be discussed.

BILIRUBIN METABOLISM AND TRANSPORT

Bilirubin Synthesis

Bilirubin is the degradative product of heme, whether from hemoglobin or from other heme compounds, including cytochromes and myoglobin (Figure 1) (Robinson, 1968). Bilirubin has a unique and very specific stereoisomeric structure which makes it virtually insoluble in water at physiologic pH (Bonnett *et al.*, 1978; Brodersen, 1979). When released into the circulation, it is transported in plasma attached to albumin. It also gains entry into red cells and other cells because of the presence of phospholipids in cell membranes. The insolubility of bilirubin requires that it be made water soluble before it can be excreted by the liver.

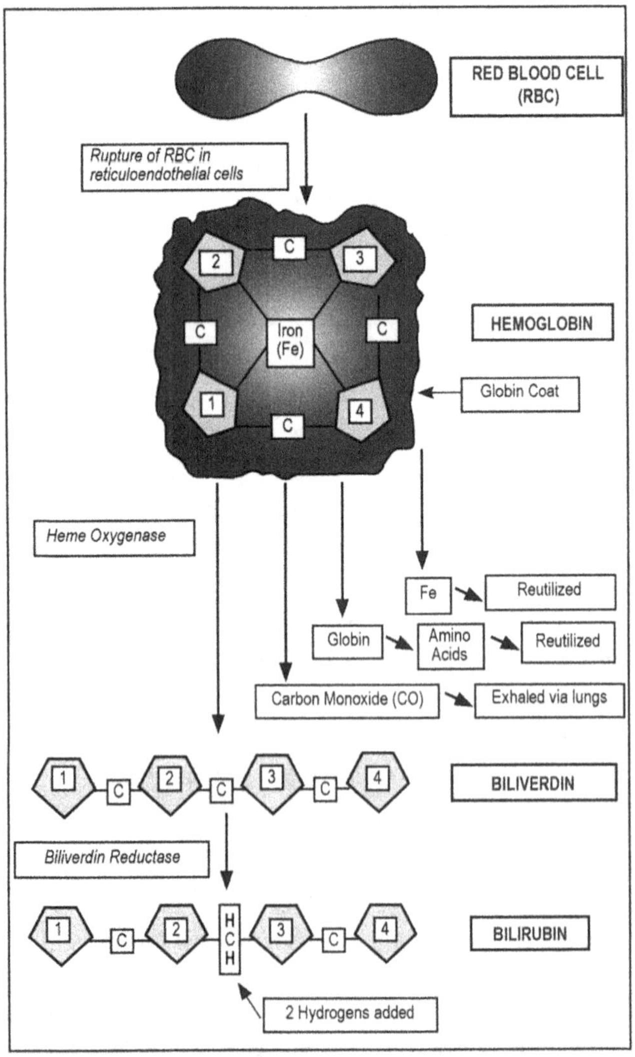

Figure 1. The synthesis of bilirublin from hemoglobin

Bilirubin is yellow-orange in color and its accumulation in skin, mucus membranes, and the sclerae of the eye produces the yellow discoloration known as jaundice or icterus.

While bilirubin is generally considered a final waste product of heme catabolism, the pigment has a biological function as a very effective antioxidant (Baranano *et al.*, 2002). When acting as an antioxidant, it is oxidized to biliverdin, a green pigment. Biliverdin, in turn, is almost instantaneously reduced by the universally available enzyme, *biliverdin reductase*, back to bilirubin. This cyclic oxidation and reduction makes bilirubin a potent antioxidant for neutralization of oxygen free radicals, which, in excess, permanently injure tissues.

The process of bilirubin production from red cells begins with the sequestration of senescent red cells in reticuloendothelial cells adjacent to the capillaries. The enzyme *heme oxygenase* splits the hemoglobin molecule, removing the iron for reuse in erythrocyte synthesis and other metabolic functions, and releases the globin coat for further degradation to amino acids and reutilization (**Figure 1**) (Tenhunen, 1976). The *heme* or pigment component of hemoglobin is a tetrapyrrole, a ring of four pyrrole rings linked by carbon bridges. Heme oxygenase removes only the *alpha* carbon bridge to convert the ring into an open chain of four pyrrole rings known as *biliverdin*, a green, water soluble, non-toxic pigment. In *non*-mammalian species, biliverdin is the final product and is then excreted via the liver into bile (Cornelius & Bruss, 1980). In mammals, however, biliverdin is completely and immediately reduced by *biliverdin reductase* to the insoluble bilirubin 9αZZ. The asymmetry of the side chains and hydrogens on bilirubin 9αZZ is responsible for the folding of the molecule into a globular form, held by intramolecular hydrogen bonds, rendering the molecule insoluble by hiding all

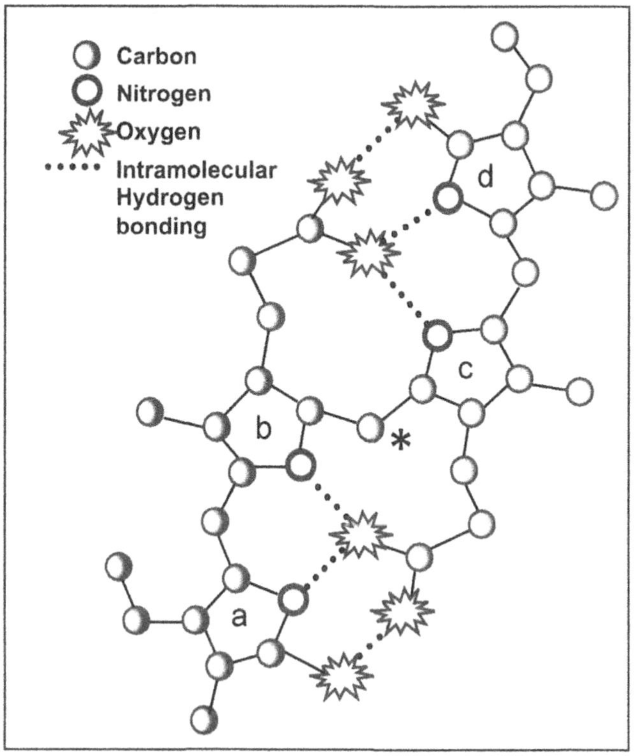

Figure 2. The structure of bilirubin 9αZZ as it occurs in nature as an insoluble molecule held in this globular structure by intramolecule hydrogen bonds (dotted lines) sequestering the polar sites internally. Redrawn from Bonnett *et al.*, 1976.

of the acid and keto side chains inside the structure, preventing these polar side chains from making contact with the aqueous medium (**Figure 2**). Even the slightest alteration of the structure of bilirubin will render it water soluble by preventing intramolecular hydrogen bonding; yet virtually all bilirubin in the body is in the insoluble form.

Bilirubin synthesis is increased many-fold in the normal newborn due to shortened erythrocyte life span, increased blood volume, and increased hemoglobin concentration compared to the older child and adult (Gartner *et al.*, 1977). In addition, a large pool of heme exists within the erythropoietic tissue in the bone marrow, spleen, and liver of the fetus and newborn. At birth, with the rise of blood oxygen saturation, erythropoietin declines precipitously, resulting in arrest of erythropoietic activity. The now inactive erythropoietic tissue is catabolized, converting large quantities of heme to bilirubin. This large production of bilirubin increases the body pool of bilirubin and contributes very significantly to the development of physiologic jaundice of the newborn.

Bilirubin Transport

Insoluble bilirubin 9αZZ is transported in plasma bound predominantly to albumin, with smaller quantities in red cell membranes (Brodersen, 1979). Very small concentrations of unbound bilirubin, known as *free bilirubin*, are also detectable (Ahlfors, 2001). With rising bilirubin concentrations in plasma, tight binding sites on albumin are saturated and the concentration of *free bilirubin* increases. Free bilirubin is believed to be the form of bilirubin which gains access to the brain (Ahlfors, 2000). Newborn albumin binding capacity and affinity are significantly lower than that of older children and adults, potentially increasing the availability of free bilirubin in the circulation. Circulating bilirubin equilibrates with tissues, gradually transferring more and more bilirubin into tissues, as becomes evident with development of cutaneous and scleral icterus. Among all of the solid tissues, the lung has the highest concentration of bilirubin, probably due to its high concentration of phospholipids (surfactants) (Gartner *et al.*, 1977). Certain drugs (sulfisoxazole and benzoate) have been shown to prevent binding of bilirubin to albumin, increasing free bilirubin and the risk of bilirubin entering the brain (Levi *et al.*, 1970).

Hepatic Bilirubin Uptake

The primary function of albumin transport of bilirubin is to bring it to the liver cell membrane where it is transferred across the liver cell membrane into the cytoplasm. In the cytoplasm, it is bound to ligandin for intracellular transport. Developmental limitations in membrane transfer and deficiency in hepatic ligandin in the newborn significantly limit the rate at which bilirubin can be transferred from the circulation into the liver, contributing to the development of physiologic jaundice of the newborn (Levi *et al.*, 1970) (**Figure 3**).

Hepatic Bilirubin Conjugation

Bilirubin can be excreted from the liver into bile only if it is rendered soluble. This is accomplished by adding glucuronic acid, a glucose derivative, to bilirubin through the action of the enzyme *glucuronyl transferase* on the smooth endoplasmic reticulum, a process known as *conjugation*. In adults, two glucuronic acid molecules are added to each bilirubin molecule (bilirubin diglucuronide), but in newborns, only *one* glucuronic acid is attached to bilirubin (bilirubin monoglucuronide).

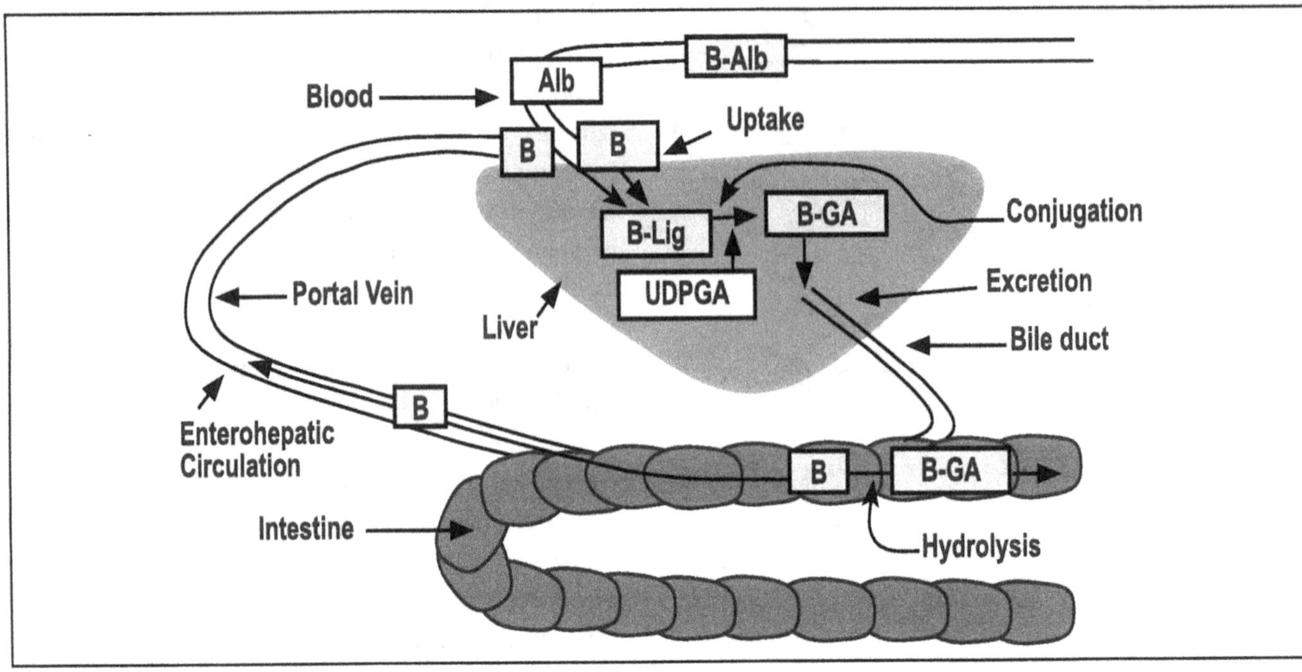

Figure 3. Transport of bilirubin from blood to the intestine. B = bilirubin; Alb = albumin; Lig = ligandin; UDPGA = uridine diphosphoglucuronic acid; GA = glucuronic acid; B-GA = bilirubin glucuronide (conjugated bilirubin or direct-reacting bilirubin). The BILIRUBIN-ALBUMIN complex in the circulation separates at the time of UPTAKE by the liver. The bilirubin then binds to LIGANDIN in the cytoplasm of the hepatocyte and is transported to the smooth endoplasmic reticulum where UDPGA transfers GA to bilirubin under the action of the enzyme, glucuronyl transferase, forming B-GA, also known as conjugated or direct-reacting bilirubin, the water soluble form of bilirubin. EXCRETION from the liver cell into bile is an active transport process moving B-GA into the bile duct and then into the small intestine. A portion of the B-GA is hydrolyzed, returning bilirubin to its prior unconjugated state (B), which is then reabsorbed across the intestinal mucosa to enter the portal circulation, returning to the liver, a process known as the enterohepatic circulation of bilirubin. This recirculated bilirubin then either enters the liver for reprocessing and excretion or it returns to the general circulation contributing to the body burden of bilirubin.

Both forms render the bilirubin water soluble; both are unstable and easily deconjugated, returning bilirubin to the insoluble, unconjugated form. However, the monoglucuronide of the newborn is more easily deconjugated, a factor of some importance in the intestine (Brodersen & Herman, 1963) (**Figure 3**).

Hepatic Bilirubin Excretion

In its conjugated, soluble state, bilirubin can be excreted by the liver into bile by an active transport system which concentrates the pigment in bile. In the normal newborn, hepatic excretion is never the rate limiting step, although it can become rate limiting under pathologic conditions of hepatitis, asphyxia, or massive hemolysis. When hepatic excretion is the rate limiting step, *direct-reacting* serum bilirubin concentrations increase to levels in excess of 1 mg/dl and greater than 10% of total bilirubin (Gartner *et al.*, 1971).

Intestinal Bilirubin Metabolism and Transport

Central to breastfeeding-related jaundice is understanding the behavior of bilirubin in the infant's intestine. Entering the intestine as water soluble bilirubin monoglucuronide, bilirubin rapidly deconjugates to unconjugated and water insoluble bilirubin. This occurs in newborns at a rate far greater than in older children and adults, not only because of the greater instability of the monoglucuronide, but also because the neonatal intestine contains a far higher concentration of the enzyme, *β glucuronidase* (Brodersen & Herman, 1963). Human milk also contains significant quantities of this same enzyme, possibly contributing further to the presence in the newborn intestine of high concentrations of unconjugated, insoluble bilirubin (Gourley & Arend, 1986). Whereas older infants, children, and adults have vast quantities of bacteria in their intestines, including clostridial species which metabolize bilirubin to urobilinogen and stercobilin, the normal brown pigment of stool, newborns have a sterile intestine or only small quantities of bacteria. This allows large quantities of bilirubin to remain in the intestine throughout its passage to the anus. Newborn and young infant stool is not brown, but is yellow, indicating the presence of bilirubin. Although counterintuitive, unconjugated bilirubin is readily absorbed across the entire length of the intestine to be returned to the liver via the portal circulation for re-excretion or distribution in the systemic circulation. This process is known as the *enterohepatic circulation* of bilirubin (Poland & Odell, 1971). In the newborn period, enterohepatic circulation of bilirubin is increased many-fold, contributing greatly to the circulating bilirubin pool and to the body's bilirubin load, adding yet another factor in the development of physiologic jaundice of the newborn (**Figure 3**).

Concept of Physiologic Jaundice of the Newborn

Physiologic jaundice of the newborn is the result of a confluence of factors which increase the load of bilirubin to such a degree that it exceeds the reduced capacity of the liver to metabolize and excrete unconjugated (indirect) bilirubin. As this imbalance in favor of bilirubin retention abates through the diminution in bilirubin synthesis and enterohepatic circulation, along with an increase in hepatic transport and metabolism, physiologic jaundice of the newborn diminishes, eventually achieving serum bilirubin concentrations which are considered the adult normal (Gartner *et al.*, 1977). The serum concentration of bilirubin varies with both chronologic and gestational age of the infant and with the mode of feeding.

PHYSIOLOGIC JAUNDICE OF THE NEWBORN AND PROLONGED PHYSIOLOGIC JAUNDICE (BREASTMILK JAUNDICE)

Serum bilirubin concentrations in newborns with physiologic jaundice of the newborn differ greatly between breastfed and artificially-fed infants after the fifth day of life (Figure 4). In artificially-fed infants, the serum bilirubin concentration falls to the adult normal range of less than 1.5 mg/dl by about the 11th day of life (Gartner *et al.*, 1977). In contrast, the great majority of normal breastfed infants have persistence of serum bilirubin concentrations greater than 1.5 mg/dl for three to, rarely, 15 weeks of life (DeAngelis *et al.*, 1980; Alonso *et al.*, 1991; Gourley *et al.*, 1999; Mauro *et al.*, 2000). While most breastfed infants will have peak serum bilirubin concentrations of less than 10 mg/dl, some will have peak values greater than 10 mg/dl and even as high as 20 to 25 mg/dl in the absence of any apparent pathologic cause. It is suspected that those with the highest values may have inherited disorders of hepatic bilirubin conjugation or mild forms of hemolysis which have not been detected or investigated (Mauro *et al.*, 2000). This pattern of prolonged, unconjugated hyperbilirubinemia in the healthy breastfed infant is called breastmilk jaundice. It is a normal and expected prolongation of physiologic jaundice seen in at least two-thirds of all newborns. Breastmilk jaundice does not begin until the appearance of significant amounts of transitional and mature milk at about the fifth day of life.

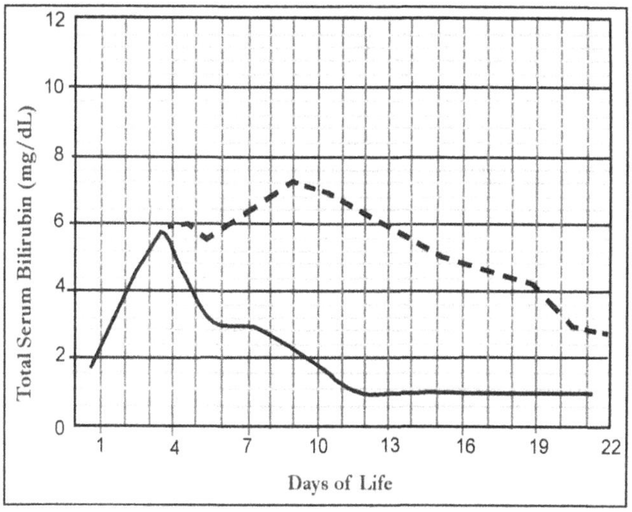

Figure 4. Patterns of physiologic jaundice of the newborn. Normal patterns of physiologic jaundice in the breastfed infant (dashed line) and in the artificially-fed infant. While these are typical patterns, individual infants vary widely in serum bilirubin concentrations and duration of hyperbilirubinemia.

Breastmilk jaundice must be distinguished from other causes of exaggerated and prolonged unconjugated hyperbilirubinemia which may or may not be associated with ingestion of human milk, including inherited disorders of hepatic bilirubin metabolism and hemolytic diseases. However, in those infants with serum bilirubin concentrations below 12 to 14 mg/dl, there is no indication to investigate the cause.

The great majority of mature human milk, unlike cow's milk and infant formulas, increase the intestinal absorption of unconjugated bilirubin, as shown in animal studies (Gartner *et al.*, 1983; Alonso *et al.*, 1991).

Colostrum does not have this effect, accounting for the fact that breastmilk jaundice does not occur in the early days of life (Gartner *et al.*, 1977). The component of human milk responsible for this enhancement of intestinal bilirubin absorption has not be defined, nor is the precise mechanism for transport of bilirubin from the intestinal lumen into the circulation understood. The degree to which human milk increases intestinal absorption of unconjugated bilirubin in animal models correlates closely with the serum bilirubin concentration reached in the infant (Alonso *et al.*, 1991). Interruption of human milk intake for one to two days results in a prompt and rapid decline in serum bilirubin concentration (Gartner & Arias, 1966). Resumption of human milk feeding results in an increase in serum bilirubin concentration or a cessation of serum bilirubin decline. After a period of rising or stable bilirubin concentrations, all infants with breastmilk jaundice have a gradual decline in serum bilirubin to eventually reach adult normal concentrations of less than 1.5 mg/dl without any treatment or interruption of breastfeeding.

Although it has been suggested that the presence of β-glucuronidase in human milk increases the hydrolysis of conjugated bilirubin, facilitating intestinal absorption of unconjugated bilirubin, other studies have indicated that this milk enzyme is not a significant factor since intestinal β-glucuronidase is already present in the infant's intestine in very high concentrations (Ince *et al.*, 1995; La Torre *et al.*, 1999; Yigit *et al.*, 2001).

Supplementation of breastfeeding with cow's milk formula results in an accelerated decline in serum bilirubin because these preparations interfere with intestinal bilirubin absorption (Gartner *et al.*, 1983). Elemental formulas are more effective in this regard than are standard infant formulas (Gourley *et al.*, 1992).

Although it is very rare for serum bilirubin concentrations in full-term infants with breastmilk jaundice alone to reach levels which can cause kernicterus (see below), it is possible that in rare infants breastmilk jaundice could result in brain damage. Therefore, it is advised that infants with breastmilk jaundice and serum bilirubin concentrations in the higher ranges be very carefully monitored, as should be practiced in all infants with significantly elevated serum bilirubin concentrations (American Academy of Pediatrics, 2004). There is no reason to believe that the potential for toxicity from bilirubin elevations due to breastmilk jaundice is any less than from other causes of severe hyperbilirubinemia.

Premature infants, even near term infants, have higher concentrations of serum bilirubin during their period of physiologic jaundice because of the delayed maturation of hepatic bilirubin conjugation and increased bilirubin production due to a shorter red cell lifespan than the term infant. It has been observed that premature infants receiving human milk feeding from their mothers or even from pooled, banked human milk, have slightly higher serum bilirubin concentrations than formula-fed infants for at least the first 50 days of life (Lucas & Baker, 1986). This is similar to that seen in term infants, but may be more prolonged because of the slower maturation of hepatic bilirubin metabolism, especially conjugation, in the premature infant. In contrast to the premature, post-mature infants have been noted to have lower serum bilirubin concentrations and briefer durations of physiologic jaundice because they begin maturation of their hepatic bilirubin transport and metabolic systems in utero (Gartner *et al.*, 1977).

The prolongation of serum unconjugated bilirubin concentrations due to human milk feeding is believed to be beneficial to the infant by providing a very potent antioxidant (bilirubin) at a time when other forms of antioxidants are markedly deficient (Dennery *et al.*, 1995; Baranano *et al.*, 2002; Hammerman *et al.*, 2002).

Breastmilk jaundice does not generally require treatment by interruption of breastfeeding or use of phototherapy unless serum bilirubin rises to potentially toxic levels, which in the full-term, healthy infant is in excess of 20 mg/dl (see section below on management).

STARVATION JAUNDICE OF THE NEWBORN

Starvation jaundice has been recognized in adult humans and animals for many years (Bloomer *et al.*, 1971; White *et al.*, 1981; Whiter & Gollan, 1983). In virtually all humans, serum unconjugated bilirubin concentrations rise to 2 or 3 mg/dl after 24 hours of complete avoidance of all caloric intake, even with ingestion of water to prevent dehydration. The mechanism has been shown in rats to be due to an enhancement of absorption of unconjugated bilirubin from the intestine. In adults with various forms of chronic unconjugated hyperbilirubinemia (Gilbert's Syndrome or mild hemolysis), serum bilirubin concentrations will usually rise more steeply and achieve higher levels during starvation. Newborns denied adequate caloric intake display the same phenomenon, but because of their developmental deficiencies in bilirubin metabolism, starvation usually results in elevations of unconjugated bilirubin which are more dramatic and can even reach levels associated with brain damage (kernicterus) (Maisels & Newman, 1995). During the initiation of breastfeeding, if nursing is not undertaken with sufficient frequency and with adequate increases in milk production and transfer to the infant, increased levels of hyperbilirubinemia are commonly seen (DeCarvalho *et al.*, 1982; Yamauchi & Yamanouchi, 1990). Thus, it is often stated that breastfed infants "normally" have elevated serum unconjugated bilirubin concentrations during the first week of life compared with artificially-fed infants (Schneider, 1986). This is not normal, however, and is a reflection of inadequate breastfeeding practices in most Western medical settings where infants are born. These deficiencies in breastfeeding practices include delays in initiation, insufficient frequency of suckling, poor positioning, and truncation of feeding sessions. Several studies have demonstrated that a breastfeeding frequency of approximately 10 to 12 sessions per day starting on the first day of life results in the lowest serum bilirubin concentrations on the third day of life and prevents early starvation jaundice in normal infants (DeCarvalho *et al.*, Yamauchi & Yamanouchi, 1990; Bertini *et al.*, 2001). Some, but not all, studies have demonstrated an association between weight loss and higher serum bilirubin concentrations (Maisels & Gifford, 1986; Bertini *et al.*, 2001). Populations receiving optimal breastfeeding have weight losses in the first week of life that are no greater than those in artificially-fed infants and also serum bilirubin concentrations that are identical (Bertini *et al.*, 2001).

Rising serum bilirubin concentrations at levels close to the toxic range often cause lethargy and poor feeding in an infant who was previously feeding well. With the reduction in breastfeeding frequency and effectiveness, the infant develops starvation jaundice, resulting in further rise in serum bilirubin concentration and even further reduction in feeding. This vicious cycle of deteriorating breastfeeding can result in bilirubin encephalopathy.

Premature infants have also been shown to manifest starvation jaundice with a negative correlation between serum bilirubin concentrations in the first week of life and total caloric intake, whether from oral or parenteral feeding (Wu *et al.*, 1985).

Starvation jaundice and breastmilk jaundice are two different but related syndromes. They share a similar mechanism in which intestinal bilirubin absorption is increased, although for different reasons. They also have a potential interrelationship in which development of starvation jaundice contributes to exaggeration of later breastmilk jaundice. Starvation jaundice of the newborn results in a progressive increase in the total body pool of bilirubin during the first week of life (or later). As hepatic excretory functions mature and excretion of bilirubin into bile and into the intestine increases, the infant with an exaggerated body burden of bilirubin will also excrete more bilirubin into the intestine. With the appearance of transitional and mature milk containing the factor responsible for breastmilk jaundice and increased intestinal bilirubin absorption, exaggerated intestinal bilirubin absorption occurs, returning larger amounts of bilirubin to the circulation, maintaining or increasing serum bilirubin concentrations and the intensity of jaundice. Thus, poor breastfeeding practices tend to increase the severity and duration of breastmilk jaundice, while optimal breastfeeding practices tend to keep bilirubin levels at lower and safer levels. This interaction of various factors to control serum bilirubin concentrations is also related to the presence of other pathologic phenomena that may be occurring in the infant during the early weeks of life. Hemolysis, internal bleeding, sepsis, and other causes of increased bilirubin synthesis, if coupled with poor breastfeeding practices and starvation, will not only further increase serum bilirubin concentrations in the first week of life, but will contribute to exaggeration of breastmilk jaundice in the later weeks, possibly even to levels requiring therapeutic intervention to prevent toxicity.

DIFFERENTIAL DIAGNOSIS OF JAUNDICE IN THE BREASTFED INFANT

While in most clinical situations of jaundice in the breastfed infant, it can be reasonably assumed that mild to moderate degrees of jaundice and hyperbilirubinemia are physiologic, diagnostic evaluation is generally recommended (Gartner & Lee, 1999; Gartner & Herschel, 2001) with:

- the onset of jaundice in the first 24 hours of life,
- elevations of total serum bilirubin into the high intermediate and high risk zones on the risk nomogram,

- significant family history of jaundice in newborns or older individuals,
- a family history of anemia,
- birth trauma,
- blood group incompatibility isoimmunization,
- prematurity.

Diagnostic investigations are primarily aimed at detecting conditions that are likely to result in progressive increases in bilirubin into the potentially toxic range, especially hemolytic disorders.

Inherited hepatic conjugating deficiencies may be suspected by progressive and otherwise unexplained rises in serum bilirubin, but they can be diagnosed only with genetic testing in specialized laboratories (Kaplan *et al.*, 2003).

The initial diagnostic workup should include infant major blood and Rh type, direct antibody test (Coombs), red blood cell smear for erythrocyte morphology, and a reticulocyte count if anemia is detected. Non-invasive measurement of expired carbon monoxide can be useful in detecting hemolysis, especially when not clinically apparent or detected by routine laboratory studies. If this new instrument is available, it may be useful to measure expired carbon monoxide in all infants with significant jaundice (Bartoletti *et al.*, 1979; Smith *et al.*, 1984).

One of the more frequently associated causes of exaggerated neonatal hyperbilirubinemia and kernicterus is glucose-6-phosphate dehydrogenase (G6PD) deficiency (Kaplan & Hammerman, 2006; Kaplan & Hammerman, 1998). Testing for this relatively common cause of hemolysis is indicated in all infants with otherwise unexplained unconjugated hyperbilirubinemia in the high ranges. The relatively high incidence of G6PD deficiency has also led to the recommendation that breastfeeding mothers avoid ingestion of fava beans and the rare medications that can precipitate hemolysis in G6PD deficient infants, since chemical components in these products can be transferred to the infant in the milk (Kaplan *et al.*, 1998; American Academy of Pediatrics, 2005). More elaborate testing for other inherited hemolytic conditions may be indicated in some rare situations, especially with a strong suspicion based on family history. There are more than 50 known red cell enzyme deficiencies associated with exaggerated neonatal jaundice.

Internal bleeding, including cephalhematoma and subgaleal hemorrhage, are the equivalent of hemolysis since extravasated erythrocytes will be rapidly metabolized to bilirubin. One gram of hemoglobin produces 37 mg of bilirubin. Even modest hemorrhage, which may not be apparent as anemia or a declining hemoglobin concentration, can produce significant increases in serum bilirubin. Many cases of kernicterus have been reported in association with such internal bleeding (Newman *et al.*, 2000). Bruising and subcutaneous bluish discoloration, especially on the head, neck, and around the ears should alert the clinician to this possibility.

Congenital thyroid deficiency is a recognized cause of early and exaggerated jaundice in the newborn (Weldon & Danks, 1972). Thyroid hormone measurements may be indicated in otherwise unexplained cases of more severe unconjugated hyperbilirubinemia and in those jaundiced infants with a family history of thyroid disease. Breastfed infants are protected from thyroid hormone deficiency to a significant degree by the absorption of thyroid hormone, a normal component in human milk (Bode *et al.*, 1978). In the breastfed infant, congenital thyroid deficiency may not become clinically apparent until partial or complete weaning.

Although sepsis and other bacterial infections can be a cause of hemolysis and increasing serum unconjugated bilirubin concentrations, in the absence of clinical evidence of infection, white blood cell counts and differentials, blood cultures, and lumbar punctures for examination of spinal fluid are generally not revealing.

Close monitoring of serum bilirubin concentrations with either serum determinations or transcutaneous measurements is recommended in these same high risk groups because pathologic states often produce the highest and most dangerous serum bilirubin concentrations (American Academy of Pediatrics, 2004).

Although both the pathologic disorders and the physiologic states we are considering here are almost always associated with serum unconjugated hyperbilirubinemia, on rare occasions, significant liver disease (e.g., hepatitis, biliary atresia), sepsis, or severe metabolic disturbance, which initially presents as unconjugated hyperbilirubinemia, can subsequently present as conjugated or direct-reacting hyperbilirubinemia (Whitington & Gartner, 1993). Therefore, the initial diagnostic workup should include not only a *total* serum bilirubin, but also a direct-reacting fraction. With persistence of significantly elevated serum bilirubin concentrations, it is best to repeat this periodically, including later in the newborn period if jaundice and hyperbilirubinemia persist into the end of the first month of life and beyond. This is particularly important in the early detection of biliary atresia, which may be amenable to surgical correction if detected in its earliest stages.

BILIRUBIN ENCEPHALOPATHY AND KERNICTERUS

The great attention paid to jaundice in the newborn and to measurement of serum bilirubin concentrations is due to the risk of development of a form of brain damage known as bilirubin encephalopathy and kernicterus under certain conditions (Volpe, 2001; Van Praagh, 1961; Harris *et al.*, 2001). The term bilirubin encephalopathy will be used for the acute or onset stages of bilirubin-related brain damage, while kernicterus will be reserved for the chronic or permanent sequelae of bilirubin-related brain injury. In recent years, between 80 and 90 percent of all infants with kernicterus had been breastfed (Ip *et al.*, 2004). Breastfeeding is the single most frequent risk factor for kernicterus. In most cases of kernicterus, the breastfeeding was either not proceeding well and had not been corrected or there were additional factors (e.g., hemolysis, internal bleeding) causing jaundice.

Bilirubin is prevented from entering cells of the central nervous system by both its tight binding to albumin in the circulation and its inability to readily cross the blood-brain barrier. When serum unconjugated bilirubin rises to concentrations at which it exceeds the tight binding capacity of albumin, the concentration of free or unbound bilirubin increases in the plasma. Free unconjugated bilirubin can then traverse the vascular barrier into the brain. The blood-brain barrier normally provides some protection against the entry of bilirubin, but appears to be more penetrable in the newborn infant, particularly the premature, and also under conditions which may damage the barrier, such as hypoxia (Hansen & Bratlid, 1986; Cashore, 1988; Brodersen, 1980; Wennberg & Hance, 1986). Administration of some anesthetic agents have also been associated with sudden development of kernicterus, possibly by altering the blood-brain barrier. Each mole of serum albumin in the adult and older child is able to tightly bind 2 moles of bilirubin. In the newborn, however, the affinity of albumin for bilirubin is weaker and its capacity reduced (Lee & Gartner, 1978). Adult albumin can tightly bind approximately 40 to 50 mg/dl of bilirubin, but newborn albumin is usually capable of only 20 to 30 mg/dl of tight binding. Therefore, the risk of development of bilirubin encephalopathy is significantly greater in the newborn period than it is in the older child or adult. At extremely high serum bilirubin concentrations (>40 mg/dl), usually only seen in individuals with inherited defects in hepatic conjugation (Crigler-Najjar Syndrome) or severe hemolysis, kernicterus has occurred in adults (Wolkoff *et al.*, 1979; Waser *et al.*, 1986). In premature infants, especially in those with low serum albumin concentrations, the risk of kernicterus is greater at even lower serum bilirubin concentrations than 20 mg/dl. Sepsis and other severe metabolic derangements increase the risk of developing kernicterus, even at serum bilirubin concentrations less than 10 mg/dl.

Conjugated bilirubin, which is more polar and water soluble, does not cross the blood-brain barrier and does not enter neurons. Only unconjugated bilirubin is responsible for the development of kernicterus. However, conjugated and unconjugated bilirubin share the same binding sites on albumin. Therefore, a high level of conjugated bilirubin in plasma may reduce the binding capacity of albumin for unconjugated bilirubin.

Certain drugs may also prevent the binding of bilirubin to albumin. Sulfisoxazole (Gantrisin), an antibiotic, and benzyl alcohol and its metabolite, benzoic acid, a preservative in intravenous fluids, have been associated with a high risk of kernicterus due to interference with albumin binding of bilirubin (Anderson *et al.*, 1956; Odell *et al.*, 1969; Jardine & Rogers, 1989). These agents should never be administered in the perinatal period to either mothers or to newborns.

The entry of small amounts of unconjugated bilirubin into neurons is normally dealt with by the cell by excretion or oxidative metabolism. If the amounts entering the cell are in excess of what it can handle, then cell death ensues. The precise mechanism of this toxicity is unknown. Only certain regions of the brain are susceptible to this injury, however. The basal ganglia of the cerebral hemispheres and the cerebellar hemispheres are the regions susceptible to bilirubin damage, although the reason for their susceptibility is unknown. Inner ear and auditory nuclei may also be damaged. The cerebral cortex is not involved. At autopsy, in those infants who have died during the acute phases of bilirubin encephalopathy, yellow staining will be seen grossly in the affected areas. After a period of time, bilirubin will

Table 1. Risk Factors for Potentially Toxic Bilirubin Concentrations

Major	Minor
Physical Examination	
Cephalohematoma Bruising Jaundice in first 24 hours of life	Jaundice prior to hospital discharge Macrosomia (? maternal diabetes) Male
History	
Sibling required phototherapy or other treatment for jaundice East Asian race Parent with jaundice (Gilbert's, etc.)	Gestational age less than 38 wks Jaundice in sibling Maternal age greater than 25 years
Hematology	
Glucose-6-Phosphate Dehydrogenase (G6PD) deficiency Blood group incompatibility (DAT Positive; Rh, ABO, other)	
Laboratory	
Bilirubin in high risk zone	Bilirubin in high intermediate risk zone
Breastfeeding	
Significant breastfeeding problems	Exclusive breastfeeding
Other	
Bacterial infection	Delayed passage of meconium

no longer be detected in those areas. Magnetic resonance imaging (MRI) demonstrates abnormalities in the basal ganglia and cerebellum which are diagnostic of bilirubin encephalopathy (Okumura *et al.*, 2006). The brain lesions are fixed and non-progressive, but the evidence of the damage evolves over time as the brain matures and potential functions are expressed.

The clinical manifestations of bilirubin encephalopathy occur in three major stages (Volpe, 2001). The first stage (stage 1) is the least specific and is generally characterized by development of lethargy and poor feeding. After a period of some hours, stage 2 begins with the infant developing an opisthotonic posture (backward arching of the neck and spine), extension of the arms and legs with increased muscle tone and rigidity, a high pitched cry, and refusal of all feeding. Seizures may also appear at this time or shortly thereafter. If no treatment is started, the child may succumb at this stage. With modern intensive care and specific treatment, nearly all infants survive, although once stage 2 has appeared, complete reversal of damage is extremely unlikely. Within one or two days, these extreme motor abnormalities disappear and for several months the infant may be considered to be normal. In many of these infants, hearing screening will reveal deafness. In the latter part of the first year of life, it begins to become apparent that the child's development is not proceeding normally and the manifestations of impending choreoathetoid cerebral palsy and deafness become apparent. Over the next year, the child will have varying degrees of disability which may include the classical writhing movements of the extremities and inability to perform controlled movements, failure to sit, stand, and walk, spasticity of the extremities with rigidity and contractures, dysarthria with inability to speak and/or swallow, and neurosensory deafness which also interferes with development of speech. In the more severe forms of kernicterus, the child may have to be fed by gastric tube. The range of severity of the sequelae of bilirubin encephalopathy is large, with some children only having mild hearing loss, others may only have the motor manifestations, but many have the complete severe set of handicaps. In nearly all cases of pure bilirubin encephalopathy, cognitive capacity appears to be normal, although it is extremely difficult to test these children because of their sensory and expressive disabilities. They also usually retain their social skills to a remarkable degree. Their lifespan is usually quite long since they have normal respiratory, intestinal, cardiac, and renal functions.

MANAGEMENT OF JAUNDICE AND HYPERBILIRUBINEMIA IN THE BREASTFED INFANT

Prevention

Since bilirubin encephalopathy is almost always irreversible once stage 2 has developed, preventive management of jaundice is essential. The principles of preventive management (American Academy of Pediatrics, 2004) include:

1) recognition of development of jaundice at the earliest time;
2) close monitoring of the infant both clinically and with serum or transcutaneous bilirubin determinations;
3) identification of all factors increasing the risk of severe hyperbilirubinemia and bilirubin encephalopathy (**Table 1**);
4) defining the total serum bilirubin concentrations at which each management step will be implemented well in advance;
5) preparing to administer management changes and treatment promptly since time is of the essence; and
6) maintaining optimal breastfeeding during and after acute management periods to the greatest degree possible.

Optimal initiation and support of exclusive breastfeeding with frequent, effective feedings and good caloric intake will prevent starvation jaundice. Prompt recognition and correction of problems with breastfeeding will avoid reduced milk intake. This will not only prevent early excessive increases in serum bilirubin, but will also minimize serum bilirubin concentrations after the first week of life when breastmilk jaundice normally appears. Even in the face of factors which may result in excessive hyperbilirubinemia, such as RH, ABO, or other hemolytic states, breastfeeding should be continued since there is no evidence that breastmilk increases the risk of hemolysis or the serum bilirubin concentration.

Routine pre-breastfeeding or supplemental administration of water, glucose water, or formula is contraindicated (American Academy of Pediatrics, 2004). Water and glucose water will not prevent hyperbilirubinemia or decrease total serum bilirubin concentrations and may increase serum bilirubin concentrations due to inhibition of breastfeeding frequency and milk transfer with resulting reduced caloric intake.

Monitoring of Jaundice in a Breastfeeding Infant

The reader is advised to review the Clinical Practice Guideline of the American Academy of Pediatrics

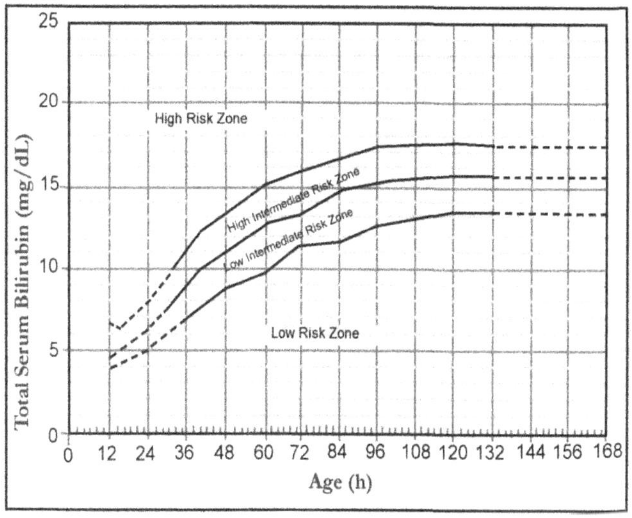

Figure 5. Nomogram for plotting neonatal total serum bilirubin concentrations to predict later serum bilirubin concentrations. From Bhutani *et al.*, 1999. Reproduced with permission by the AAP.

(AAP) entitled "*Management of Hyperbilirubinemia in the Newborn Infant 35 or more Weeks of Gestation*" (American Academy of Pediatrics, 2004). The first principle of this AAP guideline is to "Promote and support successful breastfeeding." The following recommendations are only those directly related to breastfeeding. For other guidelines and recommendations, the reader is pointed to the AAP guideline and other sources (American Academy of Pediatrics, 2004).

At the time of the recommended formal evaluation of breastfeeding to be done twice each day during the postpartum period, the observer should also examine the newborn carefully for evidence of clinical jaundice, which usually begins on the face and progresses caudally. This examination of the undressed infant is best done in daylight at the window or in a very well lit environment. The extent and degree of jaundice should be recorded in the infant's medical record.

Any jaundice which appears during the first 24 hours of life requires a prompt serum or transcutaneous bilirubin determination. Repeat determinations should be done at least once a day thereafter or more often if clinical jaundice is progressing. Total serum bilirubin values should be plotted on the nomogram (**Figure 5**) to determine the anticipated severity and to observe the rate of rise.

The appearance of jaundice *after* 24 hours, if extending below the head, requires a bilirubin determination and appropriate follow-up determinations as clinically indicated. With rapidly rising serum bilirubin concentrations, determinations may have to be performed every 4 to 6 hours.

A direct-reacting bilirubin fraction in serum should be determined at least once during the first days of life.

Prior to discharge, every infant should have a formal risk assessment for clinical factors which may increase the likelihood of severe hyperbilirubinemia in the near future (**Table 1**). Formal risk assessment should be performed at any time when there is a significant increase in serum bilirubin concentration. Breastfeeding, if not optimal, is one of the risk factors listed in the AAP guidelines (American Academy of Pediatrics, 2004). Weight loss from birth of more than 7% should also alert the clinician to the possibility of less than optimal breastfeeding and the need for more extensive study of the breastfeeding process with subsequent correction of problems. The degree of risk determines the frequency of serum bilirubin determinations, the intensity of preparation for treatment, and the time after discharge from the hospital that the infant should be scheduled for a return visit.

No breastfeeding infant and mother should be discharged from the hospital until it has been determined that breastfeeding is proceeding optimally. The great majority of breastfed infants who subsequently developed bilirubin encephalopathy had deterioration of their breastfeeding after discharge from the hospital, but there often was uncertainty about the breastfeeding *before* discharge.

Prior to discharge, parents should be given instruction about the possibility of the infant developing jaundice, both in the near future and later. With the use of color photographs and other visual aids, they should be instructed in recognition of jaundice and how it progresses. They should be told to call their physician immediately upon noticing the development or worsening of jaundice. Upon receipt of such a call, the physician or the office staff should instruct the parents to bring the child to the office or hospital without further delay. Parents can not be relied upon to evaluate the severity or extent of jaundice.

All infants, whether breastfeeding or not, should be scheduled for a visit with a knowledgeable, licensed health care provider during the period from three to five days of age (American Academy of Pediatrics, 2004; American Academy of Pediatrics, 2005). If discharged before 24 hours of age, this first visit should be no later than 72 hours of age. In addition, higher risk infants, especially if jaundiced at discharge, should be given the shortest time for the first visit, often the next day. During this first visit, the examiner should assess the presence, severity, and extent of jaundice. If there is any concern about the severity or extent of the jaundice, a serum or transcutaneous bilirubin should be determined promptly and plotted on the nomogram. The infant should be weighed and percent weight loss from birth and from discharge should be calculated. A breastfeeding session should be observed by the examiner with formal evaluation of position, latch, and milk transfer (American Academy of Pediatrics, 2005). Depending on the serum bilirubin value and the age of the infant, a repeat visit and serum bilirubin determination may be indicated, as well as a diagnostic workup. The mother should be encouraged to continue breastfeeding and any breastfeeding problems should be addressed. If serum bilirubin concentrations continue to rise, bilirubin determinations either by serum or transcutaneous route should be repeated until stable or declining. Availability of transcutaneous bilirubin technology is encouraged because it will facilitate repeat determinations with less concern about pain to the infant.

For the breastfed infant who is losing weight in excess of normal expectations and who is jaundiced, the first step in management is to increase the frequency and effectiveness of breastfeeding. In some situations, pumping after each breastfeed and feeding the additional

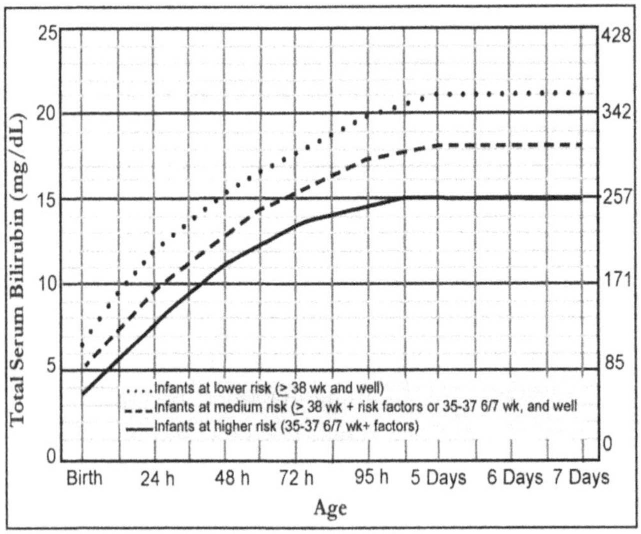

Figure 6. Indications for phototherapy in full-term and near-term newborns. Source: American Academy of Pediatrics, 2004. Reproduced with permission by AAP.

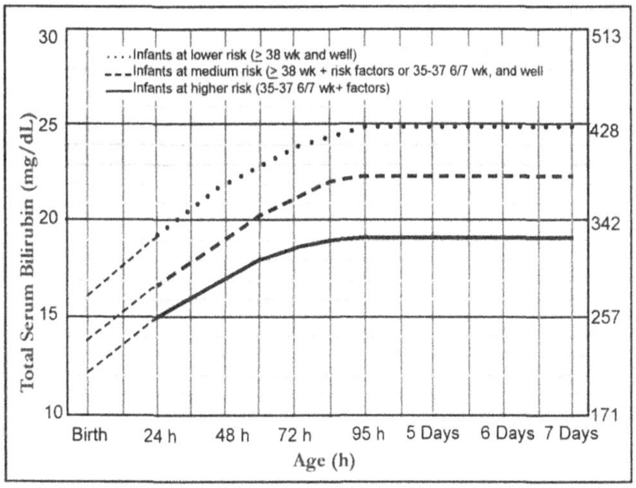

Figure 7. Indications for exchange transfusion in full-term and near-term newborns. Source: American Academy of Pediatrics, 2004. Reproduced with permission by AAP.

milk to the infant may be an effective temporary method of increasing caloric intake and mitigating the hyperbilirubinemia. In the absence of additional human milk, either from the mother or a milk bank, small quantities of formula may be given after each breastfeed either by using a nursing supplementer, cup, spoon, or bottle. The use of a nursing supplementer has the additional benefit of increasing breast stimulation and milk synthesis. A "starving" infant should always be given adequate intake and never allowed to remain with inadequate caloric intake for any period of time since this may lead to dangerously elevated serum bilirubin concentrations.

Inadequate intake of breastmilk may result in dehydration and hypernatremia due to inadequate water intake and the high sodium concentration of human milk when production has declined (Kaplan *et al.*, 1998). If clinically dehydrated or hypernatremic, intravenous fluid therapy is indicated. If neither clinically dehydrated nor hypernatremic, it is advisable to avoid intravenous therapy and use oral milk intake exclusively if the infant is able to feed. Intravenous fluid therapy will not protect against the risk of bilirubin encephalopathy even though it may appear to reduce serum bilirubin concentrations by dilution because it simultaneously dilutes the albumin concentration. Thus, the bilirubin to albumin molar ratio remains unchanged and the risk of bilirubin entering the brain has not been altered. But, the dilutional effect may falsely lead to the belief that serum bilirubin concentrations have fallen to safe levels.

Specific Therapy for Jaundice in the Breastfeeding Infant

The AAP statement provides indications for initiation of both phototherapy and exchange transfusion for full and near-term infants of low, medium, and high risk (**Figures 6 & 7**) (American Academy of Pediatrics, 2004). These guidelines are applicable to the breastfed infant. In addition, breastfeeding can be managed so as to minimize the need for these specific therapies.

If total serum bilirubin concentrations are approaching the level which indicates need for phototherapy, depending on age and risk status, the breastfed infant may be tried first on the alternative therapy of supplementing breastfeeding with infant formula, particularly with the nursing supplementer. Elemental formula is more effective than standard formula in reducing serum bilirubin concentrations because of its greater ability to prevent intestinal bilirubin absorption (Gourley *et al.*, 1999). If a 12 hour trial of this management fails to keep the total serum bilirubin below the phototherapy treatment indication level, then two additional options are available for the breastfed infant. In the first option, breastfeeding can be continued and the infant can be started on phototherapy in the hospital with the mother rooming in with the infant. In the second option, breastfeeding can be interrupted for 24 hours and the infant fed an elemental formula, with or without phototherapy, depending on the serum bilirubin concentration. Close monitoring of serum or transcutaneous bilirubin concentrations is essential during these treatments. If these fail to keep the serum bilirubin in the safe range, then it may be necessary to use phototherapy while also interrupting breastfeeding for 24 to 48 hours. Interruption of breastfeeding will be effective in those situations in which increased intestinal absorption is a significant factor in the hyperbilirubinemia (starvation jaundice, breastmilk jaundice). Interruption of breastfeeding is less effective and may not be useful in those infants with hemolysis or internal bleeding. Thus, clinical judgment and therapeutic trials may be needed to establish the best management for each infant.

If, despite the use of phototherapy and breastfeeding supplementation or interruption, the serum bilirubin continues to rise to levels which indicate the need for exchange transfusion, exchange transfusion should be initiated promptly. The need for exchange transfusion should always be anticipated through frequent monitoring of serum or transcutaneous bilirubin concentrations and plotting on a graph. Blood availability should be established well in advance and the team prepared to start the exchange transfusion on short notice. If the serum bilirubin concentration continues to rise above the indication level, the risk of developing bilirubin encephalopathy is greatly increased and every minute at these elevated levels increases the risk of brain damage. If, at any time, the infant with significant hyperbilirubinemia, even if not at the exchange transfusion indication level, demonstrates the onset of lethargy, poor feeding, or any changes in neurologic status, emergency exchange transfusion should be started immediately (American Academy of Pediatrics, 2004; Nakamura *et al.*, 1985; Nwaesei *et al.*, 1984). Stage one bilirubin encephalopathy may be reversible, avoiding permanent brain damage. Treatment early in stage 2 may minimize the severity of permanent brain damage. Breastfeeding need only be interrupted during the performance of the exchange transfusion, and it may resume upon completion of the procedure. It is also not necessary to withhold oral feedings in anticipation of exchange transfusion since there is no increased risk to the infant; failure to feed may further increase serum bilirubin concentrations.

Following completion of an exchange transfusion, it is essential that serum bilirubin concentrations continue to be monitored closely to be certain that the excessively high levels do not return. Phototherapy should either be continued or instituted after the exchange transfusion until it is clear that serum bilirubin concentrations have fallen and stabilized in the safe range.

Counseling the Family

The parents will be aware of the association of breastfeeding with the development of jaundice. This may make them fearful of breastfeeding and result in premature weaning. The care givers should hold discussions with the family so that they understand that the relationship of breastfeeding to jaundice was transient or not a major factor in the infant's jaundice and will not recur. The benefits of human milk to the health and development of the infant and health of the mother should be stressed and supported with adequate documentation so they will understand the importance of maintaining exclusive breastfeeding for as long a possible. At return visits and phone calls, these issues should be reiterated.

References

Ahlfors CE. Bilirubin-albumin binding and free bilirubin. *J Perinat.* 2001; 21:S40-S42.

Ahlfors CE. Unbound bilirubin associated with kernicterus: A historical approach. *J Pediatr.* 2000; 137:540-44.

Alonso EM, Whitington PF, Whitington SH, Rivard WA, Given G. Enterohepatic circulation of nonconjugated bilirubin in rats fed with human milk. *J Pediatr.* 1991; 118:425-30.

American Academy of Pediatrics, Clinical Practice Guideline. Management of hyperbilirubinemia in the newborn infant 35 or more weeks of gestation. *Pediatrics.* 2004; 114:297-316.

American Academy of Pediatrics, Section on Breastfeeding. Breastfeeding and the use of human milk. *Pediatrics.* 2005;115:496-506.

Anderson DH, Blanc WA, Crozier DN, *et al.* A difference in mortality rate and incidence of kernicterus among premature infants allotted to two prophylactic antibacterial regimens. *Pediatrics.* 1956; 18:614-25.

Baranano DE, Rao M, Ferris CD, Snyder SH. Biliverdin reductase: a major physiologic cytoprotectant. *Proc Nat Acad Sci.* 2002; 99:16093-98.

Barrett PVD. Hyperbilirubinemia of fasting. *JAMA.* 1971; 217:1349-53.

Bartoletti AL, Stevenson DK, Ostander CR, Johnson JD. Pulmonary excretion of carbon monoxide in the human infant as an index of bilirubin production: I. Effects of gestational age and postnatal age and some common neonatal abnormalities. *J Pediatr.* 1979; 94:952-55.

Bertini G, Dani C, Tronchin M, *et al.* Is breastfeeding really favoring early neonatal jaundice? *Pediatrics.* 2001; 107:e41-46.

Bhutani VK, Johnson L, Sivieri EM. Predictive ability of a predischarge hour-specific serum bilirubin for subsequent significant hyperbilirubinemia in healthy term and near-term newborns. *Pediatrics.* 1999; 103:6-14.

Bloomer JR, Barrett PV, Rodkey FL, Berlin NI. Studies of the mechanism of fasting hyperbilirubinemia. *Gastroenterol.* 1971; 61:479-87.

Bode HH, Vanjonack WJ, Crawford JD. Mitigation of cretinism by breast-feeding. *Pediatrics.* 1978; 62:13-16.

Bonnett R, Davies JE, Hursthouse MB, Sheldrick GM. The structure of bilirubin. *Proc Roy Soc Lond B Biol Sci.* 1978; 202:249-68.

Bonnett R, Davies JE, *et al.* The structure of bilirubin. *Nature* [London]. 1976; 262:326.

Brodersen R, Herman LS. Intestinal absorption of unconjugated bilirubin: A possible contributing factor in neonatal jaundice. *Lancet.* 1963;1:1242.

Brodersen R. Bilirubin transport in the newborn infant, reviewed with relation to kernicterus. *J Pediatr.* 1980; 96:349-56.

Brodersen R. Bilirubin. Solubility and interaction with albumin and phospholipid. *J Biol Chem.* 1979; 254:2364-69.

Cashore WJ. Kernicterus and bilirubin encephalopathy. *Sem Liver Dis.* 1988; 8:163-67.

Clarkson, JE, Cowan JO, Herbison GP. Jaundice in full term healthy neonates. A population study. *Aust. Pediatr J.* 1984; 20:303-8.

Cornelius CE, Bruss ML. Hepatic bile pigment excretion and erythrocyte turnover in various species. *Vet Clin Pathol.* 1980; 9:15-20.

DeAngelis C, Sargent J, Chun MK. Breast milk jaundice. *Wisconsin Med J.* 1980; 79:40-42.

DeCarvalho M, Klaus MH, Meerkatz RB. Frequency of breast-feeding and serum bilirubin concentration. *Am J Dis Child.* 1982; 136:737-38.

Dennery PA, McDonagh AF, Spitz DR, Rodgers PA, Stevenson DK. Hyperbilirubinemia results in reduced oxidative injury in neonatal Gunn rats exposed to hyperoxia. *Free Radical Biol & Med.* 1995; 19:395-404.

Ebbesen F. Recurrence of kenciterus in term and near-term infants in Denmark. *Acta Paediatr.* 2000; 89:1213-17.

Gartner LM, Arias IM. Studies of prolonged neonatal jaundice in the breastfed infant. *J Pediatr.* 1966; 68:54-66.

Gartner LM, Herschel M. Jaundice and breastfeeding. *Ped Clin North Amer.* 2001; 48:389-99.

Gartner LM, Lane DL, Cornelius CE. Bilirubin transport by liver in adult Macaca mulatta. *Am J Physiol.* 1971; 220:1528-35.

Gartner LM, Lee KS, Moscioni AD. Effect of milk feeding on intestinal bilirubin absorption in the rat. *J Pediatr.* 1983; 103:464-71.

Gartner LM, Lee KS, Vaisman S, Lane D, Zarafu I. Development of bilirubin transport and metabolism in the newborn rhesus monkey. *J Pediatr.* 1977; 90:513-31.

Gartner LM, Lee KS. Jaundice in the breastfed infant. *Clin Perinat.* 1999; 26:431-45.

Gartner LM, Lee, KS, Vaisman S, Lane D, Zarafu I. Development of bilirubin transport and metabolism in the newborn rhesus monkey. *J Peds.* 1977; 90:513-31.

Gourley GR, Arend RA. B-glucuronidase and hyperbilirubinemia in breast-fed and formula-fed babies. *Lancet.* 1986; 1:644-46.

Gourley GR, Kreamer B, Arend R. The effect of diet on feces and jaundice during the first 3 weeks of life. *Gastroenter.* 1992; 103:660-67.

Gourley GR, Kreamer B, Cohnen M, Kosorok MR. Neonatal jaundice and diet. *Arch Pediatr Adolesc Med.* 1999; 153:184-88.

Gronwall R, Cornelius CE. Effect of fasting on bilirubin metabolism. *N Eng J Med.* 1970; 283:204.

Hammerman C, Goldschmidt D, Caplan MS, Kaplan M, Bromiker R, *et al.* Protective effect of bilirubin in ischemia/reperfusion injury in the rat intestine. *J Ped Gastro Nutr.* 2002; 35:344-49.

Hansen TWR, Bratlid D. Bilirubin and brain toxicity. *Acta Paediatr Scand.* 1986; 75:513-22.

Harris M, Bernbaum J, Polin J, Zimmerman R, Polin RA. Developmental follow-up of breastfed term and near-term infants with marked hyperbilirubinemia. *Pediatrics.* 2001;107:1075-80.

Ince Z, Coban A, Peker I, Can G. Breastmilk beta-glucuronidase and prolonged jaundice in the neonate. *Acta Paediatr.* 1995; 84:237-39.

Ip S, Chung M, Kulig J, O'Brien R, Sege R, *et al.* An evidence-based review of important issues concerning neonatal hyperbilirubinemia. *Pediatrics.* 2004; 113:e644-72.

Jardine DS, Rogers K. Relationship of benzyl alcohol to kernicterus, intraventricular hemorrhage, and mortality in preterm infants. *Pediatrics.* 1989; 83:153-60.

Kaplan J, Stiegler R, Schmunk G. Fatal hypernatremic dehydration in exclusively breast-fed newborn infants due to maternal lactation failure. *Am J Forensic Med Pathol.* 1998; 19:19-22.

Kaplan M, Hammerman C, Maisels MJ. Bilirubin genetics for the nongeneticist: Hereditary defects of neonatal bilirubin conjugation. *Pediatrics.* 2003; 111:886-91.

Kaplan M, Hammerman C. Onset of jaundice in G6PD deficient neonates. *Indian Pediatr.* 2006; 43:459-61.

Kaplan M, Hammerman C. Severe neonatal hyperbilirubinemia: a potential complication of glucose-6-phosphate-dehydrogenase deficiency. *Clin Perinatol.* 1998; 25:575-90.

Kaplan M, Vreman HJ, Hammerman C, Schimmel MS, Abrahamov A, Stevenson DK. Favism by proxy in nursing glucose-6-phosphate dehydrogenase deficient neonates. *J Perinatol.* 1998; 18:477-79.

Kuhr M, Paneth N. Feeding practices and early neonatal jaundice. *J Ped Gastro Nutr.* 1982; 1:485-88.

La Torre A, Targioni G, Rubaltelli FF. Beta-glucuronidase and hyperbilirubinemia in breast-fed babies. *Biol Neonate.* 1999; 75:82-84.

Lee KS, Gartner LM. Bilirubin binding by plasma proteins: a criticial evaluation of methods and clinical implications. *Rev Perinatal Med.* 1978; 2:319-43.

Levi AJ, Gatmaitan Z, Arias IM. Deficiency of hepatic organic anion-binding protein, impaired organic anion uptake by the liver, and "physiologic" jaundice in newborn monkeys. *N Eng J Med.* 1970; 283:1136-39.

Lucas A, Baker BA. Breast milk jaundice in premature infants. *Arch Dis Child.* 1986; 61:1063-67.

Maisels MJ, Gifford K. Normal serum bilirubin levels in the newborn and the effect of breast-feeding. *Pediatrics.* 1986; 78:837-43.

Maisels MJ, Newman TB. Kernicterus in otherwise healthy, breast-fed term newborns. *Pediatrics.* 1995; 96:730-33.

Mauro Y, Nishizawa K, Sato H, Sawa H, Shimada M. Prolonged unconjugated hyperbilirubinemia associated with breast milk and mutations of the bilirubin uridine diphosphate-glucuronosyltransferase gene. *Pediatrics.* 2000; 106:e59-e61.

Nakamura H, Takada S, Shimabuku R, Matsuo M, Matsuo T, Megishi H. Auditory nerve and brainstem responses in newborn infants with hyperbilirubinemia. *Pediatrics.* 1985; 75:703-8.

Newman TB, Xiong B, GonzalesVM, Escobar GJ. Prediction and prevention of extreme neonatal hyperbilirubinemia in a mature health maintenance organization. *Arch Pediatr Adolesc Med.* 2000; 154:1140-47.

Nwaesei CG, Van Aerde J, Boyden M, Perlman M. Changes in auditory brain stem responses in hyperbilirubinemic infants before and after exchange transfusion. *Pediatrics.* 1984; 74:800-3.

Odell GB, Cohen SN, Kelly PC. Studies in kernicterus. II. The determination of the saturation of serum albumin with bilirubin. *J Pediatr.* 1969;74:214-30.

Okumura A, Hayakawa F, Maruyama K, Kubota T, Kato K, Watanabe K. Single photon emission computed tomography and serial MRI in preterm infants with kernicterus. *Brain Dev.* 2006; 28:348-52.

Poland RL, Odell GB. Physiologic jaundice: The enterohepatic circulation of bilirubin. *N Eng J Med.* 1971; 284:1-6.

Robinson SH. The origins of bilirubin. *N Eng J Med.*1968; 279:143-9.

Schneider AP. Breast-milk jaundice in the newborn. *JAMA.* 1986; 255:3270-74.

Smith DW, Hopper AO, Shahin SM, Cohen RS, Ostrander CR, Ariagno RL, *et al.* Neonatal bilirubin production estimated from "end-tidal" carbon monoxide concentration. *J Pediatr Gastroenterol Nutr.* 1984; 3:77-80.

Tenhunen R. The enzymatic conversion of heme to bilirubin in vivo. *Ann Clin Res.* 1976; 8(suppl 17):2-9.

Van Praagh R. Diagnosis of kernicterus in the neonatal period. *Pediatrics.* 1961;28:870-876.

Volpe JJ. *Neurology of the Newborn.* 4th Ed. Philadelphia: W.B. Saunders; 2001.

Waser M, Kleihues P, Frick P. Kernicterus in an adult. *Ann Neurol.* 1986; 19:595-98.

Weldon AP, Danks DM. Congenital hypothyroidism and neonatal jaundice. *Arch Dis Child.* 1972; 47:469-71.

Wennberg RP, Hance AJ. Experimental bilirubin encephalopathy: importance of total bilirubin, protein binding and blood-brain barrier. *Ped Res.* 1986; 20:789-92.

White GL Jr., Nelson JA, Pedersen DM, Ash KO. Fasting and gender (and altitude?) influence reference intervals for serum bilirubin in healthy adults. *Clin Chem.* 1981; 27:1140-42.

Whiter DI, Gollan JL. Mechanisms and significance of fasting and dietary hyperbilirubinemia. *Semin Liver Dis.* 1983; 3:42-51.

Whitington PF, Gartner LM. Disorders of bilirubin metabolism. In: Nathan DG, Oski FA (eds.). *Hematology of Infancy and Childhood,* 4th Ed. Philadelphia: WB Saunders, 1993. pp 98-103.

Wolkoff AW, Chowdhury JR, Gartner LM, Rose AL, Biempica L, Giblin DR, *et al.* Crigler-Najjar Syndrome (type I) in an adult male. *Gastroenterology.* 1979; 76:840-48.

Wu PYK, Hodgman JE, Kirkpatrick BV, White NB Jr, Bryla DA. Metabolic aspects of phototherapy. NICHD randomized, controlled trial of phototherapy for neonatal hyperbilirubinemia. *Pediatrics.* 1985; 75:427-33.

Yamauchi Y, Yamanouchi I. Breast-feeding frequency during the first 24 hours after birth in full-term neonates. *Pediatrics.* 1990; 86:171-75.

Yigit S, Ciliv G, Aygun C, Erdem G. Breastmilk beta-glucuronidase levels in hyperbilirubinemia. *Turk J Pediatr.* 2001; 43:118-20.

Chapter 14

Mother-Infant Cosleeping with Breastfeeding in the Western Industrialized Context

A Bio-Cultural Perspective

James J. McKenna and Lee T. Gettler

INTRODUCTION AND OVERVIEW OF ISSUES

> *"For species such as primates the mother is the environment."*
> *(Blaffer Hrdy, 1999)*
>
> *"The utero-gestate fetus, embraced, supported and rocked within the amniotic environment, as an extero-gestate requires the continued support of his mother, to be held and rocked in her arms, and in close contact with her body, swallowing colostrom and milk in place of amniotic fluid."* *(Montagu, 1986:293)*

A human infant is biologically designed to sleep next to its mother's body and to breastfeed intermittently throughout the night, at least for the first year of its life. And however distant and removed contemporary, western urban cultural environments are from the overall variable environments within which human maternal care and infant vulnerabilities co-evolved hundreds of thousands of years ago, it still remains true that nothing a human neonate can or cannot do makes sense except in light of the mother's body (Konner, 1981; Hrdy, 1999; McKenna, 1986; Granju, 1999; McKenna & McDade, 2005).

As if anticipating this view forty years earlier and consistent with recent psychobiological "skin-to-skin" infant care studies (Anderson, 1988; 1989; 1991; Goto *et al.*, 1999), Winnicott observed, "There is no such thing as a baby, there is a baby and someone." This phrase is no less applicable in describing *in utero* fetal-maternal regulatory effects than it is in characterizing the nature of regulation occurring postnatally during what Montagu (1986) calls the phase of extero-gestation for the human neonate or "...the continuation of the utero-gestative processes outside the womb" (Montagu, 1986:293).

While a major goal of this chapter is to explore scientifically the adaptive bases of breastfeeding in the context of nighttime mother-infant cosleeping, a slightly different but related goal is to illustrate continuities bridging pre- and postnatal infant sensory experiences. The reader should be alerted to the fact that much of the material in this chapter overlaps other research reviews (especially McKenna, Ball and Gettler, in press). In this chapter, however, we emphasize a developmental approach and argue that such pre- and postnatal continuities help to explain how and possibly why infants seem to be so responsive and prepared for their extero-uterine experiences which depends on sustained bodily contact with the mother, i.e., touching, being touched, smelling her, moving with her, sucking on her breasts, tasting her milk, looking at her, and hearing her voice.

Of particular heuristic relevance to many of the arguments we develop is Hofer's (1978) concept of "hidden physiological regulatory effects" in the mammalian mother-infant dyad (Gunnar, 1998). After birth, human infants appear to be pre-sensitized if not pre-adapted to particular "types" of rhythmic and arrhythmic maternal sensory stimuli involving olfaction, touch, taste, their mother's voice, heat, and movement, to name but a few. We use these data and related theories which inform us about why babies do as they do to propose why maternal proximity and contact remains as necessary and important today in promoting breastfeeding and healthy infant sleep, growth, and development in general as it was in prehistoric times. These data provide a foundation for understanding why, when practiced safely, mother-infant cosleeping with breastfeeding ordinarily provides for all of the infant's and mother's needs in just the right amounts.

Because forms of mother-infant cosleeping are so controversial and so poorly and incorrectly represented in western scientific discourse, we explore the diverse types and kinds of cosleeping, being sure to distinguish between safe and unsafe "types," and we explore their role in human evolutionary prehistory and history. We contrast important differences between breastfeeding-bedsharing and bottle-feeding-bedsharing mother-infant dyads, highlighting the relative safety of infants in each of these sleep environments, particularly as explored by Ball (2006d) in the homes of parents and in a mother-infant sleep laboratory.

We argue that only where sweeping public health recommendations acknowledge and respect maternal capacities and biologically-appropriate emotions and motivations for mothers to sleep close to their infants will there be any hope that these recommendations can be adopted and implemented in ways which promote the survival and well being of the greatest number of mother-infant dyads. According to recent studies (Ball, 2002; McKenna & Volpe, in press), where a baby ends up sleeping on any given night is the result of many intersecting factors, not the least of which involves what makes the mother and infant happy, but also the particular method of feeding (bottle, breast, or both) and the sensitivities or temperament needs of the infant and/or mother (**Figure 1**).

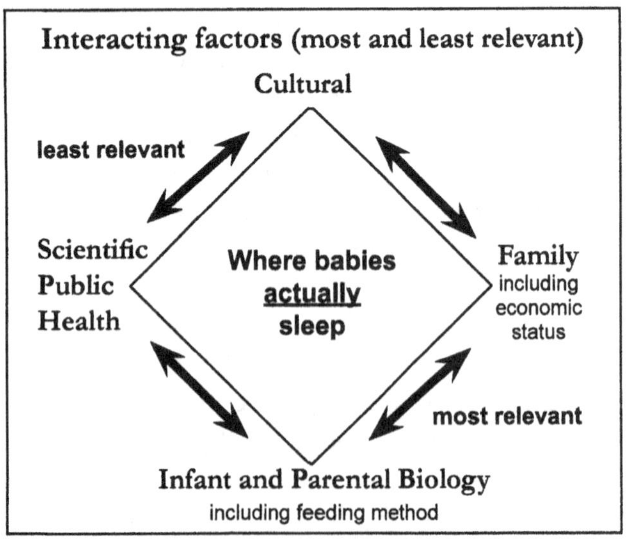

Figure 1. What determines where a baby sleeps per any given night? Most and least relevant factors.
From: Sally Baddock (New Zealand), Peter Blair and Helen Ball (Great Britan), Caroline McQuillan (Australia), James McKena and Lane Volpe (USA)

The factors and categories of influence depicted in **Figure 1** should be considered in discussions of where babies sleep and why, especially the intersection of parental and infant biology. This perspective on what determines sleeping arrangements elevates the importance of parental feelings and interpretations of infant needs contrasts with the more traditional model which employs a "one-size-must-fit-all" answer to the question: where should a baby sleep (Scheer *et al.*, 2003; AAP, 2005). A perspective which considers family goals and the imperatives and uniqueness of each family has the advantage of empowering and informing parents rather than belittling and dismissing them as they learn how best to respond to and protect their infants.

More generally, we suggest that public health policies, messages, and recommendations will greatly benefit from adopting a more holistic and comparative anthropological understanding of human infant-parent biology - a view that is at least minimally compatible with, if not appreciative of, the evolutionary-based and mostly adaptive emotional experiences and expectations of the individuals for whom the recommendations are intended. Current ways of reading and interpreting evidence on the bedsharing and breastfeeding controversies by the American Academy of Pediatrics (2005) and other medical institutions, including a governmental agency concerned with deficient products in the United States (the Consumer Product Safety Commission) (Scheer *et al.*, 2003), not only assume incorrectly that powerful factors that motivate forms of cosleeping can always be denied, but that they should be, a point of view with which we disagree, as the data we present will illustrate.

As is argued elsewhere, the choice made by medical authorities to reduce a complex, heterogeneous practice, such as bedsharing, to a simple, allegedly coherent and always "dangerous" practice without modifiable components implies little or no faith in the intellectual and less ambiguous biological capacities of mothers to successfully and safely respond to their infants' needs, no matter what. Simplistic condemnations of bedsharing ignore and dismiss the nature of the mother-infant relationship itself and ignore recent important data showing that bedsharing in the context of breastfeeding looks and functions very differently from bedsharing when bottle-feeding is involved (Ball, 2006d).

Far too often, western medical recommendations, which define and advocate for what is institutionally deemed "safe" and "proper" infant care, derive justification from highly selective, population-wide epidemiological research to the exclusion of laboratory, home, or otherwise clinical or basic research lines, particularly when those alternative data raise questions about the applicability and/or validity of singular recommendations which are supposed to apply equally well across all families and circumstances, but do not (Fleming *et al.*, 2007). In this way, medical authorities ignore the rules required to practice "evidence-based medicine" (Fleming *et al.*, 2007) and confuse their own social judgments, personal preferences, and assumptions for more broadly based and agreed upon scientific findings.

BEFORE INFANT SLEEP: THE IMPORTANCE OF "GETTING A THEORY" FOR UNDERSTANDING AND ASKING RESEARCH QUESTIONS ABOUT HUMAN INFANCY AND PARENTING

As discussed elsewhere (McKenna & Gettler, in press), an ongoing problem with much of western pediatric research is that it remains *a-theoretical*, meaning there is no accepted theory around which questions, predictions, and interpretations of data can be organized. Indeed, a powerful and appropriate theory, all but ignored in medicine in general and pediatrics in particular, is the theory of evolution. The application of evolutionary principles and reference to the human infant's unique place in nature can serve as a powerful beginning point for addressing who the infant is, what the infant needs, and why the infant responds as infants' do to certain forms of care or interventions. That the reference to evolutionary processes is missing in medical discourse is surprising. As David Brown (1993) put it: "Though medical therapies (in most cases) are constructed from the data of biology, medicine in general pays little attention to what is probably the single most important concept in biology: the theory of evolution." Without a solid empirically-based theory for understanding infancy, untested cultural assumptions rather than biological truths far too easily can appear credible and come to underlie public health policies and recommendations, cascading at times into unforeseen but nonetheless disastrous recommendations or practices.

Take, for example, the western medical assumption that solitary sleep is normal or beneficial for human infants, rather than infants should sleep in the proximity of caregivers; or that bottle feeding is superior or at least equal to breastmilk; and, worst of all, that prone infant sleep is safe even without any empirical data ever having shown it to be. After being translated into sweeping public health recommendations, these three one-time cultural-based claims were responsible for the deaths of hundreds of thousands of babies who died from SIDS and other illnesses, as breastfeeding, sleeping in a room with an adult, and sleeping on their back reduce by at least half the risk of an infant dying before its first birthday (Chen & Rogan, 2004; Carpenter *et al.*, 2004; Fleming *et al.*, 1996).

Without an organizing theory, such as evolution, understanding research findings or outcomes becomes subject to explanations which accept conventional understandings, assumptions, or stereotypes much more quickly, rather than calling forth diverse scientific studies *that potentially* explain why some factors remain so much more important and influential in determining health and behavior than do others.

Indeed, recent western interpretations of what human infants' need and why reflect far more about what the societies' values want them to be, rather than what they actually are - an infant who from an evolutionary point of view is an exceedingly unfinished (altricial) organism whose biological identity cannot be known except through its connection with the mother. In fact, the virtual absence of the use of the concept of evolution in understanding infancy helps to explain why, as a methodological research tradition, scientific reductionism, i.e., reducing and isolating smaller and smaller parts or pieces of a biological system to its minimal functional role, has not for the most part served the science of human infancy nor pediatric research very well. This is because infants continue to be defined for study relatively separate from the maternal-infant sensory micro-environments in which their bodies were designed to function. Pediatric, developmental, and clinical research continues to overstress, for example, the "amazing" competencies of the newborn infant, preferring to see the infant almost as if it can or should achieve independence rather than function as part of an age-appropriate dyad involving both the mother and infant, each sensitive and receptive to the mutual physiological regulatory effects of the other.

While contemporary infant science insists for political reasons on conceptualizing the infant as the unit of analysis, it is the mother-infant dyad that most accurately constitutes the true unit of study. In fact, diverse data show convincingly that the infant is so sensitive to changes induced by maternal contact that infant "social" care and engagement of the infant with its mother must be considered synonymous with its physiological regulation. This is because throughout human prehistory prolonged infant carrying, holding, and infant-led breastfeeding in the context of mother-infant cosleeping constituted a highly successful child care system doubtless designed by natural selection to maximize the chances of infant survival and parental reproductive success (McKenna & Gettler, in press).

Indeed, as we illustrate below, knowledge of our species' evolutionary background and characteristics, including human prehistory, greatly enriches our understanding of how and why breastfeeding and some form of mother-infant cosleeping continues to be so ubiquitous worldwide (Konner, 1981). Evolutionary-based reconstructions of parent-infant characteristics helps us to understand how and why, even without formal instructions found in local childcare manuals so familiar to the industrialized west, mother-infant breastfeeding and cosleeping in conjunction with the supine (back) infant sleep position continue to represent an integrated and predominant human universal arrangement. Reference to human evolutionary processes makes this fact not only understandable but predictable, i.e., the only way an infant can feed during the night, to get to and from its mother's breast, is by being placed on its back, the safest position.

The mother's body, in all but the industrialized western context, is thought to represent the central social-sensory protective reference point around and against which the infant's physiological and psychological development is thought to optimally develop. This is a far cry from recent American hospital policies (see below) that treat the 'mother's body as a potential lethal weapon against which both she and her infant need protection' (Model Behavior Program, First Candle & NSIDPSC, 2007).

In our (western) enthusiasm to substitute inanimate objects or technology for stimuli ordinarily provided through maternal contact and proximity, alongside social values favoring early infant autonomy and mother-infant separation, we must observe that clinical pediatric medicine pushes too far the notion of the human infant's physiological independence from its care-givers. It is easy to mistake the infant's preparedness to engage with what the mother's body provides with actual adaptation (how the infant interacts with the external conditions of the environment within which it lives...such as weather, etc.).

In this review, we employ a bio-cultural approach integrating diverse lines of evidence, including evolutionary, psycho-biological, cross-species, cross-cultural, and historical data to help illustrate the limitations of adopting first and foremost a view of infants that is more congruent with recent western social values than with the infant's evolutionary legacies. Laboratory and home bedsharing-breastfeeding studies are used to assess the biological appropriateness and functions of one form of cosleeping referred to as "bedsharing," as well as to summarize the known mutual physiological regulatory effects of mother-infant bedsharing as they relate to breastfeeding patterns and SIDS risk factors.

Although it may at first seem a distraction, a thorough discussion of our changing historical-cultural perceptions of infants in western societies is especially pertinent. This background is critical to fully understand the controversies surrounding the issue of cosleeping in the form of bedsharing in western cultures, a childcare practice that has never been considered nor discussed on anything even closely resembling a level scientific playing field. Surely, our western cultural legacy of stressing the importance of mother-infant nighttime separation helps to clarify why medical agencies choose to warn parents about the alleged inherent dangers of "cosleeping" rather than concentrating their efforts on helping parents avoid the adverse factors that can make it dangerous. An alternative approach can be seen as an important way to protect and nurture the nature of the mother-infant relationship that underlies various cosleeping practices, an important point of contention in this chapter.

INFANCY AND PARENTING IN EVOLUTIONARY PERSPECTIVE: HOW AND WHY THE HUMAN MOTHER-INFANT DYAD EVOLVED TO BE SO INTERDEPENDENT

Like scientific research itself, infant-maternal sleep and feeding biology is inseparable from the specific cultural context within which it finds expression. And while cultural factors and contexts can change relatively quickly without genetic change, including the way we think about infant sleep and feeding issues, reference to human evolutionary processes provide a less biased lens through which to examine the worldwide range of child care practices. Findings related to the evolution of the mother-infant relationship, for example, are especially useful when evaluating the reasons why some infant care practices resonate more emotionally with parents than do others as they attempt to meet both the short and long term needs of their infants.

To define an infant's biological needs and to understand to what extent more recent cultural practices might place infants (or mothers) at odds with each other and their own bodies, it is critical to examine what is biologically unique about human infants and mothers, and more specifically, the social and physical context within which the infant-maternal biological characteristics (including infant vulnerabilities) evolved alongside specific parenting responses. Insofar as human infants are born so neurologically immature (only 25% of their adult brain size at birth), it seems sensible that infant needs and parental responses to those needs constitute a dynamic, co-evolving interdependent system which continues to be subject to tremendous cultural manipulation. While it is difficult to know exactly all of the ecological factors that confronted our evolving ancestors to produce present day mother-infant characteristics, the convergence of cross-species, paleo-ecological, and comparative primate anatomical studies give us some important clues.

Why So Immature at Birth? The Effects of Bipedal Locomotion on Human Infancy and Parenting

At birth, the human infant is the least neurologically mature primate of all. It develops the most slowly and is the most dependent on the caregiver for the longest period of time. The evolutionary characteristics and

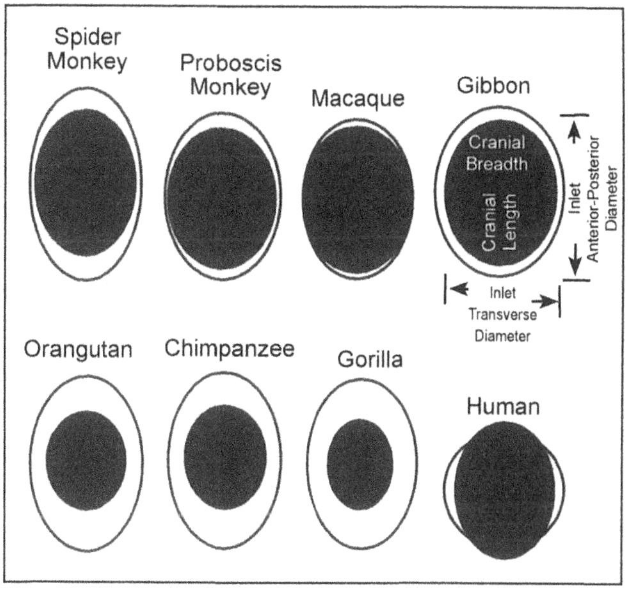

Figure 2. Comparative illustration of the relative ratio of pelvic outlet to fetal head size of different primate species. Only the human fetal cranium exceeds the diameter of its mother's pelvic outlet, complicating and making human birth more difficult.

antiquity of human upright bipedal locomotion, which developed two to six million years ago, seems an unlikely but appropriate beginning point for considering why. The evolution of upright posture cannot explain why humans breastfeed, as reference to a much earlier time period is required for that (Blaffer Hrdy, 1999). As reconstructed from the fossil record, anthropologists infer that the shift to bipedal locomotion precipitated a cascade of related developmental changes unique to human beings, which included the biological and behavioral prerequisites for culture defined here simply as a reliance on tools, language, and symbols for survival.

Consider that the pelvis of quadrupedal primates (monkeys and apes) who move on all fours is long and relatively narrow from one hip plate to the other, while the pelvis of a hominine-human primate to support bipedalism became considerably broader, flared, and more bowl-shaped in the front. The two ilia on each side of the human pelvis rotated forward to support more muscle attachment sites needed to hold the viscera in place while the body stands erect. Additionally, the hominine ischium or floor of the pelvis pushed upward a bit to accommodate the hip-femur sockets needed for efficient walking and running. But in pushing up the floor of the pelvis, the size of the outlet was diminished.

As **Figure 2** illustrates, only the human fetal head exceeds the breadth of its mother's pelvic outlet. These modifications, relative to non-human primates, made the process of human birth (parturition) on average longer in duration, more complex, certainly more risky, and ultimately more energetically costly for mothers and fathers alike (Trevathan & Rosenberg, 2003).

The concurrent morphological transformations (size and shape) of both the hominine cranium and pelvis from a quadraped to a human biped necessitated changes not only in the birth process, but also in parental postnatal survival skills and strategies aimed at keeping their vulnerable and slowly developing infants alive. Specifically, more complex learning and behavioral plasticity involving a more permanent capacity for year round sexual relations between men and women relatively committed to each other's economic survival produced for the first time what is now referred to as a "division of labor," a system which ultimately increases the survivorship of infants and children.

These changes were also required, among other things, to plan effective defense strategies against a variety of vicious predators and to find and keep high energy foods. Hence, relative to body size, both pre- and postnatally, the cerebral cortex of the human brain began to expand at the same time as the human pelvic outlet, the birth canal, was becoming smaller, creating an "obstetrical dilemma" for which the only apparent solution was to give birth to increasingly less neurologically mature human infants.

From the standpoint of comparative primate neuro-development and obstetrics, all human infants are born premature! Unlike non-human primates at birth, this developmentally early "great eviction" of the human neonate as Karp (2003) aptly describes it means that human infants are unable to cling to their mother's torso, thermoregulate (keep warm by themselves), or locomote on their own. Human infants are unable to control their bowels or their breathing underlying their vocalizations, effectively make sufficient antibodies to fight disease, or communicate, except by virtue of crying or through vegetative sounds and non-verbal cues.

Anthropologists assume that one of the positive trade-offs of upright posture involved freeing the hands to make more sophisticated tools, as well as the ability to carry them or the material resources needed to make them, which contributed to the eventual abilities of humans to organize into highly flexible but complex social coalitions.

Approximately 80% of adult brain size is achieved by two years of age or so, but full adult brain volume is not in place until approximately 18-21 years of age. These data contrast with the much faster neurological development of our closest living primate ancestors, the chimpanzees, who are born with about 45% of their adult brain weight, with 100% of it being reached by 12-14 years of age (**Figure 3**).

All of these inter-related, hominine-human changes occurred in the context of what Bowlby (1982) called the "*environment of evolutionary adaptedness*," specifically, a hunting and gathering lifestyle somewhat akin to life by contemporary gatherers living on the Kalahari, at least we pretend so (Hrdy, 1999), and a set of ecological adaptations that dominated what was to be called the human experience for well over 99% of our existence as an evolving species. The cognitive abilities that made this lifestyle (dependent on language and tools) possible was based on an ever-expanding neocortex. Indeed, brain size tripled in volume during the three million years of human evolution, therein emancipating human behavior from strict hormonal or genetic control. Continuing neurological changes in the brain produced the possibility of and an eventual reliance on language, in addition to tools and technology, all of which defines the genus Homo. It accounts for our impressive range of cultural adaptations and expansion to habitats for which humans were not necessarily biologically equipped or designed.

It is from this perspective that we can begin to understand how and why human mothers care for their

Percent of Adult Brain Size:

	Chimpanzee Infant	Human Infant
At Birth	45	25
3 months	50	35
6	60	45
9	65	50
1 year	70	60
2	75	70
4	85	80
8-9	100	95

***(100% at 14-17 years)**

Figure 3. Percent of adult brain size per developmental age achieved by the chimpanzee and human.

babies the way they do and why such an extraordinary investment is necessary. The kind of micro-environment in which such a neurologically immature, vulnerable infant could survive came to depend on the evolution of highly motivated caregivers on whose bodies after birth the infant's survival would depend as the immaturity of the neural structures controlling the infant's motor system prohibited the infant from walking, crawling, or following the mother except with its eyes. The human infant had to be carried and the duration of its biological dependence was elongated, including the period of time in which it was breastfed and educated. The evolution of parental emotions and responses provided a sensory-rich developmental context within which "extero-gestation" (Montagu, 1986) could occur.

Completing the Human Mother- Infant Adaptive Complex: The Composition of Human Milk Necessitates Nighttime Maternal-Infant Proximity Including Supine Infant Sleep

Human locomotor behavior (bipedalism) and the co-evolving behavioral sequelae are not the only characteristics that made it likely that maternal-infant carrying behavior and proximity would become so important to the human mother-infant dyad. The low amounts of fats and protein in human milk supports the idea that not just one, but a cascade of related behavioral and morphological changes associated with increased contact and carrying co-evolved to support human infant needs hundreds of thousands of years ago. Compared with other mammals, not only is human milk low in fat and protein, but it is relatively high in carbohydrates, especially lactose, a key nutrient needed, among other things, for sustained but rapid brain growth. The concentration of lactose in milk is highest among primates whose infants at birth are the least neurologically developed and need to be carried and suckled practically continuously.

Table 1. Biology of Mothers' Milk Predicts Mothering Behavior

Feed and Leave Species	Contact, Cosleeping, and Carry Species
Ungulates	**Primates and Humans**
High fat High protein Low carbohydrate	Low fat Low protein High carbohydrate
High calories = long feeding interval	Low calories = short feeding interval
To avoid predators, nested infants do not defacate or cry in mothers' absence.	Carried infants cry in absence of mother and defacate spontaneously.
Some species are designed to be "left" by their mothers in their nests or burrows; others, like humans, need to be carried and in continuous contact with their mothers due in part to the composition of breastmilk, particularly the density of calories delivered by the mother per breastfeed.	

Schoen (2007) extensively reviewed the biology of human infancy and parenting from a cultural, evolutionary, and psychobiological perspective. She points out that among non-primate mammals, such as lions and several species of deer, the young are left in nests or burrows hidden from view. These types of species are generally called "nested or cached" species with the mothers returning to them at intervals of four to twelve hours. Schoen states: "But unlike human milk, the milk of these nested or cached species remains high in fat and protein (at least a third to one–half more proteins), allowing the young to be satiated for longer periods of time and for intervals between feeds to be great." Deer mothers, Schoen expands, have about 21% fat in their milk. Human milk, with only about 3% fat, is exquisitely designed for the undeveloped infant's intestinal tract, as the milk curds are small and easily soluble (Lawrence, 1974), which also explains why sucking rates of human infants are so much more frequent per unit of time compared with nested species.

Moreover, as Blurton Jones (1974) and Schoen noted, young animals that are typically left alone for much of the day often do not defecate or urinate readily without assistance, probably in order to avoid attracting predators sensitive to scents. "Defecation is often preceded for these species by the mother generally licking her offspring's perinea region, causing the offspring to release the sphincter muscle, which in turn permits either urination, defecation, or both" (Schoen 2007) (**Table 1**).

Blurton Jones (1974) makes the case even stronger by pointing out that offspring of "nested" species never cry spontaneously during the absence of their mothers. Both crying in the absence of the mother and defecating spontaneously occur among human infants, which would attract predators to the nests, leading to the deaths of the infants. As Schoen reminds us, these responses are appropriate for a species whose biological system is designed for continuous contact and carrying. These adaptations represent evolutionary legacies unaffected by recent cultural preferences or styles of infant care that aim to separate infants from parents during the night.

In fact, the infant who cries when separated from its mother can be said to be acting on its emotions, attempting to ameliorate a potential life threatening event. This must be interpreted positively as the infant is acting in an adaptive and developmentally vigorous, if not predictive, manner. In contrast, it can be said that any western infant who quietly accepts or acquiesces to a "dangerous" situation, such as separation from its mother, might best be described as developmentally less competent. As many have argued, being alone, either during the day or at night, is a context for which human infants are not biologically designed.

How interesting it is, then, that two radically different explanations of this behavior are possible depending on the paradigm used. If infant crying in response to separation from its mother is interpreted from an evolutionary (biological) point of view, it must be deemed expectable and adaptive, i.e., beneficial. If interpreted strictly from a cultural point of view that values infant solitariness and parental separation, the protesting infant can be seen as deviant, uncooperative, and less able to control its own emotions, i.e., developmentally deficient. In this way, one's theoretical beginning point for analysis matters a great deal in understanding how and why infants behave as they do. This is why, as discussed earlier, starting with a particular theoretical foundation about who the infant is and what criteria will be used to define human infant attributes can be so important in pediatric studies.

Human Birth: Whole New Life or ...Been There, Done That? Pre-and Postnatal Continuities in Maternal Regulation of the Infant

Since especially in western cultures, the human mother's body is no longer seen to *directly* regulate the infant's physiology following parturition, western medical models of infant development typically stress that birth represents *the* moment in which the human newborn becomes a completely independent being from the mother, as opposed to a "being" still functionally interconnected in important and critical biological ways. In most hospitals, steps are taken to facilitate the infant's quick progression and development toward autonomy as early in life as possible, therein maximizing the extent to which the infant can be pushed to function outside the nutritional, social, and physical regulatory environment of the mother's body. Right from the beginning, the recommended and preferable forms of infant care are designed to promote psycho-social and physiological autonomy for the infant, i.e., physical separation from the mother for sleep (Pinilla & Birch, 1993) and breastfeeding or bottle feeding routines that encourage less continuous feeding and mutual access, in favor of more parentally controlled breastfeeds and longer sleep bouts, all of which it can be argued is not what the human is designed to experience (Schoen, 2007).

Yet, a variety of research on infants reveal that many, if not most, underlying physiological sub-systems of the neonate, especially those involved in thermo-regulation, growth, immune defenses, and maintenance, including breathing, sleep, and digestion, continue to be influenced, if not developmentally changed, *vis a vis* a variety of on-going maternal-infant (postnatal) sensory exchanges involving olfactory, auditory, tactile, kinesthetic, vestibular, and visual signals and cues with the mother.

Of course, breastfeeding behavior and the full compliment of materials found in human breastmilk function as a direct link to the mother's entero-immune system, a role played by the umbilical cord before birth. After birth, the form or experience of nutritional delivery assures the convergence of an array of sensory (skin-to-skin) experiences while receiving these critical substances not unlike what occurred in utero. Mother's milk delivered to her infant obviously includes species-specific nutritional proteins and enzymes in just the right molecular configuration and quantity, but her milk also contains anti-oxidants and unique hormonal proteins along with antibodies unique to the specific home micro-environment within which each mother-infant dyad lives. Together, maternal-infant proximity and contact bridge *in utero* prenatal experiences with postnatal ones.

Breathing behavior is generally considered independent of regulation by another person, yet liquid breathing of amniotic fluid by the human fetus occurs before birth. This "practice breathing" is affected by the mother's internal physiological status. Might there be postnatal influences that continue to regulate an infant's breathing when the mother is close? Consider that *in utero* liquid amniotic breathing has been documented among so many mammalian species that it is no longer appropriate to speak of the initiation of breathing at

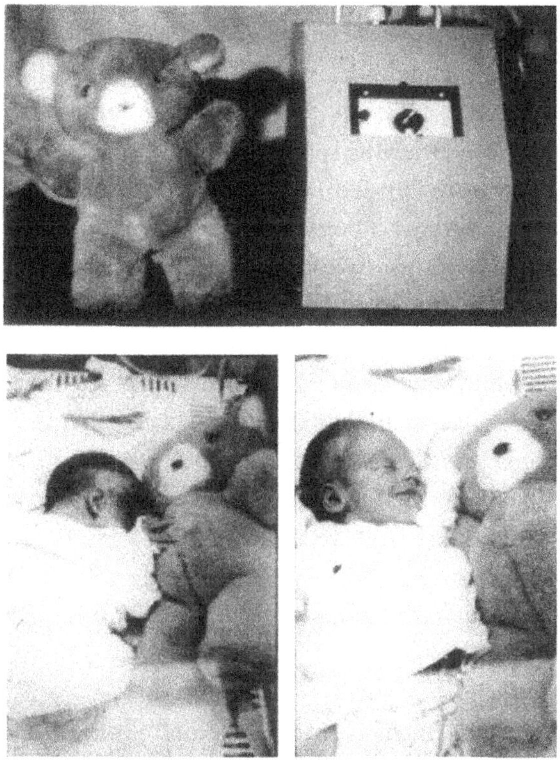

Figure 4. Thoman and Grahams' (1986) experiment with newborn infants and a breathing mechanical teddy bear illustrates the postnatal sensitivity infants maintain from prenatal experiences. The experimental infants changed their breathing patterns in relationship to the movements of their artificial breathing companion, perhaps showing a patterned response learned while breathing amniotic fluid in their mothers' womb (McKenna *et al.*, 1993). Original photo from Thoman and Graham (1986).

birth. Janzen and Chernick (1983) were the first to suggest that …"postnatal breathing may instead be viewed as a continuation of the process begun in utero." Perhaps as long as three months before birth, they suggest that "sensory stimulation alone in the absence of blood gas changes (oxygen/co2) regularly initiate rhythmic breathing (amniotic or liquid breathing) in the human fetus" (Janzen & Chernick, 1983).

Ultrasound studies reveal that fetal breathing can be identified by observing movement of the chest wall accompanied by outward movement of the abdomen. It is estimated that fetal liquid breathing occurs approximately 40% of the time during the last trimester, beginning around 30-31 weeks gestation, although its frequency varies greatly and may occur in fetuses as early as week 21 of gestation.

It appears that amniotic breathing among humans develops prenatally in conjunction with (and against) rhythmic sounds of the mother's arterial blood flow, every tenth of a second following contraction of the heart. The fetus is in close contact with the *schwooshing* sounds made by blood passing quickly through the iliac artery, which flows close to the fetus' left ear. Patrick (1978a, 1978b; 1980) monitored pregnant mothers for up to 24 hours at a time during the last ten weeks of pregnancy and found that while the frequency of fetal breathing could vary from hour to hour, it tended to peak about two to three hours after meals. There appears to be a peak between 4:00 am and 7:00 am in the morning when the mother's glucose levels are falling rapidly and the acoustic environment is quiet, permitting the fetus to be sensitized to uterine sounds and rhythms. In this way, the prenatal form of the fetus' circadian breathing rhythm is tied to, if not regulated by, the mother's rhythm through auditory and vestibular sensory stimuli.

Hence, based on breathing experiences in the womb, at least full term neonates are prepared at birth to respond to a variety of their mothers' breathing signals or cues postnatally, including her breathing sounds made as air passes through her vessels, inducing air pressure changes in the mother and infant's micro-environment, as mother exhales on or near the infant creating waves of warmed 0_2 and $C0_2$ gases.

Sensitivity to physiological regulation by the mother's breathing movements and sounds of the infant's breathing is exquisitely illustrated by studies of the effects of a sleeping companion on the human infant's breathing patterns. Thomen and Graham (1986) discovered that even mechanical breathing teddy bears placed next to apnea-prone human newborns have the effect of reducing the number of apneas (on severely apnea-prone infants) by as much as 60% (Thoman & Graham, 1986) (**Figure 4**).

In another experiment, we found that at varying distances in bed, mothers exhale amounts of CO_2 in front of their infants' faces (and under the blankets) that can shift the amount of CO_2 available for infants to breathe by two to five percent, potentially helping regulate the infant's breathing pace, since the infant's nasal chemoreceptors respond after the infant inhales (Mosko *et al.*, 1998). This is reinforced by added vestibular (movement) stimulation delivered by the mother's rising and falling chest and by stimulation of the infant's pancian cells in the skin, reacting to maternal touch and passive contact, all of which can be responded to by an infant in proximity to a parent (McKenna, 1986).

The "Social" Experiential Aspects of Learning to Breath

Perhaps this close connection between prenatal fetal breathing in the womb and the mother's physiological status also explains why the postnatal breathing of an infant is so dramatically effected by the presence of the human mother while cosleeping in the same bed. Our research team showed that it is possible to identify synchronous breathing patterns among routinely bedsharing mother-infant dyads. Infants could be associated with their mothers based on their eight-hour sleep-wake histograms and breathing traces, and by the fact that each infant seemed to breathe in respiratory cycles per minute, approximately twice the speed of its own mother (McKenna & Mosko, 1990). We also found a high number of instances in which apneas experienced by one of the partners overlapped temporally within seconds by an apnea apparently induced by the sleeping partner (McKenna & Mosko, 1990).

In a more complex and controlled study (Mosko *et al.*, 1996), we examined the differences between the physiology of breathing among routinely solitary sleeping infants and bedsharing mother-infant pairs and found that mother-infant bedsharing was associated with fewer obstructive apneas and more periodic breathing in infants than was the solitary sleep environment, where mothers and babies slept in separate rooms (Richard *et al.*, 1998). During bedsharing, irrespective of the routine sleeping arrangement at home, the infants experienced a higher frequency of short (one to three seconds) central apneas during stages 1-2 and REM (and overall). This is not surprising given that central apneas generally follow arousals. It is hard to say for certain what the functional significance is, though arousals lead to increased breaths and higher oxygen saturation readings for the infant. We can speculate that they are not harmful and might well be beneficial. Among routinely solitary sleeping infants, who slept with their mothers in the same bed in the laboratory, the increase in apneas largely consisted of the shorter variety (3-5.9 seconds) while in stage 1-2 sleep; but in routinely bedsharing infants, it reflected increases in apneas in the 6-8.9 second range during REM and in the apnea range of 9-11.9 seconds during stage 1-2 sleep. In contrast to central apneas, obstructive apneas were decreased by bedsharing, but only among routinely solitary sleeping infants (while bedsharing) who had a lower frequency overall, specifically in stages 1-2 and REM (Richard *et al.*, 1998).

> **Cultural Influences on Infant Touching**
>
> *"In the western world, it is perhaps a great advantage for an infant to have a sensitive skin or diaper rash or some other dermatological disorder, for then, at least, it can be assured of receiving something resembling an adequate amount of cutaneous stimulation."*
>
> (Montagu, 1986:247).

Figure 5. Montagu's perspective: Does diaper rash have any benefit for the western infant?

In general, the amount of periodic breathing was also significantly increased in the bedsharing environment. Routinely bedsharing infants had a higher frequency of periodic breathing and a longer mean duration over the entire night (overall) while bedsharing, specifically during REM. Routinely solitary sleeping infants exhibited more frequent periodic breathing only during stages 3-4 while bedsharing in the laboratory with their mothers (Richard *et al.*, 1998).

Maternal-Infant Contact: "Nice" Social Idea or Fundamental Infant Physiology!

Although forms of infant sleeping, including cosleeping environments, vary enormously from culture to culture, the potentially beneficial regulatory and developmental effects of contact on infants do not (**Figure 5**). Whether born in Brazil, Sweden, the United States, England, or Nepal, whether living in a hunting-gathering society or an industrialized setting, when resting on their mothers' torso, both premature and full-term infants breathe more regularly, use energy more efficiently, maintain lower blood pressure, grow faster, and experience less stress (Anderson, 1991; Ludington-Hoe, 1990; Ludington-Hoe *et al.*, 1991; Ludington-Hoe *et al.*, 1992a; Luddington-Hoe *et al.*, 1992b). These data suggest that sensory exchanges with the mother alter and potentially regulate an infant's immature physiology.

As regards infant temperature, Fardig (1980) found that among newborns up to a degree of temperature is lost when infants are removed from their mothers' torso following birth, even when the separated infants are placed in incubators with ambient temperatures set to match their mother's body temperature. Richard (1999) found that among 11- to 16-week-old infants, solitary-sleeping infants exhibited lower average axillary (under arm) skin temperatures compared with breastfeeding infants sharing a bed with their mothers.

The question of infant body temperature and the effects of varying sleep environments on it raises an interesting methodological question: under what conditions, social or solitary, is "normal" infant sleep temperature (from which notions of elevated or lowered temperatures are proposed) derived? Consider, for example, that it is not that infant skin or core temperatures are "elevated" when bedsharing (suggesting a potential SIDS risk), but that solitary sleeping infant temperatures are artificially "lower" or sub-normal. This is so, it can be argued, because the original (normal) environment is not solitary but social. Applying evolutionary models to the study of infant body temperatures during sleep suggests it is the lower and not the higher infant temperature that is potentially a variation from the norm for the infant and, thus, may be the real stress or physiological challenge.

Hundreds, perhaps thousands, of scientific studies document the important role that maternal contact plays in stimulating infant growth and development, as well as healthy psychological and cognitive development, as reviews by McKenna *et al.* (1993), Trevathan and McKenna (1994), Schoen (2007), and Ball and Klingaman (in press) clearly reveal. Indeed, there is likely no part of an infant's physiological or psychological (including neurobiological) development that is ultimately unaffected by contact, especially in the human infant's first two to four months of life, wherein brain cells are being either pruned or nurtured, depending on the infant's social and physical experiences, before the infants experience their first developmental shift, and myelinization is well under way.

Recall that Field's classic studies of the effects of massage on pre-term infants demonstrated that infants in her experimental group gained weight 47% faster per day when systematically, gently massaged (Field *et al.*, 1986; Field, 2001; 1998; 1995). She speculates that touch stimulates the vagal nerve which induces the gastrointestinal tract to absorb more calories while reducing cortisol, a stress response, which can burn calories rather than permit them to be used for immunological maintenance or growth. Touch acts as an analgesic for infants, increases axillary and core body temperatures and oxygen saturation levels (Trevathan & McKenna, 1994). Touch maintains higher glucose levels in infants, reduces crying, promotes deeper sleep among high risk infants, reduces apneas, and helps to establish not only a more secure social connection (attachment and satisfaction) as regards the mother, but sustained early contact establishes a better maternal milk supply and an enhanced breastfeeding relationship which, on average, will last a greater number of months the more the mother and infant sleep in contact, i.e., bedshare (Ball & Klingaman, in press).

Not surprisingly, even for nonhuman primates born more neurologically mature at birth than are human infants, separation from the mother, even for older infants (say six to 12 months of age), short term, hour long separations (referred to as privation experiments) are known to induce serious adverse health consequences, including anaclitic depression, cardiac arrhythmias, reduced body temperatures, higher cortisol levels, more interrupted sleep, and susceptibility to colds, breathing problems, and other illnesses. Clearly, while human infants may be on the extreme high side of a continuum of needed maternal contact, all primates depend on touch as a fundamentally critical physiological segue necessary before healthy independence can be achieved, which, for most primates, is years away.

That maternal or bodily touch and sensory exchanges play such a vital role in the infant's digestion, including calorie absorption capacities and metabolism; sleep, breathing and arousal; and heart rate (Richard & Mosko, 2004) is no longer in need of much additional documentation. Indeed, the infant's fundamental physiology is regulated by contact and the fact that the human infant's brain is so undeveloped at birth again reminds us that Winnicott was perhaps more correct than he could have imagined when he said there really "is no such thing as a baby, but a baby and someone."

Maternal Infant Nighttime Separation and SIDS

When an evolutionary and cross-cultural view of infants and infant care practices is adopted, it is hard to imagine that any health professional could seriously assume that nighttime separation for the human infant could normally be associated with intrinsic benefits, at least where benefits are not defined in terms of parental desire for independence from their infants or in terms of situations where parents pose a real danger to an infant. In fact, the only reasonable prediction for the effects of routine nighttime separation from the mother for the human infant would involve adverse consequences. Indeed, the experiences of the industrialized west, having witnessed SIDS at unprecedented worldwide rates (Nelson *et al.*, 2001), generally supports this way of thinking.

Nelson *et al.'s* (2000) cross-cultural survey of the relationship between bedsharing and SIDS rates reveals that among a variety of cultures and regions worldwide as bedsharing rates increase SIDS rates are reduced or are non-existent. Many confounding factors, such as reduced maternal smoking and increased breastfeeding, likely help explain why SIDS is either unknown or exceedingly low in cosleeping cultures. Nonetheless, these cross-cultural differences in SIDS rates as they pertain to child care practices surely argues against any simplistic notion suggesting that as bedsharing increases across all circumstances so too will SIDS risks.

Finally, it is worth mentioning that even in the United States and Great Britain, it is the sub-groups of families with the greatest increases in both breastfeeding and bedsharing over the last decade (middle class whites) who, as a class of individuals, are experiencing the most precipitous declines in SIDS. These numbers need to be compared with other less fortunate socioeconomic groups (poor African American families in the U.S.) whose bedsharing rates have traditionally remained high (about 50%), but where declines in SIDS have not occurred to the same level or degree as is true for middle class whites, many of whom bedshare for part or all of the night.

HOW CULTURAL FOLK ASSUMPTIONS ABOUT THE NORMALCY OF SOLITARY INFANT SLEEP ACHIEVED SCIENTIFIC VALIDATION

> *"Our governments recent warning that it was unsafe to ever have babies or small children in bed with parents went way too far...It should be challenged because it's bad science...Bad science sets out to make a point, looks neither to the left nor to the right but only straight ahead for evidence that supports the point it sets out to make. When it finds evidence it likes, it gathers it tenderly and subjects it to little or no testing."*
>
> (Vonnegut K, *The Boston Globe*, October 24, 1999)
>
> *"Don't sleep with your baby or put the baby down to sleep in an adult bed...The only safe place for babies to sleep is a crib that meets current safety standards and has a tight-fitting-mattress."* (Ann Brown, Commissioner, Consumer Product Safety Commission, United States of America September 29, 1999 (10/24/99)

The preceding review of the fundamental biology underlying the more universal characteristics of the human mother-infant relationship provides a background against which to consider the recent controversy over whether or not, or under what circumstances, mothers and infants should sleep together—on the same or different surfaces (nearby) in an industrialized western context. To clearly understand the direction SIDS research has taken, one must first understand the role that traditional western social values, judgments, and expectations have played and continue to play in what amounts to the "cultural production" of the infant sleep research paradigm.

That is, scientific paradigms are *supposed* to emerge from a synthesis of diverse empirically-based descriptive studies and be relatively immune from ethnocentrism and local cultural assumptions. But, in this case, concepts of how babies sleep and how to measure normal infant sleep never reflected species-wide data nor evolutionary considerations. Indeed, neither the sleep behavior of other primates nor the evolutionary history of human sleeping arrangements, or even cross-cultural infant sleep patterns, were ever considered relevant to research methods concerned with how to derive measurements of "normal" human infant sleep. The idea that throughout all of our evolution human infants slept next to their mothers and breastfed throughout the night was not considered important nor a relevant fact; perhaps it was not even known by early researchers that cosleeping with breastfeeding constitutes the universal context within which infant sleep evolved. The complete omission of important biological processes intrinsic to the evolving nighttime mother–infant relationship, especially the metabolism of breastmilk, may explain why current recommendations to place infants in a separate sleep space continue to leave western mothers confused as regards to why their bodies, emotions, and minds incline them to do otherwise in spite of what our society "approves of " or "advocates" (Ball, 2002; McKenna & Volpe, in press).

In this section, we leave behind, at least momentarily, our discussion of the evolutionary biology of mothers and infants to consider the cultural history of an ideology endemic to the industrialized west, specifically, the idea that infants sleep best and are always more safe (and healthier) when they are left by themselves and not in bodily contact with either of their parents, whether breastfeeding or not. This ideology is a central premise in a contentious debate about sleeping arrangements and fuels fierce differences in approaches, interpretations of data, opinions, and conclusions regarding the benefits and risks of bedsharing and other forms of cosleeping (McKenna, 2000).

First, be aware that only in the last century have humans anywhere asked where their babies should or would sleep. It is a very "modern" question not asked by the majority of contemporary people. Indeed, perhaps it is more pertinent to ask whether billions of people could be wrong? The overwhelming majority of contemporary parents outside the western industrialized world appreciate and accept without question the benefits and necessity, if not the inevitability, of mothers sleeping next to their infants (cosleeping), which is seen as natural and expected, if not morally appropriate. Despite medical opposition to bedsharing, an increasing number of Western parents apparently do too, as a record number of western parents are beginning to adopt various forms of cosleeping practices, whether routine or intermittent (Blair & Ball, 2004; Ball, 2000; McKenna & Volpe, in press; McCoy *et al.*, 2000; Ball & Hooker, 1999; Mccarin, 1995; Hoffmann, 1999; Seabrook, 2000; Jackson, 2000; Nix, 2000; Elias *et al.*, 1986; Cable & Rothenberg, 1984; Wright, 1998; Abbott, 1992; Werland, 1999; Goode, 1999).

Indeed, according to several recent surveys in the United States, Australia, and Great Britain, a major cultural shift is underway, leading to fewer infants being placed to sleep in rooms by themselves than ever before in recent western cultural history. It would appear that during the last decade in parallel with increasingly high rates of breastfeeding, parents in the United States and Europe increasingly "cosleep" either in the form of room sharing or sleeping together on the same surface in the form of bedsharing at least part of the night. Recent surveys and sampling suggest that between 50-75% of western infants sleep part of the night on some days of the week in the same bed with their parents (Lahr *et al.*, 2005; Ball & Blair, 2004; Kimmel, 2002; McCoy *et al.*, 2004). Surely, it appears to be "back to the future" as regards the important link between breastfeeding and forms of cosleeping, as all the studies thus far undertaken are consistent in finding that breastfeeding and bedsharing appear mutually reinforcing...that a decision to breastfeed likely means that a mother will also bedshare, as bedsharing makes breastfeeding easier and seems to just "feel right" (Ball,2004; 2005; Young, 1999; McCoy *et al.*, 2004; Baddock, 2007; Rigby *et al.*, 2001; McKenna & Volpe, in press; McKenna *et al.*, 1997).

Table 2. Historical Factors/Forces Influencing Emergence of Western Solitary Infant Sleep Ideology
Notion of infants original sin / need for imposed / self-discipline / fear of spoiling
Fear of infants / children observing sex, masturbation by wet nurses, fear of affection or touching
Catholic church bans bedsharing due to infanticide confessed (in confessionals) by starving mothers
Values favoring individualism, independence, autonomy, self discipline, and self-sufficiency
Re-location of parental decision making to outside of home to external authorities / rise of child care experts...pediatricians, as authoritative medical knowledge comes to dismiss acquired parental knowledge of infant
Emphasis on romantic nature of husband - wife conjugal relationship to exclusion of children
Emphasis on superiority of technology as a substitute for mother's body and what her body provides (cows milk rather than breastmilk, stimulating obects or swings rather than mothers sensory exchanges achieved through contact).

But Where Did The Notion of the Maternally Disconnected, Solitary Sleeping Infant Come From? Historical Roots of an Ideology

As discussed by McKenna (2000) and more recently by McKenna and McDade (2005), reference to unique western social, historical, economic, religious, and other cultural processes are necessary to fully explain the particular ideologies which underlie and enforce medical views of what constitutes healthy infant sleep, including an understanding of the willingness of the pediatric/medical community to adopt what has been proposed as invalid methods of studying "normal, healthy infant sleep." The western infants sleep research paradigm builds upon negative assumptions about the alleged devastating consequences of cosleeping behavior. Indeed, so entrenched and often hidden are unproven assumptions and false stereotypes about cosleeping, in whatever form it takes, that contemporary researchers/reviewers reading anti-bedsharing reports are not likely to spot or even notice how and where the authors' cultural assumptions, preferences, and biased interpretations are substituted and passed along as logically deducted scientific truths. These biases prevent researchers from acknowledging that the overwhelming number of deaths in the United States and other western countries involve not cosleeping, but infants sleeping alone.

For at least a century, western social and moral values have served as the basis for defining how and where infants *should* sleep, specifically, moral concerns protecting the conjugal (husband/wife) pair, enforcing social exclusivity and sexual invisibility from children, along with other cultural developments **(Table 2).** The perceived need to produce independent, self-disciplined, and secure infants through enforced nighttime separation from parents by sleeping in cribs inadvertently provided the initial basis for defining uninterrupted solitary infant sleep as "normal" and "healthy" --a desirable and beneficial way for all babies to sleep.

Indeed, the proliferation and expansion of the idea of "romantic love" throughout Europe also contributed to separating the parents, especially the father, from the children. Many European and later American households favored the role of the father as the disciplinarian, as well as the importance of his role in dispensing religious training. To display optimal moral authority, it was thought that the father should constrain from physical contact with his children in favor of functions that really mattered, i.e., providing discipline (Stone, 1977), another belief that might well have contributed to separate sleeping quarters for western children.

The exaggerated fear of suffocating an infant while cosleeping may, in part, stem from an unexpected time in western history where especially urban mothers were so destitute that in order for some of her children to live, others needed to be sacrificed in the form of being overlaid. During the last 500 years, many poor women living in Paris, Brussels, Munich, and London (to name but a few locales) confessed to Catholic priests of having murdered their infants by overlaying them in order to control family size (Flandrin, 1979; Kellum, 1979; Stone, 1977). Led by priests who threatened ex-communication, fines, or imprisonment for actual deaths, infants were banned from parental beds (Stone, 1977). The legacy of this particular historical condition in western history probably converged with other changing social mores and customs (values favoring privacy, self-reliance, and individualism) to provide yet another piece of the overall philosophical foundation at the core of our present contemporary cultural beliefs about sleeping arrangements. This particular foundation makes it far easier to find dangers associated with cosleeping than to find (or assume) hidden benefits.

As discussed by Fildes (1995), the popularity of scheduled bottle feeding in the fifties also reinforced the idea that uninterrupted solitary crib sleeping was 'normal.' In the late fifties and early sixties when electro-physiological technology became widely available to measure and quantify infant sleep, breastfeeding was at an all time low in the U.S., with less than nine percent of mothers leaving the hospital breastfeeding, usually for less than a couple of weeks. Both cows' milk and/or formula were thought to be superior to human milk. Hence, pioneering sleep researchers had no reason to question the appropriateness of quantifying infant sleep and arousal patterns under solitary sleeping conditions using bottle fed infants with little or no parental contact or nighttime feedings.

Furthermore, throughout the last century, infants sleeping separate from their parents has been argued to be ideal, certainly since Truby King, a most influential physician and author of Mothercraft in Great Britain. Manuals described by Hardyment (1983) stressed the need to keep babies on "strict feeding and sleep schedules" with parentally controlled and limited feeding. Dr. John Watson of the United States, whose overall support of any behavior toward infants which fostered infant separation and independence and who introduced behaviorism to psychology, also heavily influenced what was already a powerful cultural belief that for the infant's physical, psychological, and intellectual health, infants needed to be left alone and definitely not touched much or often.

Watson argued that no child can receive "too little affection" and that if parents insisted on any contact with their children at night at all, it should be quick and simple... no more than three pats on the forehead and a quick kiss to the head. Ferber's sleep training in the United States (though now repudiated by him) and Ford's (2002) "controlled crying" in which parents leave the infant or child alone for longer and longer periods to condition them to fall asleep on their own represent what Klingaman and Ball (in press) correctly describe as representing several of many modern descendants of Watson's authoritarian approach to the infant and what infants should be allowed to experience.

In fact, while these predecessors to Dr. Spock all argued a similar nighttime strategy, i.e., separate sleep

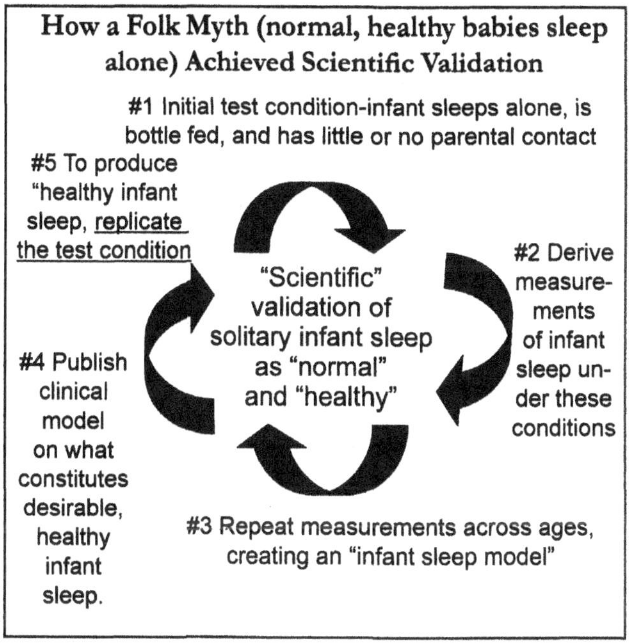

Figure 6. When infant sleep studies were first undertaken using polysomnography, not unexpectedly, the first researchers, measuring the electro-physiology of infant sleep stages and arousal patterns at various times in the first year of the infant's life, only tested the solitary sleeping, bottle-fed infant in the sleep laboratory. At the time, these experimental conditions (the infant being alone and bottle fed) were thought normal and best for the infant.

quarters for infants and children and strict, controlled, minimal nighttime feeds and contact (and certainly breastfeeding was not encouraged), their influence suggested that physicians had moral authority not only over the infants but over the parents who should do just as their doctors order…rather than relying on their own familiarity with their own unique infants. The legacy of this western medical authoritative knowledge being superior to any knowledge parents acquire or bring to their parenting experiences continues to negatively impact parents and moves them to question their own emotions and tendencies when it comes to caring for their babies—a rather strange and unique handicap associated with western cultural history.

Such ideologies and situations fail not only to consider both the biology of the infant and the parent, but such arm-chair models of infant care, rendered for the most part by men who never cared for their own babies or any babies for that matter, claim authority over a behavioral domain for which they had no special knowledge or training. Moral and cultural ideas quickly became one and the same with supposedly scientific statements and recommendations. Yet, from a human wide perspective, solitary infant sleep remains novel and abnormal, as is infant sleep that occurs after ingesting milk from a different species. Still, the solitary sleeping, bottle fed infant remains the singular source of our scientific understanding of how the healthy human infant sleeps.

The clinical and psychological problems this poses for infants and thus for parents is not trivial. This model of solitary infant sleep places parental expectations at odds with what infants are designed to biologically experience and, of course, accept! Recall that while recent lifestyles and beliefs about where and how infants should sleep can and do change relatively quickly, the physiological needs of human infants do not. Consider that for the last 10,000 years human evolution, including infant biology, has remained relatively unchanged, leading David Barash (1987) to note "...there would be little if any difficulty exchanging a Cro-Magnon and a modern infant, but great incongruity in making the same switch with adults of both cultures" (1987). Only in the last 100 to 200 years and mostly in western industrialized societies have recent cultural concepts concerning the presumed moral value of infant separateness from the mother become embedded within scientific and clinical paradigms that worked their way into popular and scientific culture. These paradigms continue to be used as a basis to limit or constrain the forms, quality,

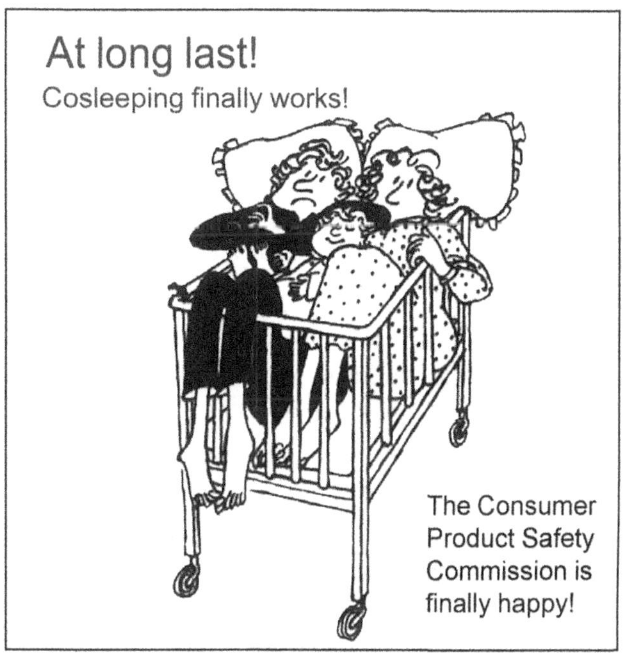
At long last!
Cosleeping finally works!
The Consumer Product Safety Commission is finally happy!

Figure 7. Sketch from Helen Jackson: Three in a Bed

and quantity of nighttime maternal-infant contact and breastfeeding.

The "science" of infant sleep, thus, became one and the same with the morals and folk beliefs of the original scientists who justified the method of measuring infant sleep in the first place—that is measuring "normal infant sleep" while infants slept alone and digested cow's milk, with little or no maternal or any parental contact. The "science" of infant sleep, meaning quantified measurements of sleep architecture and arousals over the infant's first year, and the values (both numerical and moral) that clinically defined desirable infant sleep became mutually reinforcing and mutually supportive (**Figure 6**) (McKenna & McDade, 2005).

Of course, this meant that if parents and their pediatricians wanted to produce "normal and healthy" sleeping infants, only by recreating the original environmental conditions under which "healthy" infant sleep was measured (alone and bottle fed) could anyone hope to achieve it. Thus, clinically healthy infant sleep became synonymous with solitary sleep and vice-versa, i.e., culture and science are yet again inextricably bound—a clinically healthy infant must sleep alone and be bottle fed in order to meet the proper "measurement" requirements.

Another negative consequence of these studies is that they inadvertently made infants who could not quite "measure up" to the numbers in need of remediation, either social or biological! How and where infants sleep could no longer be considered a simple relational family issue, but a serious medical one, to be assessed and monitored by authoritative sleep experts passing research information along to family pediatricians. Adherence by infants to quantified *scientific* "models" of healthy solitary infant sleep (including dire warnings to avoid cosleeping at all costs) could be used to predict, it is claimed, lifelong childhood health and sleep hygiene. Infant health could be obtained just as long as mothers, in the words of Dr. Spock, "followed the directions that *their* doctor(s) *gave them*" (McKenna & McDade, 2005).

Altogether, this chain of events explains how questions concerning what constitutes safe infant sleep environments, i.e., "the bedsharing debate," has been turned on its head: species-wide and biologically normal and protective infant sleep environments, mother-infant cosleeping with breastfeeding, are assumed to be inherently lethal while solitary crib sleeping is assumed to be healthy, beneficial, and always safer. The burden of proof concerning infant safety was left to the defenders of mother-infant cosleeping. While a Commissioner of Consumer "Product" Safety who oversees deficient products and goods and presumably knows nothing about infant sleep development, the biological significance of mother-infant cosleeping with breastfeeding, or family psychology, was encouraged by a very small cohort of anti-bedsharing researchers in the United States to make what in any other cultural context would surely be hailed as one of the most extraordinarily outrageous statements of our times: "The only safe place for an infant to sleep is in a crib…." (**Figure 7**).

In sum, socially constructed folk assumptions, not deductive, empirically-based (species-wide) science, answered the original question--how do infants sleep and, thus, how and under what conditions infant sleep must be measured. The history of infant sleep studies in western cultures illustrates how a "belief" in the moral "value" of uninterrupted solitary infant sleep remains, like religion, sacred despite recent scientific studies that seriously challenge its biological normalcy or assumed advantages. These beliefs about infant sleep continue to lead a small number of SIDS and bedsharing researchers to believe, a priori, that any violation of this artificially validated moral principle (solitary crib sleeping) is sure to lead to social or physical harm. In this way, cosleeping---and specifically bedsharing, represent both medical and moral violations---violations of cultural norms which practically assures negative physical and psychological outcomes (McKenna & McDade, 2005; McKenna & Gettler, in press).

BACK TO THE FUTURE: DEFINING COSLEEPING

What is Cosleeping?

> *"Cosleeping is a generic concept referring to the diverse ways in which a primary caregiver, usually the mother, sleeps within close proximity (arms reach) of the infant, permitting each to detect and respond to a variety of sensory stimuli (sound, movement, smells, sights) emitted by the other. Cosleeping is the universal (species-wide) human sleeping arrangement"*
> (McKenna *et al.*, 1993).

In one form or another, mother-infant cosleeping continues to represent the preferred sleeping arrangement for most of the world's parents. Based on cultures studied thus far, between 44% and 75% of the world's mothers and infants sleep in direct bodily contact (Barry & Paxson, 1971). In fact, outside of the West, there exist no ethnographic examples of industrialized countries where infants sleep outside the mother's room, away from her company.

There appears to be no "one way" to cosleep, either. Mother-infant cosleeping takes hundreds, if not thousands, of forms worldwide (Barry & Paxson, 1971; Whiting, 1981; Levine *et al.*, 1994; Mintern & Lambert, 1964; Munroe *et al.*, 1981). Infants sleep next to their mothers on floor-based futons. They sleep alongside, but not on the same surface as their mother in a crib or bassinet next to the mother's bed, but within arm's reach. Cosleeping occurs when infants sleep in a basket or a cradleboard, in a hammock above or beside the mother's sleep surface, or when mothers and infants lie beside each other on a bamboo mat. Side-by-side mother-infant sleep on the same surface, however, appears to be the most common arrangement worldwide (Barry & Paxson, 1971).

One of the problems associated with understanding differential outcomes associated with forms of cosleeping is that while a proposal to standardize a definition has been made (McKenna *et al.*, 1993; McKenna & Mosko, 2000), many researchers choose not to recognize it. By recognizing different "types" or different forms of cosleeping, one recognizes that cosleeping per se has no singular risk factor, but many, depending on how it is practiced, and this would argue against a simplistic condemnation of the practice. In other words, the diversity of cosleeping in form, function, and outcome is not generally recognized, primarily due to political and ideological reasons characteristic of those who favor the view that any and all cosleeping is dangerous.

> *"What is cosleeping? When my two lovely daughters are sleeping at the same time."* Robert Hahn, CDC

Unlike the discourse associated with crib sleeping which can be addressed in terms of safe or unsafe crib use, one can only conclude that the long history of negative thinking that all forms of "sleeping with baby" are injurious in western society has led many researchers to think of cosleeping behavior as a discrete and homogenous (coherent) behavior, rather than as being composed of many different behaviors, as discussed above. Many researchers erroneously use the terms "cosleeping" and "bedsharing" interchangeably, as a kind of "dustbin" category, lumping together dangerous forms of cosleeping, like recliner and/or couch cosleeping, in the same category as safe bedsharing, even though each carries remarkably different risk factors.

In the context of SIDS and pediatric sleep research, McKenna *et al.* (1993), McKenna and Mosko (2000), and McKenna and McDade (2005) proposed that the term cosleeping be used generically, as a beginning point, to describe a diverse, but proactive, generalized class of sleeping arrangements, and not to describe any one particular "type" of cosleeping arrangement, for example, bedsharing. One step toward standardizing a definition of safe mother-infant cosleeping that can be extended to include situations where high levels of mother or caregiver-infant body contact occurs during sleep is to apply the description safe cosleeping to particular "types" in which at least one proactive responsible adult cosleeper (whether mother or not) takes safety precautions unique to the particular "type" of cosleeping practiced. And, regardless of whether sleeping occurs on the same or a different surface or with another adult present, the cosleeping dyad are potentially able to communicate through multiple, but at least two mutually reinforcing sensory modalities, such as tactile and visual, auditory and olfactory, visual and auditory, and/or auditory and vestibular sensory channels.

Safe mother-infant cosleeping can be applied to bedsharing situations where the overall bedsharing context (physical setting and social circumstances, including triadic situations) are made as safe as current knowledge permits, and where at least one adult cosleeper/caregiver is physically capable and motivated to detect and respond to changes in the baby's status. Sleep location, such as an infant sleeping alone on an adult bed without a parent present (Drago & Dannenberg, 1999; Nakamura *et al.*, 1999), is not considered bedsharing, using this operational definition.

As proposed here and elsewhere in papers by McKenna, a safe cosleeping environment must always provide the infant with the opportunity to "sense" and respond behaviorally and/or physiologically to the caregiver's signals and cues, for example, to the mother's smells, breathing sounds, infant directed speech, sleep or breathing movements, invitations to breastfeed, touches, or to any as yet unidentified "hidden" sensory stimuli whether intended or not. In this way, bedsharing is not necessarily excluded from being considered one type of "safe cosleeping," but like the other specific "types" of cosleeping, bedsharing needs to be further taxonomically differentiated into one of two sub-types: safe or unsafe.

Although the same can be said for almost any sleeping arrangement, such as solitary crib sleeping, bedsharing is probably practiced slightly differently in each household. Yet, now we can identify specific, modifiable "bedsharing risk factors" as well as "crib risk factors" (Blaie *et al.*, 1999) that should help to eliminate unnecessary risk regardless of location or arrangement.

Cosleeping in Form, Function and Outcome: A Many Diverse Thing

> Diversity of cosleeping concept? *"I slept in the same bed with my granddaddy..and then in the same bed with my four cousins. I never slept alone until I got married."*
> Bobby Bowden, Head Football Coach, Florida State University, South Bend Tribune, 9/29/2000

An infant's sleep location is the beginning not the end point for analysis in studying sleeping arrangements for infants because so much more in the environment, including the motives of the mother herself or cosleeping adults, makes a difference in assessing safety and outcomes in general (Kelmanson, 1993; McKenna & Mosko, 2000). For example, all "types" of cosleeping must be distinguished by the condition and composition of sleeping structures or pieces of furniture or materials which are used, including characteristics of the sleep surface (hard, soft, fibrous, textured, or smooth) and by the bedding materials, including infant sleep wrappings, night clothes, and/or blankets, as well as by who and/or how many people are sleeping close to, with, or by the infant or child.

Compared with solitary infant sleep, analytically important features of the cosleeping environment are more numerous and more complex. For example, in the bedsharing environment it appears that the quality of care the infant receives from the caregiver once in bed is partially determined by the nature of their social relationship outside of the bed, which often helps to explain the parent's reasons for cosleeping. Consider that mandatory, non-elected bedsharing by smoking mothers that occurs in socially chaotic households where bedsharing is the only option leads to outcomes quite different from those situations in which bedsharing is elected by a non-smoking mother specifically to protect, nurture, and breastfeed her infant under more routinized, stable social circumstances (Kemp *et al.*, 2000; Carroll-Pankhurst & Mortimer, 2001; Clemens, 2003).

To give just a few examples, only recently have researchers begun to address in a serious way (Blair *et al.*, 1999) the impact of particular adverse circumstances on the bedsharing environment. Among parents of infants who have died unexpectedly in Great Britain, the prevalence of alcohol consumption, cigarette smoking, and the use of illegal drugs was also higher, while the infants exhibited adverse clinical features at birth (prematurity, low birth weight). Moreover, during their short lives, these doomed infants experienced more infections and lower daily weight gains, suggesting increased vulnerability from the beginning. Treating bedsharing as a starting point in which risks occur rather than as a crude end-point and a risk in and of itself, Blair *et al.* (1999) found no evidence to suggest that bedsharing was a risk among parents who did not smoke or among infants four months or older.

In another study in St. Petersberg, Russia, compromised maternal attachment was found to be associated with many babies who died while bedsharing. Physicians of the dead infants indicated that the mothers of the deceased infants had been less eager "to quiet or comfort" their infants in general. And, while their infants were being examined by the physician before their deaths, these mothers "paid less attention to the baby's responses" and were less willing or likely to touch or look at them, compared with matched control mothers whose babies lived (Kelmanson, 1993).

Bedsharing, Room Sharing, Sofa and Recliner Use, as Particular "Types" of Cosleeping

It should be increasingly clear as McKenna and Mosko (2001) previously addressed that bedsharing is just one of many forms of cosleeping, and while all bedsharing represents a more intimate type of cosleeping, not all cosleeping takes the form of bedsharing. Moreover, safe bedsharing can be distinguished from unsafe bedsharing. For these reasons, "cosleeping" and "bedsharing" are not synonymous and should not be used interchangeably, a distinction not acknowledged by Drago and Dannenberg (1999) and Nakamura *et al.* (1999) in their condemnation of "cosleeping" and "bedsharing."

Bedsharing is complicated because it involves different furniture components, sometimes articulated but sometimes not. Adult beds mostly include mattresses, usually but not always surrounded by other pieces of furniture, such as wood or metal frames. Sleeping in or on a bed represents one of the major contexts within which cosleeping among westerners is likely to take place. Bedsharers sleep on at least one cloth mattress and sometimes on a cloth mattress and a box spring in many western societies. Although cloth mattresses can sit on the floor without a frame, this can be dangerous for infants if the mattress is positioned next to a hard wall or surface. The infant's head can become wedged in the space between the wall and the mattress, leading to asphyxiation, a major category of mechanical death reported by Drago and Dannenberg (1999).

Room Sharing as a Form of Cosleeping That Helps Protect Infants from SIDS

Room-sharing between infants and parents increasingly is the norm in many western countries and is associated with increased protection against SIDS, although studies showing the protective effects of room sharing did not include data on the actual proximity of the infants to their caregivers or if their mothers were breastfeeding. Nevertheless, depending on whether or not the infant and parent can see, hear, and/or smell each other and if the caregiver intends to monitor and respond to an infant, room sharing can be considered another form of safe cosleeping. There is, of course, a spatial distance outside of which caregiver-infant sensory exchanges which define cosleeping, as proposed here, are impossible.

Roomsharing, as one form of cosleeping, is now recommended by the American Academy of Pediatrics as a way to help reduce SIDS, although statements made by the AAP Infant Sleep and SIDS sub-section following the announcement of the 2005 new SIDS guidelines seemed far more interested in publicly recommending against bedsharing, another form of cosleeping, than getting their message across that babies should sleep "proximate" to their caregivers. This recommendation constitutes an unprecedented acknowledgement. This is the first time any prestigious western medical organization has stated that a mother's presence or proximity can be critical to the survival of her infant… and that infants should never sleep alone!

Epidemiological data show that in the presence of an adult caregiver, room-sharing infants are approximately half as likely to die from SIDS as are infants sleeping either alone or in the same room with siblings (Carpenter *et al.*, 2004; Mitchell & Thompson, 1995; Blair *et al.*, 1999; Fleming *et al.*, 1996). Indeed, these findings also show that it takes a committed adult caregiver to achieve these protective effects as the findings did not generalize as to the presence of other children in the infant's room. This suggests, of course, that the mother plays a proactive role, a special protective role, involving, as has been argued elsewhere, both behavioral responses to the infant, potentially detecting risky conditions and/or dangerous sleeping situations, and inducing biological changes in the infant's body through sensory regulation which permits the infant to more easily resist SIDS (McKenna *et al.*, 1993; Mosko *et al.*, 1993; Mosko *et al.*, 1996).

BEDSHARING STUDIES: WHAT DOES IT MEAN TO BEDSHARE WITH AN INFANT AND WHAT DOES IT MEAN NOT TO? THE MOTHER-INFANT DYAD IN THE LABORATORY: SLEEPING TOGETHER AND APART

Over a 20-year period at both UC Irvine School of Medicine and the University of Notre Dame Mother-Baby Behavioral Sleep Laboratory, we have been conducting various studies of nighttime infant caregiving practices, trying to ascertain what happens when mothers and infants who usually bedshare do not and what happens when routinely solitary sleeping mother-infant pairs bedshare (McKenna *et al.*, 1990; Mosko *et al.*, 1993; McKenna *et al.*, 1999; 1997; Mosko *et al.*, 1996; 1997a; 1997b; Richard *et al.*, 1996; 1998). Our UC Irvine research team quantified differences in the sleep behavior and physiology of 70 routinely bedsharing or routinely solitary sleeping mothers and infants. This particular study was carried out over 105 separate nights and generated 155 eight-hour infrared video recordings. More than 200 separate eight-hour polysomnographic recordings were made of mothers and their infants either sharing a bed or sleeping apart in adjacent rooms over three successive nights. We specifically compared how the solitary sleep environment and the bedsharing environment affected the two kinds of mother-infant pairs – those who routinely bedshared and those who routinely slept apart.

In randomly assigned order, each mother–infant pair spent two nights sleeping in their routine (home) sleeping condition and one night sleeping in the non-routine condition; that is, routine bedsharing pairs slept in different rooms, routine solitary sleepers bedshared. All mothers and infants were healthy and nearly exclusively breastfeeding. The infants ranged in age from 11 to 15 weeks (the peak age for SIDS) (Mosko *et al.*, 1996). This is the only study ever conducted in which a full montage of recording devices monitored, filmed, and quantified a suite of physiological signals of each individual in the mother-infant pair over three successive nights, alternating between each pair's usual and imposed sleeping arrangement. Heart rates, breaths, oxygen saturation levels, and brain waves and signals were recorded, permitting us, with some accuracy, to score all nighttime sleep stage durations and progressions, including all arousals, both small transient types and epochal larger ones (Mosko *et al.*, 1997a; 1997b).

The "choice" to cosleep, specifically in the form of mother-infant bedsharing, was found to create a cascade of related changes both in terms of behavior and the physiology of each partner in the dyad (Mckenna, 2000). Most relevant to our concerns in this chapter is the fact that our laboratory studies documented a significant increase not only in the number of breastfeeds, but in the total nightly durations of breastfeeding. Different laboratories have recorded different total nightly durations of breastfeeding in the bedsharing breastfeeding dyad, but all find that when sleeping next to mother, the number of breastfeeding sessions per night increases significantly (Ball, 2003; Baddock *et al.*, 2007; Young, 1999), which likely has many benefits for the mother and infant.

Bedsharing also correlated with shorter average intervals between breastfeeding sessions. Among 70 nearly exclusively breastfeeding Latina mothers, we found that when bedsharing the average interval between breastfeeds was approximately an hour and a half. When sleeping in separate bedrooms (but still within earshot), the interval was at least twice as long. Moreover, on their bedsharing nights, babies often breastfed twice as often as they did on their solitary sleep night and had three times the total nightly duration, compared with the times they slept alone (McKenna *et al.*, 1997). Also, our studies showed that without instruction, breastfeeding mothers choose the supine infant sleep position nearly 100% of the time (Richard *et al.*, 1997; Ball, 2006a).

It should be noted that while breastfeeding babies are always under-represented in SIDS populations and fewer breastfed babies die in the first year of life compared with bottle-fed babies (Chen & Rogan, 2004), increased protection specifically from SIDS through breastfeeding is not universally recognized (Gilbert *et al.*, 1995). However, at least half the studies show it as being protective. Since no two studies use the same definition of breastfeeding, research in this area remains difficult to compare (McKenna *et al.*, 1997). In the United States, a major multi-center epidemiological study found that *not breastfeeding* was a risk factor for SIDS in both black and white populations (Hoffman *et al.*, 1988).

Only one epidemiological study has looked at whether dose-specific response effects exist and whether they are stable across races and socioeconomic groups in relationship to SIDS. This study's data support the possibility that increased breastfeeding leads to increased protection from SIDS. Fredrickson *et al.* (1993) found that for both black and white Americans, the risk of

Table 3. Potential Short Term Benefits of Cosleeping in the Form of Bedsharing when Practiced Safely

Short-Term Benefits of Cosleeping
Mother
More sleep (in minutes) and increased nightly satisfaction
Increased sensitization to infant physiological and social status
Increased comfort with and ability to interpret behavioral cues of infant
Increased sucking behavior of infant maintains milk supply
Increased prolactin levels lead to longer birth interval
Increased ability to monitor and physically manage and respond to infant needs
More time wth baby for working parents
Infant
Increased breastfeeding (total minutes and number of nightly feeding sessions)
Increased infant sleep duration
Less crying time
Increased sensitivity to mother's communication
More light (stage 1-2) sleep, less deep (stage 3-4) sleep, appropriate for age
Increase in infant heart rate
Reduction in number of obstructive apneas in stage 3-4 sleep
Practice at arousing

SIDS decreased for every month of breastfeeding. Conversely, for white mothers, the risk of SIDS increased by 1.19 for every month of not breastfeeding and 2.0 for every month of non-exclusive breastfeeding. For black mothers, the risk of SIDS increased by 1.19 for every month of not breastfeeding and by 2.3 for every month of non- exclusive breastfeeding (Jura *et al.*, 1994).

Mother-infant Interactions and Mutual Responses

In the face of no explanation of how supine sleeping might protect infants against SIDS, it is reasonable to assume that sleep position is but one factor among many. Other potential explanatory factors include arousals, sleep-stage progression and duration, body orientation, feeding, touching and movement patterns, time asleep, time awake, body temperature, and vocalizations. These physiological and behavioral changes mutually regulate each other when the breastfeeding mother-infant dyad sleeps in close proximity. Surely, as Ball (2006a) so carefully documents, almost every aspect of the infant and mother's physical orientation to each other in bed and the use of the bed and bedding by the mother (**Table 3**), in addition to physiological sensitivities, i.e., response to each other's arousals, is changed if she is a breastfeeder, as compared to a bottle feeder. It is likely the convergence of these changes that makes it safer for the breast versus bottle feeding bedsharing infant.

From our infrared video studies of mothers and infants bedsharing, it appears supine infant sleep maximizes the infant's overall ability to communicate with its mother and to control its micro-environment (McKenna *et al.*, 1994; Young, 1999). In addition to permitting the infant to move to and away from the breast, back-sleeping permits the infant to remove blankets covering its face, to turn to face toward or away from mother's face or body, to touch its own face, wipe its nose, and, without a great deal of effort, suck its fist or fingers.

Similar to Baddock *et al.* (2007), we found that in the bedsharing environment mothers interact and respond to their babies much more frequently and in more diverse ways than they do when the infant sleeps in a separate room. These interactions range from rearranging the infant's bedding and blankets, to visual inspections, to re-positioning the infant, such as pulling the infant away from pillows or uncovering the infant's head. At times, mothers just kiss or whisper to their infants, often leading to EEG identified arousals, including changes in heart rates and breathing in the infant, all potential benefits (McKenna *et al.*, 1994).

Our studies suggest that supine infant sleep in the breastfeeding/bedsharing context maximizes the chances the baby will be able to detect and respond to mother's movements, sounds, and touches, and vice versa. The supine position of the infant further promotes easy and constant communication, such as visual glancing and brief touches of the mother's breast which initiates breastfeeding sessions. This reportedly serves as the basis for growing mutual attachment between mother and infant, a prerequisite for healthy infant development (Lewis & Haviland, 1993).

Our studies have also found that, in general, small EEG-defined transient infant arousals recorded in the brain are facilitated in the bedsharing environment, albeit selectively, and that even when routinely bedsharing infants sleep alone, they continue to exhibit more transient arousals than do routinely solitary-sleeping infants sleeping alone (**Tables 2, 3**). Furthermore, bedsharing significantly shortens the amount of time per episode that infants remain in deeper stages of sleep (Stage 3-4). They spend more time in Stages 1 and 2 and more total time asleep (Mosko *et al.*, 1996). More arousals and less time in deep sleep may reduce the likelihood of an infant dying from SIDS, especially for infants born with arousal deficiencies.

We also documented an acute sensitivity on the part of the routine-bedsharing mothers to their infant's presence in bed. When sharing the bed, mothers who routinely bedshare aroused significantly more often than did routinely solitary-sleeping mothers, discounting instances in which the infant aroused first. This finding argues against the possibility that bedsharing mothers habituate to the presence of their babies and, thus, may pose a danger of overlaying them while asleep (Mosko *et al.*, 1997b).

Surprisingly, even though they awoke more often and fed their infants, routinely bedsharing mothers enjoyed as much sleep as routinely solitary-sleeping breastfeeding mothers (Mosko *et al.*, 1997a). Moreover, 84% of the routinely bedsharing mothers evaluated their sleep following their bedsharing night in the laboratory as being either good or enough, compared with 64% of the routinely solitary-sleeping mothers.

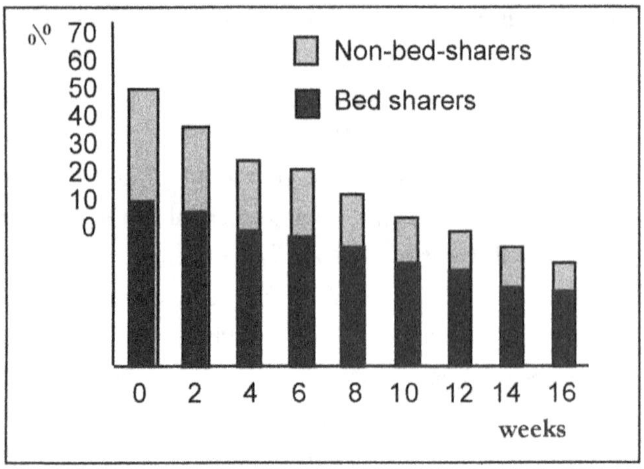

Figure 8. Ball shows here that compared with solitary sleeping breastfeeding mothers, bedsharing breastfeeding mothers were more likely to breastfeed their infants for a greater number of months.

In two earlier studies, we found that bedsharing mother-infant pairs exhibited a trend toward greater simultaneous overlap in all sleep stages, i.e., stages 1-2, 3-4, and REM. This synchronization of sleep states was not explained by chance and is not found when compared with the sleep/wake activity of randomly selected non-cosleeping infants (McKenna *et al.*, 1991; Mosko *et al.* 1993).

Researchers at the University of Otago in Dunedin, New Zealand (Baddock et al., 2007) conducted a study comparing physiologic and overnight video data from two groups of healthy infants: 40 bedsharing infants and 40 cot-sleeping infants. Bedsharing infants were defined as sleeping a minimum of five hours per night in the parental bed, whereas cot-sleeping infants regularly slept in a cot/bassinet in the parental bedroom for a minimum of five hours per night. All infants were monitored over two consecutive nights in their own homes in their normal sleep situation.

The key findings from different research papers using the same data include:

- Routinely bedsharing infants engaged in more feeding and more infant-mother interactions than cot-sleeping mother-infant dyads.
- Bedsharing infants were checked more frequently by their mothers than were cot-sleeping infants.
- Despite warmer micro-environments compared to cot-sleeping infants, bedsharing infants maintained normal rectal temperatures through increased vasodilatation.
- Total sleep time and sleep efficiency were similar for both groups.
- Five bed-sharing infants spent brief time in prone sleep. This usually followed feeding with the infant sleeping on the mother's chest. Two cot-sleeping infants spent the entire night in prone sleep.

At the University of Durham Parent Infant Sleep Laboratory, utilizing a combination of methods involving ethnographic narratives, interviews, infrared photography, and physiological monitoring devices, Dr. Helen Ball has conducted a variety studies involving various bedsharing mothers, fathers, twins, and singleton infants. Indeed, Dr. Ball also conducted the first in-home and laboratory study of co-bedded twins (Ball, 2006b; 2006c,), and the first study showing significant differences between the bedsharing, bottle feeding dyads (in bed) and the breastfeeding-bedsharing dyads (Ball, 2006a), contributing much new information to professional and scientific discourse on breastfeeding, SIDS risk factors, and sleeping arrangements, especially in the home and in hospitals (Ball, 2006d).

In one of her early studies, Ball *et al.* (1999) began with a study involving 60 mothers who were contacted in prenatal interviews at North Tees Hospital (Great Britain) regarding their intentions for child care practices.

Table 4. Characteristic Differences Among Breast and Formula Fed Infants

Orientation To Mother	Formula fed	Breastfed
Mother facing infant	59%	73%
Infant facing mother	46%	65%
Face to face	32%	47%
Infant Sleep Position		
Infant supine	83%	40%
Infant lateral	6%	54%
Infant prone	0%	0%
Height of infant in bed relative to mother		
Infant face level with mother's face or chin	71%	0%
Infant face level with mother's chest	29%	100%
Feeding frequency	**1 bout**	**2.5 bouts**
Total feeding time	9 minutes	31 minutes
Awakening frequency	**2(0-4)**	**4(3-5)**
Maternal arousals per night	2(0-4)	4(3-5)
Infant arousals per night	2(0-3)	3(2-5)
Mutual arousals	1(0-2)	3(1-4)
Source: Ball, 2006a.		

40 of these mothers were then interviewed regarding their actual child care practices two to four months following the birth of their infants. At two to four months, they found that 70% of new parents were found to bedshare at least occasionally, despite the fact that 0% intended to at the time of their prenatal interviews. Furthermore, 35% of experienced parents anticipated bedsharing, whereas 59% were actually doing so at the time of follow up. Finally, 11 of 13 babies that habitually bedshared were breastfeeders, at least initially, compared to the five infants that never bedshared and were bottle fed from birth.

Similarly, Ball (2003) focuses on postnatal interviews with 253 mothers at North Tees Hospital as well as two secondary, in-home interviews at the first and third month. Mothers were asked to complete seven sleep logs over seven consecutive days in the first and third month. Ball found that 47% of infants bedshared at least occasionally in the first month and 30% continued to do so after three to four months. Also, in this study, 87% of bedsharing mothers attempted breastfeeding in the first month compared to 50% of non-bedsharers. Finally, 46% of bedsharing infants still breastfed at three to four months versus 23% of non-bedsharers, suggesting that bedsharing may make it easier for mothers to breastfeed for a greater number of months. This finding is consistent with other studies that demonstrate that bedsharing and breastfeeding are mutually reinforcing: bedsharing promotes both a greater number of feeds per night (Baddock *et al.*, 2006; McKenna *et al.*, 1998) and a longer duration of breastfeeding in months (McCoy *et al.*, 2004).

Furthermore, Ball (2006a) observed the in-home, nighttime behaviors of 20 regular cosleeping families, comparing ten currently breastfeeding–bedsharing mothers-infant pairs with ten mother-infant pairs that had never breastfed. Her findings show that the cosleeping experience is markedly different for both the infant and the mother based on the method of feeding (**Figure 8**). Among other differences, she found prominent discrepancies between the two groups related to the positioning of the mother and infant in relation to one another and the infant's sleep position; mothers of formula fed infants faced their infants only 59% of the time, whereas breastfeeding mothers did so 73% of the time. Likewise, formula fed infants had their faces at the level of their mother's face or chin during 71% of the night and at their mothers' chest 29% of the time. This finding is significant for infant health because the risk of infant suffocation increases when the infant is positioned in and around the parent's neck or face due to blanket and pillow constriction/head covering. These findings can be juxtaposed against that of the breastfeeding infants who were found with their face at chest level 100% of the night in order to facilitate feeding as needed (**Table 4**).

Finally, in terms of infant sleep position, formula fed infants spent the night sleeping supine 83% of the time compared to six percent laterally (side sleeping). Breastfed infants slept supine 40% of the time and laterally 54%. This last figure, again, owes to the feeding method and the need for breastfeeders to have ample, frequent access, i.e., proximity, to the breast. The function of lateral sleeping in the breastfeeding, bedsharing environment is not to be conceptualized in the same way as a solitary lateral sleeping infant. The breastfeeding, lateral sleeping infant is unlikely to role into the prone position (a risk factor for SIDS) due to the fact the breastfeeding mother has positioned her body in a way, knees tucked up and often facing the infant, that prevents the infant from rolling completely prone. None of the breastfeeding-lateral sleeping infants in Ball's study rolled prone, nor did it appear that they physically could. Altogether, these data reaffirm the idea argued elsewhere that feeding method changes the functional relationship between the bedsharing mother and her infant in the direction of increased safety. This occurs by way of changes in the likely function or consequences of factors that, had the infant been sleeping alone or as reported with a formula feeding mother, they might have to be considered risky. But observations show that the mother plays an active role in mediating what might otherwise have to be considered a "risk." Other data, including feeding and awakening frequencies, which are significantly higher among breastfeeding versus formula mother-baby dyads, can be found in (**Table 4**).

Using data from Dr. Ball's sleep laboratory at the University of Durham, Leech (2006) analyzed overnight and physiological recordings of ten routine bedsharers and 11 occasional bedsharers over three consecutive nights. The first night was considered habituation, where the participants slept in their normal conditions to grow accustomed to the environment. The second and third nights were spent either bedsharing or in a cot by the bed (BTB), the order of which was randomly assigned. Leech found that infants on the BTB night spent greater time awake, less time in REM sleep, and more time in quiet sleep. Similarly, mothers spent more time awake on the BTB night and slept more overall when bedsharing. In addition, mother-infant pairs experienced more time in shared REM and total shared sleep when bedsharing, as the dyads showed 12% more simultaneous sleep time when bedsharing versus the BTB night.

Outcomes: Cosleeping Versus the Solitary-Infant-Sleep-Training Model

The ideas and comparative data justifying McKenna's original hypothesis that safe cosleeping and breastfeeding ought to reduce an infant's chances of SIDS was based on the idea that the highly neurologically immature human infant has not changed enough biologically or psychologically to accommodate the physiological challenges of sleeping alone, deprived of mother's sensory exchanges and regulation. The argument is that these mechanisms help buffer the infant from internal or external perturbations or deficits that conspire to increase SIDS risk. Expectations that infants should sleep deeply (stage 3-4) to consolidate their sleep as early in life as possible were cultural goals imposed on infants before knowing if deep sleep or more time spent in the deeper stages of sleep were safe for infants, given that arousal mechanisms, what wakes an infant up to terminate an apnea, are not on the same structural neurological time table for maturity as sleep stages are.

Aside from survival issues, it must also be remembered that emotional responses by infants and children to sleep isolation from the parent are innate and adaptive. They probably explain why anywhere between 25% and 45% of otherwise healthy infants and children in Western societies are said to suffer from "sleep disturbances" or "sleep problems" (Sadeh & Anders, 1993; Anders & Eiben, 1997). To blame infants and children for responding as they are designed, to protect themselves by crying to provoke parental retrieval if sleeping alone, is akin to blaming the victim for the crime. Not all infants and children are able to follow the cultural scripts of sleeping unattended through the night, as early in life as is possible, to accommodate parental work schedules. Indeed, it would appear that infants and children are not really supposed to do so at all when their biology is considered (Lummaa *et al.*, 1998), quite possibly because it can be dangerous, given their neurological immaturity and developmental delays.

Ancient adaptive emotions in infants probably also explain why when parents *elect* to have their infants and children sleep by their sides, i.e., non-reactive cosleeping (Madansky & Edelbrock, 1994), such pediatric sleep disturbances are greatly reduced if reported at all (Hayes *et al.*, 1994; Heron, 1994; Elias *et al.*, 1986; Latz *et al.*, 1999; Morelli *et al.*, 1992; McKenna, 1994).

THE PROFESSIONAL WORLD OF INFANT SLEEP RESEARCH .... SOCIAL VALUES MASQUERADING AS SCIENCE?

Western child-care strategies have emerged in recent decades that favor early infant autonomy. Parents have been encouraged to "train" their infants to sleep alone and to allow them to "soothe themselves back to sleep." The goal has been to eliminate nighttime feedings and/or sustained and spontaneous parental reassurances of the infant (Pinilla & Birch, 1993; Godfrey & Kilgore, 1998). Pediatric sleep "experts" and pediatricians have informed parents that infants should never be permitted to fall asleep at the breast or in the mother's arms (AAP Guide To Your Child's Sleep, 1999), even though this is the very context within which the infant's "falling asleep" evolved. As many parents will attest, this advice alone proves highly problematic.

Parents are also taught that to establish lifelong "healthy" sleep habits, infants "need" and should be "trained" to sleep alone. If the infant cannot fall back to sleep alone, it is said, the infant may have a "disorder" that can lead to sleep disabilities later in life (Ferber, 1985; AAP Guide To Your Child's Sleep, 1999). These infant-child care practices are supposed to promote early infantile independence, juvenile and adult self-assuredness, individual competence, and similar personality characteristics judged to be socially advantageous.

The problem is that it has never been shown that the "independence" achieved by the infant through learning to "soothe" itself back to sleep leads to any permanent developmental advantages or competencies later in life. No researcher has ever defined what "independence" or "autonomy" mean for an infant or young child (McKenna, 2000). Nor has "independence" been shown to correlate with any particular set of skills or talents not obtainable or more effectively acquired through other social experiences or child-care practices, including cosleeping. Indeed, according to the most recent annual report of the National Sleep Foundation in the United States, 62% of American adults – who likely were themselves reared by independence-minded caregivers – report difficulties falling and staying asleep. Sixty percent of children under the age of 18 have complained to their parents about being tired during the day and 15% admit to falling asleep in school (National Sleep Foundation Annual Report, 1999).

These data suggest that the solitary infant and childhood "sleep training" model aimed at creating "healthy sleep habits" and advocated for over 60 years have failed miserably. Yet sleep guides continue to advocate this approach (AAP Guide To Your Child's Sleep, 1999; Ferber, 1985; Godfrey & Kilgore, 1998).

Conversely, results from the first-published studies of people who coslept as infants contradict conventional Western assumptions that cosleeping leads to negative psychological, emotional, and social outcomes (Ferber, 1985; Robertiello, 1975; AAP Guide To Your Child's Sleep, 1999). Heron's (1994) recent cross-sectional study of middle-class English children shows that children who "never" slept in their parents' beds were more likely to be rated by teachers and parents as "harder to control" and "less happy," and they exhibited a greater number of tantrums. Children never permitted to bedshare were also more fearful than children who always slept in their parents' bed for all of the night.

When done safely, other research points to further advantages of cosleeping over solitary sleeping. For example:

- In their survey of adult college-age subjects, Lewis and Janda (1988) report that males who coslept with their parents between birth and five years of age had significantly higher self-esteem, experienced less guilt and anxiety, and reported greater frequency of sex. Boys who coslept between six and 11 years of age also had a higher self-esteem. For women, cosleeping during childhood was associated with less discomfort about physical contact and affection as adults.
- Crawford (1994) found that women who coslept as children had higher self-esteem than those who did not. Indeed, cosleeping appears to promote confidence, self-esteem, and intimacy, possibly by reflecting an attitude of parental acceptance (Lewis & Janda, 1988).
- A study of parents of 86 children in pediatrics and child psychiatry clinics (ages two to 13 years) on military bases (offspring of military personnel) revealed that cosleeping children received higher evaluations of their comportment from their teachers than did solitary-sleeping children, and they were *under-represented* in psychiatric-care populations, compared with children who did not cosleep. The authors state:
  Contrary to expectations, those children who had not had previous professional attention for emotional or behavioral problems coslept more frequently than did children who were known to have had psychiatric intervention and had lower parental ratings of adaptive functioning. The same finding occurred in a sample of boys one might consider "Oedipal victors" (e.g., three-year-old and older boys who sleep with their mothers in the absence of their fathers) – a finding which directly opposes traditional analytic thought (Forbes *et al.*, 1992).
- In the largest and possibly most systematic study to date – involving more than 1,400 subjects from five ethnic groups in Chicago and New York – Mosenkis (1998) found far more positive than negative adult outcomes for individuals who coslept as children. The results were the same for almost all ethnic groups (African Americans and Puerto Ricans in New York; Puerto Ricans, Dominicans, and Mexicans in Chicago). An especially robust finding cutting across all ethnic groups was that cosleepers exhibited a feeling of satisfaction with life.

Cross-cultural Perspectives on Infant Survival and Survival while Cosleeping

> *"The AAP's recommendations to advise against bedsharing and promote dummy use needs to be questioned, not for the carefully weighed evidence presented but rather the gaps in our knowledge of infant care practices and their consequences that still remain."* (Fleming *et al.*, 2006)

There is no evidence whatsoever that bedsharing is never safe, or mostly not safe, or cannot be made safe. There is only evidence that shows clearly the circumstances by which bedsharing is made dangerous and increases the risks of SIDS. This occurs when the mother smoked during or after her pregnancy, where premature babies bedshare, when the infant is positioned prone in the bed or on pillows, when drugs or alcohol are involved, or where other children are bedsharing alongside an infant.

Dangerous gaps in the furniture surrounding a mattress on which the infant sleeps or where night tables or other objects, including mattresses, are placed slightly away from a wall provide an opportunity for the infant to become wedged, all constituting modifiable factors which increase the risk of infant death (Scheer, 2000; Drago & Dannenberg, 1999; Nakamura *et al.*, 1999). However, there is no one-to one relationship between cosleeping or cosleeping in the form of bedsharing and infant mortality.

In the United States, the subgroups for which the greatest declines in SIDS rates continue to take place are precisely the groups for which bedsharing is increasing the most and reaching historic highs (Willinger *et al.*, 2002; McCoy *et al.*, 2004). Consider the Japanese data. Maternal smoking is exceedingly low (about 5%), while breastfeeding rates reach almost 95%, and forms of bedsharing represent the cultural norm in almost 90% of the population. In Japan, infant mortality in general

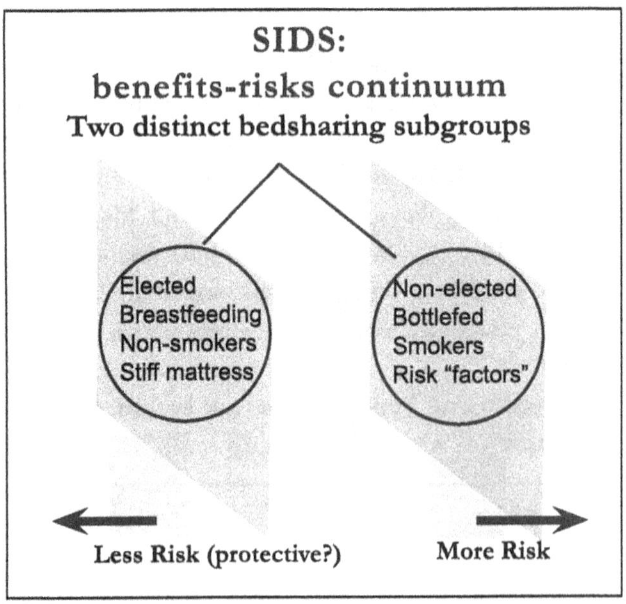

Figure 9. Outcomes associated with bedsharing, whether risky or protective, depend on the circumstances and characteristics of the sleep environment within which it occurs and, most especially, whether mothers breastfeed their infants, as breastfeeding significantly changes the functional connection and sensitivities between the mother and her infant, including the position in bed compared with bottle-feeding-bedsharing mother-infant dyads.

and SIDS in particular are among the lowest rates in the world.

In 2001, The SIDS Global Task Force Child Care Study published the results of a study in which over 56 cultures or regions were examined with particular respect to the relationship between SIDS and bedsharing rates. Contrary to what would be predicted as regards the presumed positive relationship between bedsharing and SIDS rates that some think to be inevitable, the opposite proved true: as bedsharing rates of a country, city, or region increased SIDS rates decreased. Another way to describe the findings is that as solitary infant sleep increased so did the SIDS rates! Apparently, the researchers did not expect this finding as they called it a "paradox" clearly revealing their bias… the idea that, surely, high bedsharing must correlate with high SIDS. At this point, Nelson *et al.* (2001) had no problem adopting a more complex view of the relationship between SIDS and bedsharing. Instead of concluding that bedsharing may be protective when done safely, they argue that: "Interactions with smoking may help explain this paradox, but further research is needed to understand the exact methods and complexity of bedsharing both between and within cultures."

Sankaran *et al.* (2000) present data from Saskatchewan, Canada, showing that where breastfeeding and forms of cosleeping co-exist, SIDS deaths are reduced. This finding is consistent with a study in South Africa showing that bedsharing babies have higher survival rates than solitary-sleeping babies (Kibel & Davies, 2000).

In Hong Kong, where cosleeping is the norm, SIDS rates are among the lowest in the world (Davies, 1985; Lee *et al.*,1989). In many other Asian cultures where cosleeping is also the norm (China, Vietnam, Cambodia and Thailand), SIDS is either unheard of or an unfamiliar type of infant death (Wilson, 1992; Yellend *et al.*, 1996).

Meanwhile, data collected by Grether, Schulman, and Croen (1989) looking at Asian immigrants to the United States found that the longer different Asian immigrant subgroups lived in the United States and presumably began to adopt American lifestyles, including placing infants in cribs for nighttime sleep, the traditionally low SIDS rates of these ethnic groups began to rise to match the higher rates of whites.

In contrast to studies showing the potential protective effects of bedsharing among urban, economically marginalized minority groups in which multiple relevant risk factors exist, bedsharing continues to be associated with high numbers of infant deaths, either from SIDS or accidental asphyxiations. This is especially true in the United States among African Americans living in large cities, such as Chicago, Washington, D.C., and St. Louis, the three cities that (not coincidentally) provide bedsharing critics data to argue against the safety of any and all bedsharing. Epidemiological studies also show that across marginalized sometimes indigenous groups, such as the Maori from New Zealand, Aborigines from Australia, and Cree from Canada, bedsharing or other forms of cosleeping are likewise associated with significantly increased risks. This is especially evident when associated with maternal smoking and other specific modifiable factors (Blair *et al.*, 2000; Wilson, 1992; Mitchell & Thompson, 1995).

Such disparities in outcomes associated ostensibly with the same practice are explained by looking more closely at bedsharing/cosleeping contexts and examining what is meant by the terms cosleeping, bedsharing, and a bedsharing death. The question is whether it is valid to extrapolate and infer from highly stressed and disadvantaged populations universally applicable principles concerning the relationship between SIDS risks and bedsharing. We argue it is not. Rather, these findings underscore the need to appreciate how risk factors (and general environmental factors rather than practice) can converge to make bedsharing more dangerous.

As argued elsewhere, bedsharing risks or protective factors are best conceptualized as occurring along a benefits-risk continuum (McKenna & Mcdade, 2005; McKenna & Mosko, 2001) (**Figure 9**) where, for example, breastfeeding in the context of non-smoking and highly committed mothers electing to bedshare for nurturing purposes is found, positive outcomes can be expected. Compare this situation to bedsharing as it occurs in poor environmental circumstances where mothers may have smoked before bedsharing and bottle feeding is practiced (with attendant less protective sequelae as discussed earlier). Among mothers whose economic situation provides no caregiving choice but to bedshare and cribs are not affordable, outcomes tend to be less positive.

SUMMARY, CONCLUSIONS, REFLECTIONS, CONCERNS

Where the Bedsharing Controversy Is Headed and What It Means for Breastfeeding Mothers and Infants

> *"...it would be a mistake to leap to the conclusion that because human immaturity makes possible high flexibility in later adjustment, anything is possible for the species...we would err if we assumed a priori that man's inheritance places no constraint on his power to adapt"* (Bruner,1972).

The consequences of enacting population-wide changes in infant and child care based mostly on cultural assumptions or limited science without comprehensive systematic and holistic studies carries many hidden risks. We learned this fact the hard way. It is now known that *not* breastfeeding in the United States alone leads to at least 750 infant deaths from congenital defects, birth complications, and/or primary and secondary infections (Chen & Rogan, 2004). The cultural dismantling early in the last century of what was for the most part an integrated cosleeping with breastfeeding adaptive complex contributed significantly to the deaths of hundreds of thousands of western infants from sudden infant death syndrome (SIDS). Turning infants onto their backs from their stomachs (the natural position of a breastfeeding-cosleeping infant) has reduced the SIDS rates at least by one half in most industrialized countries, while keeping babies "cosleeping" in rooms with a committed adult also cuts the chances of an infant dying by one half.

Indeed, the traditional cultural ideologies about the inherent dangers of sleeping with an infant under any circumstance continues to dominate the belief system associated with western medical institutions, including the apparent belief that mothers have no intrinsic proper sense of what is "good" or safe for their infants. Therefore, they must be taught or warned against experiencing too much contact with their infants and how and where that contact should take place. This belief is evident in a recent campaign being promoted by a national SIDS organization referred to as "First Candle." The program brochure is intended for nursery and NIC ward nurses and is entitled *"Model behavior: the most important modeling job of your life."* The set of guidelines emerges from the idea that parents tend to copy practices observed by nurses in hospital settings.

The brochure states: "As a nurse, you play a vital role in ensuring an infant's health and survival after they leave the hospital. This is the most important modeling job of your life." Judging from the tone of the brochure, the moralistic framing and text, there is no mistaking that the intent is to promote widely accepted SIDS reduction strategies, i.e., back to sleep, which is good, but also no bedsharing even for breastfeeding mothers, an issue upon which there is much less agreement professionally.

In addition, these guidelines and recommendations imply, though it is not explicitly stated, that any skin-to-skin contact should be heavily discouraged for fear that mothers will think skin-to-skin with their babies once in bed is an acceptable practice at home. Special emphasis is given, for example, on how dangerous it is to permit a mother ever to lie her infant prone on her chest, as if prone position on her chest while awake or asleep carries the same risks for SIDS as a baby lying prone on a soft or solid inert surface in a crib while sleeping alone.

Already, the AAP recommendations in the United States against any and all bedsharing with which many SIDS researchers and other scientists disagree is having a negative cascading effect in hospitals. New policies are being established to minimize the amount of contact mothers will be permitted to have with their infants and to stop practices that, for example, encourage skin-to-skin contact and/or the cobedding of twins, i.e., placing twins in the same bassinet.

One suggestion recently obtained from a U.S. government listserv associated with infant and fetal mortality review board professionals describes discussions apparently going on at hospitals in which, at least in the Washington DC area, mothers may be asked, or already are being asked, to sign contracts before their babies are permitted to be born in the hospital in which they promise never to shake their baby or to bedshare, as if bedsharing, like baby shaking, is a form of child abuse.

A salient brochure message being given on "model behavior" for NIC ward nurses mentioned above suggests that nurses have a responsibility to impress on mothers before leaving the hospital that first and foremost contact between her infant and herself is potentially dangerous. The message itself implies that "moral" nurses must all agree that bedsharing should never be permitted in a hospital or at home, and "good" nurses like "good" mothers cannot or should not disagree with the strong anti-bedsharing message.

Altogether, the heavy emphasis and uncompromising stress on denying a mother spontaneous contact with her infant and the emphasis on all the potential harm mothers can do leads us to believe that if such guidelines are adopted as endorsed by First Candle and other government-sponsored SIDS organizations under the Department of Health and Human Services rubric, breastfeeding will be negatively impacted. These guidelines, brochures, and hospital "contracts" reflect a complete dismissal of other legitimate strategies to maximize safety. These policies likewise reflect an exceedingly narrow range of scientific sources from which they are willing to draw to help formulate policies that will affect potentially millions of babies and, our guess is, many of them adversely. These kinds of messages and policies need to be challenged not only because they fail to appreciate a diverse body of scientific evidence that refutes their claims and assumptions, but they dismiss and undermine the unique qualities of each mother-infant dyad and how critical early contact can be in helping establish and facilitate optimal milk letdown and learned skills at breastfeeding, all of which are integrated with the process of mother and infant attachment.

Certainly, the emphasis on mother-infant separation and the general portrayal of potential negative effects that come with too much maternal-infant contact, with minimal attention given to the way breastfeeding changes the safety of contact, not only represents a threat to successful breastfeeding, but will no doubt further undermine maternal confidence. If the attitudes conveyed by these brochures are adopted by pediatric health personnel in general, these "programs" will no doubt significantly reduce the kinds of individual joys, experiences, and satisfaction that ordinarily come naturally as mothers and infants explore their own unique new relationship and feelings for each other in these first critical days.

It is important to realize by this example how the American Academy of Pediatrics recommendation against any and all bedsharing and the general historical negative presumptions against the practice are finding new and inappropriate applications in the neonatal and new mother nurseries. As is true in so many aspects of western infant care that involve intimate contact between an infant and its mother, sometimes knowing if, in fact, a caregiving behavior is actually dangerous or not is not as important as simply *believing* and *concluding* that it is, or that by avoiding it, infants will always benefit.

This chapter has reviewed the biological bases of increased contact and breastfeeding that generally exists between a human mother and her infant and why, when done safely, each member of the dyad benefits. For the infant, it is not untrue to say nor an exaggeration to emphasize that increased contact, especially when it begins with exclusive breastfeeding with its mother, increases and improves the infant's chances of survival and well being.

References

Abbott S. How can you expect to hold onto them later in life if you begin their lives by pushing them away? *Ethos.* 1992; 20(1):33-65.

American Academy of Pediatrics Task Force on Sudden Infant Death Syndrome. The changing concept of Sudden Infant Death Syndrome: Diagnostic coding shifts, controversies regarding the sleeping environment, and new variables to consider in reducing risk. *Pediatrics.* 2005; 116(5):1245-55.

American Academy of Pediatrics. *American Academy of Pediatrics' Guide To Your Child's Sleep.* Villard Publishing; 1999.

Anders TF, Eiben LA. Pediatric sleep disorders: a review of the past 10 years. *J Am Acad Child Adolesc Psychiatry.* 1997; 36(1):9-20.

Anderson GC. Crying, foramen ovale shunting, and cerebral volume [Letter to the editor]. *J Pediatr.* 1988; 113:411–12.

Anderson GC. Risk in mother–infant separation postbirth. *Image J Nurs Sch.* 1989; 21:196–99.

Anderson GC. Current knowledge about skin-to-skin (kangaroo) care for preterm infants. *J Perinat.* 1991; 11:216–26.

Baddock SA, Galland BC, Bolton DPG, Williams S, Taylor BJ. Differences in infant and parent behaviors during routine bed sharing compared with cot sleeping in the home setting. *Pediatrics.* 2006; 117:1599-1607.

Baddock SA, Galland BC, Taylor BJ, Bolton DPG. Sleep arrangements and behavior of bed-sharing families in the home setting. *Pediatrics.* 2007; 119(1):e200-7.

Ball HL. Babies and infants bed-sharing. Invited contribution to: *Midwifery Practice in the Post-natal Period.* Royal College of Midwives; 2000. p. 24-26.

Ball HL. Reasons to bed-share: Why parents sleep with their infants. *J Reprod Infant Psychol.* 2002; 20:207–21.

Ball HL. Breastfeeding, bedsharing, and infant sleep. *Birth.* 2003; 30(3):181-88.

Ball HL. Parent-infant bed-sharing behavior: effects of feeding type, and presence of father. *Human Nature.* 2006a; 17(3):301-18.

Ball HL. Together or apart? A behavioural and physiological investigation of sleeping arrangements for twin infants. *Midwifery.* 2007; in press (galley proofs approved 8/2006).

Ball, HL. Caring for twin infants: sleeping arrangements and their implications. *Evidence Based Midwifery.* 2006; 4(1):10-16.

Ball HL. Bed-sharing on the post-natal ward: breastfeeding and infant sleep safety. *Paediatrics and Child Health (Journal of the Canadian Paediatric Society).* 2006d; 11:43A-46A.

Ball HL, Hooker E, Kelly PJ. Where will the baby sleep? Attitudes and practices of new and experienced parents regarding cosleeping with their newborn infants. *Am Anthropol.* 1999; 10(1):143-51.

Ball HL. Evolutionary paediatrics: a case study in applying Darwinian medicine. *Medicine and Evolution.* 2007a; in press.

Ball HL, Klingaman KP. Breastfeeding and mother-infant sleep proximity: implications for infant care. In: Trevathan W, Smith EO, McKenna JJ (eds.). *Evolutionary Medicine.* 2nd Ed. New York: Oxford University Press. 2007b; in press.

Ball HL. Bed-sharing practices of initially breastfed infants in the 1st 6 months of life. In: Goldberg W, Keller M (eds.). *Infant and Child Development.* 2007c; in press.

Ball HL. Night-time infant care: cultural practice, evolution, and infant development. In: Pranee L (ed.). *Childrearing and infant care: A cross-cultural perspective.* New York: Nova Science Publishers; 2007d; in press.

Barry H III, Paxson LM. Infancy and early childhood: cross-cultural codes. *Ethology.* 1971; 10:466-508.

Blair PS, Fleming PJ, Bensley D, Smith I, Bacon C, Taylor E, *et al.* Where should babies sleep -- alone or with parents? Factors influencing the risk of SIDS in the CESDI Study. *BMJ.* 1999; 319:1457-62.

Blair P, Ball HL. The prevalence and characteristics associated with parent-infant bed-sharing in England. *Arch Dis Child.* 2004; 89:1106-10.

Blurton Jones N. Comparative aspects of mother–child contact. In: Blurton Jones N (ed.). *Ethological studies of child behaviour.* Cambridge: Cambridge University Press; 1974. p. 305–28.

Bowlby J. *Attachment and loss: Vol. 1. Attachment.* 2nd ed. New York: Basic Books; 1982.

Bruner, J. Nature and uses of immaturity. *Am Psychol.* 1972; 27:687-708.

Cable TA, Rothenberger LA. Breast-feeding behavioural patterns among La Leche League mothers: a descriptive study. *Pediatrics.* 1984; 73:830-35.

Carpenter RG, Irgens LM, Blair PS, England PD, Fleming P, Huber J, *et al.* Sudden unexplained infant death in 20 regions in Europe: case control study. *Lancet.* 2004; 363(9404):185-91.

Carroll-Pankhurst C, Mortimer A. Sudden infant death syndrome, bed-sharing, parental weight, and age at death. *Pediatrics.* 2001; 107(3):530-36.

Chen A, Rogan W. Breastfeeding and the risk of post-neonatal death in the United States. *Pediatrics.* 2004; 113:E435-39.

Clemens JD. Infant–parent bed sharing in an inner-city population. *Arch Pediatr Adolesc Med.* 2003; 157:33–39.

Crawford M. Parenting practices in the Basque country: Implications of infant and childhood sleeping location for personality development. *Ethos.* 1994; 22(1):42-82.

Davies DP. Cot death in Hong Kong: A rare problem? *Lancet.* 1985; 2:1346-48.

Drago DA, Dannenberg AL. Infant mechanical suffocation deaths in the United States, 1980-1997. *Pediatrics.* 1999; 103(5):e59.

Eaton SB, Shostak M, *et al. The Paleolithic prescription.* New York: Harper & Row; 1988.

Elias MF, Nicholson N, Bora C, Johnston J. Sleep-wake patterns of breast-fed infants in the first two years of life. *Pediatrics.* 1986; 77(3):322-29.

Elias MF, Nicholson NA, Konner M. Two sub-cultures of maternal care in the United States. In: Taub DM, King FA (eds.). *Current perspectives in primate social dynamics.* New York: Van Nostrand Reinhold; 1986. p. 37–50.

Färdig JA. A comparison of skin-to-skin contact and radiant heaters in promoting neonatal thermoregulation. *J Nurse Midwifery.* 1980; 25(1):19–28.

Ferber R. *Solve your child's sleep problems.* New York: Simon and Schuster; 1985.

Field T. *Touch in early development.* Malwah, NJ: Lawrence Earlbaum Associates; 1995a.

Field T. Infant massage therapy. In: Field TM (ed). *Touch in early development.* Malwah, NJ: Lawrence Erlbaum Associates; 1995b. p. 105–14.

Field TM. Touch therapy effects on development. *Int J Behav Dev.* 1998; 22:779–97.

Field T. Massage therapy facilitates weight gain in preterm infants. *Curr Dir Psychol Sci.* 2001; 10:51–54.

Field TM, Schanberg SM, Scafidi F, Bauer CR, Vega-Lahr N, Garcia R, *et al.* Tactile/kinesthetic stimulation effects on preterm neonates. *Pediatrics.* 1986; 77:654–58.

Flandrin JL. *Families in former times: Kinship, household and sexuality.* New York: Cambridge University Press; 1979.

Fleming PJ, Blair PS, Bacon C, Bensley D, Smith I, Taylor E, *et al.* Environments of infants during sleep and risk of sudden infant death syndrome: results of 1993-1995 case control study for confidential inquiry into stillbirths and deaths in infancy. *BMJ.* 1996; 313:191-95.

Fleming P, Blair P, McKenna J. New knowledge, new insights, new recommendations. *J Arch Dis Child.* 2006; 91:799-801.

Forbes JF, Weiss DS, Folen RA. The cosleeping habits of military children. *Mil Med.* 1992; 157:196-200.

Ford RPK, Mitchell EA, Scragg R, Stewart AW, Taylor BJ, Allen EM. Factors adversely associated with breast feeding in New Zealand. *Journal of Paediatric Child Health.* 1994; 30:483-89.

Fredrickson DD, Sorenson JF, Biddle AK, *et al.* Relationship of sudden infant death syndrome to breast-feeding duration and intensity. *Am J Dis Child.* 1993; 147:460.

Gilbert RE, Wigfield RE, Fleming PJ, Berry PJ, Rudd PT. Bottle feeding and the sudden infant death syndrome. *BMJ.* 1995; 310:88-90.

Godfrey AB, Kilgore A. An approach to help young infants sleep through the night. *Zero To Three.* 1998; 19(2):15-21.

Goode E. Baby in parents' bed in danger? U.S. says yes, but others demur. *New York Times.* September 30, 1999.

Goto K, Mirmiran M, Adams M, Longford R, Baldwin R, Boeddiker M, *et al.* More awakenings and heart rate variability during sleep in preterm infants. *Pediatrics.* 1999; 103(3):603-9.

Granju KA. *Attachment parenting: Instinctive care for your baby and young child.* New York: Pocket Books; 1999.

Grether JK, Schulman J, Croen LA. Sudden infant death syndrome among Asians in California. *J Pediatr.* 1990; 116(4):525-28.

Gunnar MR. Quality of early care and buffering of neuroendocrine stress reactions: Potential effects on the developing human brain. *Prev Med.* 1998; 27:208–11.

Hardyment C. *Dream babies: Child care from Locke to Spock.* London: Jonathan Cape Ltd; 1983.

Hayes MJ, Roberts SM, Stowe R. Early childhood cosleeping: parent-child and parent-infant interactions. *Int Men Health J.* 1996; 17:348-57.

Heron P. Non-reactive cosleeping and child behavior: Getting a good night's sleep all night every night. Masters Thesis: University of Bristol, Department of Psychology; 1994.

Hofer M. Parental contributions to the development of offspring. In: Gubernick D, Klopfer P (eds.). *Parental Care in Mammals.* New York: Academic Press; 1981. p. 77-115.

Hoffman H, Damus K, Hillman L, Krongrad E. Risk factors for SIDS: Results of the Institutes of Child Health and Human Development SIDS cooperative epidemiological study. In: Schwartz P, Southall D, Valdes-Dapena M (eds.). Sudden infant death syndrome: Cardiac and respiratory mechanisms. *Annals of the New York Academy of Sciences.* Vol. 533. 1988. p. 13-30.

Hoffman J. Sleep Like A Baby: What Does That Really Mean? *Today's Parent.* 1999; 16 (7): 34-40.

Hrdy SB. *Mother nature.* New York: Pantheon Press; 1999.

Jackson D. Three in a bed: How attitudes toward cosleeping have evolved over the last ten years. *Mothering Magazine.* 1999; 98:40-44.

Jura J, Olejar V, Dluholucky S. Epidemiological risk factors of SIDS in Slovakia, 1993, 1994 (Abstract). *Program and Abstracts Third SIDS International Conference, Stavanger, Norway.* July 31-August 4. Oslo: Holstad Grafisk; 1994. p. 98.

Kellum BA. Infanticide in England in the later Middle Ages. History of Childhood Quarterly. *J Psychohist.* 1974; 1(3):367-88.

Kemp JS, Unger B, Wilkins D, Psara RM, Ledbetter TL, Graham MA, *et al.* Unsafe sleep practices and an analysis of bed sharing among infants dying suddenly and unexpectedly: Results of a four year, population-based, death-scene investigation study of sudden infant death syndrome and related deaths. *Pediatrics.* 2000; 106(3):e41.

Kibel MA, Davies MF. Should the infant sleep in mother's bed? Auckland, New Zealand: SIDS International Conference; Feb. 8-11, 2000.

Konner MJ. Evolution of human behavior development. In: Munroe RH, Munroe RL, Whiting JM (eds.). *Handbook of Cross-Cultural Human Development.* New York: Garland STPM Press; 1981. p. 3-52.

Lawrence RA. *Breastfeeding: A guide for the medical profession* (4th ed.). St. Louis, MO: Mosby; 1994.

Lahr MB, Rosenberg KD, Lapidus JA. Bedsharing and maternal smoking in a population-based survey of new mothers. *Pediatrics.* 2005; 116 (4):e530-42.

Latz S, Wolf A, Lozoff B. Cosleeping in context: Sleep practices and problems in young children in Japan and the United States. *Arch Pediatr Adolesc Med.* 1999; 153:339–46.

Leach P. Beware of the parenting police. *New York Times* (Op Ed). October 1, 1999.

Lee NY, Chan YF, Davies DP, Lau E, Yip DCP. Sudden infant death syndrome in Hong Kong: confirmation of low incidence. *Br Med J.* 1989; 298:721.

LeVine R, Dixon S, LeVine S, *et al. Child care and culture: Lessons from Africa.* Cambridge, England: Cambridge University Press; 1994.

Lewis RJ, Janda LH. The relationship between adult sexual adjustment and childhood experience regarding exposure to nudity, sleeping in the parental bed, and parental attitudes toward sexuality. *Arch Sex Behav.* 1988; 17:349-63.

Lewis M, Havilland J. *The Handbook of Emotion.* New York: Gulford Press; 1993.

Ludington-Hoe SM. Energy conservation during skin-to-skin contact between premature infants and their mothers. *Heart Lung.* 1990; 19:445-51.

Ludington-Hoe SM, Hadeed AJ, Anderson GC. Physiological responses to skin-to-skin contact in hospitalized premature infants. *J Perinat.* 1991a; 11:19-24.

Ludington-Hoe SM, Hadeed A, Anderson GC. Randomized trials of cardiorespiratory, thermal and state effects of kangaroo care for preterm infants. Seattle, WA: Society for Research in Child Development Biennial Meeting; April 19, 1991b.

Ludington-Hoe SM, Hosseini RB, Hashemi MS, Argote LA, Medellin G, Rey H. Selected physiologic measures and behavior during paternal skin contact with Colombian preterm infants. *J Dev Physiol.* 1992; 18:223-32.

Lummaa V, Vurisalo T, Barr R, Lehtonen L. Why cry? Adaptive significance of intensive crying in human infants. *Evol Hum Behav.* 1998; 19:193-202.

Mandansky D, Edelbrock C. Cosleeping in a community of 2- and 3-year-old children. *Pediatrics.* 1990; 86:1987-2003.

McCarin Julie. Bed sharing and non bed-sharing preschool children and selected emotional variables. New York University: Ph.D. Dissertation, Department of Psychology; 1995.

McCoy RC, Hunt CL, Lesko SM. Population-based study of bedsharing and breastfeeding. *Pediatr Res.* 2000; program abstract.

McCoy RC, Hunt CL, Lesko SM, Vezina R, Corwin M, Willinger M, *et al.* Frequency of bed sharing and its relationship to breast feeding. *J Dev Behav Pediatr.* 2004; 25(3):141-49.

McKenna JJ, Ball, Gettler LT. *Yearbook of Phys Anthropol.* 2007; in press.

McKenna JJ. An anthropological perspective on the sudden infant death syndrome (SIDS): The role of parental breathing cues and speech breathing adaptations. *Med Anthropol.* 1986; 10:9-53.

McKenna J. Cultural influences on infant and childhood sleep biology and the science that studies it: Toward a more inclusive paradigm. In: Loughlin J, Carroll J, Marcus C, Dekker M. *Sleep in development and pediatrics.* New York: Marcel Dekker, Inc.; 2000. p. 99-130.

McKenna JJ, McDade T. Why babies should never sleep alone: a review of the cosleeping controversy in relation to SIDS, bedsharing and breastfeeding. *Paediatr Respir Rev.* 2005; 6:134-52.

McKenna JJ, Mosko S. Evolution and the sudden infant death syndrome (SIDS). Part III: Infant arousal and parent–infant cosleeping. *Hum Nat.* 1990; 1:291–330.

McKenna J, Mosko S. Breast feeding and mother-infant cosleeping in relation to SIDS prevention. In: Trevathan W, Smith N, McKenna J (eds.). *Evolutionary Medicine.* New York: Oxford University Press; 1999.

McKenna JJ, Mosko S. Mother-infant cosleeping: Toward a new scientific beginning. In: Byard R, Krous H (eds.). *Sudden infant death syndrome: Problems, puzzles, possibilities.* New York: Arnold Publishing; 2001.

McKenna JJ, Volpe LE. Sleeping with baby: An internet-based sampling of parental experiences, choices, perceptions, and interpretations in a Western industrialized context. *Infant Child*. [in press].

McKenna JJ, Mosko S, Dungy C, McAninch P. Sleep and arousal patterns of cosleeping human mother/infant pairs: A preliminary physiological study with implications for the study of Sudden Infant Death Syndrome (SIDS). *Am J Phys Anthropol.* 1990; 83:331-47.

McKenna JJ, Mosko S, Dungy C, McAnninch J. Sleep and arousal patterns among cosleeping mother-infant pairs: Implications for SIDS. *Am J Phys Anthropol.* 1991; 83:331-347.

McKenna JJ, Thoman E, Anders T, Sadeh A, Schechtman V, Glotzbach S. Infant-parent cosleeping in evolutionary perspective: Implications for understanding infant sleep development and the Sudden Infant Death Syndrome (SIDS). *Sleep.* 1993; 16:263-82.

McKenna JJ, Mosko S, Richard C, Drummond S, Hunt L, Cetal M, *et al.* Mutual behavioral and physiological influences among solitary and cosleeping mother-infant pairs; implications for SIDS. *Early Hum Dev.* 1994; 38:182-201.

McKenna J, Mosko S, Richard C. Bedsharing promotes breast feeding. *Pediatrics.* 1997; 100:214-19.

Minturn L, Lambert WW. *Mothers of six cultures: Antecedents of child rearing.* New York: John Wiley and Sons; 1964.

Mitchell EA, Thompson JMD. Cosleeping increases the risks of the sudden infant death syndrome, but sleeping in the parent's bedroom lowers it. In: Rognum TO. *Sudden infant death syndrome in the nineties.* Oslo: Scandinavian University Press; 1995. p. 266-69.

Montagu A. *Touching: The human significance of the skin.* 3rd ed. New York: Harper & Row; 1986.

Morelli GA, Rogoff B, Oppenheim D, Goldsmith D. Cultural variation in infants' sleeping arrangements: questions of independence. *Dev Psychol.* 1992; 28:604-13.

Mosenkis Jeff. The effects of childhood cosleeping on later life development. The University of Chicago: Masters Thesis, Department of Cultural Psychology; 1998.

Mosko S, McKenna JJ, Dickel M, Hunt L. Parent-infant cosleeping: the appropriate context for the study of infant sleep and implications for SIDS research. *J Behav Med.* 1993; 16(3):589-610.

Mosko S, Richard C, McKenna J, Drummond S. Infant sleep architecture during bedsharing and possible implications for SIDS. *Sleep.* 1996; 19:677-84.

Mosko S, Richard C, McKenna J. Infant arousals during mother-infant bedsharing; implications for infant sleep and SIDS research. *Pediatrics.* 1997a; 100:5;841-49.

Mosko S, Richard C, McKenna J. Maternal sleep and arousals during bedsharing with infants. *Sleep.* 1997b; 20(2):142-50.

Mosko S, Richard C, McKenna J, Drummond S, Mukai D. Maternal proximity and infant CO2 environment during bedsharing and possible implications for SIDS research. *Am J Phys Anthropol.* 1997; 103:315-28.

Munroe RH, Munroe RL, Whiting BB. *Handbook of cross-cultural development.* New York: Garland Press; 1981.

Nakamura S, Wind M, Danello MD. Review of hazards associated with children placed in adult beds. *Arch Pediatr Adolesc Med.* 1999; 153:1018-23.

Nelson EA, Taylor BJ, Jenik A, Vance J, Walmsley K, Pollard K, *et al.* International child care practices study: infant sleeping environment. *Early Hum Dev.* 2001; 62(1):43-55.

Nelson EAS, Schiefenhoevel W, Haimerl F. Child care practices in nonindustrialized societies. *Pediatrics.* 2000; 105(6):e75.

Nix S. Confessions of a bed lizard. *Mothering Magazine.* 2000; 98:48-50.

Pinilla T, Birch LL. Help me make it through the night: behavioral entrainment of breast-fed infants' sleep patterns. *Pediatrics.* 1993; 91(2):436-44.

Quillin SI, Glenn L. Interaction between feeding method and cosleeping on maternal-newborn sleep. *J Obstet Gynecol Neonatal Nurs.* 2004; 33(5):580-88.

Richard C, Mosko S, McKenna J. Sleeping position, orientation, and proximity in bedsharing infants and mothers. *Sleep.* 1996; 19:667-84.

Richard C, Mosko S, McKenna J. Apnea and periodic breathing in the bedsharing infant. *Am J Applied Phys.* 1998; 84(4):1374-80.

Richard CA, Mosko SS. Mother-infant bedsharing is associated with an increase in infant heart rate. *Sleep.* 2004; 27(3):507-11.

Rigda RS, McMillen IC, Buckley P. Bed sharing patterns in a cohort of Australian infants during the first six months after birth. *J Paediatr Child Health.* 2000; 36(2):117-21.

Robertiello RC. *Hold them very close, then let them go.* New York: The Dial Press; 1975.

Sadeh A, Anders TF. Infant sleep problems: origins, assessment, interventions. *Infant Ment Health J.* 1993; 14(1):17-34.

Sankaran AH, Koravangattu PO, Dhananjayan, A, *et al.* Sudden infant death syndrome (SIDS) and infant care practices in Saskatchewan Canada. Auckland, New Zealand: Sixth SIDS International Meeting (abstract); 2000.

Scheer NJ. Safe sleeping environments for infants: A CPSC perspective. Auckland, New Zealand: Sixth SIDS International Meeting (abstract); 2000.

Scheer NJ, Rutherford GW, Kemp JS. Where should infants sleep? A comparison of risk for suffocation of infants sleeping in cribs, adult beds, and other sleeping locations. *Pediatrics.* 2003; 112(4):883-89.

Seabrook J. Sleeping with the baby. *The New Yorker.* Nov 1999. p. 56-65.

Stone L. *The family, sex and marriage in England, 1500-1800.* New York: Harper & Row; 1977.

Trevathan WR, McKenna JJ. Evolutionary environments of human birth and infancy: Insights to apply to contemporary life. *Children's Environments.* 1994; 11(2): 88-104.

Thoman EB, Graham SE. Self-regulation of stimulation by premature infants. *Pediatrics.* 1986; 78:855-60.

Vonnegut M. Beware of bad science. *The Boston Globe.* Oct 24, 1999.

Werland R. Tossing and turning on the issue of the family bed. *Chicago Tribune.* Oct 17, 1999.

Whiting JWM. Environmental constraints on infant care practices. In: Munroe RH, Munroe RL, Whiting BB (eds). *Handbook of cross-cultural human development.* New York: Garland STPM Press; 1981. p. 155-179.

Willinger M, Ko CW, Hoffman HJ, Kessler RC, Corwin MJ. Trends in infant bed sharing in the United States, 1993–2000: The National Infant Sleep Position Study. *Arch Pediatr Adoles Med.* 2003; 157:43–49.

Wilson E. Sudden infant death syndrome (SIDS) and environmental perturbations in cross-cultural context. University of Calgary: Masters Thesis; 1990.

Wright R. Why Johnny can't sleep. *Time.* April 14, 1997.

Yelland J, Gifford S, MacIntyre M. Explanatory models about maternal and infant health and sudden infant death syndrome among Asian-born mothers. Monash University. 1996; p. 175-89.

Young J. Night-time behavior and interactions between mothers and their infants of low risk for SIDS: a longitudinal study of room sharing and bed sharing. University of Bristol: Doctoral Thesis; 1999.

SECTION IV

MANAGEMENT - MOTHER

Chapter 15

Breastfeeding, Birth Spacing, and Family Planning

Miriam Labbok

INTRODUCTION

There are multiple biomedical, social, and cultural relationships between breastfeeding, fertility, birth spacing, and family planning method, selection, and use. This chapter addresses the biomedical and public health considerations in the sociocultural context.

Should Breastfeeding be Included and Considered in Discussions of Reproductive Health?

Reproduction is a physiological continuum and is the quintessential intergenerational health issue. Maternal health and nutrition may influence conception as well as the development of a future child's reproductive organs during fetal development; the health of the germ cells in the developing fetus can have impact on future grandchildren. Given this interface of at least three generations, it is not surprising that there are close biological relationships, and certain redundancy, among the many factors that lead to the successful achievement of producing a child that will live and procreate.

The primary hormones associated with ovulation and pregnancy – estrogens and progesterones – are also the major hormones of maturation of mammary tissue. Other hormones, such as gonadotropin-releasing hormone (GnRH), are inseparable components of successful pregnancy and birth (Schneider *et al.*, 2006). Many stimuli are known to affect reproductive function by influencing either GnRH release from the hypothalamus or pituitary gland responsiveness to GnRH. Advances in the understanding of the multiple functions and details of interactions of reproductive hormones are occurring regularly, contributing to the ability of the biomedical field to support reproductive functions.

Disruption of these hormones impacts negatively on reproduction and on the establishment and duration of lactation. Clinical correction once disruption has occurred can be difficult. Maternal neurophysiological production, interactions, and metabolism of hormones and related factors can be disrupted with the use of anesthesia and other obstetric interventions. Therefore, decisions to intervene during labor and birth should take into consideration the potential negative impact on the perinatal hormonal feedback systems and, hence, on establishment of lactation (Kroger & Smith, 2003).

The hormones of breastfeeding also contribute to maternal recovery, possible reduction in certain cancers and chronic diseases, and perhaps to the mother's ability to nurture and bond with her infant. The oxytocin of let-down (milk release from the breast without suckling) is considered a "bonding" hormone, and prolactin (the hormone most associated with early postpartum milk production) responds to stress, helping to ensure survival of the next generation.

What is clearly evident is that the physiological intimacy of reproduction, lactation, and fertility in mammals, including humans, is indisputable. The ovarian- hypothalamic-pituitary axis is intimately connected to fertility, lactation, and maternal recovery postpartum. Due to this intimate continuum, establishment of lactation is sometimes referred to as the fourth stage of labor.

Is Birth Spacing Necessary for Health?

Adequate birth spacing has implications for the health of both mother and child. The child born after an adequate inter-birth interval will have a reduced risk of neonatal, infant, and child mortality. A multivariate analysis, controlling for a wide variety of potential confounders and using data from 17 developing countries, identified 36-59 months as optimal (Rutstein, 2005). Presented as adjusted odds ratios, the risk of neonatal mortality and infant mortality was found to decrease with increasing birth interval lengths up to 36 months, at which point the risk plateaus. For child mortality, the analysis indicated that the longer the birth interval, the lower the risk, even for intervals of 48 months or more. In addition, this study found a clear pattern of increasing chronic and general under-nutrition as the birth interval is shorter, as indicated by the averages of the adjusted odds ratios for all 14 countries with anthropometric data. The optimal interval for maternal health outcomes, including decreased maternal death, third trimester bleeding, premature rupture of membranes, puerperal endometritis, eclampsia, and anemia, has been shown in various studies to allow for shorter or longer intervals, from about 15 to 68 months (Conde-Agudelo & Belizan, 2000), 8 to 23 months (Zhu, 2005), and, in some studies, up to 59 months (Conde-Agudelo *et al.*, 2006).

However, when we bring optimal breastfeeding into this equation, we must also consider what timing is associated with optimal maternal nutrition. An interesting study carried out in Guatemala examined maternal and fetal responses to the stress of concurrent lactation and pregnancy (Merchant *et al.*, 1990). Although women often continue breastfeeding into a next pregnancy, the nutritional requirements are increased. They found that short recuperative periods (less than six months) from the end of lactation to the beginning of the next pregnancy, resulted in increased maternal nutritional needs. The maternal stores buffer the impact on the fetus; however, the mother has increased need for supplements, and her own energy stores will be depleted. Since optimal infant feeding includes six months of exclusive breastfeeding with up to two years or longer of continued breastfeeding, the logical minimal birth interval would be at least two years plus six months for recuperation before pregnancy or at least 39 months between births.

Many experts are concerned that, at older ages, prolonging the birth interval may cause the mother to experience increased risks with increased age. This factor is extremely important in the clinical setting.

Breastfeeding Protects Against Pregnancy: Old Wives' Tale or Human Physiology?

The understanding that breastfeeding contributes to the delay in the return of fertility is not new. Although often referred to as an 'old wives' tale,' virtually all societies have a shared understanding that there is indeed a relationship. The decline of breastfeeding rates in the last century in concert with the increase in availability of family planning methods led to loss of this understanding. From traditional and historic fertility rates of up to 12 children, with perhaps two to four surviving to adulthood, mankind has progressed to the stage where more children survive, contributing to a population explosion in the last century or two. With the advent of modern contraception, the understanding that the reason women tended to have 12 children--rather than a theoretically possible 24 or more--during their reproductive lives was due to the fact that there had been intensive breastfeeding. The World Fertility Surveys of the 1970s sparked renewed interest and analyses confirmed that there was a clear and dose related association between breastfeeding and reduced fertility. Modeling by Jain and Bongaarts and others (Jain & Bongaarts, 1981) supported this association, generally using duration of amenorrhea as a proxy for fertility return. Jain and Bongaarts concluded that, on average, each month of continued breastfeeding contributed about 0.4 months to birth spacing. At the same time, the links between development, breastfeeding, and fertility were being explored (Butz, 1981). This work and the more sophisticated modeling that followed allowed for projection of possible increases in fertility at the national level that would occur if breastfeeding levels were not maintained (Becker *et al.*, 2003).

Is Family Planning Needed During Lactation?

The old wives' tales concerning inability to conceive during lactation is a good basis for exploration.

Table 1. Percent of Sexually Active Women Who Will Become Pregnant Under Various Conditions When No Contraceptive Method Is Used

Approximate annualized pregnancy rate if:	In percent
Non-lactating interval	40-60
Lactating	15-40
Lactating and amenorrheic	5-15
Fully lactating and amenorrheic	5
Fully lactating, amenorrheic, <6 months pp	2
LAM is used	0 <2

However, lactation, or lactational amenorrhea alone, do not have contraceptive efficacy that is acceptable to most women (**Table 1**).

While it was clear that breastfeeding contributed significantly to birth-spacing at the population level, much work remained to establish its impact at the individual level. The research of the last few decades of the 20th century led to the development of the Lactational Amenorrhea Method and a better understanding of the impact of contraceptive use in the lactating woman.

THE LACTATIONAL AMENORRHEA METHOD

What are the Basics of the Physiology of Lactational Infertility?

The multiple subtle interactions and different feedback that occurs during cycling and during lactational amenorrhea are not as yet fully elucidated; however, the basic feedback systems are evident (**Figure 1**). A review by McNeilly offers an explanation of the mechanisms and feedback known to exist, but also raises questions that remain (McNeilly, 2001). In sum, the review notes that breastfeeding suppresses fertility via suckling for variable durations after birth. After postpartum recovery of GnRH from the hormone levels of pregnancy, there is a period of suppressed ovarian activity with limited follicle growth. The pulsatility of luteinizing hormone (LH) is erratic and slower than the one pulse per hour required in the normal follicular phase of the menstrual cycle to drive follicle growth. When the suckling stimulus declines or drops precipitously, there is a resumption of pulsatile LH secretion, associated development of follicles, and some steroid secretion. However, McNeilly notes the positive feedback of estradiol which triggers the preovulatory LH surge and ovulation appears to be initially blocked by continued suckling.

Possible Paradoxical Feedback Stimulated During Lactation

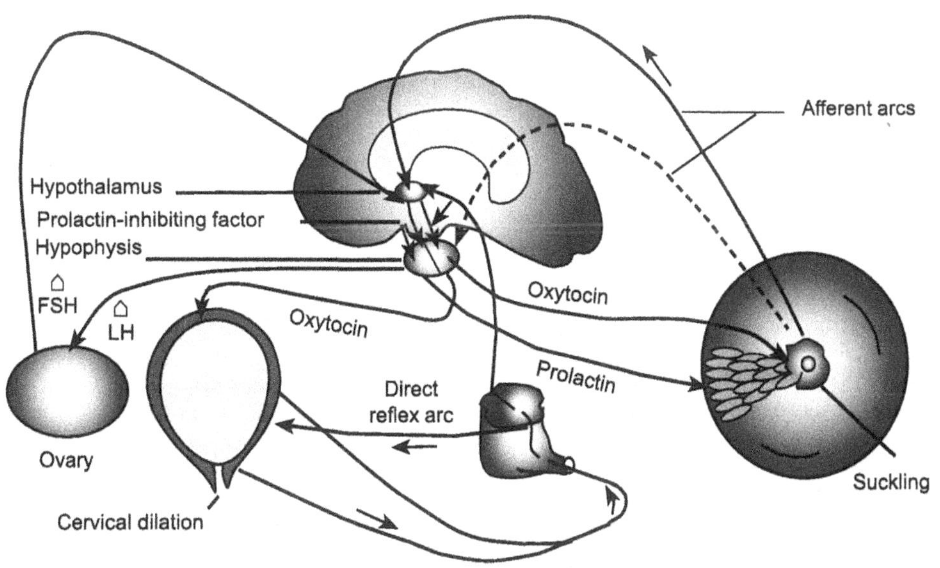

Figure 1. Production of milk and suppression of fertility rely on hormonal responses to breast stimulation and interaction within the mammary / hypothalamic / pituitary / ovarian axes. Adapted from Lawrence & Lawrence, 2005.

The hypothalamus is central in these feedback loops (**Figure 1**). The hypothalamic gonadotropin-releasing hormone (GnRH) is a key regulator of the reproductive system, mainly through its effects on pituitary luteinizing hormone (LH) and follicle-stimulating hormone (FSH) release. GnRH is also a factor in prolactin release. Prolactin is released in response to suppression of GnRH (Cavagna *et al.*, 2005). When prolactin levels are high, there is feedback suppression of GnRH (Page-Wilson *et al.*, 2006). Although these interactions have been under study for decades, the full details of these interactions in the human remain to be elucidated.

Once lactation is established and continuing without any long intervals, there is a paradoxical increase in the suppression of ovarian function if estrogens begin to rise. There is now some evidence that this may occur at the follicular level (Velasquez *et al.*, 2006a). Possibly due to this paradoxical re-suppression of ovulation, if women continue intensive breastfeeding, the first few ovulations and menses are associated with inadequate corpus luteum development and function, reducing the likelihood of pregnancy (Gray *et al.*, 1990). Eventually, normal menstrual cycles resume when breast stimulation declines further. The duration of amenorrhea and its association with return of luteal function varies greatly between mother-baby pairs and in different societies, probably in association with subtle differences in breastfeeding patterns, individual physiological responsiveness of end organs, and possible mediated variance in hormones, such as induced microheterogeneity (Velasquez *et al.*, 2006b) and ratios between levels of a mix of hormones (Campino *et al.*, 2001).

Is What is Best for the Child also Best for Fertility Suppression?

Full breastfeeding (responding to frequent cues from the infant, with no long intervals, day and night) is the pattern of feeding most often associated with lactational infertility and with best child health outcomes. Another factor that has emerged as important to lactational infertility and to child survival is the early establishment of lactation. Immediate contact, skin-to-skin, is key to early initiation of feeding, lactation, and infant homeostasis, including thermal regulation. The immediate onset of feeding postpartum is associated with survival in all mammalian species. While humans have sought substitutes for the nutritional components of milk, the risks of not feeding colostrum, the first milk richest in immune factors, remains for humans as well. Edmond *et al.* (Edmond *et al.*, 2006) report on a prospective study of 10,947 breastfed infants in Sub-Saharan Africa. There was a clear dose response in that risk of neonatal mortality increased with longer delay in initiation of breastfeeding, from one hour to day seven. Late initiation (after day one) was associated with a 2.4-fold increase in risk. This effect was similar when the model controlled for infants at high risk or experiencing death in the first week. They also found that the risk of neonatal death was fourfold higher in children given milk-based fluids or solids in addition to breastmilk. They concluded that 16% of neonatal deaths could be avoided if all infants were breastfed from day one and 22% of the deaths could be avoided if breastfeeding started within the first hour.

These same patterns of early contact and feeding and frequent feeding as indicated by infant hunger cues are the patterns most likely to delay fertility return.

How was the Lactational Amenorrhea Method for Family Planning developed?

In the 1970s and 1980s, there was an increase in the study of the physiology of fertility, some seeking new methods of family planning and others seeking to better understand physiology and pathologies (Tyson, 1980; Tyson *et al.*, 1976). Data published in the early

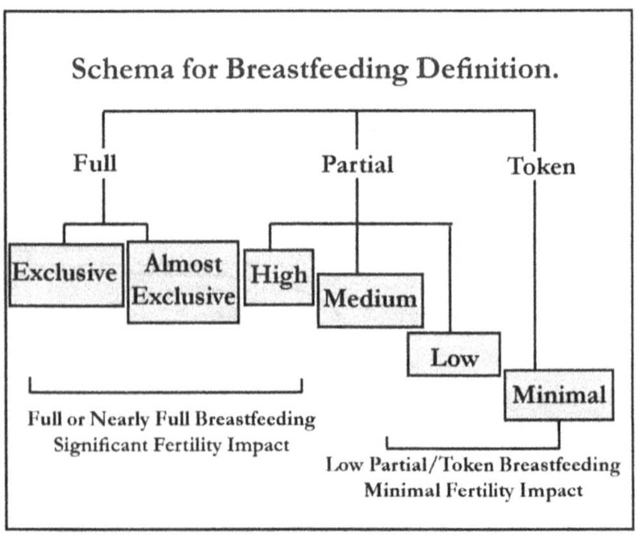

Figure 2. Under the conditions of Full or Nearly Full Breastfeeding, the return of menses will be delayed and the risk of an adequate ovulation preceding the first menses will be very low. Clinically, it is appropriate to strive for exclusive breastfeeding to ensure best outcomes. Source: Labbok & Krasovec, 1989.

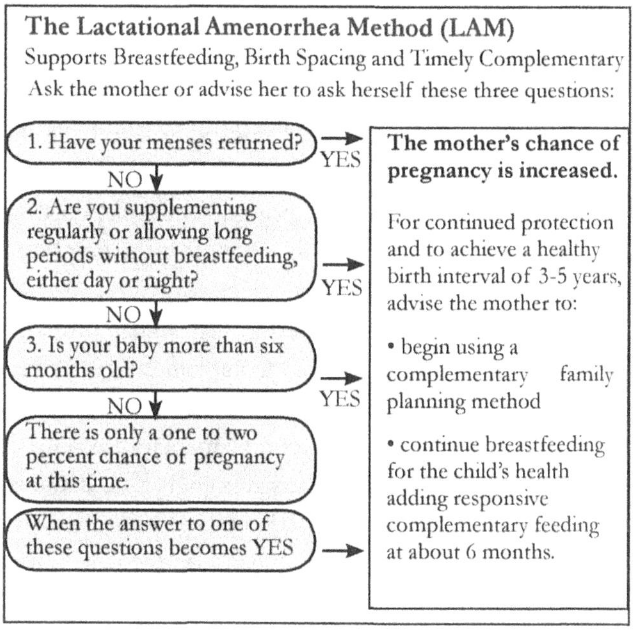

Figure 3. The parameters that encompassed the physiology of full lactational infertility were codified as a method of postpartum family planning known as the Lactational Amenorhea Method.

1970s had shown that women who breastfed were less likely to ovulate early postpartum, and if breastfeeding were more intensive, they were less likely than partial or non-breastfeeders to experience a normal ovulation prior to the first menstrual-like bleed (Perez *et al.*, 1972). Following this, several research groups examined the relationship between breastfeeding and fertility return prospectively in individuals (Tyson, 1977), eventually using hormonal assays and/or ultrasound to assess return to ovulation (Gray *et al.*, 1987; Diaz *et al.*, 1988).

Several of these groups met in the Rockefeller Bellagio Conference Center in 1988 to consider the parameters associated with fertility suppression among lactating women. The group concluded that: "Women who are not using family planning, but who are fully or nearly fully breastfeeding and amenorrheic, are likely to experience a risk of pregnancy of less than 2% in the first six months after delivery (Kennedy *et al.*, 1989)."

During the same period, researchers and policy makers alike became concerned that the definitions of breastfeeding used in research were highly variable and were contributing to the poor understanding of the findings. Therefore, a group of experts gathered at UNICEF to formulate breastfeeding definitions that would describe maternal as well as child physiology (**Figure 2**) (Labbok & Krasovec; 1990).

All of the above findings were then presented to a group of family planning service providers at Georgetown University, resulting in the codification of LAM as a family planning method (**Figure 3**) (Labbok *et al.*, 1994).

In 1995, a second Bellagio meeting reviewed subsequent work and included studies of Lactational Amenorrhea Method (LAM) in use (Perez *et al.*, 1992). The studies presented confirmed the findings of the first meeting and demonstrated the potential efficacy and usefulness of the LAM (Kennedy *et al.*, 1996). Several studies carried out subsequently have continued to support these initial findings (WHO, 1999a; WHO, 1999b; Labbok *et al.*, 1997; Hight-Laukaran *et al.*, 1997; Bongiovanni *et al.*, 2005). Bellagio II as this meeting has come to be known:

Confirmed efficacy of LAM: >98% by six month life table,

Suggested further study might enable "relaxing" the fully breastfeeding and six month requirements,

Defined menses return as two consecutive days of bleeding **or** a vaginal bleed that the woman perceives as a menses (after eight weeks postpartum),

Encouraged worldwide implementation of LAM for all of its positive impacts.

The Lactational Amenorrhea Method (LAM) was developed and has been most often studied and used as an algorithm (**Figure 3**) and includes three criteria for defining the period of lowest pregnancy risk.

Furthermore, it advises the immediate commencement of other methods if any one of the three criteria is not met. Clinically, the mother is asked:

- Have you had a menstrual bleed?
- Are you giving any supplementary foods or fluids in addition to breastfeeding?
- Is your infant older than six months of age?

If she answers negatively to all three criteria, she meets the requirements for LAM efficacy. She should be advised to initiate another form of contraception if **any** of the above three questions are answered affirmatively to achieve adequate efficacy for birth spacing or fertility limitation. If the mother is interested in and qualifies for LAM, she is advised to ask herself the same three questions in an ongoing manner. It is advisable to ensure that she has her next method on hand and initiates its use whenever her answer to any of the three questions changes. She should be advised to contact her health care professional immediately if she has any questions as to whether or not the method still applies.

To use LAM correctly, it is important that the patient understand each of the three criteria. Menses return for the purposes of LAM use is defined as any bleeding that occurs after 56 days postpartum that is perceived by the patient as a menses or any two consecutive days of bleeding. Full or nearly full breastfeeding includes exclusive or nearly exclusive breastfeeding, but also allows for occasional supplemental feedings, as long as they do not disrupt the frequency of breastfeeds. This method of family planning is now used in more than 30 countries, including recent reaffirmation by ACOG (ACOG Clinical Review, 2007), and has been included in the family planning and Maternal and Child Health policy in several countries. It has been widely accepted as a natural family planning method that demands no abstinence. It is used as an introductory method for the postpartum period or for the woman who hesitates to use a commodity-based method. It has the added benefit of encouraging optimal breastfeeding behavior, providing synergistic support for the primary health of mother and child.

LAM has been found to be 98% effective (**Figure 4**) (Labbok, 2000), and it has been used in a wide variety of settings, including different cultures, socioeconomic groups, and health care venues. **Figure 4** illustrates the LAM efficacy in a variety of studies.

The three questions used in ascertaining whether the method is in place are in descending order of importance. Amenorrhea is the most important of the three questions, as it alone is associated with a significant reduction in fertility. The intensity of the breastfeeding is also very important since it contributes both to the duration of amenorrhea and to the suppression of normal ovulation in the first postpartum cycle, creating the physiological conditions to ensure that the first bleed will tend to precede the first adequate ovulation.

The "six months" criterion is added primarily because this is the time that complementary feeding should begin. However, if breastfeeding continues at a high level even after complementary feeding is started, efficacy apparently remains high. In Rwanda, the LAM method was used up to nine months, maintaining breastfeeding frequency by feeding before each complementary feeding. In a study (Valdes, 2000) involving working women expressing milk after separation at least as often as breastfeeding would occur when together, LAM was found to be 96.5% effective. Although this finding is not statistically different from the results of other studies, it suggests a small increased risk of conception in women separated from their infants. This information should be given to the affected women so that they may make informed decisions. The World Health Organization (WHO) carried out a prospective trial on lactational amenorrhea and fertility return. Although this was not a study of women selecting and using LAM, the findings confirmed the high efficacy of the LAM trials (Kennedy, 2002).

A Cochrane literature review on efficacy in 2003 (Van der Wijden *et al.*, 2003) was carried out using a MEDLINE and EMBASE search from 1966-2002, as well as other publications and data sources on lactational amenorrhea. The selection of dates is of note as LAM was not developed and tested as a method until 1990. Nonetheless, thirteen publications reporting on nine intervention and two control groups met the inclusion criteria. The reviewers concluded that LAM is a viable contraceptive method, available and accessible to many women, with life table pregnancy rates at six months among LAM users ranging from 0.45 to 2.45 percent.

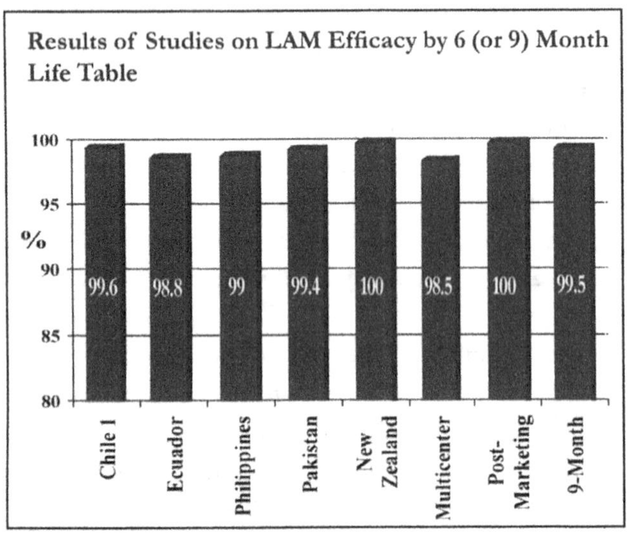

Figure 4. Early clinical studies of the Lactational Amenorrhea Method consistently demonstrated life table rates of unplanned pregnancy to vary around 99%, even when method use was extended to nine months by encouraging women to breastfeed before any complementary feeding.

Clinical Counseling and Postpartum Options for the Breastfeeding Mother

Postpartum contraception, like breastfeeding, should be discussed with patients during prenatal visits. The contraceptive choice a woman makes, with or without her partner's input, depends on factors such as previous experience with contraceptives, future childbearing plans, husband or partner's attitude, and her lactation status. If a patient is not comfortable with a method, she may use it ineffectively or not at all, even if she does not wish to become pregnant.

There are several common reasons why a woman may choose LAM: she may prefer a period of time without taking medicine or using any devices, she may prefer more time for selection of a long-term or permanent method, or she may wish to try something based on her natural physiology.

Frequent nursing and milk expression alters the hypothalamic pulsatility of gonadotropin releasing hormone (GnRH) production, which in turn mediates follicle stimulating and luteinizing hormones, so that effective ovulation is less likely to occur. Several milk expression studies have confirmed that the hormonal response is not identical to breastfeeding, so if the milk expression is a regular occurrence, some of the physiological responses may be modified. This is not directly mediated by prolactin. A patient who has had a spontaneous or induced abortion prior to 20 weeks usually will have spontaneous ovulation that results in the secretory portion of the menstrual cycle leading to menses. The patient will usually ovulate before any vaginal bleeding. If she delivers at term and is fully breastfeeding, however, vaginal bleeding (once the six weeks of lochia has stopped) nearly always occurs prior to first adequate ovulation during the first six months. Once regular feeding begins, there is an increase in fertile first cycles. Ovulation in the non-lactating woman may occur as early as three weeks postpartum.

There are several suggested behaviors that contribute to method success and duration. For example, LAM is not meant for patients who are giving regular supplemental feedings.

However, the one study (Valdes, 2000) of LAM in women who expressed their milk and provided it to the baby's caregiver during their absence found the efficacy was not significantly lower than among women not separated from their infants. Since most pregnancies in this study occurred after regular separation had commenced, further research is needed on this issue to better establish efficacy. Nonetheless, if this is the only method a woman is willing to accept and if she is well informed of the possibly increased pregnancy risk, LAM should remain an option.

It has been suggested that the duration of last postpartum amenorrhea could be used as a marker for fertility return. While duration of amenorrhea is statistically associated with the duration following the

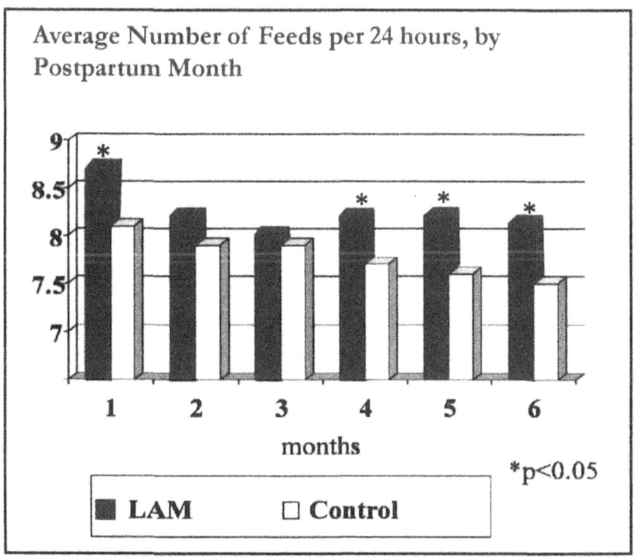

Figure 5. **LAM may achieve higher efficacy than lactational amenorrhea as LAM users would appear to practice a slightly more frequent pattern of feeding than fully lactating amenorrheic non-users. (Data from Santiago Study. Presented at ISRHML meeting, 2002)**

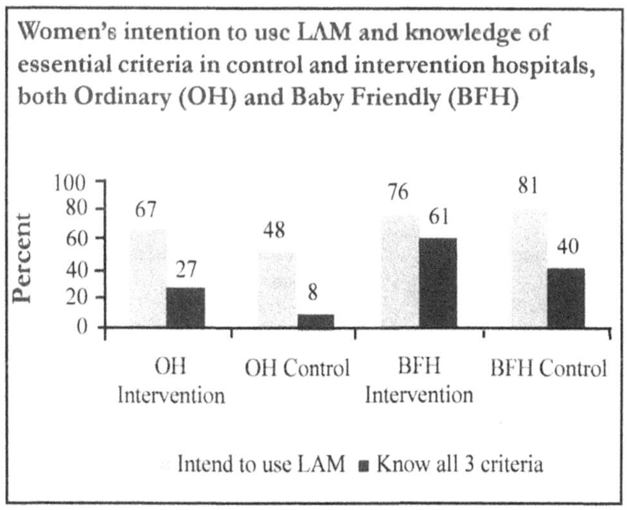

Figure 6. **Where breastfeeding support is in place, more women state an intention to use LAM. With LAM support in place, the rate of LAM knowledge increases from 40 of 81 (49%) to 61 of 76 (80%). Where there is no breastfeeding support, among the percentage with the intention to use LAM, the rate of LAM knowledge increases from 8 of 48 (17%) to 27 of 67 (40%). The impact of LAM programing is seen both in BFHI and non-BFHI settings, but is more successful overall in settings with BFHI. Sources: Frontiers Publications, 2006; Bongiovanni *et al.*, 2005.**

Table 2. Family Planning Methods Presented by Relative Impact on Lactation
For each method, efficacy, risks, benefits for lactation, and special considerations are presented.

Method	Description	Efficacy[1]	Risks to lactation	Benefits for lactation	Clinical/counseling suggestions and special considerations
No known impact on lactation					
LAM	Defined by three criteria that reflect reliable physiology for fertility delay	2/0.45	None	The required breastfeeding behaviors benefit maternal and child health and nutrition.	When any one of the criteria no longer applies, immediate transition to another method is recommended.
Abstinence/ Periodic Abstinence/ NFP Methods • Complete Abstinence • Calendar • Ovulation Method • Sympto-Thermal • Post Ovulation	Signs, symptoms, or timing of presumptive ovulation are used to identify periods of time when abstinence is necessary to avoid conception.	 0 25 9 3 2	None, however, most methods may demand substantial periods of abstinence during lactation due to difficulty in assessing signs of ovulation.	None	Even experienced users of these methods will benefit from special counseling for their use during lactation as the signs and symptoms will vary and may be difficult to properly interpret during the hormonal changes that may occur during lactation.
Barrier Methods: Condoms: • Male • Female Diaphragms Cervical caps w/o spermicide Spermicides alone Sponge	Condoms: Provides barrier to prevent ejaculum from coming in contact with cervical mucus. Diaphragms/caps: Generally used with spermicide, so provides elements of both physical and chemical barriers. Spermicides: Provide chemical barrier.	 15/2 21/5 16/6 32/26 29/18 32/20	Some spermicides may provide lubrication, however, some varieties may cause additional sensitivity in some individuals.	Condoms: Lubricated varieties may be useful with lactational suppression of estrogenic vaginal lubricants.	Subject to user error; some individuals have allergies to ingredients; some couples may find methods inconvenient. Few side effects. Highly effective if used consistently and correctly. The condom can provide some protection against sexually transmitted diseases. If a patient has previously used a diaphragm or cervical cap, it should be refitted at the six-week postpartum visit.
Little to no known impact on lactation					
IUD Non copper/non hormonal IUD Copper IUD: 7-10 yrs	IUD functions as a foreign body in the uterus, provoking hormonal changes that reduce the possibility of fertilization of the egg and implantation of an embryo.	0.8/0.6 0.1/0.1	Some women may have excess lochia or contraction-associated uterine discharge.	Once inserted, no further action or intervention is needed during lactation.	An IUD should be inserted within the first 48 hours after delivery or delayed for at least 4 weeks as lactating women have strong uterine contractions. This also requires that IUD insertion be high in the uterus to decrease risk of expulsion.
Surgical Sterilization • Male-vasectomy • Female-tubal ligation	Surgical blockage of path of gametes by bisecting, separating ends, and ligation of vas/fallopian tubes	0.15/0.10 0.5/0.5	Tubal ligation may necessitate temporary interruption in breastfeeding while surgery takes place. Milk should be expressed in advance for feeding during the procedure.	Once performed, no further intervention is needed. Both may be outpatient procedures.	Permanent decision. Reversal is expensive, requires surgical expertise, and may not be successful. Highly effective. Male: If coupled with postpartum infertility, simplifies contraception during the months necessary for healing. Male sterilization is easier and safer and may be performed in an office setting.

Method	Description	Efficacy[1]	Risks to lactation	Benefits for lactation	Clinical/counseling suggestions and special considerations
Some reports of negative impact on lactation					
Progestin-only • Pills • Injectables [e.g., DMPA 3 months; norethisterone 2 months] • Implants [e.g., Number, size, and content of implanted rods offer different lengths of protection in years) • Levonorgestrel IUD: up to 5 yrs	Mechanism of action includes some disruption of lactation and modification of intra-uterine milieu and readiness for implantation. Progestin-only contraception during lactation does not suppress gonadotropins nor affect growth of ovarian follicles during breastfeeding. Thus, the contraceptive effect of POP is likely mediated through local actions at the endometrium and cervix in a manner similar to that in menstruating women (Perheentupa *et al.*, 2003).	5/0.5 3/0.3 0.05/0.05 0.1/0.1	May decrease milk supply if started before milk supply is well established. Anecdotal reports of immediate negative impact even when initiated after lactation is well established. Progestin IUD typically has minimal impact, but has the potential to have the same impact as other progestin-only methods.	Some studies report increased milk production with injectables.	Common side effects include: irregular bleeding (less common in predominantly breastfeeding women), weight gain, and headaches. Return to fertility with injections may be delayed beyond expected duration--of potential concern for some women. Must develop routine for taking daily pills. Implants require procedure for placement and removal.
Expected to have negative impact on lactation					
• Combined pill • Contraceptive patch (e.g., ethinyl estradiol/norelgestromin) • Combined vaginal ring (e.g., ethinyl estradiol/ etonogestrel) • Combined injectables (e.g., estradiol/medroxy-progesterone)	Exogenous estrogen serves to suppress ovulation	8/0.3 8/0.3 8/0.3 3/0.05	Significant risk of reducing milk supply. It is suggested that initiation be delayed until 6 months postpartum. Reduction in supply appears dose dependent. Injectables more difficult to stop if problems arise.	None	Several good noncontraceptive effects, e.g., reduced risk of ovarian and endometrial cancers, decreased anemia, and regular menses. Not suitable for women with history of clotting problems, estrogen-dependent cancers, severe migraines, or women over 35 who smoke.

[1] Percent Pregnant by Life Table in use/in research evaluation (12 month life table; LAM efficacy based on 6 month life table). Efficacy for most methods has not been fully studied during lactation, therefore, the life-table estimates presented here, except for LAM, do not reflect efficacy during lactation. Source: WHO Medical Eligibility Criteria, 2002.

last pregnancy, more than 50% of subsequent durations differ by more than three months (Labbok *et al.*, 2002). Perhaps this is in part due to changing patterns of breastfeeding. One set of studies found that exclusively breastfeeding women using LAM are more likely to be amenorrheic at six months than exclusively breastfeeding controls (84% vs. 69.7%, respectively) (Valdes, 1998). Women who actively used LAM had a higher feeding frequency and, hence, shorter inter-feeding intervals than other exclusive breastfeeders (**Figure 5**). However, even with short inter-feeding intervals, some women still experience earlier menses return. While we do not know whether these cycles are adequate for conception, whether or not breastfeeding continues to be frequent, another method is recommended for birth spacing whenever menses return.

After women practice LAM for six months, they continue very low pregnancy rates as long as they continue breastfeeding and are amenorrheic. At least three studies (Kazi *et al.*, 1995; Cooney *et al.*, 1996; Kennedy, 2002) have indicated that the efficacy of LAM can be maintained during the six to 12 month period, provided the mother who originally followed this method continues to breastfeed before giving complementary foods at less than four hour intervals during the day and six hour intervals at night and remains amenorrheic. However, studies of LAM continuation and acceptability have shown that more than 80% of LAM acceptors do begin another family planning method in a timely manner (Hight-Laukaran *et al.*, 1997; Bongiovanni *et al.*, 2005).

LAM use and success has been shown to be independent of level of education, religion, geographic location, and presence or absence of active breastfeeding support. Education concerning the criteria for LAM use results in increased efficacious use of LAM, both in the context of breastfeeding support and in settings where it is presented without special breastfeeding support. (**Figure 6**), from a study in Jordan (Bongiovanni *et al.*, 2005), illustrates that LAM education can be successful whether or not in a BFHI setting of support for breastfeeding.

CONTRACEPTIVE USE DURING LACTATION

This section draws heavily on protocol for the use of contraception during lactation that was recently developed by the Academy of Breastfeeding Medicine, the professional organization of physicians interested in improving education and physician capacity related to breastfeeding (Labbok *et al.*, 2006), and on WHO Medical Eligibility Criteria (WHO/CDC/USAID, 2004).

All family planning choices are available to the postpartum lactating woman; however, her choice and the clinical ramifications of that choice merit special counseling. **Table 2** includes a method by method explanation of risks and benefits of their use in terms of lactation, and any special considerations. Methods are grouped to reflect impact on lactation rather than contraceptive efficacy. For many methods, the efficacy of use during different patterns of breastfeeding has not been established, but is generally assumed to be

Table 3. Family Planning Counseling for the Breastfeeding Woman Should Include Consideration of Several Factors

When counseling a breastfeeding mother in choosing a method of family planning, discuss and consider:	The responses will have implications in selecting:
1. Feeding patterns, status, and plans	LAM, hormonal methods
2. Child's age	LAM, hormonal methods, IUD insertion, barrier sizing
3. Maternal age	Hormonal methods
4. Previous contraceptive experience	Social and use issues, as well as sensitivities
5. Husband's (partner's) opinions on various methods	Social and use issues
6. Childbearing plans	Spacing versus limiting methods
7. Health status	Spacing versus limiting methods, hormonal methods
8. Accessibility and acceptability of methods	Periodic abstinence, LAM, barriers
9. Health care system, healthworker training, and reimbursement payment plans	All
10. Prevalence of sexually transmitted disease, including HIV	Condoms, abstinence

Source: Labbok et al., 2006

enhanced by the overall reduced risk of conception during any breastfeeding.

In general, the first choice methods would be those that either support lactation or would have no direct impact on lactation. These include LAM, barrier methods, and periodic abstinence/natural family planning methods. Other methods that would not interfere with lactation over time, but which merit special clinical attention include IUDs and sterilization.

Second choice methods are those that have demonstrated a negative impact on lactation. These include hormonal methods. Progestin-only methods may not have the same degree of impact on lactation as is seen with estrogenic methods. Although Koetsawang (Koetsawang, 1987) reported an increase in milk supply with these methods, Tankeyoon (Tankeyoon *et al.*, 1984) noted a 12% decline in milk supply with progestin-only contraception compared to a placebo. A recent Cochrane review indicated that evidence from randomized controlled trials on the effect of hormonal contraceptives during lactation is limited and of poor quality: "Evidence is inadequate to make recommendations regarding hormonal contraceptive use for lactating women" (Truitt *et al.*, 2003). Since that time, a study of the progestin-only ring found no difference between users and controls in a variety of parameters related to lactation (Massai *et al.*, 2005). Stress may also be a factor, as stress impairs the ovarian cycle through activation of the hypothalamus pituitary adrenal axis (Edozien, 2006). Some women will choose to initiate contraceptive use secondary to other life changes and stresses, compounding the potential to disrupt lactation.

However, given the high level of anecdotal reports of the association of hormonal contraception with milk supply, it would be reasonable to consider that all hormonal contraceptive methods may have some risk of decreasing mother's milk supply and/or passing into the infant through active absorption or through passive passage across the gut wall in the youngest children. Given this, hormonal methods, including progestin-only methods, should be discouraged where there is:

1) a young infant: less than six weeks for progestin-only, less than six months for combined,
2) existing low milk supply or history of lactation failure,
3) history of breast surgery,
4) multiple birth (twins, triplets),
5) preterm birth, or
6) compromised health of mother and/or baby.

The increasingly common practice of immediate postpartum injection of depot-type contraceptives has not been adequately studied in lactating women to allow for the conclusion that any benefit for the lactating woman would outweigh the potential risks.

Table 3 offers some ideas for counseling the breastfeeding mother concerning her choice of methods. In addition to issues that should be included in counseling all women, there are special issues and some unique methods for the lactating woman.

Is it possible to stay current with new findings?

With ongoing research on contraceptive efficacy and increasing trends in breastfeeding and exclusive breastfeeding in all countries, it is reasonable to expect that the knowledge base on this issue will increase. Thus, no text or chapter can be fully up to date by the time of publication. However, WHO, CDC,

Table 4. WHO Medical Eligibility Criteria: Guidance for Use of Contraceptive Methods during Breastfeeding

Duration of breastfeeding method	Progestin-only pills	Progestin-only depots	Progestin-only implants	Combined injectable contraceptives	Combined patch	Combined ring	Low dose combined
<6 weeks postpartum	3	3	3	4	4	4	4
≥ 6 weeks to < 6 months postpartum (primarily breastfeeding)	1	1	1	3	3	3	3
≥6 months postpartum	1	1	1	2	2	2	2

and USAID collaborated to produce the WHO/CDC/USAID Medical Eligibility Criteria, currently available in the third edition (WHO/CDC/USAID Medical Eligibility Criteria, 2004), with a fourth edition pending in 2006. In addition, WHO offers selected practice recommendations for contraceptive use (Department of Reproductive Health and Research, 2004). These documents provide information about the appropriateness of use of each method under specified conditions. One of the conditions consistently explored is the impact of the method on lactation. The conditions affecting eligibility for use of each contraceptive method are classified under one of the following four categories with clinical implications:

1. A condition for which there is no restriction for use of the contraceptive method: Use method in any circumstance.
2. A condition where the advantages of using the method generally outweigh the theoretical or proven risks: Generally use the method.
3. A condition where the theoretical or proven risks usually outweigh the advantages of using the method: Use of method not usually recommended unless other more appropriate methods are not available or not acceptable.
4. A condition which represents an unacceptable health risk if the contraceptive method is used: Method not to be used.

These categories for method use during lactation are included in **Table 4**.

For updates, the ABM Clinical Protocols, including "#13: Contraception during Breastfeeding" (Labbok *et al.*, 2005), are updated regularly and published in *Breastfeeding Medicine*, the journal of the Academy of Breastfeeding Medicine, as well as on the ABM web site: www.bfmed.org. WHO updates and adds to the recommendations in the WHO/CDC/USAID Medical Eligibility Criteria at appropriate intervals through expert Working Group meetings every three to four years and through input from its Family Planning Guidelines Steering Group on an as-needed basis. Contraceptive Eligibility Checklists are available from WHO as well. The last Contraceptive Eligibility Checklist was produced in 2000 (Stang *et al.*, 2000), specifically for provision of combined oral contraceptives and depot-medroxyprogesterone acetate; however, additional checklists are expected.

CONCLUSIONS AND THE WAY FORWARD

Can We Ensure That Health Care Providers Respect and Support Breastfeeding During Contraception?

Despite the clear recommendations of the WHO eligibility criteria, not all clinicians are aware of the potential risks to successful breastfeeding that can be caused by poor choice of contraceptive method. This may be compounded by lack of continuity of care in many settings, where the clinician who prescribes the method is rarely the same individual who later must deal with the issue of compromised breastfeeding.

With the increasing trends in breastfeeding initiation and exclusivity worldwide, the need for proper counseling and prescription of contraceptives during lactation is an important issue. The Lactational Amenorrhea Method can provide a lactation-supportive introductory method, which also indicates when it is necessary to begin the next method.

In sum, it is the responsibility of the clinician to remain informed, up-to-date, and attentive to the needs of lactating women, their breastfeeding intentions, and their need for family planning to achieve appropriate birth intervals.

References

Becker S, Rutstein S, Labbok MH. Estimation of births averted due to breast-feeding and increases in levels of contraception needed to substitute for breast-feeding. *J Biosoc Sci.* 2003; 35(4):559-74.

Bongiovanni A, Samam'he M, Al Sarabi R, Masri S, Zehner E, Huffman S. *Promoting the Lactational Amenorrhea Methods (LAM) in Jordan-Increases Modern Contraceptive Use in the Extended Postpartum Period.* Washington DC: Linkages/ Academy for Educational Development; October 2005.

Butz WP. The changing role of breastfeeding in economic development: a theoretical exposition. *Res Hum Cap Dev.* 1981; 2:95-117.

Campino C, Torres C, Rioseco A, Poblete A, Pugin E, Valdes V, *et al.* Plasma prolactin/oestradiol ratio at 38 weeks gestation predicts the duration of lactational amenorrhoea. *Hum Reprod.* 2001; 16(12):2540-45.

Cavagna M, Mantese JC, Freitas GD, Dzik A, Soares JB, Hameiry Y, *et al.* Pattern of prolactin secretion after administration of gonadotropin-releasing hormone agonist at the preovulatory phase of intrauterine insemination cycles. *Sao Paulo Med J.* 2005; 123(6):295-97. [Epub 2006 Jan 20].

Committee on Health Care for Underserved Women and Committee on Obstetric Practices. Special Report from

ACOG - Breastfeeding: Maternal and Infant Aspects. *ACOG Clinical Review.* 2007; 12(1):1S-16S.

Conde-Agudelo A, Belizan JM. Maternal morbidity and mortality associated with interpregnancy interval: cross sectional study. *BMJ.* 2000; 321(7271):1255-59.

Conde-Agudelo A, Rosas-Bermudez A, Kafury-Goeta AC. Birth spacing and risk of adverse perinatal outcomes: a meta-analysis. *JAMA.* 2006; 295(15):1809-23.

Cooney KA, Nyirabukeye T, Labbok MH, Hoser PH, Ballard E. An assessment of the nine-month lactational amenorrhea method (MAMA-9) in Rwanda. *Stud Fam Plann.* 1996; 27(3):102-71.

Department of Reproductive Health and Research (RHR). *Selected practice recommendations for contraceptive use.* World Health Organization; 2004. Available from: http://whqlibdoc.who.int/publications/2004/9241562846.pdf.

Diaz S, Rodriguez G, Peralta O, Miranda P, Casado ME, Salvatierra AM, *et al.* Lactational amenorrhea and the recovery of ovulation and fertility in fully nursing Chilean women. *Contraception.* 1988; 38(1):53-67.

Edmond K, Zandoh C, Quigley M, Amenga-Etego S, Owusu-Agyei S, Kirkwood B. Delayed breastfeeding initiation increases risk of neonatal mortality. *Pediatrics.* 2006; 117(3):e380-86.

Edozien LC. Mind over matter: psychological factors and the menstrual cycle. *Curr Opin Obstet Gynecol.* 2006; 18(4):452-56.

Frontiers Publications/Resources. *Kazakhstan: Promote LAM for Postpartum Family Planning and Birth Spacing.* OR Summary no. 56. Oct 19, 2006.

Gray RH, Campbell OM, Apelo R, Eslami SS, Zacur H, Ramos RM, *et al.* Risk of ovulation during lactation. *Lancet.* 1990; 335(8680):25-29.

Gray RH, Campbell OM, Zacur HA, Labbok MH, MacRae SL. Postpartum return of ovarian activity in nonbreastfeeding women monitored by urinary assays. *J Clin Endocrinol Metab.* 1987; 64(4):645-50.

Hight-Laukaran V, Labbok M, Peterson A, Fletcher V, von Hertzen H, Van Look P, *et al.* Multicenter Study of the Lactational Amenorrhea Method (LAM) II. Acceptability, Utility, and Policy Implications. *Contraception.* 1997; 55:337-46.

Jain A, Bongaarts J. Breastfeeding: patterns, correlates, and fertility effects. *Stud Fam Plann.* 1981; 12(3):79-99.

Kazi A, Kennedy KI, Visness CM, Khan T. Effectiveness of the lactational amenorrhea method in Pakistan. *Fertil Steril.* 1995; 64(4):717-23.

Kennedy K, Labbok M, Van Look P. Consensus statement: Lactational amenorrhea method for family planning. *Int J Gynaecol Obstet.* 1996; 54:55-57.

Kennedy KI, Rivera R, McNeilly AS. Consensus statement on the use of breastfeeding as a family planning method. *Contraception.* 1989; 39(5):477-96.

Kennedy KI. Efficacy and effectiveness of LAM. *Adv Exp Med Biol.* 2002; 503:207-16.

Koetsawang S. The effects of contraceptive methods on the quality and quantity of breast milk. *Int J Gynaecol Obstet.* 1987; 25 Suppl:115-27.

Kroger M, Smith L. *Impact of birthing practices on breastfeeding: Protecting the mother and baby continum.* Boston: Jones & Bartlett; 2004.

Labbok M, Krasovec K. Towards consistency in breastfeeding definitions. *Stud Fam Plann.* 1990; 21(4):226-30.

Labbok M, Hight-Laukaran V, Peterson A, Fletcher V, von Hertzen H, Van Look P, *et al.* Multicenter study of the Lactational Amenorrhea Method (LAM) I. Efficacy, duration, and implications for clinical application. *Contraception.* 1997; 55:327-36.

Labbok M, Nichols-Johnson V, Valdes-Anderson V. ABM Clinical Protocol #13: Contraception during breastfeeding. *Breastfeeding Medicine.* 2006; 1(1):43-51. Available from: http://www.bfmed.org/ace-files/protocol/finalcontraceptionprotocolsent2.pdf.

Labbok M, Perez A, Valdes V, Sevilla F, Wade K, Laukaran V, *et al.* The Lactational Amenorrhea Method: A new postpartum introductory family planning method with program and policy implications. *Advances in Contraception.* 1994; 10:93-109.

Labbok M. Breastfeeding, fertility and family planning. In: Sciarra J, editor. *Gynecology and Obstetrics.* Lippincott; 2000.

Lawrence RA, Lawrence RL. *Breastfeeding: A Guide for the Medical Profession.* Mosby; 2005.

Massai R, Quinteros E, Reyes MV, Caviedes R, Zepeda A, Montero JC, *et al.* Extended use of a progesterone-releasing vaginal ring in nursing women: a phase II clinical trial. *Contraception.* 2005; 72(5):352-57.

McNeilly AS. Neuroendocrine changes and fertility in breast-feeding women. *Prog Brain Res.* 2001;133:207-14.

Merchant K, Martorell R, Haas J. Maternal and fetal responses to the stresses of lactation concurrent with pregnancy and of short recuperative intervals. *Am J Clin Nutr.* 1990; 52(2):280-88.

Page-Wilson G, Smith PC, Welt CK. Prolactin suppresses GnRH but not TSH secretion. *Horm Res.* 2006;65(1):31-38. Epub 2005 Dec 16.

Perez A, Labbok M, Queenan J. A clinical study of the Lactational Amenorrhea Method for family planning. *Lancet.* 1992; 339:968-70.

Perez A, Vela P, Masnick GS, Potter RG First ovulation after childbirth: the effect of breast-feeding. *Am J Obstet Gynecol.* 1972; 114(8):1041-7.

Perheentupa A, Critchley H, Illingworth P, McNeilly A. Effects of progestin-only pill on pituitary-ovarian axis activity during lactation. *Contraception.* 2003; 67: 467-71.

Rutstein SO. Effects of preceding birth intervals on neonatal, infant and under-five years mortality and nutritional status in developing countries: evidence from the demographic and health surveys. *Int J Gynaecol Obstet.* 2005; 89 Suppl 1: S7-24. Epub 2005 Jan 26.

Schneider F, Tomek W, Grundker C. Gonadotropin-releasing hormone (GnRH) and its natural analogues: A review. *Theriogenology.* 2006 Apr 28; [Epub ahead of print].

Stang A, Schwingl P, Rivera R. Contraceptive eligibility checklists for provision of combined oral contraceptives and depot-medroxyprogesterone acetate. *Bull World Health Organ.* 2000; 78(8):1015-23.

Tankeyoon M, Dusitsin N, Chalapati S, Koetsawang S, Sas M, *et al.* Effects of hormonal contraceptives on milk volumes and infant growth. WHO Special Programme of Research, Development and Research Training in Human Reproduction. Task force on oral contraceptives. *Contraception.* 1984; 30(6):505-22.

The World Health Organization Task Force on Methods for the Natural Regulation of Fertility. The World Health Organization multinational study of breast-feeding and lactational amenorrhea. III. Pregnancy during breast-feeding. *Fertil Steril.* 1999a; 72(3):431-40.

The World Health Organization Task Force on Methods for the Natural Regulation of Fertility. Fertil Steril. The World Health Organization multinational study of breast-feeding and lactational amenorrhea. IV. Postpartum bleeding and lochia in breast-feeding women. 1999b; 72(3):441-47.

Truitt ST, Fraser AB, Grimes DA, Gallo MF, Schulz KF. Combined hormonal versus nonhormonal versus progestin-only contraception in lactation. *Cochrane Database Syst Rev.* 2003; (2):CD003988.

Tyson J. Neuroendocrine control of female fertility: role of prolactin. *Adv Biochem Psychopharmacol.* 1980; 23:199-207.

Tyson J. Mechanisms of puerperal lactation. *Med Clin North Am.* 1977; 61(1):153-63.

Tyson JE, Perez A, Zanartu J. Human lactational response to oral thyrotropin releasing hormone. *J Clin Endocrinol Metab.* 1976; 43(4):760-68.

Valdes V, Labbok MH, Pugin E, Perez A. The efficacy of the lactational amenorrhea method (LAM) among working women. *Contraception.* 2000; 62(5):217-19.

Valdes V. *Oaxaca Proceedings.* Washington: Wellstart EPB; 1998.

Van der Wijden C, Kleijnen J, Van den Berk T. Lactational amenorrhea for family planning. *Cochrane Database Syst Rev.* 2003;(4):CD001329.

Velasquez E, Trigo R, Creus S, Campo S, Croxatto H. Pituitary-ovarian axis during lactational amenorrhoea. I. Longitudinal assessment of follicular growth, gonadotrophins, sex steroids and inhibin levels before and after recovery of menstrual cyclicity. *Human Reprod.* 2006; 21(4):909-15.

Velasquez EV, Creus S, Trigo RV, Cigorraga SB, Pellizzari EH, Croxatto HB, *et al.* Pituitary-ovarian axis during lactational amenorrhoea. II. Longitudinal assessment of serum FSH polymorphism before and after recovery of menstrual cycles. *Hum Reprod.* 2006;21(4):916-23. Epub 2005 Dec 16.

WHO/CDC/USAID. *Medical Eligibility Criteria.* 3rd edition. Geneva: WHO; 2004.

Zhu BP. Effect of interpregnancy interval on birth outcomes: findings from three recent US studies. *Int J Gynaecol Obstet.* 2005; 89 Suppl 1:S25-33.

Chapter 16

Reproductive Bioenergetics, Infertility, and Ovulation Induction in the Lactating Female

Robert P. Kauffman

INTRODUCTION

Human reproduction and lactation are physiologic functions vital for procreation and survival of the species. Although development of infant supplements has impacted the frequency and duration of breastfeeding in developed nations, breastfeeding remains fundamental to infant survival in underdeveloped nations. In addition to infant nutrition, health, and disease prevention, human lactation plays a pivotal role in family planning and population control (McNeilly, 1997; Ellison, 2003; Hanson *et al.*, 2003). By spacing children apart, the prospect for infant survival is enhanced, particularly in underdeveloped countries where food supplies may be scarce (Diaz *et al.*, 1995). A birth interval of fewer than two years boosts the probability of prematurity, low birth weight (fetal growth restriction), perinatal infectious morbidity, and neonatal death (Miller, 1994; Miller, 1991).

Postpartum amenorrhea is highly influenced by the duration and pattern of breastfeeding (McNeilly, 1997; Prema & Ravindranah, 1982; Jones & Palloni, 1994; Gross, 1988). In industrialized nations, evolving breastfeeding patterns and the introduction of infant dietary supplements have provoked a greater need for contraceptive measures which do not rely upon lactational amenorrhea.

The desire to delay fertility until later reproductive life, coupled with the intent to breastfeed between pregnancies, necessitates a need to search for effective methods of ovulation induction under these circumstances. Furthermore, the advent of assisted reproductive technologies (ART), most notably *in vitro* fertilization (IVF), has extended the limits of genetically determined reproductive potential.

Within this complex interface of societal demands and biological limitations, this chapter will examine the energetics of reproduction, principles of human infertility and reproductive failure, the physiology of human lactational amenorrhea, and ovulation induction in the lactating woman.

REPRODUCTION AND BIOENERGETICS

Physiologic stress and starvation play an important modulatory role in the process of human reproduction. Exercise induced menstrual irregularities (particularly in ballet dancers and distance runners) are due, in part, to an interruption of normal gonadotropin releasing hormone (GnRH) pulsatility at the hypothalamus. Under these conditions, pituitary luteinizing hormone (LH) secretion is suppressed more so than follicle stimulating hormone (FSH) (Warren & Perlroth, 2001). Up to 79% of ballet dancers (where lean body composition is desirable) experience oligomenorrhea or secondary amenorrhea (Abraham *et al.*, 1982). Although excessive physical exertion has been suggested as a cause of exercise-induced hypothalamic amenorrhea, Loucks *et al.* identified caloric restriction as the primary stressor (Loucks *et al.*, 1989). The effect of compromised energy resources on GnRH secretion is regulated by a complex network of neuroendocrine and peripheral signaling mechanisms. Leptin, a product of the obesity (ob) gene and primarily secreted by the adipocytes, plays a major role in reproductive physiology (Henson & Castracane, 2003). Leptin levels correlate with body mass index (BMI) and adipose stores, and prolonged fasting and/or starvation lower circulating leptin levels and suppress leptin's normal diurnal secretory pattern (Henson & Castracane, 2003; Macut *et al.*, 1998). Leptin receptors are found at hypothalamic neurons regulating GnRH production, and leptin assumes a key role in providing feedback to GnRH-secreting neurons during starvation and stress (Henson & Castracane, 2003). Other gut, central nervous system (CNS), and adipocyte hormones are also involved in this intricate feedback system, and more detailed discussions of the subject can be found elsewhere (Morales *et al.*, 1996; Kageyama *et al.*, 2005; Smith & Grove, 2002).

Breastfeeding confers a state of negative energy balance. The role of leptin in reactivation of LH secretion in lactating women appears to be minor, if any. In contrast to rodent models where leptin levels are decreased during lactation (similar to the starvation model), leptin levels do not vary between lactating and non-lactating ovulatory women, and therefore, leptin itself does not appear to be the sentinel regulator of postpartum hypothalamic-pituitary-ovarian (HPO) axis reactivation (Henson & Castracane, 2003; Sir-Petermann *et al.*, 2001; Brogan *et al.*, 1999; Butte *et al.*, 1999; Tennekoon *et al.*, 2005). Re-establishment of a positive energy balance in well nourished breastfeeding individuals is one of the critical determinants influencing the duration of postpartum amenorrhea (Tennekoon *et al.*, 2005; Valeggia & Ellison, 2004).

The allocation of maternal energy resources to support gestational and lactational demands is vital to reproductive success (Ellison, 2003). Following birth, the mother must meet neonatal metabolic needs. Somatic and neurological growth exact further energy demands on the mother. The metabolic cost of lactation is approximately 750 kcal/day during the first five postpartum months (Dewey, 1997; Butte & King, 2005). The ability of the mother to meet these demands diverts energy resources necessary for successful reproductive effort (Ellison, 2003). Maternal metabolic resources appear dedicated to infant nutritional needs even in the face of relative maternal malnutrition. As supplemental foods are introduced to the infant during the weaning process, maternal metabolic resources can now be reallocated to the reproductive process (Ellison, 2003; Valeggia & Ellison, 2004).

From a bio-ecological standpoint, the duration of postpartum amenorrhea is the primary determinant of birth spacing in populations without ready access to contraceptive technologies (Ellison, 1994). The frequency and pattern of infant suckling play critical roles in modulating the re-emergence of ovulation following childbirth (Delvoye *et al.*, 1978; Konner & Worthman, 1980).

In impoverished regions of the world, exclusive long-term breastfeeding conveys a survival advantage by affording longer intervals between births, which, in turn, confers a protective effect on survival of future children (Miller, 1994; Miller, 1991; Diaz *et al.*, 1997). A three year inter-birth interval appears to be optimal. Even maternal morbidity and mortality is diminished when inter-birth intervals extend two years or greater (Conde-Agudelo & Belizan, 2000).

The pattern of infant suckling, the primary stimulus for milk letdown, independently regulates postpartum ovulatory function (Tay *et al.*, 1996; Rogers, 1997). Mothers with inadequate nutritional resources require more intense nipple stimulation to produce adequate milk supplies than those under better economic and nutritional circumstances (Valeggia & Ellison, 2004; Ellison, 1994; Lunn, 1992). In one study, the inter-birth interval in Bangladeshi women was prolonged when food intake was limited, independent of lactation status. Similar results have been recorded in other cultures as well (Konner & Worthman, 1980; Carneio, 1988; Worthman *et al.*, 1993). Women with lower body mass indices (BMIs) demonstrate longer durations of amenorrhea than those who are overweight or obese (Valeggia & Ellison, 2004; Ford & Huffman, 1988).

PREGNANCY LOSS AND HUMAN INFERTILITY

Before beginning a discussion of human infertility, it is appropriate to review factors governing ovarian development and early pregnancy loss (also referred to as spontaneous abortion and miscarriage).

The rise and fall of the oocytes

Human reproduction is a wasteful process. The human fetus produces approximately six to seven million oocytes by gestational week 16-20, declining to one to two million at birth. At menarche, the number diminishes to approximately 300,000 oocytes, and by the onset of menopause, the oocyte supply is nearly exhausted (Baker, 1963; Gondos *et al.*, 1975; Santoro, 2005). During the course of reproductive life, only 400-500 ova complete the follicular maturation process and are released by the dominant (Graafian) follicle into the peritoneal cavity for tubal transport (Richardson *et al.*, 1987). Most follicles undergo apoptosis (programmed cell death) and atresia during fetal, pre-pubertal, and reproductive life (Richardson *et al.*, 1987; Faddy *et al.*, 1992; Gougeon *et al.*, 1994; Skinner, 2005).

Ovarian aging accelerates the tempo of follicular loss (Santoro, 2005; Faddy *et al.*, 1992; Gougeon *et al.*, 1994; Warburton, 2005). As menopause nears, the serum concentration of circulating inhibin B produced by the follicular granulosa cells decreases. Since inhibin B is the principle regulator of pituitary follicle stimulating hormone (FSH) production, serum FSH levels rise reflexively as the ovarian oocyte supply diminishes (Santoro, 2005). Clinically, high FSH (and lower inhibin B and anti-mullerian hormone) levels reflect a reduction in the number and the quality of the remaining oocytes (Faddy *et al.*, 1992; Klein *et al*, 1996; Laven & Fauser, 2004; Santoro *et al.*, 2003).

Early Pregnancy Loss

Following conception, about 15-20% of clinically recognized pregnancies undergo spontaneous abortion before the end of the second trimester with most occurring by the end of the first trimester. If all fertilized oocytes are considered, then only 50% progress to a viable pregnancy (Wramsby *et al.*, 1987; Warburton, 1987; Wilcox *et al.*, 1988).

About 20% of newly developed embryos are aneuploid, and the vast majority of these end as early miscarriages (Eichenlaug-Ritter, 1998). The frequency of spontaneous abortion increases with chronological aging, and by the age of 40, the incidence of early pregnancy loss (realized and unrealized) may be as high as 70% (Gougeon *et al.*, 1994). Paternal age also influences the rate of early miscarriage, but less dramatically than that of the female partner. Chromosomal anomalies (particularly trisomy disorders) are primarily responsible for the increased incidence of fetal wastage as women age (Harlap & Ghiono, 1980). Defective spindle formation during meiosis I is more prevalent in aging oocytes, culminating in impaired chromosomal migration following fertilization (Warburton, 2005; Battaglia *et al.*, 1996).

Infertility

Infertility is a disease defined as 12 or more months of unprotected intercourse without successful conception (Practice Committee of the American Society for Reproductive Medicine, 2004). The true incidence of infertility in any given population is unknown since many couples never seek (or have access to) medical evaluation and treatment. About 15% of couples attempting pregnancy fail to conceive by the end of one year and about five to seven percent remain childless at two years. Failure of a couple to achieve pregnancy spontaneously after three years is associated with a poor prognosis for success without medical or surgical intervention (Mosther & Pratt, 1991; Homburg, 2005; Guttmacher, 1956; Wang *et al.*, 2003). Pregnancies conceived by previously infertile couples are more likely to end as miscarriage than couples with normal fertility (Winter *et al.*, 2002). The reasons behind this phenomenon are incompletely understood, but genetic, endocrine, immunologic, oocyte aging, and chronic disease factors contribute to the observed differences (Christiansen *et al.*, 2005).

Over the past half century, biomedical research has elucidated many of the pathophysiologic processes associated with infertility. Despite this, fertility rates in the United States continue to fall, mostly owing to a deferment of marriage and pregnancy until later in life (Mosher & Pratt, 1991); however, a number of other conditions and circumstances play an important, albeit smaller, role (**Table 1**).

Table 1. Explanations for Declining Fertility Rates in the United States

- Postponement of marriage
- Desire to delay childbearing
- Career opportunities for women
- Voluntary childlessness
- Availability and safety of effective contraceptive methods
- Increased incidence of sexually transmitted diseases, especially *Chlamydia trachomatis*
- Legalization and safety of elective abortion

Table 2. Human Infertility: Diagnostic Categories and Frequencies

Category	Frequency (%)
Ovulatory Dysfunction	15-40%
Tubo-Peritoneal Disease*	30-40%
Utero-Cervical Factors†	5%
Male Factors	30-40%
Unknown Etiology	25%

* Endometriosis, pelvic adhesive disease, tubal obstruction, etc.
† Mullerian (structural) anomalies, uterine leiomyomata, DES in utero exposure, Asherman's syndrome, endometrial polyps, cervicitis, abnormal cervical mucus, etc.

A detailed discussion of the clinical investigation and treatment of the infertile couple is beyond the scope of this book, but a brief summary of conditions associated with infertility, the clinical work up, and current treatment options follows below. An understanding of these concepts will illustrate some of the unique challenges associated with ovulation induction in the lactating woman.

Causative factors which require investigation in the infertile couple are listed in (**Table 2**). The incidence of these disorders may vary substantially between populations and age groups.

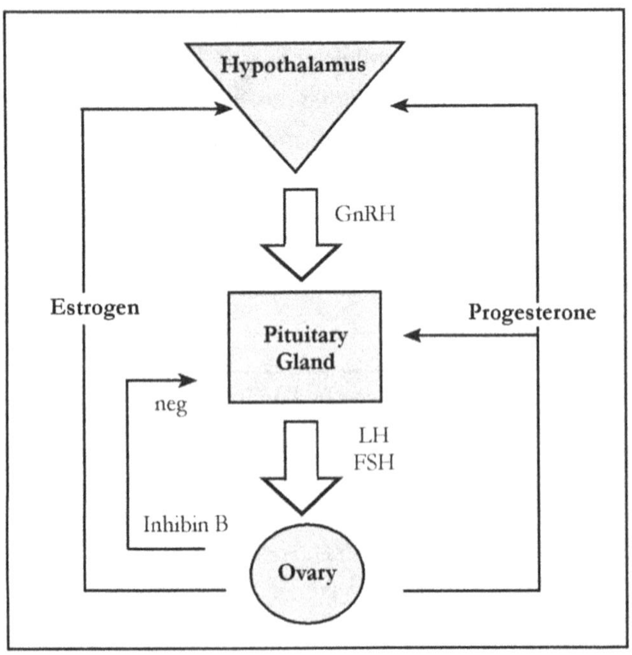

Figure 1. The hypothalamic-pituitary-ovarian (HPO) axis and major feedback loops. (GnRH = gonadotropins releasing hormone, LH = luteinizing hormone, FSH = follicles stimulating hormone.)

Ovulatory dysfunction

Depending on the population studied, 15-40% of those undergoing infertility investigation present with the absence of regular and cyclic menses, indicative of a disruption in the HPO axis (**Figure 1**).

The World Health Organization (WHO) has devised a practical classification for disorders of ovulation which is useful for guiding therapeutic interventions (World Health Organization Scientific Group, 1976). A description of these categories is found in **Table 3**.

Anovulatory women may experience secondary amenorrhea (bleeding episodes >6 months apart), oligomenorrhea (menses >35 and <180 days apart), or polymenorrhea (frequent vaginal bleeding episodes of varying amount and duration). Still others experience "regular" bleeding episodes despite the absence of ovulation. (Obviously, clinical assessment for ovulation is an essential component of the infertility investigation.) The presence of moliminal symptoms —perimenstrual bloating, dysmenorrhea, mastalgia, peripheral edema, mood changes, etc.—before or during vaginal bleeding episodes is suggestive of ovulation earlier in the cycle, and clinical verification by a well timed serum progesterone level is recommended. From a clinical standpoint, qualitative home urinary luteinizing hormone (LH) tests are useful to detect the preovulatory LH surge. False positives and negatives occur but are relatively infrequent, and some of the errors are simply due to misinterpretation by patients (Chiu *et al.*, 1990; McGovern *et al.*, 2004).

The single most common cause of oligomenorrhea and secondary amenorrhea is polycystic ovary syndrome (PCOS) which is found in approximately 70% of women with ovulatory dysfunction. The etiology of the remaining 30% presenting with oligomenorrhea or secondary amenorrhea is scattered among diverse pathologic conditions: hypothalamic amenorrhea (10%), hyperprolactinemia (10%), and premature ovarian failure (10%) (Reindollar & Novak, 1986; Knochenhauer *et al.*, 1998). Exhaustion of the oocyte supply in women over 40 years of age is consistent with menopause (Nelson *et al.*, 2005). Two random elevated FSH levels in the presence of secondary amenorrhea are sufficient to make the diagnosis of menopause. Serum FSH levels are usually higher than LH levels at menopause due to the absence of an inhibin-like feedback inhibition of LH. A more rapid clearance of LH from the circulatory system (about 20 minutes for LH and three to four hours for

Table 3. World Health Organization (WHO) Classification of Ovulatory Disorders

WHO Class	Category	Incidence	Laboratory Findings	Physiologic Conditions Or Disease States	Comments
I	Hypogonadotropic hypogonadism (Hypothalamic-pituitary failure)	5-10%	Low or low normal FSH and LH levels Low estradiol levels Normal prolactin levels	Pre-puberty Kallman's syndrome Isolated gonadotropin deficiency Inadequate caloric intake or malnutrition Anorexia nervosa (but not bulimia nervosa) Stress or exercise induced Head trauma CNS irradiation Chronic diseases (including HIV)	Variety of presentations. Potential remedies include weight gain, treatment of underlying disease state, pulsatile GnRH, or injectable gonadotropins. Anti-estrogens (*i.e.*, clomiphene citrate) inappropriate for ovulation induction.
II	Normogonadotropic normogonadism (Hypothalamic-pituitary dysfunction)	80-85%	Normal FSH and estradiol levels Normal or elevated LH levels	Hypothalamic-pituitary dysfunction Polycystic ovary syndrome (PCOS)	May present with secondary amenorrhea, oligomenorrhea, or abnormal uterine bleeding. Variety of treatments available: injectable gonadotropins, anti-estrogens, aromatase inhibitors, corticosteroids, metformin (PCOS only).
III	Hypergonadotropic hypogonadism (Ovarian failure)	10-30%	Elevated LH and FSH Low estradiol levels	Premature ovarian failure (POF) Perimenopause and menopause	Usually present with amenorrhea. Unresponsive to ovulation induction protocols. Candidates for donor oocytes (with *in vitro* fertilization).

NB: Diseases or conditions associated with hyperprolactinemia (including human lactation) do not easily fit into this classification system. Manifestations will vary from secondary amenorrhea with low FSH, LH, and estradiol levels (Class I) to dysfunctional uterine bleeding with relatively normal gonadotropins and estradiol concentrations (Class II). Source: WHO Scientific Group, 1976.

Table 4. Rotterdam ESHRE/ASRM diagnostic criteria for PCOS

Two of three criteria must be met:

1. Oligo- or anovulation
   - Menses ≥ 35 days apart
2. Clinical and/or biochemical signs of hyperandrogenism
   - Hirsutism, acne, seborrhea, or frank virilization
   - Elevations of total or free testosterone, free androgen index, androstenedione, or dihydroepiandrosterone sulfate (DHEAS)
3. Polycystic ovaries by ultrasound
   - Twelve or more follicles between 2 and 9 mm on either ovary [or] ovarian volume > 10 mL

NB: Other etiologies of androgen excess (Cushing's syndrome, congenital adrenal hyperplasia, androgen-secreting tumors, etc.) must be excluded. Source: Rotterdam ESHRE/ASRM-Sponsored PCOS Consensus Committee, 2004.

FSH) is another contributing factor) (Speroff & Fritz, 2005).

A long-awaited international consensus conference was convened in Rotterdam in 2003, and participants formulated criteria for the diagnosis of PCOS (**Table 4**) (Rotterdam ESHRE/ASRM-Sponsored PCOS Consensus Committe, 2004).

Contrary to Irving Stein and Michael Leventhal's original description of the syndrome now known as PCOS (Stein & Levinthal, 1935), the presence of obesity and infertility are not part of the contemporary Rotterdam diagnostic criteria.

In the past, a multicystic ovarian appearance (**Figure 2**) has not been included in the diagnostic criteria used by most American studies of PCOS, but was commonly used in Europe (Kauffman & Kauffman, 2003). The Rotterdam consensus statement has attempted to bridge this disagreement, but the Rotterdam consensus definition is not without its critics (Carmina, 2004).

The most commonly utilized drug for ovulation induction in the U.S. for women with normogonadotropic ovulatory dysfunction (WHO Class II) is the selective estrogen receptor modulator, clomiphene citrate, which is technically a racemic mixture of zuclomiphene and enclomiphene (Ernst *et al.*, 1976). A related anti-estrogenic drug, tamoxifen, is used with greater frequency outside of the United States, but no pharmaceutical company has pursued FDA approval for this indication in the U.S. Clomiphene citrate and tamoxifen inhibit the negative feedback action of circulating estradiol at the hypothalamus, and in response, hypothalamic GnRH secretion is enhanced (a more detailed explanation is offered later in this chapter). Clomiphene and tamoxifen are equally successful in inducing ovulation and generate similar pregnancy rates (Steiner *et al.*, 2005; Beck *et al.*, 2005). The aromatase inhibitor, letrozole, may be a better choice for ovulation induction in women with PCOS. Letrozole has produced comparable pregnancy rates to clomiphene citrate, but has been associated with a reduced risk of multiple gestation (Mitwally *et al.*, 2005). The shorter half-life of letrozole (2 days vs. 5 days for clomiphene) may be another advantage since putative clomiphene associated anti-estrogenic effects at the cervix and endometrium would be unlikely with letrozole (Fatemi *et al.*, 2003). Neither letrozole nor another aromatase inhibitor, anastrozole, has undergone the FDA approval process as ovulatory agents. Because of their primary use as chemotherapeutic agents for breast cancer, it is unlikely that the manufacturers will consider the FDA application process to be a financially prudent decision.

Metformin, an oral biguanide insulin sensitizing agent, may re-establish ovulation in approximately 20% of those with PCOS. When combined with

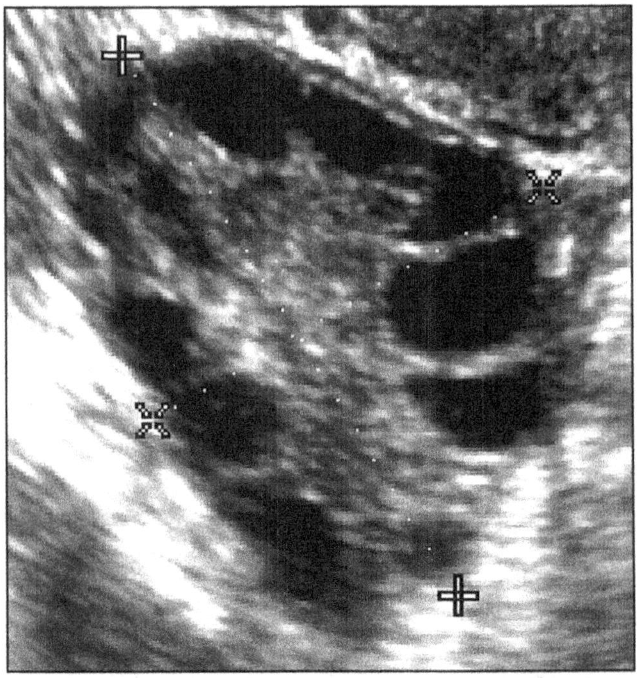

Figure 2. Typical ultrasonographic appearance of a polycystic ovary (one of three diagnostic criteria for PCOS). Note peripheral distribution of follicles. Ultrasound image courtesy of the author.

clomiphene citrate, ovulation rates are even higher than when metformin or clomiphene citrate are used alone (Homburg, 2003). Metformin increases insulin receptor sensitivity at the liver, adipocytes, and skeletal muscle leading to lower circulating insulin levels (via decreased pancreatic β-cell insulin production). Excessive circulating serum insulin levels stimulate ovarian theca cells to produce testosterone in excess (Kauffman & Kauffman, 2003; Pugeat *et al.*, 2000).

Metformin also acts as a direct inhibitor of 17α-hydroxylase activity necessary for the production of testosterone precursors. Testosterone is converted to estradiol by the enzyme aromatase (Lord *et al.*, 2003). This pharmacologic action by metformin explains the drug's success in restoring ovulation in PCOS patients who do not demonstrate insulin resistance by homeostatic or minimal model analyses (Checa *et al.*, 2005). The endocrine pathways for testosterone and estradiol production are illustrated in **Figure 3.**

The PPAR-γ agonists (thiazolidinediones), pioglitazone and rosiglitazone, which also increase insulin receptor site sensitivity, are promising alternatives to metformin in hyperinsulinemic women with PCOS. Unlike metformin, weight gain can be problematic with these agents, but pioglitazone and rosiglitazone tend to cause few gastrointestinal side-effects (Lord *et al.*, 2003; Stout & Fugate, 2005). The thiazolidinediones neither inhibit 17α-hydroxylase enzymatic activity nor inhibit carbohydrate uptake from the GI tract. In obese women with PCOS, weight loss remains the mainstay of therapy. Even five to ten percent weight loss tends to improve insulin sensitivity and responses to medical therapy (Kauffman & Kauffman, 2003).

In PCOS cases refractory to oral antiestrogens and insulin sensitizers, exogenous purified urinary or recombinant FSH (with or without LH) administration have produced high ovulation rates. Gonadotropin therapy is more expensive than oral pro-ovulatory agents, requires more comprehensive monitoring, and is associated with a higher multiple pregnancy rate. Perhaps the greatest potential risk to the patient during gonadotropin stimulation is the development of ovarian

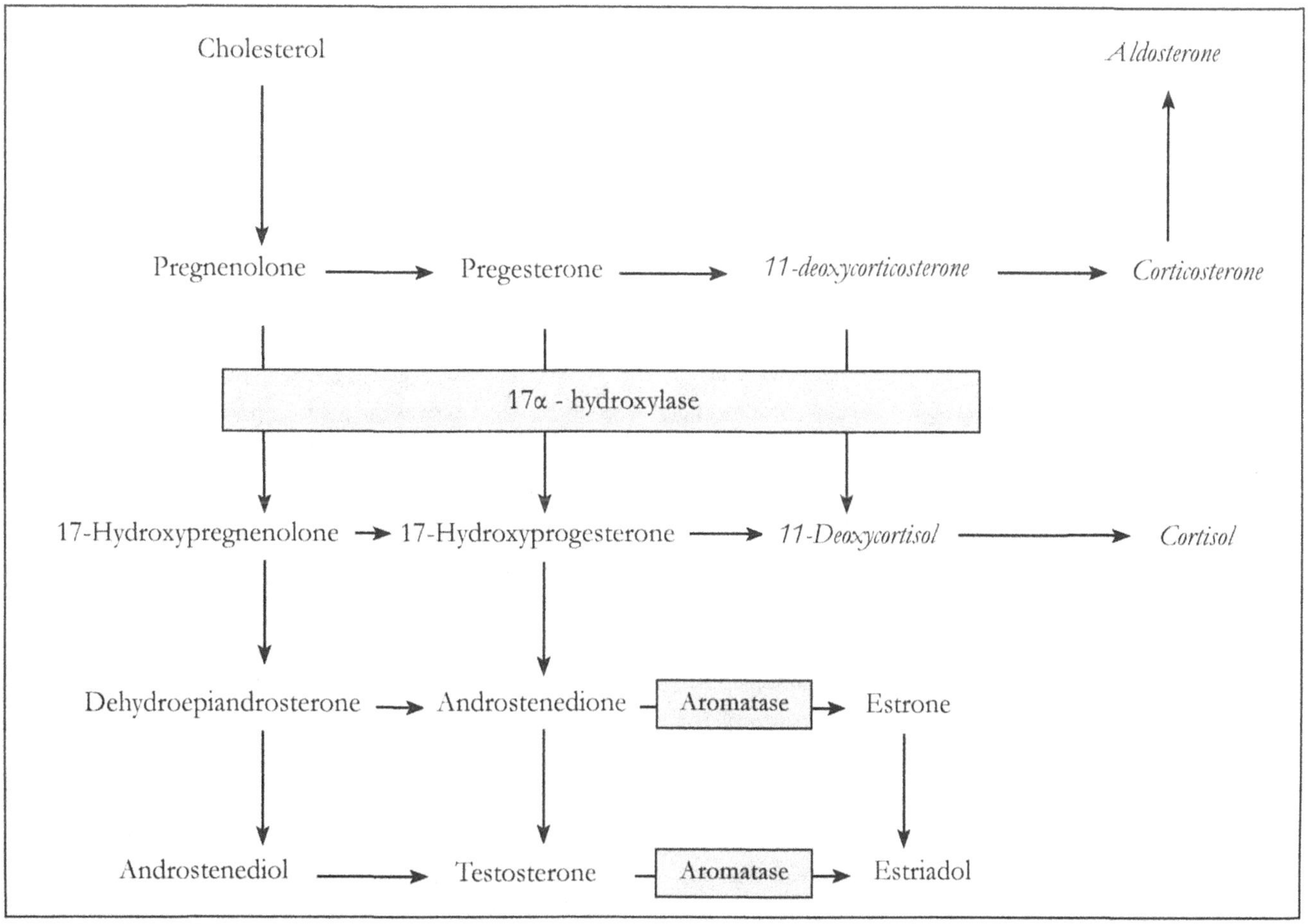

Figure 3. Adrenal and gonadal steroidogenic pathways with localization of the enzymes 17-hydroxyprogesterone and aromatase. Italicized substances are produced solely by the adrenal gland.

hyperstimulation syndrome (OHSS) which, in serious cases, may require hospital admission. Fortunately, severe OHSS is relatively rare (Delvigne & Rozenberg, 2002). Laparoscopic bilateral ovarian diathermy (Laser or electrosurgical drilling of ten or more "windows" into the ovarian cortex) is another viable option in refractory cases and is associated with fewer multiple births than clomiphene citrate and gonadotropin therapy (Farquhar *et al.*, 2005).

Primary hypothyroidism is a relatively uncommon cause of abnormal uterine bleeding, particularly in asymptomatic women. A Finnish study detected elevated thyroid stimulating hormone (TSH) concentrations in only 6.3% of a group of infertile women with ovulatory dysfunction (Arojoki *et al.*, 2000). Pituitary production of TSH and prolactin is regulated by hypothalamic release of thyrotropin releasing factor (TRF), and hence, excess secretion of TRF can trigger rises in pituitary prolactin production. Serum prolactin levels are usually <50 ng/mL in most cases (Roberts & Landenson, 2004; Kleinberg *et al.*, 1977). In patients with primary hypothyroidism, physiologic thyroid hormone replacement usually restores hypothalamic release of TRF to normal levels, and prolactin production returns to baseline levels if no other pathophysiologic process is present (Meier *et al.*, 2003).

In non-pregnant women, excess prolactin production disrupts the normal pulsatile hypothalamic secretion of GnRH, which, in turn, disturbs the normal process of follicular maturation and release. The differential diagnosis of hyperprolactinemia should consider pituitary adenomas, primary hypothyroidism, and use of antidopaminergic drugs including metoclopramide, domperidone, tricyclic antidepressants, and major tranquilizers (particularly the phenothiazines, thioxanthenes, and butyrophenones) (Grubb *et al.*, 1987; Gsponer *et al.*, 1999; Biller *et al.*, 1999; Massara *et al.*, 1981; Ferrari *et al.*, 1983). Other established causes are listed in **Table 5**.

The dopamine (D2) receptor agonists, bromocriptine and cabergoline, are considered first line treatment for most benign prolactin-secreting pituitary adenomas. Bromocriptine and cabergoline bind to D2 receptors of normal and tumor cells alike (Ivan *et al.*, 2005). Dopamine originating from the arcuate nucleus directly inhibits prolactin secretion thereby allowing physiologic secretion of hypothalamic GnRH to resume (Verhelst *et al.*, 1999; Weil, 1986). Approximately 80% with pituitary adenomas will ovulate with dopamine receptor agonists, and treatment should be discontinued upon the diagnosis of pregnancy in the majority of cases (Weil, 1986). A neurosurgical approach is usually unnecessary for the primary treatment of most microadenomas, but has a place in the treatment of large tumors (microadenomas) and those unresponsive to medical therapy (Liu & Couldwell, 2004).

Whether or not luteal phase deficiency (insufficiency) represents a true pathologic entity in female infertility is arguable (Bukulmex & Arici, 2004). A luteal phase deficiency is usually assumed when late luteal phase endometrial histologic dating lags greater than two days behind chronological dating (Murray *et al.*, 2004). Unfortunately, considerable intra- and inter-examiner variability exists amongst experienced gynecologic pathologists performing histologic endometrial dating. Furthermore, the accuracy of the Noyes criteria, the "gold standard" for endometrial dating for more than 50 years, has been challenged (Murray *et al.*, 2004; Coutifaris *et al.*, 2004; Noyes *et al.*, 1950). The existence of luteal phase deficiency as a diagnostic entity has been further eroded by the finding of a greater than two day difference in endometrial maturation in up to 50% of normal fertile women (Bukulmez & Arici, 2004; Coutifaris *et al.*, 2004; Davis *et al.*, 1989; Balasch *et al.*, 1992). Elevations of serum progesterone at 7 days post-ovulation is a sensitive marker of ovulation, but is unable to predict endometrial histology (Bukulmez & Arici, 2004).

Women undergoing GnRH downregulation during an IVF cycle represent an exception to this discussion; GnRH agonist and antagonist therapy may create a luteal phase deficiency (by suppressing postovulatory secretion of gonadotropins), and luteal phase administration of exogenous progesterone improves pregnancy rates in these women (Pritts & Atwood, 2002).

Hypogonadotropic hypogonadism (hypothalamic anovulation) is most commonly encountered in thin women with body mass indices <20 kg/m^2 and in those with anorexia nervosa, Kallman's Syndrome, intensive exercising, and caloric malnutrition. (Other conditions are listed in **Table 3**. When applicable, treatment of the underlying disorder (i.e., modification of exercise, psychotherapy for anorexia nervosa, etc.) is the management of choice, but administration of exogenous

Table 5. Known Etiologies of Hyperprolactinemia

Physiologic
• Pregnancy
• Lactation
• Stress
• Exercise
• Nipple stimulation
Pharmacologic
• Dopamine receptor antagonists (phenothiazines, metoclopramide, domperidone, major tranquilizers)
• Dopamine-depleting agents (α-methyldopa, reserpine)
• Estrogens and anti-androgenic agents (oral contraception pills)
• Opiates
• Tri-cyclic antidepressants
• Selective serotonin reuptake inhibitors
• H_2 antagonists (cimetidine, ranitidine)
Pathologic
• Pituitary tumors
• Hypothalamic and pituitary stalk diseases (sarcoidosis, cranyopharygiomas, empty sella syndrome, lymphocytic hypothesitis, metastatic carcinomas, etc.)
• Primary hypothyroidism
• CNS irradiation
• Chronic renal failure
• Cirrhosis
• Chest wall trauma (including surgery and herpes zoster)
• Seizure disorders
• Polycystic ovary syndrome

gonadotropins may be successful in inducing ovulation in selected cases of Kallman's syndrome and idiopathic hypogonadotropic hypogonadism (Shoham *et al.*, 1991). Exogenous GnRH (gonadorelin) administration is also another effective therapy, but the need for periodic administration by a pump device (similar to an insulin pump) has diminished patient and physician enthusiasm for this modality (Malo *et al.*, 1985; Aharoni *et al.*, 1989). Administration of gonadorelin will be discussed in greater detail later in this chapter.

The diagnosis of premature ovarian failure (POF) is made when estrogen deficiency symptoms and amenorrhea are associated with hypergonadotropic hypogonadism before the age of 40 in the absence of surgical bilateral oophorectomy, ootoxic chemotherapy, or radiotherapy (Nelson *et al.*, 2005; Kauffman & Castracane, 2003; van Kasteren & Schoemaker, 1999). The etiology of the majority of POF cases remains obscure, but infectious, genetic, cytogenetic, and autoimmune causes have been described (van Kasteren & Schoemaker, 1999). Autoantibodies to the thyroid and adrenal glands should be assayed when an ovarian autoimmune process is suspected or confirmed (Nelson *et al.*, 2005; Kauffman & Castracane, 2003). Turner syndrome and a premutation of the FMR1 gene (Fragile X syndrome) have also been linked to POF (Nelson *et al.*, 2005; Kauffman & Castracane, 2003; Bakalov *et al.*, 2005).

Referral to a reproductive endocrinologist is highly recommended when POF is suspected or encountered. In approximately five to ten percent of reported cases, spontaneous pregnancies have occurred following the diagnosis, suggesting that oocyte destruction may not always be complete (Nelson *et al.*, 2005; van Kasteren & Schoemaker, 1999). In most documented cases, IVF using a donated oocyte is the only viable option left for women with POF short of adoption.

Tuboperitoneal Factors

Sexually transmitted diseases (particularly *Chlamydia trachomatis*), adhesive disease secondary to prior abdominopelvic surgery, and endometriosis are established risk factors for impaired tubal motility and obstruction. The presence of serum *Chlamydia trachomatis* IgG antibodies is highly associated with tubal pathology (tubal adhesions and/or obstruction), and the absence these antibodies greatly diminishes the likelihood of inflammatory tubal pathology (Land *et al.*, 2003). Hysterosalpingography (HSG) remains the primary diagnostic modality for tubal obstruction, and abnormalities by HSG should be verified by hysteroscopy and laparoscopy in most instances (Swart *et al.*, 1995).

Tubal adhesions and distal occlusions may be amenable to surgical treatment by a competent reproductive surgeon. A laparoscopic approach is generally preferred, but the final decision should rest with the surgeon's judgment and experience. Although proximal fallopian tube obstruction may be treatable by selective salpingography and tubal catheterization in experienced hands, IVF remains the most successful treatment option for those with surgically uncorrectable conditions or prior surgical failures (ESHRE Capri Workshop Group, 2004). Contrary to conventional wisdom, HSG is infrequently associated with a "fertility enhancing effect" (Johnson *et al.*, 2005).

Endometriosis

Endometriosis is characterized by the presence of functioning endometrial tissue outside the confines of the endometrial cavity. Although the presence of endometriosis can be suspected on a clinical basis, the definitive diagnosis is made by laparoscopy or laparotomy with histologic confirmation by surgical excision or biopsy (Farquhar, 2000). A puckered blue-gray lesion (**Figure 4**) is the typical gross appearance of an endometriosis lesion, but endometriosis implants may also be red, white, or clear in appearance (Donnez *et al.*, 2003). A unique serological marker for endometriosis has yet to be identified.

The presence of endometriosis has been reported in 20-50% of infertile women (a higher incidence than in women with proven fertility), but the specific pathophysiologic role played by endometriosis is not fully understood (ESHRE Capri Workshop Group, 2004; Farquhar, 2000; Schlindler, 2004; Mahmood & Templeton, 1991). Many women with documented endometriosis conceive without further treatment. Endometriosis-related pelvic adhesions and scarring may impair tubal motility and occlude the distal portion of the fallopian tube. Endometriosis of the cornuo-isthmic portion of the fallopian tube can mechanically obstruct the tubal lumen (Speilvogel *et al.*, 2000). Myometrial and tubal dysperistalsis secondary to release of inflammatory cytokines by endometriosis implants have also been implicated to play a role in infertility. Endometrial implantation of the blastocyst appears to be interrupted in some women with co-existing endometriosis, possibly due to pro-inflammatory cytokine production by endometriosis (ESHRE Capri Workshop Group, 2001; Halis & Arici, 2004).

Medical therapy with GnRH analogs (leuprolide, naferelin, and goserelin) without surgical excision or obliteration of endometriosis lesions does not appear to increase pregnancy rates in subfertile women, although an improvement in pain associated with endometriosis is common (Fedele *et al.*, 1992). Surgical excision of all visible implants and adhesions by laparoscopy improves pregnancy rates, although not to normal levels (Marcoux *et al.*, 1997). IVF is indicated when other treatment modalities have been exhausted.

Utero-Cervical Factors

Diseases of the uterus and cervix are relatively uncommon causes of human infertility, accounting for less than five percent in most case series. The finding of a uterine anomaly on evaluation, per se, does not necessitate surgical treatment since many women with uterine anomalies will conceive and deliver without difficulty.

Studies of IVF failures in women with transmural and submucosal leiomyomata have demonstrated that distortion of the uterine cavity by leiomyomata may cause endometrial implantation failure (Rice *et al.*, 1989; Berkovitz *et al.*, 1999; Farhi *et al*, 1995). Surgical removal of leiomyomata may increase fertility rates by 40-60%, but surgical intervention may also create pelvic tubal adhesions. Adhesions can be minimized by careful surgical technique, minimizing tissue trauma, and use of anti-adhesion surgical barrier materials (Sudik *et al*, 1996; Stovall *et al.*, 1998; Surrey *et al.*, 2005). Hysteroscopic resection is the preferred surgical modality for submucosal leiomyomata while an abdominal approach is usually selected for intramural myomas. Laparoscopic myomectomy can be performed by skilled laparoscopic surgeons, but the risk of uterine rupture during a subsequent pregnancy may be higher than with the multilayer closure techniques used with open approaches (Advincula & Song, 2005). Following surgery, new myomas may develop, and women with multiple myomas and an enlarged uterus at the time of the original surgery appear to have the greatest risk (Hanafi, 2005).

Presence of an avascular uterine septum is the most common congenital mullerian anomaly associated with

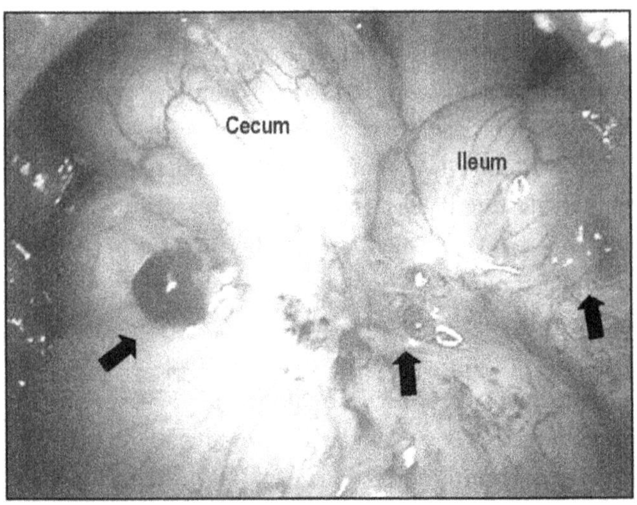

Figure 4. Endometriosis at the ileocecal junction. Note dark lesions with local scarring and secondary puckering (see arrows). The appendix is not visible in this photograph. Photograph courtesy of the author.

infertility and recurrent pregnancy loss. Fortunately, the midline septum is amenable to outpatient hysteroscopic resection. Fertility rates are improved and pregnancy losses diminished with successful surgical excision (Heinonen, 1982; March & Israel, 1987). A hysteroscopic approach is also ideal for excision of endometrial polyps and intrauterine synechiae (adhesions).

Diethylstilbesterol (DES), an estrogen analog, was widely prescribed in the 1950's and 1960's as a "preventive" measure against spontaneous abortion (Rheingold, 1976). At least four million women were exposed in utero prior to the FDA advisory issued in 1971 (Herbst, 1981). A substantial number of these women (as high as 43% in one series) developed structural uterine and fallopian tube abnormalities, clearly establishing DES as a known teratogen (Senekjian *et al.*, 1988). Women exposed to DES in utero are also at risk for clear cell adenocarcinoma of the cervix and vagina, although the risk is only about 0.1% (Herbst *et al.*, 1977). The classical radiographic appearance of a DES exposed uterus is found in **Figure 5.** IVF has yielded limited successes in those with DES associated structural abnormalities. Surgical procedures designed to "expand" the small uterine cavity characteristic of DES exposure are mentioned only to be condemned (Aubriot *et al.*, 2001). Because antenatal administration of DES essentially ceased in 1971, DES-related infertility should become a historical footnote in the near future.

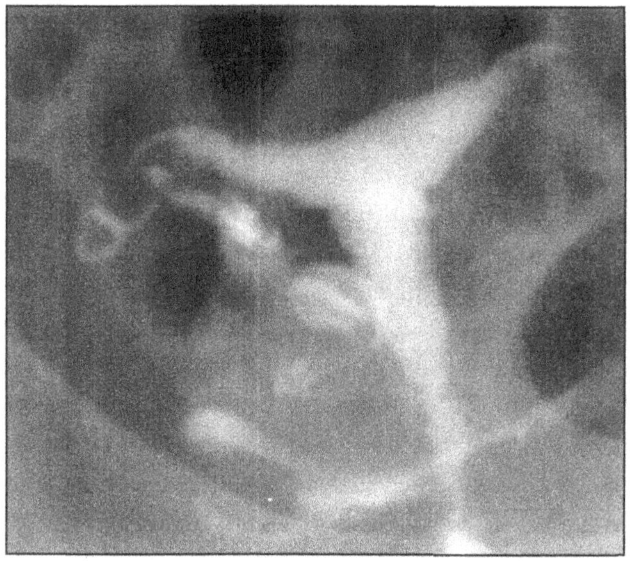

Figure 5. Hysterosalpingogram (HSG) performed on a 35 year old infertile female exposed to DES in utero. Note the abnormal uterine "T" shape, dilation of the tubal cornua, irregular endometrial borders, long cervix, and distal tubal (fimbrial) phimosis ("rosebud" appearance). X-ray courtesy of the author.

Conservative treatments for cervical dysplasia (cone biopsy, loop excision procedures, and cryosurgery) excise or destroy many of the endocervical glands responsible for the production of cervical mucus. Cervical stenosis is another known complication of these procedures. Enthusiasm for the postcoital test (PCT) as a useful assessment of midcycle cervical mucus-sperm interaction has diminished over the past decade, primarily due to a lack of consensus on the definition of an abnormal study. Also, the abnormal PCT seems to poorly predict impaired fertility (Grimes & Schulz, 2005). Exogenous estrogen administration in the late follicular phase to enhance cervical mucus production has failed to demonstrate a benefit on pregnancy rates (Bateman *et al.*, 1990). The potential value of the mucolytic drug, guaifenesin, on thickened cervical mucus requires study under more rigorous conditions before an evidence-based recommendation can be made (Check *et al.*, 1982). At the present time, washed intrauterine insemination (IUI) is the preferred treatment for women with cervical mucus abnormalities, although the efficacy of this procedure remains to be verified by prospective, adequately powered trials (te Velde *et al.*, 1989; Helmerhorst *et al.*, 2005).

Male Factor Infertility

Since an abnormal male factor may be found in 30-40% of infertile couples (Guttmacher, 1956; Baker, 1994; World Health Organization, 1987), evaluation of the male partner is an essential element of the clinical investigation.

Counseling the male partner to substitute boxer shorts for briefs has no scientifically proven benefit and only tends to delay appropriate investigation (Munkelwitz & Gilbert, 1998). The potential for dietary supplements to diminish seminal levels of reactive oxidative species has merit, but until the exact nature of the defect is identified in the laboratory, such treatments should be considered entirely empiric (Agarwal & Said, 2005).

In addition to a history and physical examination of the male partner, a semen analysis should be submitted to a qualified andrology laboratory rather than a community based clinical lab since quality assurance has been problematic in the latter (Keel, 2004). A one to three day abstinence period (and no greater than ten days) is preferable before a semen specimen is submitted (Levitas *et al.*, 2005). An abnormal semen analysis should always be repeated after a six week (or more) hiatus since many semen parameters may vary considerably from day to day (Keel, 2006). An endocrine evaluation (LH, FSH, total testosterone, and prolactin) and analysis of the Y-chromosome for micro-deletions may yield vital information when the semen analysis is consistently subnormal (ESHRE Capri Workshop Group, 2004; Marmar, 2001). Referral to a specialist with expertise in the diagnosis and treatment of the subfertile male is recommended in difficult cases.

A history of undescended testes (cryptorchidism) and varicocele are the most commonly encountered conditions associated with an abnormal semen analysis. At the present time, a clear-cut etiology for male subfertility is evasive in over 50% of all cases (ESHRE Capri Workshop Group, 2004; Dohl *et al.*, 2002).

Known and suspected causes of male factor subfertility are listed in **Table 6**.

An abnormal semen analysis is not synonymous with male subfertility since many of these men demonstrate little or no difficulty fathering a child. The converse of this statement is also true (Nikolettos *et al.*, 1999).

Treatment of the subfertile male is generally based on the underlying etiology (if known). Surgical repair of the varicocele is commonly associated with improved semen parameters, but unfortunately, varicocelectomy appears to have little or no effect on pregnancy rates despite improvement in semen parameters (Evers & Collins, 2004; Evers & Collins, 2003; Nabi *et al.*, 2004). For the large number of males with an abnormal semen analysis without an established explanation following comprehensive investigation, intrauterine insemination (IUI) or in vitro fertilization with intracytoplasmic sperm injection (ICSI) should be considered (Crosignani *et al.*, 1993; Dohle *et al.*, 1998). Donor insemination is another effective option which should be presented in the discussion of male factor infertility (McLaughlin, 2002).

Unexplained infertility

The fact that up to 25% of infertile couples have no apparent etiology to explain their condition or fail to conceive with conventional treatments (including IVF) indicates a critical need to fill several gaps in the current knowledge base. Disorders of endometrial implantation and neo-angiogenesis may explain some hereunto unexplained cases (Horcajades *et al.*, 2004; Minas *et al.*, 2005). Unfortunately, many conditions commonly associated with infertility (low grade endometriosis, pelvic adhesions, varicocele, etc.) may simply represent incidental findings.

When no etiology can be found, treatments are mostly empiric. A stair-step approach may be offered, although good clinical trial data to support some of the empiric treatment options are either lacking or inconclusive (Balasch, 2004; Cantineau *et al.*, 2004; Practice Committee of the American Society for Reproductive Medicine, 2004, Isaksson & Tiitinen, 2004). Gonadotropin administration with IUI (up to four cycles) has been proven effective in cases of endometriosis, cervical factor, and unknown infertility

Table 6. Established Causes of Male Factor Subfertility

Condition	Incidence (%)	% Associated with a Genetic Anomaly
Cryptorchidism	13.3	21.7
Varicocele	10	20
Congenital absence of the vas deferens (CAVD)	4	66.6
Genital infections	5.3	0
Endocrinopathies	2	0
Chronic diseases	2.6	0
Malignancy	1.3	0
Prior inguinal or scrotal surgery	2.6	0
Unexplained	56.6	31.7

Adapted from Dohle *et al.*, 2002.

(Dodson & Haney, 1991; Guzick *et al.*, 1998). A treatment algorithm for couples with infertility of unknown origin or who have failed evidence-based treatments is presented in **Figure 6.**

At some point, a discussion of medical futility is inevitable in selected cases. Adoption should be one of the treatment options presented to all prospective parents. In addition, psychological support should be incorporated into any comprehensive infertility treatment plan.

PHYSIOLOGY OF POSTPARTUM AND LACTATION INDUCED AMENORRHEA

A complex network of central and peripheral hormone signaling mechanisms and neural connections governs the hypothalamic-pituitary-ovarian axis. Dramatic changes in this system characterize the transition from the non-pregnant state to pregnancy and lactation.

Suckling, Prolactin, and Gonadotropin Suppression

Prolactin pays a crucial role in mammary gland development during pregnancy, milk production during lactation, and in neurohypotheseal release of oxytocin (a nanopeptide essential for milk letdown) (Speroff & Fritz, 2005; Andrews, 2005; Parker *et al.*, 1991). Prolactin production and secretion is under a short inhibition feedback loop between the hypothalamic arcuate nucleus and pituitary lactotrophs. When dopamine binds at lactotrophic receptors in the anterior pituitary gland, prolactin release is tonically inhibited (Andrews, 2005; Li, 2005). Opioid peptides binding at *mu* and *kappa* opioid receptors appear to downregulate dopamine inhibition of prolactin production in late pregnancy and during lactation (Arobogast & Voogt, 1998; Selmanoff & Gregerson, 1986).

Infant suckling initiates a series of neuroendocrine events. Suckling elicits the secretion of one or more prolactin releasing factors (PRF) via spinal afferents from the nipple to the hypothalamic paraventricular nucleus. There are several PRF candidates, most notably TRF, vasoactive intestinal polypeptide (VIP), and oxytocin (Cone *et al.*, 2003). One or more PRF's enter the portal-hypophyseal circulation prompting prolactin release from the lactotrophs. Suckling also causes oxytocin release from the neurohypothesis, stimulating the myoepithelial ductal cells of the breast (Zarate & Canales, 1987).

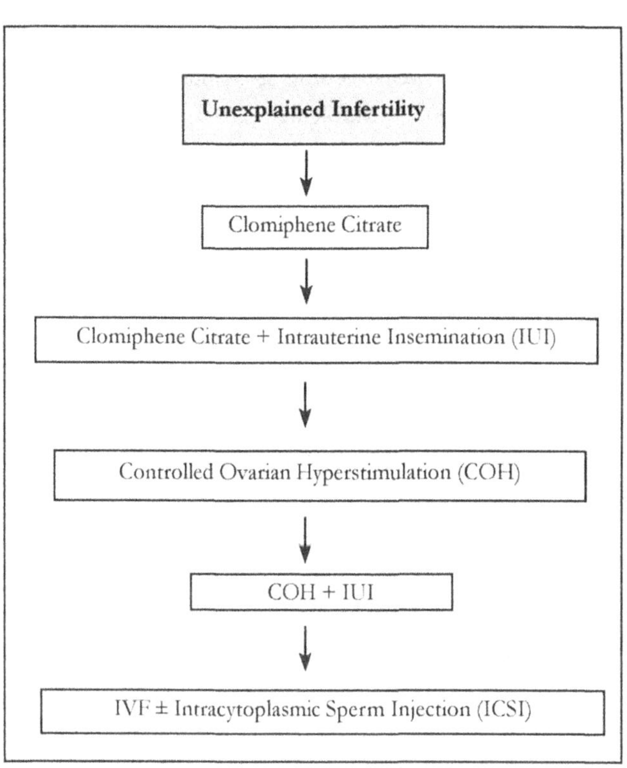

Figure 6. Algorithm for empiric therapy of unexplained infertility (Guzick et al., 1998). Individual protocols should be individualized to patient needs, desires, and resources. Controlled ovarian hyperstimulation (COH) involves use of exogenous gonadotropins. Tamoxifen and letrozole can be substituted for clomiphene citrate.

Finally, suckling sustains relative GnRH suppression via afferent neural connections from the breast to the spinal cord, finally terminating in the hypothalamus. The precise mechanism of action is unknown, but it appears to be independent of circulating prolactin concentrations (Tay *et al.*, 1996; McNeilly, 2001).

Baseline serum prolactin levels are elevated in term pregnant women (200-400 ng/mL), decline in the newly postpartum (to approximately 100 ng/mL), and gradually diminish over the ensuing weeks (to the 40-50 ng/mL range) even in the presence of frequent newborn suckling (Tyson *et al.*, 1972). Suckling induces transient elevations in prolactin release above baseline levels. In the first few weeks, the response is ten to twenty-fold over baseline, falling to a two-fold rise with extended breastfeeding (Stern *et al.*, 1986; Battin *et al.*, 1985). By implication, high prolactin levels appear to be necessary for the initiation of lactation, but lower concentrations can maintain the neuroendocrine and enzymatic systems crucial for lactation maintenance.

The frequency and duration of suckling appears to be the primary factor regulating lactational amenorrhea and continues to play a pivotal role in HPO axis regulation until breastfeeding is limited or terminated (McNeilley, 2003; McNeilly, 2001; Short, 1993). Prolactin appears to have little effect, if any, on GnRH regulation. Women who remain amenorrheic for long durations during exclusive lactation tend to exhibit higher mean circulating prolactin levels than those who experience shorter durations of amenorrhea (Diaz *et al.*, 1989; Diaz *et al.*, 1991), but this observation is probably a reflection of the strength of suckling (McNeilly, 2001). Tay and colleagues found no relationship between 24 hour prolactin concentrations and the duration of amenorrhea (Tay *et al.*, 1996).

Elevated prolactin concentrations inhibit the positive feedback action of estradiol on the HPO axis, preventing the pre-ovulatory LH surge (Diaz *et al.*, 1995; Zinaman *et al.*, 1995; McNatty *et al.*, 1974; Liu & Park, 198; Baird *et al.*, 1979). Prolactin also works peripherally by interfering with corpus luteal production of progesterone, and hence, a transient luteal phase deficiency during the first one or two ovulatory cycles is not uncommon (McNeilly, 2003; Speroff & Fritz, 2005; Diaz *et al.*, 1992).

Hyperprolactinemia cannot explain lactational amenorrhea in its entirety since ovarian suppression may persist well beyond normalization of serum prolactin levels in breastfeeding mothers (Diaz *et al.*, 1991). As previously stated, intense suckling blunts (but does not totally inhibit) hypothalamic secretion of GnRH, an action independent of prolactin (McNeilly, 2001; Zinaman *et al.*, 1995; McNeilly *et al.*, 1994). Serotonin, dopamine, GABA, β-endorphin, and corticotropin releasing factor are released in response to suckling and serve to further inhibit GnRH production (Cone *et al.*, 2003; Campbell & Gray, 1993). Zinaman and colleagues administered pulsatile GnRH to lactating women experiencing amenorrhea and were able to demonstrate pituitary and ovarian responsiveness resulting in ovulation (similar to the response seen when GnRH is administered to women with prolactin-secreting microadenomas)(Zinaman *et al.*, 1995; Leyendecker *et al.*, 1980; Tay *et al.*, 1993). As the frequency and duration of infant suckling dwindles over time, GnRH pulsatility returns to a physiologic pattern and normal LH production is restored.

Gonadotropin levels are practically non-detectable for the first few days postpartum. The pulsatile release of GnRH is low amplitude and low frequency during active breastfeeding favoring low to normal FSH production and lower levels of LH (Zarate & Canales, 1987; Perheentupa *et al.*, 2000; Tay *et al.*, 1992; Illingworth, 1995; Glasier *et al.*, 1984). Dopamine receptor antagonists (metoclopramide, domperidone, trycyclic antidepressants, traditional antipsychotics, etc.) and endogenous opioids do not consistently increase GnRH production in the early puerperium (Tay *et al.*, 1993; Gabay, 2002).

The hypothalamus is more sensitive to the negative feedback of circulating estradiol during lactation compared to the non-pregnant state, and as a result, relatively low estradiol concentrations inhibit GnRH pulsatility in lactating individuals. In contrast, the anterior pituitary gland remains relatively responsive to GnRH during this time (McNeilly, 2001; Zinaman *et al.*, 1995; Perheentupa *et al.*, 2000; Illingworth, 1995; Glasier & McNeilly, 1986). Despite the fact that LH production is essentially nil in early breastfeeding and remains low during lactational amenorrhea, pituitary FSH remains at low to normal levels, stimulating small follicle production of estradiol (Zarate & Canales, 1987; Perheentupa *et al.*, 2000; Tay *et al.*, 1992; Illingworth, 1995; Glasier *et al.*, 1984). As estradiol production increases, the hypothalamus remains relatively insensitive to positive feedback by estradiol which promotes the pre-ovulatory LH surge. Subsequently, further follicular development (and ovulation) is arrested. This represents the principal mechanism behind lactation induced amenorrhea over extended periods (Perheentupa *et al.*, 2000). Unlike non-lactating women, recent data suggest that dopamine and endogenous opioids do not play a major role in the GnRH regulatory process (Ililngworth, 1995; Tay *et al.*, 1993).

Issues for Bottle-Feeding Mothers

In the newly postpartum women electing to bottle feed, the shortest interval reported from delivery to date of first ovulation is 25 days, but this interval is typically longer, averaging around 45 days. In one small prospective study of non-breastfeeding women, 50% ovulated by the sixth week postpartum (Campbell & Gray, 1993). Administration of dopamine receptor agonists (i.e., bromocriptine and cabergoline) to suppress lactation following delivery accelerates return of ovulation. GnRH secretory patterns may normalize in fewer than two weeks, particularly if dopamine agonist therapy is initiated immediately after parturition (Kremer *et al.*, 1989; Haartsen *et al.*, 1992).

In the absence of dopamine agonist administration, pulsatile production of GnRH usually normalizes somewhere between three and eight weeks, corresponding with the return of serum prolactin to pre-pregnancy levels (McNeilly, 2001; Gray *et al.*, 1987). Campbell and Gray observed ovulation in 100% of non-breastfeeding mothers by 12 weeks following childbirth (**Figure 7**) (Campbell & Gray, 1993). Initiation of supplemental feedings accelerates the return of spontaneous ovulation (Diaz *et al.*, 1991).

Women intermittently breastfeeding or who bottle feed only should be offered contraceptive counseling no later than the third postpartum week (Speroff & Fritz, 2005). Logically, contraceptive education should be offered while in the hospital or delivery setting.

Issues for Breastfeeding Mothers

Natural restoration of ovulatory menses in breastfeeding women can be hastened by four mechanisms: (a) voluntary weaning, (b) newborn death (abrupt or involuntary weaning), (c) introduction of oral feedings, and (d) restoration of a positive nutrition and energy balance (McNeilly, 1997; Ellison, 2003; Jones & Palloni, 1994; Smith & Grover, 2002; Valeggia & Ellison, 2004; Delvoye *et al.*, 1978; Konner & Worthman, 1980; Ford & Huffman, 1988; Gross *et al.*, 2002).

Breastfeeding patterns affect the re-emergence of postpartum ovulation (Ellison, 2003; Prema & Ravindranath, 1982; Speroff & Fritz, 2005; McNeilly, 2001; Diaz & Croxatto, 1993). Complete cessation of breastfeeding usually restores normal HPO axis functioning within 30 days.

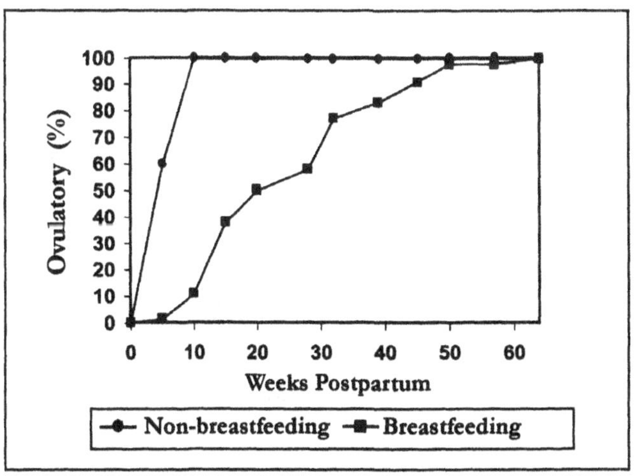

Figure 7. Cumulative ovulation rates in breastfeeding and non-breastfeeding populations (U.S. study). (Reprinted from the American Journal of Obstetrics and Gynecology, volume 169(1), Campbell OM and Gray RH, Characteristics and determinants of postpartum ovarian function in the United States, pp. 55-60, 1993, with permission from Elsevier.)

Exclusive breastfeeding affords total contraceptive benefits for at least the first ten weeks postpartum (Visness *et al.*, 1997), and hence, all breastfeeding women should be offered contraceptive counseling in some form by the tenth postpartum week (Speroff & Fritz, 2005). Mothers who exclusively breastfeed and remain amenorrheic for the first six months postpartum have contraceptive benefits similar to those using combination oral contraceptive pills (Campbell & Gray, 1993; Labbok *et al.*, 1997). A contraceptive success rate as high as 92% has been reported in exclusively breastfeeding women during the first year, although few women in developed countries maintain exclusive breastfeeding (without supplementary feeding) for this length of time. Exclusive long term breastfeeding has been reported to delay return of ovulatory cycles for up to four years (McNeilly, 2001).

Only 40-70% of regularly (but not exclusively) breastfeeding mothers remain amenorrheic for six months, and 0-37% do so until one year (Campbell & Gray, 1993; Gross *et al.*, 2002; Labbok *et al.*, 1997).

Maternal nutritional status, cultural factors, and socio-economic status play lesser, albeit important, roles in the return of ovulation (Rogers, 1997; Truitt *et al.*, 2003; IPPF International Advisory Committee, 1990). In any event, all breastfeeding mothers should be warned that the re-emergence of ovulation is unpredictable.

OVULATION INDUCTION DURING LACTATION: AN OXYMORON?

Prolongation of the interbirth interval afforded by human breastfeeding is an evolutionary benefit shared with most mammals and a reflection of Darwinian selection (Cuthberson, 1999). On occasion, women with lactational amenorrhea may present in the outpatient setting seeking ovulation induction coupled with the desire to continue breastfeeding. (In the author's experience, most are approaching the latter stages of the normal reproductive lifespan.) In the strictest sense, this demand would appear "unnatural," but in the industrialized world, biotechnological advances are negating genetically determined human potential, and perhaps defying normal bioecological safeguards.

This scenario presents the practitioner with several vexing questions. Is the pharmacotherapeutic regimen for ovulation induction safe for the existing infant? Will breastmilk suffer in quantity or quality? Which pro-ovulatory agents are effective and under what circumstances? At present, the answer to these questions is clouded by more uncertainties than unassailable truths

Antiestrogens

Clomiphene citrate is indicated for ovulation induction in women with normogonadotropic anovulation (WHO Class II defect). Since suckling induces a transient spike in prolactin secretion and disruption of GnRH pulsatility (i.e., a hypogonadotropic, hypoestrous milieu similar to the WHO Class I ovulation disorders), administration of conventional antiestrogens, such as clomiphene and tamoxifen, to promote folliculogenesis and LH surge would seem counterintuitive.

The use of clomiphene citrate and tamoxifen in breastfeeding women for induction of ovulation has undergone relatively limited scientific scrutiny. In non-breastfeeding individuals, clomiphene citrate occupies CNS estrogen receptors at a greater affinity than estradiol, and subsequently, the number of hypothalamic intracellular estrogen receptors is reduced. In the absence of negative feedback by estrogen at the hypothalamus, GnRH production is activated (Kerin *et al.*, 1985). Clomiphene also has direct pituitary and ovarian effects, although its primary mode of action is at the hypothalamus (de Moura *et al.*, 1992; Kessel & Hsueh, 1987). Clomiphene does not directly trigger ovulation at the ovary. Unfortunately, clomiphene citrate and other anti-estrogens appear to suppress lactation in newly postpartum women. Clomiphene citrate reduces pituitary prolactin secretion induced by nipple stimulation and, in fact, may be used for therapeutic lactation suppression if administered in doses of 100 mg/day for five days (Masala *et al.*, 1978; Zuckerman & Carmel, 1973; Weinstein *et al.*, 1976; Kalir *et al*,. 1975). Canales *et al.* failed to demonstrate significant suppression of circulation prolactin levels or milk production during and following a seven-day course of clomiphene citrate 100 mg in a series of ten newly postpartum women, but this contrasts with essentially all other published reports (Masala *et al.*, 1978; Zuckerman & Carmel, 1973; Weinstein *et al.*, 1976; Kalir *et al.*, 1975; Canales *et al.*, 1977). Tamoxifen also appears to limit milk production (Masala *et al.*, 1978). Theoretically, antiestrogens may be capable of effecting ovulation in breastfeeding women distant from delivery with relatively normalized GnRH pulsatility, but no randomized clinical trials have been undertaken to study this hypothesis. In addition, the unfavorable consequences on breastmilk production would likely persist.

Aromatase Inhibitors

Letrozole, in contrast to clomiphene citrate and tamoxifen, reduces circulating estradiol levels by inhibition of cytochrome P450 aromatase (**Figure 3**). In murine models, an inhibitory effect on lactation has been found (Luthra *et al.*, 2003), but no published human studies exist to date. The effect of letrozole on the developing infant is unknown (PDR, 2005).

Gonadotropins

Administration of exogenous gonadotropins (FSH or FSH/LH by subcutaneous or intramuscular injection) for ovulation induction in lactating women has not received systematic study, but limited case series has reported successes (and viable pregnancies) (Nakano *et al.*, 1975). Responsiveness to gonadotropin therapy appears to be diminished in mothers with higher circulating prolactin levels (Zarate & Canales, 1987; Zarate *et al.*, 1974). As with non-lactating women receiving gonadotropin therapy, the pre-ovulatory LH surge must be simulated with recombinant LH or human chorionic gonadotropin (hCG) administration (the α-subunits of hCG and LH are identical). Compared to oral antiestrogens, gonadotropin stimulation cycles are relatively expensive due to medication costs, necessity for ultrasound monitoring, and measurement of serial serum estradiol levels. Also, patients must be instructed on drug self-administration by injection since gonadotropin therapy is administered by the subcutaneous or intramuscular route. Multifetal pregnancy is a recognized and undesired complication. Gonadotropins should be prescribed only by physicians who have been specifically trained in their use since serious and even life-threatening side-effects can occur.

Whether lactating women receiving gonadotropin therapy routinely benefit from luteal phase support with intramuscular or intravaginal progesterone is unclear, but since excess prolactin production may diminish progesterone production from the corpus luteum (McNeilly, 1997;Speroff & Fritz, 2005; Diaz *et al.*, 1992), luteal phase support should be strongly considered.

Table 7. Approach to Ovulation Induction in Breastfeeding Women Experiencing Lactational Amenorrhea

- Review prior pregnancies and conception history. Has the patient experienced difficulty conceiving in the past?
- Rule out other causes of infertility (including male factor). History and physical examination should guide this evaluation.
- Baseline assessment of LH, FSH, prolactin, TSH (the first three should be measured on two or more separate occasions.) Prolactin assessments should not be drawn immediately after breastfeeding.
- Patient education: benefits of initiating a weaning schedule.

Pulsatile Gonadotropin Releasing Hormone

In the follicular phase of an ovulatory woman, LH is released preferentially over FSH from the pituitary gland when GnRH pulsatility is frequent and greater in amplitude. Under normal conditions, LH is secreted every 90-120 minutes, diminishing to every three to four hours in the luteal phase. FSH is secreted in smaller amounts and less frequently than LH, but proper synchrony of LH and FSH release is essential for successful follicular development and ovulation (Homburg, 2005; Marshall *et al.*, 2001).

A portable pump device can be programmed to release intravenous or subcutaneous GnRH (gonadorelin) in a physiologic manner. Continuous administration of GnRH by infusion pump will result in anovulation by downregulating pituitary gland GnRH receptors and suppressing FSH and LH release. Essentially, this is the mechanism by which the GnRH analogs leuprolide, naferilin, and buserelin inhibit ovulation and potentiate a hypoestrous environment. When exogenous GnRH is administered in a pulsatile fashion (ordinarily every 60-90 minutes in clinical practice) to women with hypothalamic amenorrhea, follicular maturation and ovulation can occur (Homburg *et al.*, 1989). Amenorrhea associated with Kallman's syndrome, excessive exercise, calorie malnutrition, low body weight (including anorexia nervosa), and idiopathic hypogonadotropic hypogonadism are also responsive to GnRH pump therapy with reported pregnancy rates as high as 80% (Warren & Perlroth, 2001; Homburg *et al.*, 1989; Shoham *et al.*, 1990). Monitoring can be less tedious than with injectable gonadotropins since ovarian hyperstimulation syndrome (OHSS) and multiple follicle release (associated with multiple births) are less common with gonadorelin administration compared to gonadotropin usage; nevertheless, ultrasonographic and serum estradiol monitoring are necessary for dosage adjustment. Widespread use of the GnRH pump has been limited by low patient acceptability of the pump device and the relatively small number of women with hypogonadotropic hypogonadism in the infertile population (Homburg, 2005).

Glasier *et al.* administered pulsatile gonadorelin by pump infusion to four fully lactating women at six weeks postpartum and found follicular development and luteinization in three out of four subjects, but ovum release from the dominant follicle did not occur (Glasier *et al.*, 1986). Another group of investigators demonstrated successful ovulation by using intravenous synthetic GnRH delivered by a controlled infusion in a limited number of breastfeeding women, but it should be noted that ovulation (and not pregnancy) was the primary endpoint of this study (Zinaman *et al.*, 1995). Kastin *et al.* reported a single pregnancy following infusion of porcine GnRH (Kastin *et al.*, 1971). Obviously, clinical experience with GnRH induced ovulation in lactating women is limited.

CONCLUSIONS

Specific recommendations for ovulation induction in the breastfeeding mother experiencing lactational amenorrhea are difficult to formulate due to a scarcity of high quality studies in the peer-reviewed literature. A logical approach to the pre-treatment assessment is listed in **Table 7**.

Gonadotropin administration with FSH/LH or pure FSH has proven effective and represents the most sensible approach. Alternatively, pulsatile GnRH infusion can be considered, although there is considerably less experience with this approach.

Antiestrogens and aromatase inhibitors may generate a sudden drop in milk production and are best avoided. As luteal phase insufficiency may accompany early spontaneous (non-stimulated) ovulatory cycles, luteal phase support with exogenous progesterone makes sense for gonadotropin and gonadorelin stimulated cycles. A "cookbook" approach is discouraged, and treatment should be individualized.

From a biological perspective, exclusively breastfeeding women desiring pregnancy are best served by initiation of a weaning schedule and introduction of supplemental feedings to the infant. Breastfeeding need not be terminated altogether except in refractory cases.

References

Abraham SF, Beumont PJ, Fraser IS, Llewellyn-Jones JD. Body weight, exercise and menstrual status among ballet dancers in training. *BJOG.* 1982; 89:507-10.

Advincula AP, Song A. Endoscopic management of leiomyomata. *Semin Reprod Med.* 2005; 22(2):149-55.

Agarwal A, Said TM. Oxidative stress, DNA damage and apoptosis in male infertility: a clinical approach. *BJU Int.* 2005; 95:503-6.

Aharoni A, Tal J, Paltieli Y, Porat N, Liebowitz Z, Sharf M. Kallmann syndrome: a case of twin pregnancy and review of the literature. *Obstet Gynecol Surv.* 1989; 44(7):491-4.

Andrews ZB. Neuroendocrine regulation of prolactin secretion during late pregnancy: easing the transition into lactation. *J Neuroendocrinol.* 2005; 17:466-73.

Arbogast LA, Voogt JL. Endogenous opioid peptides contribute to suckling-induced prolactin release by suppressing tyrosine hydroxylase activity and messenger ribonucleic acid levels in tuberoinfundibular dopaminergic neurons. *Endocrinology.* 1998; 139:2857-62.

Arojoki M, Jokimaa V, Koskinen P, Irjala K, Antilla L. Hypothyroidism among infertile women in Finland. *Gynecol Endocrinol.* 2000; 14(2):127-31.

Aubriot FX, Hamou J, Dubuisson JB, Frydman R, Fernandez H. Hysteroplasty for enlargment: apropos of the results. *Gynecol Obstet Fertil.* 2001; 29(12):888-93.

Baird DR, McNeilly AS, Sawers SR, Sharpe RM. Failure of estrogen-induced discharge of luteininzing hormone in lactating women. *J Clin Endocrinol Metab.* 1979; 49:500-6.

Bakalov VK, Anasti JM, Calis KA, Vanderhoof VH, Premkaumar A, Chen S, *et al.* Autoimmune oophoritis as a mechanism of follicular dysfunction in women with 46,XX spontaneous premature ovarian failure. *Fertil Steril.* 2005; 84(4):958-65.

Baker HW. Clinical male infertility. II. Critical evaluation of the prospects for therapy. *Reprod Fertil Dev.* 1994; 6(1):9-12.

Baker TG. A quantitative and cytological study of germ cells in human ovaries. *Proc R Soc Lond B Biol Sci.* 1963; 158:417-33.

Balasch J, Fabregues F, Creus M, Vanrell JA. The usefulness of endometrial biopsy for luteal phase evaluation in infertility. *Hum Reprod.* 1992; 7:973-77.

Balasch J. Gonadotrophin ovarian stimulation and intrauterine insemination for unexplained infertility. *Reprod Biomed Online.* 2004; 6:664-72.

Bateman BG, Nunley WC, Jr., Kolp LA. Exogenous estrogen therapy for treatment of clomiphene citrate-induced cervical mucus abnormalities: is it effective? *Fertil Steril.* 1990; 55(4):849-50.

Battaglia S, Goodwin P, Klein NA, Soules MR. Influence of maternal age on meiotic spindle assembly in oocytes from naturally cycling women. *Hum Reprod.* 1996; 11(10):2217-22.

Battin DA, Marrs R, Fleiss PM, Mishell DR, Jr. Effect of suckling on serum prolactin, luteinizing hormone, follicle-stimuilating hormone, and estradiol during prolonged lactation. *Obstet Gynecol.* 1985; 65(6):785-88.

Beck JI, Boothroyd C, Proctor M, Farquhar C, Hughes E. Oral anti-oestrogens and medical adjuncts for subfertility associated with anovulation. *Cochrane Database Syst Rev.* 2005; (1):CD002249.

Berkovitz A, Eltes F, Soffer Y, Zabludovsky N, Beyth Y, Farhi J, *et al.* ART success and in vivo sperm cell selection depend on the ultramorphological status of spermatozoa. *Andrologia.* 1999; 31(1):1-8.

Biller BM, Luciano A, Crosignani PG, Molitch M, Olive D, Rebar R, *et al.* Guidelines for the diagnosis and treatment of hyperprolactinemia. *J Reprod Med.* 1999; 44(12 Suppl):1075-84.

Brogan RS, Michell SE, Trayhurn P, Smith MS. Suppression of leptin during lactation: contribution of the suckling stimulus versus milk production. *Endocrinology.* 1999; 140:2621-27.

Bukulmez O, Arici A. Luteal phase defect: myth or reality. *Obstet Gynecol Clin North Am.* 2004; 31:727-44.

Butte NF, Hopkinson JM, Nicolson MA. Leptin in human reproduction: serum leptin levels in pregnant and lactating women. *J Clin Endocrinol Metab.* 1999; 82:585-89.

Butte NF, King JC. Energy requirements during pregnancy and lactation. *Public Health Nutr.* 2005; 8(7A):1010-27.

Campbell OM, Gray RH. Characteristics and determinants of postpartum ovarian function in women in the United States. *Am J Obstet Gynecol.* 1993; 169(1):55-60.

Canales ES, Lasso P, Soria J, Zarate A. Effect of clomiphene on prolactin secretion and lactation in puerperal women. *BJOG.* 1977; 84(10):758-59.

Cantineau AE, Heineman MJ, Al-Inany H, Cohlen BJ. Intrauterine insemination versus Fallopian tube sperm perfusion in non-tubal subfertility: a systematic review based on a Cochrane review. *Hum Reprod.* 2004; 19(12):2721-29.

Carmina E. Diagnosis of polycystic ovary syndrome: from NIH criteria to ESHRE-ASRM guidelines. *Minerva Ginecol.* 2004; 56(1):1-6.

Carneiro P. Breast-feeding patterns and lactational amenorrhoea among the Warli tribals: a socioanthropological inquiry. *Int J Fertil.* 1988; 33 Suppl:35-39.

Checa MA, Requena A, Salvador C, Tur R, Callejo J, Espinos JJ, *et al.* Insulin-sensitizing agents: use in pregnancy and as therapy in polycystic ovary syndrome. *Hum Reprod Update.* 2005; 11(4):375-90.

Check JH, Adelson H, Wu CH. Improvement of cervical factor with guafenesin. *Fertil Steril.* 1982; 37(5):707-8.

Chiu TT, Tam PP, Mao KR. Evaluation of a semiquantitative urinary LH assay for ovulation detection. *Int J Fertil.* 1990; 35(2):120-24.

Christiansen OB, Nybo Andersen AM, Bosch E, Daya S, Delves PJ, Hviid TV, *et al.* Evidence-based investigations and treatments of recurrent pregnancy loss. *Fertil Steril.* 2005; 83(4):821-39.

Conde-Agudelo A, Belizan JM. Maternal morbidity and mortality associated with interpregnancy interval: cross section study. *BMJ.* 2000; 321(7271):1255-59.

Cone RD, Low MJ, Elmquist JK, Cameron JL. Neuroendocrinology. In: Larsen PR, Kronenberg HM, Melmed S, Polonsky KS (eds.). *Williams Textbook of Endocrinology.* 10th Ed. Philadelphia: Saunders; 2003. p. 81-176.

Coutifaris C, Myers ER, Guzick DS, Diamond MP, Carson SA, Legro RS, *et al.* Histological dating of timed endometrial biopsy tissue is not related to fertility status. *Fertil Steril.* 2004; 82(5):1264-72.

Crosignani PG, Collins J, Cooke ID, Diczfalusy E, Rubin B. Recommendations of the ESHRE workshop on "unexplained infertility." *Hum Reprod.* 1993; 8(6):977-80.

Cuthberson WF. Evolution of infant nutrition. *Br J Nutr.* 1999; 81(5):359-71.

Davis OK, Berkeley AS, Naus GJ, Cholst IN, Freedman KS. The incidence of luteal phase defect in normal, fertile women determined by serial endometrial biopsies. *Fertil Steril.* 1989; 51(4):582-86.

de Moura MD, Ferriani RA, de Sa MF. Effects of clomiphene citrate on pituitary luteinizing hormone and follicle-stimulating hormone release in women before and after treatement with ethinyl estradiol. *Fertil Steril.* 1992; 58(3):504-7.

Delvigne A, Rozenberg S. Epidemiology and prevention of ovarian hyperstimulation syndrome (OHSS): a review. *Hum Reprod Update.* 2002; 8(6):559-77.

Delvoye P, L'Hermite A, Vis HL, Robyn C. Interrelationship between breast feeding, nutritional state, and reproduction. *J Gynecol Obstet Biol Reprod.* (Paris) 1978; 7(2):285-94.

Dewey KG. Energy and protein requirements during lactation. *Ann Rev Nutr.* 1997; 17:19-36.

Diaz S, Aravena R, Cardenas H, Casado ME, Miranda P, Schiappacasse V, *et al.* Contraception efficacy of lactational amenorrhea in urban Chilean women. *Contraception.* 1991; 43(4):335-52.

Diaz S, Cardenas H, Brandeis A, Miranda P, Miranda P, Salvatierra AM, *et al.* Relative contributions of anovulation and luteal phase defect to the reduced pregnancy rate of breastfeeding women. *Fertil Steril.* 1992; 58(3):498-503.

Diaz S, Cardenas H, Brandeis A, Miranda P, Schiappacasse V, Salvatierra AM, *et al.* Early difference in the endocrine profile of long and short lactational amenorrhea. *J Clin Endocrinol Metab.* 1991; 72(1):196-201.

Diaz S, Croxatto HB. Contraception in lactating women. *Curr Opin Obstet Gynecol.* 1993; 5(6):815-22.

Diaz S, Seron-Ferre M, Cardenas H, Schiappacasse V, Brandeis A, Croxatto H. Circadian variation of basal plasma prolactin, prolactin response to suckling, and length of amenorrhea in nursing women. *J Clin Endocrinol Metab.* 1989; 68(5):946-55.

Diaz S, Seron-Ferre M, Croxatto H, Veldhuis JD. Neuroendocrine mechanisms of lactational infertility in women. *Biol Res.* 1995; 28(2):155-63.

Diaz S, Zepeda A, Maturana X, Reyes MV, Miranda C, Casado ME, *et al.* Fertility regulation in nursing women. IX. Contraceptive performance, duration or lactation, infant growth, and bleeding patterns during use of progesterone vaginal rings, progestin-only pills, Norplant injections, and Copper T 380-A intrauterine devices. *Contraception.* 1997; 56(4):223-32.

Dodson WC, Haney AF. Controlled ovarian hyperstimulation and intrauterine insemination for treatment of infertility. *Fertil Steril.* 1991; 55(3):478-80.

Dohle GR, Halley DJJ, Van Hemel JO, van den Ouwel AMW, Pieters MHEC, Weber RFA, *et al.* Genetic risk factors in infertile men with severe oligozoospermia and azoospermia. *Hum Reprod.* 2002; 17(1):13-16.

Dohle GR, Ramos L, Pieters MH, Braat DD, Weber RF. Surgical sperm retrieval and intracytoplasmic sperm injection as treatment of obstructive azoospermia. *Hum Reprod.* 1998; 13(3):620-23.

Donnez J, Squifflet J, Casanas-Roux F, Pirard C, Jadoul P, Van Langendonckt A. Typical and subtle atypical presentations of endometriosis. *Obstet Gyncol Clin North Am.* 2003; 30(1):83-93.

Eichenlaub-Ritter U. Genetics of oocyte aging. *Maturitas.* 1998; 30(2):143-69.

Ellison PT. Advances in human reproductive ecology. *Annu Rev Anthropol.* 1994; 23(255):275.

Ellison PT. Energetics and reproductive effort. *Am J Hum Biol.* 2003; 3:342-51.

Ernst S, Hite G, Cantrill J, Richardson A, Benson H. Stereochemistry of geometric isomers of clomiphene: a correction of the literature and a reexamination of structure-activity relationships. *J Pharm Sci.* 1976; 65(1):148-50.

ESHRE Capri Workshop Group. Diagnosis and management of the infertile couple: missing information. *Hum Reprod Update.* 2004; 10(4):295-307.

Evers JL, Collins JA. Assessment of efficacy of varicocele repair for male subfertility: a systematic review. *Lancet.* 2003; 361(9372):1849-52.

Evers JL, Collins JA. Surgery or embolisation for varicocele in subfertile men. *Cochrane Database Syst Rev.* 2004;(3): CD000479.

Faddy MJ, Gosden R, Gougeon A, Richardson SJ, Nelson JF. Accelerated disappearance of ovarian follicles in the mid-life: implications for forecasting menopause. *Hum Reprod.* 1992; 7(10):1342-46.

Farhi J, Ashkenazi J, Feldberg D, Dicker D, Orvieto R, Ben Rafael Z. Effect of uterine leiomyomata on the results of in-vitro fertilization. *Hum Reprod.* 1995; 10(10):2576-78.

Farquhar C, Lilford R, Marjoribanks J, Vandekerckhove P. Laparoscopic "drilling" by diathermy or laser or ovulation induction in anovulatory polycystic ovary syndrome. *Cochrane Database Syst Rev.* 2005; 2005(3):CD001122.

Farquhar CM. Extracts from "Clinical Evidence": Endometriosis. *BMJ.* 2000; 320(7247):1449-52.

Fatemi HM, Kolibianakis EM, Tournaye H, Camus M, Van Steirteghem AC. Clomiphene citrate versus letrozole for ovarian stimulation: a pilot study. *Reprod Biomed Online.* 2003; 7(5):543-46.

Fedele L, Parazzini F, Radici E, Bocciolone L, Bianchi S, Bianchi C. Buserelin acetate versus expectant management in the treatment of infertility associated with minimal or mild endometriosis: a randomized clinical trial. *Am J Obstet Gynecol.* 1992; 166(5):1345-50.

Ferrari C, Scarduelli C, Rampini P, Brambilla G, Benco R, Pistolesi E, *et al.* Prolactin response to the dopamine antagonists sulpirimide and domperidone. Further evidence for pituitary dopamine deficiency in hyperprolactinemic disorders of different etiology. *Gynecol Obstet Invest.* 1983; 16(5):299-306.

Ford K, Huffman S. Nutrition, infant feeding and postpartum amenorrhea in rural Bangladesh. *J Biosoc Sci.* 1988; 20(4):461-69.

Gabay MP. Galactogogues: medications that induce lactation. *J Hum Lact.* 2002; 18(3):274-79.

Glasier A, McNeilly AS, Baird DT. Induction of ovarian activity by pulsatile infusion of LHRH in women with lactational amenorrhoea. *Clin Endocrinol.* (Oxf) 1986; 24(3):243-52.

Glasier A, McNeilly AS, Howey WP. Pulsatile secretion of LH in relation to the resumption of ovarian activity post partum. *Clin Endocrinol.* (Oxf) 1984; 20:415-26.

Gnoth C, Godehardt D, Godehardt E, Frank-Herrmann P, Freundl G. Time to pregnancy: results of the German prospective study and impact on the management of infertility. *Hum Reprod.* 2003; 18(9):1959-66.

Gondos B, Bhiraleus P, Hobel C. Ultrastructural observations on germ cells in human fetal ovaries. *Am J Obstet Gynecol.* 1975; 110(5):644-52.

Gougeon A, Echochard R, Thalabard JC. Age-related changes of the population of human ovarian follicles: increase in the disappearance rate of non-growing and early-growing follicles in aging women. *Biol Reprod.* 1994; 50:653-63.

Gray RH, Campbell OM, Zacur H, Labbok M, MacRae SL. Postpartum return of ovarian activity in nonbreastfeeding women monitored by urinary assays. *J Clin Endocrinol Metab.* 1987; 64(4):645-50.

Grimes DA, Schulz K. Surrogate end points in clinical research: hazardous to your health. *Obstet Gynecol.* 2005; 105(5 Pt 1):1114-8.

Gross BA, Burger H, WHO Task Force on Methods for Natural Fertility Regulation. Breastfeeding patterns and return to fertility in Australian women. *Aust N Z J Obstet Gynecol.* 2002; 42(2):148-54.

Gross BA. Breast-feeding and natural family planning. *Int J Fertil.* 1988; 33 Suppl:24-31.

Grubb MR, Chakeres D, Malarkey WB. Patients with primary hypothyroidism presenting as prolactinomas. *Am J Med.* 1987; 83(4):765-69.

Gsponer J, DeTribolet N, Deruaz J, Janzer R, Uske A, Mirimanoff RO, *et al.* Diagnosis, treatment, and outcome of pituitary tumors and other abnormal intrasellar masses: retrospective analysis of 353 patients. *Medicine.* (Baltimore) 1999; 78(4):236-69.

Guttmacher AF. Factors affecting normal expectancy of conception. *JAMA.* 1956; 161(9):855-60.

Guzick DS, Sullivan MW, Adamson GD, Cedars MI, Falk RJ, Peterson EP, *et al.* Efficacy of treatment for unexplained infertility. *Fertil Steril.* 1998; 70(2):207-13.

Haartsen JE, Heineman MJ, Elings M, Evers JL, Lancranjan I. Resumption of pituitary and ovarian activity postpartum: endocrine and ultrasonic observations in bromcriptine-treated women. *Hum Reprod.* 1992; 78:746-50.

Halis G, Arici A. Endometriosis and inflammation in infertility. *Ann NY Acad Sci.* 2004; 1034:300-15.

Hanafi M. Predictors of leiomyomata recurrence after myomectomy. *Obstet Gynecol.* 2005; 105(4):877-81.

Hanson LA, Korotkova IV, Lundin S, Haversen L, Silfverdal SA, Mattsby-Baltzer I, *et al.* The transfer of immunity from mother to child. *Ann NY Acad Sci.* 2003; 987:199-206.

Harlap S, Shiono PH. Alcohol, smoking, and incidence of spontaneous abortions in the first and second trimester. *Lancet.* 1980; 2(8187):173-76.

Heinonen PK. Longitudinal vaginal septum. *Eur J Obstet Gynecol Reprod Biol.* 1982; 13(4):253-58.

Helmerhorst FM, Van Vliet HA, Gornas T, Finken M, Grimes D. Intrauterine insemination of washed husband's spermatozoa: a controlled study. *Cochrane Database Syst Rev.* 2005; 4(CD002809).

Henson MC, Castracane VD. *Leptin and reproduction.* New York: Kluwer Academic; 2003.

Herbst AL, Cole P, Colton T, Robboy SJ, Scully RE. Age-incidence and risk of diethylstilbestrol-related clear cell adenocarcinoma of the vagina and cervix. *Am J Obstet Gynecol.* 1977; 128(1):43-50.

Herbst AL. Diethylstilbestrol and other sex hormones during pregnancy. *Obstet Gynecol.* 1981; 58(5 Suppl):35S-40S.

Homburg R, Eshel A, Armar NA, Tucker M, Mason PW, Adams J, *et al.* One hundred pregnancies after treatment with pusatile luteinsing hormone releasing hormone to induce ovulation. *BMJ.* 1989; 298:809-12.

Homburg R. *Ovulation induction and controlled ovarian hyperstimulation.* Abingdon, U.K.: Taylor and Francis; 2005.

Homburg R. The management of infertility associated with polycystic ovary syndrome. *Reprod Biol Endocrinol.* 2003; 1:109-18.

Horcajades JA, Riesewilk AN, Dominguez FR, Cervero AN, Pellucier RA, Simon CA. Determinants of endometrial receptivity. *Ann NY Acad Sci.* 2004; 1034(1):166-75.

Illingworth DR. Low dose transdermal oestradiol suppresses gonadotropin secretion in breast-feeding women. *Hum Reprod.* 1995; 10(7):1671-77.

IPPF International Advisory Committee. New IPPF statement on breastfeeding, fertility and post-partum contraception. *IPPF Med Bull.* 1990; 24(2):2-4.

Isaksson R, Tiitinen A. Present concept of unexplained infertility. *Gynecol Endocrinol.* 2004; 18(5):278-90.

Ivan G, Szigeti-Csucs N, Olah M, Nagy GM, Goth M. Treatment of pituitary tumors: dopamine agonists. *Endocrine.* 2005; 28(1):101-10.

Jiroutek MR, Chen MH, Johnston CC, Longcope C. Changes in reproductive hormones and sex hormone-binding globulin in a group of postmenopausal women measured over 10 years. *Menopause.* 1998; 5(2):90-94.

Johnson N, Vandekerckhove P, Watson A, Lilford R, Harada T, Hughes E. Tubal flushing for subfertility. *Cochrane Database Syst Rev.* 2005; (2):CD003718.

Jones RE, Palloni A. Investigating the determinants of postpartum amenorrhea using a multistate hazards approach model. *Ann NY Acad Sci.* 1994; 709:227-30.

Kageyama H, Takenoya F, Kita T, Hori T, Guan JL, Shioda S. Galanin-like peptide in the brain: effects on feeding, energy metabolism, and reproduction. *Regul Pept.* 2005; 126(1-2):21-26.

Kalir R, David MP, Kraicer PF. Clomiphene citrate in suppression of puerperal lactation. *Am J Obstet Gynecol.* 1975; 122(5):570-72.

Kastin AJ, Zarate A, Midgley AR, Jr., Canales ES, Schally AV. Ovulation confirmed by pregnancy after infusion of porcine LH-RH. *J Clin Endocrinol Metab.* 1971; 33(6):980-82.

Kauffman MM, Kauffman RP. Polycystic ovary syndrome--a complex disorder among women. *JAAPA.* 2003;16(8):39-47.

Kauffman RP, Castracane VD. Premature ovarian failure associated with autoimmune polyglandular syndrome: pathophysiological mechanisms and future fertility. *J Womens Health.* 2003; 12(5):513-20.

Keel BA. How reliable are results from the semen analysis? *Fertil Steril.* 2004; 82(1):41-44.

Keel BA. Within- and between-subject variation in semen parmeteres in infertile men and normal semen donors. *Fertil Steril.* 2006; 85(1):128-34.

Kerin JF, Liu JH, Phillipou G, Yen SSC. Evidence for a hypothalamic site of action of clomiphene citrate in women. *J Clin Endocrinol Metab.* 1985; 61(2):265-68.

Kessel B, Hsueh AJ. Clomiphene citrate augments follicle-stimulating hormone-induced luteinizing hormone receptor content in cultured rat granulosa cells. *Fertil Steril.* 1987; 47(2):334-40.

Klein NA, Battaglia S, Fujimoto VY, Davis GS, Bremner WJ. Reproduction aging: accelerated ovarian follicular development associated with a monotropic follicle-stimulating hormone rise in older women. *J Clin Endocrinol Metab.* 1996; 81(3):1038-45.

Kleinberg DL, Noel GL, Frantz AG. Galactorrhea: a study of 235 cases, including 48 with pituitary tumors. *N Engl J Med.* 1977; 296(11):589-600.

Knochenhauer ES, Key TJ, Kahsar-Miller MD, Waggoner W, Boots LR, Azziz R. Prevalence of polycystic ovary syndrome in unselected black and white women of the southeastern United States: a prospective study. *J Clin Endocrinol Metab.* 1998; 83(9):3078-82.

Konner M, Worthman C. Nursing frequency, gonadal function, and birth spacing among Kung hunter-gatherers. *Science.* 1980; 207(4432):788-91.

Kremer J, Rolland R, van der Heijden PF, Thomas CF. Return of gonadotropic function in pstpartum women during bromocriptine treatment. *Fertil Steril.* 1989;51:622-7.

Labbok MH, Hight-Laukaran V, Peterson AE, Fletcher V, von HH, Van Look PF. Multicenter study of the Lactational Amenorrhea Method (LAM): I. Efficacy, duration, and implications for clinical application. *Contraception.* 1997; 55(6):327-36.

Land JA, Gijsen AP, Kessels AG, Slobbe MEP, Bruggeman CA. Performance of five serological chlamydia antibody tests in subfertile women. *Hum Reprod.* 2003; 18(12):2621-7.

Laven J, Fauser BC. Inhibins and adult ovarian function. *Mol Cell Endocrinol.* 2004; 225(1-2):37-44.

Levitas E, Lunenfeld E, Weiss N, Friger M, Har-Vardi I, Koifman A, *et al.* Relationship between the duration of sexual abstinence and semen quality: analysis of 9,489 semen samples. *Fertil Steril.* 2005; 83(6):1680-86.

Leyendecker G, Struve T, Plotz EJ. Induction of ovulation with chronic intermittent (pulsatile) administration of LHRH in women with hypothalamic and hyerprolactinemic amenorrhea. *Arch Gynecol.* 1980; 229(3):177-90.

Li C, Chen P, Smith MS. Neuropeptide Y and tuberoinfundibular dopamine activities are altered during lactation: role of prolactin. *Endocrinology.* 1999; 140:118-23.

Liu JH, Park KH. Gonadotropin and prolactin secretion increases during sleep during the puerperium in nonlactating women. *J Clin Endocrinol Metab.* 1988; 66(4):839-45.

Liu JK, Couldwell WT. Contemporary management of prolactinomas. *Neurosurg Focus.* 2004; 16(4):E2.

Lord JM, Flight I, Norman RJ. Insulin-sensitizing drugs (metformin, troglitazone, rosiglitazone, pioglitazone, D-chiro-inositol) for polycystic ovary syndrome. *Cochrane Database Syst Rev.* 2003; 3(CD003053).

Lord JM, Flight I, Norman RJ. Metformin in polycystic ovary syndrome: systematic review and meta-analysis. *BMJ.* 2003; 327(7421):951.

Loucks AB, Mortola JF, Girton L, Yen SSC. Alterations in the hypothalamic-pituitary-ovarian and hypothalamic-pituitary-adrenal axes in athletic women. *J Clin Endocrinol Metab.* 1989; 68:402-11.

Lunn PG. Breast-feeding patterns, maternal milk output and lactational infecundity. *J Biosoc Sci.* 1992; 24(3):317-24.

Luthra P, Kirma N, Jones J, Tekmal RR. Use of letrozole as a chemopreventive agent in aromatase overexpressing transgenic mice. *J Steroid Biochem Mol Biol.* 2003; 86(3-5):461-67.

Macut D, Micic D, Pralong FP, Bischof P, Campana A. Is there a role for leptin in human reproduction? *Gynecol Endocrinol.* 1998; 12:321-26.

Mahmood TA, Templeton A. Prevalence and genesis of endometriosis. *Hum Reprod.* 1991; 6(4):544-49.

Malo JW, Bezdicek B, Campbell E, Pavelka DA, Covato T. Ovulation induction with pulsatile intravenous GnRH. *J Reprod Med.* 1985; 30(12):902-6.

March CM, Israel R. Hysteroscopic management of recurrent abortion caused by septate uterus. *Am J Obstet Gynecol.* 1987; 156(4):834-42.

Marcoux S, Maheux R, Berube S. Laparoscopic surgery in infertile women with minimal or mild endometriosis. *N Engl J Med.* 1997; 337(4):217-24.

Marmar JL. The diagnosis and treatment of male infertility in the new millennium. *Int J Fertil Womens Med.* 2001; 46(3):116-36.

Marshall JC, Eagleson CA, McCartney CR. Hypothalamic dysfunction. *Mol Cell Endocrinol.* 2001; 183(1-2):29-32.

Masala A, Delitala G, Alagna S, Devilla L, Stoppelli I, Lo DG. Clomiphene and puerperal lactation. *Panminerva Med.* 1978; 20(3):161-63.

Masala A, Delitala G, Lo Dico G, Stoppelli I, Alagna S, Devilla L. Inhibition of lactation and inhibition of prolactin release after mechanical breast stimulation in puerperal women given tamoxifen or placebo. *BJOG.* 1978; 85(2):134-37.

Massara F, Camanni F, Amoroso A, Molinatti GM, Muller EE. Increased thyrotripin and prolactin secretion induced by domperidone in hypothyroid patients. *Acta Endocrinol.* (Copenh) 1981; 97(1):48-53.

McGovern PG, Myers ER, Silva S, Coutifaris C, Carson SA, Legro RS, *et al.* Absence of secretory endometrium after false-positive home urine luteinizing hormone testing. *Fertil Steril.* 2004; 82(5):1273-77.

McLaughlin EA. Cryopreservation, screening and storage of sperm: the challenges for the twenty-first century. *Hum Fertil.* (Camb) 2002; 5(1 Suppl)(S61):S65.

McNatty KP, Sawers SR, McNeilly AS. A possible role for prolactin in control of steroid secretion by the human graafian follicle. *Nature.* 1974; 250:653-55.

McNeilly AS, Tay CC, Glasier A. Physiological mechanisms underlying lactational amenorrhea. *Ann N Y Acad Sci.* 1994; 709:145-55.

McNeilly AS. Lactation and fertility. *J Mammary Gland Biol Neoplasia.* 1997; 2(3):291-98.

McNeilly AS. Lactational control of reproduction. *Reprod Fertil Dev.* 2001; 13(7-8):583-90.

McNeilly AS. Neuroendocrine changes and fertility in breast-feeding women. In: Russell JA (ed.). *Progress in Brain Research.* Elsevier Science; 2001.

Meier C, Christ-Crain M, Guglielmetti M, Huber P, Staub JJ, Muller B. Prolactin dysregulation in women with subclinical hypothyroidism: effect of levothyroxine replacement therapy. *Thyroid.* 2003; 13(10):979-85.

Miller JE. Birth intervals and perinatal health: an investigation of three hypotheses. *Fam Plann Perspect.* 1991; 23(2):62-70.

Miller JE. Birth order, interpregnancy interval and birth outcomes among Filipino infants. *J Biosoc Sci.* 1994; 26(2):243-49.

Minas V, Loutradis D, Makrigiannis A. Factors controlling blastocyst implantation. *Reprod Biomed Online.* 2005; 10(2):205-16.

Mitwally MF, Biljan MM, Casper RF. Pregnancy outcomes after the use of an aromatase inhibitor for ovarian stimulation. *Am J Obstet Gynecol.* 2005; 192(2):381-86.

Morales AJ, Laughlin GA, Butzow T, Maheshwari H, Baumann G. Insulin, somatotropic, and luteinizing hormone axes in lean and obese women with polycystic ovary syndrome: common and distinct features. *J Clin Endocrinol Metab.* 1996; 81(8):2854-64.

Mosher WD, Pratt WF. Fecundity and infertility in the United States: incidence and trends. *Fertil Steril.* 1991; 56(2):192-93.

Munkelwitz R, Gilbert BR. Are boxer shorts really better? A critical analysis of the role of underwear type in male subfertility. *J Urol.* 1998; 160(4):1329-33.

Murray MJ, Meyer WR, Zaino RJ, Lessey BA, Novotny DB, Ireland K, *et al.* A critical analysis of the accuracy, reproducibility, and clinical utility of histologic endometrial dating in fertile women. *Fertil Steril.* 2004; 81(5):1333-43.

Nabi G, Asterlings S, Greene DR, Marsh RL. Percutaneous embolization of varicoceles: outcomes and correlation of semen improvement with pregnancy. *Urology.* 2004; 63(2):359-63.

Nakano R, Mori A, Kayashima F, Washio M, Tojo S. Ovarian response to exogenously administered human gonadotropins during the postpartum period. *Am J Obstet Gynecol.* 1975; 121(2):187-92.

Nelson LM, Covington SN, Rebar R. An update: spontaneous premature ovarian failure is not an early menopause. *Fertil Steril.* 2005; 83(5):1327-32.

Nikolettos N, Kupker W, Demirel C, Schopper B, Blasig C, Sturm R, *et al.* Fertilization potential of spermatozoa with abnormal morphology. *Hum Reprod.* 1999; 14(Suppl 1):47-70.

Noyes RM, Hertig A, Rock JA. Dating the endometrial biopsy. *Fertil Steril.* 1950; 1:3-25.

Parker SL, Armstrong WE, Sladek CD, Grosvenor CE, Crowley WR. Prolactin stimulates the release of oxytocin in lactating rats: evidence for a physiological role via an action at the neural tube. *Neuroendocrinology.* 1991; 53:503-10.

PDR. *Physicians' Desk Reference.* 59th Ed. Montvale, NJ: Thomson PDR; 2005.

Perheentupa A, Critchley HO, Illingworth PJ, McNeilly AS. Enhanced sensitivity to steroid-negative feedback during breast-feeding: low-dose estradiol (transdermal estradiol supplementation) suppresses gonadotropins and ovarian activity assessed by inhibin B. *J Clin Endocrinol Metab.* 2000; 85(11):4280-86.

Practice Committee of the American Society for Reproductive Medicine. Definition of "infertility." *Fertil Steril.* 2004; 82(Supp 1):S206.

Practice Committee of the American Society for Reproductive Medicine. Effectiveness and treatment for unexplained infertility. *Fertil Steril.* 2004; 82(Suppl 1):S160-S163.

Prema K, Ravindranath M. The effect of breastfeeding supplements on the return of fertility. *Stud Fam Plann.* 1982; 13(10):293-96.

Pritts EA, Atwood AK. Luteal phase support in infertility treatment: a meta-analysis of the randomized trials. *Hum Reprod.* 2002; 17(9):2287-99.

Pugeat M, Ducluzeau PH, Mallion-Donadieu M. Association of insulin resistance with hyperandrogenemia in women. *Horm Res.* 2000; 54(5-6):322-26.

Reindollar RH, Novak M, Tho SP, McDonough PG. Adult-onset amenorrhea: a study of 262 cases. *Am J Obstet Gynecol.* 1986; 155(3):531-43.

Rheingold PD. Litigation involving DES. *Women Health.* 1976; 1(5):26-27.

Rice JP, Kay HH, Mahony BS. The clinical significance of uterine leiomyomas in pregnancy. *Am J Obstet Gynecol.* 1989; 160(5 Pt 1):1212-16.

Richardson SJ, Senikas V, Nelson JF. Follicular depletion during the menopausal transition: evidence for accelerated loss and ultimate exhaustion. *J Clin Endocrinol Metab.* 1987; 65(6):1231-37.

Roberts C, Landenson PW. Hypothyroidism. *Lancet.* 2004; 363(9411):793-803.

Rogers IS. Lactation and fertility. *Early Hum Dev.* 1997; 49 Suppl:S185-S190.

Rotterdam ESHRE/ASRM-Sponsored PCOS Consensus Committee. Revised 2003 consensus on diagnostic criteria and long-term health risks related to polycystic ovary syndrome. *Fertil Steril.* 2004; 81(1):19-25.

Santoro N, Isaac B, Neal-Perry G, Adel T, Weingart L, Nussbaum A, *et al.* Impaired folliculogenesis and ovulation in older reproductive age women. *J Clin Endocrinol Metab.* 2003; 88(11):5502-9.

Santoro N. The menopausal transition. *Am J Med.* 2005; 118(12 Suppl 2):8-13.

Schlindler AE. Pathophysiology, diagnosis, and treatment of endometriosis. *Minerva Ginecol.* 2004; 56(5):419-35.

Selmanoff M, Gregerson KA. Sucking-induced prolactin release is suppressed by naloxone and stimulated by beta-endorphin. *Neuroendocrinology.* 1986; 42:255-59.

Senekjian EK, Potkul RK, Frey K, Herbst AL. Infertility among daughters either exposed or not exposed to diethylstilbestrol. *Am J Obstet Gynecol.* 1988; 158(3 Pt 1):493-98.

Shibata K, Hosoda H, Kojima M, Kangawa K, Makino Y, Makino I, *et al.* Regulation of ghrelin secretion during pregnancy and lactation in the rat: possible involvment of hypothalamus. *Peptides.* 2004; 25(2):279-87.

Shoham Z, Balen A, Patel A, Jacobs C. Results of ovulation induction using human menopausal gonadotropin or purified follicle stimulating hormone in hypogonadotropic hypogonadism. *Fertil Steril.* 1991; 56(6):1048-53.

Shoham Z, Homburg R, Jacobs HS. Induction of ovulation with pulsatile GnRH. *Baillieres Best Pract Res Clin Obstet Gynaecol.* 1990; 4(3):589-608.

Short RV. Lactational infertility in family planning. *Ann Med.* 1993; 25(2):175-80.

Sir-Petermann T, Devoto L, Maliqueo M, Peirano P, Recabarren SE, Wildt L. Resumption of ovarian function during lactational amenorrhoea in breastfeeding women with polycystic ovarian syndrome: endocrine aspects. *Hum Reprod.* 2001; 16(8):1603-10.

Sir-Petermann T, Recabarren SE, Lobos A, Maliqueo M, Wildt L. Secretory pattern of leptin and LH during lactational amenorrhoea in breastfeeding normal and polycystic ovarian syndrome women. *Hum Reprod.* 2001; 16(2):244-49.

Skinner MK. Regulation of primordial follicle assembly and development. *Hum Reprod Update.* 2005; 11(5):461-71.

Smith MS, Grove KL. Integration of the regulation of reproductive function and energy balance: lactation as a model. *Front Neuroendocrinol.* 2002; 23(3):225-56.

Speilvogel K, Shwayder JM, Coddington CC. Surgical management of adhesions, endometriosis, and tubal pathology in the woman with infertility. *Clin Obstet Gynecol.* 2000; 43(4):916-28.

Speroff L, Fritz MA. *Clinical Gynecologic Endocrinology and Infertility.* 7th Ed. Philadelphia: Lippincott Williams & Wilkins; 2005.

Stein IF, Leventhal ML. Amenorrhea associated with bilateral polycystic ovaries. *Am J Obstet Gynecol.* 1935; 29:188-91.

Steiner AZ, Terplan M, Paulson RJ. Comparison of tamoxifen and clomiphene citrate for ovulation induction: a meta-analysis. *Hum Reprod.* 2005; 20(6):1511-15.

Stern JM, Konner M, Herman TN, Reichlin S. Nursing behaviour, prolactin and postpartum amenorrhea during prolonged lactation in American and !Kung mothers. *Clin Endocrinol.* (Oxf) 1986; 25(3):247-58.

Stout DL, Fugate SE. Thiazolidinediones for treatment of polycytic ovary syndrome. *Pharmacotherapy.* 2005; 25(2):244-52.

Stovall DW, Parrish SB, Van Voorhis BJ, Hahn SJ, Sparks AE. Uterine leiomyomas reduce the efficacy of assisted reproduction cycles: results of a matched follow-up study. *Hum Reprod.* 1998; 13(1):192-97.

Sudik R, Husch K, Steller J, Daume E. Fertility and pregnancy outcome after myomectomy in sterility patients. *Eur J Obstet Gynecol Reprod Biol.* 1996; 65(2):209-14.

Surrey E, Minjarez DA, Stevens J, Schoolcraft WB. Effects of myomectomy on the outcome of assisted reproductive technologies. *Fertil Steril.* 2005; 83(5):1473-79.

Swart P, Mol BW, van d V, van BM, Redekop WK, Bossuyt PM. The accuracy of hysterosalpingography in the diagnosis of tubal pathology: a meta-analysis. *Fertil Steril.* 1995; 64(3):486-91.

Tay CC, Glasier A, McNeilly AS. The 24 h pattern of pulsatile luteinizing hormone, follicle stimulating hormone and prolactin release during the first 8 weeks of lactational amenorrhea in breastfeeding women. *Hum Reprod.* 1992; 7(7):951-58.

Tay CC, Glasier A, McNeilly AS. Twenty-four hour patterns of prolactin secretion during lactation and the relationship to suckling and the resumption of fertility in breast-feeding women. *Hum Reprod.* 1996; 11(5):950-55.

Tay CC, Glasier AF, Illingworth DR, Baird DT. Abnormal twenty-four hour pattern of pulsatile luteinizing hormone secretion and the response to naloxone in women with hyperprolactinemic amenorrhea. *Clin Endocrinol.* (Oxf) 1993; 39(5):599-606.

Tay CC, Glasier AF, McNeilly AS. Effect of antagonists of dopamine and opiates on the basal and GnRH-induced secretion of luteinizing hormone, follicle stimulating hormone and prolactin during lactational amenorrhoea in breastfeeding women. *Hum Reprod.* 1993; 8(4):532-39.

te Velde ER, van Kooy RJ, Waterreus JJ. Intrauterine insemination of washed husband's spermatozoa: a controlled study. *Fertil Steril.* 1989; 51(1):182-85.

Tennekoon KH, Wasalathanthri S, Jeevathayaparan S, Karunanayake EH. Serum leptin and lactational amenorrhea in well-nourished and under-nourished lactating women. *Fertil Steril.* 2005; 83(4):988-94.

Truitt ST, Fraser A, Grimes D, Gallo M, Schulz K. Hormonal contraception during lactation: systemic review of randomized controlled trials. *Contraception.* 2003; 68(4):233-38.

Tyson JE, Hwang P, Guyda H, Friesen H. Factors influencing the secretion of human prolactin and growth hormone in menstrual and gestational women. *Am J Obstet Gynecol.* 1972; 113(1):14-20.

Valeggia C, Ellison PT. Lactational amenorrhea in well-nourished Toba women of Formosa, Argentina. *J Biosoc Sci.* 2004; 36:573-95.

van Kasteren YM, Schoemaker J. Premature ovarian failure: a systematic review on therapeutic interventions to restore ovarian function and achieve pregnancy. *Hum Reprod Update.* 1999; 5(5):483-92.

Verhelst J, Abs R, Maiter D, van den Brule AJ, Vandeweghe M, Velkeniers B, *et al.* Cabergoline in the treatment of hyperprolactinemia: a study in 455 patients. *J Clin Endocrinol Metab.* 1999; 84(7):2518-22.

Visness CM, Kennedy KI, Gross BA, Parenteau-Carreau S, Flynn AM. Fertility of fully breast-feeding women in the early postpartum period. *Obstet Gynecol.* 1997; 89(2):164-67.

Wang X, Chen C, Wang L, Chen D, Guang W, Franch J. Conception, early pregnancy loss, and time to clinical pregnancy. *Fertil Steril.* 2003; 79(3):577-84.

Warburton D. Biological aging and the etiology of aneuploidy. *Cytogenet Genome Res.* 2005; 111(3-4):266-72.

Warburton D. Reproductive loss: how much is preventable? *N Engl J Med.* 1987; 316(3):158-60.

Warren MP, Perlroth NE. The effects of intense exercise on the female reproductive system. *J Endocrinol.* 2001; 170:3-11.

Weil C. The safety of bromocriptine in hyperprolactinemic female infertility: a literature review. *Curr Med Res Opin.* 1986; 10(3):172-95.

Weinstein D, Ben-David M, Polishuk WZ. Serum prolactin and the suppression of lactation. *Br J Obstet Gynaecol.* 1976; 83(9):679-82.

Wilcox AJ, Weinberg CR, O'Connell FJ, Baird DD, Schlatterer JP. Incidence of early loss of pregnancy. *N Engl J Med.* 1988; 319(4):189-94.

Winter E, Wang J, Davies M, Norman R. Early pregnancy loss following assisted reproductive technology treatment. *Hum Reprod.* 2002; 17(12):3220-23.

World Health Organization Scientific Group. *Agents stimulating gonadal function in the human.* 1976. Report No: 514.

World Health Organization. Towards more objectivity in diagnosis and managment of male infertility. *Int J Androl.* 1987; 7(Suppl):1.

Worthman C, Jenkins CL, Stallings JF, Lai D. Attenuation of nursing-related ovarian suppression and high fertility in well-nourished, intensively breast-feeding Amele women of lowland Papau New Guinea. *J Biosoc Sci.* 1993; 25(4):425-43.

Wramsby H, Fredga K, Liedholm P. Chromosome analysis of human oocytes recovered from preovulatory follicles in stimulated cycles. *N Engl J Med.* 1987; 316(3):121-24.

Zarate A, Canales ES, Soria J, Leon C, Garrido J, Fonseca E. Refractory postpartum ovarian response to gonadal stimulation in non-lactating women. *Obstet Gynecol.* 1974; 44(6):819-22.

Zarate A, Canales ES. Endocrine aspects of lactation and postpartum fertility. *J Steroid Biochem.* 1987; 27(4-6):1023-28.

Zinaman M, Cartledge TP, Tomai T, Tippett P, Merriam GR. Pulsatile GnRH stimulates normal cyclic ovarian function in amenorrheic lactating postpartum women. *J Clin Endocrinol Metab.* 1995; 80(7):2088-93.

Zuckerman H, Carmel S. The inhibition of lactation by clomiphene. *J Obstet Gynaecol Br Commonw.* 1973; 80(9):822-23.

Chapter 17

Polycystic Ovary Syndrome: Pathophysiology, Endocrinopathy, Treatment, and Lactation

Charles J. Glueck, Marzieh Salehi, Dawit Aregawi, Luann Sieve, and Ping Wang

INTRODUCTION

Polycystic ovary syndrome (PCOS), characterized by oligo-amenorrhea and clinical and biochemical hyperandrogenism, is the most common endocrinopathy in women. Insulin resistance and compensatory hyperinsulinemia are major pathoetiologies of PCOS. Insulin-sensitizing drugs, metformin and thiazolidinediones, effectively resolve the endocrinopathy of PCOS, to a large degree restoring normal ovulation and improving fertility. During pregnancy, metformin sharply reduces the frequency of first trimester miscarriage, reduces the likelihood of gestational diabetes, reduces development of fetal macrosomia, and is not teratogenic. Metformin is commonly continued throughout lactation, given its continuing resolution of endocrinopathy. During the first six months of life, we have assessed 61 breastfed and 50 formula-fed infants born to 92 PCOS mothers, all of whom took metformin throughout pregnancy and continued through lactation. Growth, motor-social development, and intercurrent illnesses in breastfed and formula-fed infants from metformin-treated PCOS mothers did not differ. Metformin during lactation appears to be safe and effective in the first six months of infancy.

PATHOPHYSIOLOGY, ENDOCRINOPATHY

In 1935, Stein and Leventhal described seven women with amenorrhea, hirsutism, obesity, and a characteristic polycystic appearance to their ovaries – one of the first descriptions of a complex phenotype today known as the polycystic ovary syndrome (PCOS) (Stein and Leventhal, 1935). PCOS is the most common endocrinopathy in women, affecting about six percent of Caucasians and a larger percentage of African-Americans and Hispanics (Knochenhauer *et al.*, 1998). The 2003 Rotterdam consensus conference on the diagnosis of PCOS (2004a) required the presence of two of the following three findings to make a secure diagnosis of PCOS: clinical hyperandrogenism (hirsutism, severe acne), biochemical hyperandrogenism (high testosterone, androstenedione, DHEAS), and polycystic ovaries by pelvic ultrasound or laparoscopy. Very rarely, delayed onset congenital adrenal hyperplasia can mimic PCOS, as can idiopathic or acquired hyperprolactinemia (Ehrmann, 2005; Glueck *et al.*, 2002b), or hyperinsulinemia induced by valproic acid (Wood *et al.*, 2005).

Insulin resistance appears to be at the pathophysiologic heart of PCOS (Glueck *et al.*, 1999a; 2001b; 2002b; Ehrmann, 2005; Nestler *et al.*, 1997a; 1997b; 2000; 2003) leading to compensatory hyperinsulinemia (**Figures 1-3**). Hyperinsulinemia then promotes a panoply of adverse outcomes, with obesity (Glueck *et al.*, 2005; Nestler *et al.*, 1989; 2000) being a prominent early development of the PCOS phenotype (**Figure 1**). Obesity, by stimulating the release of TNF-alpha (**Figure 1**), contributes to arterial inflammation (Kaiser & Schunkert, 2001). TNF-alpha activates hypofibrinolytic plasminogen activator

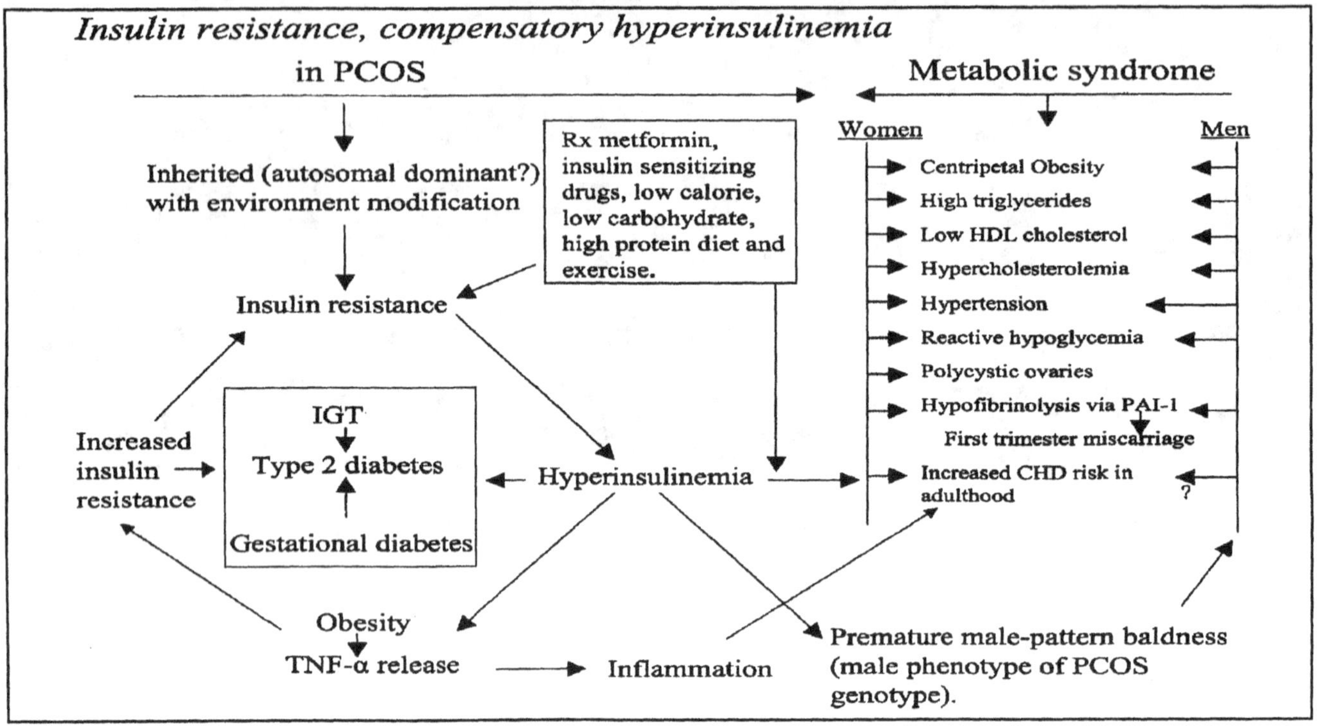

Figure 1. Insulin resistance, compensatory hyperinsulinemia, and its ramifications in polycystic ovary syndrome.

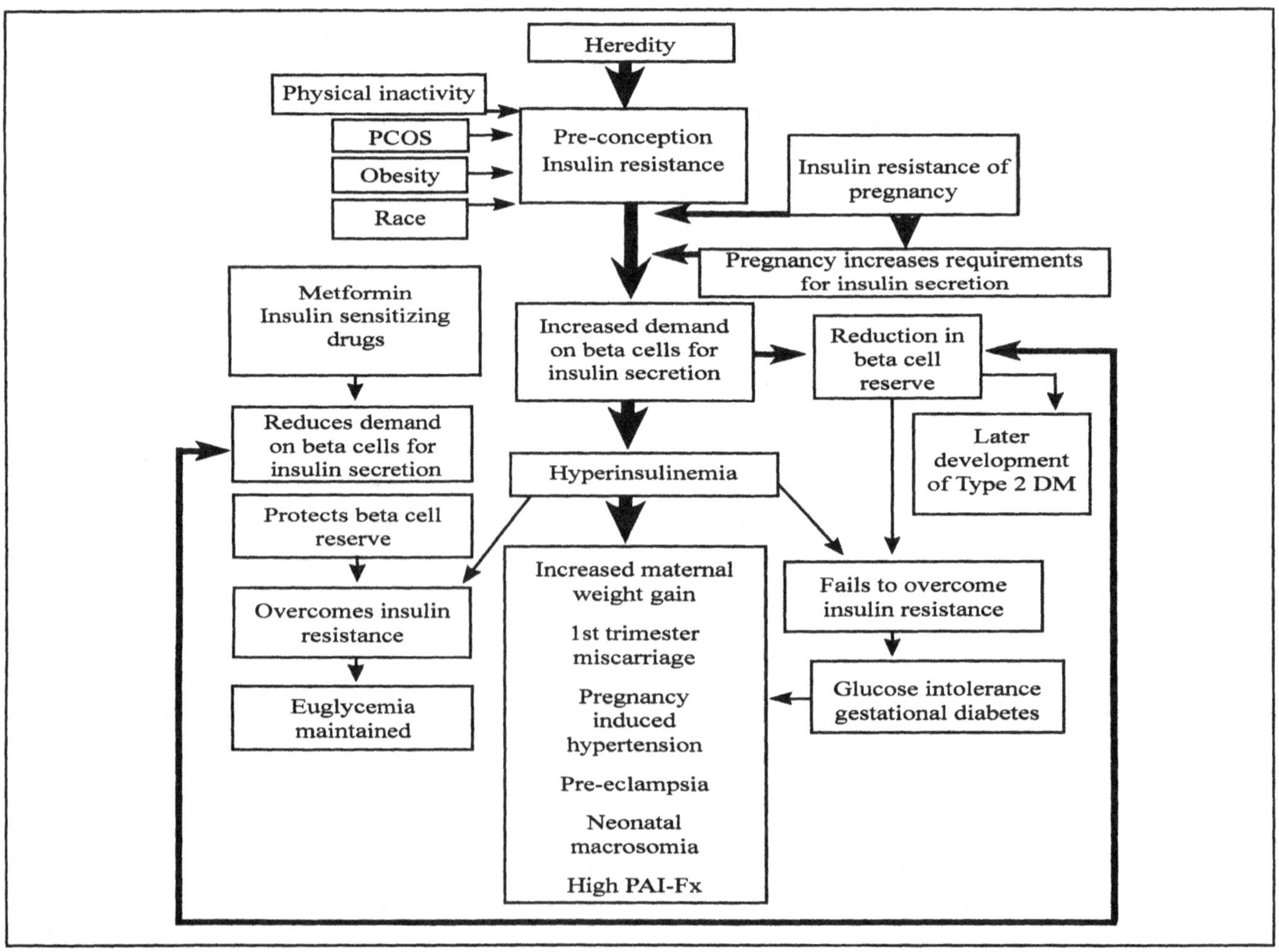

Figure 2. Insulin resistance, polycystic ovary syndrome, pregnancy, and gestational diabetes.

inhibitor activity (PAI-Fx), with subsequent increased risk of atherothrombotic arterial disease (Araya *et al.*, 2002; Gyongyosi *et al.*, 2004). Obesity, by making adipocytes and muscle cells more insulin resistant (Nestler *et al.*, 1989; 2000), promotes further increases in insulin resistance, leading to more compensatory hyperinsulinemia, completing a vicious cycle of more obesity and more insulin resistance (**Figure 1**). Under circumstances where a meal or two is missed, the hyperinsulinemia often overcomes peripheral insulin resistance, leading to recurrent hypoglycemic episodes (**Figure 1**) (Glueck *et al.*, 1999a; 2002b). Over time, despite heightened insulin secretion, as the beta cells fail to overcome insulin resistance, impaired fasting glucose, impaired glucose tolerance, and Type 2 diabetes mellitus (DM) develop (**Figure 1**). When pregnancy occurs in women with PCOS, itself an insulin resistant event (Glueck *et al.*, 2002d; 2003a; 2004c), about 40% of the time, the beta cells cannot overcome the pregnancy-augmented hyperinsulinemia and gestational diabetes occurs (**Figures 1, 2**). Exhaustion of beta cell reserves (Buchanan *et al.*, 2002; Glueck *et al.*, 2003a; 2004c) during development of gestational diabetes also has downstream adverse effects, leading to development of type 2 diabetes in 70% of women with previous gestational diabetes (**Figures 1, 2**). Hyperinsulinemia also stimulates hepatic production of triglyceride and VLDL cholesterol (**Figure 1**) (Glueck *et al.*, 1999a; 2002b; Slowinska-Srzednicka *et al.*, 1991; Talbott *et al.*, 1998). Hyperinsulinemia promotes development of thrombophilic, atherogenic homocystinemia (Bulgan Kilicdag *et al.*, 2004; Glueck *et al.*, 2001b; 2002b). Hyperinsulinemia stimulates production of aldosterone (Engeli *et al.*, 2003; Goodfriend *et al.*, 1999), which facilitates development of hypertension (**Figure 1**). Hyperinsulinemia increases production of hypofibrinolytic PAI-Fx (Velazquez *et al.*, 1994; 1997) (**Figure 1**), which is an independent cause of the common (~50%) first trimester miscarriage in women with PCOS (Glueck *et al.*, 1999b). High PAI-Fx can also contribute to increased risk of atherothrombotic coronary heart disease and ischemic stroke, probably through promotion of unstable, ulcerated plaque (Gyongyosi *et al.*, 2004). The aggregate of centripetal obesity, hyperinsulinemia, high triglycerides, low HDL cholesterol, hypertension, and high PAI-Fx comprise the

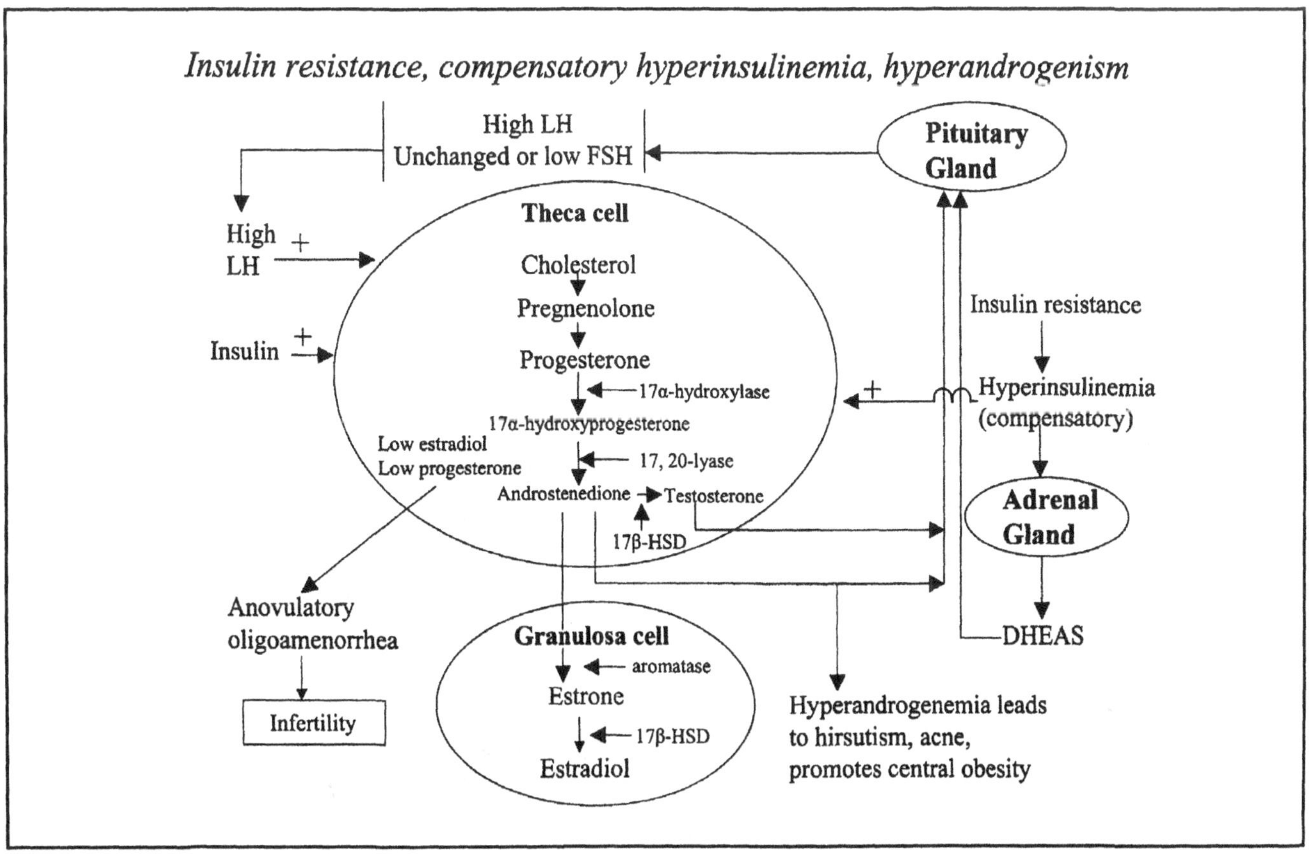

Figure 3. **Insulin resistance and hyperinsulinemia: effects on the ovary, adrenal, and pituitary.**

Adolescence	Adulthood	Metformin Effect
Obesity: Onset and progression →	Progression of obesity →	>5% Weight loss
Oligo - Amenorrhea →	Oligo - Amenorrhea →	Resolution in ~ 90%
Clinical Hyperandrogenism Hirsute, acne, balding	Clinical Hyperandrogenism Hirsute, acne, balding →	Improved, but slow ~ 1 year
Biochemical Hyperandrogenism High testosterone, and rostenendione, DHEAS, low SHBG, low estrogen and progesterone, abnormal LH/FSH ratio →	Biochemical Hyperandrogenism High testosterone, and rostenendione, DHEAS, low SHBG, low estrogen and progesterone, abnormal LH/FSH ratio →	Improved in <6 months
Polycystic Ovaries →	Polycystic Ovaries →	Improved, normalized
Infertility →	Infertility →	Improved, often resolved
Hyperinsulinemia →	Hyperinsulinemia, more severe →	Improved, usually resolved
Hyperlipidemia →	Hyperlipidemia →	Usually resolved
Hypertension →	Hypertension, more severe →	Improved
Impaired fasting glucose Impaired fasting tolerance →	Impaired fasting tolerance →	Usually resolved
Gestational Diabestes →	Gestational Diabestes, more severe →	Largely prevented
Type 2 Diabetes →	Type 2 Diabetes	Development slowed, prevented
	Myocardial Infarct, stroke → Enometrial Carcinoma →	To a large degree, prevented or reduced

Figure 4. Clinical and biochemical characteristics of polycystic ovary syndrome during adolescence and adulthood, and metformin effect.

metabolic syndrome, which, along with type 2 diabetes, is associated with an apparent seven-fold increase in coronary heart disease and ischemic stroke risk in women with PCOS (**Figure 1)** (Talbott *et al.*, 1998; 2000; 2001; 2004a; 2004b; 2004c).

Hyperinsulinemia stimulates ovarian production of testosterone and androstenedione (Nestler, 1997a; 1998) and the adrenal production of DHEAS (**Figure 3**) (Adams *et al.*, 2004). High levels of these male hormones produce hirsutism and acne (clinical hyperandrogenism) that is a hallmark of the PCOS phenotype (**Figure 3**) (Rotterdam Consensus Conference, 2004b). Hyperandrogenemia also leads to development of male pattern baldness, and, along with hyperinsulinemia, promotes centripetal fat distribution (**Figures 1, 3**). Hyperinsulinemia-driven high levels of testosterone, androstenedione, and DHEAS cycle back to the pituitary, affecting the normal production and cycling of LH and FSH, so that their trophic signals do not properly stimulate normal ovarian production of estradiol and progesterone, and inhibit ovulation, leading to oligo-amenorrhea and infertility, characteristic of the PCOS phenotype (**Figure 3**) (Rotterdam Consensus Conference, 2004a). The inability to have a normal ovarian luteal phase, caused by the high male hormones, promotes the development of ovarian cysts, an anatomic characteristic of PCOS (Rotterdam Consensus Conference, 2004a).

In aggregate, during the childbearing years, PCOS is characterized by obesity, oligo-amenorrhea, clinical and biochemical hyperandrogenism, polycystic ovaries, infertility, hyperinsulinemia, hyperlipidemia, hypertension, impaired fasting glucose, gestational diabetes and type 2 diabetes (**Figures 1-5**) (Glueck *et al.*, 1999a; 2001b; 2002b). During the adult years, women with PCOS frequently develop Type 2 diabetes and appear to be at increased risk for coronary heart disease and ischemic stroke (**Figure 4**) (Talbott *et al.*, 1995; 1998; 2000; 2001; 2004a; 2004b; 2004c). In women with PCOS having chronic oligo-amenorrhea, there is also increased risk of endometrial carcinoma (**Figure 4**) (Hardiman *et al.*, 2003). Early diagnosis of PCOS, close follow-up, and serial screening for diabetes and cardiovascular diseases are warranted.

TREATMENT WITH METFORMIN AND THIAZOLIDINEDIONES

Resolution of insulin resistance is the key to successful treatment of the clinical and biochemical abnormalities of PCOS (**Figures 1-5**). Reduction of hyperinsulinemia, particularly by insulin sensitizing drugs, facilitates weight loss, reduction of blood pressure, amelioration of hyperlipidemia, reduction of PAI-Fx, and will reduce the likelihood of beta cell burnout and both gestational and type 2 diabetes mellitus (**Figures 2, 4, 5**) (Buchanan *et al.*, 2002; Glueck *et al.*, 2002b; 2003a). Reduction of hyperinsulinemia, by reducing hyperandrogenism, reduces hirsutism and acne, and uninhibits the pituitary so that it can normally produce LH and FSH, with normal stimulation of the ovary to produce estradiol and progesterone, ovulation, and conception (**Figures 3, 5**) (Glueck *et al.*, 2002b). Although difficult, major weight loss (>5%) and exercise (lifestyle intervention) without concurrent insulin-sensitizing drugs are therapeutic in PCOS (**Figure 5**) (De Leo *et al.*, 2003; Norman *et al.*, 2002; Olszanecka-Glinianowicz *et al.*, 2004).

Coupled with diet, metformin largely ameliorates the endocrinopathy of PCOS (**Figures 1-5**) (Ehrmann, 2005; Glueck *et al.*, 1999a; Velazquez *et al.*, 1994; 1997). In PCOS, metformin facilitates more regular ovulation and facilitates conception (Baillargeon *et al.*, 2004; 2005; Ehrmann, 2005; Glueck *et al.*, 1999a; Homburg, 2005; Kumari *et al.*, 2005; Orio *et al.*, 2005; Velazquez *et al.*, 1994; 1997). When continued throughout pregnancy in PCOS, metformin may reduce severe pregnancy and postpartum complications (Vanky *et al.*, 2004), reduces first trimester miscarriage and gestational diabetes (Glueck *et al.*, 2001a; 2002a; 2002c; 2002d; 2003a; 2004a; 2004d; Jakubowicz *et al.*, 2002), reduces macrosomia (Glueck *et al.*, 2004a), does not increase likelihood of pre-eclampsia or eclampsia (Glueck *et al.*, 2004a), and does not appear to be teratogenic (Coetzee and Jackson, 1979; Glueck *et al.*, 2001a; 2002a; 2002c; 2002d; 2003a; 2004a; 2004b; 2004c; 2004d; Jakubowicz *et al.*, 2002; Vanky *et al.*, 2004).

Insulin-sensitizing drugs, metformin and thiazolidinediones (pioglitazone, rosiglitazone), are all therapeutic in PCOS (**Figures 1, 4, 5**), with metformin being the most widely studied and accepted (Lord *et al.*, 2003; 2004). Thiazolidinediones have also effectively been used to treat the endocrinopathy of PCOS (Brettenthaler *et al.*, 2004; Coffler *et al.*, 2003; Glueck *et al.*, 2003b; Guido *et al.*, 2004; Iuorno and Nestler, 2001; Lord *et al.*, 2003; Mehta *et al.*, 2005; Ortega-Gonzalez *et al.*, 2004; 2005; Romualdi *et al.*, 2003; Seli and Duleba,

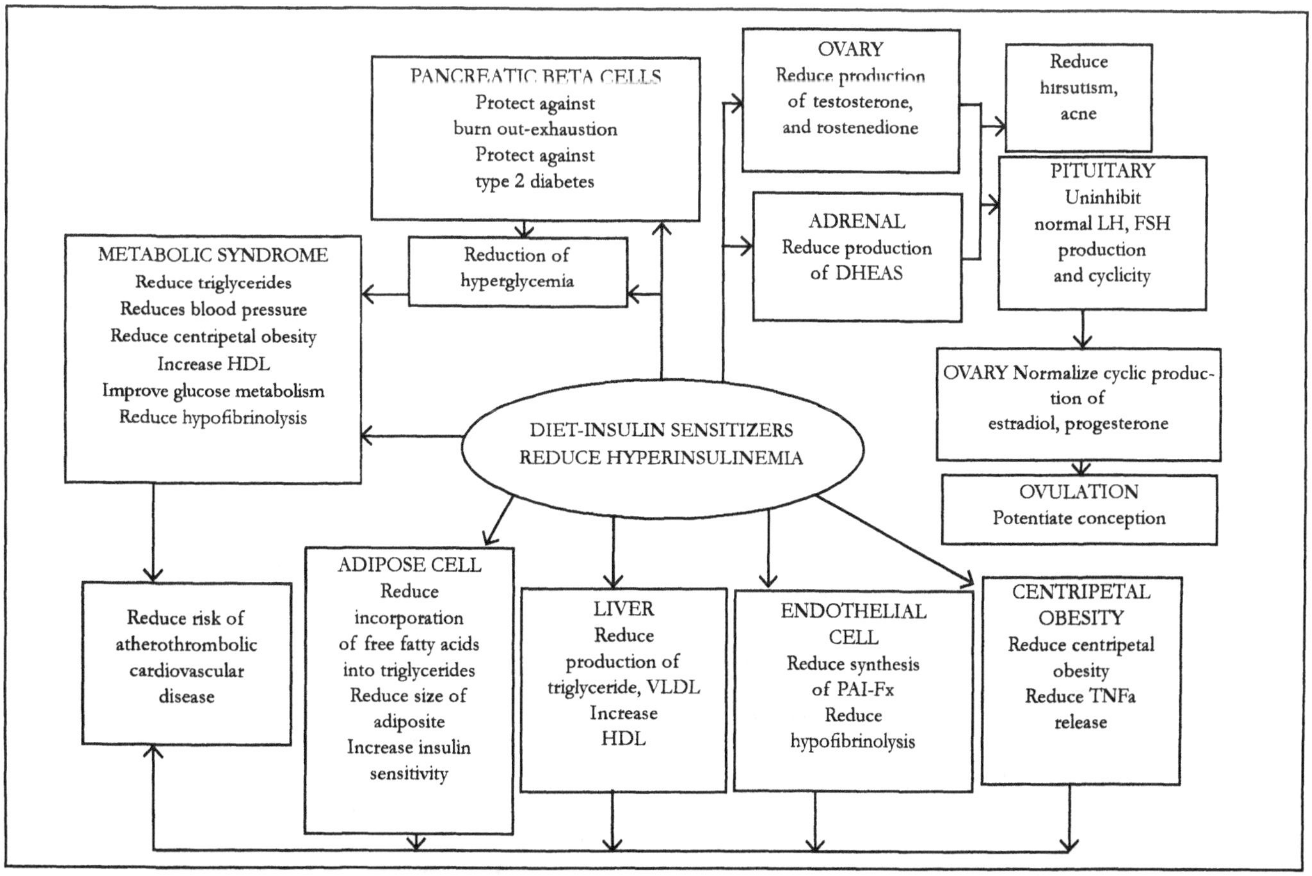

Figure 5. Clinical and biochemical outcomes of treatment of polycystic ovary syndrome with insulin-sensitizing drugs.

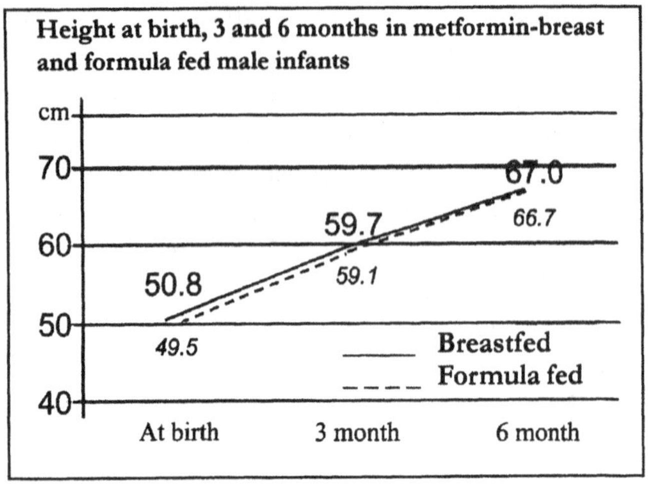

Figure 6. **Height at birth, 3, and 6 months in metformin-breast (n=21) and formula-fed (n=19) male infants born to mothers with PCOS who continued metformin throughout pregnancy.**

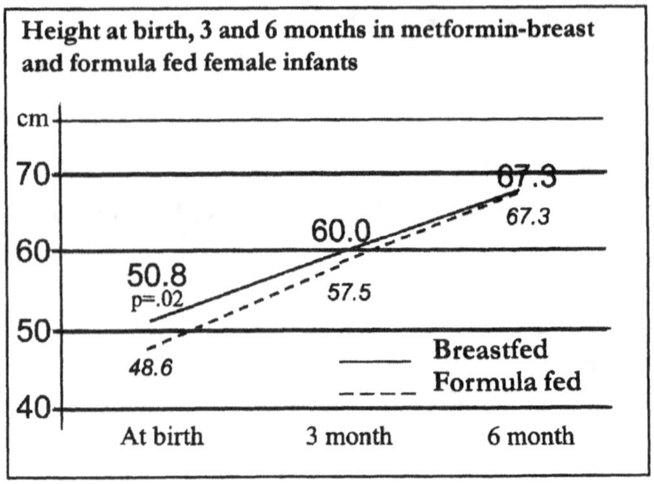

Figure 7. **Height at birth, 3, and 6 months in metformin-breast (n=40) and formula-fed (n=30) female infants born to mothers with PCOS who continued metformin throughout pregnancy.**

2004). Pioglitazone and rosiglitazone both reduce hyperinsulinemia and its sequelae in PCOS, but, unlike metformin, are generally weight neutral, or even promote weight gain. The safety of thiazolidinediones in pregnancy is not documented, nor is its safety during lactation. Based on currently published data, thiazolidinediones should be stopped when pregnancy is first documented and should not be used during lactation. We have had ten women with PCOS conceive while taking combined metformin-pioglitazone without adverse maternal or fetal outcomes, but the pioglitazone was stopped immediately after conception (Glueck *et al*, personal communication, 2005). When metformin alone does not successfully ameliorate PCOS, addition of pioglitazone (Glueck *et al*, 2003b) or rosiglitazone (Baillargeon *et al.*, 2004; 2005; Cataldo *et al.*, 2001) will ameliorate PCOS by providing incremental reversal of insulin resistance.

LACTATION

Metformin is increasingly used during pregnancy in women with PCOS (Glueck *et al.*, 2004b; 2004c; Jakubowicz *et al.*, 2002; Vanky *et al.*, 2004) because it promotes regular ovulation and conception, reduces

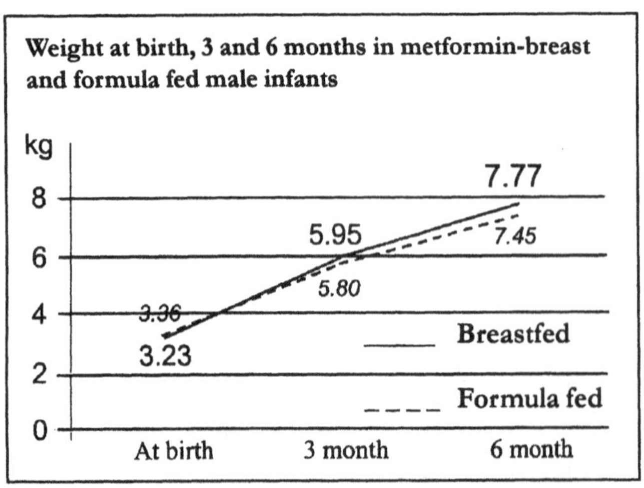

Figure 8. **Weight (kg) at birth, 3, and 6 months in metformin-breast (n=21) and formula-fed (n=19) male infants born to mothers with PCOS who continued metformin throughout pregnancy.**

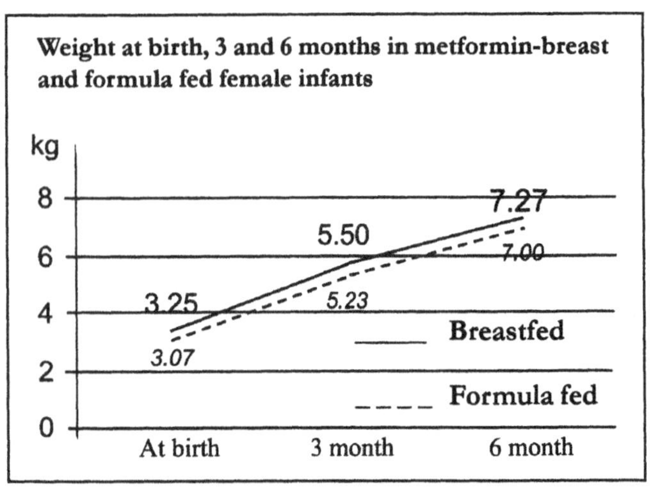

Figure 9. **Weight (kg) at birth, 3, and 6 months in metformin-breast (n=40) and formula-fed (n=31) female infants born to mothers with PCOS who continued metformin throughout pregnancy.**

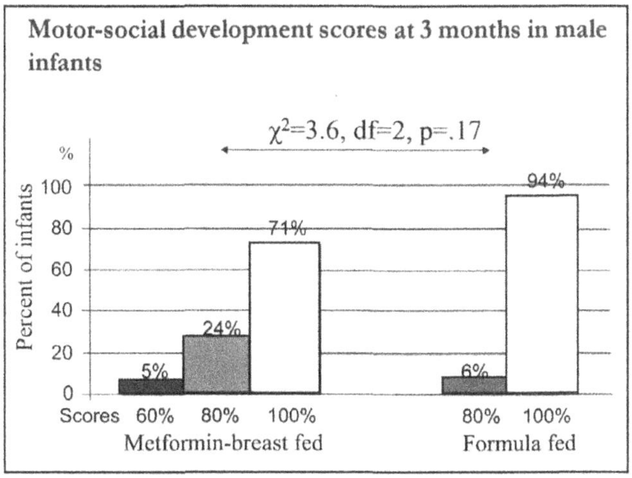

Figure 10. Motor-social development scores at 3 months in male infants, metformin-breast fed (n=21) and formula-fed (n=18). Maximum motor-social development score = 100%.

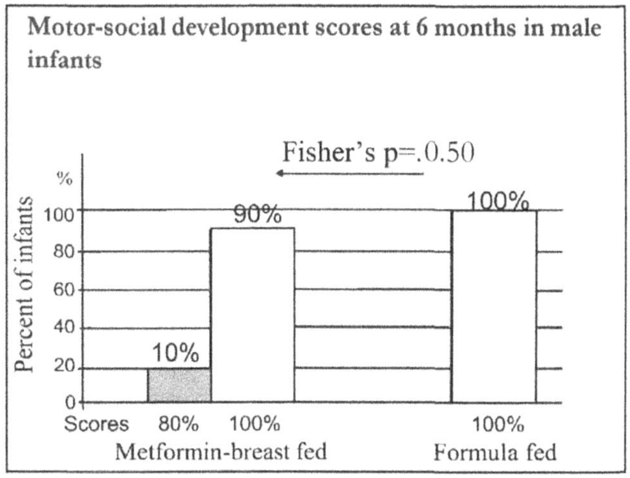

Figure 11. Motor-social development scores at 6 months in male infants, metformin-breast fed (n=21) and formula-fed (n=15). Maximum motor-social development score = 100%.

first trimester miscarriage, gestational diabetes, and macrosomia, and is not, apparently, teratogenic (Coetzee & Jackson, 1979; Glueck *et al.,* 2001a; 2002a; 2002c; 2002d; 2003a; 2004a; 2004b; 2004c; 2004d; Jakubowicz *et al.,* 2002; Vanky *et al.,* 2004). Because metformin ameliorates the endocrinopathy of PCOS (Baillargeon *et al.,* 2003; 2005; Ehrmann, 2005; Glueck *et al.,* 1999a; Velazquez *et al.,* 1994; 1997), it has been continued after delivery during lactation (Glueck *et al.,* 2004b). Metformin has also been used in type 2 diabetics during lactation (Briggs *et al.,* 2005).

Metformin therapy during lactation continues resolution of the endocrinopathy of PCOS (Glueck *et al.,* 1999a; 2004a). Studies available to date and summarized below suggest that metformin is safe and effective for lactating women and their infants. In a pilot study of 30 women with gestational diabetes randomized to insulin or metformin, there were no differences in cord blood c-peptide levels or in neonatal outcomes (Hague et al, 2003). Metformin is excreted into breastmilk (Briggs *et al.,* 2005; Gardiner *et al.,* 2003; 2004; Hale *et al.,* 2002), but in amounts which appear to be clinically insignificant, albeit with only 13 infants very briefly studied and without prospective longitudinal follow-up.

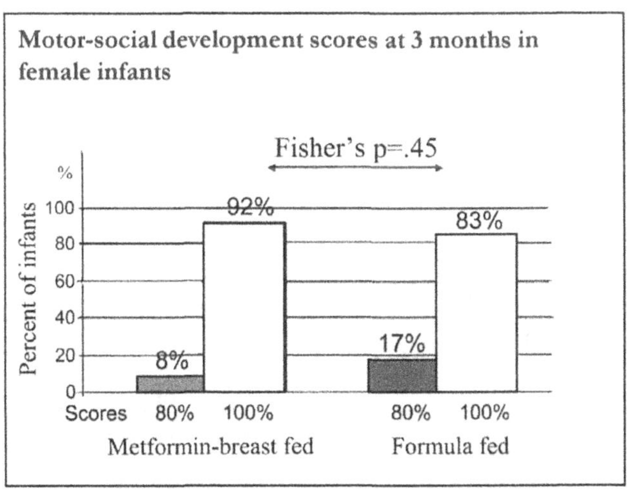

Figure 12. Motor-social development scores at 3 months in female infants, metformin-breast fed (n=37) and formula-fed (n=30). Maximum motor-social development score = 100%.

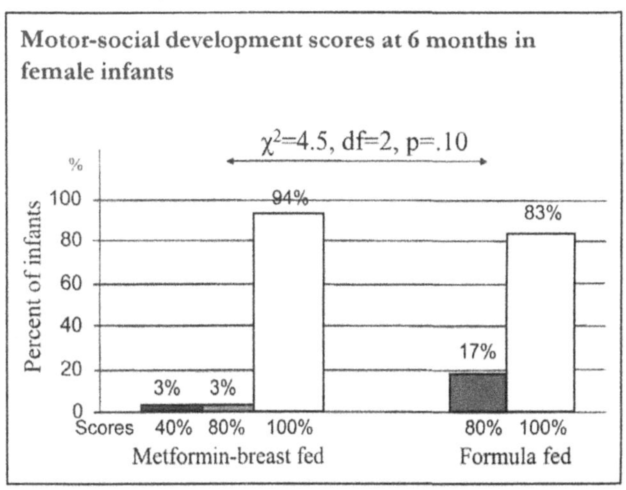

Figure 13. Motor-social development scores at 6 months in female infants, metformin-breast fed (n=36) and formula-fed (n=30). Maximum motor-social development score = 100%.

In three infants whose mothers were taking metformin 1 g/day, blood glucose concentrations four hours after feeding were within normal limits (Briggs *et al.*, 2005). Similarly, metformin does not induce hypoglycemia in adults (Derosa *et al.*, 2004; Glueck *et al.*, 1999a; Velazquez *et al.*, 1994; 1997).

Hale (Hale *et al.*, 2002) evaluated seven women taking metformin 1500 mg/day and four of their infants, finding metformin in very low or undetectable concentrations in their plasma. Hale (Hale *et al.*, 2002) found no "health problems" in the six infants who were evaluated. Gardiner (Gardiner *et al.*, 2004), reviewing metformin therapy and diabetes in pregnancy, concluded "...we believe that there is sufficient evidence for metformin to be considered a safe therapeutic option in the treatment of diabetes or polycystic ovary syndrome in breastfeeding mothers, with the usual caveat of weighing up the risk-benefit ratio in each case." Simons (Simmons *et al.*, 2004), also assessing metformin therapy and diabetes in pregnancy, noted "...in some circumstances (e.g., severe insulin resistance), metformin therapy during pregnancy may be warranted."

In our recent (Glueck *et al*, 2006) large, six month prospective study of 61 breastfed and 50 formula-fed infants born to 92 PCOS mothers, all of whom took metformin throughout pregnancy, our hypothesis was that PCOS women's metformin treatment during lactation, compared to formula, would be both safe and effective for infants, having no adverse effects on infants' growth, motor and social development, and development of intercurrent illness at ages three and six months. Growth, motor-social development, and intercurrent illnesses were prospectively studied at ages three and six months in 111 infants, 61 breastfed and 50 formula-fed (**Figures 6-13**), born to 92 metformin-treated PCOS women, who had taken metformin (1.5-2.55 g/day) throughout pregnancy (Glueck *et al.*, 2004a; 2004b; 2004c) and continued metformin (1.5-2.55 g/day) during lactation (Glueck *et al*, 2006). The simple, descriptive 1993 American Academy of Pediatrics motor and social development questionnaire (Pediatrics, 1993) was completed by the infant's parents at well-baby visits at three and six months and reviewed in detail with the pediatricians and with a principal investigator. At months three and six, the Academy's questionnaire (Pediatrics, 1993) included five questions. Each question was given an equivalent score of one, and entirely normal motor and social development had a score of 100% (**Figures 10-13**). At three and six months, history was taken of any intercurrent illness requiring a visit to a pediatrician in the antecedent three months. We had previously reported that maternal metformin use throughout pregnancy did not have adverse effects on infants' height, weight, and motor and social development during the first 18 months of life (Glueck *et al.*, 2004b). However, our previous prospective studies did not separate and compare breastfed and bottle-fed infants, as has our most recent study (Glueck *et al*, 2006).

During lactation, the mean ±SD and median maternal metformin dose was 2.2 ±0.5 and 2.55 g/day (Glueck *et al.*, 2006). Within gender, at three and six months of age, weight and height and motor-social development did not differ between breastfed and formula-fed infants (**Figures 6-9**) (Glueck *et al.*, 2006). No infants were identified by their pediatricians as having retardation of growth or of motor-social development (Glueck *et al.*, 2006). Mean motor-social development scores ranged from 93% to 100% at three and six months, and within gender, did not differ between breastfed and formula-fed infants (**Figures 10-13**). Neither the mode of feeding (breast, formula) nor gestational week at birth were significant explanatory variables for height or weight at ages three and six months (Glueck *et al.*, 2006). There was no difference in the development of any intercurrent illnesses requiring a pediatrician visit, occurring in 22% of formula fed and 30% of breastfed infants by three months ($p = 0.4$), and in 34% of formula-fed and 46% of breastfed infants by six months ($p = 0.2$) (Glueck *et al.*, 2006).

Our recent prospective study (Glueck *et al.*, 2006) and other small, short-term studies of metformin in breastmilk (Briggs *et al.*, 2005; Gardiner *et al.*, 2003; 2004; Hale *et al.*, 2002) suggest that metformin can safely be used during lactation, whether in women with type 2 diabetes (Briggs *et al.*, 2005; Coetzee *et al.*, 1979; Gardiner *et al.*, 2003; 2004; Hale *et al.*, 2002), or continued during lactation in women with PCOS who had taken metformin throughout pregnancy.

References

Adams JM, Taylor AE, Crowley WF Jr, Hall JE. Polycystic ovarian morphology with regular ovulatory cycles: insights into the pathophysiology of polycystic ovarian syndrome. *J Clin Endocrinol Metab.* 2004; 89:4343-50.

American Academy of Pediatrics. Your child's growth: developmental milestones. AAP Pamphlet 1-3. 1993.

Araya AV, Aguirre A, Romero C, Miranda C, Molina MC, Ferreira A. Evaluation of tumor necrosis factor alpha production in ex vivo short term cultured whole blood from women with polycystic ovary syndrome. *Eur Cytokine Netw.* 2002; 13:419-24.

Baillargeon JP, Iuorno MJ, Nestler JE. Insulin sensitizers for polycystic ovary syndrome. *Clin Obstet Gynecol.* 2003; 46:325-40.

Baillargeon JP, Jakubowicz DJ, Iuomo MJ, Jakubowicz S, Nestler JE. Effects of metformin and rosiglitazone, alone and in combination, in nonobese women with polycystic ovary syndrome and normal indices of insulin sensitivity. *Obstet Gynecol Surv.* 2005; 60:178-79.

Baillargeon JP, Jakubowicz DJ, Iuorno MJ, Jakubowicz S, Nestler JE. Effects of metformin and rosiglitazone, alone and in combination, in nonobese women with polycystic ovary syndrome and normal indices of insulin sensitivity. *Fertil Steril.* 2004; 82:893-902.

Brettenthaler N, De Geyter C, Huber PR, Keller U. Effect of the insulin sensitizer pioglitazone on insulin resistance, hyperandrogenism, and ovulatory dysfunction in women with polycystic ovary syndrome. *J Clin Endocrinol Metab.* 2004; 89:3835-40.

Briggs GG, Ambrose PJ, Nageotte MP, Padilla G, Wan S. Excretion of metformin into breast milk and the effect on nursing infants. *Obstet Gynecol.* 2005; 105:1437-41.

Buchanan TA, Xiang AH, Peters RK, Kjos SL, Marroquin A, *et al.* Preservation of pancreatic beta-cell function and prevention of type 2 diabetes by pharmacological treatment of insulin resistance in high-risk hispanic women. *Diabetes.* 2002; 51:2796-2803.

Bulgan Kilicdag E, Bagis T, Zeyneloglu HB, Tarim E, Aslan E, *et al.* Homocysteine levels in women with polycystic ovary syndrome treated with metformin versus rosiglitazone: a randomized study. *Hum Reprod.* 2005; 20(4):894-99. Epub 2004 Dec 23.

Cataldo NA, Abbasi F, McLaughlin TL, Lamendola C, Reaven GM. Improvement in insulin sensitivity followed by ovulation and pregnancy in a woman with polycystic ovary syndrome who was treated with rosiglitazone. *Fertil Steril.* 2001; 76:1057-59.

Coetzee EJ, Jackson WP. Diabetes newly diagnosed during pregnancy: A 4-year study at Groote Schuur Hospital. *S Afr Med J.* 1979; 56:467-75.

Coffler MS, Patel K, Dahan MH, Yoo RY, Malcom PJ, *et al.* Enhanced granulosa cell responsiveness to follicle-stimulating hormone during insulin infusion in women with polycystic ovary syndrome treated with pioglitazone. *J Clin Endocrinol Metab.* 2003; 88:5624-31.

De Leo V, la Marca A, Petraglia F. Insulin-lowering agents in the management of polycystic ovary syndrome. *Endocr Rev.* 2003; 24:633-67.

Derosa G, Franzetti I, Gadaleta G, Ciccarelli L, Fogari R. Metabolic variations with oral antidiabetic drugs in patients with Type 2 diabetes: comparison between glimepiride and metformin. *Diabetes Nutr Metab.* 2004; 17:143-50.

Ehrmann DA. Polycystic ovary syndrome. *N Engl J Med.* 2005; 352:1223-36.

Engeli S, Schling P, Gorzelniak K, Boschmann M, Janke J, Ailhaud G, *et al.* The adipose-tissue renin-angiotensin-aldosterone system: role in the metabolic syndrome? *Int J Biochem Cell Biol.* 2003; 35:807-25.

Gardiner SJ, Begg, EJ, Kirkpatrick CM, Buckham RB. Metformin therapy and diabetes in pregnancy. *Med J Aust* 2004; 181:174-75; author reply 175.

Gardiner SJ, Kirkpatrick CM, Begg EJ, Zhang M, Moore MP, *et al.* Transfer of metformin into human milk. *Clin Pharmacol Ther.* 2003; 73:71-77.

Glueck CJ. Normal pregnancies in women with PCOS who conceived while taking pioglitzone-metformin. Personal observation. 2005.

Glueck CJ, Bornovali S, Pranikoff J, Goldenberg N, Dharashivkar S, *et al.* Metformin, pre-eclampsia, and pregnancy outcomes in women with polycystic ovary syndrome. *Diabet Med.* 2004a; 21:829-36.

Glueck CJ, Dharashivkar S, Wang P, Zhu B, Gartside PS, *et al.* Obesity and extreme obesity, manifest by ages 20-24 years, continuing through 32-41 years in women, should alert physicians to the diagnostic likelihood of polycystic ovary syndrome as a reversible underlying endocrinopathy. *Eur J Obstet Gynecol Reprod Biol.* 2005; 122:206-12.

Glueck CJ, Goldenberg N, Pranikoff J, Loftspring M, Sieve L, *et al.* Height, weight, and motor-social development during the first 18 months of life in 126 infants born to 109 mothers with polycystic ovary syndrome who conceived on and continued metformin through pregnancy. *Hum Reprod.* 2004b; 19:1323-30.

Glueck CJ, Goldenberg N, Streicher P, Wang P. The contentious nature of gestational diabetes: diet, insulin, glyburide and metformin. *Expert Opin Pharmacother.* 2002a; 3:1557-68.

Glueck CJ, Goldenberg N, Streicher P, Wang P. Metformin and gestational diabetes. *Curr Diab Rep.* 2003a; 3:303-12.

Glueck CJ, Goldenberg N, Wang P, Loftspring M, Sherman A. Metformin during pregnancy reduces insulin, insulin resistance, insulin secretion, weight, testosterone and development of gestational diabetes: prospective longitudinal assessment of women with polycystic ovary syndrome from preconception throughout pregnancy. *Hum Reprod.* 2004c; 19:510-21.

Glueck CJ, Moreira A, Goldenberg N, Sieve L, Wang P. Pioglitazone and metformin in obese women with polycystic ovary syndrome not optimally responsive to metformin. *Hum Reprod.* 2003b; 18:1618-25.

Glueck CJ, Phillips H, Cameron D, Sieve-Smith L, Wang P. Continuing metformin throughout pregnancy in women with polycystic ovary syndrome appears to safely reduce first-trimester spontaneous abortion: a pilot study. *Fertil Steril.* 2001a; 75:46-52.

Glueck CJ, Salehi M, Sieve L, Wang P. Growth, motor, and social development in breast and formula fed infants of metformin treated women with polycystic ovary syndrome. *J Pediatr.* 2006; 148:628-32.

Glueck CJ, Streicher P, Wang P. Treatment of polycystic ovary syndrome with insulin-lowering agents. *Expert Opin Pharmacother.* 2002b; 3:1177-89.

Glueck CJ, Wang P, Fontaine R, Tracy T, Sieve-Smith L. Metformin-induced resumption of normal menses in 39 of 43 (91%) previously amenorrheic women with the polycystic ovary syndrome. *Metabolism.* 1999a; 48:511-19.

Glueck CJ, Wang P, Fontaine R, Tracy T, Sieve-Smith L. Metformin to restore normal menses in oligo-amenorrheic teenage girls with polycystic ovary syndrome (PCOS). *J Adolesc Health.* 2001b; 29:160-69.

Glueck CJ, Wang P, Fontaine RN, Sieve-Smith L, Tracy T, *et al.* Plasminogen activator inhibitor activity: an independent risk factor for the high miscarriage rate during pregnancy in women with polycystic ovary syndrome. *Metabolism.* 1999b; 48:1589-95.

Glueck CJ, Wang P, Goldenberg N, Sieve-Smith L. Pregnancy outcomes among women with polycystic ovary syndrome treated with metformin. *Hum Reprod.* 2002c; 17:2858-64.

Glueck CJ, Wang P, Goldenberg N, Sieve L. Pregnancy loss, polycystic ovary syndrome, thrombophilia, hypofibrinolysis, enoxaparin, metformin. *Clin Appl Thromb Hemost.* 2004d; 10:323-34.

Glueck CJ, Wang P, Kobayashi S, Phillips H, Sieve-Smith, L. Metformin therapy throughout pregnancy reduces the development of gestational diabetes in women with polycystic ovary syndrome. *Fertil Steril.* 2002d; 77:520-25.

Goodfriend TL, Kelley DE, Goodpaster BH, Winters SJ. Visceral obesity and insulin resistance are associated with plasma aldosterone levels in women. *Obes Res.* 1999; 7:355-62.

Guido M, Romualdi D, Suriano R, Giuliani M, Costantini B, *et al.* Effect of pioglitazone treatment on the adrenal androgen response to corticotrophin in obese patients with polycystic ovary syndrome. *Hum Reprod.* 2004; 19:534-39.

Gyongyosi M, Glogar D, Weidinger F, Domanovits H, Laggner A, *et al.* Association between plasmin activation system and intravascular ultrasound signs of plaque instability in patients with unstable angina and non-st-segment elevation myocardial infarction. *Am Heart J.* 2004; 147:158-64.

Hague WM, Davoren PM, Oliver J, Rowan J. Contraindications to use of metformin. Metformin may be useful in gestational diabetes. *BMJ.* 2003; 326:762.

Hale TW, Kristensen JH, Hackett LP, Kohan R, Ilett KF. Transfer of metformin into human milk. *Diabetologia.* 2002; 45:1509-14.

Hardiman P, Pillay OC, Atiomo W. Polycystic ovary syndrome and endometrial carcinoma. *Lancet.* 2003; 361:1810-12.

Homburg R. Polycystic ovary syndrome in adolescence. *Endocr Dev.* 2005; 8:137-49.

Iuorno MJ, Nestler JE. Insulin-lowering drugs in polycystic ovary syndrome. *Obstet Gynecol Clin North Am.* 2001; 28:153-64.

Jakubowicz DJ, Iuorno MJ, Jakubowicz S, Roberts KA, Nestler JE. Effects of metformin on early pregnancy loss in the polycystic ovary syndrome. *J Clin Endocrinol Metab.* 2002; 87:524-29.

Kaiser T, Schunkert H. [Cardiovascular changes in obesity]. *Herz.* 2001; 26:194-201.

Knochenhauer ES, Key TJ, Kahsar-Miller M, Waggoner W, Boots LR, *et al.* Prevalence of the polycystic ovary syndrome in unselected black and white women of the southeastern United States: a prospective study. *J Clin Endocrinol Metab.* 1998; 83:3078-82.

Kumari AS, Haq A, Jayasundaram R, Abdel-Wareth LO, Al Haija SA, *et al.* Metformin monotherapy in lean women with polycystic ovary syndrome. *Reprod Biomed Online.* 2005; 10:100-104.

Lord J, Wilkin T. Metformin in polycystic ovary syndrome. *Curr Opin Obstet Gynecol.* 2004; 16:481-86.

Lord JM, Flight IH, Norman RJ. Insulin-sensitising drugs (metformin, troglitazone, rosiglitazone, pioglitazone, D-chiro-inositol) for polycystic ovary syndrome. *Cochrane Database Syst Rev.* 2003; 3:CD003053.

Mehta RV, Patel KS, Coffler MS, Dahan MH, Yoo RY, *et al.* Luteinizing hormone secretion is not influenced by insulin infusion in women with polycystic ovary syndrome despite improved insulin sensitivity during pioglitazone treatment. *J Clin Endrocrinol Metab.* 2005; 90: 2136-41.

Nestler JE. Insulin regulation of human ovarian androgens. *Hum Reprod.* 1997a; 12 Suppl. 1:53-62.

Nestler JE. Role of hyperinsulinemia in the pathogenesis of the polycystic ovary syndrome, and its clinical implications. *Semin Reprod Endocrinol.* 1997b; 15:111-22.

Nestler JE. Obesity, insulin, sex steroids and ovulation. *Int J Obes Relat Metab Disord.* 2000; 24 Suppl 2:S71-73.

Nestler JE. Insulin resistance syndrome and polycystic ovary syndrome. *Endocr Pract.* 2003; 9 Suppl 2:86-89.

Nestler JE, Clore JN, Blackard WG. The central role of obesity (hyperinsulinemia) in the pathogenesis of the polycystic ovary syndrome. *Am J Obstet Gynecol.* 1989; 161:1095-97.

Nestler JE, Jakubowicz DJ, de Vargas AF, Brik C, Quintero N, *et al.* Insulin stimulates testosterone biosynthesis by human thecal cells from women with polycystic ovary syndrome by activating its own receptor and using inositolglycan mediators as the signal transduction system. *J Clin Endocrinol Metab.* 1998; 83:2001-05.

Norman RJ, Davies MJ, Lord J, Moran LJ. The role of lifestyle modification in polycystic ovary syndrome. *Trends Endocrinol Metab.* 2002; 13:251-57.

Olszanecka-Glinianowicz M, Zahorska-Markiewicz B, Jochemczyk-Banek U, Banas M, Zurakowski A. [Sibutramine administration in polycystic ovary syndrome treatment]. *Ginekol Pol.* 2004; 75:470-74.

Orio F Jr, Palomba S, Cascella T, Di Biase S, Manguso F, *et al.* The increase of leukocytes as a new putative marker of low-grade chronic inflammation and early cardiovascular risk in polycystic ovary syndrome. *J Clin Endocrinol Metab.* 2005; 90:2-5.

Ortega-Gonzalez C, Cardoza L, Coutino B, Hidalgo R, Arteaga-Troncoso G, *et al.* Insulin sensitizing drugs increase the endogenous dopaminergic tone in obese insulin-resistant women with polycystic ovary syndrome. *J Endocrinol.* 2005; 184:233-39.

Ortega-Gonzalez C, Luna S, Hernandez L, Crespo G, Aguayo P, *et al.* Responses of serum androgen and insulin resistance to metformin and pioglitazone in obese, insulin-resistant women with polycystic ovary syndrome. *J Clin Endocrinol Metab.* 2005; 90:1360-65. Epub 2004 Dec 14.

Radon PA, McMahon MJ, Meyer WR. Impaired glucose tolerance in pregnant women with polycystic ovary syndrome. *Obstet Gynecol.* 1999; 94:194-97.

Romualdi D, Guido M, Ciampelli M, Giuliani M, Leoni F, *et al.* Selective effects of pioglitazone on insulin and androgen abnormalities in normo- and hyperinsulinaemic obese patients with polycystic ovary syndrome. *Hum Reprod.* 2003; 18:1210-18.

Rotterdam ESHRE/ASRM-Sponsored PCOS Consensus Workshop Group. Revised 2003 consensus on diagnostic criteria and long-term health risks related to polycystic ovary syndrome. *Fertil Steril.* 2004a; 81:19-25.

Rotterdam ESHRE/ASRM-Sponsored PCOS Consensus Workshop Group. Revised 2003 consensus on diagnostic criteria and long-term health risks related to polycystic ovary syndrome (PCOS). *Hum Reprod.* 2004b; 19:41-47.

Seli E, Duleba AJ. Treatment of PCOS with metformin and other insulin-sensitizing agents. *Curr Diab Rep.* 2004; 4:69-75.

Simmons D, Walters BN, Rowan JA, McIntyre HD. Metformin therapy and diabetes in pregnancy. *Med J Aust.* 2004; 180:462-64.

Slowinska-Srzednicka J, Zgliczynski S, Wierzbicki M, Srzednicki M, Stopinska-Gluszak U, *et al.* The role of hyperinsulinemia in the development of lipid disturbances in nonobese and obese women with the polycystic ovary syndrome. *J Endocrinol Invest.* 1991; 14:569-75.

Stein IF, Leventhal ML. Amenorrhea associated with bilateral polycystic ovaries. *Am J Obstet Gynecol.* 1935; 29:181-91.

Talbott E, Clerici A, Berga SL, Kuller L, Guzick D, *et al.* Adverse lipid and coronary heart disease risk profiles in young women with polycystic ovary syndrome: results of a case-control study. *J Clin Epidemiol.* 1998; 51:415-22.

Talbott E, Guzick D, Clerici A, Berga S, Detre K, *et al.* Coronary heart disease risk factors in women with polycystic ovary syndrome. *Arterioscler Thromb Vasc Biol.* 1995; 15:821-26.

Talbott EO, Guzick DS, Sutton-Tyrrell K, McHugh-Pemu KP, Zborowski JV, *et al.* Evidence for association between polycystic ovary syndrome and premature carotid atherosclerosis in middle-aged women. *Arterioscler Thromb Vasc Biol.* 2000; 20:2414-21.

Talbott EO, Zborowski JV, Boudreaux MY, McHugh-Pemu KP, Sutton-Tyrrell K, *et al.* The relationship between C-reactive protein and carotid intima-media wall thickness in middle-aged women with polycystic ovary syndrome. *J Clin Endocrinol Metab.* 2004a; 89:6061-67.

Talbott EO, Zborowski JV, Rager JR, Boudreaux MY, Edmundowicz DA, *et al.* Evidence for an association between metabolic cardiovascular syndrome and coronary and aortic calcification among women with polycystic ovary syndrome. *J Clin Endocrinol Metab.* 2004b; 89:5454-61.

Talbott EO, Zborowski JV, Sutton-Tyrrell K, McHugh-Pemu, KP, Guzick DS. Cardiovascular risk in women with polycystic ovary syndrome. *Obstet Gynecol Clin North Am.* 2001; 28:111-33.

Talbott EO, Zborowskii JV, Boudraux MY. Do women with polycystic ovary syndrome have an increased risk of cardiovascular disease? Review of the evidence. *Minerva Ginecol.* 2004c; 56:27-39.

Vanky E, Salvesen KA, Heimstad R, Fougner KJ, Romundstad P, *et al.* Metformin reduces pregnancy complications without affecting androgen levels in pregnant polycystic ovary syndrome women: results of a randomized study. *Hum Reprod.* 2004; 19:1734-40.

Velazquez EM, Mendoza S, Hamer T, Sosa F, Glueck CJ. Metformin therapy in polycystic ovary syndrome reduces hyperinsulinemia, insulin resistance, hyperandrogenemia, and systolic blood pressure, while facilitating normal menses and pregnancy. *Metabolism.* 1994; 43:647-54.

Velazquez EM, Mendoza SG, Wang P, Glueck CJ. Metformin therapy is associated with a decrease in plasma plasminogen activator inhibitor-1, lipoprotein(a), and immunoreactive insulin levels in patients with the polycystic ovary syndrome. *Metabolism.* 1997; 46:454-57.

Wood JR, Nelson-Degrave VL, Jansen E, McAllister JM, Mosselman S, *et al.* Valproate-induced alterations in human theca cell gene expression: clues to the association between valproate use and metabolic side effects. *Physiol Genomics.* 2005; 20:233-43.

Chapter 18

Management of Lactation in the Puerperium

Pamela Berens

INTRODUCTION

Optimal management of lactation begins well before the puerperium. The well prepared mother will have received anticipatory guidance during the pregnancy to assist her in making well informed decisions regarding hospital routines which can subsequently impact lactation. Ideal management of the healthy mother-infant dyad includes practices such as skin to skin contact at the time of delivery, transitioning the well baby in the delivery room with the family, early initiation of breastfeeding, and the avoidance or postponement of elective procedures, such as tubal ligation sterilization procedures during the immediate postpartum period.

The puerperium is defined as the time from delivery of the infant through approximately six to eight weeks postpartum. Many physiologic changes return to a condition similar to pre-pregnancy during this time, though some changes are more gradual and continue well beyond eight weeks after delivery. Other pregnancy changes never truly revert back to their pre-pregnant state.

IMPACT OF PAIN MANAGEMENT

Some concerns regarding lactation are more common during the early puerperium than others, which more typically arise later during lactation. Early in the puerperium, the effects of various labor and delivery routines may linger and potentially impact lactation. All presently used medical methods of pain relief during labor have potential effects on the breastfeeding dyad. Unmedicated birth has the least adverse impact on successful lactation; however, not all mothers choose to have an unmedicated birth. The health care provider should be aware of the potential impact of different forms of labor pain control on lactation and avoid imposing additional risks to successful breastfeeding with the addition of unnecessary routines. An example of this might be unnecessarily delaying skin-to-skin contact or early initiation of breastfeeding due to the use of a particular analgesia/anesthesia. It is also important for the care provider to remain optimistic regarding the mother's success with breastfeeding despite her choice to have a medicated labor (**Table 1**).

Table 1. Best Practices for Breastfeeding Support in the Delivery Suite.

- Limit unnecessary invasive procedures during labor and delivery.
- Encourage participation of significant other / companionship during the birthing process.
- Initiate skin-to-skin contact at delivery. Allow uninterrupted maternal-infant contact in first hour of life.
- Delay routine newborn procedures, such as vitamin K injection, eye ointment, infant bath, until after initial maternal-infant contact (1st hour).
- Encourage breastfeeding within first hour of delivery.
- Transition newborn in delivery room with family.

LABOR SUPPORT

The support of a doula or trained labor coach during childbirth has been associated with increased rates of breastfeeding initiation and improved exclusivity (Scott *et al.*, 1999; Langer *et al.*, 1998; Hoymeyr *et al.*, 1991). Langer *et al.* performed a randomized trial in 724 Mexican women and found that the doula supported group had better exclusive breastfeeding rates at one month (12% verses 7%). Hofmeyr similarly found an improved exclusive breastfeeding rate at six weeks postpartum in women who received labor companionship (51% verses 29%). A systematic review in the Cochrane database found that continuous labor support of the expectant mother resulted in a reduced likelihood of requiring pain medications (Hodnett *et al.*, 2003). Doula support also increases breastfeeding rates during the initial postpartum period. Barron *et al.* provided doula support in the initial two week period after delivery to 41 low income first time mothers and found an increased mean duration of breastfeeding in those women receiving doula support (23.4 weeks verses 12.3 weeks) (Barron *et al.*, 1988).

Narcotic Analgesia

The use of intravenous narcotics has a potential negative effect on infant state and suckling behavior in addition to potentially delaying breastfeeding initiation. A small study done by Crowell *et al.* compared the time to first effective breastfeeding of the newborn in the first 48 hours of life using the IBFAT (Infant Breast-feeding Assessment Tool)(Crowell et al., 1994). This tool scores four behaviors on a 0-3 point scale with a maximal score of 12. Infants from 26 mothers who received either butorphanol (Stadol®) or nalbuphine (Nubain®) in labor were compared to 22 infants whose mothers received no labor analgesia. The time to first effective breastfeeding (defined as three consecutive IBFAT scores of 10-12) was 46.5 hours in the analgesia group compared to 35.4 hours in the no analgesia group. This eleven hour difference was not statistically significant. An additional interesting finding of this study was that the group of infants delivered to mothers receiving analgesia less than one hour prior to delivery had a similar mean time to effective feeding (34.4 hours) as the group not receiving analgesia.

Another researcher did a similar study assessing time to effective feed with the IBFAT tool comparing alphaprodine (Nisentil®) to a non-medicated group (Matthews, 1988). This study found that the narcotic delayed the time to effective feeding by approximately six hours. The unmedicated mothers' infants established effective feeding at a mean of 10.88 hours compared to 16.95 hours (defined as the first of three consecutive IBFAT scores of 10-12). Again, this did not reach statistical significance and no difference was found in the subgroup of infants whose mothers received the narcotic within one hour of delivery and the unmedicated group. Mothers who received the narcotic between one and three hours prior to delivery had infants who required longer time after delivery to achieve effective feeding by the IBFAT tool.

Nissen *et al.* studied the use of 100 mg of pethidine (meperidine) intramuscularly in 13 primiparous women in labor (Nissen *et al.*, 1977). Infants of mothers who had received the narcotic between 1.1 and 5.3 hours prior to delivery had depressed sucking behavior compared to those whose mothers had received the drug between 8.1 and 9.9 hours prior to delivery. Rajan also noted the use of pethidine in labor to be adversely associated with breastfeeding success six weeks post-delivery in a subset analysis of a questionnaire assessing the impact of obstetrical procedures on breastfeeding (Rajan, 1994). Additional information regarding meperidine used for post-cesarean pain suggests that it has an adverse effect on infant feeding behavior. This will be discussed further in the following section on post-operative pain control.

Epidural Anesthesia

The potential effects of labor anesthesia on breastfeeding success are contentiously debated. Multiple different medications and techniques can be used for labor management, and most studies do not delineate groups based on specific drug regimes. The confounding that results makes comparisons between studies and optimization of knowledge for establishing a best practice difficult. Many researchers have attempted to look at this intervention and the impact it may have on lactation. Some have even attempted unsuccessfully to randomize women to either receiving epidural anesthesia or a non-medicated birth. Population differences may play a significant role as well.

Albani *et al.* found no difference in breastfeeding rates at hospital discharge between those delivering vaginally with epidural anesthesia (96.5%) and those without analgesia (97.8%) (Albani *et al.*, 1999). Riordan *et al.* looked at suckling assessment using the IBFAT. They compared those women delivering vaginally with unmedicated births to those who received either intravenous narcotics or epidural alone to those receiving both (Riordan *et al.*, 2000). The infants of women with unmedicated births had the highest mean score (11.1). Those with intravenous narcotics alone had a mean score of 8.5, the same as did those with an epidural only. Infants exposed to both narcotics and epidural during labor had the lowest mean score at 6.4. Interestingly, there was no difference in breastfeeding rates between medicated and unmedicated births at six weeks postpartum with 72% continuing to breastfeed. Those dyads with low IBFAT scores (0-4) did wean earlier than those with higher scores.

An observational study performed by Halpern *et al.* enrolled women intending to breastfeed with complete data available on 171 patients (Halpern *et al.*, 1999). Fifty-nine percent received epidural anesthesia: 79 via combined spinal epidural (CSE) and 34 via epidural. At six weeks postpartum, 72% were fully breastfeeding and 20% continued to partially breastfed. There was no correlation noted between labor analgesia and breastfeeding success. In subgroup analysis, this study did delineate the agents used in the epidural anesthetic and the duration and timing of exposure. The authors additionally comment that only six participants in the study received parental opiates within five hours of delivery.

Baumgarder *et al.* compared 115 consecutive vaginally delivered dyads receiving epidural anesthesia with 116 that did not receive an epidural (Baumgarder *et al.*, 2003). They assessed the incidence of two successful LATCH scores in the first 24 hours after delivery defined as a score of 7+ on a 10 point scale. This occurred in 69.9% in the epidural group and 81% of the no epidural group, though the finding did not reach statistical significance. The researchers did find that the epidural group did not have fewer attempts at breastfeeding, and there was a trend toward greater likelihood of initiation within an hour of delivery in the epidural group. Despite these findings, there was an increased risk of bottle supplementation in the epidural group. This suggests a different potential association related to epidural anesthesia and breastfeeding success as bottle supplementation in the labor ward itself may account for an important effect.

A study by Radzyminski compared breastfeeding behavior of 56 vaginally delivered dyads using the Premature Infant Breastfeeding Behavior Scale after birth and at 24 hours (Radzminski, 2003). The mothers had received either an epidural using ultra low dose bupivacaine and fentanyl or no pain medication. There was no statistically significant difference between groups in newborn behavior.

Torvaldsen *et al.* conducted a study on breastfeeding in the first week postpartum and cessation during 24 weeks after delivery (Torvaldsen *et al.*, 2006). Women were divided into five categories: 1) non-pharmacologic, 2) nitrous oxide, 3) pethidine (+/- nitrous), 4) epidural (+/- pethidine), (+/- nitrous), and 5) general anesthesia (+/- any 1-4 prior). The breastfeeding rates in this population were high with 93% breastfeeding in the first week and 60% continuing at 24 weeks. Those women receiving epidurals were less likely to be breastfeeding at either time point. The authors found that women in this study with epidurals were more likely to stop breastfeeding than those using non-pharmacologic pain control methods with a hazard ratio of 2.02. Though this data is interesting, it is concerning that woman in the epidural group also received pethidine (a medication previously discussed as potentially adversely impacting lactation). This may cause significant confounding of effects.

IMPACT OF DELIVERY ROUTE

Influence of Cesarean Delivery

Cesarean delivery may add a challenge to breastfeeding success. The impact of cesarean delivery has been researched in different settings with varying results. Again, these differences likely reflect differences in populations and confounding influences which often present in the context of cesarean delivery. Many hospital routines differ for the vaginally delivered dyad compared to those delivered by cesarean. Cesarean may unnecessarily lead to routines which separate mother and infant. Breastfeeding initiation may be delayed, feeding frequency decreased, different anesthetics employed, and additional pain medications and narcotics may be required. In addition to hospital routines, often the maternal or fetal circumstance leading to the decision to deliver by surgical means is itself a risk to successful lactation. The premature infant is more likely to present in labor with malpresentation. The infant who is otherwise ill is more likely to be delivered via cesarean due to evidence suggesting a non-reassuring fetal status. Many underlying factors such as these may lead to cesarean, but also, independently, to breastfeeding adversity. Beyond all of these considerations, the concept of cesarean at patient request is becoming more popularized. The woman who may choose the controlled experience of cesarean by request may have different expectations of motherhood which may also influence her decision and commitment to breastfeeding.

When reviewing literature about cesarean delivery and breastfeeding, it is important to keep all of the above considerations and confounders in mind as well as the particular patient population which is being studied.

A study by Vestermark *et al.* was performed in Denmark with a population in which breastfeeding was a normative behavior (Vestermark *et al.*, 1990). In this cohort study, 231 women spontaneously delivered vaginally (SVD), 37 had vacuum assisted vaginal deliveries (VAVD) and 102 underwent cesarean delivery (CD). There was a delay in the "milk coming in" and an increased use of supplement in the first four days after delivery in the cesarean group. There was, however, no statistical difference in the breastfeeding rate at day four or after discharge. The risk of not breastfeeding on day four was approximately 1% for SVD, 3% for VAVD, and 4% for CD. At six months, 56% of those delivered by SVD and 47% delivered by CD were still breastfeeding. The influence of cesarean delivery may be different in a population with lower breastfeeding rates.

A number of studies suggest that the conditions under which cesarean delivery occurs may be of prognostic importance to breastfeeding success. A Brazilian birth cohort study of 4912 dyads found similar breastfeeding initiation rates between groups of women delivered vaginally (92%), by elective cesarean (92%), or by emergent cesarean (93%) (Victora *et al.*, 1990). However, continuation at six months occurred in 26% of those delivered vaginally, 29% of those undergoing elective cesarean, but only 22% of those who had an emergent cesarean ($p < 0.05$). A study of 100 dyads from India looked at initiation rates only and found that initiation in the elective cesarean group was 65.7% compared to 53.7% for the emergent group (Mathur *et al.*, 1993).

In an attempt to look at some of the influences which may go along with cesarean delivery, Kearney *et al.* evaluated the average time to first breastfeed (Kearney *et al.*, 1990). They evaluated breastfeeding outcomes in 121 primiparas of which 23% were delivered by cesarean. On average, mothers delivered by cesarean first breastfed 11.1 hours after delivery compared to 4.5 hours for the vaginally delivered group. There was, however, no difference in weaning at 12 weeks or six months noted between these groups. Rowe-Murray and Fisher had similar findings in their Australian study of 203 primiparous women (Rowe-Murray & Fisher, 2002). Participants were interviewed at two days postpartum and again at eight months. Twenty-four percent of patients underwent cesarean section which was associated with a delay in breastfeeding initiation ($p < 0.001$). However, there was no statistical difference in continued breastfeeding.

A study by Patel *et al.* looked at the breastfeeding outcome of women who had reached full dilation, but then required either cesarean delivery or instrumented vaginal delivery (Patel *et al.*, 2003). Thus, all of the women in this study had experienced labor. There was no difference in exclusive breastfeeding rates based on method of delivery. Seventy percent of women were exclusively breastfeeding at hospital discharge and 44% at six weeks postpartum. They did find that women delivered by cesarean were more likely to be exclusively breastfeeding at discharge with a longer hospital stay (66% discharged day 0-4 verses 78% discharged day 5+).

One possible mechanism that may influence the impact cesarean delivery has on breastfeeding success involves the possible delay in onset of lactation. The previously mentioned study by Vestermark did not find a difference in breastfeeding success related to cesarean delivery, but did find a delay in onset of lactation and increased use of supplement in the first four days (Vestermark *et al.*, 1990). Other studies have noted similar findings. Grajeda *et al.* evaluated the timing of the onset of lactation (Grajeda & Perez-Escamilla, 2002). This was experienced, on average, on day 2.9 for primiparous women delivered vaginally and on day 3.4 for those delivered by emergent cesarean. For multiparous women, the mode of delivery was not significant with onset of lactation occurring, on average, at day 2.5. Dewey *et al.* followed 280 mother–infant pairs during the first two weeks of life (Dewey *et al.*, 2003). They used the IBFAT and defined suboptimal infant breastfeeding behavior (SIBB) as a score ≤ 10. Infants delivered by cesarean section had both an increased risk of delayed onset of lactation (defined as > 72 hours) and an increased risk of SIBB on day of life zero.

Excessive infant weight loss was defined as ≥ 10% from birth weight by 72-96 hours. Delayed onset of lactation increased the risk of excessive weight loss 7.1 times and SIBB on day of life 0 increased the risk of weight loss 2.6 times. Therefore, cesarean delivery increased the risk of excessive infant weight loss by both mechanisms. Detailed information about specific characteristics is described in this study. This study noted delayed onset of lactation in 16% of women delivered vaginally, 27% delivered by elective cesarean delivery, and 56% of those delivered by urgent cesarean.

Evans *et al.* studied the milk volume transferred to the infant in the first week of life related to cesarean delivery (Evans *et al.*, 2003). Eighty-eight dyads delivered vaginally were compared to 97 delivered by cesarean. Milk transfer was assessed using test weights prior to and after all feeds during the first six days. The first breastfeed occurred at less than one hour in 18.6% of cesarean delivered dyads compared to 64.8% of vaginal deliveries. The mean breastmilk transfer (in mL/kg body weight) was consistently less during days 2-5 for dyads experiencing cesarean delivery compared to vaginal delivery. By day six, there was no difference between groups. As would be expected from the above data, birth weight was regained by day six more commonly for vaginally delivered infants (40%) compared to cesarean delivered infants (20%).

Some research has attempted to evaluate if the delayed onset of lactation which may be associated with cesarean delivery can be overcome. Chapman *et al.* designed a study using a bilateral electric breast pump to provide extra breast stimulation three times daily from 24 to 72 hours after delivery (Chapman *et al.*, 2001). There was no improvement in milk supply found with this technique.

Less information is available about the impact on breastfeeding success from instrumented vaginal delivery. A population birth cohort study from China following 7825 mother-infant pairs did find cesarean delivery to be a risk for both not initiating breastfeeding and shorter breastfeeding duration (Leung *et al.*, 2002). In addition, this study also noted instrumented vaginal delivery with either vacuum or forceps to be a risk for shorter breastfeeding duration, though there was no difference in breastfeeding initiation rates.

The above information suggests that to best support breastfeeding in the patient requiring cesarean delivery, hospital routines should reflect preservation of normal routines which would otherwise surround vaginal delivery. Limit separation of mother and infant to what is medically necessary. Allow the healthy newborn to remain with the mother at the time of cesarean section and in recovery areas. Encourage breastfeeding in the first hours after delivery and assist the new family with techniques that are cognizant of the abdominal incision. Placement of pillows can be done in such a way as to avoid contact between the newborn and the incision during breastfeeding. Often, in the recovery area, the epidural anesthetic is still effective which makes this a comfortable time for learning positioning for breastfeeding. The father or other family members can be instructed on how to help with positioning as well. Rooming-in should be encouraged. Frequent breastfeeding should be recommended as it should be in the setting of a vaginal delivery. If possible, experienced breastfeeding personnel should be available to assist with latch and milk transfer as prior research has suggested that cesarean delivery may put the infant at risk for difficulty with milk transfer and excessive weight loss and the mother at risk for delayed onset of lactation.

Emergent cesarean may put the dyad at even further risk of breastfeeding failure or early cessation. If the infant is otherwise ill or premature, it is important that hospital policy reflect the availability of a breast pump for initiation of pumping soon and frequently after delivery rather than broaching the subject when hospital discharge is anticipated days later and milk supply may be jeopardized.

Anesthesia & Analgesia for Cesarean Delivery

A regional anesthetic is preferred for cesarean delivery which is not emergent and when patient circumstances do not dictate otherwise. Regional anesthesia is preferable for breastfeeding and bonding and is also safer for the mother and infant. The previously mentioned study by Albani found breastfeeding initiation rates to be higher with regional anesthesia (95%) than general anesthesia (85%) (Albani *et al.*, 1999). Similar findings were noted in a small prospective matched study with 96% of those with epidural anesthesia (EA) establishing breastfeeding by day seven compared to 89% of those with general anesthesia (GA) (Lie & Juul, 1988). At three months, the breastfeeding rates were 89% EA and 61% GA ($p=0.025$) and at six months - 71% EA and 39% GA ($p=0.025$).

Various options may be available for post-operative pain control depending on anesthetic expertise in your particular area. Wittles *et al.* (1997) performed a randomized controlled trial involving 47 infants of mothers delivered by cesarean. All mothers received 4 mg of epidural morphine after umbilical cord clamping. They were then randomly assigned to receive meperidine (Demerol®) or morphine by patient controlled analgesia (PCA) intravenous route. The infants were assessed each day during the first four days of life using the Brazelton Neonatal Behavioral Assessment Scale (NBAS). Bottle fed infants were used as the comparison group. Infants in the PCA morphine group were found to be more alert on days three and four than the infants of mothers who were receiving meperidine. In addition, maternal PCA narcotic use was decreased 66-74% with the use of 4 mg of epidural morphine after cord clamping. A recent study compared pain management in 1256 women delivered by cesarean using a visual analogue pain scale and breastfeeding (Yost *et al.*, 2004). The women were separated into four groups based on pain relief: 1) meperidine intramuscularly, 2) PCA meperidine, 3) morphine intramuscularly, and 4) PCA morphine. Women in the morphine group reported less pain. They were also less likely to stop breastfeeding ($p=0.02$) and more likely to room-in with their infants.

Hirose *et al.* performed a randomized trial on 30 dyads receiving spinal anesthesia either with or without continuous infusion of 0.25% bupivacaine for three days after delivery (Hirose *et al.*, 1996). Diclofenac was available if needed for pain in all patients. They found that the group treated with continuous infusion bupivacaine had lower visual analogue pain scales (suggesting better pain control), a higher weight of milk fed to the infant, and a higher infant weight. Measurements of the milk and infants were taken for 11 days after cesarean. A similar study was undertaken by the same author using extradural buprenorphine (an opioid) in addition to the bupivacaine, and this added medication was found to suppress lactation (Hirose *et al.*, 1997).

Particular choices for pain control to optimize successful breastfeeding will continue to depend on safe and available options at the particular facility the practitioner works. Further investigation into the potential impact these choices have on the mother-infant dyad is needed and will ideally shape future care. Regional anesthesia appears to be the optimal choice for the surgical procedure itself in most circumstances. If possible, it appears that the use of regional morphine after cord clamping may reduce later narcotic requirements for the mother. The use of PCA morphine appears to be preferable to meperidine in the initial post-operative period. The mother can then be transitioned to oral codeine derivatives and non-steroidal medications, such as ibuprofen. It also appears to be optimal care to have experienced lactation personnel available to give support and assistance to women undergoing cesarean delivery and to extend the hospital stay if feasible until effective exclusive breastfeeding is established. It is suggested from the literature that infants delivered by cesarean may be at increased risk of excessive weight loss, especially in circumstances where the mother notes delayed onset of lactation. Education about assessing adequacy of milk supply and who to notify if the mother has not experienced her milk coming in by day five may be beneficial. Early infant follow-up after discharge in circumstances where onset of lactation and reversal of the initial trend of infant weight loss have not been experienced prior to hospital discharge is also prudent (**Table 2**).

Table 2. Best Practices for Breastfeeding Support Following Cesarean Delivery

- Early mother-infant contact. Avoidance of separation unless dictated by medical indications
- Early breastfeeding <1 hour after delivery. Can occur in delivery suite or recovery room.
- Regional anesthesia for cesarean delivery.
- Infant positioning to minimize incisional discomfort. Use of side lying or football breastfeeding positions. Use of pillow to protect incision site.
- Use of regional medication after cord clamping to decrease the need for post-operative narcotics
- Preferential use of narcotics with less adverse effects on neonatal behavior, such as morphine rather than meperidine.
- Frequent breastfeeding and rooming-in such as would be routine for vaginal delivery.
- Protocols for early breast pumping, expression if infant separation is dictated due to medical indication, such as prematurity. Should be initiated day of delivery.
- Easy availablilty of lactational expert for further support and assistance if needed.
- Monitoring for delayed onset of lactation in mother and excessive weight loss in the newborn.
- Education and encouragement of family members in methods of supporting breastfeeding in the new family.

MATERNAL HEMORRHAGE

Postpartum hemorrhage (PPH) remains a significant cause of maternal morbidity and mortality. Various factors may predispose women to postpartum hemorrhage, such as an over distended uterus which accompanies multiple gestations or polyhydramnios; disorders which affect clotting, such as pre-eclampsia and the syndrome of hemolysis; low platelets and elevated liver enzymes (HELLP); multiparity; lacerations; prolonged labor; and prior postpartum hemorrhage. The most common cause of PPH is uterine atomy in the immediate postpartum period. Management of this complication frequently involves the use of various uterotonic medications to abate the hemorrhage. Other causes of hemorrhage should be excluded, such as vaginal or cervical lacerations which require surgical repair and retained placental fragments which require removal with possible surgical therapy, such as uterine curettage. Provided the hemorrhage is consistent with atony and uterine massage has been unsuccessful, attention should be given to both medical therapy to cause uterine contraction and minimize further blood loss and supporting maternal hemodynamics with intravenous fluids and possibly blood transfusion. Hemorrhage and hypotension can rarely result in pituitary hypoperfusion with ischemic necrosis and Sheehan's syndrome. This could subsequently result in lactation failure and amenorrhea in addition to other medical complications.

Multiple uterotonic medications are available, such as oxytocin (Pitocin®), ergot alkaloids (Methergine®), and prostaglandins- 15-methyl prostaglandin F2-alpha (Hemabate®), or a prostaglandin E1 analogue (Misoprostol®). Oxytocin is an endogenous nonapeptide hormone naturally produced from the posterior pituitary. It stimulates contraction of uterine muscle and myoepithelial cells in the alveoli of breast tissue in addition to other actions. The half-life of the hormone is quite brief at three to five minutes. Oxytocin has been used as a traditional uterotonic in obstetrics for management of postpartum hemorrhage. Additionally, it has been used for prevention of hemorrhage given near the time of delivery. A recent study by Fujimoto *et al.* found intravenous injection of oxytocin after delivery of the anterior shoulder reduced postpartum blood loss and the frequency of blood loss >500cc (Fujimoto *et al.*, 2006). Choy et *al.* also documented a reduction in postpartum blood loss ($p < 0.001$) with the use of 10 U of intravenous oxytocin after delivery of the anterior shoulder (Choy *et al.*, 2002).

Ergot derivatives, such as ergometrine, have also been found to be effective in prevention and treatment of postpartum hemorrhage. A systemic review comparing oxytocin alone to a combination of oxytocin with ergometrine found the combination to be associated with a small further reduction in postpartum hemorrhage compared to oxytocin alone (McDonald *et al.*, 2004). More side effects were noted, however, with the combination product. Ergot derivatives cause vasoconstriction and should be avoided in the setting of hypertension. The drug is usually administered intramuscularly as the oral absorption is very poor. Breastmilk exposure from a single dose given around the time of delivery is probably minimal. Continued administration during the postpartum period is not typical and breastfeeding in the setting of continued use should be temporarily discouraged. Due to the potential for adverse side effects of ergot derivatives compared to oxytocin, they are often reserved for treatment of postpartum hemorrhage with oxytocin more commonly used for prevention.

Prostaglandin medications have also been used for treatment of postpartum hemorrhage (Lokugmage *et al.*, 2001; O'Brien *et al.*, 1998). Due to the low cost and easy administration, there has been recent enthusiasm for the use of misoprostol for prevention of postpartum hemorrhage, especially in resource poor areas (Derman *et al.*, 2006). Common side effects include chills and fever. Prostaglandin medications have a relatively short half-life: hemabate less than one hour and misoprostol approximately 20-40 minutes. Again, due to the potential side effects, the use of prostaglandin medications in modern maternity settings is primarily reserved for treatment of hemorrhage rather than prevention.

A prospective study compared the use of 200 μg of misoprostol to 250 μg of methylergometrine in lactating women (ten in each group) (Vogel *et al.*, 2004). The study was done postpartum day three to six and breastmilk levels were collected during the initial five hours after the medication was dosed. Milk to plasma ratios were calculated and the ratio for misoprostol was approximately one-third of that for methylergometrine at both one and two hours after the dose. The mean half-life of the misoprostol was 1.1 hours compared to 2.33 hours for the methylergometrine, suggesting that the misoprostol may be cleared from breastmilk much faster. This study suggests that if effectiveness of these medications for managing postpartum hemorrhage is similar, the infant may receive less medication exposure with the use of misoprostol. The finding that misoprostol is cleared from the milk rather quickly is supportive of a prior study looking at breastmilk concentrations in 12 women after a 600 μg dose. This study found that the level of misoprostol in colostrum was negligible (<1 pg/mL) five hours after dosing (Abdel-Aleem *et al.*, 2003). Further study regarding the use of optimal uterotonic medications and their potential impact on both the mother and breastfeeding infant is warranted.

MATERNAL ANEMIA

Insufficient maternal milk supply has anecdotally been reported in situations of maternal hemorrhage, but without resulting Sheehan's syndrome. Ten cases were reported by Willis and Livingstone with maternal blood loss ranging between 500 and 1500 cc (Willis & Livingstone, 1995). All infants in this report were failure to thrive and many had electrolyte abnormalities. Though this does not provide information regarding the frequency of such occurrences related to postpartum hemorrhage, it does suggest that hemorrhage may be a risk factor for establishing an adequate milk supply.

Additionally, information also suggests that the infant of an anemic mother may be at risk for anemia in situations of prolonged, exclusive breastfeeding without the introduction of iron supplementation. Maternal anemia was found to be a risk factor for anemia in the infant at nine months, as was exclusive breastfeeding for greater than six months (Meinzen-Derr *et al.*, 2006).

BREAST ENGORGEMENT

Breast engorgement is a common occurrence in the postpartum period. The literature suggests that few treatments are adequately supported by scientific investigation. The ideal situation in the delivery setting suggests optimal support of early and effective infant feeding as the primary focus of attention in order to prevent the occurrence of severe engorgement. Many nursing mothers will notice some breast discomfort in the early postpartum period. An observational study done by Hill and Humenick noted that 72% of nursing mothers noticed breast tenderness with the peak occurring on day five after delivery (Hill & Humenick, 1994). Some research has suggested the early initiation of breastfeeding and increased cumulative time spent breastfeeding in the first 48 hours after delivery were negatively correlated with subsequent engorgement (Moon & Humenick, 1989). This relationship appeared to be most evident in primiparous women. Interestingly, in this study, the engorgement was also noted to occur later in the women who were delivered by cesarean.

Severe engorgement presents difficulty for breastfeeding mothers, not just due to the associated pain, but also due to the potential problems it may cause with respect to successful infant latch and milk transfer. Unfortunately, there is a large body of scientific research on suppression of lactation, but little research into prevention and treatment of breast engorgement to aid in successful lactation. Different techniques have been suggested in a few studies for the prevention of engorgement, though little research from well designed clinical trials is available to support their use. Some techniques which have been suggested for prevention of engorgement include breast massage, alternate breast emptying (Evans *et al.*, 1995), nipple conditioning (Storr, 1988), prospective counseling regarding proper breastfeeding technique (De Olivera *et al.*, 2006), and cabbage leaves (Nikodem *et al.*, 1993). Neither cabbage leaves nor prospective counseling noted any significant difference in frequency of engorgement between groups. The differences between groups in the other studies were small.

Various treatments for engorgement have also been suggested. Cabbage leaves have been studied for treating engorgement. An unblinded study using cabbage leaves found a difference in pain scale score after treatment with cabbage leaves of 37-38%. This difference was not statistically significant, and there was no difference between treatment groups (either chilled or room temperature cabbage leaves) (Roberts *et al.*, 1995). Another study compared chilled cabbage leaves on one breast to a chilled gel pack on the other (Roberts, 1995). Both treatments reduced pain scores, but there was no significant difference between groups (30% reduction for cabbage and 39% reduction for gel packs). A double blinded study was attempted comparing cabbage leaf extract to a placebo cream with no difference in pain scale noted between treatment groups (Roberts *et al.*, 1998). A study of an anti-inflammatory medication, serrapeptase (Danzen), found a reduction in engorgement as rated by an independent observer with 85% of the treated group and 60% of the untreated group having either a marked or moderate improvement of symptoms (Kee *et al.*, 1989). Though this was a statistically significant difference ($p < 0.05$), few women in this study were actually breastfeeding. This study also reveals that a significant percentage of women had improvement without intervention. A systematic review of treatments for breast engorgement in 2001 identified only eight trials with 424 women. It concluded that cabbage leaves, cabbage leaf extract, oxytocin, cold packs, and ultrasound performed no better than placebo (Snowden *et al.*, 2001). The only therapies which outperformed placebo in the conclusion of this review were the previously mentioned Danzen and bromelain/trypsin complex.

As demonstrated from the above information, there is limited scientific evidence regarding effective prevention and treatment strategies for breast engorgement. It appears prudent to encourage early and effective milk transfer. This should be achieved during postpartum hospitalization with routine and repeated breastfeeding assessments. Appropriate positioning and latch of the infant and milk transfer should also be routinely documented prior to hospital discharge by personnel knowledgeable in lactation. If the engorgement prohibits successful infant latch, the use of manual expression, breast massage, relaxation, a warm shower, or a breast pump to soften the nipple-areolar complex and facilitate infant attachment can also be attempted. If symptomatic engorgement is bothersome for the new mother, comfort measures should be instituted and consideration of a non-steroidal pain medication, such as ibuprofen, may be appropriate.

SORE NIPPLES

Another common difficulty which may be encountered during the postpartum period is nipple pain and trauma. The foremost consideration in the new mother experiencing sore nipples should be assessment of infant positioning and latch. Again, the ready availability of lactation experts who can assess and educate the new dyad in breastfeeding technique is optimal. Unresolved nipple pain is a leading cause of premature breastfeeding discontinuation.

The differential diagnosis for nipple pain is extensive. Lacerations and fissuring on the nipples may suggest infection with either a bacterium, such as *Staphylococcus*, or a fungal infection, such as *Candida*. Hormonal changes may affect nipple sensitivity. There is typically a rapid fall in hormones after delivery unless there is retained placental tissue. Later during lactation, return of menstrual cycles may change sensitivity related to hormonal fluctuation, and a new pregnancy can cause increased sensitivity as well. Many dermatologic conditions can occur on the nipple which can cause sensitivity, though this typically occurs in women with known dermatologic conditions. Dermatitis on the breast or nipple in a patient that lacks such a history should prompt investigation by the clinician. Herpes infection can occur on the nipple and cause exquisitely painful lesions which typically begin as vesicles and progress through ulcerations. This would indicate that breastfeeding temporarily be suspended from the affected nipple until the lesions are resolved. Nipple vasoconstriction (Raynaud's phenomenon) can cause pain and typically is associated with changes of color or blanching of the nipple. Often, women will have other evidence of this condition, having noticed it in fingers or toes as well. This condition may be triggered by exposure to cold temperature. Biting can also cause pain and trauma, but the history should provide the definitive diagnosis.

Treatment of nipple pain should be guided to appropriately treat the underlying etiology of the pain. If the cause is believed to be related to latch and positioning and trauma or fissuring are not yet present, often the focus of therapy is directed to improving breastfeeding technique. Cadwell *et al.* (2004) performed a study which randomized 94 breastfeeding women with nipple pain into one of three intervention groups. All groups received assessment of their breastfeeding practice followed by education. Group one received no other intervention, group two also received breast shells and lanolin cream, and group three also received glycerin gel. Nipple pain was self assessed using a five point scale. No statistical difference was noted between the groups.

When positioning and latch are not adequately addressed, the new mother is at risk for developing trauma and fissures on the nipple. If this occurs, she is then put at further risk of secondary infections and mastitis. *Candida* breast infections are typically described as excruciatingly painful, with radiation of the pain to the chest wall and axilla, though the appearance of the nipple may not be that abnormal. Many predisposing factors have been reported, such as antibiotic use, the use of nursing pads, diabetes, steroids, vaginal yeast infections, and immune deficiency in the mother. Risk factors reported in the infant include antibiotics, the use of pacifiers, and candidal diaper rash. The impact of the pain associated with sore nipples was investigated by Amir *et al.* (1996a). Forty-eight women with reported nipple pain and 65 women without were given the Edinburgh Postnatal Depression Scale. A score greater than 12 was considered consistent with depression. The mean score was 12.4 for the group with nipple pain compared to 7.3 for the group without pain ($p < 0.0001$). Those women with nipple pain were more likely to score in the range consistent with depression (38%) compared to only 14% of those without pain scoring in the same range. After resolution of the nipple pain, the percentage returned to a rate similar to the group without pain (16%).

Studies in women with nipple pain attempting to identify the infectious cause have suggested that both *Candida* and bacteria are often cultured. Thomassen *et al. (1998)* studied 20 breastfeeding women with deep pain, 20 with superficial pain, and 20 without pain. Swabs were taken from the infant's mouth, the nipple, and expressed breastmilk. Fissures were present in ten of 20 women with deep pain and 13/20 with superficial pain. Maternal cultures for *Candida* were positive in 5/20 women with deep pain, 10/20 with superficial pain, and 3/20 controls. Maternal cultures were positive for skin bacteria nearly twice as often in the group with deep pain. Amir did a similar study and found maternal cultures were positive for *candida* in 19% of those with and 3% of those without nipple pain (Amir *et al.*, 1996b). In this study, none of the 31 non-lactating women had a positive culture. *Staphylococcus aureus (S. aureus)* was cultured from 42% of those with pain and five percent of those without. If fissures were present, 62% of women with pain were culture positive for *S. aureus.* Livingstone *et al.*, (1996) also researched this topic performing nipple swabs on 112 women without pain and 115 with pain. Twenty-eight percent of women in this study had a break in the skin. Twenty-one percent of women with pain and 15% without pain were culture positive for *Candida.* If the pain was described as moderate or severe, 41% cultured *Candida* and 34% cultured *Staphylococcus aureus.* If there was a break in the skin, 47% cultured *Candida* and 36% cultured *Staphylococcus aureus.* These research studies suggest that both organisms may be involved when infection is suspected as a cause of nipple pain, though present technology does not provide a useful technique for clinical testing. Often topical therapy is aimed at potentially covering both organisms. Livingstone and Stringer (1999) performed a randomized clinical trial in 84 mothers. They were assigned to four treatment groups for sore, cracked nipples: "optimal" breastfeeding technique alone, topical mupiricin, topical fusidic acid, or oral antibiotics. Improvement after five to seven days of therapy occurred in 8% treated with "optimal technique," 16% with mupiricin, 29% with fusidic acid, and 79% of those treated with oral antibiotics ($p < 0.0001$). Additionally, only five percent of those treated with systemic antibiotics developed mastitis compared to 12-35% of those who did not receive oral antibiotics.

POSTPARTUM IN THE HOSPITAL

Many other influences to successful breastfeeding are present during the hospitalization for childbirth. The Baby-Friendly Hospital Initiative makes recommendations for a supportive environment. In addition to rooming-in, early breastfeeding initiation, and on demand feeding schedules, many other hospital routines can have an impact. A systematic review of the literature on infant feeding schedules found that a restrictive feeding schedule of every four hours was associated with an increased risk of maternal

Table 3. Best Practices for Breastfeeding Support During Postpartum Hospitalization

- Allow infant transitioning in the delivery room
- Encourage rooming-in
- Suggest delay of elective procedures until breastfeeding is established
- Provide adequate availability of lactation expertise for consultation with new mothers
- Encourage infant rounds in room with family
- Refer new families to support groups after discharge, such as La Leche League
- Suggest infant follow-up 24-48 hours after discharge

Table 4. Best practices for breastfeeding support following preterm delivery

- If infant is vigorous at delivery, consider delayed cord clamping for 30-60 seconds after delivery
- Initiate breastpumping or expression soon after delivery unless infant is able to attempt breastfeeding
- When infant is stabilized, allow skin-to-skin exposure/ kangaroo care
- Encourage pumping mothers to pump or express at frequencies similar to full term routines, 8-12 times daily. Long term pumping may be benefited by bilateral, electric pump
- Discourage interval > 6 hours between any two episodes of breast stimulation
- Advise relaxation techniques for pumping, maintaining supply while away from the infant
- Provide support breastfeeding services, lactation consultation if needed. Support groups such as La Leche League
- Begin direct breastfeeding as soon as infant is capable to facilitate transition to breast
- Encourage use of care by parent rooms prior to discharge to allow new family to "practice" home routines, including infant feeding prior to discharge home
- Maintain close follow up with pediatrics for monitoring infant growth while converting to exclusive breastfeeding

breast engorgement and an increased likelihood of breastfeeding discontinuation by four to six weeks postpartum (Renfrew *et al.*, 2000). Pacifier use prior to established, effective breastfeeding is another reported obstacle which should be discouraged during hospitalization. The use of supplemental infant feeding during hospitalization is a significant adverse predictor of breastfeeding success (Howard *et al.*, 2003). The use of artificial infant feedings or supplement should be discouraged unless there is a medical indication or a contraindication to the use of mother's own milk. Hospital routines for minor infant procedures, such as heel sticks or circumcision, should not interfere with regular breastfeeding. If circumcision is to be performed, some method of pain control should be implemented.

Education of the new parents and family in normal infant feeding and voiding/stooling patterns is imperative. Reasons to contact the infant's health care provider and an easily accessible contact number should be provided. Support service for lactation assistance in your community should be given to the mother prior to hospital discharge. Resources such as local lactation consultants and La Leche League are valuable if they are available in your area. Close follow-up of the infant after discharge to assure adequate weight gain and lack of significant jaundice should also be routine.

Many different influences on successful lactation occur during hospitalization for childbirth. Some of these are amenable to change while others are dictated by circumstance. The hospital environment should be patient and family focused. Routines should be altered to reflect the best interests of the mother-infant dyad. Education should be a routine part of all personnel and patient interactions and should be encouraged. For those influences which cannot be changed, focus should be on providing the best breastfeeding support to limit any negative influence on successful lactation. This can be accomplished with adequate support and training of the staff and administration caring for maternity and pediatric patients (**Table 3, Table 4**).

References

Abdel-Aleem H, Villar J, Gulmezoglu AM, Mostafa SA, Youssef AA, Shokry M, *et al.* The pharmacokinetics of the prostaglandin E1 analogue misoprostol in plasma and colostrum after postpartum administration. *Eur J Obstet Gynecol Reprod Biol.* 2003; 108:25-28.

Albani A, Addamo P, Renghi A, Voltolin G, Peano L, Ivani G. The effect on breastfeeding rates of regional anesthesia technique for cesarean and vaginal childbirth. *Minerva Anestesiol.* 1999; 65(9): 625-30.

Amir LH, Dennerstein L, Garland SM, Fisher J, Farish SJ. Psychological aspects of nipple pain in lactating women. *J Psyhosom Obstet Gynaecol.* 1996a; 17(1):53-58.

Amir LH, Garland SM, Dennerstein L, Farish SJ. Candida albicans: is it associated with nipple pain in lactating women? *Gynecol Obstet Invest.* 1996b; 41(1):30-34.

Barron SP, Lane HW, Hannan TE, Struempler B, Williams JC. Factors influencing duration of breast feeding among low-income women. *J Am Diet Assoc.* 1988; 88(12):1557-61.

Baumgarder DJ, Muehl P, Fischer M, Pribbenow B. Effect of labor epidural anesthesia on breast-feeding of healthy full-term newborns delivered vaginally. *J Am Board Fam Pract.* 2003; 16(1):7-13.

Cadwell K, Turner-Maffei C, Blair A, Brimdyr K, Maja McInerney Z. Pain reduction and treatment of sore nipples in nursing mothers. *J Perinat Educ.* 2004; 13(1):29-35.

Chapman DJ, Young S, Ferris AM, Perez-Escamilla R. Impact of breast pumping on lactogenesis stage II after cesarean delivery: A randomized clinical trial. *Pediatrics.* 2001; 107(6) e94: 1-7.

Choy CM, Lau WC, Tam WH, Yuen PM. A randomized controlled trial of intramuscular syntometrine and intravenous oxytocin in the management of the third stage of labour. *BJOG.* 2002; 109(2):173-77.

Crowell MK, Hill PD, Humenick SS. Relationship between obstetric analgesia and time of effective breast feeding. *J Nurse Midwifery.* 1994; 39(3): 150-56.

De Olivera LD, Giugliani ERJ, Santo LCE, Franca MCT, Weigert EML, Kohler F. Effect of intervention to improve breastfeeding technique on the frequency of exclusive breastfeeding and lactation related problems. *J Hum Lact.* 2006; 22(3):315-21.

Derman RJ, Kodkany BS, Goudar SS, Geller Se, Naik VA, Bellad MB, *et al.* Oral misoprostol in preventing postpartum haemorrhagia in resource-poor communities: a randomized controlled trial. *Lancet.* 2006; 368(9543):1248-53.

Dewey KG, Nommsen-Rivers MS, Heinig MJ, Cohen RJ. Risk factors for suboptimal infant breastfeeding behavior, delayed onset of lactation, and excess neonatal weight loss. *Pediatrics.* 2003; 112:607-19.

Evans K, Evans R, Simmer K. Effect of the method of breastfeeding on breast engorgement, mastitis and infantile colic. *Acta Paediatr.* 1995; 84(8):849-52.

Evans KC, Evans RG, Royal R, Esterman AJ, James SL. Effect of caesarean section on breast milk transfer to the normal term newborn over the first week of life. *Arch Dis Child Fetal Neonatal Ed.* 2003; 88:F380-82.

Fujimoto M, Takeuchi K, Sugimoto M, Mauro T. Prevention of postpartum hemorrhage by uterotonic agents: comparison of oxytocin and methyl ergotamine in the management of the third stage of labor. *Acta Obstet Gynecol Scand.* 2006; 85(11):1310-14.

Grajeda R, Perez-Escamilla R. Stress during labor and delivery is associated with delayed onset of lactation among urban Guatemalan women. *J Nutr.* 2002; 132:3055-60.

Halpern SH, Levine T, Wilson D, MacDonell J, Katsiris SE, Leighton BL. Effect of labor analgesia on breastfeeding success. *Birth.* 1999; 26(2):83-88.

Hill PD, Humenick SS. The occurrence of breast engorgement. *J Hum Lact.* 1994; 10(2):79-86.

Hirose M, Hara Y, Hosokawa T, Tanaka Y. The effect of postoperative analgesia with continuous epidural bupivacaine after cesarean section on the amount of breast feeding and infant weight gain. *Anesth Analg.* 1996; 82:1166-69.

Hirose M, Hosokawa T, Tanaka Y. Extradural buprenorphine suppresses breast feeding after cesarean section. *Br J Anaesth.* 1997; 79:120-21.

Hodnett ED, Gates S, Hofmeyr GJ, Sakala C. Continuous support for women during childbirth. *Cochrane Database of Systematic Reviews.* 2003; 3:CD003766. DOI: 10.1002/14651858.CD003766.

Hofmeyr GJ, Nikodem VH, Wolman WL, Chalmers BE, Kramer T. Companionship to modify the clinical birth environment: effects of progress and perceptions of labour, and breastfeeding. *Br J Obstet Gynecol.* 1991; 98:756-64.

Howard CR, Howard FM, Lanphear B, Eberly S, deBlieck EA, Oakes D, *et al.* Randomized clinical trial of pacifier use and bottle-feeding or cup feeding and their effect on breastfeeding. *Pediatrics.* 2003; 111:511-18.

Kearney MH, Cronenwett LR, Reinhardt R. Cesarean delivery and breastfeeding outcomes. *Birth.* 1990; 17(2): 97-103.

Kee WH, Tan SL, Lee V, Salmon YM. The treatment of breast engorgement with Serrapeptase (Danzen): a randomized double-blind controlled study. *Singapore Med J.* 1989; 30(1):48-54.

Langer A, Campero L, Garcia D, Reynoso S. Effects of psychosocial support during labour and childbirth on breastfeeding, medical interventions, and mothers' wellbeing in a Mexican public hospital: a randomized clinical trail. *Br J Obstet Gynaecol.* 1998; 105(10):1056-63.

Leung GM, Lam TH, Ho LM. Breast-feeding and its relation to smoking and mode of delivery. *Obstet Gynecol.* 2002; 99(5 pt 1):785-94.

Lie B, Juul J. Effect of epidural vs. general anesthesia on breastfeeding. *Acta Obstet Gynecol Scand.* 1988; 67(3):207-9.

Livingstone V, Stringer LJ. The treatment of Staphylococcus aureus infected sore nipples: a randomized comparative study. *J Hum Lact.* 1999; 15(3):241-46.

Livingstone VH, Willis CE, Berkowitz J. Staphylococcus aureus and sore nipples. *Can Fam Physician.* 1996; 42:654-59.

Lokugmage AU, Sullivan KR, Niculescu I, Tigere P, Onyangunga F, El-Refaey H, *et al.* A randomized study comparing rectally administered misoprostol verses Syntometrine combined with an oxytocin infusion for the cessation of primary post partum hemorrhage. *Acta Obstet Gynecol Scand.* 2001; 80:835-39.

Mathur GP, Pandey PK, Mathur S, Sharma S, Agnihotri M, Bhalla M, *et al.* Breastfeeding in babies delivered by cesarean section. *Indian Pediatr.* 1993; 30:1285-90.

Matthews MK. The relationship between maternal labour analgesia and delay in the initiation of breastfeeding in healthy neonates in the early neonatal period. *Midwifery.* 1988; 5(1):3-10.

McDonald S, Abbott JM, Higgins SP. Prophylactic ergometrine-oxytocin verses oxytocin for the third stage of labour. *Cochrane Database Syst Rev.* 2004; (1):CD000201.

Meinzen-Derr JK, Guerrero ML, Altaye M, Ortega-Gallegos H, Ruiz-Palacios GM, Morrow AL. Risk of infant anemia is associated with exclusive breast-feeding and maternal anemia in a Mexican cohort. *J Nutr.* 2006; 136(2): 452-58.

Moon JL, Humenick SS. Breast engorgement: contributing variables and variables amenable to nursing interventions. *JOGNN.* 1989; 18(4):309-15.

Nikodem VC, Danzinger D, Gebka N, Gulmezoglu AM, Hofmeyr GJ. Do cabbage leaves prevent breast engorgement? A randomized, controlled study. *Birth.* 1993; 20(2):61-64.

Nissen E, Wildstrom AM, Lilja G, Matthiesen AS, Uvnas-Moberg K, Jacobsson G, *et al.* Effects of routinely given pethidine during labour on infants' developing breastfeeding behavior. Effects of dose-delivery time interval and various concentrations of pethidine/nor pethidine in cord plasma. *Acta Paediatr.* 1977; 86(2): 201-8.

O'Brien P, El-Refaey H, Gordon A, Geary M, Rodeck CH. Rectally administered misoprostol for the treatment of postpartum hemorrhage unresponsive to oxytocin and ergometrine: a descriptive study. *Obstet Gynecol.* 1998; 92(2):212-14.

Patel RR, Liebling RE, Murphy DJ. Effect of operative delivery in the second stage of labor on breastfeeding success. *Birth.* 2003; 30(4):255-60.

Radzyminski S. The effect of ultra low dose epidural analgesia on newborn breastfeeding behaviors. *J Obstet Gynecol Neonatal Nurs.* 2003; 32(3):322-31.

Rajan L The impact of obstetric procedures and analgesia/ anaesthesia during labour and delivery on breast feeding. *Midwifery.* 1994; 10(2):87-103.

Renfrew MJ, Lang S, Martin L, Woolridge MW. Feeding schedules in hospitals for newborn infants. *Cochrane Database Syst Rev.* 2000; 2:CD000090.

Riordan J, Gross A, Angeron J, Krumwiede B, Melin J. The effect of labor pain relief medication on neonatal suckling and breastfeeding duration. *J Hum Lact.* 2000; 16(1):7-12.

Roberts KL, Reiter M, Schuster D. A comparison of chilled and room temperature cabbage leaves in treating breast engorgement. *J Hum Lact.* 1995; 11(3):191-94.

Roberts KL, Reiter M, Schuster D. Effects of cabbage leaf extract on breast engorgement. *J Hum Lact.* 1998; 14(3):231-36.

Roberts KL. A comparison of chilled cabbage leaves and chilled gel paks in reducing breast engorgement. *J Hum Lact.* 1995; 11(1):17-20.

Rowe-Murray HJ, Fisher JRW. Baby friendly hospital practices: cesarean section is a persistent barrier to early initiation of breastfeeding. *Birth.* 2002; 29(2):124-31.

Scott KD, Klaus PH, Klaus MH. The obstetrical and postpartum benefits of continuous support during childbirth. *J Womens Health Gend Based Med.* 1999; 8(10):1257-64.

Snowden HM, Renfrew MJ, Woolridge MW. Treatments for breast engorgement during lactation. *Cochrane Database Syst Rev.* 2001; (2):CD000046.

Storr G. Prevention of nipple tenderness and breast engorgement in the postpartal period. *J Obstet Gynecol Neonatal Nurs.* 1988; 17(3):203-9.

Thomassen P, Johansson VA, Wassberg C, Petrini B. Breast-feeding, pain and infection. *Gynecol Obstet Invest.* 1998; 46(2):73-74.

Torvaldsen S, Roberts CL, Simpson JM, Thompson JF, Ellwood DA. Intrapartum epidural analgesia and breastfeeding: a prospective cohort study. *Int Breastfeed J.* 2006; 1(24):1-7.

Vestermark V, Hogdall CK, Birch M, Plenov G, Toftager-Larsen K. Influence of the mode of delivery on initiation of breast-feeding. *Eur J Obstet Gynecol Reprod Biol.* 1990; 38:33-38.

Victora CG, Huttly SRA, Barros FC, Vaughan JP. Caesarean section and duration of breastfeeding among Brazilians. *Arch Dis Child.* 1990; 65:632-34.

Vogel D, Burkhardt T, Rentsch K, Schweer H, Watzer B, Zimmermann R, *et al.* Misoprostol verses methylergometrine: pharmacokinetics in human milk. *Am J Obstet Gynecol.* 2004; 191(6):2168-73.

Willis CE, Livingstone V. Infant insufficient milk syndrome associated with maternal postpartum hemorrhage. *J Hum Lact.* 1995; 11(2):123-26.

Wittles B, Glosten B, Faure EAM, Moawad AH, Ismail M, Hibbard J, *et al.* Postcesarean analgesia with both epidural morphine and intravenous patient-controlled analgesia: neurobehavioral outcomes among nursing neonates. *Anesth Analg.* 1997; 85:600-6.

Yost NP, Bloom SL, Sibley MK, Lo JY, McIntire DD, Leveno KJ. A hospital-sponsored quality improvement study of pain management after cesarean delivery. *Am J Obstet Gynecol.* 2004; 190(5):1341-46.

Chapter 19

Nutrition in Lactation

Judy Hopkinson

NUTRITION IN LACTATION

Nutritional recommendations for lactating women vary with maternal status prior to and during pregnancy. Women who are well nourished prior to pregnancy can draw on body stores to meet nutrient requirements. Both they and their infants are relatively insulated from the potential detrimental effects of a poor quality diet during lactation. In contrast, poorly nourished women with inadequate nutrient stores are at greater risk. Both they and their infants are more likely to exhibit deficiency symptoms when diet during lactation is inadequate. If health professionals wish to insure the nutritional well being of mothers and infants, careful attention to diet should begin well before the mother becomes pregnant in order to optimize not only fetal growth and development, but also maternal health and milk composition.

In this chapter, we will discuss nutrient requirements of lactating women and the impact of maternal diet on milk composition in the context of maternal nutritional status.

ENERGY REQUIREMENTS

Energy requirements increase during lactation to cover the cost of milk production. Mean milk output during the first six months of lactation is 780 mL/day for American mothers of term infants (Allen *et al.*, 1991; Heinig *et al.*, 1993). The energy density of human milk is approximately 67 kcal/100 mL (Institute of Medicine, 2005). This translates into an output of 523 kcal/day during the first six months of full lactation. The energy efficiency of milk production is approximately 80% (Butte & King, 2005), thus the total energy requirement for milk production may be estimated from the following equation:

$$780 \text{ mL/day} \times (67 \text{ kcal} / 100 \text{ mL}) / 0.8 = 653 \text{ kcal/day}$$

Milk production varies for individual women and an average requirement of 650 kcal/day is a reasonable estimate. In well nourished women, a portion of this energy is derived from body stores deposited during gestation. Allowing 150 kcal per day for energy contributed from body stores leaves a net requirement of 500 kcal/day. Actual needs of individual women will vary depending on the volume of milk produced. Basal metabolic rate, efficiency of work performance, and total energy expenditure differ little between lactating and non-lactating postpartum women (Butte & King, 2005).

Conversely, undernourished women and those who deposit insufficient body stores during lactation must conserve energy during lactation for their own well being and the well being of the infant. For these women, the full energy requirements for lactation must be provided in the diet. Accordingly, mean desirable increases in energy intake to support lactation would be lower in developed countries where the majority of women are well nourished or overweight than in underdeveloped countries where a higher percentage of women are undernourished.

Importantly, energy requirements decrease in the second six months of lactation following the introduction of complementary foods. The extent of the decrease will vary depending on the volume of milk produced.

During pregnancy, fat is deposited preferentially at the thigh and to a lesser extent at the suprailiac, subscapular, costal, biceps, and triceps sites (Taggart *et al.*, 1967). During lactation, the pattern is reversed and fat is mobilized from the trunk and thighs (Butte *et al.*, 1984; Butte & Hopkinson, 1998; Sohlstrom & Forsum, 1995).

Exercise, Calorie Restriction, and Weight Loss During Breastfeeding

In the U.S. and the developed world, each pregnancy increases the risk of overweight by 60% and the risk of obesity by 110% (Keppel & Taffel, 1993; Rooney & Schauberger, 2005). In countries where food is abundant, breastfeeding has relatively little impact on short term postpartum weight loss (Fraser & Grimes, 2003). Rather, energy required for lactation is derived from increased intake in preference to body fat mobilization (Butte *et al.*, 2001). The impact of lactation on long term weight loss in developed countries is unclear. A recent study by Rooney and Schauberger (Rooney & Schauberger, 2005) followed 540 women for ten years after delivery and found that breastfeeding for at least three months was associated with reduced net weight gain over the next 8.5 years compared to not breastfeeding. During the early postpartum period, well-nourished women and undernourished women lost an average of 0.8 and 0.1 kg/month, respectively (Butte & Hopkinson, 1998). In well nourished women, this represents a calorie deficit of 170 kcal/day. Greater weight loss can be achieved by further restricting energy intake and/or increasing voluntary energy expenditure. In reality, weight loss patterns are highly variable and many women gain weight during the postpartum period, even during lactation.

Women who have not returned to pre-pregnancy weight by six months postpartum are at significantly increased risk for long term development of obesity (Rooney & Schauberger, 2005). Pre-pregnancy weight and pregnancy weight gain (Butte & Hopkinson, 1998) are also important predictors of long term weight gain in postpartum women (Boardley *et al.*, 1995).

On average, well nourished postpartum women lose about 0.5 – 1.0 kg per month after postpartum diuresis (Butte & Hopkinson, 1998; Prentice & Prentice, 1988). However, individual weight loss varies greatly. The myth that breastfeeding assures postpartum weight loss is prevalent, and prenatal as well as postnatal education regarding the realities of postpartum weight management is advisable.

Fortunately, both exercise and moderate calorie restriction are compatible with exclusive breastfeeding, and combining lactation with regular exercise and a balanced, calorie restricted diet is a reasonable and prudent strategy for reducing body weight in most circumstances. In randomized controlled trials, calorie restriction (500 kcal/day below estimated requirements) and regular exercise did not impair milk production or infant growth (Dewey *et al.*, 1994; Larson-Meyer, 2002; Lovelady *et al.*, 2000; Lovelady *et al.*, 2001; Lovelady, 2004; McCrory *et al.*, 1999). Moreover, exercise benefited mothers by increasing weight loss and by improving cardiovascular fitness, blood lipid profiles, and insulin response (Lovelady *et al.*, 1995; Lovelady *et al.*, 2004).

Exercise alone does not promote weight loss (Butte & Hopkinson, 1998; Dewey *et al.*, 1994; Lovelady, 2004; Dewey & McCrory, 1994). Programmed physical activity and diet increase weight loss for exclusively breastfeeding overweight women (BMI 25-30) without impacting infant growth (Lovelady *et al.*, 2000). In the study by Lovelady *et al.*, mothers were randomly assigned to exercise 45 minutes per day with a daily energy deficit of 500 kcal. Over a ten week period, the intervention group lost 4.4 $\pm$ 0.4 kg compared to 0.9 $\pm$ 0.5 kg ($p<.01$) in the control group. There were no differences in infant growth. McCrory *et al.* (McCrory *et al.*, 1999) conducted a short-term (11 day) randomized controlled trial of the impact of diet, diet plus exercise, and no intervention on weight loss, milk production, and milk composition in 67 lactating women. Diet with exercise resulted in greater fat loss and retention of lean tissue than either diet alone or no intervention.

Extreme dieting during breastfeeding can undermine milk production (Prentice & Prentice, 1988; Tully & Dewey, 1985). In well-nourished women consuming less than 1,500 calories/day for one week, milk production was temporarily decreased by 15% (Dusdieker *et al.*, 1994). Early warning signs of low milk production can include infant loss of appetite, irritability or restlessness, and maternal fatigue. In all cases, infants should be closely monitored for adequate growth.

Overweight breastfeeding women who want to accelerate weight loss may be advised to initiate moderate caloric restriction (500 kcal/day) and regular exercise after breastfeeding is well established. Trials examining the impact of regular exercise and moderate energy restriction have been conducted only during established lactation and not during the initial four to six weeks.

Actual energy requirements for lactating women are estimated as the sum of total energy expenditure (TEE) plus the energy of milk output minus energy mobilized from tissue stores. Four studies have measured TEE of lactating women (Butte *et al.*, 2000; Lovelady *et al.*, 1993; Forsum *et al.*, 1992; Goldberg *et al.*, 1991), and measurements vary significantly with maternal physical activity level (PAL). Reductions in physical activity (PAL) have been reported in early lactation (four to five weeks) (Butte & King, 2005; Goldberg *et al.*, 1991; van Raaij *et al.*, 1991), with gradual resumption of pre-pregnancy PAL thereafter (Butte & King, 2005, van Raaij *et al.*, 1991).

Because obese women have lower breastfeeding initiation rates (Baker *et al.*, 2004; Donath & Amir, 2000; Kugyelka *et al.*, 2004; Li *et al.*, 2003) and breastfeed for a shorter time than women of normal weight, greater weight loss goals should not be expected or encouraged.

Exercise, Weight Loss, and Milk Composition

Exercise has no apparent impact on milk composition with the exception of a temporary rise in milk lactate after prolonged, heavy exercise (Larson-Meyer, 2002; Prentice, 1994). Although infants have been reported to exhibit more negative facial expressions when offered drops of post exercise breastmilk compared with pre-exercise breastmilk (Wallace & Rabin, 1991), no controlled trials have documented an exercise-induced reduction in milk intake during breastfeeding. No increase in lactic acid was observed following moderate exercise (Carey *et al.*, 1997). Milk mineral content was not influenced by maternal exercise in a randomized crossover trial comparing phosphorus, calcium, magnesium, sodium, and potassium content of milk from women during a rest period with milk from the same women before and 10, 30, and 60 minutes after maximal graded exercise (Fly *et al.*, 1998).

VITAMIN AND MINERAL REQUIREMENTS OF LACTATING WOMEN

Dietary Reference Intakes

In addition to energy requirements, protein and selected macronutrient and micronutrient requirements increase during lactation.

Dietary Reference Intakes (Dri)

Recommended Dietary Allowance (RDA): the average daily dietary nutrient intake level sufficient to meet the nutrient requirement of nearly all (97 to 98 percent) healthy individuals in a particular life stage and gender group.

Adequate Intake (AI): the recommended average daily intake level based on observed or experimentally determined approximations or estimates of nutrient intake by a group (or groups) of apparently healthy people that are assumed to be adequate -- used when an RDA cannot be determined.

Tolerable Upper Intake Level (UL): the highest average daily nutrient intake level that is likely to pose no risk of adverse health effects to almost all individuals in the general population. As intake increases above the UL, the potential risk of adverse effects may increase.

Estimated Average Requirement (EAR): the average daily nutrient intake level estimated to meet the requirement of half the healthy individuals in a particular life stage and gender group.

Source: Institute of Medicine, 2005.

Protein

During the first six months of lactation, the RDA for protein is increased by 25 grams/day above non-pregnant, non-lactating levels for all age groups to compensate for secretory losses. Thus a total RDA for all lactating women is 71 grams of protein/day during exclusive breastfeeding (Institute of Medicine, 2005). For non-pregnant, non-lactating women, in contrast, the RDA is 46 grams/day. Intake should vary with weight and the corresponding incremental intakes recommended are 0.8 g/kg/day for non-pregnant, non-lactating women and 1.3 g/kg/day during lactation.

Table 1. Dietary Reference Intakes: Elements

Element	Unit	Age	Non-pregnant Non-lactating RDA[1]/AI[1]*	Pregnancy RDA/AI*	Lactation RDA/AI*	UL[1] for Lactation
Boron	mg/d	14-18	ND	ND	ND	17
		>18	ND	ND	ND	20
Calcium	mg/d	14-18	1300*	1300*	1300*	2500
		19-50	1000*	1000*	1000*	2500
		>50	1200*	--	--	--
Chromium	µg/d	14-18	24*	29*	44*	ND
		19-50	25*	30*	45*	ND
		>50	20*	--	--	--
Copper	µg/d	14-18	890	1000	1300	8000
		19-50	900	1000	1300	10000
		>50	900	--	--	--
Flouride	mg/d	>14	3*	3*	3*	10
Iodine	µg/d	14-18	150	220	290	900
		>18	150	220	290	1100
Iron[2]	mg/d	14-18	15	27	10	45
		19-50	18	27	9	45
		>50	8	--	--	--
Magnesium	mg/d	14-18	360	400	360	350**
		19-30	310	350	310	350**
		30-50	320	360	320	350**
		>50	320	--	--	--
Manganese	mg/d	14-18	1.6*	2.0*	2.6*	9
		> 18	1.8*	2.0*	2.6*	11
Molybdenum	µg/d	14-18	43	50	50	1700
		> 18	45	50	50	2000
Nickel	mg/d	>9	ND	ND	ND	1.0
Phosphorus	mg/d	14-18	1250	1250	1250	4000
		>18	700	700	700	4000
Selenium	µg/d	>14	55	60	70	400
Zinc	mg/d	14-18	9	12	13	34
		> 18	8	11	12	40

[1]**RDA** = Recommended Dietary Allowance; AI* = adequate intake; UL = tolerable upper limit. Values were extracted in Aug. 2006 from the National Academy of Sciences. Institute of Medicine. Food and Nutrition Board DRI reports.
* Indicates adequate
** Upper limit for supplemental intake over and above food sources
[2] Assumes 75% of iron is from heme sources. Recommended intake for vegetarians is approximately double indicated values.

Minerals

Dietary recommended intakes of minerals for women before and during pregnancy and during lactation are listed in **Table 1.**

Calcium

Approximately 210 mg of calcium are secreted into breastmilk daily during exclusive breastfeeding. Accumulated losses exceed those of pregnancy within six months. Calcium required for milk production is obtained through mobilization of trabecular bone and decreased urinary losses (Kent *et al.*, 1990; Specker *et al.*, 1994; Vargas Zapata *et al.*, 2004; O'Brien *et al.*, 2003; Moser-Veillon *et al.*, 2001; Ritchie *et al.*, 1998). In contrast, calcium needs for fetal growth during pregnancy are met primarily through increased intestinal absorption (Vargas Zapata *et al.*, 2004; O'Brien *et al.*, 2003; Ritchie *et al.*, 1998). Lactation induced bone loss is not appreciably affected by increased dietary calcium intake (Specker *et al.*, 1994; Cross *et al.*, 1995; Kalkwarf *et al.*, 1999; Kalkwarf *et al.*, 1997; Jarjou *et al.*, 2006; Laskey *et al.*, 1998; Prentice *et al.*, 1995), and is reversed following resumption of menses and weaning (Cross *et al.*, 1995; Kalkwarf *et al.*, 1997; Laskey *et al.*, 1998; Hopkinson *et al.*, 2000; Kalkwarf *et al.*, 1996; Sowers *et al.*, 1995). In a cross sectional study including 245 women who gave birth as adolescents, those who breastfed had higher bone mineral density of the proximal femur at 20-25 years of age than their peers who did not breastfeed (Chantry *et al.*, 2004). Thus, teenage women should not be discouraged from breastfeeding out of concern for their own continued bone development.

Because supplemental calcium intake has little impact on maternal calcium balance, maternal bone density following lactation, or milk calcium concentrations, the DRI for calcium (1000 mg/day) is the same for lactating and non-lactating adult women. Teenage mothers should consume higher amounts of calcium (1300 mg/day) in both lactating and non-lactating states (Institute of Medicine, 1997).

Blood calcium levels are tightly controlled independently of calcium intake, and there are no acute measures of calcium status. Moreover, there are no data identifying levels of calcium intake least likely to be associated with bone fracture in later life. Therefore, the DRI for calcium is presented as an adequate intake level or AI rather than an RDA.

The primary source of calcium in most diets is dairy products. Vegans and other individuals who do not consume dairy products must find alternate sources of calcium to insure bone health. Women who curtail their intake of dairy products during lactation because of infant sensitivity to cow milk protein or associated IgE antibodies in milk will also need assistance in choosing foods rich in calcium. It is important to recognize that fractional absorption of calcium varies between food sources and with total intake as well as with individual differences and physiological states. Calcium bioavailability from plant sources is inversely related to the oxalate and phytate content. Calcium is poorly absorbed from plants with high levels of oxalic acid, such as spinach, and very easily absorbed from those with low oxalate contents, such as bok choy and broccoli. Beans, on the other hand, are a poor source of calcium because they contain high levels of phytates (Weaver *et al.*, 1999). Comparative calcium content and bioavailability of a variety of foods are listed in **Table 2.**

Calcium may also be consumed as a dietary supplement. Bioavailability of calcium consumed as supplements varies with the size of the dose and with the milieu in which it is consumed. The type of supplement can influence absorption to a minor extent. Under similar conditions, intake of 250 mg elemental calcium with breakfast resulted in fractional absorption of 35% for calcium citrate malate, 27% for calcium carbonate, and 25% for tricalcium phosphate (Institute of Medicine, 1997). Solubility of the supplement is less important than whether or not the tablet disintegrates readily to increase surface area. Absorption efficiency of calcium supplements decreases when doses exceed 500 mg (Institute of Medicine, 1997; Heaney *et al.*, 1975).

Iron

Relatively small amounts of iron are secreted into breastmilk (1.5-3.0 mg/day), and losses are more than offset by prolonged amenorrhea. No increase in iron intake above pre-pregnant levels is required, and iron needs are lower during lactation than during and before pregnancy (Institute of Medicine, 2001). Lactational amenorrhea constitutes a natural period of recovery from the high iron demands of pregnancy. Iron requirements for teenagers are only minimally higher (10 mg/day compared to 9 mg/day) than those for adults during full lactation. Following resumption of menses, iron requirements increase to offset menstrual losses.

Other Minerals

Incremental increases in intake of zinc (4 mg/day), iodine (140 µg/day) (Institute of Medicine, 2001), and selenium (15 µg/day) (Institute of Medicine, 2001; Institute of Medicine, 2000) are recommended during breastfeeding compared to the non-pregnant, non-lactating state. The upper limit for iodine is slightly lower for adolescents than for adult women. Phosphorus and magnesium balances are not affected by dietary supplements, and recommended intakes for these minerals are the same for lactating and non-lactating women (Institute of Medicine, 1997). While no adverse effects have been documented from consumption of foods containing high levels of magnesium, diarrhea and gastrointestinal disturbances are associated with intake of high levels of magnesium salts. Therefore, an upper limit for supplemental, but not dietary magnesium is provided. Dietary recommended intakes for minerals for women of different age groups and reproductive states are listed in **Table 1.**

Vitamins

Recommended intakes of vitamins for women of different ages and different reproductive states are listed in **Table 3**. With the exception of vitamins D and K, recommended intakes increase during lactation. The AI for vitamin D is 5 µg (200 IU) for lactating adolescent and adult women up to the age of 50. For lactating women 51 years of age or older, the AI is 10 µg/day (400 IU). Vitamin D insufficiency is common in older adults and may be relatively common among children and younger adults in more northern latitudes, including the U.S.-Canadian border (Hanley & Davies, 2003). Studies by Heaney and colleagues provide evidence that intake of 1000 IU/day (25 µg) maintains, but does not increase serum 25(OH)D over time (Heaney *et al.*,

Table 2. Comparison of Sources of Absorbable Calcium with Milk

Food	Serving size[1]	Calcium content[2]	Fractional absorption[3]	Estimated absorbable calcium[4]	Servings needed to equal 240 mL milk
	g	mg	%	mg	n
Milk	240	300	32.1	96.3	1.0
Pinto beans	86	44.7	26.7	11.9	8.1
Red beans	172	40.5	24.4	9.9	9.7
White beans	110	113	21.8	24.7	3.9
Bok choy	85	79	53.8	42.5	2.3
Broccoli	71	35	61.3	21.5	4.5
Cheddar cheese	42	303	32.1	97.2	1.0
Cheese food	42	241	32.1	77.4	1.2
Chinese cabbage flower leaves	85	239	39.6	94.7	1.0
Chinese mustard greens	85	212	40.2	85.3	1.1
Chinese spinach	85	347	8.36	29	3.3
Fruit punch with calcium citrate malate	240	300	52.0	156	0.62
Kale	85	61	49.3	30.1	3.2
Spinach	85	115	5.1	5.9	16.3
Sweet potatoes	164	44	22.2	9.8	9.8
Rhubarb	120	174	8.54	10.1	9.5
Tofu with calcium	126	258	31.0	80.0	1.2
Yogurt	240	300	32.1	96.3	1.0

[1]Based on half-cup serving size (85 g for green leafy vegetables) except for milk and fruit punch (1 cup or 240 mL) and cheese (1.5 oz).
[2]Averaged for beans and broccoli processed in different ways, except for the Chinese vegetables, which were analyzed in authors' laboratory.
[3]Adjusted for load using the equation for milk [fractional absorption = 0.889-0.0964 in load] then adjusted for the ratio of calcium absorption of the test food relative to milk tested at the same load, the absorptive index. The absorptive index was taken from the literature for beans, bok choy, broccoli, Chinese vegetables, fruit punch with calcium citrate malate, kale, sweet potatoes, rhubarb, tofu, and dairy products.
[4]Calculated as calcium content x fractional absorption.
Source: Weaver *et al.*, 1999; reproduced with permission from *The American Journal of Clinical Nutrition.*

Table 3. Dietary Reference Intakes: Vitamins RDA[1] / AI[1]* UL[1]

Vitamin	Unit	Age	Non-pregnant Non lactating RDA/AI*	Pregnant RDA/AI*	Lactating RDA/AI*	Lactating UL
Biotin	µg/d	>14	30*	30*	35*	ND**
Choline	mg/d	14-18	425*	450*	550*	3000
		>18	425*	450*	550*	3500
Folate	µg/d	14-18	400	600	500	800
		> 18	400	600	500	1000
Niacin	mg/d	14-18	14	18	17	30
		> 18	14	18	17	35
Pantothenic acid	mg/d	>14	5*	6*	7*	ND
Riboflavin	mg/d	>14	1.1	1.4	1.4	ND
Thiamine	mg/d	>14	1.1	1.4	1.4	ND
Vitamin A	µg/d	14-18	700	750	1200	2800
		> 18	700	770	1300	3000
Vitamin B-6	mg/d	14-18	1.2	1.9	2.0	80
		19-50	1.3	1.9	2.0	100
		> 50	1.5	--	--	--
Vitamin B-12	µg/d	>14	2.4	2.6	2.8	ND
Vitamin C	mg/d	> 18	75	85	120	2000
		14-18	65	80	115	1800
Vitamin D	µg/d	14-50	5*	5*	5*	50
		50-70	10*	10*	10*	50
		>70	15*	--	--	--
Vitamin E	mg/d	14-18	15	15	19	800
		> 18	15	15	19	1000
Vitamin K	µg/d	14-18	75*	75*	75*	ND
		> 18	90*	90*	90*	ND

[1]RDA = Recommended Dietary Allowance; AI* = adequate intake; UL = tolerable upper limit. Values were extracted in Aug of 2006 from the National Academy of Sciences. Institute of Medicine. Food and Nutrition Board DRI reports.
* indicates adequate ** UL not determined

2003). Supplementing lactating women with 2000 IU of vitamin D/day elevated maternal levels in at least one study (Hollis & Wagner, 2004). In another report, pharmacologic doses of ergocalciferol (2500 µg) resulted in toxic levels in milk (Greer *et al.*, 1984). The recommended upper limit for vitamin D is 50 µg/day (2000 IU), well above the AI. Therefore, intakes slightly above the AI should not cause concern.

Vitamin K requirements are difficult to establish, and therefore no recommended intake can be defined. The adequate intake for vitamin K is set at 75 µg/day for teenage girls and 90 µg/day for women 18 and older regardless of reproductive status. No upper limit is set for intake of vitamin K as toxicity has not been reported. Intakes are generally believed to exceed requirements in healthy children and adults. Neonatal requirements are high to prevent hemorrhagic disease of the newborn. In contrast, deficiency symptoms have not been demonstrated in adults. Feeding healthy individuals diets restricted in vitamin K to levels almost impossible to achieve in a self-selected nutritionally adequate diet did not impair normal haemostatic control in healthy subjects (Institute of Medicine, 2001).

Additional vitamin A (500 µg retinol palmitate/day) and vitamin E (4 mg alpha-tocopherol equivalents/day) are recommended for lactating women to compensate for milk losses and to maintain maternal stores (Institute of Medicine, 2001).

Increased intake of vitamin C is recommended to replace amounts secreted into milk. In a study of 47 lactating women (Salmenpera, 1984), three women consuming less than 100 mg/day of vitamin C had plasma ascorbate values below the lower limit of normal. Women with intakes between 100 and 199 mg/day had plasma ascorbate levels in the normal range and no dose – response relationship was detected. In another study, intake of over 200 mg/day resulted in increased urinary excretion of the vitamin without impacting milk content (Byerley & Kirksey, 1985).

Increased intake of B vitamins are also recommended to compensate for losses in milk and to allow for metabolic inefficiencies (Institute of Medicine, 1998). Increased anabolic activity during pregnancy and lactation elevate the risk for maternal folate deficiency. Severe folate deficiency results in megaloblastic anemia. In the absence of supplementation, plasma folate concentrations generally decrease during lactation (Bruinse *et al.*, 1985; Bates *et al.*, 1986; Mackey & Picciano, 1999). Maternal blood folate levels of lactating women can be maintained with dietary supplements (Bates *et al.*, 1986; Willoughby & Jewell, 1968). Women of child bearing age are advised to consume 400 μg/day of folate to reduce the risk of neural tube defects in offspring. During pregnancy and lactation, recommended intakes increase to 600 and 500 μg/day, respectively. In women with chronic deficiencies, higher intakes may be required to overcome deficits (Lonnerdal, 1986). However, supplemental folic acid intake should not exceed 1,000 micrograms (μg) per day to prevent triggering symptoms of vitamin B_{12} deficiency (Institute of Medicine, 1998).

IMPACT OF MATERNAL DIET ON MILK COMPOSITION

The influence of maternal diet on milk composition cannot be adequately addressed without considering maternal nutritional status prior to and during pregnancy. Mothers can and do produce adequate milk in sufficient quantities to support infant growth and development, even on very inadequate diets (Lawrence & Lawrence, 2005). Yet, fluctuations in milk composition do occur in response to dietary inadequacies particularly among malnourished women. Moreover, nutritional deficiencies can occur in breastfed infants if maternal diets are restricted and/or mothers become severely malnourished prior to, during, or after pregnancy (Allen, 2005). Allen categorizes thiamine, riboflavin, vitamins B_6 and B_{12}, vitamin A, and iodine as "priority" nutrients for lactating women. When milk levels of these nutrients are low secondary to malnutrition, they can be readily increased by maternal supplementation. In well nourished women, on the other hand, milk nutrient content is more stable in response to dietary fluctuations. In general, providing complicated "rules" about diet during lactation without considering maternal nutritional status and dietary preferences can undermine breastfeeding and should be avoided (Lawrence & Lawrence, 2005). In the section below, the influence of variations in maternal dietary intake of protein, fat, vitamins, and minerals will be addressed.

Protein

Milk protein concentrations are not associated with maternal protein intakes, even in malnourished populations (Villalpando *et al.*, 1992; Lonnerdal *et al.*, 1976). However, increasing maternal protein intake from 8% to 20% of dietary energy increased milk nitrogen over a four day period in a study of three women (Forsum & Lonnerdal, 1980). Concentrations of urea, free amino acids, and protein increased significantly, but the increase in protein was small and unlikely to be of clinical significance since 24 hour output of individual proteins was not increased significantly.

Fat

To a first approximation, total milk fat content is unaffected by maternal dietary fat intake. The cholesterol level in breastmilk is also independent of maternal intake. In general, the fatty acid profile of breastmilk is responsive to maternal intake. Women who consume very little dietary fat utilize depot fat to maintain milk levels and the fatty acid content of their milk reflects this source. In women with normal fat intake, the fatty acid profile of milk more closely reflects the types of fats consumed in the diet such that women who consume large amounts of polyunsaturated fats will have higher polyunsaturated/saturated fat ratios in their milk.

A diet rich in fish oil or consumption of cod liver oil supplements alters milk fatty acid profile and increases the content of DHA and other polyunsaturated fats (Olafsdottir *et al.*, 2006). In a study of 24 breastfeeding women randomly assigned to receive no supplement or one of three levels of DHA supplements daily (170-260 mg/day) between two and eight weeks postpartum, DHA supplementation increased maternal plasma phospholipid and breastmilk DHA concentrations and resulted in higher plasma phospholipid DHA concentrations in infants. Breastmilk DHA increased in proportion to the supplement received (32- 91%) and decreased by 17% in the control group. Mean infant plasma phospholipid DHA increased by 11-42% in the supplement groups, but only by five percent in the control group (Jensen *et al.*, 2000).

Docosahexaenoic acid (DHA; 22:6 n-3) and arachidonic acid (AA; 20:4 n-6) are important for development of the central nervous system. Deposition of these fats is pronounced in the last trimester of pregnancy and the first few months postpartum. In a randomized controlled trial of women followed from pregnancy through nine (n = 262) or forty-eight (n = 90) months postpartum, mothers were assigned to receive 10 mL of corn oil (4747 mg/10 mL linoleic acid and 92 mg/10 mL alpha-linolenic acid) or cod liver oil (1183 mg/10 mL DHA, 803 mg/10 mL eicosapentaenoic acid, and a total of 2494 mg/10 mL summation operator n 3 PUFAs) from 18 months of pregnancy through three months postpartum. Children born to mothers in the cod liver oil group scored higher on the Mental Processing Composite of the Kaufman Assessment Battery for Children at four years of age than did children born to women in the corn oil group (Helland *et al.*, 2003). In multiple regression analyses, maternal intake of DHA during pregnancy was the only variable of statistical significance for the children's mental processing scores at four years of age. The Mental Processing Composite score correlated significantly with head circumference at birth (r = 0.23). This study suggests that maternal intake of DHA during pregnancy may be more significant for infant outcome than intake during lactation.

In another randomized control trial of breastfeeding mothers supplemented with DHA during the first four months after delivery, the Bayley Psychomotor Development Index, but not the Mental Development Index, of children of the supplemented women was higher (P < 0.01) at 30 months of age than that of children of unsupplemented mothers (Jensen *et al.*, 2005). In contrast, increasing DHA content of breastmilk through maternal supplementation was associated with a temporary delay in early language development in Danish infants (Lauritzen *et al.*, 2005). Considerable research will be required to clarify precisely how providing DHA supplements to lactating women impacts the development of their infants.

VITAMINS

Vitamin content of milk is generally responsive to increased maternal intake among malnourished women, and less so among well nourished women.

Milk from well nourished women may contain insufficient quantities of vitamin K and vitamin D (Olafsdottir *et al.*, 2001) to optimize infant health. High levels of vitamin K are most critical during and immediately after birth to reduce the risk of bleeding. Routine intramuscular injection of vitamin K_1 at birth provides all the vitamin K needed to reduce the risk of hemorrhagic disease of the newborn, and no further supplementation is required. Both breast and formula-fed infants receive this injection. The recommendation for supplemental vitamin D for breastfed infants is recent and reflects environmental degradation of the ozone layer and subsequent need for avoidance of sun exposure. The primary natural source of vitamin D is internal production rather than dietary intake. Vitamin D is a hormone produced in the skin through the action of ultraviolet light. Sunlight exposure required for vitamin D production varies with skin color, latitude, altitude, and season. Depletion of the ozone layer by accumulated greenhouse gas has increased the risk of skin cancer from ultraviolet radiation. Contrary to popular misconception, use of sun block has not been shown to reduce the risk of skin cancer, and parents are advised to minimize that risk by reducing infant exposure to direct sunlight. A resurgence of vitamin D deficiency rickets has been observed in the United States, particularly among African American breastfed infants (Weisberg *et al.*, 2004). Consequently, the American Academy of Pediatrics recommends both minimal sunlight exposure during infancy and a supplement of 200 IU per day of vitamin D to all breastfed and non-breastfed infants unless they consume at least 500 ml per day of vitamin-D-fortified formula or milk (Gartner *et al.*, 2005). Vitamin D supplementation should begin within the first two months of life. Evidence suggests that higher levels of vitamin D in early childhood may afford long term risk reduction for type I diabetes (Hanley & Davison, 2005; Hypponen *et al.*, 2001).

Concentrations of fat soluble vitamins are decreased in maternal deficiency and can be increased by supplementation. In one study, vitamin D levels were initially undetectable in milk from vitamin D deficient women, but increased following supplementation and exposure to ultraviolet light (Greer *et al.*, 1984). Mothers who are deficient in vitamin D should receive supplements for their own sake. General recommendations to give supplemental vitamin D to the infant rather than the mother are based in part on concern for potential for toxicity to the mother when sufficient quantities of vitamin D are consumed to assure that milk levels will be high enough to meet infant needs in the absence of sunlight exposure. Studies in lactating women fail to demonstrate increases in infant vitamin D status with maternal supplements of 700 IU/day (Greer & Marshall, 1989), but do show improvements in infant status with maternal supplements of 1000 (Ala-Houhala, 1985), 2000 (Hollis & Wagner, 2004; Ala-Houhala *et al.*, 1986), and 4000 IU/day (Hollis & Wagner, 2004). Toxic levels of vitamin D have been reported in milk following maternal intake of pharmacological doses of vitamin D_2 (Greer *et al.*, 1984).

Vitamin K

Vitamin K levels in human milk can also be increased with maternal supplementation prior to delivery. However, given the standard administration of vitamin K to newborns, this has received relatively little attention.

Vitamin E

Few and somewhat conflicting data are available regarding the impact of maternal vitamin E supplementation on milk composition. It is generally believed that maternal supplementation does not increase milk vitamin E content (Lonnerdal, 1986; Allen, 2005; Helland *et al.*, 1998; Ali *et al.*, 1986). In one study, milk levels of γ-tocopherol (but not α-tocopherol) were reduced in women who consumed cod liver oil supplements (Olafsdottir *et al.*, 2001). It is likely that maternal stores of vitamin E are mobilized to maintain milk levels during lactation (Ali *et al.*, 1986).

Water-Soluble Vitamins

In maternal deficiency states, water soluble vitamins are decreased in human milk and respond readily to maternal supplementation.

Maternal status or dietary intake of the B vitamins (with the exception of folate) strongly influence levels of these nutrients in breastmilk (Lonnerdal, 1986; Allen, 2005; Chang & Kirksey, 2002; Greer, 2001). If maternal intakes are chronically low, this can result in infant intakes below recommended amounts and depletion of infant body stores. These vitamins are all present in relatively large amounts in standard multivitamin tablets given to lactating mothers. There appears to be an upper limit on the concentration of at least some water soluble vitamins in human milk. Upper limits for vitamin C and thiamine (vitamin B_1) are approximately 160 mg/L and 200 μg/L, respectively (Byerley & Kirksey, 1985; Kang-Yoon *et al.*, 1995; Pratt *et al.*, 1951). Folate levels in milk are preferentially maintained at the expense of maternal stores. Therefore, supplementation has less impact on milk composition of well nourished women. Supplementation with pantothenic acid, biotin, folate, and vitamin B_{12} has little impact on milk composition of well nourished women while vitamin C and thiamine concentrations respond only to a limited extent.

Vitamin C

Maternal vitamin C intake in excess of 1000 mg/day did not impact milk levels, but significantly elevated maternal urinary excretion, suggesting a regulatory mechanism for control of vitamin C levels (Byerley & Kirksey, 1985).

Vitamin B_{12}

Symptoms of vitamin B_{12} (cobalamine) deficiency include neurological problems, hypotonia, and cerebral atrophy. This vitamin is found only in animal products and supplements. Strict vegetarians who do not consume supplements will eventually develop B_{12} deficiencies and produce B_{12} deficient milk (Specker *et al.*, 1990). In addition to strict vegans, lacto-ovo vegetarians and individuals who consume little meat are also at elevated risk for low vitamin B_{12} status (Helman & Darnton-Hill, 1987). Breastfed infants may become symptomatic before their mothers. Although infant symptoms can be partially reversed with B_{12} shots, neurologic deficits can be irreversible (Weiss *et al.*, 2004; Casella *et al.*, 2005; Codazzi *et al.*, 2005; Graham *et al.*, 1992; Kuhne *et al.*, 1991). All strict vegetarians should consume vitamin B_{12} supplements, and those who consume few animal products are also well advised to do so.

Gastric bypass surgery and severe malnutrition increase the risk for producing vitamin B_{12} deficient breastmilk. When malnutrition is accompanied by the presence of intestinal parasites, the resulting nutrient malabsorption exacerbates the risk (Allen, 2005; Casterline, 1997). Gastric bypass surgery or partial gastrectomy (Grange & Finley, 1994) reduce B_{12} absorption by reducing absorptive surfaces. These surgeries may also seriously reduce production of vitamin B_{12} transporter, intrinsic factor, by gastric parietal cells (Wardinsky *et al.*, 1995) making dietary supplementation ineffective. In these cases, intravenous vitamin B_{12} administration may be required (Grange & Finlay, 1994).

Folate

In well nourished women, milk folate levels are believed to be maintained independently of dietary intake at the expense of maternal stores (Mackey & Picciano, 1999; Metz *et al.*, 1968; O'Connor *et al.*, 1997; Smith *et al.*, 1983; Tamura *et al.*, 1980). However, Tamura and Picciano have suggested that this data needs to be updated using improved methodology (Tamara & Picciano, 2006). In women with severe folate deficiency, milk concentrations are reduced and increase after folate supplementation (Metz *et al.*, 1968).

Vitamin B_6

The B_6 content of human milk is correlated with maternal intake and increases readily with maternal supplementation (Lovelady *et al.*, 2001; Chang & Kirksey, 2002; Chang & Kirksey, 1990; Kang-Yoon *et al.*, 1995; Kang-Yoon *et al.*, 1992). Chang and Kirksey (Chang & Kirksey, 2002) demonstrated maternal supplements of 2.5 mg/day of pyridoxine HCl provided an adequate amount of vitamin B_6 in breastmilk for normal vitamin B_6 status and growth of breastfed infants. Maternal supplements of 10.0 mg/day HCl were associated with infant intake of the Recommended Dietary Allowance from four to six months of age. In a study by Chang and Kirksey (Chang & Kirksey, 1990), supplements between 2.5 and 4.0 mg/day pyridoxine ensured vitamin B_6 adequacy of the mother and maintained relatively saturated concentrations of vitamin B_6 in breastmilk, and vitamin B_6 supplementation during pregnancy was associated with increased vitamin B_6 in colostrum ($p<.001$).

Although exercise is believed to increase vitamin B_6 losses, in a randomized controlled trial, regular exercise did not adversely affect vitamin B_6 status of overweight mothers or their breastfed infants between four and 14 weeks lactation. Mothers in this study consumed 2.0 mg/day of supplemental vitamin B_6 (Lovelady *et al.*, 2001). Pyridoxine use in higher doses (>50 mg/day) has been associated with various dermatologic, gastrointestinal, and even neuropathic syndromes. Chronic high doses should be avoided.

Vitamin Losses During Breastmilk Storage and Processing

Concentrations of vitamins in expressed human milk are affected by storage and handling. Holder pasteurization significantly lowered the concentrations of vitamins C (36%), folacin (31%), and B_6 (15%). Tube feeding of premature infants significantly lowered the concentrations of vitamins C (44%) and B_6 (19%) (van Zoeren-Grobben *et al.*, 1987).

MILK MINERALS AND MATERNAL DIET

For the most part, human milk is remarkably stable with respect to mineral content irrespective of variations in maternal intake. Exceptions to this general rule include selenium, iodine, and magnesium as well as heavy metals, such as lead, cadmium, and mercury, to which women may be exposed as a result of industrial or agricultural pollution. Concentrations of selenium, iodine, and manganese (Vuori *et al.*, 1980) in human milk have been reported to correspond to maternal dietary intake of these minerals. Other minerals including calcium, sodium, potassium, chlorine, iron, zinc, phosphorous, magnesium, copper, chromium, and fluoride appear to be independent of maternal dietary intake in the majority of cases. Specific minerals are discussed below.

Iron

Neither maternal iron intake nor maternal serum iron levels are associated with iron content of breastmilk. Thus, even women who suffer from iron deficiency anemia produce breastmilk with normal iron levels. Concentrations of iron are relatively low in all breastmilk, but readily absorbed by infants. During the first half of infancy, iron needs of term infants are met through a combination of breastmilk iron and mobilization of infant iron stores. In the second half of infancy, iron is the most likely limiting nutrient in the diet of an exclusively breastfed infant (Krebs, 2000; Krebs & Westcott, 2002). Premature infants with low iron stores at birth require supplementation earlier. For fully breastfed term infants, addition of meat products early in the second half of infancy has been recommended to provide a complementary source of bioavailable iron (Ali *et al.*, 1986; Butte *et al.*, 2004). Iron fortified cereals are a poor source of this nutrient in comparison to the heme iron found in red meat.

Zinc

Zinc in human milk is also highly bioavailable and generally meets the needs of healthy breastfed infants during the first half of infancy with the exception of small for gestational age and low birth weight infants (Krebs, 2000; Krebs & Westcott, 2002). Zinc deficient breastmilk has been reported in severely malnourished Ethiopian women on low zinc diets (Urrieta *et al.*, 2003). While some investigators have suggested that low zinc levels in breastmilk may limit growth of older breastfed infants, Heinig *et al.* found that zinc supplementation had no effect on growth or development between four and ten months of age (Heinig *et al.*, 2006).

Selenium

Maternal dietary intake of selenium influences selenium content of human milk. Both selenium deficiencies and selenium toxicity can occur, but deficiencies are more common. The content of selenium in plants varies with soil content in the region where the plants are grown. The daily selenium intake of breastfed infants in the western part of Poland is lower than the recommended daily requirement – apparently due to low selenium in the soil, and consequently in the foodstuffs from this region (Zachara & Pilecki, 2001).

Iodine

Iodine deficiency in infancy can result in developmental brain damage. Use of iodized salt is a critical international intervention to prevent iodine deficiency during pregnancy and to maintain adequate iodine levels in human milk. The iodine content of human milk has been found to vary with maternal iodine consumption, and concentrations range from 5.4 – 2170 μg/L (median 62 μg/L) around the world (Dorea, 2002). There is some controversy, however, regarding the influence of dietary intake on milk iodine content when maternal status is adequate and intakes are within normal ranges. Chierici *et al.*, for example, found no relationship between milk iodine and maternal intake among a group of Italian women (Chierici *et al.*, 1999). Very high milk iodine levels were observed in colostrum of Korean women. In the Korean culture, seaweed is normal part of the diet and new mothers are traditionally served seaweed soup. The iodine content of their milk decreased rapidly to 892 μg/L by four weeks (Moon & Kim, 1999). In healthy populations, milk iodine is reduced in mothers who smoke cigarettes (Laurberg *et al.*, 2004), and is inversely related to milk perchlorate levels (an environmental contaminant) (Kirk *et al.*, 2005).

Calcium, Sodium, Potassium, Phosphorus, Chlorine, Magnesium, Copper, and Chromium

Calcium, sodium, potassium, phosphorus, chlorine, magnesium, copper, and chromium concentrations in human milk do not respond to dietary supplementation. This is not to say that variations in these minerals do not occur. Sodium, for example is increased during mastitis and is higher in colostrum and during weaning than in mature milk as a result of disruptions in tight junctions between alveolar cells. This cannot be altered by diet.

SUMMARY

Good nutrition is vital throughout the life cycle, and attention to diet should not be limited to the period of lactation. Maternal stores of a variety of nutrients are depleted during pregnancy and lactation and must be replenished in order to insure maternal health and infant well being. If the mother is well nourished with good body nutrient stores, the composition of her milk during lactation is relatively, but not entirely, impervious to temporary fluctuations in diet quality. On the other hand, if the mother is poorly nourished in general or has limited stores of particular nutrients, both her health and the health of her nursing infant are more susceptible to dietary shortcomings during pregnancy and lactation. It is also the case that many women have exaggerated concerns regarding the impact of their diet on the quality of their breastmilk and the safety of breastfeeding. For this reason, it is particularly important to consider the mother's history and nutritional status when providing dietary guidance for lactation. A realistic and balanced approach must be adopted so that women feel validated in their breastfeeding goals and empowered to adopt appropriate dietary habits which will optimize their individual milk quality. As discussed above, women at risk for low levels of particular nutrients in their milk should be encouraged to consume dietary supplements. Conversely, women pre-disposed to consume megadoses of vitamins and minerals should be made aware of potential toxicities both to themselves and to their infants when those compounds accumulate in breastmilk.

References

Ala-Houhala M, Koskinen T, Terho A, Koivula T, Visakorpi J. Maternal compared with infant vitamin D supplementation. *Arch Dis Child.* 1986; 61:1159-63.

Ala-Houhala M. 25-Hydroxyvitamin D levels during breast-feeding with or without maternal or infantile supplementation of vitamin D. *J Pediatr Gastroenterol Nutr.* 1985; 4:220-26.

Ali J, Kader HA, Hassan K, Arshat H. Changes in human milk vitamin E and total lipids during the first twelve days of lactation. *Am J Clin Nutr.* 1986; 43:925-30.

Allen JC, Keller RP, Archer P, Neville MC. Studies in human lactation: milk composition and daily secretion rates of macronutrients in the first year of lactation. *Am J Clin Nutr.* 1991; 54:69-80.

Allen LH. Multiple micronutrients in pregnancy and lactation: an overview. *Am J Clin Nutr.* 2005; 81:1206S-12S.

Baker JL, Michaelsen KF, Rasmussen KM, Sorensen TI. Maternal prepregnant body mass index, duration of breastfeeding, and timing of complementary food introduction are associated with infant weight gain. *Am J Clin Nutr.* 2004; 80:1579-88.

Bates CJ, Fuller NJ, Prentice AM. Folate status during pregnancy and lactation in a West African rural community. *Hum Nutr Clin Nutr.* 1986; 40:3-13.

Bates CJ, Prentice AM, Prentice A, Lamb WH, Whitehead RG. The effect of vitamin C supplementation on lactating women in Keneba, a West African rural community. *Int J Vitam Nutr Res.* 1983; 53:68-76.

Boardley DJ, Sargent RG, Coker AL, Hussey JR, Sharpe PA. The relationship between diet, activity, and other factors, and postpartum weight change by race. *Obstet Gynecol.* 1995; 86:834-38.

Bruinse HW, van der BH, Haspels AA. Maternal serum folacin levels during and after normal pregnancy. *Eur J Obstet Gynecol Reprod Biol.* 1985; 20:153-58.

Butte N, Cobb K, Dwyer J, Graney L, Heird W, Rickard K. The start healthy feeding guidelines for infants and toddlers. *J Am Diet Assoc.* 2004; 104:442-54.

Butte NF, Garza C, Stuff JE, Smith EO, Nichols BL. Effect of maternal diet and body composition on lactational performance. *Am J Clin Nutr.* 1984; 39:296-306.

Butte NF, Hopkinson JM. Body composition changes during lactation are highly variable among women. *J Nutr.* 1998; 128:381S-85S.

Butte NF, King JC. Energy requirements during pregnancy and lactation. *Public Health Nutr.* 2005; 8:1010-27.

Butte NF, Wong WW, Hopkinson JM, Heinz CJ, Mehta NR, Smith EO. Energy requirements derived from total energy expenditure and energy deposition during the first 2 y of life. *Am J Clin Nutr.* 2000; 72:1558-69.

Butte NF, Wong WW, Hopkinson JM. Energy requirements of lactating women derived from doubly labeled water and milk energy output. *J Nutr.* 2001; 131:53-58.

Byerley LO, Kirksey A. Effects of different levels of vitamin C intake on the vitamin C concentration in human milk and the vitamin C intakes of breast-fed infants. *Am J Clin Nutr.* 1985; 41:665-71.

Carey GB, Quinn TJ, Goodwin SE. Breast milk composition after exercise of different intensities. *J Hum Lact.* 1997; 13:115-20.

Casella EB, Valente M, de Navarro JM, Kok F. Vitamin B12 deficiency in infancy as a cause of developmental regression. *Brain Dev.* 2005; 27:592-94.

Casterline JE, Allen LH, Ruel MT. Vitamin B-12 deficiency is very prevalent in lactating Guatemalan women and their infants at three months postpartum. *J Nutr.* 1997; 127:1966-72.

Chang SJ, Kirksey A. Pyridoxine supplementation of lactating mothers: relation to maternal nutrition status and vitamin B-6 concentrations in milk. *Am J Clin Nutr.* 1990; 51:826-31.

Chang SJ, Kirksey A. Vitamin B6 status of breast-fed infants in relation to pyridoxine HCl supplementation of mothers. *J Nutr Sci Vitaminol* (Tokyo). 2002; 48:10-17.

Chantry CJ, Auinger P, Byrd RS. Lactation among adolescent mothers and subsequent bone mineral density. *Arch Pediatr Adolesc Med.* 2004; 158:650-56.

Chierici R, Saccomandi D, Vigi V. Dietary supplements for the lactating mother: influence on the trace element content of milk. *Acta Paediatr Suppl.* 1999; 88:7-13.

Codazzi D, Sala F, Parini R, Langer M. Coma and respiratory failure in a child with severe vitamin B(12) deficiency. *Pediatr Crit Care Med.* 2005; 6:483-85.

Cross NA, Hillman LS, Allen SH, Krause GF. Changes in bone mineral density and markers of bone remodeling during lactation and postweaning in women consuming high amounts of calcium. *J Bone Miner Res.* 1995; 10:1312-20.

Dewey KG, Lovelady CA, Nommsen-Rivers LA, McCrory MA, Lonnerdal B. A randomized study of the effects of aerobic exercise by lactating women on breast-milk volume and composition. *N Engl J Med.* 1994; 330:449-53.

Dewey KG, McCrory MA. Effects of dieting and physical activity on pregnancy and lactation. *Am J Clin Nutr.* 1994; 59:446S-52S.

Donath SM, Amir LH. Does maternal obesity adversely affect breastfeeding initiation and duration? *J Paediatr Child Health.* 2000; 36:482-86.

Dorea JG. Iodine nutrition and breast feeding. *J Trace Elem Med Biol.* 2002; 16:207-20.

Dusdieker LB, Hemingway DL, Stumbo PJ. Is milk production impaired by dieting during lactation? *Am J Clin Nutr.* 1994; 59:833-40.

Fly AD, Uhlin KL, Wallace JP. Major mineral concentrations in human milk do not change after maximal exercise testing. *Am J Clin Nutr.* 1998; 68:345-49.

Forsum E, Kabir N, Sadurskis A, Westerterp K. Total energy expenditure of healthy Swedish women during pregnancy and lactation. *Am J Clin Nutr.* 1992; 56:334-42.

Forsum E, Lonnerdal B. Effect of protein intake on protein and nitrogen composition of breast milk. *Am J Clin Nutr.* 1980; 33:1809-13.

Fraser AB, Grimes DA. Effect of lactation on maternal body weight: a systematic review. *Obstet Gynecol Surv.* 2003; 58:265-69.

Gartner LM, Morton J, Lawrence RA, Naylor AJ, O'Hare D, Schanler RJ, *et al.* Breastfeeding and the use of human milk. *Pediatrics.* 2005; 115:496-506.

Goldberg GR, Prentice AM, Coward WA, Davies HL, Murgatroyd PR, *et al.* Longitudinal assessment of the components of energy balance in well-nourished lactating women. *Am J Clin Nutr.* 1991; 54:788-98.

Graham SM, Arvela OM, Wise GA. Long-term neurologic consequences of nutritional vitamin B12 deficiency in infants. *J Pediatr.* 1992; 121:710-14.

Grange DK, Finlay JL. Nutritional vitamin B12 deficiency in a breastfed infant following maternal gastric bypass. *Pediatr Hematol Oncol.* 1994; 11:311-18.

Greer FR, Hollis BW, Cripps DJ, Tsang RC. Effects of maternal ultraviolet B irradiation on vitamin D content of human milk. *J Pediatr.* 1984; 105:431-33.

Greer FR, Hollis BW, Napoli JL. High concentrations of vitamin D2 in human milk associated with pharmacologic doses of vitamin D2. *J Pediatr.* 1984; 105:61-64.

Greer FR, Marshall S. Bone mineral content, serum vitamin D metabolite concentrations, and ultraviolet B light exposure in infants fed human milk with and without vitamin D2 supplements. *J Pediatr.* 1989; 114:204-12.

Greer FR. Do breastfed infants need supplemental vitamins? *Pediatr Clin North Am.* 2001; 48:415-23.

Hanley DA, Davison KS. Vitamin D insufficiency in North America. *J Nutr.* 2005; 135:332-37.

Heaney RP, Davies KM, Chen TC, Holick MF, Barger-Lux MJ. Human serum 25-hydroxycholecalciferol response to extended oral dosing with cholecalciferol. *Am J Clin Nutr.* 2003; 77:204-10.

Heaney RP, Saville PD, Recker RR. Calcium absorption as a function of calcium intake. *J Lab Clin Med.* 1975; 85:881-90.

Heinig MJ, Brown KH, Lonnerdal B, Dewey KG. Zinc supplementation does not affect growth, morbidity, or motor development of US term breastfed infants at 4-10 mo of age. *Am J Clin Nutr.* 2006; 84:594-601.

Heinig MJ, Nommsen LA, Peerson JM, Lonnerdal B, Dewey KG. Energy and protein intakes of breast-fed and formula-fed infants during the first year of life and their association with growth velocity: the DARLING Study. *Am J Clin Nutr.* 1993; 58:152-61.

Helland IB, Saarem K, Saugstad OD, Drevon CA. Fatty acid composition in maternal milk and plasma during supplementation with cod liver oil. *Eur J Clin Nutr.* 1998; 52:839-45.

Helland IB, Smith L, Saarem K, Saugstad OD, Drevon CA. Maternal supplementation with very-long-chain n-3 fatty acids during pregnancy and lactation augments children's IQ at 4 years of age. *Pediatrics.* 2003; 111:e39-e44.

Helman AD, Darnton-Hill I. Vitamin and iron status in new vegetarians. *Am J Clin Nutr.* 1987; 45:785-89.

Hollis BW, Wagner CL. Vitamin D requirements during lactation: high-dose maternal supplementation as therapy to prevent hypovitaminosis D for both the mother and the nursing infant. *Am J Clin Nutr.* 2004; 80:1752S-58S.

Hopkinson JM, Butte NF, Ellis K, Smith EO. Lactation delays postpartum bone mineral accretion and temporarily alters its regional distribution in women. *J Nutr.* 2000; 130:777-83.

Hypponen E, Laara E, Reunanen A, Jarvelin MR, Virtanen SM. Intake of vitamin D and risk of type 1 diabetes: a birth-cohort study. *Lancet.* 2001; 358:1500-3.

Institute of Medicine, Panel on Macronutrients, Panel on the Definition of Dietary Fiber, Subcommittee on Upper Reference Levels of Nutrients, Subcommittee on Interpretation and Uses of Dietary Reference Intakes, Standing committee on the Scientific Evaluation of Dietary Reference Intakes. *DRIs for energy, carbohydrate, fiber, fat, fatty acids, cholesterol, protein, and amino acids.* Washington, DC: National Academy Press, 2005.

Institute of Medicine, Standing Committee on the Scientific Evaluation of Dietary Reference Intakes, Food and Nutrition Board. *DRIs: Vitamin C, vitamin E, selenium, and carotenoids.* Washington, DC: National Academy Press, 2000.

Institute of Medicine. *DRI, Dietary reference intakes: For calcium, phosphorus, magnesium, vitamin D, and flouride.* Washington, DC: National Academy Press, 1997.

Institute of Medicine. *DRIs for thiamine, riboflavin, niacin, vitamin B6, folate, vitamin B12, pantothenic acid, biotin, and choline.* Washington, DC: National Academy Press, 1998.

Institute of Medicine. *DRIs for vitamin A, vitamin K, arsenic, boron, chromium, copper, iodine, iron, manganese, molybdenum, nickel, silicon, vanadium, and zinc.* Washington, DC: National Academy Press, 2001.

Jarjou LM, Prentice A, Sawo Y, Laskey MA, Bennett J, *et al.* Randomized, placebo-controlled, calcium supplementation study in pregnant Gambian women: effects on breast-milk calcium concentrations and infant birth weight, growth, and bone mineral accretion in the first year of life. *Am J Clin Nutr.* 2006; 83:657-66.

Jensen CL, Maude M, Anderson RE, Heird WC. Effect of docosahexaenoic acid supplementation of lactating women on the fatty acid composition of breast milk lipids and maternal and infant plasma phospholipids. *Am J Clin Nutr.* 2000; 71:292S-99S.

Jensen CL, Voigt RG, Prager TC, Zou YL, Fraley JK, *et al.* Effects of maternal docosahexaenoic acid intake on visual function and neurodevelopment in breastfed term infants. *Am J Clin Nutr.* 2005; 82:125-32.

Kalkwarf HJ, Specker BL, Bianchi DC, Ranz J, Ho M. The effect of calcium supplementation on bone density during lactation and after weaning. *N Engl J Med.* 1997; 337:523-28.

Kalkwarf HJ, Specker BL, Heubi JE, Vieira NE, Yergey AL. Intestinal calcium absorption of women during lactation and after weaning. *Am J Clin Nutr.* 1996; 63:526-31.

Kalkwarf HJ, Specker BL, Ho M. Effects of calcium supplementation on calcium homeostasis and bone turnover in lactating women. *J Clin Endocrinol Metab.* 1999; 84:464-70.

Kang-Yoon SA, Kirksey A, Giacoia G, West K. Vitamin B-6 status of breast-fed neonates: influence of pyridoxine supplementation on mothers and neonates. *Am J Clin Nutr.* 1992; 56:548-58.

Kang-Yoon SA, Kirksey A, Giacoia GP, West KD. Vitamin B-6 adequacy in neonatal nutrition: associations with preterm delivery, type of feeding, and vitamin B-6 supplementation. *Am J Clin Nutr.* 1995; 62:932-42.

Kent GN, Price RI, Gutteridge DH, Smith M, Allen JR, *et al.* Human lactation: forearm trabecular bone loss, increased bone turnover, and renal conservation of calcium and inorganic phosphate with recovery of bone mass following weaning. *J Bone Miner Res.* 1990; 5:361-69.

Keppel KG, Taffel SM. Pregnancy-related weight gain and retention: implications of the 1990 Institute of Medicine guidelines. *Am J Public Health.* 1993; 83:1100-3.

Kirk AB, Martinelango PK, Tian K, Dutta A, Smith EE, Dasgupta PK. Perchlorate and iodide in dairy and breast milk. *Environ Sci Technol.* 2005; 39:2011-17.

Krebs NF, Westcott J. Zinc and breastfed infants: if and when is there a risk of deficiency? *Adv Exp Med Biol.* 2002; 503:69-75.

Krebs NF. Dietary zinc and iron sources, physical growth and cognitive development of breastfed infants. *J Nutr.* 2000; 130:358S-60S.

Kugyelka JG, Rasmussen KM, Frongillo EA. Maternal obesity is negatively associated with breastfeeding success among Hispanic but not Black women. *J Nutr.* 2004; 134:1746-53.

Kuhne T, Bubl R, Baumgartner R. Maternal vegan diet causing a serious infantile neurological disorder due to vitamin B12 deficiency. *Eur J Pediatr.* 1991; 150:205-8.

Larson-Meyer DE. Effect of postpartum exercise on mothers and their offspring: a review of the literature. *Obes Res.* 2002; 10:841-53.

Laskey MA, Prentice A, Hanratty LA, Jarjou LM, Dibba B, *et al.* Bone changes after 3 mo of lactation: influence of calcium intake, breast-milk output, and vitamin D-receptor genotype. *Am J Clin Nutr.* 1998; 67:685-92.

Laurberg P, Nohr SB, Pedersen KM, Fuglsang E. Iodine nutrition in breast-fed infants is impaired by maternal smoking. *J Clin Endocrinol Metab.* 2004; 89:181-87.

Lauritzen L, Jorgensen MH, Olsen SF, Straarup EM, Michaelsen KF. Maternal fish oil supplementation in lactation: effect on developmental outcome in breast-fed infants. *Reprod Nutr Dev.* 2005; 45:535-47.

Li R, Jewell S, Grummer-Strawn L. Maternal obesity and breast-feeding practices. *Am J Clin Nutr.* 2003; 77:931-36.

Lonnerdal B, Forsum E, Gebre-Medhin M, Hambraeus L. Breast milk composition in Ethiopian and Swedish mothers. II. Lactose, nitrogen, and protein contents. *Am J Clin Nutr.* 1976; 29:1134-41.

Lonnerdal B. Effects of maternal dietary intake on human milk composition. *J Nutr.* 1986; 116:499-513.

Lovelady CA, Fuller CJ, Geigerman CM, Hunter CP, Kinsella TC. Immune status of physically active women during lactation. *Med Sci Sports Exerc.* 2004; 36:1001-7.

Lovelady CA, Garner KE, Moreno KL, Williams JP. The effect of weight loss in overweight, lactating women on the growth of their infants. *N Engl J Med.* 2000; 342:449-53.

Lovelady CA, Meredith CN, McCrory MA, Nommsen LA, Joseph LJ, *et al.* Energy expenditure in lactating women: a comparison of doubly labeled water and heart-rate-monitoring methods. *Am J Clin Nutr.* 1993; 57:512-18.

Lovelady CA, Nommsen-Rivers LA, McCrory MA, Dewey KG. Effects of exercise on plasma lipids and metabolism of lactating women. *Med Sci Sports Exerc.* 1995; 27:22-28.

Lovelady CA, Williams JP, Garner KE, Moreno KL, Taylor ML, *et al.* Effect of energy restriction and exercise on vitamin B-6 status of women during lactation. *Med Sci Sports Exerc.* 2001; 33:512-18.

Lovelady CA. The impact of energy restriction and exercise in lactating women. *Adv Exp Med Biol.* 2004; 554:115-20.

Mackey AD, Picciano MF. Maternal folate status during extended lactation and the effect of supplemental folic acid. *Am J Clin Nutr.* 1999; 69:285-92.

McCrory MA, Nommsen-Rivers LA, Mole PA, Lonnerdal B, Dewey KG. Randomized trial of the short-term effects of dieting compared with dieting plus aerobic exercise on lactation performance. *Am J Clin Nutr.* 1999; 69:959-67.

Metz J, Zalusky R, Herbert V. Folic acid binding by serum and milk. *Am J Clin Nutr.* 1968; 21:289-97.

Moon S, Kim J. Iodine content of human milk and dietary iodine intake of Korean lactating mothers. *Int J Food Sci Nutr.* 1999; 50:165-71.

Moser-Veillon PB, Mangels AR, Vieira NE, Yergey AL, Patterson KY, *et al.* Calcium fractional absorption and metabolism assessed using stable isotopes differ between postpartum and never pregnant women. *J Nutr.* 2001; 131:2295-99.

O'Brien KO, Nathanson MS, Mancini J, Witter FR. Calcium absorption is significantly higher in adolescents during pregnancy than in the early postpartum period. *Am J Clin Nutr.* 2003; 78:1188-93.

O'connor DL, Green T, Picciano MF. Maternal folate status and lactation. *J Mammary Gland Biol Neoplasia.* 1997; 2:279-89.

Olafsdottir AS, Thorsdottir I, Wagner KH, Elmadfa I. Polyunsaturated fatty acids in the diet and breast milk of lactating Icelandic women with traditional fish and cod liver oil consumption. *Ann Nutr Metab.* 2006; 50:270-76.

Olafsdottir AS, Wagner KH, Thorsdottir I, Elmadfa I. Fat-soluble vitamins in the maternal diet, influence of cod liver oil supplementation and impact of the maternal diet on human milk composition. *Ann Nutr Metab.* 2001; 45:265-72.

Ortega RM, Martinez RM, Andres P, Marin-Arias L, Lopez-Sobaler AM. Thiamine status during the third trimester of pregnancy and its influence on thiamine concentrations in transition and mature breast milk. *Br J Nutr.* 2004; 92:129-35.

Ortega RM, Quintas ME, Martinez RM, Andres P, Lopez-Sobaler AM, Requejo AM. Riboflavin levels in maternal milk: the influence of vitamin B2 status during the third trimester of pregnancy. *J Am Coll Nutr.* 1999; 18:324-29.

Pratt JP, Hamil BM, Moyer EZ, Kaucher RM, Roderuck C, *et al.* Metabolism of women during the reproductive cycle. XVIII. The effect of multivitamin supplements on the secretion of B vitamins in human milk. *J Nutr.* 1951; 44:141-57.

Prentice A, Jarjou LM, Cole TJ, Stirling DM, Dibba B, Fairweather-Tait S. Calcium requirements of lactating Gambian mothers: effects of a calcium supplement on breast-milk calcium concentration, maternal bone mineral content, and urinary calcium excretion. *Am J Clin Nutr.* 1995; 62:58-67.

Prentice A. Should lactating women exercise? *Nutr Rev.* 1994; 52:358-60.

Prentice AM, Prentice A. Energy costs of lactation. *Annu Rev Nutr.* 1988; 8:63-79.

Ritchie LD, Fung EB, Halloran BP, Turnlund JR, Van L, Cann CE, *et al.* A longitudinal study of calcium homeostasis during human pregnancy and lactation and after resumption of menses. *Am J Clin Nutr.* 1998; 67:693-701.

Rooney BL, Schauberger CW. Excess pregnancy weight gain and long-term obesity: One decade later. *Obstet Gynecol.* 2005; 100:245-52.

Salmenpera L. Vitamin C nutrition during prolonged lactation: optimal in infants while marginal in some mothers. *Am J Clin Nutr.* 1984; 40:1050-56.

Smith AM, Picciano MF, Deering RH. Folate supplementation during lactation: maternal folate status, human milk folate content, and their relationship to infant folate status. *J Pediatr Gastroenterol Nutr.* 1983; 2:622-28.

Sohlstrom A, Forsum E. Changes in adipose tissue volume and distribution during reproduction in Swedish women as assessed by magnetic resonance imaging. *Am J Clin Nutr.* 1995; 61:287-95.

Sowers M, Eyre D, Hollis BW, Randolph JF, Shapiro B, Jannausch ML, *et al.* Biochemical markers of bone turnover in lactating and nonlactating postpartum women. *J Clin Endocrinol Metab.* 1995; 80:2210-16.

Specker BL, Black A, Allen L, Morrow F. Vitamin B-12: low milk concentrations are related to low serum concentrations in vegetarian women and to methylmalonic aciduria in their infants. *Am J Clin Nutr.* 1990; 52:1073-76.

Specker BL, Vieira NE, O'Brien KO, Ho ML, Heubi JE, Abrams SA, *et al.* Calcium kinetics in lactating women with low and high calcium intakes. *Am J Clin Nutr.* 1994; 59:593-99.

Taggart NR, Holliday RM, Billewicz WZ, Hytten FE, Thomson AM. Changes in skinfolds during pregnancy. *Br J Nutr.* 1967; 21:439-51.

Tamura T, Picciano MF. Folate and human reproduction. *Am J Clin Nutr.* 2006; 83:993-1016.

Tamura T, Yoshimura Y, Arakawa T. Human milk folate and folate status in lactating mothers and their infants. *Am J Clin Nutr.* 1980; 33:193-97.

Tully J, Dewey KG. Private fears, global loss: a cross-cultural study of the insufficient milk syndrome. *Med Anthropol.* 1985; 9:225-43.

Umeta M, West CE, Verhoef H, Haidar J, Hautvast JG. Factors associated with stunting in infants aged 5-11 months in the Dodota-Sire District, rural Ethiopia. *J Nutr.* 2003; 133:1064-69.

van Raaij JM, Schonk CM, Vermaat-Miedema SH, Peek ME, Hautvast JG. Energy cost of lactation, and energy balances of well-nourished Dutch lactating women: reappraisal of the extra energy requirements of lactation. *Am J Clin Nutr.* 1991; 53:612-19.

van Zoeren-Grobben D, Schrijver J, Van den BH, Berger HM. Human milk vitamin content after pasteurisation, storage, or tube feeding. *Arch Dis Child.* 1987; 62:161-65.

Vargas Zapata CL, Donangelo CM, Woodhouse LR, Abrams SA, Spencer EM, *et al.* Calcium homeostasis during pregnancy and lactation in Brazilian women with low calcium intakes: a longitudinal study. *Am J Clin Nutr.* 2004; 80:417-22.

Villalpando SF, Butte NF, Wong WW, Flores-Huerta S, Hernandez-Beltran MJ, Smith EO, *et al.* Lactation performance of rural Mesoamerindians. *Eur J Clin Nutr.* 1992; 46:337-48.

Vuori E, Makinen SM, Kara R, Kuitunen P. The effects of the dietary intakes of copper, iron, manganese, and zinc on the trace element content of human milk. *Am J Clin Nutr.* 1980; 33:227-31.

Chapter 20

Maternal Obesity and the Outcome of Breastfeeding

Kathleen M. Rasmussen

INTRODUCTION

Obesity has recently reached "epidemic" proportions in the United States, and other countries are all too rapidly following suit. This increase in the proportion of obese individuals affects women and men, young, middle-aged and elderly. Although it would be preferable to express obesity in terms of some direct measure of body fatness, this is often impractical. Therefore, much of the scientific literature has used body mass index (BMI, kg/m^2) as a proxy for body fatness. BMI affords a reasonable approximation of body fatness in individuals whose lean body mass is in the normal range (World Health Organization, 1998). Two different definitions of obesity have been used for women of reproductive age. The Institute of Medicine (IOM), in its report on weight gain during pregnancy (Institute of Medicine, 1990), defined overweight as a BMI of 26.0-29.0 kg/m^2 and obesity as a BMI of >29.0 kg/m^2. In contrast, the World Health Organization (WHO) defines overweight as a BMI of 25 kg/m^2 and obesity as a BMI of 30.0 kg/m^2 (WHO, 1998). Women of reproductive age are not immune to these population trends in obesity. In fact, among American women 20-39 years old, 28.9% were obese and 8.0% were extremely obese (BMI 40 kg/m^2) in the most recent nationally representative data (Ogden *et al.*, 2006).

At the same time as women of reproductive age have become fatter, it has only become more apparent how important it is for them to breastfeed–not only for their babies' health but also for their own (Section on Breastfeeding, 2005; Lawrence & Lawrence, 2005; Breastfeeding Handbook for Physicians, 2006). As a result, public health goals in the United States are for 75% of women to attempt breastfeeding (i.e., ever put the baby to the breast), 50% of women to continue to breastfeed for at least six months, and for 25% to breastfeed for one year or more (U.S. Department of Health and Human Services, 2000). In addition, it is recommended that women exclusively breastfeed their babies for six months (Section on Breastfeeding, 2005; Anonymous, 2005). Although there has been some improvement in the rates of breastfeeding among American women in recent years, particularly for the proportion of those who attempt to breastfeed, the proportion who are still breastfeeding at six and 12 months after delivery remains low (Ryan *et al.*, 2002; Li *et al.*, 2005), with values about half those recommended by health authorities.

As a result, it is important to identify and ameliorate factors that might make it difficult for women to succeed at breastfeeding. We have recently shown that maternal overweight and obesity before pregnancy are associated with failure of both the initiation and continuation of breastfeeding among white (Hilson *et al.*, 1997) and Hispanic (Kugyelka *et al.*, 2004) but not black (Kugyelka *et al.*, 2004) women who ever put their babies to the breast. Similar findings have been reported by others (Rutishauser & Carlin, 1992, Li *et al.*, 2003; Donath & Amir, 2000). To understand how maternal fatness could affect the success of breastfeeding, the development of the mammary gland, the role of maternal fatness in reproductive success generally, and what is known about the mechanisms behind the association between maternal fatness and the success of breastfeeding will be reviewed in this chapter.

ROLE OF BODY FATNESS IN THE DEVELOPMENT OF THE MAMMARY GLAND

A woman who is obese at the time of conception has gained her excess fat during one or more periods of her earlier life. Inasmuch as development of the mammary glands takes place before, during, and after pregnancy, the role of excess fatness in each period must be considered. As reviewed by Lawrence and Lawrence (Lawrence & Lawrence, 2005), development of the mammary glands begins early in embryonic life. For elongation of the mammary ducts to occur, the mammary epithelial tissue must be closely associated with an adipocyte-containing stroma. "Human mammary ducts proliferate in a stoma containing considerably more fibrous tissue than rodents" (Sheffield, 1988). Before puberty, growth of the human mammary gland is proportional to growth in general, with a rapid expansion just before puberty that is estrogen-dependent (Lawrence & Lawrence, 2005). Age at menarche has declined a few months over the last several decades while a progressively higher proportion of girls have experienced early (< 11.0 years) menarche (Freedman *et al.*, 2002). Those who are the heaviest at seven years of age have an earlier menarche than those who are lightest (Cooper *et al.*, 1996). In addition, menarche is occurring at progressively higher BMI values (Demerath *et al.*, 2004). Whether these trends are related is controversial as the higher proportion of childhood overweight may be contributing to earlier menarche (Anderson *et al.*, 2003) or these trends may be simultaneous yet independent (Demerath *et al.*, 2004). What either of these trends mean for development of the mammary gland is unknown at present.

In human beings, lipids begins to accumulate in the adipocytes of the mammary gland at puberty. The hormonal changes associated with the menstrual cycle are associated with cyclic changes in the mammary glands of adult, non-pregnant women (Lawrence & Lawrence, 2005). Obesity is one of the predictors of differences among individuals in the amount of adipose tissue within the breast (Hovey *et al.*, 1999).

ASSOCIATION OF MATERNAL OBESITY WITH DIFFICULTIES IN CONCEPTION

Although a minimal amount of body fat seems to be necessary for menarche to occur (Frisch, 1984), it has been known since the 1950's that women who are too heavy experience menstrual disturbances (Rogers & Mitchell, 1952). "Overweight women have a higher incidence of menstrual dysfunction and anovulation, possibly because of altered secretion of pulsatile gonadotropin releasing hormone, sex hormone binding globulin, ovarian and adrenal androgen, and luteinising hormone, and also because of altered insulin resistance" (Wang *et al.*, 2000). Wang and colleagues (Wang *et al.*, 2000) have shown that overweight, obese and "very obese" (BMI 35 kg/m^2) women also have a reduced probability of becoming pregnant during assisted reproductive treatment. Nonetheless, some women are still able to conceive at very high BMI values [55 kg/m^2 in our study (Hilson *et al.*, 2006)]. Weight loss causes resumption of menstruation among anovulatory, obese women and improves their probability of conception (Clark *et al.*, 1995).

Paradoxically, obese women who use contraception to prevent pregnancy are at increased risk of unintended pregnancy. This finding comes from a case-control study of 18,445 women within the 1999 Pregnancy Risk Assessment Monitoring System in the US (Huber & Hogue, 2005). It appears that obesity may affect the biological effectiveness of the contraceptives being used, but data on the actual type of contraception used by these women were not collected.

THE ASSOCIATION OF MATERNAL OBESITY BEFORE OR DURING PREGNANCY WITH THE OUTCOME OF PREGNANCY

To understand the observed association between maternal obesity and reduced success in breastfeeding, it is important to recognize that the conditions that make breastfeeding difficult may have begun before delivery. In this section, the association between maternal prepregnant obesity and the progress and outcome of pregnancy is reviewed. In addition, prepregnant obesity affects the condition of the infant at birth and, potentially, the baby's ability to nurse, so this possibility is also considered.

Maternal Outcomes

Health care professionals and researchers have known for decades that women who are too heavy experience a variety of complications of pregnancy [see, for example, (Edwards *et al.*, 1978)]. In the older studies (as well as some recent ones), BMI was not used to classify subjects and there was no agreed-upon definition of obesity, either as an absolute body weight or as a percentage of a reference value. In a recent report that described the outcome of 287,213 pregnancies in London, Sebire and his colleagues (Sebire *et al.*, 2001) compared obese (BMI > 30 kg/m^2) and normal-weight women (BMI 20-25 kg/m^2). This large study serves as a convenient summary of many other, smaller investigations with similar conclusions but lower statistical power. The obese women studied by Sebire *et al.* (Sebire *et al.*, 2001) were at significant excess risk of gestational diabetes mellitus (GDM), preeclampsia, genital and urinary tract infections, wound infection, induction of labor, emergency and elective cesarean section, and both postpartum hemorrhage and major postpartum hemorrhage (**Figure 1**), top and middle panels). In another large sample, 62,127 women in the Danish National Birth Cohort, Nøhr and colleagues (Nøhr *et al.*, 2006) found that maternal obesity was associated with a higher risk of premature rupture of membranes as well as early induced preterm delivery.

In addition, compared to babies born to normal-weight women, Sebire *et al.* (Sebire *et al.*, 2001) observed that babies born to obese women were significantly

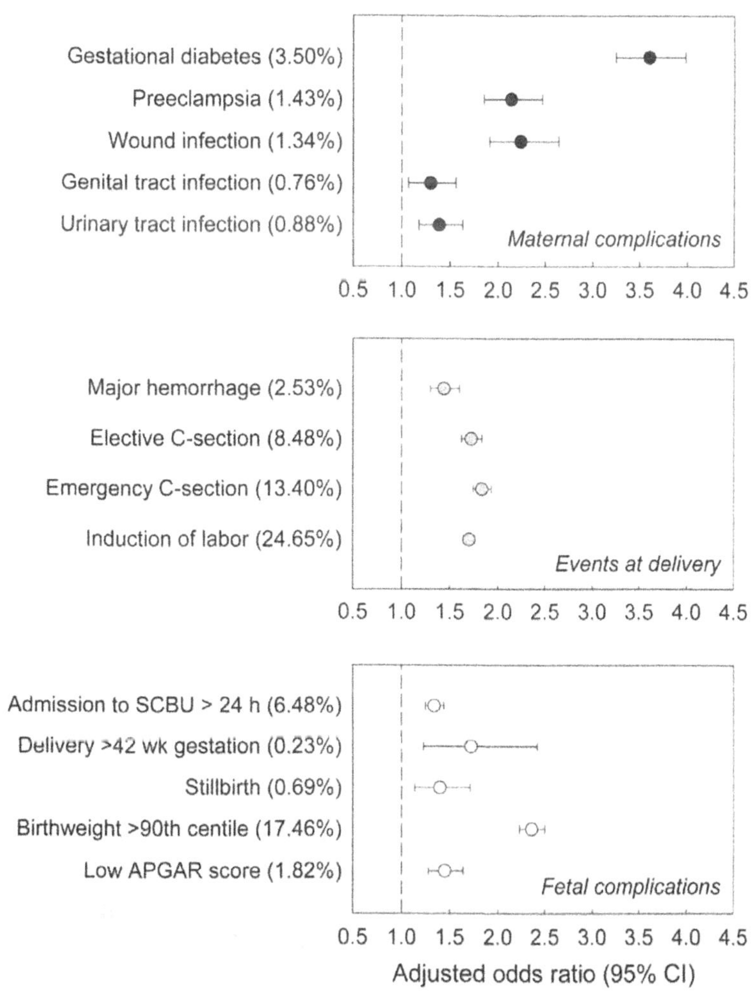

Figure 1. Association between prepregnant maternal obesity (body mass index >30 kg/m^2) and selected maternal and fetal outcomes of 282,213 pregnancies in London. Data are graphed from Sebire *et al.* (Sebire *et al.*, 2001) and show adjusted odds ratios and 95% confidence intervals (CI) compared to normal-weight women. The factors used for adjustment differ as appropriate for each outcome; see Sebire *et al.*, 2001 for details.

more likely to be born after 42 week gestation, to be stillborn, to have a birthweight > 90th percentile (large-for-gestational age, LGA), to have a low or a very low APGAR score, and to be admitted to a special care unit (**Figure 1**), bottom panel). Babies born to obese women were significantly less likely to be born before 32 weeks gestation, to have a birthweight < 5th percentile, and to breastfeed. Unfortunately, obese women were also at excess risk of having a fetus who dies before the 28th week of gestation (Nøhr *et al.*, 2005), after the 28th week of gestation (Nøhr *et al.*, 2005; Cnattingius *et al.*, 1998; Kristensen *et al.*, 2005), and in the neonatal period (Kristensen *et al.*, 2005) in studies in Denmark and Sweden with very large samples (~25,000 - ~165,000 women). In the Danish National Birth Cohort, researchers also observed an increased risk of fetal death before 28 weeks of gestation among obese women after 14 weeks gestational age (Nøhr *et al.*, 2005). In contrast to normal-weight women, among whom the risk of early fetal death declines as gestation progresses, the risk increased as gestation progressed among obese women.

Although obesity is a risk factor for GDM, investigators have found that both obesity and GDM are independently associated with an increased risk of delivering an LGA infant at term (Ehrenberg *et al.*, 2004; Ray *et al.*, 2001). Although the risk of having an LGA infant is higher for diabetic than for obese women, there are so many more obese than diabetic women that Ehrenberg and coworkers (Ehrenberg *et al.*, 2004) calculated that the attributable risk of delivering a LGA infant was about three times higher for obese than for diabetic women in the urban population that they studied in Ohio.

It is noteworthy that the excess risks of undesirable maternal and fetal outcomes of pregnancy get progressively worse as women get heavier. To establish this association, Cedergren (Cedergren, 2004) used data from pregnancies in Sweden over a ten year period (1992-2001) that were identified through the Swedish Medical Birth Registry. Her study included the 805,275 pregnancies for which data on maternal height and weight in early pregnancy were available. With such high statistical power, she was able to divide the obese women into three BMI groups: 29.1-35, 35.1-40, and > 40 kg/m^2. The risk of preeclampsia, cesarean delivery, shoulder dystocia, induction of labor, delivery at 42 weeks gestation, and birth of a large-for-gestational age baby all increased with increasing BMI values within the obese range (**Figure 2**). Similar findings are available from a multicenter study in the U.S. of over 16,000 women (Weiss *et al.*, 2004). This dose-response relationship between increasing degrees of maternal adiposity and cesarean delivery in particular was also evident in the 1999-2000 data from the Pregnancy Risk Assessment Monitoring System (Dietz *et al.*, 2005).

In recent years, many investigators have reported that obese women have an excessive risk of delivering

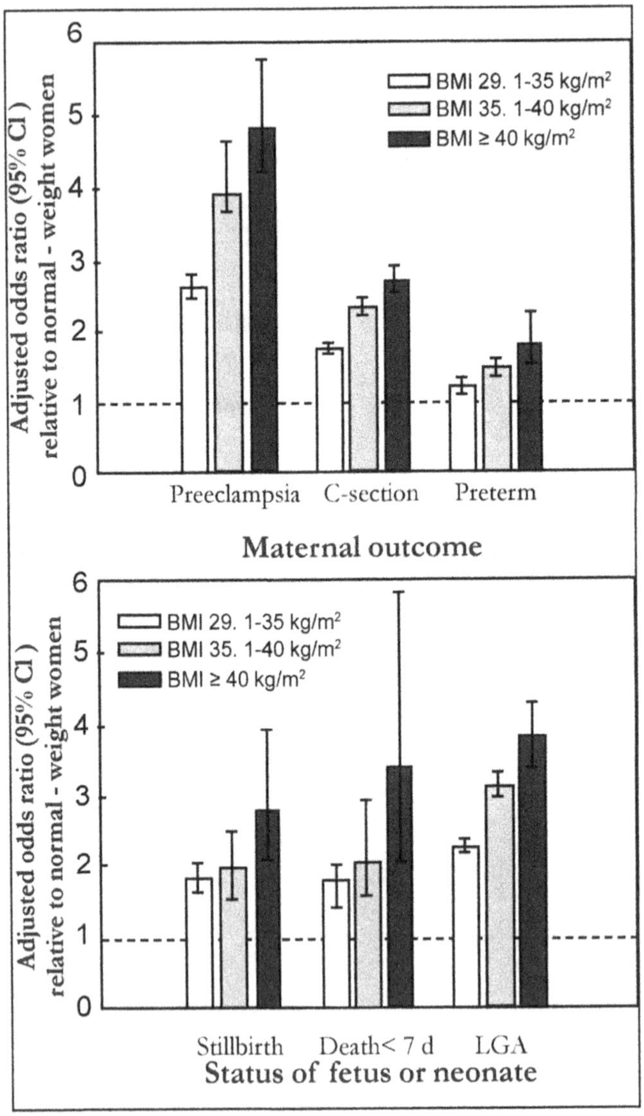

Figure 2. Association between increasing degrees of maternal prepregnant obesity and selected maternal, fetal, and neonatal outcomes of 621,221 singleton pregnancies in Sweden from 1992-2001. Data are graphed from Cedergren (Cedergren, 2004) and show adjusted (for maternal age, parity, smoking in early pregnancy, and year of birth) odds ratios and 95% confidence intervals (CI) compared to normal-weight women. Stillbirths occurred >28 weeks of gestation; LGA, large-for-gestational age (birthweight >2 standard deviations above the mean).

infants with major congenital malformations, including heart defects and multiple anomalies (Watkins *et al.*, 2003) as well as neural tube defects [see (Watkins *et al.*, 2003) for a summary of the findings of these studies]. The mechanism for this is unclear, but inasmuch as type I diabetes is associated with congenital defects and obese women are at high risk of GDM, it is of interest to know if obesity amplifies the association. Anderson *et al.* (Anderson *et al.*, 2005) found that this was the case: obese women had an excess risk of delivering babies with central nervous system defects (such as anencephaly and spinal bifida) and that risk was multiplied in women with GDM. This suggests that the conditions that cause congenital abnormalities occur at glucose values below our current screening thresholds for GDM.

In most of the studies of the association between prepregnant obesity and the outcome of pregnancy, the investigators either did not account for weight gain during pregnancy or did not examine its contribution directly. Obese women are at excess risk for low gestational weight gain (GWG) (Naeye, 1990) and are, at the same time, highly likely to exceed the IOM guidelines for GWG (Hilson *et al.*, 2006), which are lower for obese than for women in other categories of prepregnant BMI (Institute of Medicine, 1990). Excessive GWG can add to the adverse effects of prepregnant BMI on the outcome of pregnancy, and this possibility has received some attention in the literature. For example, Edwards and her associates (Edwards *et al.*, 1996) showed that although obese (BMI > 29 kg/m^2) women were more likely to have complications of pregnancy than normal-weight women, the incidence of complications (such as GDM, hypertension, cesarean delivery, or preeclampsia) was not associated with GWG. However, GWG was positively associated with birthweight in this case-control study and almost one quarter of the obese women who gained > 16 kg delivered babies who weighed 4,000 g regardless of their gestational age at birth. In Denmark, Jensen *et al.* (Jensen *et al.*, 2005) observed a trend toward higher birthweight with increasing weight gain among glucose-tolerant, obese women. Those who gained 15 kg were much more likely [adjusted odds ratio (AOR) 4.7 (2.0-11.0)] to deliver a LGA baby than those who gained < 5 kg.

Infants of Obese Mothers

In the most recent (2001-2002) US national data, infants who weighed 4000 g at birth represented 12.7% of the births > 3000 g (Boulet *et al.*, 2005). This proportion has decreased significantly since 1989-1992, when it was 14.4% (Boulet *et al.*, 2005). This may be because of a tendency to induce labor in women who are carrying a fetus who is thought to be large. In contrast, the proportion of babies who weighed 4000 g at birth increased from 16.6% in 1990 to 20.7% in 1999 in a series of 36,265 births in Aarhus, Denmark (Ørskou *et al.*, 2003). During this period maternal weight, height, age, and education increased while cigarette smoking decreased.

A more meaningful statistic is the proportion of LGA babies because this is independent of decisions made by physicians or mothers about when to deliver. There are good data on this from Canada, where Wen *et al.* (Wen, *et al.*, 2003) showed that the proportion of LGA babies has increased significantly from 8.7 to 10.0% from 1981-83 until 1995-97. This increase occurred primarily among babies born at 37 week of gestation; the proportion of LGA infants decreased over this period at earlier stages of gestation. The determinants of this trend were studied by Kramer and his colleagues (Kramer *et al.*, 2002) in a hospital-based cohort that included 61,437 non-malformed singleton infants who were born alive at 22-43 week gestational age between 1978 and 1996. They found that the observed increase in LGA births over this period was largely the result of increases that had also been occurring in prepregnant BMI, GWG and GDM along with decreases in maternal cigarette smoking and post-term delivery.

Inasmuch as large infants may be treated differently than lighter infants after delivery, it is important to understand the predictors and consequences of having such a large baby. This issue has also been studied by Sebire and his colleagues (Jolly *et al.*, 2003) among 350,311 births in the North West Thames Region in the United Kingdom between 1988 and 1997. Regardless of whether the infant was classified as being macrosomic by absolute (> 4000 g) or relative (> 90th percentile of weight-for-gestational age) size, the predictors of being large at birth were similar: maternal overweight or obesity, parity 2+, age of 35-40 year and either preexisting or GDM (Jolly *et al.*, 2003). Having such an infant was associated with substantial maternal morbidity, including anemia, prolonged labor, emergency cesarean section, second- and third-degree tears, postpartum hemorrhage and prolonged hospital stay (Jolly *et al.*, 2003). These babies were more likely to have a low or a very low APGAR score and to be admitted to a special-care nursery (Jolly *et al.*, 2003). Interestingly, these large babies were not less likely to be breastfed in the hospital than normal-weight babies (Jolly *et al.*, 2003).

In other studies of macrosomic infants, researchers have found that macrosomia itself, rather than maternal obesity, was the strongest predictor of shoulder dystocia (Robinson *et al.*, 2003). Shoulder dystocia is a problem not only because it can create an obstetric emergency but also because it can injure or kill the baby (Mehta *et al.*, 2006). When delivered vaginally, macrosomic babies had higher rates of asphyxia, birth trauma, clavicular injury, brachial or Erb palsy and seizures than normal-weight infants in a study of 68,911 births in Washington state in 1990 (Gregory *et al.*, 1998). When delivered by cesarean section, macrosomic babies were not at higher risk of these complications (Gregory *et al.*, 1998). Using U.S. national data for 1995-97, Boulet and her colleagues (Boulet *et al.*, 2003) showed that the heavier the baby within the macrosomic range, the more likely it was to have been born to a woman who experienced obstetric complications and procedures, such as induced labor and cesarean delivery, and to have had a low APGAR score, assisted ventilation and birth injuries (Boulet *et al.*, 2003). Moreover, the heavier the macrosomic baby, the more likely it was to have been delivered by a woman with abnormal glucose tolerance tests in pregnancy and to have high umbilical cord insulin values itself (Wollschlaeger *et al.*, 1999). However, maternal obesity–not diabetes–was associated with an increased risk of neonatal injury among babies with shoulder dystocia in a recent study (Mehta *et al.*, 2006).

In summary, these statistics indicate that women who are obese before they conceive are likely to suffer from medical complications of pregnancy and delivery that can be expected to impair their ability to nurse their infants in the immediate postpartum period. Moreover, obese women deliver infants who themselves may have physical characteristics that could make nursing difficult. Increasing degrees of prepregnant obesity are associated with additional complications of pregnancy, and excessive GWG among women who are obese before conception is associated with the delivery of an even-larger infant.

ASSOCIATION OF THE CONDITION OF THE MOTHER AND INFANT AT BIRTH WITH BREASTFEEDING

Cesarean Section And the Success of Breastfeeding

The rates of cesarean section have been increasing in the U.S. and elsewhere in recent years, and reached 27.5% in the U.S. in 2003, the highest ever reported (Martin *et al.*, 2003). As described above, obese women are more likely than normal-weight women to have this procedure. For some women, this is a life-saving procedure for them and/or their fetuses. For others, the need for operative delivery is less clear, and various trade-offs, including those relative to breastfeeding, then come into play. Cesarean section is a more difficult procedure in an obese than in a normal-weight woman. These difficulties include correctly determining the amount of anesthetic needed and giving it correctly, intraoperative blood loss, and post-operative infection (Andreasen *et al.*, 2004). Regardless of their prepregnant BMI, women who have experienced a cesarean section have a longer recovery postpartum and a delay in breastfeeding their babies for the first time (Chen *et al.*, 1998) compared to those who have not had an operative delivery. It has long been known that a delay in putting the baby to the breast for the first time is associated with a shorter total duration of breastfeeding (Salariya *et al.*, 1978). Cesarean delivery may (Dewey *et al.*, 2003; Evans *et al.*, 2003) or may not (Kulski *et al.*, 1981; Patel *et al.*, 2003) be associated with a significant delay in milk "coming in." There is evidence from one small study that women who delivered by cesarean and offered the breast sooner were able to feed colostrum sooner and their milk came in sooner than women who offered their infants the breast later (Sözmen, 1982).

It is also possible that cesarean delivery affects whether the mother executes her choice to breastfeed and, if she does so, whether she is able to initiate breastfeeding successfully. However, few studies have been conducted that have provided this level of detail. One exception to this is the work of Pérez-Escamilla *et al.* (Pérez-Escamilla *et al.*, 1996), who used data collected as part of the Demographic and Health Survey in Mexico in 1987. In this study, 2,487 women reported on how their children, who were greater than five years old, had been fed as infants. Cesarean delivery was significantly and negatively associated with ever putting the newborn to the breast [AOR 0.64 (0.50, 0.82)] and breastfeeding for less than one month [AOR 0.58 (0.37, 0.91)].

The Postnatal Characteristics of Infants of Obese Mothers

After birth, all newborns must adapt to extrauterine life by mobilizing glucose and fatty acids from their stores to meet energy needs until adequate feeding begins. Fuels are mobilized in response to hormonal signals and the expression of key genes (Cornblath *et al.*, 2000). In appropriate-for-gestational age infants born to normal-weight mothers, there is a transient decrease in plasma glucose values before a new steady state is reached two to three hours after birth (Cornblath *et al.* 2000; Kliegman *et al.*, 1984). Concentrations of plasma insulin decrease during this period, while concentrations of plasma triglycerides, free fatty acids, and glycerol rise. In the period before the milk "comes in" (lactogenesis II), concentrations of plasma glucose will continue to be lower and concentrations of ketone bodies will be higher in breastfed than in formula-fed infants. In reviewing this information, Cornblath *et al.* (Cornblath *et al.*, 2000) concluded that "the provision of alternate fuels constitutes a normal adaptive response [of the infant] to transiently low nutrient intake during the establishment of breastfeeding." Moreover, "[breastfed] infants may well tolerate lower plasma glucose levels without any significant clinical manifestations or sequelae."

Of concern here is whether the metabolic characteristics of infants of obese mothers differ from those born to normal-weight women. Kliegman and colleagues (Kliegman *et al.*, 1984) showed that although the infants of obese women were hypoglycemic, their plasma insulin values remained higher than those of infants born to normal-weight women in the first four hours after delivery. Their values for plasma triglycerides, free fatty acids, and glycerol were also higher than those of infants born to normal-weight mothers. Neonatal hypoglycemia is a concern because, if sustained, it can cause seizures and permanent brain injury (Stanley & Baker, 1999). In contrast to infants born to diabetic women, who may have hyperinsulinemia and, as a result, persistent hypoglycemia, infants born to nondiabetic, obese women are not hyperinsulinemic (Kliegman *et al.*, 1984). Infants of diabetic women have more adipose tissue at a given birthweight than do babies of normal-weight mothers (Catalano *et al.*, 2003); it is not known whether this is also true of infants of obese mothers.

LGA infants whose mothers do not have diabetes should not be considered a high-risk group for hypoglycemia according to de Rooy and Hawdon (de Rooy & Hawdon, 2002) because "although low blood glucose levels did occur" in their sample of breastfed newborns who were 98th percentile of weight-for-gestational age, "this was offset by a normal [ketone body] response. . ." They argue that "neonatal ketogenesis. . .is a normal adaptive response that enables the transition from fetal to infant metabolism." They speculate that there may be a factor that is present in human milk but absent from infant formula that augments ketogenesis in breastfed babies. However, hypoglycemia in LGA babies may reveal maternal diabetes that was not previously diagnosed (R.J. Schanler, pers. comm., 2006). Therefore, whether to screen LGA babies for hypoglycemia remains controversial.

This finding of a normal ketone-body response among breastfed newborns is important because it is routine practice in many hospitals to screen all LGA babies for hypoglycemia regardless of whether their mothers are diabetic (C.L. Kjolhede and R.J. Schanler, pers. comm. 2005). Babies who have blood glucose values below a cutoff are given a dextrose and water solution or infant formula even though the Academy of Breastfeeding Medicine recommends that breastfed neonates be put directly to the breast (Lawrence & Lawrence, 2005). Unfortunately, use of these solutions may interfere with establishing breastfeeding (Michaelson *et al.*, 1984; Martin-Calama *et al.*, 1997; Bloomquist *et al.*, 1994). Inasmuch as a wide range of cutoff values for plasma glucose are in use (McGowan, 1999) and "there is no single value for plasma glucose concentration which determines absolute clinical risk or predicts sequelae" (Williams, 2005), it seems prudent to follow the advice of Williams (Williams, 2005) and base treatment on "operational thresholds and clinical assessment, and not plasma glucose concentration alone." It is noteworthy that the list of risk factors that indicate the need for screening for neonatal hypoglycemia given by Williams (Williams, 2005) and Deshpande and Platt (Deshpande & Platt, 2005) in their recent reviews did not include large size at birth by itself.

Those who care for newborn infants note that LGA babies can be difficult to feed. They are often born near term and are sleepy, they may be difficult to hold because they are so large, and there may be a discrepancy between how hungry they are and how much milk their mothers can produce in the first few days after delivery. These factors may lead to what has been called the "big baby blues" (C.L. Kjolhede and R.J. Schanler, pers. comm. 2005). Such babies would fall into the groups that Gagnon *et al.* (Gagnon *et al.*, 2005) identified as likely to be given formula supplementation in the hospital. Although there is ample information in the medical literature about infants of diabetic women and their unique needs, there is a corresponding lack of information about the infants of obese women and their own unique needs.

In summary, both operative delivery and the birth of a LGA baby represent potential challenges for breastfeeding among obese women. At a minimum, cesarean section delays the first breastfeeding and may contribute to delayed lactogenesis II. At least one blood sample is taken from most LGA babies for the determination of their blood glucose concentrations, and many of these infants receive glucose water or infant formula as a result. These supplements may be unnecessary and may interfere with establishing breastfeeding. LGA babies born to obese, nondiabetic women may be difficult to feed, but little is known about their specific needs.

DEVELOPMENT OF THE MAMMARY GLANDS DURING PREGNANCY AND LACTATION

The human breast changes profoundly during pregnancy, with marked expansion of the ducts and formation of additional lobules (Lawrence & Lawrence, 1995). These structural changes are associated with an increase in breast size that, in turn, is associated with an increase in milk production postpartum (Hytten, 1954). The hormonal control of this process includes human placental lactogen, prolactin, and human chorionic gonadotropin; estrogen mediates the increase in prolactin concentration during pregnancy (Lawrence & Lawrence, 1995). Information on how maternal obesity before conception might affect these processes in unavailable from women.

However, information is available from experimental species that provides evidence for a negative effect of maternal overfeeding or overfatness before and during pregnancy on aspects of lactational performance. Rats fed a high-fat diet before conception (Shaw *et al.*, 1997) made an inadequate metabolic transition from pregnancy to lactation (i.e., plasma insulin did not decrease nor did plasma prolactin increase as much

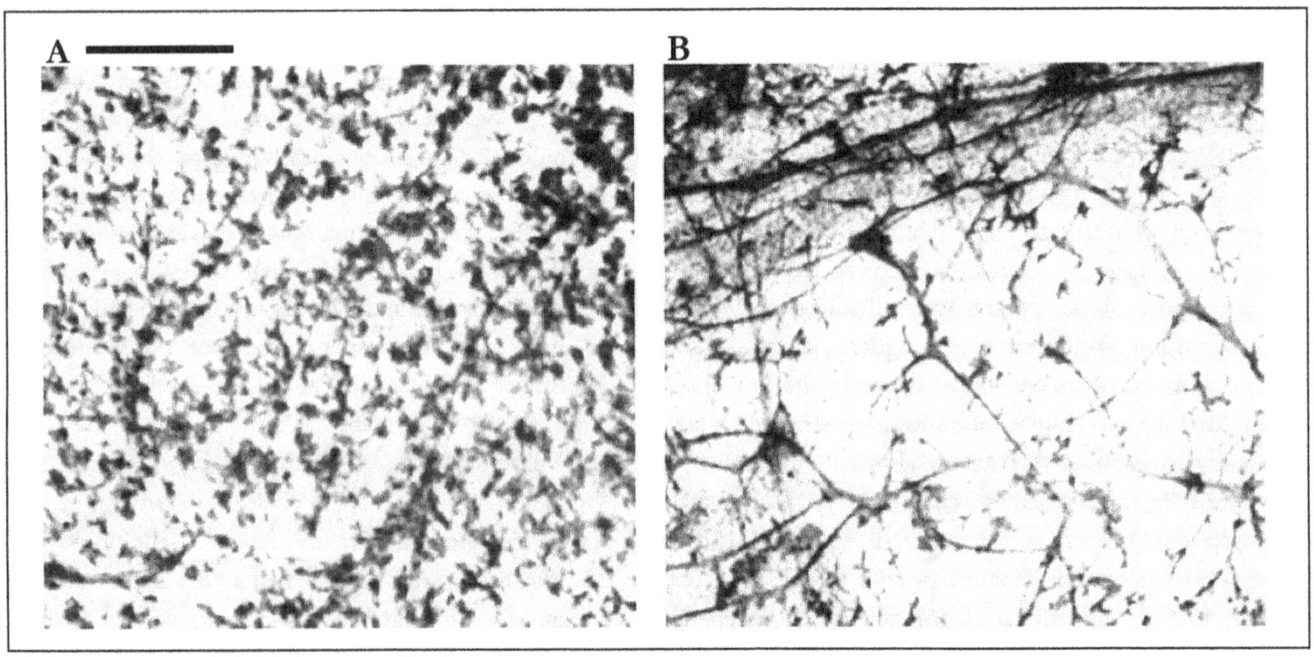

Figure 3. Association between diet-induced obesity in mice and mammary gland development at day 14 of pregnancy. Whole mounts of mammary glands from lean (panel A, left) and obese (panel B, right) mice are shown. Scale bar represents 1 mm. From Flint *et al.*, 2005; used with permission from AJP- Endocrinology and Metabolism.

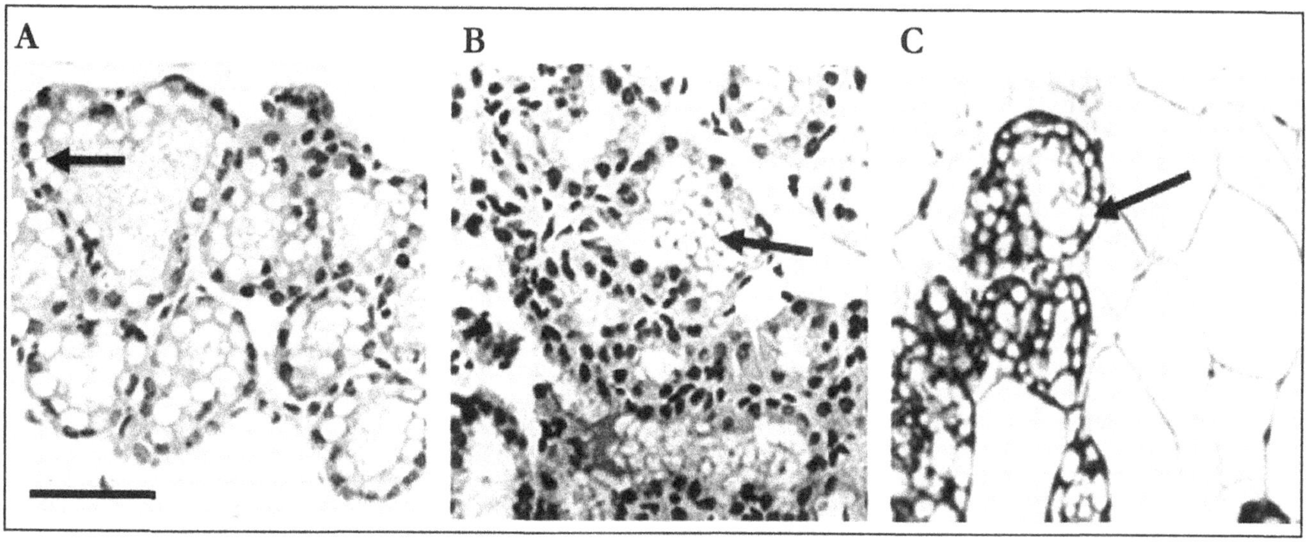

Figure 4. Association between diet-induced obesity in mice and lipid accumulation in mammary gland alveoli during late pregnancy and early lactation. Accumulation of triglycerides in alveolar epithelium of a lean mouse on day 18 of pregnancy (panel A, left) and an obese mouse on day 1 of lactation (panel C, right) can be seen from the single lipid droplets (arrow) within numerous cells of the alveoli. In contrast, in a lean mouse on day 1 of lactation (panel B, middle), lipid secretion has occurred as evidenced by the large number of lipid droplets present in the alveolar lumen (arrow). Scale bar represents 1 mm. From Flint *et al.*, 2005; used with permission of AJP - Endocrinology and Metabolism.

during this transition in obese as in normal animals). These changes could result in both inadequate availability of the glucose that is necessary for milk production as well as an inadequate hormonal signal to produce milk. Overfeeding of singleton-bearing ewes resulted in a reduction in the length of gestation and also in the production of colostrum (Wallace *et al.*, 2005). Feeding mice a "cafeteria-style" high-fat diet resulted in impaired lactogenesis as indicated by poor pup weight gain immediately after birth and changes in mRNA expression that were consistent with a decrease in milk synthesis (Flint *et al.*, 2005). The mice fed the high-fat diet exhibited impaired alveolar development in their mammary glands as early as day 14 of pregnancy, giving them a reduced parenchymal mass (**Figure 3**). The mammary glands of these animals were heavier, but did not have more secretory cells. Lipid accumulated in the secretory cells early in lactation, which indicated an absence of copious milk secretion (**Figure 4**). The authors noted that this accumulation of lipid was "reminiscent of late pregnancy" (Flint *et al.*, 2005).

Taken together, these findings suggest that excess maternal fat during pregnancy impairs the development of the mammary glands that must occur during pregnancy. As a result, such individuals may begin the breastfeeding period still needing to complete this developmental process before they can begin the additional development that must occur to get to lactogenesis II and later to lactogenesis III.

ASSOCIATION OF MATERNAL OBESITY WITH THE INITIATION AND CONTINUATION OF BREASTFEEDING

Ever Breastfeeding

Many factors are associated with whether a woman ever gives her infant a chance to breastfeed. In large samples of American women from national pregnancy and pediatric surveillance systems and the National Immunization Survey, Li and her coworkers (Li *et al.*, 2005; Li *et al.*, 2003) found that maternal age, education, marital status, race or ethnicity, smoking status, and poverty status were all associated with ever breastfeeding. It is noteworthy that maternal prepregnant BMI was not on this list, although Li *et al.* (Li *et al.*, 2003) found that prepregnant BMI interacted with GWG as a determinant of ever breastfeeding.

Initiation of Breastfeeding

The picture is different for successful initiation of breastfeeding (defined as still breastfeeding at the time of hospital discharge), however. We observed that rats that were fed a high-fat diet beginning before conception, continuing through pregnancy, and into lactation not

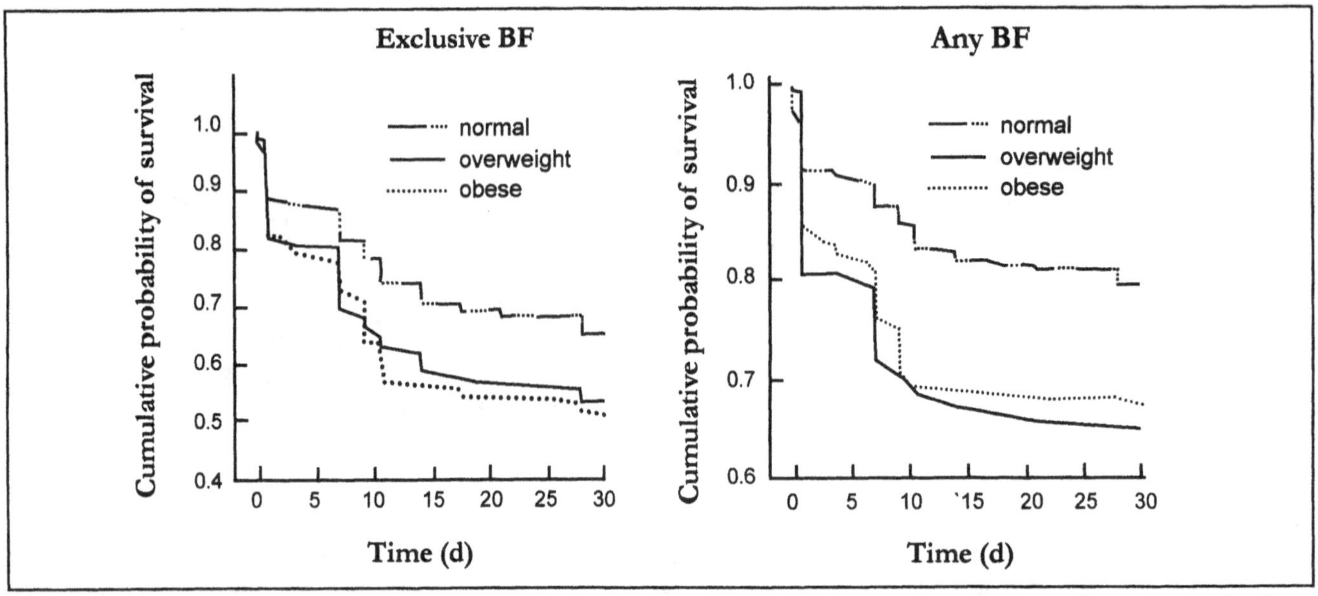

Figure 5. Association between maternal overweight or obesity and the probability of continuing to breastfeed. The IOM categories were used to characterize maternal prepregnant BMI values. Both prepregnant overweight and obesity were negatively associated with exclusive breastfeeding (left panel) (overweight: relative risk = 1.42, P < 0.04; obesity: relative risk = 1.42, P < 0.02) and any breastfeeding (right panel) (overweight: relative risk = 1.68, P < 0.006; obesity: relative risk = 1.73, P < 0.001). From Hilson *et al.*, 1997; reproduced with permission from The American Journal of Clinical Nutrition.

infrequently failed to nurse their newborn pups, who died shortly thereafter (Shaw *et al.*, 1997). This finding suggested a primary failure of lactogenesis, so we examined this possibility among white women who lived in a rural area of the U.S. We found that, among women who had ever put their baby to the breast, the odds ratio for failure to continue to breastfeed through the time of hospital discharge was significantly higher among overweight (AOR 2.54, P < 0.05) and obese women (AOR 3.65, P < 0.001) than among normal-weight women (Hilson *et al.*, 1997). In this study, most of the women were discharged before their milk "came in." We have also examined this possibility among black and Hispanic women who lived in an urban area of the U.S. (Kugyelka *et al.*, 2004). For Hispanic women, we saw the same general pattern as among white women: the heavier women were more likely than normal-weight women to have stopped exclusive breastfeeding. For black women, this trend was not observed.

The period–albeit short–while the woman is hospitalized is an opportunity for staff members, particularly nurses and lactation consultants (if they are available), to assist mothers in learning to breastfeed, including helping them with proper positioning of the infant and latching on. There is evidence from a relatively informal study that health-care providers do not treat obese women differently than normal-weight women (Rasmussen *et al.*, 2006). Health-care providers perceived that large breasts were more of a problem than obesity itself. There is only limited information with which to address this possibility. Pisacane *et al.* (Pisacane *et al.*, 2004) recently observed that while obesity was associated with reduced frequency of breastfeeding, breast size before pregnancy (measured as bra cup size) was not. The increase in breast size during pregnancy, because of its association with milk production (Hytten, 1954), and breast size early in lactation, because of the association of large breast size with the difficulty in latching on by the newborn, are likely to be more important than breast size before pregnancy.

Continuation of Breastfeeding

After the time of hospital discharge, continuation of breastfeeding is affected by the timing of lactogenesis and the mother's perception that she is able to provide enough milk to meet her infant's needs, as well as many psychosocial and sociocultural factors, some of which affect obese women differentially (**Figure 5**).

Maternal obesity is one of the factors that is associated with delayed onset of lactogenesis II (Dewey *et al.*, 2003; Chapman & Perez-Escamilla, 2000; Hilson *et al.*, 2004), although it is less important that nulliparity as a predictor of this problem. Parous women produce more milk at day seven of lactation than nulliparous women (Hytten, 1959) and they also may have had prior experience with breastfeeding. A delay in the onset of lactogenesis II not only leads to frustration and reduced satisfaction with the process of breastfeeding, it is also associated with reduced milk transfer to the infant at the time lactogenesis is expected (Chapman & Pérez-Escamilla, 2000) and a shortened total duration of breastfeeding (Chapman & Pérez-Escamilla, 1999).

Several factors may contribute to a delay in lactogenesis II among obese women. First, mechanical problems with positioning the baby and latching on may be stressful to the mother and may result in poor suckling stimulus by the baby. Both stress and poor suckling stimulus interfere with lactogenesis (Chen *et al.*, 1998; Dewey, 2001), but this possibility has not been studied in obese compared to normal-weight women. Second, one of the triggers for lactogenesis II is the postpartum decrease in progesterone concentration that occurs with the delivery of the placenta (Neville, 2001). We proposed that this might occur more slowly in obese women, and the trend was in this direction from two to seven days postpartum, but the difference between obese and normal-weight women was not statistically significant (Rasmussen & Kjolhede, 2004). Third, prolactin secretion is blunted in response to various stimuli among obese subjects (Kopelman, 2000) and adequate prolactin values necessary for lactogenesis II to occur (Neville, 2001). Therefore, we proposed that prolactin values would be reduced in response to suckling in obese women. Indeed, this is what we observed at both day two and day seven postpartum (Rasmussen & Kjolhede, 2004). Lovelady (Lovelady, 2005) has proposed an alternative explanation for these findings, namely that difficulties in latching-on and positioning of the infants of the heavier mothers are solely responsible for the observed poor prolactin response to suckling. This explanation cannot be excluded with the available data. And finally, we observed that rats fed a high-fat diet made an inadequate metabolic and physiologic transition from late pregnancy to early lactation; their plasma insulin values did not decrease as much nor did their prolactin values increase as much as those of rats fed a control diet (Shaw *et al.*, 1997). Women make this same kind of metabolic transition (Lind & Harris, 1976). The difference between obese and normal-weight women was in the proposed direction at day two postpartum, but it was not statistically significant (Rasmussen & Kjolhede, 2004). Given the low level of statistical power in our study (Rasmussen & Kjolhede, 2004), the hypotheses about progesterone and insulin cannot yet be rejected.

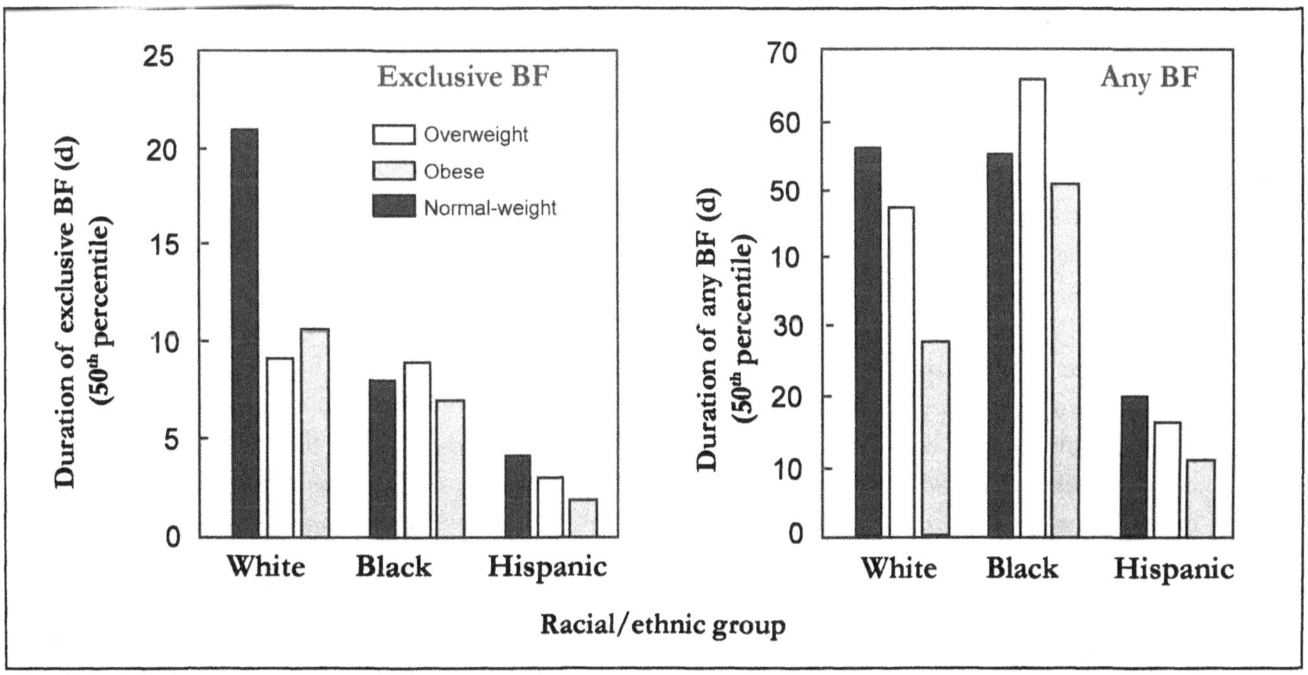

Figure 6. Association among racial/ethnic group, maternal prepregnant BMI, and the duration of breastfeeding. Left panel, exclusive breastfeeding; right panel, any breastfeeding. Data are graphed as the 50th percentile of the distribution. Data for white women are derived from Hilson *et al.* (1997) and for black and Hispanic women from Kugyelka *et al.* (2004).

The behavior of breastfeeding is, of course, embedded in a psychosocial and sociocultural milieu and a substantial body of research has contributed to our understanding of these issues. At present, little is known about how these factors might interact with maternal obesity. In a study of the psychosocial factors that might have an impact on the success of breastfeeding, Hilson *et al.* (Hilson *et al.*, 2004) found that only their shorter planned duration of breastfeeding and lower satisfaction with their appearance distinguished obese from normal-weight women. The maternal BMI groups did not differ in their plans to return to work or school, in self-efficacy for breastfeeding, or beliefs about breastfeeding, and none of these factors modified the association between maternal obesity and later onset of lactogenesis II.

Several researchers have now observed that maternal obesity is associated with a shorter duration of exclusive (Hilson *et al.*, 1994; Kugyelka *et al.*, 2004; Li *et al.*, 2002) and any breastfeeding (Hilson *et al.*, 1997; Kugyelka *et al.*, 2004; Rutishauser & Carlin, 1992; Donath & Amir, 2000, Li *et al.*, 2002). This finding is not completely uniform, however. Riva *et al.* (Riva *et al.*, 1999) found a negative association between maternal prepregnant BMI (as a continuous variable) and the duration of exclusive breastfeeding [(relative risk 1.02 (1.00, 1.04)]. For the white and Hispanic obese women studied in upstate New York, the drop-off in "survival" of breastfeeding was particularly rapid in the first ten days after delivery (Hilson *et al.*, 1997; Kugyelka *et al.*, 2004). Two additional findings are striking in these data. First, the durations of exclusive (**Figure 6**, left panel) and any (**Figure 6**, right panel) breastfeeding were quite short among white women from a rural area as well as black and Hispanic women from an urban area. Second, there was a dose-response–as women became heavier, the shorter their breastfeeding duration–among white and Hispanic, but not black, women. The reason for the difference among these racial ethnic groups is unknown (Kugyelka *et al.*, 2004). When interviewed during pregnancy, white women intended to breastfeed for a much longer period (months instead of weeks) (Hilson *et al.*, 2004), so this early termination of breastfeeding may not necessarily signal a lack of desire to breastfeed or commitment to breastfeeding. There is a strong possibility that, in addition to the biological factors discussed above, this early termination of breastfeeding is related in part to a lack of adequate support for breastfeeding–among health-care personnel, families, communities, and American society itself.

In nearly all of these studies of the association between maternal obesity and the duration of breastfeeding, prepregnant BMI was used to capture a woman's relative fatness at delivery. Of course, this ignores the contribution of GWG to maternal fatness during pregnancy and at delivery, which may be as or more important to the success of lactation than the woman's condition at conception. This possibility has been explored in two studies in which GWG was characterized as below, within or above the IOM recommendations for GWG (Institute of Medicine, 1990). In our study of 2783 white women living in a rural area of the US who gave their newborns a chance to nurse, we found that both normal-weight and obese women who gained in excess of the IOM recommendations had a higher likelihood of unsuccessful initiation of breastfeeding (Hilson *et al.*, 2006). For obese women, gaining in excess of the IOM recommendations just made the likelihood of early termination of exclusive or any breastfeeding worse (Hilson *et al.*, 2006). In their study of 13,234 low-income women in the U.S., Li *et al.* (Li *et al.*, 2003) found that both maternal prepregnant obesity and excessive GWG were independently associated with a shorter duration of breastfeeding than that of normal-weight women and those who gained within the IOM guidelines. Although it is impossible to change a woman's prepregnant BMI once she conceives, it is theoretically possible to moderate her weight gain during pregnancy.

In summary, there are numerous reasons why obese women who wish to breastfeed and actually give their newborns a chance to suckle might not be able to achieve their own or society's goals for breastfeeding. These include their condition or that of their infant at delivery, how members of the medical staff treat them and their infants while they are hospitalized after delivery, difficulty positioning the newborn to nurse and the newborn's difficulty in latching on the breast, the physiological effects of obesity on aspects of breast development and milk production that result in delayed lactogenesis and reduced milk production and, finally, inadequate support to overcome these challenges.

WAYS TO IMPROVE LACTATIONAL PERFORMANCE AMONG OBESE WOMEN

For many reasons beyond those presented here, it would be ideal if women were able to plan their pregnancies and prepare themselves nutritionally for pregnancy, including achieving a normal weight before conception. In addition, it would also be desirable for women to limit their GWG to the amounts recommended by the IOM. This is a point of intervention, albeit difficult to achieve (Olson *et al.*, 2004; Polley *et al.*, 2002).

It may also be possible to improve the success of lactation in women who remain too heavy at delivery. We have previously suggested that pediatricians could "help overweight/obese women to succeed at breastfeeding by targeting them for contact with a lactation consultant before discharge from the hospital to be sure that they have received optimal advice on breastfeeding techniques. Additionally, early contact with the mother after discharge–by calling her at home to offer her support and counseling for breastfeeding, by scheduling the first pediatric visit earlier than for other patients, or by enlisting the assistance of public health nurses for a home visit if this is possible–would help overweight/obese women to continue to breastfeed" (Rasmussen & Kjolhede, 2004). These kinds of interventions would help women to continue to breastfeed through the period of lactogenesis II.

It may also be reasonable to think about longer-term treatments that include changes in diet or physical exercise. There is evidence from our small study in obese rats that changing from a high-fat to a low-fat diet after parturition increased milk production and pup growth (Rasmussen *et al.*, 2001). In postpartum women, additional aerobic exercise (45 min/day, five days/week for 12 weeks) alone did not compromise milk production or infant growth among women who were still exclusively breastfeeding at six to eight weeks postpartum (Dewey *et al.*, 1994). The effects of dieting (35% energy deficit), additional physical exercise, or both have been studied in women with a mean BMI of 31-32 kg/m^2 at eight to 16 weeks postpartum (McCrory *et al.*, 1999). In this short (11-day) study, women lost about 1 kg of weight without a compromise in lactational performance or infant growth. It is unknown whether such interventions could be started sooner and last longer so as to help obese women continue to breastfeed for longer than they do at present.

CONCLUSIONS AND IMPLICATIONS

Sufficient evidence is now available to show that maternal prepregnant obesity is negatively associated with the initiation and duration of breastfeeding. Studies from experimental species and limited information from women provide a biological basis for this association. However, it is likely that additional factors also contribute to the difficulty that obese women experience in breastfeeding their babies. Clinicians cannot change an obese woman's prepregnant BMI, GWG, experience during delivery, or the condition of her baby at birth once she has delivered. However, it is important to recognize that obese women and their babies have unique needs and may require additional support while in the hospital and in the days immediately following discharge to maximize the possibility that they will succeed at breastfeeding.

References

Anderson JL, Waller DK, Canfield MA, Shaw GM, Watkins ML, Werler MM. Maternal obesity, gestational diabetes, and central nervous system birth defects. *Epidemiology.* 2005; 16:87-92.

Anderson SE, Dallal GE, Must A. Relative weight and race influence average age at menarche: results from two nationally representative surveys of US girls studied 25 years apart. *Pediatrics.* 2003; 111:844-50.

Andreasen KR, Andersen ML, Schantz AL. Obesity and pregnancy. *Acta Obstet Gynecol Scand.* 2004; 83:1022-29.

Anonymous. Position of the American Dietetic Association: Promoting and supporting breastfeeding. *J Am Diet Assoc.* 2005; 105(5):810-18.

Bloomquist HK, Jonsbo F, Serenius F, Persson LÅ. Supplementary feeding in the maternity ward shortens the duration of breast feeding. *Acta Pædiatr.* 1994; 83:1122-26.

Boulet SL, Alexander GR, Salihu HM. Secular trends in cesarean delivery rates among macrosomic deliveries in the United States, 1989 to 2002. *J Perinatol.* 2005; 25:569-76.

Boulet SL, Alexander GR, Salihu HM, Pass M. Macrosomic births in the United States: determinants, outcomes, and proposed grades of risk. *Am J Obstet Gynecol.* 2003; 188:1372-78.

Breastfeeding Handbook for Physicians. Elk Grove, IL: American Academy of Pediatrics and American College of Obstetricians and Gynecologists; 2006.

Catalano PM, Thomas A, Huston-Presley L, Amini SB. Increased fetal adiposity: a very sensitive marker of abnormal in utero development. *Am J Obstet Gynecol.* 2003; 189:1698-704.

Cedergren MI. Maternal morbid obesity and the risk of adverse pregnancy outcome. *Obstet Gynecol.* 2004; 103:219-24.

Chapman DJ, Pérez-Escamilla R. Does delayed perception of the onset of lactation shorten breastfeeding duration? *J Hum Lact.* 1999; 15:107-11.

Chapman DJ, Perez-Escamilla R. Maternal perception of the onset of lactation is a valid, public health indicator of lactogenesis stage II. *J Nutr.* 2000; 130:2972-80.

Chen DC, Nommsen-Rivers L, Dewey KG, Lönnerdal B. Stress during labor and delivery and early lactation performance. *Am J Clin Nutr.* 1998; 68:335-44.

Clark AM, Ledger W, Galletly C, Tomlinson L, Blaney F, Wang X, *et al.* Weight loss results in significant improvement in pregnancy and ovulation rates in anovulatory obese women. *Hum Reprod.* 1995; 10:2705-12.

Cnattingius S, Bergström R, Lipworth L, Kramer MS. Prepregnancy weight and the risk of adverse pregnancy outcomes. *New Engl J Med.* 1998; 338:147-52.

Cooper C, Kuh D, Egger P, Wadsworth M, Barker D. Childhood growth and age at menarche. *Br J Obstet Gynæcol.* 1996; 103:814-17.

Cornblath M, Hawdon JM, Williams AF, Aynsley-Green A, Ward-Platt MP, Schwartz R, *et al.* Controversies regarding definition of neonatal hypoglycemia: suggested operational thresholds. *Pediatrics.* 2000; 105:1141-45.

de Rooy L, Hawdon J. Nutritional factors that affect the postnatal metabolic adaptation of full-term small- and large-for-gestational-age infants. *Pediatrics.* 2002; 109:e42.

Demerath EW, Li J, Sun SS, Chumlea WC, Remsberg KE, Czerwinski SA, *et al.* Fifty-year trends in serial body mass index during adolescence in girls: the Fels Longitudinal Study. *Am J Clin Nutr.* 2004; 80:441-46.

Demerath EW, Towne B, Chumlea WC, Sun SS, Czerwinski SA, Remsberg KE, *et al.* Recent decline in age at menarche: the Fels Longitudinal Study. *Am J Hum Biol.* 2004; 16:453-7.

Deshpande S, Platt WM. The investigation and management of neonatal hypoglycaemia. *Semin Fetal Neonatal Med.* 2005; 10:351-61.

Dewey KG. Maternal and fetal stress are associated with impaired lactogenesis in humans. *J Nutr.* 2001; 131:3012S-15S.

Dewey KG, Lovelady CA, Nommsen-Rivers LA, McCrory MA, Lönnerdal B. A randomized study of the effects of aerobic exercise by lactating women on breast-milk volume and composition. *N Engl J Med.* 1994; 330:449-53.

Dewey KG, Nommsen-Rivers LA, Heinig MJ, Cohen RJ. Risk factors for suboptimal infant breastfeeding behavior, delayed onset of lactation, and excess neonatal weight loss. *Pediatrics.* 2003; 112:607-19.

Dietz PM, Callaghan WM, Morrow B, Cogswell ME. Population-based assessment of the risk of primary cesarean delivery due to excess prepregnancy weight among nulliparous women delivering term infants. *Mat Child Health.* 2005; 9:237-44.

Donath SM, Amir LH. Does maternal obesity adversely affect breastfeeding initiation and duration? *J Paediatr Child Health.* 2000; 36:482-86.

Edwards LE, Dickes WF, Alton IR, Hakanson EY. Pregnancy in the massively obese: course, outcome, and obesity prognosis of the infant. *Am J Obstet Gynecol.* 1978; 131:479-83.

Edwards LE, Hellerstedt WL, Alton IR, Story M, Himes JH. Pregnancy complications and birth outcomes in obese and normal-weight women: effects of gestational weight change. *Obstet Gynecol.* 1996; 87:389-94.

Ehrenberg HM, Mercer BM, Catalano PM. The influence of obesity and diabetes on the prevalence of macrosomia. *Am J Obstet Gynecol.* 2004; 191:964-68.

Evans KC, Evans RG, Royal R, Esterman AJ, James SL. Effect of caesarean section on breast milk transfer to the normal term newborn over the first week of life. *Arch Dis Child Fetal Neonatal Ed.* 2003; 88:F380-F382.

Flint DJ, Travers MT, Barber MC, Binart N, Kelly PA. Diet-induced obesity impairs mammary development and lactogenesis in murine mammary gland. *Am J Physiol Endocrinol Metab.* 2005; 288:e1179-e1187.

Freedman DS, Khan LK, Serdula MK, Dietz WH, Srinivasan SR, Berenson GS. Relation of age at menarche to race, time period, and anthropometric dimensions: the Bogalusa Heart Study. *Pediatrics.* 2002; 110:e43.

Frisch RE. Body fat, puberty and fertility. *Biol Rev.* 1984; 59:161-88.

Gagnon AJ, Leduc G, Waghorn K, Yang H, Platt RW. In-hospital formula supplementation of healthy breastfeeding newborns. *J Hum Lact.* 2005; 21:397-405.

Gregory KD, Henry OA, Ramicone E, Platt LD. Maternal and infant complications in high and normal weight infants by method of delivery. *Obstet Gynecol.* 1998; 92:507-13.

Hilson JA, Rasmussen KM, Kjolhede CL. Maternal obesity and breastfeeding success in a rural population of Caucasian women. *Am J Clin Nutr.* 1997; 66:1371-78.

Hilson JA, Rasmussen KM, Kjolhede CL. High prepregnant body mass index is associated with poor lactation outcomes among white, rural women independent of psychosocial and demographic correlates. *J Hum Lact.* 2004; 20:18-29.

Hilson JA, Rasmussen KM, Kjolhede CL. Excessive weight gain during pregnancy is associated with earlier termination of breast-feeding among white women. *J Nutr.* 2006; 136:1-7.

Hovey RC, McFadden TB, Akers RM. Regulation of mammary gland growth and morphogenesis by the mammary fat pad: a species comparison. *J Mammary Gland Biol Neoplasia.* 1999; 4:53-68.

Huber LRB, Hogue CJ. The association between body weight, unintended pregnancy resulting in a livebirth, and contraception at the time of conception. *Mat Child Health.* 2005; 9:413-20.

Hytten FE. Clinical and chemical studies in human lactation. VI. The functional capacity of the breast. *Br Med J.* 1954; i:912-5.

Hytten FE. Differences in yield and composition between first and second lactations. *Proc Nutr Soc.* 1959; 18:xxi-xxii.

Institute of Medicine (Subcommittees on Nutritional Status and Weight Gain During Pregnancy and Dietary Intake and Nutrient Supplements During Pregnancy, Committee on Nutritional Status During Pregnancy and Lactation, Food and Nutrition Board). *Nutrition during pregnancy: Part I, Weight gain; Part II, Nutrient supplements.* Washington, DC: National Academy Press; 1990.

Jensen DM, Ovesen P, Beck-Nielsen H, Molsted-Pedersen L, Sorensen B, Vinter C, *et al.* Gestational weight gain and pregnancy outcomes in 481 obese glucose-tolerant women. *Diabetes Care.* 2005; 28:2118-22.

Jolly MC, Sebire NJ, Harris JP, Regan L, Robinson S. Risk factors for macrosomia and its clinical consequences: a study of 350,311 pregnancies. *Eur J Obstet Gynecol Reprod Biol.* 2003; 111:9-14.

Kliegman R, Gross T, Morton S, Dunnington R. Intrauterine growth and postnatal fasting metabolism in infants of obese mothers. *J Pediatr.* 1984; 104:601-7.

Kopelman PG. Physiopathology of prolactin secretion in obesity. *Int J Obes.* 2000; 24 (Suppl 2):S104-S108.

Kramer MS, Morin I, Yang H, Platt RW, Usher R, McNamara H, *et al.* Why are babies getting bigger? Temporal trends in fetal growth and its determinants. *J Pediatr.* 2002; 141:538-42.

Kristensen J, Vestergaard M, Wisborg K, Kesmodel U, Secher NJ. Pre-pregnancy weight and the risk of stillbirth and neonatal death. *Br J Obstet Gynæcol.* 2005; 112:403-8.

Kugyelka JG, Rasmussen KM, Frongillo EA Jr. Maternal obesity negatively affects breastfeeding success among Hispanic but not Black women. *J Nutr.* 2004; 134:1746-53.

Kulski JK, Smith M, Hartmann PE. Normal and caesarian section delivery and the initiation of lactation in women. *Aust J Exp Biol Med Sci.* 1981; 59:405-12.

Lawrence RA, Lawrence RM. *Breastfeeding: A guide for the medical profession.* 6th Ed. Philadelphia: Elsevier Mosby; 2005.

Li R, Darling N, Maurice E, Barker L, Grummer-Strawn LM. Breastfeeding rates in the United States by characteristics of the child, mother, or family: The 2002 National Immunization Survey. *Pediatrics.* 2005; 115:e31-e37.

Li R, Jewell S, Grummer-Strawn LM. Maternal obesity and breast-feeding practices. *Am J Clin Nutr.* 2003; 77:931-36.

Li R, Ogden C, Ballew C, Gillespie C, Grummer-Strawn LM. Prevalence of exclusive breastfeeding among US infants: The Third National Health and Nutrition Examination Survey (Phase II, 1991-1994). *Am J Public Health.* 2002; 92:1107-10.

Li R, Zhao Z, Mokdad A, Barker L, Grummer-Strawn L. Prevalence of breastfeeding in the United States: the 2001 National Immunization Survey. *Pediatrics.* 2003; 111:1198-201.

Lind T, Harris VG. Changes in the oral glucose tolerance test during the puerperium. *Br J Obstet Gynæcol.* 1976; 83:460-63.

Lovelady CA. Is maternal obesity a cause of poor lactation performance? *Nutr Rev.* 2005; 63:352-55.

Martin JA, Hamilton BE, Sutton PD, Ventura SJ, Menacker F, Munson ML. Births: final data for 2003. *Nat Vital Stat Rep.* 2005; 54:1-116.

Martin-Calama J, Buñuel J, Valero MT, Labay M, Lasarte JJ, Valle F, *et al.* The effect of feeding glucose water to breastfeeding newborns on weight, body temperature, blood glucose and breastfeeding duration. *J Hum Lact.* 1997; 13:209-13.

McCrory MA, Nommsen-Rivers LA, Molé PA, Lönnerdal B, Dewey KG. Randomized trial of the short-term effects of dieting compared with dieting plus aerobic exercise on lactation performance. *Am J Clin Nutr.* 1999; 69:959-67.

McGowan JE. Neonatal hypoglycemia. *NeoReviews.* 1999; e6-e15.

Mehta SH, Blackwell SC, Bujold B, Sokol RJ. What factors are associated with neonatal injury following shoulder dystocia? *J Perinatol.* 2006; 26:85-88.

Michaelsen KF, Larsen PS, Thomsen BL, Samuelsen G. The Copenhagen cohort study on infant nutrition and growth: duration of breast feeding and influencing factors. *Acta Pædiatr.* 1984; 83:565-71.

Naeye RL. Maternal body weight and pregnancy outcome. *Am J Clin Nutr.* 1990; 52:273-79.

Neville MC, Morton S. Physiology and endocrine changes underlying human lactogenesis II. *J Nutr.* 2001; 131:3005S-8S.

Nøhr EA, Bech BH, Davies MJ, Frydenberg M, Henriksen TB, Olsen J. Prepregnancy obesity and fetal death: a study within the Danish National Birth Cohort. *Obstet Gynecol.* 2005; 106:250-59.

Nøhr EA, Bech BH, Væth M, Rasmussen KM, Henricksen TB, Olsen J. Obesity, gestational weight gain and preterm birth. A study within the Danish National Birth Cohort. *Pædiatr Perinat Epidemiol.* 2007; 21(1):5-14.

Ogden CL, Carroll MD, Curtin LR, McDowell MA, Tabak CJ, Flegal KM. Prevalence of overweight and obesity in the United States, 1999-2004. *JAMA.* 2006; 295:1549-55.

Olson CM, Strawderman MS, Reed RG. Efficacy of an intervention to prevent excessive gestational weight gain. *Am J Obstet Gynecol.* 2004; 191:530-36.

Ørskou J, Henriksen TB, Kesmodel U, Secher NJ. Maternal characteristics and lifestyle factors and the risk of delivering high birth weight infants. *Obstet Gynecol.* 2003; 102: 115-20.

Patel RR, Liebling RE, Murphy DJ. Effect of operative delivery in the second stage of labor on breastfeeding success. *Birth.* 2003; 30:255-60.

Pérez-Escamilla R, Maulén-Radovan I, Dewey KG. The association between cesarean delivery and breast-feeding outcomes among Mexican Women. *Am J Public Health.* 1996; 86:832-36.

Pisacane A, Continisio P, on behalf of the Italian Working Group on Breastfeeding. Breastfeeding and perceived changes in the appearance of the breasts: a retrospective study. *Acta Pædiatr.* 2004; 93:1346-48.

Polley BA, Wing RR, Sims CJ. Randomized controlled trial to prevent excessive weight gain in pregnant women. *Int J Obes.* 2002; 26:1494-502.

Rasmussen KM, Kjolhede CL. Prepregnant overweight and obesity diminish the prolactin response to suckling in the first week postpartum. *Pediatrics.* 2004; 113:e465-e471.

Rasmussen KM, Lee VE, Ledkovsky TB, Kjolhede CL. A description of lactation counseling practices that are used with obese mothers. *J Hum Lact.* 2006; 22:322-27.

Rasmussen KM, Wallace MH, Gournis E. A low-fat diet but not food restriction improves lactational performance in obese rats. In: Newberg DS (ed.). *Bioactive substances in human milk.* New York: Kluwer Academic/Plenum Publishers; 2001. p. 101-5.

Ray JG, Vermeulen MJ, Shapiro JL, Kenshole AB. Maternal and neonatal outcomes in pregestational and gestational diabetes mellitus, and the influence of maternal obesity and weight gain: the DEPOSIT study. Diabetes Endocrine Pregnancy Outcome Study in Toronto. *QJM.* 2001; 94:347-56.

Riva E, Banderali G, Agostini C, Silano M, Radaelli G, Giovannini M. Factors associated with initiation and duration of breastfeeding in Italy. *Acta Pædiatr.* 1999; 88:411-15.

Robinson H, Tkatch S, Mayes DC, Bott N, Okun N. Is maternal obesity a predictor of shoulder dystocia? *Obstet Gynecol.* 2003; 101:24-27.

Rogers J, Mitchell GW Jr. The relation of obesity to menstrual disturbances. *New Engl J Med.* 1952; 247:53-55.

Rutishauser IHE, Carlin JB. Body mass index and duration of breast feeding: a survival analysis during the first six months of life. *J Epidemiol Comm Health.* 1992; 46:559-65.

Ryan AS, Wenjun Z, Acosta A. Breastfeeding continues to increase into the new millennium. *Pediatrics.* 2002; 110:1103-9.

Salariya EM, Easton PM, Cater JI. Duration of breast-feeding after early initiation and frequent feeding. *Lancet.* 1978; ii:1141-43.

Sebire NJ, Jolly M, Harris JP, Wadsworth J, Joffe M, Beard RW, *et al.* Maternal obesity and pregnancy outcome: a study of 287,213 pregnancies in London. *Int J Obes Relat Metab Disord.* 2001; 25:1175-82.

Section on Breastfeeding. Breastfeeding and the use of human milk. *Pediatrics.* 2005; 115:496-506.

Shaw MA, Rasmussen KM, Myers TR. Consumption of a high-fat diet impairs reproductive performance in Sprague-Dawley rats. *J Nutr.* 1997; 127:64-69.

Sheffield LG. Organization and growth of mammary epithelia in the mammary gland fat pad. *J Dairy Sci.* 1988; 71:2855-74.

Sözmen M. Effects of early suckling of cesarean-born babies on lactation. *Biol Neonate.* 1982; 62:67-68.

Stanley CA, Baker L. The causes of neonatal hypoglycemia. *N Engl J Med.* 1999; 340:1200-1.

U.S. Department of Health and Human Services. *Healthy People 2010.* Washington, DC: Department of Health and Human Services; 2000.

Wallace JM, Milne JS, Aitken RP. The effect of overnourishing singleton-bearing adult ewes on nutrient partitioning to the gravid uterus. *Br J Nutr.* 2005; 94:533-39.

Wang JX, Davies M, Norman RJ. Body mass and probability of pregnancy during assisted reproduction treatment: retrospective study. *BMJ.* 2000; 321:1320-21.

Watkins ML, Rasmussen SA, Honein MA, Botto LD, Moore CA. Maternal obesity and risk for birth defects. *Pediatrics.* 2003; 111:1152-58.

Weiss JL, Malone FD, Emig D, Ball RH, Nyberg DA, Comstock CH, *et al.* Obesity, obstetric complications and cesarean delivery rate-a population-based screening study. *Am J Obstet Gynecol.* 2004; 190:1091-97.

Wen SW, Kramer MS, Platt R, Demissie K, Joseph KS, Liu S, *et al.* Secular trends of fetal growth in Canada, 1981 to 1997. *Paediatr Perinat Epidemiol.* 2003; 17:347-54.

Williams AF. Neonatal hypoglycaemia: clinical and legal aspects. *Semin Fetal Neonatal Med.* 2005; 10:363-68.

Wollschlaeger K, Nieder J, Köppe I, Härtlein K. A study of fetal macrosomia. *Arch Gynecol Obstet.* 1999; 263:51-55.

World Health Organization. *Obesity: Preventing and managing the global epidemic.* Geneva: World Health Organization; 1998.

Chapter 21

Chemical Senses and the Development of Flavor Preferences in Humans

Julie A. Mennella

INTRODUCTION

Breastfeeding, a defining feature of all mammals, is a biological process in which the mother continues to nourish her infant after birth with a secretion produced by her mammary glands. In his writings, Hippocrates reasoned that breastmilk was best suited for infants because it was made from the same converted blood as was amniotic fluid and thus was a familiar source of nourishment (Hippocrates in Lloyd, 1983). In this chapter, the insights gleaned from scientific research that revealed that amniotic fluid and breastmilk share a commonality in their flavor profiles with the foods eaten by the mother are summarized. Thus, components of breastmilk are indeed familiar to the infant and help bridge the experiences with flavors *in utero* with those in solid foods. The types and intensity of flavors experienced in amniotic fluid and mother's milk may be unique for each infant and help to identify the culture to which they belong. These early flavor experiences contribute to adaptive responses in the postnatal environment and provide transnatal chemosensory continuity (Marlier *et al.*, 1998) and may 'program' later food preferences (Mennella *et al.*, 2001). But first, the current knowledge on the ontogeny of the sensory systems underlying flavor perception and the literature that describes one of the first ways in which mammalian young learn about foods available in the environment will be reviewed.

ONTOGENY OF FLAVOR PERCEPTION

The Chemical Senses

The chemical senses of taste and smell evolved to reject that which is harmful and to seek out that which is beneficial and pleasurable (Cowart, 2005). Flavor, a powerful determinant of human consummatory behavior throughout the lifespan, is a product of these two sensory systems. Although there are only a small number of primary taste qualities (e.g., sweet, salty, bitter, sour, and savory tastes) which can be perceived in all areas of the tongue, olfactory sensations result from the activation of a thousand or more distinct types of chemical receptor proteins located on millions of receptor cells lining the upper recesses of the nose. The receptors for the olfactory system are stimulated during inhalation through the nose (orthonasal route) as well as when molecules reach the receptors by passing from the oral cavity through the nasal pharynx during sucking in infants and deglutition in both children and adults. This latter route, often referred to as retronasal olfaction, contributes more significantly than does taste to the complexity of flavor (Rozin, 1976). To demonstrate this, if you pinch your nostrils closed while eating you will interrupt retronasal olfaction and thereby eliminate many of the subtleties of food, leaving the taste components remaining. This is clearly noted by head cold sufferers who lose the ability to discriminate common foods when their olfactory receptors are blocked by a head cold. Similarly, foods often 'taste' better after a person quits smoking, perhaps because their sense of smell has improved, allowing them to detect more subtleties of flavor (Frye *et al.*, 1990).

During the past century, research has revealed that the chemical senses develop and function before birth, but continue to mature postnatally. For example, taste buds and olfactory receptors are capable of conveying information to the central nervous system by the last trimester of pregnancy, and this information is available to systems organizing changes in sucking, facial expressions, and other affective behaviors (for review see Ganchrow & Mennella, 2003). However, although responsiveness to tastes and flavors is evident very early in development, infants are not merely miniature adults since these chemosensory systems (e.g., salt taste perception) continue to develop during infancy and childhood and are influenced by experiences in ways in which are only beginning to be understood.

Taste and Olfactory Development

A fundamental question related to the topic of early flavor learning in humans is when do the systems underlying flavor perception develop? Taste here refers to the sensation that occurs when chemicals stimulate taste receptors located on a large portion of the tongue's dorsum and other parts of the oropharynx, such as the larynx, pharynx, and epiglottis. Taste receptors are localized in taste buds and are innervated by branches of three cranial nerves: facial (VIIth), glossopharyngeal (IXth), and the vagal (Xth) nerves. The taste stimuli that interact with these receptors are often separated into a small number of "primary" tastes that include sweet, salty, bitter, sour, and savory tastes which can be perceived in all areas of the tongue (Bartoshuk & Beauchamp, 1994). Taste buds make their first appearance around the seventh or eighth week of gestation. By 13 to 15 weeks, the taste bud morphologically resembles the adult bud, except for the cornification overlying the papilla. Taste pores, which provide the access for taste stimuli to interact with taste receptor cells, are present in fetal fungiform papillae before the end of the fourth month of gestation (Bradley & Mistretta, 1975).

Olfaction occurs when chemicals stimulate olfactory receptors located on a relatively small patch of tissue high in the nasal cavity. Unlike that observed for taste, there are many different classes of odor stimuli, as suggested by the identification of a large family of genes that codes for a large number of receptor proteins located on membranes of the cilia of olfactory neurons. In fact, the olfactory receptor genes are encoded by the largest mammalian gene superfamily consisting of more than a thousand genes (Buck & Axel, 1991). During fetal life, the olfactory bulbs and receptor cells attain adult-like morphology by the eleventh week of gestation. Because the epithelial plugs that obstruct the external nares resolve by the second trimester (Schaffer, 1910), there is a continual turnover of amniotic fluid through the nasal passages. Because even in air-breathing organisms, volatile molecules must penetrate the aqueous mucus layer covering the olfactory epithelium to reach receptor sites on the cilia, it is important to note that there is no fundamental distinction between olfactory detection of airborne versus water-borne stimuli.

Taken together, this body of research demonstrates that the machinery needed to detect tastants and retronasal odors is operating as early as late fetal and neonatal life. One source of early stimulation of olfactory and taste receptors is the maternal diet. The environment in which the fetus lives, the amniotic sac, changes as a function of the food choices of the mother since dietary flavors are transmitted to and flavor amniotic fluid (Mennella *et al.*, 1995). Some of these same flavors find their way to and flavor mothers' milk. In the next section, the literature that demonstrates that learning about the dietary choice of the mother through flavor cues in amniotic fluid and mothers' milk is evident in a wide variety of mammalian species and thus may be a common feature of mammalian flavor learning is summarized. The more recent findings that flavors are also transmitted to human milk and that these early flavor experiences lead to increased enjoyment and preference for these flavors then follow.

FLAVOR PROGRAMMING

Mammalian Flavor Learning

By definition of being a mammal, the mammalian mother can produce milk to nourish her young. Invariably, the time must come for the young animal to accept plants or animal foods or both. Thus, developmental processes must act to insure that young mammals learn not only what to eat but how to forage. One of the first (not the only) ways young mammals learn about the dietary choices of the mother is through transmitted flavor cues. All else being equal, these are the flavors that are associated with nutritious foods or at least foods she has access to and hence the foods to which the infant most likely will have the earliest exposure.

Research in dairy cows gave us one of the first glimpses on how flavor cues in milk may be a potential source of chemosensory information for the suckling animal, enabling it to learn about the dietary choices of the mother. For example, a variety of odors from various feeds and weeds (e.g., wild onion, garlic) eaten by the cow or from the air it breathes can be transmitted to the milk while it is in the udder (Babcock 1938; Bassette *et al.*, 1986; Shipe *et al.*, 1978). Perhaps the most common and readily recognized transmitted flavor is that which results when the cow grazes on wild garlic or onions. To determine the mechanisms underlying such flavor transmission, milk samples were obtained before and after onion odors were introduced directly into the cow's lungs or rumen by means of tracheal and ruminal fistulae, respectively. An evaluation of the milk samples by a trained sensory panel of adults revealed that volatiles are transferred to the udder via vascular routes from either the digestive system or respiratory system (Dougherty *et al.*, 1962; Shipe *et al.*, 1962). These transmitted volatiles altered the flavor of the milk.

Table 1 illustrates the wide variety of transmitted flavors and the number of mammalian species studied.

Flavor memories can form during milk feedings that, in turn, facilitate the transition to solid foods. For example, the growth rate of weanling pigs improved when a flavor that had been incorporated into the sow's feed during lactation was added to the weanling's feed (Campbell, 1976). Moreover, weanling animals actively seek and prefer the flavors of the foods eaten by their mother during nursing (Bilko *et al.*, 1994; Capretta & Rawls, 1974; Chotro *et al.*, 1991; Chotro & Molina, 1990; Dominguez *et al.*, 1993; Galef *et al.*, 1994; Galef & Clark, 1972; Galef & Henderson, 1972; Galef & Sherry, 1973; Mainardi *et al.*, 1989; Morrill & Dayton, 1978; Nolte & Provenza, 1991; Nolte *et al.*, 1990; Wuensch, 1978) and are more likely to accept unfamiliar flavors

Table 1. Experimental Studies on Flavor Transmission to Mothers' Milk and Effect on Subsequent Preferences in Non-Human Mammals.

Type of Flavors	Species	References
butterscotch, maple, and ethyl butyrate	*Bos taurus*	Morrill & Dayton, 1978
fennel	*Mus musculus*	Mainardi *et al.*, 1989
lab chow	*Rattus norvegicus*	Galef & Clark, 1972 Galef & Henderson, 1972 Galef & Sherry, 1973
garlic	*Rattus norvegicus*	Capretta & Rawls, 1974
chocolate, vanilla, rum, and walnut	*Rattus norvegicus*	Capretta *et al.*, 1975
alcohol	*Rattus norvegicus*	Phillips & Stainbrook, 1976 Chotro *et al.*, 1991 Chotro & Moloina, 1990
onion	*Rattus norvegicus*	Wuensch, 1978
citric acid	*Rattus norvegicus*	London *et al.*, 1979
caffeine	*Rattus norvegicus*	Gullberg *et al.*, 1986
Firanor #3	*Sus scrofa*	Campbell, 1976
juniper berry	*Oryctolagus cuniculus*	Bilko *et al.*, 1994
onion	*Ovis aries*	Nolte & Provenza, 1991
garlic	*Ovis aries*	Nolte & Provenza, 1991
cumin	*Ovis aries*	Desage *et al.*, 1996

if they experience a variety of different flavors during the nursing period (Capretta *et al.*, 1975). This learning results from exposure to flavors in mother's milk rather than from other sensory cues present in the mother's breath, body odor, or from food particles clinging to the mother's fur or vibrissae (Babcock, 1938; Bradley & Mistretta, 1975; Shipe *et al.*, 1978). **Table 1** illustrates the research on a number of mammalian species that demonstrated that young animals are learning about the flavor cues in mothers' milk.

One striking example of the plasticity and stability of the flavor memories formed comes from research on the European rabbit (*Oryctolagus cuniculus*). Learning occurred when flavors were experienced in either amniotic fluid or mothers' milk (Bilko *et al.*, 1994). By feeding pregnant and lactating does aromatic juniper berries, newborn, weanling, and even adult animals demonstrate a preference for juniper flavor without subsequent postnatal experience (Bilko *et al.*, 1994). This increased preference for juniper flavor was associated with enhanced peripheral sensitivity of the olfactory system to juniper odor as measured by electro-olfactogram, a finding which is consistent with mechanisms underlying olfactory imprinting in salmon (Hudson & Distel, 1998). Such redundancy of dietary information may be important biologically because it provides complementary routes of transferring information on the types of foods available in the environment should the mothers' diet change during the course of pregnancy and lactation.

The research of Provenza and colleagues puts this early learning from the mother in an ecological perspective (Provenza *et al.*, 2003). Learned food preferences are transmitted from mothers to their offspring, resulting in greater biodiversity that benefits the solid, plants and animals. Experiences early in life cause a variety of neurological, morphological, and physiological changes that influence subsequent behaviors. There is some evidence that suggests that dietary learning may be more pronounced during early life, and there may be sensitive periods for such learning. Through such early experiences, young animals learn how to forage, acquire preferences for particular foods, and their bodies adapt to using particular arrays of foods.

One factor influencing the young animals' food choices appears to be exposure to the diet of conspecifics, especially the mother (Provenza, 1995). Lambs that ate certain foods (e.g., wheat, mountain mahogany) with their mothers formed more persistent and long-lasting (e.g., 3 years) preferences for these foods (Green *et al.*, 1984; Nolte *et al.*, 1990). Similarly, lambs that ate novel foods with their mothers consumed approximately twice as much of these foods after weaning than did lambs that ate the foods with a non-lactating ewe (Thorhallsdottir *et al.*, 1990). Exposure to flavors in mother's milk also teaches the young what foods are safe (Nolte & Provenza, 1991). Consequently, young animals may tend to choose a diet similar to that of their mothers when faced with their first solid meal.

Although experiences in utero and early in life are critical, it is important to emphasize that animals continue to adapt to their environment. Moreover, the presence of a food in the environment does not ensure that the animal will learn to eat this particular food (Villalba & Provenza, 2005). Rather, food preferences increase with repeated exposures and are strongly influenced by the conditions in which the exposure occurs. The following section reviews the literature that revealed that, like other mammals, human infants are gradually introduced and exposed to food flavors through flavor cues in amniotic fluid and mothers' milk.

The Transfer of Dietary Volatiles to Human Milk and Amniotic Fluid

In the 1970's, Elizabeth Barker, a graduate student in the laboratory of Dr. Mina McDaniel at the University of Manitoba, collected foremilk and hindmilk samples from lactating women during the morning hours on three consecutive days (Barker, 1980). Within three hours of expression, a trained sensory panel tasted the milk samples and evaluated them for taste, quality of sweetness, and textural properties, such as viscosity and mouth coating. Each of these sensory attributes varied from mother to mother and from foremilk to hindmilk supporting the contention that each breastfed infant's sensory experience is unique and highly varied. The sensory panel also reported that off-flavors were present in approximately one-third of the samples. Of particular interest was the finding that panelists described the milk of one woman who had consumed a "spicy" meal during the test period as hot, spicy, and peppery.

In the late 1980's, Gary Beauchamp and this author developed a research program that aimed to systematically study the transfer of dietary volatiles to human milk and determine what effects, if any, this has on the breastfed infant's behavior. However, taste panel work on human milk could not be conducted because the human immunodeficiency virus had been isolated in human milk (Thiry *et al.*, 1985), and there was some evidence at that time that it could be transmitted from mother to infant via infected breastmilk (Seltzer & Benjamin, 1990). Thus, panelists evaluated the milk samples on the basis of odor, the primary component of flavor.

To conduct psychophysical studies on human milk, several procedures and methodologies were developed, some of which are summarized here (Mennella & Beauchamp, 1991a). First, mothers were required to avoid wearing perfumes or scented products and eating the dietary volatile under study (e.g., garlic) for several days prior to testing to minimize the amount of such volatiles in the milk at the beginning of testing. Second, a within-subject design study was conducted such that women were tested on two days separated by one week. Foremilk samples were obtained at fixed intervals before and after she ingested the particular food or beverage on one testing day and placebo during the other. Third, the order of testing was counterbalanced. This allowed us to control for the effects of time of day on the flavor profile of the milk. Third, a sensory panel of adults who were screened for normal olfactory functioning was trained on the psychophysical methods used in the testing. The sensory panel analyzed the milk samples shortly after the last collection. To this end, milk samples were placed individually in plastic squeeze bottles with a plastic flip-up cap to minimize any visual differences in the milk samples. Using a forced-choice procedure, the panelists, who were blind to the experimental condition, were presented with all possible pairs of samples and asked to indicate which of the pair 'smelled stronger' or like the volatile (e.g., garlic) under study.

This research revealed that human milk is not a food of invariant flavors. Rather, it has the potential to provide the infant with a rich source of varying chemosensory experiences. To date, a wide variety of volatiles either ingested (e.g., alcohol, garlic, mint, cheese, vanilla, carrot) or inhaled (e.g., tobacco) by the lactating mother are transmitted to her milk (Mennella & Beauchamp, 1991a; Mennella & Beauchamp, 1991b; Mennella & Beauchamp, 1993a; Mennella & Beauchamp, 1996; Mennella & Beauchamp, 1998; Mennella *et al.*, 2001). No such changes occurred on the days the mothers consumed the placebos. In general, there were significant increases in the intensity of the milk odor within a half hour to an hour after consumption and the intensity of the flavor decreased thereafter. For all cases, the flavor change in the milk after an acute dosage of the flavor was transient. **Figure 1** highlights some of the flavors studied and the time course of the flavor changes in the milk. Whether the flavor of human milk changes due to the transmission of volatiles from the ambient environment is an important area of future research. As shown in **Figure 1**, data was collected that suggests that some of the volatiles in the perfume worn by the mother get transmitted to and significantly alter the odor of her milk.

When studying the effects of drinking alcohol or smoking a cigarette on the flavor of human milk, alcohol (Mennella & Beauchamp, 1991b; Mennella & Beauchamp, 1993b) and nicotine (Mennella & Beauchamp, 1998), respectively, were measured in the milk. In both cases, the sensory change paralleled the changing concentrations of ethanol or nicotine,

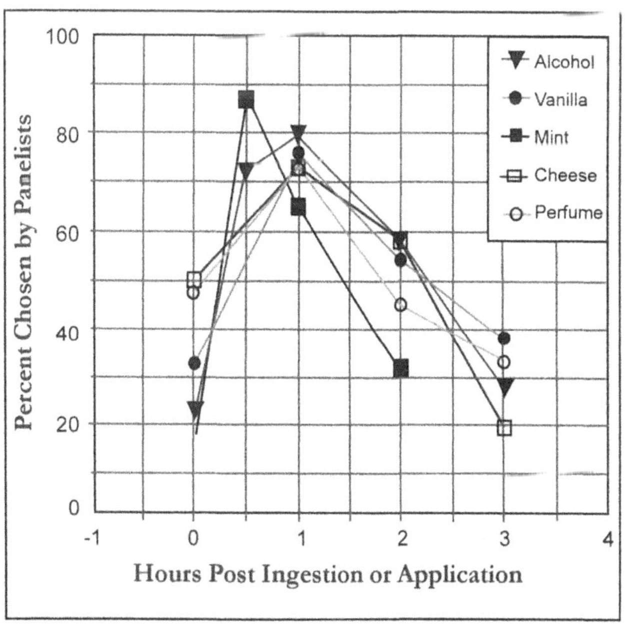

Figure 1. Percentage of time panelists chose milk samples as smelling stronger or more like the particular flavor or smell. Samples were taken at fixed intervals before and following ingestion of a 0. 3g/kg dose of alcohol (closed inverted triangles); vanilla (closed circles); Altoid™ mints (closed squares); or 60 grams of bleu cheese (open squares); or after the inhalation of perfume and its application on pulse points on neck and wrists (Pheromone™, Marilyn Miglin, Chicago, IL; open diamonds).

respectively, in the milk. During more recent years, additional psychophysical techniques have been employed (see Mennella, 1999) and focused on the perception of the milk flavor in the mouth. To this aim, nursing women, who had experience expressing and freezing their milk and subsequently tasting their milk before feeding it to their infants, were trained in sensory evaluation techniques. In one study, each woman expressed milk before and one hour after drinking a 0.3g/kg body weight dose of alcohol in orange juice. Approximately three hours later, they were presented with equal amounts of both of their own milk samples and asked to determine which tasted stronger or more like alcohol. The results were unambiguous. Mothers could detect the alcohol flavor in their mouth.

It is interesting to note that lactating mothers are often advised to avoid cruciferous vegetables, garlic, onion, and chocolate since consumption of these foods has been shown to be associated with colic symptoms in young infants (Lust *et al.*, 1996). Often, it is believed that the baby is rejecting the flavor in the milk. However, the data suggests that this rejection most likely is not due to the flavor change if the colic symptoms occurred several hours after the mother ingested the food. Moreover, for those infants whose mothers had been eating these foods (e.g., garlic) throughout pregnancy, data suggest that they may have experienced these flavors previously since, like that observed for breastmilk, garlic ingestion altered the flavor of amniotic fluid (Mennella *et al.*, 1995).

That amniotic fluid and breastmilk have the potential to share a commonality in flavor profiles with the foods eaten by the mother suggests that breastmilk may 'bridge' experiences with flavors *in utero* to those in solid foods. Moreover, the sweetness and textural properties of human milk, such as viscosity and mouth coating, vary from mother to mother (Barker, 1980), thus suggesting that breastfeeding, unlike formula feeding, provides the infant with the potential for a rich source of variety. The types and intensity of flavors experienced in breastmilk may be unique for each infant and serve to identify the culture to which the child is born. The next section reviews the literature that revealed that experiences with flavors in amniotic fluid and mother's milk lead to increased enjoyment and preference for these flavors at birth and during weaning and how the duration since exposure plays an important role in how the infant responds to the flavor.

Pre-natal and Post-natal Flavor Memories in Humans

Emerging evidence suggests that the taste and olfactory systems are operating before birth and that prenatal sensory experiences bias the newborn's behavior and preferences. Within days of birth, human infants will orient toward the odor of their own amniotic fluid (Marlier *et al.*, 1998). That they are learning about flavors of foods eaten by their mother was suggested by studies conducted in France (Schaal *et al.*, 2000) and Northern Ireland (Hepper, 1988). Newborns whose mothers regularly consumed an anise-flavored beverage or ate garlic-containing foods displayed less negative facial responses and more mouthing and orienting responses to anise and garlic odors, respectively, during the immediate postpartum period.

The retronasal perception of odors in amniotic fluid and mothers' milk may provide the infant with the potential for a rich source of varying chemosensory experiences and a possible route for the development of preferences for a diet similar to that of the mother. This is due, in part, to the fact that the context in which the flavor is experienced, with the mother and during feeding, consists of a variety of elements (e.g., tactile stimulation, warmth, milk, mothers' voice) which have been shown to be reinforcers for early learning. To test the hypothesis that prenatal and postnatal flavor experiences enhance the acceptance and enjoyment of flavors during weaning, an experimental study was conducted in which pregnant women, who planned on breastfeeding their infants, were randomly assigned to one of three groups (Mennella *et al.*, 2001). Women in one group drank carrot juice for several days per week during the last trimester of pregnancy; mothers in a second group drank the carrot juice for a similar time period during lactation, whereas those in the control group drank water during both pregnancy and lactation. All mothers refrained from eating carrots or drinking carrot juice during and between the two exposure periods. Approximately four weeks after the mothers began complementing their infants' diet with cereal and before the infants had ever been fed foods or juices containing the flavor of carrots, the infants were videotaped as they were fed, in counterbalanced order, cereal prepared with water during one test session and cereal prepared with carrot juice during another. Infants who had exposure to the flavor of carrots in either amniotic fluid or mothers' milk behaved differently in response to carrot-flavored cereal than did non-exposed control infants. Specifically, previously exposed infants displayed fewer negative facial expressions while feeding the carrot-flavored cereal when compared to the plain cereal. Moreover, those infants who were exposed to carrots prenatally were perceived by their mothers as enjoying the carrot-flavored cereal more when compared to the plain cereal. Postnatal exposure had similar consequences thus highlighting the importance of a healthy and varied diet for both pregnant and lactating women.

When an infant experiences a flavor in amniotic fluid or breastmilk and is tested sometime later, the exposed infant accepts the flavor more than infants without such experience. Presumably, learning (e.g., elimination of neophobia, conditioning, "mere exposure") has occurred. Teleologically, one can argue that the infant has acquired information that the food associated with the flavor is not dangerous, is nutritionally valuable, or both. It is important for the infant to accept and be particularly attracted to the flavors consumed by the mother. As stated earlier, these are the flavors that are associated with nutritious foods, or at least, foods the mother has access to, and hence the foods to which the infant will have the earliest exposure.

In support of this contention, it was found that at the time of weaning, breastfed infants' acceptance of their first solid food, cereal, was enhanced when it was flavored with mothers' milk (Mennella & Beauchamp, 1997). That is, breastfed infants, who were fed cereal for approximately two weeks, but had only experienced cereal prepared with water, readily accepted and preferred the cereal when it was prepared with their mothers' milk. They not only consumed more of the cereal flavored with mothers' milk, but they displayed a series of behaviors signaling their preferences. In addition, the more varied the mothers' diet, the greater the acceptance of the cereal prepared with mothers' milk. Because the infants' first flavor experience occurs before birth in amniotic fluid, breastmilk may bridge the experiences of flavors in utero to those in solid foods. It is also possible that experience with a variety of flavors (e.g., in amniotic fluid, mothers' milk) may predispose the infant to be more willing to accept novel flavors during the weaning process (Sullivan & Birch, 1994).

Indeed, there is some evidence that the exposure needed to enhance later acceptance may not require experience with the actual flavor. Rather, research in humans infants (Gerrish & Mennella, 2001) and animal models (Capretta *et al.*, 1975) suggests that experience with flavor variety enhances the acceptance of novel foods during weaning. Of interest is the finding that breastfed infants are more willing to accept a novel vegetable upon first presentation than are formula-fed infants (Sullivan & Birch, 1994). The breastfed infants' enhanced acceptance of the vegetables could be due to the breastfed infants' familiarity with specific flavors associated with the vegetables in mothers' milk, the fact that they had much more experience with flavor variety than did the formula-fed infants, or both. Unlike the formula-fed infant who experiences a monotony of flavors in infant formula, the breastfed infant is exposed to a variety of flavors in breastmilk, setting the pattern for a diversified diet.

Effects of Exposure: Short-term and Long-term Effects

The time since exposure to a flavor in milk plays an important role in how infants respond to that particular flavor. Infants can clearly detect the flavors in the milk as evidenced by changes in their patterning and duration of feeding and suckling at the breast (Mennella & Beauchamp, 1991a; Mennella & Beauchamp, 1993a; Mennella & Beauchamp, 1996) as well as taking the bottle (Mennella, 1997; Mennella & Beauchamp, 1996). For the majority of flavors, they will respond to a flavor by suckling more at the breast or bottle, especially if they haven't experienced that flavor in the recent past.

When studying how flavor changes in milk affects infants' behaviors at the breast, it is important to emphasize that it is difficult to separate the direct effects on the infant from other possible influences the consumed flavors could have on the mother (e.g., changes in the odor of the mother's breath or sweat) (Mennella & Beauchamp, 1991a). Consequently, one cannot unequivocally conclude that the flavor change caused the alteration in the infants' suckling behavior. To examine the effects of flavoring directly, a flavor was added (i.e., vanilla) to infant formula and tested formula-fed infants (Mennella & Beauchamp, 1996). Consistent with that observed in breastfed infants, the bottle-fed infants' response to the vanilla-flavored formula was altered relative to their response to the unflavored formula. In the first, short-term preference test, the infants sucked more vigorously when feeding the vanilla-flavored formula, and in the second test that encompassed an entire feeding, they spent more time feeding on the first bottle when it contained the vanilla flavor. Similar findings were observed in breastfed infants who were fed alcohol-flavored breastmilk in a bottle (Mennella, 1997).

Why do infants respond to flavored milk by enhanced suckling? In the studies demonstrating enhanced suckling response to a flavor in breastfed infants (e.g., vanilla, garlic), the nursing mothers were asked to eat bland diets devoid of these flavors during the three days preceding each testing day. In the study with formula-fed infants, their mothers clearly were providing a very monotonous diet since formula is virtually unchanging (Mennella & Beauchamp, 1996). Perhaps the novelty was sufficient to induce increased suckling because these flavors are inherently positive or arousing, or like sweet taste, a hard-wired (innate) response. When aroused, mammalian infants will suck more and exhibit a variety of other oral behaviors (Korner *et al.*, 1968).

Following repeated exposure to the vanilla-flavored formula, the infants' suckling response to the flavor diminished, however (Mennella & Beauchamp, 1996). Similarly, repeated exposure to a flavor in breastmilk modified the breastfed infants' responsiveness to that particular flavor (Mennella & Beauchamp, 1993a; Mennella & Beauchamp, 1999). Infants of lactating mothers who had repeatedly consumed garlic, breastfed for similar periods of time during the four-hour testing session in which their mothers' consumed garlic as compared with the session in which their mothers ingested the placebo. In contrast, the infants who had no recent exposure to garlic volatiles in their mother's milk spent more time breastfeeding when their mothers ingested garlic than when their mothers ingested the placebo. Similar patterns of findings were observed after exposure to carrot flavor in mothers' milk. During the immediate days after exposure, infants responded by eating less of and spent less time feeding carrot-flavor cereal (Mennella & Beauchamp, 1999). In contrast, infants tended to eat more carrot-flavored cereal and showed signs of enjoying the cereal several months after the exposure (Mennella *et al.*, 2001).

Taken together, these data suggest that infants may be exhibiting a form of sensory-specific satiety when recently exposed to a flavor in milk. Perhaps the flavor becomes monotonous to those infants who were repeatedly exposed to it in milk. In the short term, children (Birch & Deysher, 1986) and adults (Rolls, 2000) report that the palatability of a food and the amount consumed declines following repeated consumption of that food, whereas less recently consumed foods are considered more palatable and stimulate food intake. Moreover, the flavor (e.g., garlic-flavored milk) may have aroused the infants exposed to a diet of mother's milk relatively low in flavor, garlic-like compounds, or both (Mennella & Beauchamp, 1993a). In the long-term, preferences develop for the exposed flavor and infants will enjoy eating foods that have a flavor previously experienced in mothers' milk (Mennella *et al.*, 2001) or formula (Mennella *et al.*, 2004; Mennella & Beauchamp, 2002).

Transfer of Alcohol to Human Milk: Effects on Infant Behaviorand Lactational Performance

As discussed previously, infants can detect flavors in mothers' milk as evidenced by increased suckling behavior at the breast, especially if they had not been exposed to that flavor in the recent past. However, when studying the infants' breastfeeding response following maternal alcohol consumption, it was found that, unlike other flavors, they consumed less milk (Mennella & Beauchamp, 1991b; Mennella & Beauchamp, 1991b; Mennella & Beauchamp, 1993b). That is, they consumed approximately 23% less milk during the four hours that followed their mothers' drinking of an alcoholic beverage that was coincident with flavor change in the milk. The diminished intake at the breast was not due to shorter periods of breastfeeding following maternal ethanol consumption since there was no significant difference in the number of feedings. Nor was it due to infants rejecting the altered flavor in their mother's milk that also resulted from maternal ethanol consumption. Rather, this diminished intake was due to a direct effect of alcohol on milk production (Mennella, 1998) and hormonal responsiveness (e.g., decreased oxytocin) (Mennella *et al.*, 2005) by the mother.

To determine whether infants were rejecting the flavor of alcohol in the milk, they were observed feeding their mothers' milk from a bottle (Mennella, 1997). No rejection occurred. Rather, the infants consumed significantly more and sucked more frequently when drinking the alcohol-flavored milk as compared with the unaltered milk. That experience with the flavor of alcohol in mothers' milk modified the infants' responses to alcohol flavor was suggested by the relationship between the reported frequency of mothers' drinking during lactation and the infants' rhythm and frequency of sucking when feeding the alcohol-flavored milk. Consistent with that observed for other flavors, more experience with alcohol as assessed by maternal frequency of drinking was associated with a diminished suckling response to alcohol-flavored milk when feeding from a bottle. These findings indicate that infants can readily detect the flavor of alcohol in mother's milk and experience will modify how they respond to it in subsequent feedings.

CONCLUSIONS

The notion of the individuality of each woman's milk is ingrained in the traditional wisdom of many cultures. Nursing women are often told to consume certain herbs, foods, and beverages while avoiding others because there is a strong belief that the mother can optimize the quality and quantity of her milk to meet the needs of her child through her own diet and psychological well being. As a consequence of the traditional food practices evident in many cultures, it is now known that the type of foods and herbs eaten by women, and hence the flavor principles of the culture, are experienced by the infants before their first taste of solid foods. Flavors of foods eaten by the mother transmit to amniotic fluid and mother's milk. These flavors are not only detected by the infant, but they serve to modulate feeding and acceptance of these foods at weaning and beyond.

The long-term consequences of breastfeeding on the development of aspects of food and flavor preferences have been the subject of a few studies in recent years. In an eight-year longitudinal study conducted in the United States, fruit and vegetable consumption by school-aged children was predicted by either breastfeeding duration, food-related experiences during early life, or mothers' preferences (Skinner *et al.*, 2002a; Skinner *et al.*, 2002b). Similar findings have been recently reported in the United Kingdom (Cooke *et al.*, 2004) and France (Nicklaus, 2004, Nicklaus *et al.*, 2005). Clearly, more research in this area is needed, but the findings that infants are learning via flavor cues in breastmilk suggests one (but not the only) mechanism underlying these associations.

References

Babcock CJ. Feed flavors in milk and milk products. *J Dairy Sci.* 1938; 21:661-67.

Barker E. *Sensory evaluation of human milk.* M.S. Thesis, University of Manitoba. Manitoba, Canada; 1980.

Bartoshuk LM, Beauchamp GK. Chemical senses. *Annual Review of Psychology.* 1994; 45:419-49.

Bassette R., Fung DYC, Mantha VR. Off-flavors in milk. *CRC Crit Rev Food Sci Nutr.* 1986; 24:1-52.

Bilkó A, Altbacker V, Hudson R.) Transmission of food preference in the rabbit: the means of information transfer. *Physiol Behav.* 1994; 56:907-12.

Birch LL, Deysher M. Caloric compensation and sensory specific satiety: evidence for self regulation of food intake by young children. *Appetite.* 1986; 7:323-31.

Bradley RM, Mistretta CM. Fetal sensory receptors. *Physiol Rev.* 1975; 55:352-82.

Buck L, Axel R. A novel multigene family may encode odorant receptors: a molecular basis for odor recognition. *Cell.* 1991; 65:175-87.

Campbell RG. A note on the use of feed flavour to stimulate the feed intake of weaner pigs. *Animal Production.* 1976; 23:417-19.

Capretta PJ, Petersik JT, Steward DJ. Acceptance of novel flavours is increased after early experience of diverse taste. *Nature.* 1975; 254:689-91.

Capretta PJ, Rawls LH. Establishment of a flavor preference in rats: importance of nursing and weaning experience. *J Comp Physiol Psychol.* 1974; 86:670-73.

Chotro MG, Cordoba NE, Molina JC. Acute prenatal experience with alcohol in the amniotic fluid: interactions with aversive and appetitive alcohol orosensory learning in the rat pup. *Dev Psychobiol.* 1991; 24:431-51.

Chotro MG, Molina JC. Acute ethanol contamination of the amniotic fluid during gestational day 21: postnatal changes in alcohol responsiveness in rats. *Dev Psychobiol.* 1990; 23:535-47.

Cooke LJ, Wardle J, Gibson EL, Sapochnik M, Sheilham A, *et al.* Demographic, familial and trait predictors of fruit and vegetable consumption by pre-school children. *Public Health Nutrition.* 2004; 7:295-302.

Cowart BJ. Taste, our body's gustatory gatekeeper. *Cerebrum.* 2005; 7:7-22.

Dominguez HD, Chotro MG, Molina JC. Alcohol in the amniotic fluid prior to cesarean delivery: effects of subsequent exposure to the drug's odor upon alcohol responsiveness. *Behav Neural Biol.* 1993; 60:129-38.

Dougherty RW, Shipe WF, Gudnason GV, Ledford RA, Peterson RD, *et al.* Physiological mechanisms involved in transmitting flavors and odors to milk. I. Contribution of eructated gases to milk flavor. *J Dairy Sci.* 1962; 45:472-76.

Frye RE, Schwartz BS, Doty RL. Dose-related effects of cigarette smoking on olfactory function. *JAMA*. 1990; 263:1233-36.

Galef BG, Mainardi M, Valsecchi P. *Behavioral aspects of feeding: basic and applied research in mammals.* Langhorne, PA: Harwood Academic Publishers; 1994.

Galef BG Jr, Clark MM. Mother's milk and adult presence: two factors determining initial dietary selection by weanling rats. *J Comp Physiol Psychol.* 1972; 78:220-25.

Galef BG Jr, Henderson PW. Mother's milk: a determinant of the feeding preferences of weaning rat pups. *J Comp Physiol Psychol.* 1972; 78:213-19.

Galef BG Jr, Sherry DF. Mother's milk: a medium for transmission of cues reflecting the flavor of mother's diet. *J Comp Physiol Psychol.* 1973; 83:374-78.

Ganchrow JR, Mennella JA. In: Doty RL (ed.). *The ontogeny of human flavor perception.* New York: Marcel Dekker, Inc.; 2003. pp. 823-946.

Gerrish CJ, Mennella JA. Flavor variety enhances food acceptance in formula-fed infants. *Am J Clin Nutr.* 2001; 73:1080-85.

Green GC, Elwin RL, Mottershead BE, Lynch LL. Long-term effects of early experience to supplementary feeding in sheep. *Proceedings for the Australian Society on Animal Production.* 1984; 15:373-75.

Hepper PG. Adaptive fetal learning: prenatal exposure to garlic affects postnatal preferences. *Animal Behavior.* 1988; 36:935-36.

Hippocrates. Embryology and anatomy. The seed and the nature of the child. Translated by I. M. Lonie. In: Lloyd GER (ed.). *Hippocratic Writings.* London, England: Penguin Books; 1983. pp. 317.

Hudson R, Distel H. Induced peripheral sensitivity in the developing vertebrate olfactory system. *Ann N Y Acad Sci.* 1998; 855:109-15.

Korner AK, Chuck B, Dontchos S. Organismic determinants of spontaneous oral behavior in neonates. *Child Dev.* 1968; 39:1147-57.

Lust KD, Brown JE, Thomas W. Maternal intake of cruciferous vegetables and other foods and colic symptoms in exclusively breast-fed infants. *J Am Diet Assoc.* 1996; 96:46-48.

Mainardi M, Poli M, Valsecchi P. Ontogeny of dietary selection in weaning mice: effects of early experience and mother's milk. *Biology of Behaviour.* 1989; 14:185-94.

Marlier L, Schaal B, Soussignan R. Neonatal responsiveness to the odor of amniotic and lacteal fluids: a test of perinatal chemosensory continuity. *Child Dev.* 1998; 69:611-23.

Mennella JA. Infants' suckling responses to the flavor of alcohol in mothers' milk. *Alcohol Clin Exp Res.* 1997; 21:581-85.

Mennella JA. Short-term effects of maternal alcohol consumption on lactational performance. *Alcohol Clin Exp Res.* 1998; 22:1389-92.

Mennella JA. The transfer of alcohol to human milk: Sensory implications and effects on mother-infant interaction. In: Hannigan JH, Spear N, Spear L, Goodlett CR (eds.). *Alcohol and alcoholism: Brain and development.* New Jersey: Lawrence Erlbaum Associates, Inc.; 1999. p. 177-98.

Mennella JA, Beauchamp GK. Maternal diet alters the sensory qualities of human milk and the nursling's behavior. *Pediatrics.* 1991a; 88:737-44.

Mennella JA, Beauchamp GK. The transfer of alcohol to human milk. Effects on flavor and the infant's behavior. *N Engl J Med.* 1991b; 325:981-85.

Mennella JA, Beauchamp GK. The effects of repeated exposure to garlic-flavored milk on the nursling's behavior. *Pediatric Research.* 1993a; 34:805-8.

Mennella JA, Beauchamp GK. Beer, breastfeeding, and folklore. *Dev Psychobiol.* 1993b; 26:459-66.

Mennella JA, Beauchamp GK. The human infants' responses to vanilla flavors in human milk & formula. *Infant Behavior and Development.* 1996; 19:13-19.

Mennella JA, Beauchamp GK. Mothers' milk enhances the acceptance of cereal during weaning. *Pediatr Res.* 1997; 41:188-92.

Mennella JA, Beauchamp GK. Smoking and the flavor of breastmilk. *N Engl J Med.* 1998; 339:1559-60.

Mennella JA, Beauchamp GK. Experience with a flavor in mother's milk modifies the infant's acceptance of flavored cereal. *Dev Psychobiol.* 1999; 35:197-203.

Mennella JA, Beauchamp GK. Flavor experiences during formula feeding are related to preferences during childhood. *Early Hum Dev.* 2002; 68:71-82.

Mennella JA, Griffin CE, Beauchamp GK. Flavor programming during infancy. *Pediatrics.* 2004; 113:840-45.

Mennella JA, Jagnow CP, Beauchamp GK. Prenatal and postnatal flavor learning by human infants. *Pediatrics.* 2001; 107:E88.

Mennella JA, Johnson A, Beauchamp GK. Garlic ingestion by pregnant women alters the odor of amniotic fluid. *Chem Senses.* 1995; 20:207-9.

Mennella JA, Pepino MY, Teff KL. Acute alcohol consumption disrupts the hormonal milieu of lactating women. *J Clin Endocrinol Metab.* 2005; 90:1979-85.

Morrill JL, Dayton AD. Effect of feed flavor in milk and calf starter on feed consumption and growth. *J Dairy Sci.* 1978; 61:229-32.

Nicklaus S, Boggio V, Chabanet C, Issanchou S. A prospective study on food variety seeking in childhood, adolescence and early adult life. *Appetite.* 2005; 44:289-97.

Nicklaus S. *Etude longitudinale des preferences et de la variete alimentaires de la petite enfance a l'age adulte - These de Doctorat.* Dijon, France: Universite de Bourgogne; 2005.

Nolte DL, Provenza FD. Food preferences in lambs after exposure to flavors in milk. *Applied Animal Behavior Science.* 1991; 32:381-89.

Nolte DL, Provenza FD, Balph DF. The establishment and persistence of food preferences in lambs exposed to selected foods. *J Anim Sci.* 1990; 68:998-1002.

Provenza FD. Tracking variable environments: there is more than one kind of memory. *J Chem Ecol.* 1995; 21:911-23.

Provenza FD, Villalba JJ, Dziba LE, Atwood SB, Banner RE. Linking herbivore experience, varied diets, and plant biochemical diversity. *Small Rumin Res.* 2003; 49: 257-74.

Rolls BJ. Sensory specific satiety and variety in the meal. In: Meiselman HL (ed.). *Dimensions of the meal: the science, culture, business and art of eating.*. Gaithersburg, MD: Aspen Publishers, Inc.; 2000. p. 107-16.

Rozin P. The selection of food by rats, humans and other animals. In: *Advances in the study of behaviors.* New York: Academic Press; 1976. p. 21-76.

Schaal B, Marlier L, Soussignan R. Human foetuses learn odours from their pregnant mother's diet. *Chem Senses.* 2000; 25:729-37.

Schaffer JP. The lateral wall of the cavum nasi in man with special reference to the various developmental stages. *J Morphol.* 1910; 21:613-17.

Seltzer V, Benjamin F. Breast-feeding and the potential for human immunodeficiency virus transmission. *Obstet Gynecol.* 1990; 75:713-15.

Shipe WF, Bassette R, Deane DD, Dunkley WL, Hammond EG, *et al.* Off-flavors of milk: nomenclature, standards and bibliography. *J Dairy Sci.* 1978; 61:855-68.

Shipe WF, Ledford RA, Peterson RD, Scanlan RA, Geerken HF, *et al.* Physiological mechanisms involved in transmitting flavors and odors to milk. II. Transmission of some flavor components of silage. *J Dairy Sci.* 1962; 45:477-80.

Skinner JD, Carruth BR, Bounds W, Ziegler P, Reidy K. Do food-related experiences in the first 2 years of life predict dietary variety in school-aged children? *J Nutr Educ Behav.* 2002a; 34:310-15.

Skinner JD, Carruth BR, Wendy B, Ziegler PJ. Children's food preferences: a longitudinal analysis. *J Am Diet Assoc.* 2002b; 102:1638-46.

Sullivan S, Birch LL. Infant dietary experience and acceptance of solid foods. *Pediatrics.* 1994; 93: 271-77.

Thiry L, Sprecher-Goldberger S, Jonckheer T, Levy J, Van de Perre P, *et al.* Isolation of AIDS virus from cell-free breastmilk of three healthy virus carriers. *Lancet.* 1985; 2:891-92.

Thorhallsdottir AG, Provenza FD, Balph DF. Ability of lambs to learn about novel foods while observing or participating with social models. *Applied Animal Behavior Science.* 1990; 25:25-33.

Villalba JJ, Provenza FD. Foraging in chemically diverse environments: energy, protein, and alternative foods influence ingestion of plant secondary metabolites by lambs. *J Chem Ecol.* 2005; 31:123-38.

Wuensch KL. Exposure to onion taste in mother's milk leads to enhanced preference for onion diet among weanling rats. *J Gen Psychol.* 1978; 99:163-67.

Chapter 22

Nutrition, Growth, and Complementary Feeding of the Breastfed Infant

Kathryn G. Dewey

INTRODUCTION

There is little argument that human milk is the ideal food for young infants. Although infant formulas are designed to mimic human milk as much as possible, it is very difficult to duplicate all of its unique nutritional characteristics (Institute of Medicine, 1991; Picciano, 2001). For example, in terms of protein content, human milk has a high ratio of whey to casein, a relatively high proportion of non-protein nitrogen, and high concentrations of certain specific proteins (Dewey *et al.*, 1996). These components serve both nutritional and non-nutritional functions (Institute of Medicine, 1991). In addition, human milk is rich in certain fatty acids essential for brain development and contains several non-lactose carbohydrates that play a role in resistance to infection. Furthermore, human milk changes in composition as the infant matures.

After a certain age, however, human milk alone can no longer supply all of the infant's nutritional requirements, and complementary foods are needed to assure adequate nutrition and growth. The term "complementary foods" is preferred rather than "weaning foods" because weaning implies the cessation of breastfeeding, whereas the goal is that such foods should complement breastmilk, not replace it. It is sometimes assumed that an increased need for energy and protein is the primary factor dictating complementary feeding, but in fact some of the micronutrients are likely to become limiting sooner than the macronutrients. If the mother nurses in response to the infant's cues and is herself well-nourished, her milk supply can probably keep pace with the infant's energy needs for considerably longer than six months. By contrast, the amount of iron provided by breastmilk may become insufficient even before six months if the infant has suboptimal iron reserves at birth.

This chapter will review the contribution of human milk to nutritional needs during the first two years of life, growth patterns of breastfed infants, and recommendations regarding the age of introduction and optimal nutrient content of complementary foods. The focus will be on healthy, term infants, as the needs of preterm infants are somewhat unique.

CONTRIBUTION OF HUMAN MILK TO NUTRIENT NEEDS DURING THE FIRST TWO YEARS OF LIFE

Nutrient needs during the first six months can normally be met by human milk alone (Butte *et al.*, 2002). Iron is one possible exception, as iron deficiency may occur prior to 6 months in infants whose iron reserves at birth are low (Griffin & Abrams, 2001). Risk factors for iron deficiency in exclusively breastfed infants include relatively low birth weight (e.g., <3000 g), maternal prenatal iron deficiency, and immediate clamping of the umbilical cord, which deprives the newborn of the placental transfusion of blood (Chaparro *et al.*, 2006). Vitamin D may also be needed prior to six months in populations with inadequate exposure to sunlight or

Table 1. Recommended Nutrient Intakes, Average Amount Provided by Breastmilk, and Amount Needed from Complementary Foods at 6-8, 9-11, and 12-23 months.

	6-8 month			
	RNI[a]	Amount from breastmilk[b]	Amount needed from CF[c]	% from CF[c]
Energy (kcal/d)	615	413;486	202;129	33;21
Protein (g/d)	9.1	7.2	1.9	21
Vitamin A (µg RE/d)	400	337;461	63;0	16;0
Folate (µg/d)	80	58	22	28
Niacin (mg/d)	4	1	3.0	75
Riboflavin (mg/d)	0.40	0.24	0.16	40
Thiamine (mg/d)	0.30	0.14	0.16	53
Vitamin B_6 (mg/d)	0.30	0.06	0.24	80
Vitamin B_{12} (µg/d)	0.50	0.66	0	0
Vitamin C (mg/d)	30	28	2	7
Vitamin D (µg/d)	5	0.4	4.6	92
Calcium (mg/d)	270	191	79	29
Copper (mg/d)	0.20	0.17	0.03	15
Iodine (µg/d)	90	75	15	17
Iron[d] (mg/d)	9.3	0.2	9.1	98
Magnesium (mg/d)	54	24	30	56
Phosphorus (mg/d)	275	95	180	65
Selenium (µg/d)	10	14	0	0
Zinc (mg/d)	3	0.6	2.4	80

[a] Recommended Nutrient Intakes, from FAO/WHO (Joint FAO/WHO Expert Consultation on Human Vitamin and Mineral Requirements, 2004) except for energy and protein (from Dewey and Brown, 2003) and calcium, copper, phosphorus and zinc (from the U.S. Dietary Reference Intakes).

[b] Based on average milk volumes of 674, 616 and 549 mL/d in developing countries and 688, 529, and 448 mL/d in industrialized countries for 6-8, 9-11 and 12-23 mo respectively (World Health Organization, 1998), and milk nutrient concentrations from the Institute of Medicine (Institute of Medicine, 1991), except for vitamin A in milk of women from developing countries (World Health Organization, 1998) and

inadequate maternal vitamin D intake (Greer, 2001). If the mother is malnourished, concentrations of certain nutrients in breastmilk may be lower than normal (e.g., some of the B vitamins, iodine, selenium), but this can be rectified by providing vitamin-mineral supplements to the mother. Maternal deficiency does not affect the concentrations of most of the minerals in human milk (e.g., iron, zinc, calcium).

The amounts of nutrients provided by breastmilk can be estimated by multiplying average breastmilk intake by the concentration of each nutrient in human milk. By subtracting these values from total recommended nutrient intakes, one can derive estimates of the amounts of nutrients needed from complementary foods after six months of age. Using this approach, **Table 1** provides these estimates for three age ranges: 6-8, 9-11 and 12-23 months. In this table, the recommended nutrient intakes (RNI) for energy and protein are taken from current recommendations for complementary feeding (Dewey & Brown, 2003) and the RNIs for micronutrients are taken from the most recent FAO/WHO estimates (Joint FAO/WHO Expert Consultation on Human Vitamin and Mineral Requirements, 2004) or the U.S. Dietary Reference Intakes. The estimated amount of each nutrient provided by breastmilk is based on average milk intake during each of the age intervals, calculated separately for infants in developing countries and in industrialized countries (World Health Organization,

9-11 month				12-23 month			
RNI[a]	Amount from breastmilk [b]	Amount needed from CF[c]	% from CF[c]	RNI[a]	Amount from breastmilk [b]	Amount needed from CF[c]	% from CF[c]
686	379;375	307;311	45	894	346;313	548;581	61;65
9.6	6.5;5.6	3.1;4.0	32;42	10.9	5.8;4.7	5.1;6.2	47;57
400	308;354	92;46	23;12	400	275;300	125;100	31;25
80	52;45	28;35	35;44	160	47;38	113;122	71;76
4	0.9;0.8	3.1;3.2	78;80	6	0.8;0.7	5.2;5.3	87;88
0.40	0.22;0.19	0.18;0.21	45;53	0.50	0.19;0.16	0.31;0.34	62;68
0.30	0.12	0.18	60	0.50	0.11	0.39	78
0.30	0.06	0.24	80	0.50	0.05	0.45	90
0.50	0.60;0.51	0	0	0.90	0.53;0.47	0.37;0.43	41;48
30	25;21	5;9	17;30	30	22;18	8;12	27;40
5	0.3	4.7	94	5	0.3;0.2	4.7;4.8	94;96
270	172;148	172;148	36;45	500	154;125	346;375	69;75
0.20	0.14	0.06	30	0.30	0.14;0.11	0.16;0.19	53;63
90	68;58	22;32	24;36	90	60;49	30;41	33;46
9.3	0.2	9.1	98	5.8	0.2;0.1	5.6;5.7	97;98
54	22;19	32	59	60	19;16	41;44	68;73
275	86;74	189;201	69;73	460	77;63	383;397	83;86
10	12	0	0	17	11	6	35
3	0.5;0.4	2.5;2.6	83;87	3	0.4;0.3	2.6;2.7	87;90

zinc (Krebs et al., 1995). For each nutrient, the first value refers to developing countries and the second value (after the semi-colon) refers to industrialized countries, whenever there is a difference between the two.

[c] CF=Complementary foods. For each nutrient, the first value refers to developing countries and the second value (after the semi-colon) refers to industrialized countries, whenever there is a difference between the two.

[d] Assuming medium bioavailability of iron

1998). Because of differences between developing and industrialized countries in average milk intake and in the assumed breastmilk concentration of vitamin A, the estimated amount of each nutrient provided by breastmilk may vary. Within each column of **Table 1**, the first value listed refers to developing countries and the second value refers to industrialized countries (if the values are very close, only one value is shown).

The first row of **Table 1** shows the total energy requirements and the estimated amounts of energy from breastmilk and complementary foods at each age. It should be noted that the values for breastmilk consumption are based on intakes of infants who were already receiving complementary foods. Because such foods tend to displace breastmilk intake, at least partially, it is somewhat circular to describe the gap between breastmilk intake and total energy requirements as the energy "required" from complementary foods. Infants exclusively breastfed beyond six months are likely to have considerably higher breastmilk intakes, but because there are very few data available for such cases, it is not possible to calculate the true energy "gap" (if any) under these circumstances. Thus, the values for energy shown in the column for the "amount needed from complementary foods" should be considered as descriptive of usual patterns rather than as prescriptive of what should be consumed. With this caveat in mind, the average expected energy intake from complementary foods in developing countries is approximately 200 kcal (837 kJ) at six to eight months, 300 kcal (1256 kJ) at nine to 11 months, and 550 kcal (2302 kJ) at 12-23 months. These values represent 33%, 45%, and 61% of total energy needs, respectively. In industrialized countries, the corresponding values are approximately 130 kcal (544 kJ) at six to eight months, 310 kcal (1298 kJ) at nine to 11 months, and 580 kcal (2428 kJ) at 12-23 months (21%, 45%, and 65% of total energy needs, respectively). Of course, these values will differ if the child is consuming more or less breastmilk than the average.

The second row of **Table 1** shows the same estimates for protein. Assuming average breastmilk intake, the amount of protein needed from complementary foods increases from about 2 g/d at six to eight months to 5-6 g/d at 12-23 months, with the percentage from complementary foods increasing from 21% to about 50%. The remaining rows show the estimates for the key vitamins and minerals. For vitamin B_{12} and selenium, the amount needed from complementary foods prior to 12 months is zero because human milk contains generous amounts of these nutrients if the mother is adequately nourished. For the other micronutrients, the percentage of the RNI needed from complementary foods ranges widely. At six to eight months, for example, complementary foods need to provide <30% of the RNI for vitamin A, folate, vitamin C, copper, and iodine, but >70% of the RNI for niacin, vitamin B_6, vitamin D, iron, and zinc. The values for niacin needed from complementary foods are high in all age intervals (75-88% of the RNI), but because niacin needs can also be met by the contribution of tryptophan in the diet, niacin is not likely to be a limiting nutrient among infants who receive adequate protein. Similarly, the percentage of vitamin D needed from other sources is very high (>92%) because there is relatively little vitamin D in human milk; however, it should be noted that adequate exposure to sunlight can meet the child's needs for vitamin D even if complementary foods are not rich in this nutrient.

Complementary foods need to provide relatively large amounts (≥ 80% of the RNI in all age intervals) of iron, zinc, and vitamin B_6. Because the amount of iron in human milk is very low (even though what is present is well absorbed), it is likely to be one of the first limiting nutrients in the diets of infants who rely predominantly on breastmilk.

Fat is not listed in **Table 1** because there is uncertainty about the optimal intake of fat during the first two years of life. Dietary lipids are important not only as a source of essential fatty acids, but also because they influence dietary energy density and sensory qualities. Breastmilk is generally rich in fat (~30-50% of energy) compared to most complementary foods, so as breastmilk intake declines with age, total fat intake is also likely to decline. If one assumes that the percentage of energy from fat in the total diet should be at least 30% and that breastmilk fat concentration averages 38 g/L, the amount of fat needed from complementary foods (assuming average breastmilk intake) is 0 at six to eight months, ~3 g/d at nine to 11 months, and 9-13 g/d at 12-23 months, or 0%, 5-8%, and 15-20% of the energy from complementary foods, respectively. As infants decrease their intake of breastmilk, they also need other good sources of essential fatty acids, such as fish, egg, liver, nut pastes, and most vegetable oils.

GROWTH PATTERNS OF BREASTFED INFANT

Assessing the growth of the breastfed infant is a commonly used method for advising when to introduce complementary foods and for evaluating the adequacy of the diet. However, the conclusions drawn from plotting the growth of a breastfed infant on a standard growth chart may be erroneous if the growth chart does not adequately reflect normal growth. For this reason, it is useful to review this issue herein.

Until 2006, the most widely used growth reference data were the growth charts that were based on data compiled by the U.S. National Center for Health Statistics (NCHS) in 1977, and subsequently adopted for international use by the World Health Organization (WHO). For children under 24 months of age, the 1977 NCHS charts were based on data from a single community (Yellow Springs, Ohio), collected between 1929 and 1975 as part of the Fels Longitudinal Study. These reference data had a number of limitations (Garza & de Onis, 1999): 1) the sample was relatively homogeneous with regard to ethnic and racial background; 2) measurements were made only every three months, which is too infrequent to adequately characterize the pattern of growth in early infancy; 3) there were technical problems related to variable sample sizes and outdated curve-fitting procedures; and 4) very few infants in the Fels study were breastfed for more than three months. When growth of a breastfed infant was compared against the 1977 NCHS growth chart, the typical pattern observed was a relatively rapid gain in the first two to three months, followed by a downward trend in percentile ranking thereafter (Dewey *et al.*, 1995). The downward trend after the first few months caused some health care providers to conclude that there was growth faltering due to inadequate breastmilk intake, leading to the premature introduction of supplementary formula or complementary foods.

Some of the technical problems in the 1977 charts were subsequently rectified by NCHS, and new CDC growth charts were released in 2000 which were based primarily on national child growth surveys. However, the CDC 2000 growth charts still have a number of serious limitations. The most important of these is the lack of growth survey data for the first three months of life, which required the use of modeling procedures that may not have adequately captured the growth pattern during this critical age interval. Furthermore, the national survey data used for the CDC 2000 growth charts included relatively few infants who were breastfed for more than a few months. As a result, there are still notable differences in the growth patterns of breastfed infants when plotted against the CDC 2000 charts, especially after six months of age (de Onis & Onyango, 2003).

In 2006, the World Health Organization released new growth charts that are based on the growth of breastfed children in six different countries with widely differing ethnic backgrounds (WHO Multicentre Growth Reference Study Group, 2006a; WHO Multicentre Growth Reference Study Group, 2006b). The WHO Multicentre Growth Reference Study collected data on growth and other outcomes from 8440 children zero to five years of age from families with high socioeconomic status living in environments supportive of unconstrained growth. For the longitudinal component (zero to two years of age), all children included in the growth curves were breastfed for at least 12 months. The principle underlying the new curves is that they are intended to reflect how children should grow under optimal conditions, based on the premise that the growth pattern of the breastfed infant is the biological "norm." There was remarkable similarity in child growth among the six sites, confirming the hypothesis that when young children are fed optimally and live in healthy environments, they achieve their genetic growth potential regardless of their ethnicity or cultural background. These new charts are recommended because they accurately depict the growth of breastfed children. The WHO 2006 curves differ considerably from the CDC 2000 growth charts, particularly during the first two years of life.

Regardless of the growth chart utilized, there is considerable evidence of differences in growth rates between breastfed and formula-fed infants. When growth of breastfed and formula-fed infants in affluent populations is compared directly (Dewey, 1998), nearly all of the studies show greater weight gain among the latter than among the former. The difference in average attained weight at 12 months is approximately 600-650 g. Differences in length gain are generally less than those for weight gain. As a result, most studies show that breastfed infants are lower in weight-for-length and other indices of fatness than formula-fed infants after the first six months (Dewey *et al.*, 1993). There is no evidence that individuals who were breastfed are shorter as adults than those who were formula-fed (Dewey, 2007a), but there is growing evidence that breastfeeding may be protective against obesity later in life (Dewey, 2007b).

The finding that breastfed infants do not show "maximal" growth has raised questions regarding the adequacy of breastmilk intake and/or nutrient content. However, in affluent populations, breastmilk intake is not associated with maternal characteristics such as nutritional status, but rather is determined primarily by infant demand (Institute of Medicine, 1991; Dewey *et al.*, 1991). Furthermore, the most striking deviation in growth relative to formula-fed infants occurs during the latter part of infancy, when breastfed infants are receiving complementary foods. If these infants were receiving insufficient breastmilk, they presumably could compensate for this by consuming more energy from other foods, yet the data indicate that breastfed infants regularly leave a portion of the complementary food offered to them unconsumed. These and other data suggest that breastfed infants self-regulate their energy intake at a lower level than formula-fed infants (Butte, 1990; Dewey, 1991). The reasons for this are unclear, but it is known that body temperature and minimal observable metabolic rate are lower in breastfed than formula-fed infants (Butte *et al.*, 1990). It could be argued that the greater weight gain of formula-fed infants represents excessive growth, given that there are no deleterious functional outcomes associated with the slower weight gain of breastfed infants (Dewey *et al.*, 1991). In certain circumstances, however, the combination of breastmilk and complementary foods offered (even in affluent populations) may be inadequate in certain nutrients, which could lead to suboptimal growth in some infants.

AGE OF INTRODUCTION OF COMPLEMENTARY FOODS

In 2001, the World Health Organization adopted the policy of recommending exclusive breastfeeding for six months (World Health Assembly, 2001). This recommendation followed a report by a WHO Expert Consultation on the Optimal Duration of Exclusive Breastfeeding (World Health Organization, 2001), which considered the results of a systematic review of the evidence (Kramer & Kakuma, 2002). The Expert Consultation concluded that waiting until six months to introduce complementary foods to breastfed infants confers several benefits on the infant and the mother. Prior to 2001, the WHO recommendation had been to introduce complementary foods at "four to six months" of age, but by the time of the systematic review, enough evidence had accumulated to warrant changing the wording to "six months." In some countries, however, there is a difference of opinion among professionals about whether to recommend "six months" or "four to six months" as the optimal age of introduction of complementary foods. For example, in the most recent American Academy of Pediatrics Pediatric Nutrition Handbook (Kleinman, 2004), both views are expressed. Thus, it is useful to briefly review the evidence on this issue.

The WHO Expert Consultation concluded that the principal advantage of exclusive breastfeeding for six months was a reduced risk of gastrointestinal infection. Even in industrialized countries, there is evidence of less infection among infants breastfed exclusively for six months (Kramer & Kakuma, 2002; Chantry *et al.*, 2006). On a population basis, there is no evidence for any deficit in weight or length gain among infants who are exclusively breastfed for six months, compared to those given complementary foods (Dewey, 2006). This is probably because the energy provided by complementary foods largely displaces breastmilk during the four to six month age interval (Dewey, 2006). As a result, total energy intake (from both breastmilk and complementary foods) does not differ significantly at six months between breastfed infants receiving complementary foods and those who do not. However, the type of complementary food consumed may influence the nature of the growth response. Kramer *et al.* (2004) found that formula and other milks had a growth-accelerating effect on weight and length gain throughout infancy (a result that is consistent with the differences in growth observed between breastfed and formula-fed infants (Dewey *et al.*, 1995), whereas intake of cereal at three to six months was associated with substantially lower weight, length, and head circumference gain among infants in Belarus during that interval, compared to exclusively breastfed infants.

As mentioned in a previous section, the nutrient needs of a full-term, normal birth weight infant can generally be met by breastmilk alone for the first six months if the mother is well-nourished. However, in certain circumstances some of the micronutrients may become limiting prior to six months. In the case of iron, for example, the reserves present at birth are a critical factor determining the risk of anemia during infancy, as the iron concentration of human milk is low. In normal birth weight infants, who generally have adequate liver iron reserves, there is little risk of anemia with exclusive breastfeeding prior to nine months of age, although biochemical indices of low iron status may occur in some between six and nine months (Griffin & Abrams, 2001). The risk of iron deficiency is much greater in low birth weight infants because their iron stores at birth are much smaller, and for this reason, it is advised that low birth weight infants receive medicinal iron drops beginning at two months of age (International Nutritional Anemia Consultative Group *et al.*, 1998). The evidence suggests that iron deficiency can be prevented more effectively by iron supplementation to high risk infants than by introducing complementary foods prior to six months (Dewey, 2006).

As is the case for iron, the zinc concentration of human milk is relatively low, and it is thought that low stores of zinc at birth may predispose certain subgroups of infants to zinc deficiency (Krebs, 2002). In well-nourished breastfed infants, there is little evidence that additional zinc is needed (Heinig *et al.*, 2006), but in disadvantaged populations, zinc supplementation during infancy has generally had positive effects on growth and morbidity (Osendarp *et al.*, 2002). Nonetheless, there is no evidence that complementary feeding prior to six months, even with zinc-rich foods, enhances zinc status (Dewey, 2006). High-risk infants, however, may benefit from zinc supplementation.

In some circumstances, exclusively breastfed infants may have low intakes of certain vitamins: a) vitamin D deficiency may occur among infants who do not receive much exposure to sunlight, b) signs of vitamin B_{12} deficiency may be exhibited in infants of mothers with poor vitamin B_{12} status (e.g., complete vegetarians), c) vitamin A status may be low among infants whose mothers' vitamin A reserves are depleted, and d) riboflavin and vitamin B_6 status may be low in infants of mothers with very low intakes of these vitamins. Otherwise, vitamin deficiencies are very unlikely in exclusively breastfed infants during the first six months. In all of these situations, improving the mother's diet or giving her supplements (for vitamin A, B_6, B_{12}, and riboflavin) or giving vitamin drops directly to the infant (for vitamin D) is the recommended treatment, rather than providing complementary foods to the infant.

Apart from reduced risk of infection, there are several other potential benefits of exclusive breastfeeding for six months. For the infant, there is some evidence that motor development is more advanced in those who are breastfed exclusively for six months (Dewey, 2006). For the mother, a longer duration of exclusive breastfeeding is associated with prolonged lactational amenorrhea (which can be beneficial for birth spacing and maternal iron status) and greater weight loss postpartum (which may help prevent obesity) (Dewey, 2006). Thus, the evidence to date supports the WHO recommendation to introduce complementary foods at six months. In developing countries, the reduced risk of infant gastrointestinal illness and increased duration of maternal lactational amenorrhea associated with exclusive breastfeeding for six months make the benefit-risk ratio of this recommendation highly favorable. In industrialized countries, the case is less clear-cut, but the benefit-risk ratio is also likely to be favorable. In these settings, waiting until six months to introduce complementary foods is likely to be of benefit with regard to outcomes such as infectious morbidity and maternal weight loss postpartum.

MEETING NUTRIENT NEEDS DURING THE PERIOD OF COMPLEMENTARY FEEDING

As shown in **Table 1**, breastfed infants need considerable amounts of certain nutrients from complementary foods after six months of age. It is a challenge to meet nutrient needs at this age because the amount of food consumed is relatively small, yet nutrient requirements during infancy (per unit of body weight) are very high because of the rapid rate of growth. Thus, nutrient-dense complementary foods are needed. The desired nutrient density (e.g., amount of nutrient per 100 kcal of food) can be calculated by dividing the amount of each nutrient needed from complementary foods by the amount of energy expected to come from complementary foods (as shown in **Table 1**). When the desired nutrient densities are compared with actual nutrient densities of the typical complementary food diets consumed in various populations, protein density is generally adequate, but several micronutrients are "problem nutrients." In most developing countries, iron, zinc, and vitamin B_6 are problem nutrients, and even in industrialized countries these nutrients may be limiting. Intake of iron is likely to be marginal in all populations unless iron-fortified products or substantial amounts of meat are consumed. Riboflavin, niacin, thiamin, folate, calcium, vitamin A, and vitamin C may also be problem nutrients, depending on the local mix of complementary foods. At present, there is insufficient information to determine the extent to which some of the other micronutrients, such as vitamin E, iodine, and selenium, may be problem nutrients.

What guidelines can be offered to caregivers with regard to meeting nutrient needs of breastfed infants during the period of complementary feeding? The first is to continue to breastfeed as often as the infant desires, if possible. This is important to avoid excessive displacement of breastmilk by other foods and to ensure that the nutritional and immunological benefits of breastfeeding are maximized. As shown in **Table 1**, breastmilk remains an excellent source of protein, fat, and most vitamins and can make a valuable nutritional contribution well beyond the first year of life. The second is to aim for a variety of complementary foods, with fruits, vegetables, and animal products (e.g., meat, fish, poultry, or egg) offered daily (Pan American Health Organization/World Health Organization, 2003). Iron-fortified infant cereals are a good source of iron, but meats can also provide adequate iron if consumed in large enough quantities, and they have the added advantage of being rich in zinc. Predominantly vegetarian diets cannot meet nutrient needs of breastfed infants unless nutrient supplements or fortified products are used. Part of the reason for this is that plant-based diets are often high in phytate, which greatly reduces the bioavailability of iron and zinc. Adequate calcium can be obtained via cheese, yogurt, and other dairy products. Some vegetables can also provide modest amounts of calcium, but the bioavailability of calcium from foods with high amounts of oxalate (such as spinach) is very low. Beverages with low nutrient density (e.g., sugary drinks) should be avoided and the amount of juice should be limited because such beverages can displace more nutrient-dense foods and potentially contribute to child obesity. Caregivers should also be alert to any signs that the child's appetite, growth, or development is impaired. These are often the first indicators of subtle nutritional deficits (such as zinc deficiency). When a child refuses to eat a varied diet, or eats little or no animal products (e.g., if the parents are vegetarians), a balanced vitamin-mineral supplement is advisable. The standard chewable formulations are usually well accepted and can be crushed into a powder and mixed with foods. Lastly, it is important for parents to make mealtimes an enjoyable experience and avoid force-feeding or coercion. Modeling enjoyment of a varied, nutritious diet is the best way to ensure good dietary practices throughout childhood and beyond.

References

Butte NF, Lopez-Alarcon MG, Garza C. *Nutrient adequacy of exclusive breastfeeding for the term infant during the first six months of life.* Geneva: World Health Organization; 2002.

Butte NF, O'Brian Smith E, Garza C. Energy utilization of breast-fed and formula fed infants. *Am J Clin Nutr.* 1990; 51:350-58.

Butte NF. Energy requirements of infants. *Eur J Clin Nutr.* 1996; 50:S24-S36.

Chantry C, Howard C, Auinger P. Full breastfeeding and associated decrease in respiratory tract infection in US children. *Pediatrics.* 2006; 117:425-32.

Chaparro CM, Neufeld LM, Tena Alavez G, Eguia-Líz Cedillo R, Dewey KG. Effect of the timing of umbilical cord clamping on iron status in 6-month-old Mexican infants: a randomized controlled trial. *Lancet.* 2006; 367:1997-2004.

de Onis M, Onyango AW. The Centers for Disease Control and Prevention 2000 growth charts and the growth of breastfed infants. *Acta Paediatr.* 2003; 92:413-19.

Dewey KG. Growth characteristics of breast-fed compared to formula-fed infants. *Biol Neonate.* 1998; 74:94-105.

Dewey KG. Breastfeeding and other infant feeding practices that may influence child obesity. In: Dietz W, Birch L (eds.). *Eating behaviors in the young child.* Johnson & Johnson Pediatric Institute Pediatric Round Table Series; 2007b.

Dewey KG. Infant feeding and growth. In: Goldberg G, *et al.* (eds.). *Breastfeeding: Early influences on later health.* London: Springer; 2007a.

Dewey KG. What is the optimal age of introduction of complementary foods? In: Rigo J, Ziegler EE (eds.). *Protein and energy requirements in infancy and childhood.* Nestle Nutr Workshop Ser Pediatr Program. Vevey: Nestec Ltd.; 2006. p. 161-175.

Dewey KG, Beaton G, Fjeld C, Lonnerdal B, Reeds P. Protein requirements of infants and children. Proceedings of the International Dietary Energy Consultative Group. *Eur J Clin Nutr.* 1996; Supplement 1:S119-S150.

Dewey, KG, Brown, K.H. Update on technical issues concerning complementary feeding of young children in developing countries and implications for intervention programs. *Food Nutr Bull.* 2003; 24:5-28.

Dewey KG, Heinig MJ, Nommsen LA, Lonnerdal B. Adequacy of energy intake among breast-fed infants in the DARLING study: relationships to growth velocity, morbidity, and activity levels. *J Pediatr.* 1991; 119:538-47.

Dewey KG, Heinig MJ, Nommsen LA, Lonnerdal B. Maternal versus infant factors related to breast milk intake and residual milk volume: the DARLING study. *Pediatrics.* 1991; 1987:829-37.

Dewey KG, Heinig MJ, Nommsen LA, Peerson JM, Lonnerdal B. Breast-fed infants are leaner than formula-fed infants at 1 y of age: the DARLING study. *Am J Clin Nutr.* 1993; 57:140-45.

Dewey KG, Peerson JM, Brown KH, Krebs NF, Michaelsen KF, Persson LA, *et al.* WHO Working Group on Infant Growth. Growth of breastfed infants deviates from current reference data: a pooled analysis of U.S., Canadian and European data sets. *Pediatrics.* 1995; 96:495-503.

Garza D, de Onis M. A new international growth reference for young children. *Am J Clin Nutr.* 1999; 70:169S-72S.

Greer FR. Do breastfed infants need supplemental vitamins? *Pediatr Clin North Am.* 2001; 48:415-23.

Griffin IJ, Abrams SA. Iron and breastfeeding. *Pediatr Clin North Am.* 2001; 48:401-13.

Heinig MJ, Brown KH, Lonnerdal B, Dewey KG. Zinc supplementation does not affect growth, morbidity, or motor development of U.S. term breastfed infants at 4 to 10 mo of age. *Am J Clin Nutr.* 2006; 84(3):594-601.

Heinig MJ, Nommsen LA, Peerson JM, Lonnerdal B, Dewey KG. Energy and protein intakes of breast-fed and formula-fed infants during the first year of life and their association with growth velocity: the DARLING study. *Am J Clin Nutr.* 1993; 58:152-61.

Institute of Medicine. *Nutrition during lactation.* Washington, DC: National Academy Press; 1991.

International Nutritional Anemia Consultative Group, World Health Organization, UNICEF (Stoltzfus RJ, Dreyfuss ML (eds.). *Guidelines for the use of iron supplements to prevent and treat iron deficiency anemia.* Washington, DC: ILSI Press; 1998.

Joint FAO/WHO Expert Consultation on Human Vitamin and Mineral Requirements. *Vitamin and mineral requirements in human nutrition.* 2nd Ed. Geneva: World Health Organization; 2004.

Kleinman RE (ed.). *Pediatric nutrition handbook.* 5th Ed. Chicago, IL: American Academy of Pediatrics; 2004.

Kramer MS, Guo T, Platt RW, *et al.* Feeding effects on growth during infancy. *J Pediatr.* 2004; 145:600-5.

Kramer MS, Kakuma R. *The optimal duration of exclusive breastfeeding. A systematic review.* Geneva, Switzerland: World Health Organization; 2002.

Krebs NF, Reidinger CJ, Hartley S, Robertson AD, Hambidge KM. Zinc supplementation during lactation: effects on maternal status and milk zinc concentrations. *Am J Clin Nutr.* 1995; 61:1030-36.

Krebs NF. Zinc and breastfed infants: if and when is there a risk of deficiency? In: Davis MK, Isaacs CE, Hanson LA, Wright AL (eds.). *Integrating population outcomes, biological mechanisms and research methods in the study of human milk and lactation.* Kluwer Academic Publishers; 2002. p. 69-75.

Osendarp SJM, Santosham M, Black RE, Wahed MA, van Raaij JMA, Fuchs GJ. Effect of zinc supplementation between 1 and 6 mo of life on growth and morbidity of Bangladeshi infants in urban slums. *Am J Clin Nutr.* 2002; 76:1401-8.

Pan American Health Organization/ World Health Organization. *Guiding principles for complementary feeding of the breastfed child.* Washington DC: PAHO; 2003.

Picciano MF. Nutrient composition of human milk. *Pediatr Clin North Am.* 2001; 48:53-67.

WHO Multicentre Growth Reference Study Group. *WHO child growth standards. Length/height-for-age, weight-for-age, weight-for-length, weight-for-height and body mass index-for-age. Methods and development.* Geneva: World Health Organization; 2006a.

WHO Multicentre Growth Reference Study Group. WHO child growth standards. *Acta Paediatr.* 2006b; Suppl 450.

World Health Assembly. *Infant and young child nutrition.* Geneva, Switzerland: World Health Organization; 18 May 2001. Resolution 54.2.

World Health Organization. *Complementary feeding of young children in developing countries: a review of current scientific knowledge.* WHO/NUT/98.1.Geneva: World Health Organization; 1998.

World Health Organization. *The optimal duration of exclusive breastfeeding. Report of an expert consultation.* Geneva, Switzerland: World Health Organization; 2001.

Chapter 23

Vitamin D and the Breastfed Infant

Daniel S. Hirsch

INTRODUCTION

Vitamin D is a unique essential nutrient in that its biological requirement is met by a combination of exogenous sources and endogenous production, via exposure to ultraviolet B (UVB) light (Raiten & Picciano, 2004). Until recently, vitamin D was thought to only be important for bone health and calcium and phosphorus homeostasis. In light of this understanding, the primary benefit of ensuring vitamin D sufficiency in the pediatric arena was the treatment and prevention of rickets; while in adults, the principal benefits were felt to be the treatment and prevention of osteoporosis. It is now appreciated that vitamin D is a substance with a wide range of functions throughout the body. Additionally, vitamin D can regulate the proliferation and differentiation of a wide variety of normal and abnormal cell types. Its actions are primarily mediated via binding of the active metabolite 1,25 dihydroxyvitamin D_3 (1,25-vitaminD) to the intranuclear vitamin D receptor (VDR). The VDR is present in many different tissues and cell types, most of which do not participate in bone, calcium, or phosphorus physiology. Human, animal, and in vitro data suggest that mild asymptomatic vitamin D deficiency may also play a role in the pathogenesis of hypertension, certain autoimmune disorders, and cancers (Zittermann, 2003). In a recent review on vitamin D, Michael Holick concluded: "*Vitamin D can no longer be thought of as a nutrient necessary for the prevention of rickets among children. Vitamin D should be considered essential for overall health and well-being* (Holick, 2004)."

Breastfeeding is the optimal method of infant feeding. Extensive research documents "*diverse and compelling advantages for infants, mothers, families, and society from breastfeeding and use of human milk for infant feeding* (Gartner *et al.*, 2005)." The 2005 policy statement of the American Academy of Pediatrics (AAP), Section on Breastfeeding states: "*Exclusive breastfeeding is the reference or normative model against which all alternative feeding methods must be measured with regard to growth, health, development, and all other short- and long-term outcomes* (Gartner *et al.*, 2005)." Despite its benchmark status, it is well-recognized that human milk contains low levels of vitamin D (Butte *et al.*, 2002; Gartner & Greer, 2003). Over the past 30 years, there have been numerous published reports of vitamin D deficient rickets in breastfed children throughout the world. Breastfeeding is also associated with asymptomatic vitamin D deficiency. Large-scale investigations of vitamin D status in nursing children have not been performed. Because mild vitamin D deficiency is silent, it has been hypothesized that underlying the relatively small number of instances of rickets is a much larger population who are vitamin D deficient (Calikoglu & Davenport, 2003). Given the scenario of a widespread deficiency of a substance involved in a wide range of bodily processes and functions, researchers and clinicians are actively debating the merits of various approaches to enhancing the vitamin D status of the breastfeeding child.

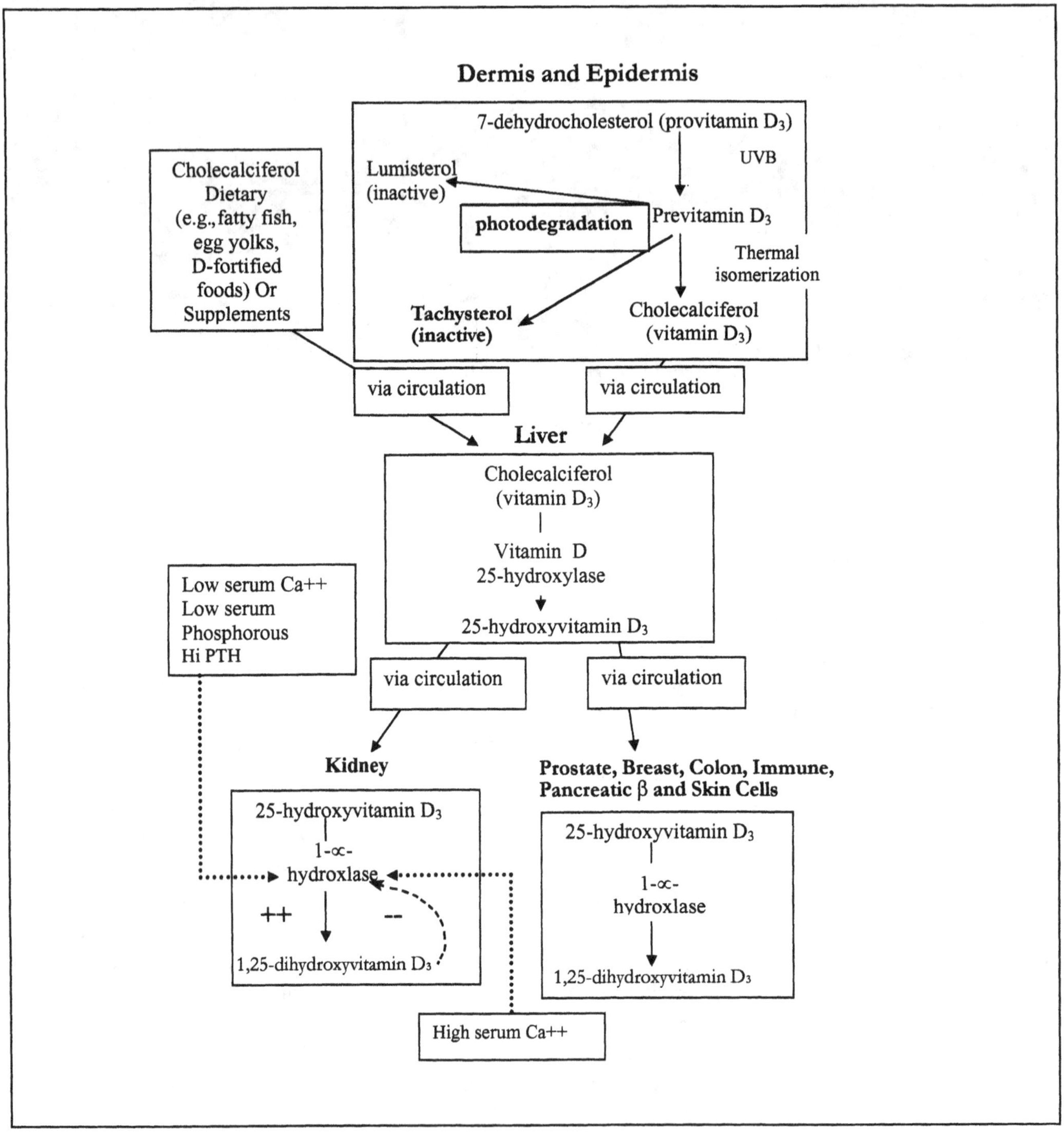

Figure 1. UVB photons trigger the conversion, via a nonenzymatic photochemical reaction, of 7-dihydrocholesterol (provitamin D_3) to previtamin D_3. Previtamin D_3 is unstable and, in the lipid bilayer, is rapidly isomerized to vitamin D_3 by thermal energy. This conformational change can deliver the vitamin D_3 into the circulation where it is bound to vitamin D binding protein and transported to the liver for further processing. Previtamin D_3 is very photosensitive and significant amounts are photodegraded to inactive sterols, lumisterol and tachysterol. It is estimated that a maximum of 10-15% of 7-dihydrocholesterol (provitamin D_3) will be converted to vitamin D. Sunlight-induced melanin synthesis, acting as a natural sunscreen, provides additional protection against vitamin D intoxication.

In the liver, both exogenous vitamin D_3 and endogenous vitamin D_3 (generated in the skin) are converted to 25-hydroxyvitamin D_3 via the enzyme vitamin D 25-hydroxylase. In the final step of vitamin D bioactivation, 25-hydroxyvitamin D_3 undergoes a second hydroxylation via the enzyme 1-∞-hydroxlase, resulting in the active metabolite, 1,25-dihydroxyvitamin D_3. This second hydroxylation occurs in the kidney and in numerous extrarenal sites (immune cells, keratinocytes, parathyroid, breast, colon, prostate and pancreatic βcells).

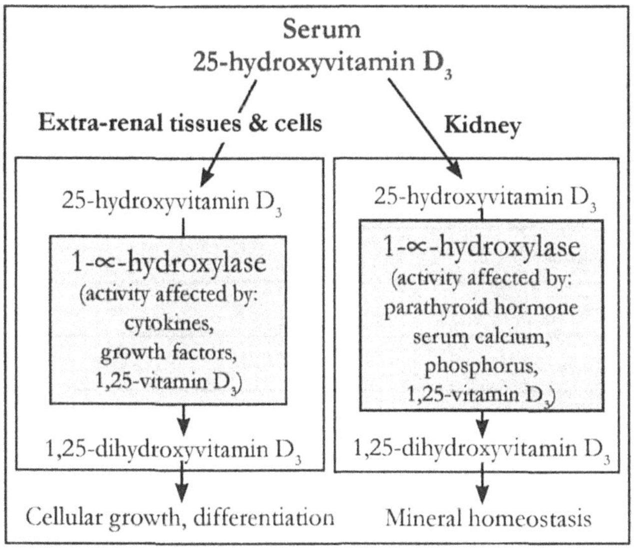

Figure 2. Regulation of renal and extrarenal 1-∝-hydroxylase

BASIC BIOCHEMISTRY, PHOTOBIOLOGY AND METABOLISM

Vitamin D is a family of fat-soluble biologically active secosteroids. The best-known examples of vitamin D are cholecalciferol (vitamin D_3), which is produced in the skin and can be obtained via the diet (primarily from animal sources), and ergocalciferol (vitamin D_2), which is derived from plants. When skin cells in the dermis and epidermis are briefly exposed to sunlight that contains a sufficient level of ultraviolet B (UVB) photons with energies between 290 and 315nm, a photochemical reaction converts 7-dehydrocholesterol (provitamin D_3) to previtamin D_3 (Figure 1) (Holick *et al.*, 1977). Previtamin D_3 then either undergoes a temperature-dependent thermal isomerization to become vitamin D_3 or photodegradation into biologically inactive compounds (Holick *et al.*, 1980; Holick *et al.*, 1981). Once vitamin D_3 is formed, it can either enter into the circulation or is degraded by UV light (Webb *et al.*, 1989). Because sunlight degrades significant amounts of both previtamin D_3 and vitamin D_3, it is believed that excessive chronic exposure to sunlight will not lead to vitamin D intoxication (Holick, 1994). Biological activation of vitamin D_3 requires two hydroxylations. The initial hydroxylation of vitamin D_3 is catalyzed in the liver by the enzyme vitamin D_3 25-hydroxylase to produce 25-hydroxyvitamin D_3 (25-OH-vitaminD_3). Because there are animal and plant forms of vitamin D, one's vitamin D status is assessed by measuring total serum 25-hydroxyvitamin D levels (Heaney, 2003). This parameter consists of the circulating concentrations of both 25-OH-vitaminD_3 and 25-hydroxyvitamin D_2 and reflects exogenous and endogenous sources of vitamin D. 25-OH-vitaminD_3 is hydroxylated primarily in the kidney by the enzyme 25-hydroxyvitamin D-1α-hydroxylase (1α-hydroxylase) to yield the active metabolite, 1,25-dihydroxyvitamin D_3 (1,25-vitaminD_3) (Figure 1). Serum levels of 1,25-vitaminD_3 are carefully regulated by several feedback mechanisms. While PTH and low serum calcium and phosphorous will increase renal 1-∝-hydroxylase activity, 1,25-vitaminD_3 and high serum calcium will suppress the enzyme's expression.

Relevant to vitamin D's diverse functions, 1α-hydroxylase is also present in many other cells and tissues. The extrarenally produced 1,25-vitaminD_3 mainly serves as an autocrine and paracrine factor with local cell-specific functions (such as cell growth, replication, and differentiation). Extrarenal 1α-hydroxylase is largely under the control of local input, such as cytokines and growth factors, optimizing the levels of 1,25-vitamin D_3 for local cell-specific functions (**Figure 2**) (Dusso *et al.*, 2005). Because renal production of 1,25-vitamin D_3 is largely independent of 25-OH-vitamin

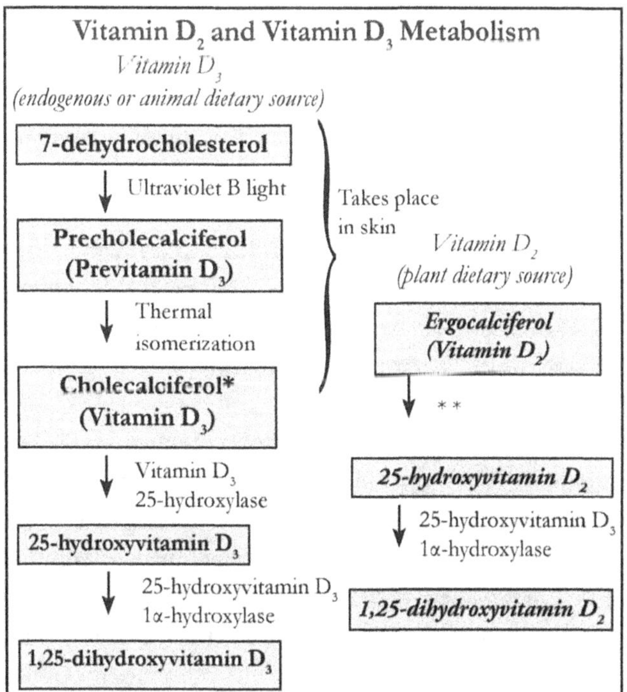

Figure 3.

* Cholecalciferol (animal form of vitamin D) can also be obtained via the diet.

** Vitamin D_3 25-hydroxylase does not 25-hydroxylate ergocalciferol (vitamin D_2)

Table 1. Maternal Vitamin D Status and Total Mean Breastmilk Antirachitic Activity

Study	Country	Stage of Lactation	Mean Maternal Serum [25-OH-Vitamin D] in ng/ml (SD)	Total Mean Breastmilk Antirachitic Activity in IU/liter (SD)
Hollis, 1981	USA	1 day to 3 wks	not reported	25
Hollis, 1982	USA	"Mid-lactation"	not reported	30
Reeve, 1982	USA		not reported	40-50
Hollis, 1986	USA	2 wks to 3 mo	not reported	68
Ala-Houhala, 1988	Finland	20 wks	not reported	44
		8 wks	not reported	124
		20 wks	not reported	51
		8	not reported	35
Hollis, 2004	USA	1 month (baseline)	low dose: 27 (3) high dose: 33(2)	low dose: 36 (4) high dose: 40 (4)
*primarily used D_2 supplements		4 months	low dose: 36 (2) high dose: 45(4)	low dose: 70 (3) high dose: 135 (48)
Wagner, 2006	USA	1 month (baseline)	controls: 32 experimental subjects: 34	controls: 60 experimental subjects: 82
*only used D_3 supplements		6 months	controls: 38 experimental subjects: 59	controls: 76 experimental subjects: 874

Daily supplementation regimens-Hollis, 2004: Low dose received 1600 IU D2 & 400 IU D3, High dose 3600 IU D2 & 400 IU D3; Wagner, 2006: Controls received 400 IU D3, Experimentals received 6400 IU D3

D concentrations, it is believed that mild to moderate degrees of hypovitaminosis D (defined as low 25-OH-vitamin D levels) will only attenuate extrarenal synthesis of the active metabolite (Peterlik & Cross, 2005). It is theorized that a deficiency of extrarenal 1,25-vitamin D_3 contributes to the development of autoimmune and inflammatory disorders and malignancies (Peterlik & Cross, 2005).

Exogenously acquired vitamin D_2 may contribute significantly to the vitamin D status of humans and other mammals. However, recent investigations have found that in humans, as in other mammals, vitamin D_2 has a significantly lower nutritional value (Armas *et al.*, 2004; Trang *et al.*, 1998). Compared to vitamin D_3, it is metabolized in a similar fashion into the active metabolite 1,25-dihydroxyvitamin D_2 (1,25-vitamin D_2) (**Figure 3**). Data suggest that the active metabolites, 1,25-vitamin D_2 and 1,25-vitamin D_3 have similar biological potency (Horst *et al.*, 2005).

Most of the biological activities of 1,25-vitamin D are mediated via the 48-kilodalton nuclear receptor, vitamin D receptor (VDR) (Dusso *et al.*, 2005). The VDR is present in an extensive range of organs, tissues, and cell types including: the brain, heart, lung, liver, pancreas, kidney, thyroid, small and large intestine, bone, skin, testis, ovary, and immune and hematopoietic cells (Pike *et al.*, 2005). Its detection in tumor cells has helped stimulate interest in vitamin D and vitamin D analogs as potential therapies for cancer. The binding of 1,25-vitamin D_3 to the VDR triggers a complex sequence of events resulting in changes in the transcription of vitamin D-responsive genes. Alteration of gene transcription directly mediates the physiological actions of vitamin D (Dusso *et al.*, 2005; Pike *et al.*, 2005). In addition to the local concentration of 1,25-vitamin D_3, the response by vitamin D target tissues may also be modified by the concentration and phosphorylation of the VDR. Vitamin D-dependent rickets type II, an autosomal recessive disease, is probably the most well known example of the VDR's physiologic significance. As a result of a mutation-induced inactivation of the VDR, there is an end-organ resistance to 1,25-vitamin D_3. Patients with the disorder develop severe, early-onset postnatal rickets accompanied by hypocalcemia, secondary hyperparathyroidism, and alopecia (Bouillon, 2006).

SOURCES OF VITAMIN D

For nearly every infant, breastmilk is the best form of nutrition. Employing sensitive assay technology since the 1980's, researchers have been able to accurately assess the vitamin D content of human milk. Its vitamin D content, also referred to as antirachitic activity, consists primarily of vitamin D_3 and 25-OH-vitamin D_3 (Basile *et al.*, 2006). A nursing woman who is consuming vitamin D_2, via either supplements or a plant source, will produce breastmilk with a portion of antirachitic activity also attributable to vitamin D_2 and 25-OH-vitamin D_2. The vitamin D content of human milk is affected by diet, sunlight exposure, and race (Hollis & Wagner, 2004; Specker *et al.*, 1985). With the exception of a small subset of subjects from one study, research has shown that breastmilk has a relatively low level of antirachitic activity, ranging between 25 and 82 international units (IU) per liter (Table 1). In 1997, the United States Food and Nutrition Board of the Institute of Medicine recommended a daily adequate intake (AI) of 200 IU of vitamin D (Standing Committee on Dietary Reference Intakes, 1997). Therefore, in order to meet the AI for vitamin D, an exclusively nursing infant would need to consume as little as 2.5 liters or as much as eight liters of human milk per day (this assumes a breastmilk antirachitic activity of 80 or 25 IU, respectively).

There are very few foods that are naturally rich in vitamin D (Calvo & Whiting, 2006). Cholecalciferol (vitamin D_3) is found in animal sources and is the main form of vitamin D in food. Ergocalciferol (vitamin D_2), of plant origin, is primarily found in wild mushrooms (Lamberg-Allardt, 2006). The best natural sources of vitamin D_3 are fatty fish (e.g., eel, herring, whitefish, salmon, sardines, mackerel, and tuna) and egg yolks (National Public Health Institute, 2006; USDA, 2005). In the United States, several foods are currently vitamin D-fortified, including cow's milk, breakfast cereals, some orange juices, and yogurts (USDA, 2005). Contrary to popular belief, because dairy products are not routinely fortified with vitamin D, they are not a good source of vitamin D (Calvo *et al.*, 2004). In Canada, all fluid milks and margarines must be fortified with vitamin D. However, with the exception of some egg products, no other vitamin D fortification is permitted in food (Calvo *et al.*, 2004). In several other countries (e.g., the United Kingdom, Ireland, Scotland, and Australia) fortification is not required, but is allowed in a number of staple foods, such as margarine and breakfast cereals (Calvo *et al.*, 2005). However, in Europe and most other countries, vitamin D fortification is restricted (Calvo *et al.*, 2005). Analyzing vitamin D intake data from nationally representative surveys as well as small focused studies, Calvo *et al.* concluded that throughout the world current fortification practices are inadequate to sustain a 'healthy' vitamin D status (Calvo *et al.*, 2005).

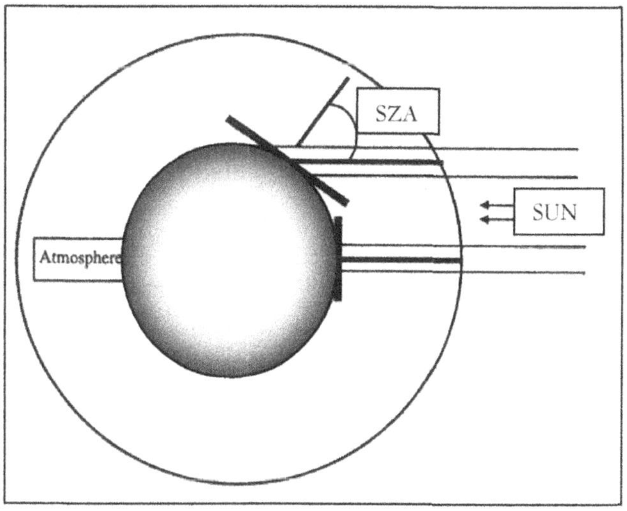

Figure 4. Solar zenith angle is the angle between the local vertical and the direct solar beam. At a large SZA the radiation traverses a longer pathlength through the atmosphere, which can greatly attenuate shorter wavelengths, and the attenated power is spread over a larger area of surface. Source: Webb, 2006; reprinted with permission from Elsevier.

Traditionally for humans, the primary source of vitamin D has been vitamin D_3 produced in response to exposure of the skin to UVB radiation (Holick, 1994; Hollis, 2005). Humans have the capacity to produce large amounts of vitamin D_3. For example, an untanned Caucasian individual wearing a bathing suit who, in the middle of a cloudless July day in Boston (latitude 42° north), is exposed to sunlight for ten to 12 minutes will generate approximately 10,000 to 20,000 IU of vitamin D_3 (Hollis, 2005). Unfortunately, there are many factors which significantly affect the probability and amount of cutaneous vitamin D_3 synthesis.

Webb has classified the influences on vitamin D_3 production into two categories: environmental or external variables and intrinsic or personal variables (Webb, 2006). The external factors impact the amount of solar UVB available to an individual. Examples of external factors include latitude, altitude, season, time of day, cloud cover, air pollution, ozone level, and direct versus indirect sunlight. Additionally, because glass blocks out a high percentage of UVB photons, exposure to sunlight that has passed through a glass window will not yield any vitamin D_3 (Holick, 1994). Personal factors affect whether the UVB radiation present is able to generate vitamin D. Examples of personal factors include skin color, exposed body surface area, sunscreen (sunscreen with a sunscreen protection factor of eight will reduce vitamin D production by 97.5%), time spent outdoors, and age (Matsuoka *et al.*, 1990). The amount of vitamin D_3 produced by the skin varies according to the combination of external and personal factors unique to each individual.

The importance of several of the environmental variables affecting cutaneous vitamin D synthesis is dependent upon the solar zenith angle (SZA). The SZA is defined as the angle between the local vertical and the sun (**Figure 4**) (Webb, 2006). At a small SZA, the sun's UVB rays have a shorter path through the atmosphere and less attenuation will occur. At a large SZA, the UVB rays have a longer path through the atmosphere and greater attenuation will occur. The smallest SZA exists during the summer, in the middle of the day, and at low latitudes, while the largest SZA occurs during the winter, the beginning and end of the day, and at high latitudes. Utilizing an in vitro model of cutaneous vitamin D synthesis, it has been determined that in Boston (latitude 42° north) and Edmonton (latitude 52° north) there is an insufficient quantity of UVB photons reaching the earth's surface for four months and six months of the year, respectively (Webb *et al.*, 1988). By contrast, in Buenos Aires (latitude 34° south), even in the middle of winter, enough UVB radiation is present to affect endogenous vitamin D synthesis (Ladizesky *et al.*, 1995). In other words, at increased latitudes during the winter, the greater SZA will significantly attenuate the quantity of UVB rays reaching the Earth's surface. As a result, at increased latitudes during the winter months, sunlight exposure in the middle of a clear sunny day will not result in vitamin D production.

The most thoroughly studied personal variables effecting cutaneous vitamin D synthesis is skin color. Skin color is largely determined by the quantity of melanin in the skin (Webb, 2006). Melanin is a molecule that blocks a substantial proportion of UVB photons from reaching the lower layers of the skin where vitamin D synthesis occurs (Kollias, 1995). Compared to lightly pigmented Caucasian adults, darkly pigmented African-Americans exposed to a fixed dose of UVB radiation produced significantly lower amounts of vitamin D_3 and had significantly lower total 25-OH-vitamin D levels (Matsuoka *et al.*, 1991). These findings are consistent with data from several small and large population-based studies which noted that African-American adolescents and adults had significantly lower 25-OH-vitamin D levels and greater incidences of vitamin D deficiency (Harris & Dawson-Hughes, 1998; Harkness & Cromer, 2005; Looker *et al.*, 2002; Nesby-O'Dell *et al.*, 2002). Another clinically relevant personal factor is one's style of dress. It is well-documented that, compared to females who wear clothing which exposes their face, arms, and legs, those who wear concealing clothing have significantly lower vitamin D levels (Andiran *et al.*, 2002; Gannagé-Yared *et al.*, 2000; Hatun *et al.*, 2005). Yet another illustration of the importance of personal factors on endogenous vitamin D_3 production is continued reports of vitamin D deficient rickets in infants and children and the relatively high incidence of vitamin D deficiency amongst children and adults residing at latitudes affording year-round exposure to sufficient levels of UVB radiation (Atiq *et al.*, 1998; Dawodu *et al.*, 2003; Ghannam *et al.*, 1999; Goswami *et al.*, 2000; Robinson *et al.*, 2006).

Vitamin D can be obtained via the diet or endogenously produced upon exposure to sufficient levels of UVB radiation. Research has shown that breastmilk is a poor source of vitamin D. Few foods contain significant amounts of vitamin D. The best natural dietary sources of vitamin D include fatty fish, egg yolks, and some species of wild mushrooms. In order to enhance one's vitamin D intake, some countries have either mandated or permitted the fortification of several food stuffs. However, in most countries throughout the world, vitamin D fortification is severely restricted. Traditionally, for humans, the primary source of vitamin D has been cutaneously produced vitamin D_3. This supply of vitamin D is modified by a host of environmental and personal variables such as latitude, season, time of day, skin color, body surface area exposure, and time spent outdoors. The literature suggests that throughout the world many people are deprived of an adequate supply of endogenous and/or exogenous vitamin D.

BIOLOGICAL ACTIONS OF VITAMIN D

For years, vitamin D has been known to have a central role in bone health and calcium and phosphorus homeostasis. In the late 1970's, Stumpf *et al.* noted that rats possessed the VDR in several sites not involved in vitamin D's established functions, including the stomach, epidermis, and pituitary and parathyroid glands (Stumpf *et al.*, 1979). Further work ascertained the VDR to exist in numerous organs, tissues, and cell types (Pike *et al.*, 2005). Additionally, this nuclear receptor has been demonstrated in over 25 different tumors and cancer cells (van Leeuwen & Pols, 2005). The widespread distribution of the VDR in normal and abnormal cells helped trigger a search, which continues even today, for 'new' roles for vitamin D. Based on a large body of knowledge derived from molecular, cellular, animal, and human studies, it is now appreciated that vitamin D possesses both classical (bone health and calcium and phosphorous metabolism) and non-classical functions in a wide range of systems and processes (Dusso *et al.*, 2005).

Vitamin D's classical functions (maintaining skeletal integrity and serum calcium and phosphorus levels) are mediated by effects on the intestine, kidney, parathyroid gland, and bone (Dusso *et al.*, 2005). Maintaining serum calcium within a narrow range is tightly regulated by parathyroid hormone (PTH) and 1,25-vitamin D. When serum ionized calcium declines, the calcium sensors of the parathyroid gland initiate an increase in PTH production and secretion by the parathyroid gland. This results in increased phosphorus clearance and conversion of 25-OH-vitamin D to 1,25-vitamin D by the kidney, as well as increased calcium mobilization from bone. 1,25-vitamin D raises calcium levels by optimizing PTH-mediated osteoclast production and by enhancing calcium absorption in the small intestine and reabsorption in the kidney (Dusso *et al.*, 2005; Holick, 2003). By dissolving bone, osteoclasts help release calcium and phosphorus into the circulation. Once calcium levels have been corrected, calcium sensors in the parathyroid suppress PTH release. Additionally, in the presence of normocalcemia, 1,25-vitamin D exerts negative feedback on both its own production and PTH secretion (Dusso *et al.*, 2005; Bouillon, 2006). Vitamin D's role in phosphorus homeostasis consists primarily of 1,25-vitamin D's ability to increase the small intestine's absorptive efficiency of phosphorus and decrease renal phosphorus losses (Dusso *et al.*, 2005). Vitamin D influences bone health and development by direct and indirect means. Recent experiments in VDR knockout mice demonstrate that, via the VDR, 1,25-vitamin D exerts a direct anabolic effect on bone formation (Goltzman, 2004). By helping to simultaneously maintain serum calcium and phosphorus levels in the normal range, vitamin D facilitates the passive mineralization of the collagen matrix laid down by osteoblasts (Holick, 2003).

One of the most noteworthy non-classical actions of vitamin D is its impact on the cell cycle. Cell replication, the result of progression through all four phases of the cell cycle, is important for normal growth and development of the entire organism. It is tightly controlled in normal tissues, but poorly regulated in pathologic processes, such as cancer. 1,25-vitamin D regulates proliferation and differentiation in keratinocytes, osteoblasts, and hematopoietic cells (Bohnsack & Hirschi, 2004). In vitro studies have shown that, via multiple mechanisms, 1,25-vitamin D arrests the cell cycle of a variety of human cancer cells. Because these actions are seen at concentrations too low to activate the VDR, researchers speculate that they may be mediated via both paracrine and endocrine processes (Dusso *et al.*, 2005).

Another area of active investigation is the role of vitamin D in the immune system. The VDR is expressed by many cells of the immune system, including lymphocytes and antigen-presenting cells, such as macrophages and dendritic cells (Dusso *et al.*, 2005). Moreover, macrophages and dendritic cells express 25-hydroxyvitamin D-1-α-hydroxylase (1-α-hydroxylase), the enzyme responsible for the final step in the synthesis of 1,25-vitamin D. The presence of both the VDR and 1-α-hydroxylase in immune cells suggests that vitamin D affects the immune system in a local or paracrine fashion. The detection of the VDR in immune cells has facilitated the discovery that 1,25-vitamin D impacts the production of several important cytokines. Regulatory T cells and helper T cells, Th1 and Th2, are central to all antigen-specific immune responses. A balance of these three subtypes characterizes a 'normal' tolerant immune system. In autoimmune disorders, Th1 cells, activated by the cytokines interleukin-2 (IL-2) and interferon gamma (IFN-γ), are misdirected against self proteins. The finding that 1,25-vitamin D induces regulatory T cells, increases the production of Th2 cytokines IL-4, IL-5, and IL-10, and inhibits the production of the Th1 cytokines IL-2 and IFN-γ suggests that it may have an important role in the development and maintenance of self-tolerance, as well as in the pathogenesis of autoimmune disorders (Cantorna & Mahon, 2004; van Etten & Mathieu, 2005). In addition to its influence on immunologic tolerance, evidence has been uncovered suggesting that Vitamin D is involved in the immune system's ability to fight infection (Liu *et al.*, 2006).

Additional nonclassical functions of vitamin D have been discovered such as:

- skeletal muscle development (Endo *et al.*, 2003),
- mammary gland biology throughout the reproductive cycle (Zinser *et al.*, 2004),
- negative endocrine regulation of the renin-angiotensin system (Li *et al.*, 2004),
- hair and skin development (Dusso *et al.*, 2005),
- cardiac function and development (Achinger & Ayus, 2005),
- insulin secretion (Zeitz *et al.*, 2003),
- brain development (Feron *et al.*, 2005).

In these and other areas, investigators are attempting to further elucidate the actions of vitamin D.

Vitamin D is well known for its physiological roles in calcium and phosphorus balance and bone health. Over the last 20 years, vitamin D has been found to possess a number of additional nonclassical functions including cell proliferation and differentiation, immune regulation, insulin secretion, feedback inhibition of the renin-angiotensin system, and development of the brain, breast, heart, skin, and skeletal muscle.

DEFINING VITAMIN D SUFFICIENCY

Although it is widely accepted that one's vitamin D status is best defined by the serum concentration of 25-OH-vitamin D, the range of values of 25-OH-vitamin D which delineate pediatric and adult vitamin D sufficiency are being actively debated (Hollis & Wagner, 2005; Katz *et al.*, 2005). Humans evolved in hot tropical climates without clothing and sunlight exposure of virtually 100% of their skin surface would have been normal (Vieth, 2006). As the result of significant regular exposure to UVB radiation, it is believed that our species habituated to relatively elevated vitamin D levels (Hollis, 2005; Vieth 2006). It is only in the last few thousand years that we have started to shield ourselves from the sun, a timeframe too short to change the fundamental nature of our biology (Vieth, 2006). Unfortunately, traditional normative adult vitamin D levels were derived from population studies or from healthy subjects who, for the most part, experienced low amounts of sunshine exposure, causing them to be vitamin D deficient. Therefore, it is now believed that traditional normative adult vitamin D levels are invalid (Hollis, 2005; Lips, 2005). Currently, several experts in the field believe that an upward revision of normative vitamin D levels is a key step in optimizing the numerous physiologic processes impacted by the active vitamin D metabolite, 1,25-vitamin D (Hollis, 2005; Vieth, 2006; Holick, 2002; Heaney, 2005; Grant, 2005). In order to generate biologically valid reference data with which to define normal vitamin D status, Hollis has proposed that vitamin D measurements ought to be derived from healthy subjects who spend a lot of time outdoors (e.g., field and construction workers) (Hollis, 2005). Compared to subjects with limited regular sunlight exposure, those in sun-rich environments in which clothing or cultural practices do not preclude sun exposure have significantly higher serum 25-OH-vitamin D levels (54-90 ng/mL) (Hollis, 2005). More recently, investigators have been trying to define normal vitamin D status by employing biological markers and clinical outcomes associated with serum 25-OH-vitamin D concentrations (Hollis, 2005; Lips, 2005).

Until relatively recently in adults, most vitamin D experts relied upon population studies to define vitamin D sufficiency as a serum 25-OH-vitamin D concentration of at least 10 or 20 nanograms/mL (ng/mL) [25 or 50 nanomols/liter (nmol/L)]. In the last ten years as the result of trials which have examined the relationship between 25-OH-vitamin D levels and various biological markers and clinical outcomes, including PTH levels, bone mineral density, occurrence of osteoporotic fractures, and intestinal calcium absorption, many investigators have questioned this definition of normal vitamin D status. According to a recent, informal consensus of investigators, optimal PTH levels (PTH is an indirect measure of intestinal calcium absorptive efficiency) are associated with a serum 25-OH-vitamin D of 30 ng/mL or higher (Heaney, 2005). These concentrations have also been found to be associated with reduction in fracture risk and optimal bone mineral density as well as with superior lower extremity neuromuscular indices, insulin sensitivity in non-diabetic individuals, and periodontal attachment (Hollis, 2005; Heaney, 2005; Whiting, 2005). Moreover, two prospective case-control studies noted that 25-OH-vitamin D concentration below 25 ng/mL was associated with an increase in the risk of colon and rectal cancer (Garland, 1989; Feskanich *et al.*, 2004). Given that optimal health outcomes, other than cancer, are strongly associated with 25-OH-vitamin D levels of at least 30-32 ng/mL, several investigators have recommended that vitamin D status in adults should be maintained above this threshold (Hollis, 2005; Vieth, 2006; Holick, 2002; Heaney, 2005; Grant, 2005; Whiting 2005). While maintaining a serum 25-OH-vitamin D level of 20 ng/mL or even as low as 10 ng/mL may prevent osteoporosis and significant osteomalacia, there is a growing body of evidence suggesting that optimal long-term health is promoted by maintaining 25-OH-vitamin D concentrations above 30-32 ng/mL.

Surprisingly, little has been published concerning vitamin D sufficiency for the lactating woman. Hollis *et al.* are the only investigators who have documented that what many currently consider to be a normal maternal vitamin D status is associated with producing breastmilk possessing a low antirachitic content (**Table 1**). At one month postpartum, prior to commencement of daily supplementation with either vitamin D_2 1,600 IU and vitamin D_3 400 IU or vitamin D_2 3,600 IU and vitamin D_3 400 IU, one group of subjects had a mean serum 25-OH-vitamin D level of 27 ng/mL and mean breastmilk antirachitic activity of only 36 IU/L, while the other group had a mean serum 25-OH-vitamin D level of 33 ng/mL and mean breastmilk antirachitic activity of only 40 IU/L (Hollis & Wagner, 2004). At the conclusion of the three month trial, only the high dose subjects, with a mean serum 25-OH-vitamin D concentration of 45 ng/mL, produced breastmilk with a robust level of antirachitic activity. In a second study, 19 subjects who at baseline had a 'normal' vitamin D status also had relatively low levels of antirachitic activity in their milk (Wagner, 2006). Other than the relationship between maternal vitamin D status and breastmilk vitamin D content, no other biomarkers or clinical outcome measures have been assessed to define vitamin D sufficiency in the lactating female.

The basis and definition of vitamin D sufficiency in infants and children have been aptly characterized by Frank Greer, MD, chairman of the AAP's Committee on Nutrition. He writes, "According to the IOM (Institute of Medicine), the lower limit of the normal range may be as low as 20 nmol/L (8 ng/mL) or as high as 37.5 nmol/L (15 ng/mL). In general, a serum $25(OH)2D_3$ concentration of <27.5 nmol/L (11 ng/mL) is considered deficient for children (Greer, 2004)." In contrast to the use of several biomarkers and clinical outcomes to establish a more valid definition of adult vitamin D sufficiency, prevention of vitamin D deficient rickets has been the only outcome measure utilized to define pediatric vitamin D sufficiency. However, it is now appreciated that "... many cells in the body have vitamin D receptors, and vitamin D likely is functionally important in other ways (Greer, 2004)." Given the multiple functions of vitamin D and that biomarkers and clinical outcomes (other than rickets) associated with serum 25-OH-vitamin D concentrations have not been examined in the pediatric population, the true normal range of 25-OH-vitamin D levels and definition of pediatric vitamin D sufficiency is not known (Greer, 2004).

Currently, there is no consensus regarding the definitions of pediatric and adult vitamin D sufficiency. Humans evolved in hot tropical climates without clothing and experienced significant regular sunshine exposure. In this environment, our species is believed to have habituated to relatively high systemic vitamin D concentrations. Traditional normative pediatric and adult ranges (≥11 ng/mL or 27.5 nmol/L) have been derived from cohorts of 'healthy' sun-deprived subjects who, in retrospect, are now thought to have had a high proportion of vitamin D deficiency. In lactating women, 'normal' vitamin D levels are associated with producing breastmilk with low levels of antirachitic activity (Hollis & Wagner, 2004; Wagner, 2006). Pediatric vitamin D sufficiency was also based upon the level of 25-OH-vitamin D associated with prevention of vitamin D

Table 2. Vitamin D Intake Guidelines of the Scientific Committee on Food 1993 (European Commission)

Age Group	PRI (IU)
6-11 months	400-1000
1-3 yr	400
4-6 yr	0-400
7-10 yr	0-400
11-14 yr	0-600
15-17 yr	0-600
18-64 yr	0-400
Lactation	400
Pregnancy	400

Abbreviations: PRI = population reference intake
IU = international units.
Source: Scientific Committee for Food, 1993

deficient rickets (Greer, 2004). It is now appreciated that vitamin D has numerous biological functions and, in addition to rickets and osteoporosis, its deficiency is associated with several other clinical conditions. In the last ten years, research in adults examining the relationship between vitamin D levels, biomarkers (PTH levels), and clinical outcomes (bone mineral density, fracture risk, insulin sensitivity, and cancer risk) has brought about a re-examination of the conventional definition of vitamin D sufficiency. Recently, several investigators have recommended that the lower limit of adult vitamin D sufficiency be readjusted to a threshold of 30-32 ng/mL (75-80 nmnol/L). Similar work in children regarding biomarkers and clinical outcomes associated with vitamin D levels has yet to be published.

VITAMIN D REQUIREMENTS AND GUIDELINES

For nearly all nutrients, biological requirements are met solely by an adequate dietary intake. By contrast, our need for vitamin D may be satisfied via the diet and/or endogenous cutaneous synthesis. Because it is difficult to estimate the quantity of vitamin D generated upon exposure to UVB rays, experts have long acknowledged the challenges of establishing appropriate intake levels for the general population.

The complexities of establishing vitamin D guidelines are further appreciated when viewed in an evolutionary context. Humans evolved in the presence of limited dietary sources of vitamin D in the sun-rich environment on or near the Equator. In this setting, Vieth has speculated that diet could not have played a significant role in meeting our vitamin D needs. Rather, they were satisfied by regular sunshine exposure (Vieth, 2005). However, over recent millennia, due to geographic factors (living far from the Equator) and living conditions (living and working indoors), the vast majority of individuals have been deprived of a sufficient supply of UVB rays with which to synthesize vitamin D.

Table 3. Vitamin D Intake Guidelines for North America, Europe and the WHO

Country or Organization	Recommended Daily Intake Vitamin D (IU per day)		
	6-12 m	1-3 or 1-4 yr	Adults
World Health Organization, 2002	200	200	200
European Union, 1992 & 2003	400-1000	400	0-400
FNB, North America, 1997	200	200	200
Belgium, 2000	400-600	200-400	100-400
France, 2001	800-1000	400	200
Germany, Austria, Switzerland, 2000	400	200	200
Ireland, 1999	280	400	0-400
Italy, 1996	400-1000	400	0-400
Netherlands, 2003	200-400	200-400	100-200
Nordic Countries, 1996	400	400	200
Spain, 1994-8	400	400	100
United Kingdom, 1991	400	400	-

Sources: Standing Committee on the Scientific Evaluation of Dietary References Intakes, 1997; Scientific Committee for Food, 1993; Scientific Committee on Food, 2003

In the absence of sufficient endogenous production, exogenous sources of the vitamin are needed to compensate for the "biological consequences of modern life (Vieth, 2005)."

Given that vitamin D may be obtained exogenously and synthesized endogenously, nutritional adequacy is not based on intake, but on one's overall vitamin D status as reflected by the serum 25-OH-vitamin D concentration (Vieth, 2006). In setting the current adult and pediatric vitamin D intake guidelines in Europe and North America, both the Scientific Committee on Food (SCF) and the Food and Nutrition Board (FNB), respectively, defined vitamin D deficiency for all groups as a serum 25-OH-vitamin D level of <11 ng/mL (27.5 nmol/L) (Standing Committee, 1997; SCF, 1993). Vitamin D measurements above this value are associated with an absence of vitamin D deficient rickets and adult osteomalacia.

In 1997, North America's FNB established the current Dietary Reference Intakes (DRI) for each nutrient. The DRI includes the following parameters: Estimated Average Requirement (EAR), Recommended Daily Allowance (RDA), Adequate Intake (AI), and the Tolerable Upper Intake Level (UL). However, because the committee believed that insufficient scientific data for vitamin D were available at this time, the Committee only set an AI and UL. The AI for individuals ages 0 to 50 years, including during pregnancy and lactation, was set at 200 IU per day. Underlying this recommended level of intake was the assumption that a substantial portion of the population would be exposed to minimal amounts of sunlight (Standing Committee, 1997). In establishing the AI during lactation, the Committee concluded that although the minimum vitamin D intake necessary to maintain normal serum 25-OH-vitamin D levels during lactation had not been determined, "there is no evidence that lactation increases a mother's AI for vitamin D."

Similar to an RDA, in 1993 the European Commission's SCF unveiled a population reference intake (PRI) for each nutrient, representing the level of intake sufficient for virtually all healthy people (SCF, 1993). In contrast to the single value put forth by the FNB, the SCF introduced, for nearly every age group, a recommended range for vitamin D intake (**Table 2**).

They stated that while "many individuals maintain their circulating 25(OH)D concentrations in the desirable range by endogenous synthesis," others, due to factors such as latitude and climate, will need a certain level of dietary intake to compensate for "... the shortfall of exposure to effective UV radiation (SCF, 1993)."

Table 4. Estimated Daily Dose of Vitamin D_3

Baseline Serum 25-OH-Vitamin D	Daily Oral Dose Vitamin D 3 in IU
ng/ml (nmol/L)	
8-16 (20-40)	2200
16-24 (40-60)	1800
24-32 (60-80)	1160
>32 (>80)	0

IU= international units
Source: Heaney, 2005. Reprinted with permission of Elsevier.

Furthermore, as opposed to the homogeneous intake levels put forth by the FNB (200 IU between the ages of 0-50 years), the SCF suggested a significantly higher PRI for infants ages six to 11 months (400-1000 IU) and that all children aged one to three years receive 400 IU per day. Interestingly, despite vitamin D deficiency and vitamin D deficient rickets being well-documented in infants <6 months of life, no PRI was delineated for this age group. Another important difference between the European and North American guidelines is their approach to vitamin D supplementation during pregnancy and lactation. In setting a specific PRI of 400 IU, as opposed to a range of intake for all other adults under 65 years of life, the SCF affirmed that "numerous studies" have revealed that during pregnancy and lactation "customary exposure to sunlight in Europe may be insufficient to cover the needs for vitamin D (SCF, 1993)."

Current vitamin D intake guidelines of other countries as well as those of the World Health Organization (WHO) are listed in (**Table 3**).

In 2003 and 2005, the AAP's Section on Breastfeeding and Committee on Nutrition concurred with the FNB's guidelines that all children, from the newborn period through adolescence, receive a daily vitamin D intake of 200 IU (Gartner *et al.*, 2003; Gartner & Freer, 2005). The basis of this affirmation consisted of data showing that this amount of vitamin D will *"prevent physical signs of vitamin D deficiency and maintain serum 25-hydroxy-vitamin D at or above 27.5 nmol/L (11 ng/mL)."* Additionally, for the first time, the AAP recommended that, beginning in the first two months of life, all breastfed infants be given supplemental vitamin D.

Recently, many vitamin D experts have questioned the validity and adequacy of the current intake guidelines for adults and children (Zittermann, 2003; Hollis & Wagner, 2004; Hollis, 2005; Greer, 2004; SCF, 1993; Dawson-Hughes *et al.*, 2005; Whiting, 2005; Bischoff-Ferrari, 2006; Vieth, 2004). For example, Heaney stated that the FNB's current recommended dietary input levels for adults *"fall into a curious zone between irrelevance and inadequacy (Heaney, 2003)."* These reservations derive from data published over the past decade which strongly support a significant upward revision of the definition of adult vitamin D sufficiency, the foundation of all existing vitamin D intake recommendations. A number of adult clinical trials examining the relationship between serum 25-OH-vit-D levels and several biomarkers (e.g., PTH, bone mineral density, and intestinal calcium absorption) as well as clinical outcomes (e.g., occurrence of osteoporotic fractures and risks of colon and rectal cancer) have found optimal results to be associated with a vitamin D concentration of at least 25 ng/mL (62 nmol/L), while others support a minimal level of 30-32 ng/mL (75-80 nmol/L) (Hollis, 2005; Heaney, 2005; Whiting, 2005; Feskanich *et al.*, 2004). Whiting *et al.* and others have theorized that the improved outcomes associated with higher serum vitamin D levels is due to an enhanced availability of 25-OH-vitamin D for localized, extrarenal synthesis of 1,25-vitamin D, the active metabolite (Whiting, 2005). The enhanced supply of 1,25-vitamin D facilitates optimal execution of vitamin D's important non-classical autocrine functions in numerous organs, tissues, and cell types. Because these studies have not been performed in the pediatric population, Greer has stated that the true normal range of 25-OH-vitamin D levels and the definition of pediatric vitamin D deficiency have not been defined (Greer, 2004). (Note: For a more detailed discussion of the upward revision of vitamin D sufficiency, refer to the section, "Defining Vitamin D Sufficiency.")

If sunshine exposure levels were to remain constant, the only way to raise one's 25-OH-vitamin D concentration to meet the higher definition of vitamin D sufficiency (at least 32 ng/mL or 80 nmol/L) would be to significantly increase one's daily vitamin D consumption. In a formal oral pharmacokinetic trial involving healthy young- and middle-aged adult subjects in Omaha, Nebraska, the dose of vitamin D_3 required to reach and maintain a given 25-OH-vitamin D level was inversely proportional to the initial or starting 25-OH-vitamin D measurement (Barget-Lux, 1998). Investigators also noted, for a given dose of vitamin D_3, a significant inverse relationship between one's body mass index and the rise in 25-OH-vitamin D. Except for vitamin D replete subjects, the necessary estimated daily oral doses (**Table 4**) far exceed all current intake guidelines (Heaney, 2005).

Another approach used to determine vitamin D requirements is to estimate the level of intake that will prevent a reduction in serum 25-OH-vitamin D levels during winter. In a later pharmacokinetic trial involving 67 healthy men, whose baseline mean 25-OH-vitamin D levels ranged between 65 and 72 nmol/L (26 and 29 ng/mL), Heaney calculated that, in addition to utilizing 3300 IU per day from tissue stores, a daily oral input of 500 IU of vitamin D_3 was required to maintain a stable vitamin D level (Heaney, 2003). Similarly, in a randomized, open-label study involving subjects with mean baseline 25-OH-vitamin D concentrations of 30 ng/ml (75 nmol/L), Meier *et al.* noted that daily supplementation with 500 IU of vitamin D_3 and 500 mg of elemental calcium during the winter months was associated with a stable vitamin D status (Meier, 2004). Thus, these data suggest that in the absence of cutaneous vitamin D synthesis, non-lactating vitamin D replete adults should be receiving at least 500 IU of vitamin D_3 per day.

In delineating a healthy level of vitamin D consumption for the breastfeeding dyad, the conventional approach is to view the vitamin D status of the mother and her infant as separate. In a randomized double-blind pilot study of vitamin D supplementation during lactation, Wagner *et al.* found that during the first four months, the vitamin D levels of those mothers receiving 400 IU of vitamin D_3 per day decreased slightly. Only with increased sun exposure over the final two months of the trial did their vitamin D status improve (Wagner, 2006). Although these subjects' breastmilk mean antirachitic content remained relatively low throughout the study (60-76 IU per liter), provision of their nursing infants with 300 IU of vitamin D_3 per day was associated, compared to baseline, with a significant improvement in 25-OH-vitamin D levels (baseline: 13 ng/mL, 6-months: 43 ng/mL). These and other data indicate that while the current vitamin D intake guidelines during lactation require significant revision, those for breastfeeding infants are appropriate.

However, development of more authoritative evidence-based guidelines for this population will also require large clinical trials which examine the association between serum 25-OH-vitamin D and various biological markers and clinical outcomes.

Because vitamin D requirements may be met by endogenous production and exogenous intake, it has been difficult to establish appropriate vitamin D intake guidelines. Additionally, rather than being defined by the level of dietary intake, nutritional adequacy for vitamin D is judged by one's serum 25-OH-vitamin D concentration. In setting the current adult and pediatric dietary guidelines in North America and Europe, the FNB, AAP, and SCF defined vitamin D deficiency for all age groups as a serum 25-OH-vitamin D level <11 ng/mL (27.5 nmol/L). Vitamin D measurements above this value are associated with an absence of vitamin D deficient rickets and adult osteomalacia. In North America, the FNB set an AI of 200 IU of vitamin D for all individuals ages zero to 50 years. However, in Europe, the SCF established, for nearly every age group, a recommended range of vitamin D intake with the highest range for infants ages six to 11 months (400-1000 IU per day). Furthermore, only during pregnancy and lactation did the SCF endorse a specific level of intake (400 IU) because "customary exposure to sunlight in Europe may be insufficient to cover the needs for vitamin D (SCF, 1993). However, recent adult studies examining the relationship between 25-OH-vitamin D levels and various biomarkers and clinical outcomes support a significant upward revision of the definition of vitamin D deficiency to a threshold of at least 30-32 ng/mL (75-80 nmol/L). Given a similar amount of sunshine exposure, in order to raise one's vitamin D status to the new lower limit of normal requires a substantial increase in vitamin D consumption. Except in vitamin D replete subjects, adult pharmacokinetic studies suggest that the necessary daily level of intake far exceeds all current guidelines. In a randomized double blind study of vitamin D supplementation during lactation published in 2006, Wagner *et al.* found a daily maternal vitamin D_3 intake of 400 IU (equal to the SCF's PRI and to twice the FNB's AI) to be inadequate. On the other hand, during the six-month trial, an intake of 300 IU by their breastfeeding infants was associated with a robust increase in mean 25-OH-vitamin D concentrations (Wagner, 2006). Formulation of more authoritative evidence-based vitamin D supplementation guidelines for all individuals will require investigations which bear in mind and evaluate the classical and non-classical functions of vitamin D.

EFFECTS AND IMPLICATIONS OF VITAMIN D DEFICIENCY

Throughout the world, Vitamin D deficiency is not uncommon in children and adults (Holick, 2005). Until recently, the consequences of hypovitaminosis D were thought to be restricted to impairment of bone health (e.g., vitamin D deficient rickets and osteoporosis) and calcium and phosphorus homeostasis (Peterlik *et al.*, 2005). It is now appreciated that, via the active metabolite, 1,25-vitamin D_3 (also known as calcitriol), vitamin D affects the functioning of a diverse range of cells, tissues, and organs (Dusso *et al.*, 2005). There is a vast body of data derived from in vitro, in vivo, and animal model research as well as from interventional and observational studies which suggests that vitamin D deficiency is detrimental to a wide range of physiological processes and contributes to the pathogenesis of several classes of chronic diseases (Holick, 2005; Heaney, 2003; Peterlik *et al.*, 2005; Zittermann, 2003).

The classic short term consequence of vitamin D deficiency is vitamin D deficiency rickets (vitamin D rickets). Rickets is a clinical syndrome characterized by a failure or delay in mineralization of the growth plate and preformed osteoid of growing bones (Pettifor, 2005). Clinically apparent vitamin D rickets is believed to develop after vitamin D deficiency has existed for many months (Greer, 2003). The clinical manifestations of rickets are numerous and varied and depend on the age at presentation and duration and severity of vitamin D deficiency. In the first year of life, the most common manifestations are hypocalcemic seizures, craniotabes, delayed closure of the fontanelles, palpable and visible enlargement of the long bones (e.g., wrists and ankles), as well as the costochondral junctions of the thorax (rachitic rosary). In the second year of life when weight bearing has begun, children with vitamin D rickets may present with poor growth, motor delay, genu varum (bow legs), or genu valgum (knock knees). Additionally, there may be delayed eruption of teeth and enamel hypoplasia. Older children may complain of bone pain and fatigue (Shaw, 2003).

In the absence of formal reporting mechanisms, the true prevalence and incidence of vitamin D rickets is unknown. Judging from published case reports and larger case series, most cases of the disorder are diagnosed between the ages of six and 30 months (Bachrach, 1979; Kreiter, 2000; Mylott; 2004; Robinson, 2005; Weisberg, 2004). Vitamin D rickets is relatively uncommon in the first four to six months of life because many newborns will have transplacentally acquired adequate vitamin D stores from a vitamin D sufficient mother. Given the three week half life of 25-OH-vitamin D, the insidious nature of vitamin D deficiency and relatively prolonged interval between onset of deficiency and manifestations of vitamin D rickets, the vitamin D sufficient newborn who, during infancy, is deprived of adequate vitamin D will not be diagnosed with rickets until after several months of life (Pettifor, 2005). However, if a pregnant woman is significantly vitamin D deficient, her neonate will also be vitamin D deficient. The most severely affected fetuses will present in the immediate newborn period with craniotabes, fractures, swollen ribs, and/or hypocalcemic seizures (Pettifor, 2005). Presumably, those born with more mild degrees of vitamin D deficiency, in the presence of continued postnatal vitamin D deprivation, may develop vitamin D rickets later in infancy.

Arnaud and Kruse have proposed a three stage pathophysiological progression for vitamin D rickets (Arnaud, 1991; Kruse, 1995). It is believed that, initially, hypovitaminosis D affects a reduction of 1,25-vitamin D levels, resulting in intestinal calcium malabsorption and hypocalcemia. This initial hypocalcemia has been labeled stage I rickets. In response to hypocalcemia, a compensatory or secondary hyperparathyroidism occurs. The elevated level of PTH enhances 1α-hydroxylase activity, raising 1,25-vitamin D levels. Together, PTH and 1,25-vitamin D increase bone resorption and intestinal calcium absorption thereby correcting the hypocalcemia. The resulting secondary hyperparathyroidism, normal or elevated 1,25-vitamin D levels, hypophosphatemia, normocalcemia, and bone resorption characterize stage II rickets. The mineralization defect noted at this phase is felt to be caused by the hypophosphatemia. Despite persistent hyperparathyroidism, progression of the vitamin D deficiency results in a drop in 1,25-vitamin D levels. This impairs intestinal calcium absorption and calcium mobilization from bone, producing hypocalcemia. In stage III, the combination of hypocalcemia and hypophosphatemia increases the severity of the bone disease.

In addition to rickets, other short term complications of vitamin D deficiency have been reported. English and Norwegian investigators have described several infants with severe cardiomyopathy and hypovitaminosis D without rickets (Brunvand, 1995; Maiya, 2006). Additionally, Namgung *et al.* and Weiler *et al.* both found that compared to vitamin D sufficient newborns, those who were vitamin D deficient had a significantly lower neonatal bone mineral content (Namgung *et al.*, 1995; Weiler *et al.*, 2005).

Although the immediate complications of overt vitamin D deficiency have long been widely recognized, there is a growing body of evidence suggesting that mild-to-moderate degrees of deficiency contribute to the pathogenesis of long-latency disorders, such as malignancies, autoimmune disorders, and cardiovascular disease (Zittermann, 2003; Peterlik *et al.*, 2005). In nutritional science, there has been a tendency to link, via a single mechanism, a nutrient deficiency to a single disease (e.g., thiamine to beriberi and iodine to goiter) (Heaney, 2003). Additionally, given the relative ease of detecting a disorder resulting from a dramatic short-term nutrient deficiency, compared to one resulting from

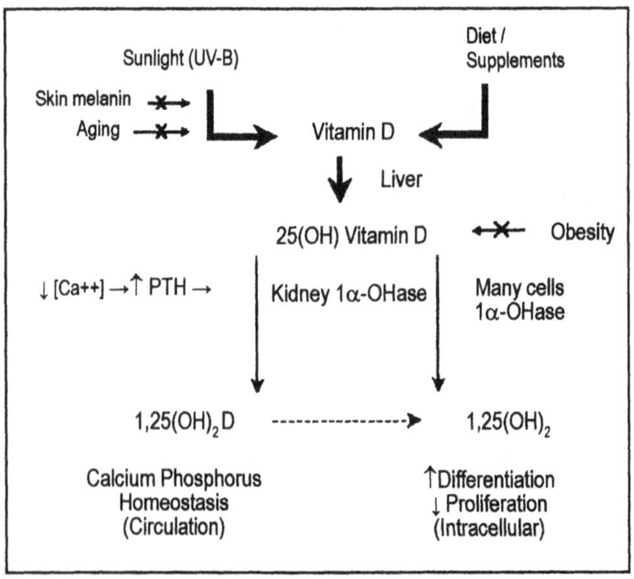

Figure 5. Proposed mechanism for vitamin D and cancer. The main sources of vitamin D are sunlight and diet or supplements. Darker skin, older age, and obesity are associated with lower 25(OH)D. Anti-cancer effects may be largely due to conversion of 25(OH)D to 1,25(OH)$_2$D within cells, although circulating 1,25(OH)$_2$D may contribute. Source: Giovannucci, 2005; reprinted with kind permission of Springer Science and Business Media.

an asymptomatic long-term deficiency, there has been a primary focus on preventing and treating conditions resulting from the former scenario (Heaney, 2003). With respect to vitamin D, scientists and clinicians have, for decades, been primarily concerned with the scenario in which a severe and relatively brief deficiency of this nutrient impairs calcium and phosphorus homeostasis, resulting in osteomalacia or vitamin D rickets. Because mild chronic hypovitaminosis D does not cause a clinical bone disorder and is associated with calcium and 1,25-vitamin D_3 levels in the normal range, it was traditionally thought to have little clinical import (Peterlik *et al.*, 2005). In other words, in the absence of rickets or osteomalacia, it was presumed that a 'significant' vitamin D deficiency did not exist (Heaney, 2005). Both renal and non-renal cells synthesize 1,25-vitamin D_3 from its immediate precursor, 25-OH-vitamin D_3. Whereas mild-to-moderate vitamin D deficiency will not impair the renal production of 1,25-vitamin D_3, investigators theorize it will compromise the extrarenal generation of 1,25-vitamin D_3. This extrarenal 1,25-vitamin D_3 is needed for autocrine and paracrine control of many cell types (Peterlik *et al.*, 2005). The realization that vitamin D possesses a host of nonclassical functions and actions in many organs and tissues, along with data from a number of epidemiological, clinical, and experimental studies has shifted our outlook and concerns beyond the traditional solitary focus on short-term implications of severe vitamin D deficiency.

The pathogenesis of type 1 diabetes mellitus (type 1 DM) consists of a chronic autoimmune destruction of the pancreatic beta cells. The disease results from a combination of genetic and environmental factors. In light of vitamin D's suppression of Th1 cytokine (IL-2 and IFN-γ) production and its effects on regulatory T-cell activity and dendritic cell maturation, it has been hypothesized that one's vitamin D status will influence the risk of developing type 1 DM (Hypponen, 2004). In 2001, Hypponen *et al.* published a birth-cohort study noting an association between vitamin D intake in the first year of life and the risk of type 1 DM (Hypponen *et al.*, 2001). The cohort consisted of all women and their newborns who, in 1966, were living in two municipalities in northern Finland. Both the frequency and dose of supplementary vitamin D in the first year of life were recorded. Over 30 years later, 10,366 or 86% of the subjects were surveyed for the occurrence of type 1 DM. Children suspected of having rickets in the first year of life were three times more likely to have later developed type 1 DM compared to those without such a suspicion. Moreover, compared to children who regularly received less than the current daily recommended dose of 2000 international units (IU) of vitamin D, those who regularly received the recommended amount were one-fifth as likely to be diagnosed with type 1 DM. The protective effect of supplemental vitamin D during infancy noted by Hypponen *et al.* was similar to that shown in an earlier large retrospective multicentered European study (EURODIAB, 1999). Results of human observational studies are supported by in vitro data and findings from a murine model of type 1 DM (Hypponen, 2004). In genetically susceptible individuals, it is theorized that suboptimal vitamin D levels during infancy and possibly fetal life impair immune system self-tolerance and lead to pancreatic beta cell destruction (Mathieu, 2005). Furthermore, vitamin D supplementation may suppress the autoimmune process directed against the beta cells (Hypponen, 2001).

There is also mounting scientific evidence that vitamin D deficiency may contribute to the risk and development of other long-latency autoimmune disorders, such as multiple sclerosis, rheumatoid arthritis, and inflammatory bowel disease (Cantorna & Mahon, 2004; Holick, 2005; Peterlik *et al.*, 2005; Zittermann, 2003). The VDR is present in many cells of the immune system (Cantorna, 2005). Autoimmune diseases are driven by T helper cells (Th1) and are characterized by the targeted self-destruction of tissue by the immune system. By modulating Th1 and dendritic cell function while inducing regulatory T-cell function, the active vitamin D metabolite, 1,25-vitamin D_3, fosters the development of self-tolerance (Cantorna & Mahon, 2004). In experimental models of multiple sclerosis, rheumatoid arthritis, and inflammatory bowel disease, vitamin D deficiency has been shown to accelerate the development of these disorders (Cantorna & Mahon, 2004). In large observational studies, vitamin D intake is inversely associated with rates of multiple sclerosis and rheumatoid arthritis (Cantorna, 2005). Despite the encouraging data accumulated thus far, additional clinical data are needed to confirm the connection between vitamin D and autoimmune disorders.

Cancer is another class of long-latency diseases in which chronic asymptomatic vitamin D deficiency is proposed to play a role. The VDR is present in numerous types of normal and cancer cells (Pike *et al.*,

2005; van Leeuwen *et al.*, 2005). In vitro and in vivo data from multiple cancer models (animal and human) and cell types have shown that 1,25-vitamin D_3 inhibits growth and induces differentiation, cell cycle arrest, and/or apoptosis (Beer & Myrthue, 2004; Giovannucci, 2005; Trump, 2004). Mild degrees of vitamin D deficiency may impair local concentrations of 1,25-vitamin D_3 and thus compromise the ability of 1,25-vitamin D_3 to exert its favorable effects (Giovannucci, 2005). Almost 70 years ago, Peller *et al.* noted that in American men, increased sunlight exposure was associated with a lower morbidity and mortality from cancer of the "inner organs" (Peller & Stephenson, 1937). Although the relationship between sunlight exposure and vitamin D production was known at this time, no connection was proposed between vitamin D status and cancer rates to explain these observations. Similarly, several decades later other researchers found an inverse relationship between mean daily solar radiation values for the contiguous United States and geographic mortality from colon cancer (Garland & Garland, 1980). Since sunlight exposure affects cutaneous vitamin D synthesis and given the direct relationships between latitude and sunlight exposure as well as between latitude and vitamin D status, the authors hypothesized that "the strong inverse association of sunlight and colon cancer raises the possibility that vitamin D, which prevents rickets, may also act in the prevention of colon cancer (Garland & Garland, 1980)." Since the publication of the "Garland hypothesis," a number of other American and European investigators have observed a significant inverse correlation between sunlight exposure or latitude and other nondermatologic malignancies including breast, prostate, and ovarian cancers and non-Hodgkin's lymphoma (Giovannucci, 2005; Grant, 2003; John *et al.*, 1999). One of the most dramatic examples of this association is an inverse correlation between UVB radiation and cancer mortality in men and women between 1970 and 1994 for 13 different malignancies (Grant, 2002). In light of the importance of sunlight exposure on vitamin D status, antineoplastic properties of vitamin D and the inverse association between UVB radiation levels and the geographic variation of multiple types of cancer, Giovannucci has speculated that deficient sunlight exposure results in chronic asymptomatic hypovitaminosis D. This leads to a shortage of extrarenally generated 1,25-vitamin D_3, allowing cancer cells to express their carcinogenic potential (Giovannucci, 2005).

Classically, it has been taught that vitamin D deficiency merely produced derangements in calcium and phosphorus metabolism and bone mineralization. It is now established that vitamin D has a wide range of actions including immune cell function and regulation of cell replication and differentiation. Mild-to-moderate vitamin D deficiency, a worldwide problem, is asymptomatic and associated with adequate renal synthesis of the active vitamin D metabolite, 1,25-vitamin D_3, and normocalcemia. Researchers speculate that this asymptomatic vitamin D deficiency leads to an extrarenal shortage of 1,25-vitamin D_3 needed for autocrine and paracrine functions in many cell types. Based on an impressive combination of in vitro and in vivo data and observations from animal models and human cohorts, it is now believed that vitamin D deficiency plays a role in the development of various long-latency disorders such as malignancies, autoimmune disorders, and cardiovascular disease (**Figure 5**). The possible link between insidious degrees of hypovitaminosis D and chronic diseases has helped prompt a reevaluation of current vitamin D intake guidelines and the definition of vitamin D deficiency (Heaney, 2003).

VITAMIN D DEFICIENT RICKETS AND VITAMIN D DEFICIENCY IN UNSUPPLEMENTED BREASTFED INFANTS AND TODDLERS

For many years, it was widely believed that human milk protected infants from developing rickets and was an adequate source of vitamin D (Hollis & Roos, 1981; Hollis *et al.*, 2004). Before the discovery of vitamin D, both McCollum and Park attributed rickets to a lack of sunlight and a dietary factor X. They asserted that factor X was found in "good breastmilk" and cod liver oil. Moreover, it was observed that although rickets occurred in breastfed children, it was rarely as severe as that seen in artificially fed infants (McCollum *et al.*, 1922; Park, 1923). Researchers at the Massachusetts Institute of Technology proclaimed, "For the prevention and cure of rickets in infants, human breastmilk is admittedly superior to cow's milk (Harris *et al.*, 1939)." In 1961, in attempting to elucidate the cause of the high incidence of rickets in the "colored" community of Cape Town, South Africa, it was concluded that the most significant etiological factors were breastfeeding for less than three months and insufficient sunlight exposure (Dancaster & Jackson, 1961). One of the few researchers who found a strong association between breastfeeding and rickets in New Haven, Connecticut, remarked, "It is an uncommon thing to find a healthy vigorous breastfed infant who does not show rickets by roentgen-ray examination (Eliot, 1925)."

Over the past 30 years, a wealth of evidence has been amassed which undermines the long-held conviction that exclusive breastfeeding without supplemental infant vitamin D will sustain a normal vitamin D status for the infant. The refutation of this belief is based upon the numerous retrospective reports of breastfed infants and toddlers diagnosed with vitamin D deficient rickets. In a recent review of the disorder, Chesney grouped these instances of the disorder into two major "epidemics." The first wave of cases occurred in the 1960's through 1980's while the second current wave began in the mid-1990's (Chesney, 2003). In addition to the sheer number of cases, it is the tremendous variation in the subjects' demographic profiles which also suggests that nursing children require supplemental vitamin D. During this era, rickets has emerged in nearly every continent, latitude, climate, social and economic stratum, race, and ethnicity. Not only has nutritional rickets resurfaced in both developed and undeveloped countries, it has also appeared in populations receiving daily prenatal and postnatal vitamin D-containing supplements and who consume vitamin D-fortified foods. One of the most compelling retrospective reports of rickets in breastfed children consists of a group of 24 otherwise healthy, urban African-American subjects who were identified with the disorder at the Children's Hospital of Philadelphia between January, 1974, and June, 1978. At presentation, patients' ages ranged between four and 58 months. In every instance, the diagnosis was established both biochemically and radiographically. All 24 infants lived in Philadelphia (latitude 39° north), were breastfed, and, at the time of diagnosis, half of them were still nursing. Only two of the subjects received multivitamin supplements for more than three months, while none of the mothers recalled taking supplements during pregnancy and lactation. An atypical factor, which was thought to contribute to the development of vitamin D deficiency and rickets in 11 of these individuals, was that all meat, fish, and dairy products were excluded from their diet. Although maternal vitamin D status was not formally assessed, limited biochemical testing on seven of the 20 mothers noted elevations of parathyroid hormone and alkaline phosphatase lending the investigators to believe that maternal vitamin D deficiency was present and contributed to the development of the disorder. They speculated this outbreak of vitamin D deficient rickets was the result of a multitude of factors including: maternal vitamin D deficiency, breastfeeding with little or no vitamin D supplementation, dietary restrictions, dark skin color, and urban environment (e.g., air pollution and decreased sunlight exposure) (Bachrach, 1979).

Weisberg *et al.* recently summarized the persistence of rickets among infants and children in the United States. Via the MEDLINE database, between 1986 and 2003, 24 published retrospective reports involving 166 individuals were identified. The authors of nearly all case reports indicated that rickets was the result of severe vitamin D deficiency. All patients were four to 54 months old. However, in 17 of the papers, the maximal age was <30 months. The cases were diagnosed in 17 states from all regions of the country. Similar to the Bachrach *et al.* cohort, only six percent of the subjects were Caucasian and 96% were breastfed. Among those breastfed, only five percent received a vitamin D supplement while nursing. The age range, ethnic make-up, and dietary history of the 166 subjects with vitamin D deficiency reported between 1986 and 2003 was strikingly similar to those of an earlier review of the literature on "nutritional" rickets (Weisberg, 2004). Cosgrove *et al.* found that of the 63 American cases of rickets between 1975 and 1985, 91% were African-American, all had or were still nursing at the time of diagnosis, and were between the ages of two and 45 months (Cosgrove & Dietrich, 1985). Therefore, it appears that over the past 30 years, despite the profound advancements in our understanding of vitamin D physiology and photobiology, as well as our knowledge of the factors affecting vitamin D sufficiency, the epidemiology of vitamin D deficient rickets in the United States has not changed.

One of the largest and perhaps most widely known cohorts included in Weisberg's review of nutritional rickets in the United States is the report of Krieter *et al.* They reviewed 30 cases of rickets referred to two regional medical centers in North Carolina (population in 2000 of approximately 8,000,000, latitude 33-37°north) during a nine-year period. Interestingly, over half of the cases (17) presented in the final 18 months of the study. The age at diagnosis ranged from five to 25 months of life. All subjects had laboratory evidence of long-standing vitamin D deficiency and classic radiologic findings of rickets, were of African-American background, and breastfed without vitamin D supplementation (average duration 12.5 months). It was speculated that this 'outbreak' of cases in the last 18 months may have been caused by the recent increase in breastfeeding rates among the state's African-American population. Other factors posited to have contributed to the situation were the low antirachitic activity of human milk, lack of infant vitamin D supplementation, decreased exposure to sunlight, and the increased sunlight exposure required by dark-skinned individuals to produce a given amount of vitamin D (Kreiter, 2000). In an accompanying editorial, Welch *et al.* emphasized that cholecalciferol is not a vitamin, but rather a steroid hormone whose production is dependent upon exposure levels to UVB radiation. However, the "realities of modern living" (e.g., working and dwelling indoors and the use of sunscreen) deprive humankind of a significant portion of its exposure to these photons, resulting in breastmilk with low levels of vitamin D. The provision of supplemental vitamin D should be viewed as a way of compensating for these effects. Given the efficacy, safety, and minimal cost of daily vitamin D supplementation, as well as the reemergence of this disorder, they advocated supplemental vitamin D for all nursing infants (Welch *et al.*, 2000).

At a latitude of 33° south, Sydney, Australia, is blessed with abundant sunshine. Not only are daytime levels of UVB radiation sufficient to affect cutaneous vitamin D synthesis throughout the year, but also being in the southern hemisphere, the ambient levels of UV radiation are 12-15% higher than for similar locations in the northern hemisphere (Gies *et al.*, 2004). Puzzled by a recent anecdotal resurgence of vitamin D deficient rickets in Sydney, Australia, Robinson *et al.* conducted a retrospective descriptive study of cases diagnosed at three of the city's major teaching hospitals. In these three facilities alone, from 1993 through 2003, 126 children ages 15 years and under were found to have the disorder. Furthermore, 66% of all subjects were less than two years of age. Unfortunately, the rate of breastfeeding in this subgroup was not specified. Only four percent of the individuals were Caucasian, with the remainder having emigrated from the Middle East, Africa, the Indian subcontinent, and several regions of Asia (Note: 79% of the cohort was born in Australia). Given that sunny Sydney is a "modern city with good nutritional and health standards," researchers were surprised to have uncovered the largest case series of vitamin D deficient rickets reported from a developed country. It was theorized that limited dietary sources of vitamin D, inadequate or absent vitamin D supplementation, sun avoidance, sunscreen use, and darkly pigmented skin all contributed to the problem. It was recommended that supplementation, education, and screening of at risk immigrant groups be initiated (Robinson *et al.*, 2006).

Further undermining the assertion that vitamin D supplementation is unnecessary during lactation has been the publication of several prospective studies which have uncovered a significant incidence among breastfed infants and toddlers of asymptomatic vitamin D deficiency. Vitamin D deficient rickets arises after a severe and long-standing vitamin D deficiency. In light of a 1986 retrospective report of 48 infants and toddlers diagnosed with vitamin D deficient rickets in Manitoba, Canada (latitude 50° north), during the summer of 1987, a random, prospective, cross-sectional survey to assess the vitamin D status of 67 of the region's mothers and babies, aged three to 24 months, was initiated. Via a questionnaire, it was discovered that 91% of the children had been breastfed. After weaning, only 64% of subjects were fed either formula or cow's milk. Although 60% had been given vitamin supplements, the majority of children who took supplements, received them irregularly. Vitamin D deficiency, defined as a serum 25-OH-vitamin D <10 ng/mL, was detected in 43% of the children and 76% of the mothers. Investigators speculated that the high prevalence of vitamin D deficiency in the region was caused by climate and lifestyle, resulting in minimal cutaneous vitamin D synthesis, compounded by the low vitamin D content of human milk. In order to prevent rickets, they suggested that consumption of vitamin D-fortified dairy products and infant and maternal vitamin D supplementation be promoted (Lebrun *et al.*, 1993).

Much closer to the equator, in Karachi, Pakistan (latitude 24° north), investigators theorized that the continued reporting of vitamin D deficient rickets among the country's infants and children merely represented the proverbial "tip of the iceberg." They speculated that underlying the small number of cases of rickets was a large number of individuals with undiagnosed vitamin D deficiency. To test their assertion, they prospectively measured, over a two-year period, serum 25-OH-vitamin D levels in 62 healthy breastfed infants (ages six weeks to 11 months) and their mothers. In order to enroll individuals from both the lower and upper classes, subjects were recruited from a government-sponsored facility and a private "Well-Baby Clinic" in Karachi. Neither infants nor mothers received any vitamin D supplements. The mean serum 25-OH-vitamin D concentrations of the mothers and infants were 12.8±9 and 13.9±10.6 respectively. There was a significant correlation between the 25-OH-vitamin D measurements of infants less than three months old and those of their mothers. Hypovitaminosis D (defined as a serum 25-OH-vitamin D <10 ng/mL) was noted in 45% of mothers and 55% of infants. Significantly lower infant vitamin D levels were associated with the following variables: age less than six months, winter season, higher level of maternal education, upper social class, and decreased sunlight exposure (Atiq *et al.*, 1998). The association between class and infant vitamin D levels was reminiscent of findings from an earlier retrospective study of 65 breastfed infants in Karachi diagnosed with vitamin D deficient rickets. In this earlier paper, a majority of the D-deficient subjects belonged to the middle and upper classes (Ahmed *et al.*, 1995).

At a similar latitude, Bahijri assessed the vitamin D status of infants and children in sunny Jeddah, Saudi Arabia (latitude 21° north). He randomly surveyed 739 subjects between the ages of four and 72 months. Except for one child, all 25-OH-vitamin D_3 values ranged between 1 and 31 ng/mL. The only child with a level >31 ng/mL was a 4.5 month old infant delivered to a mother who "was over dosing herself with vitamins and minerals all through pregnancy." In the four to six and six to 12 month subgroups, 17% and 15.5% of infants, respectively, were classified as vitamin D deficient (definition: <10 ng/mL). By maternal report, none of the four to six month old subjects were exposed to sunlight and only 21% had a dietary intake of >77% of the World Health Organization's (WHO) Recommended Daily Allowance (RDA) for vitamin D. Among the six to 12 month old infants, the mean sunlight exposure was a mere 16 minutes per week and only 28% consumed >77% of the WHO RDA for vitamin D. Given the well-established social custom of women staying inside the home and the low vitamin D content of breastmilk, the author suggested that fortification of infant foods and infant vitamin D supplementation would enhance the vitamin D status of infants in Saudi Arabia (Bahijri, 2001).

The assumption that living at low-to-moderate latitudes in a sunny climate will ensure vitamin D sufficiency in an unsupplemented breastfeeding infant has been further weakened by a recent prospective investigation into the vitamin D status of 90 Arab and South Asian exclusively nursing infants in Al Ain, United Arab Emirates (UAE) (latitude 24° north). During the summer, subjects were recruited consecutively from local maternal child health clinics. Their ages ranged between four and 16 weeks. Neither the infants nor their mothers were receiving vitamin D supplements. Most women did not consume fortified milk, while 40%, according to dietary recall, had an average daily vitamin D intake of only 88 IU. The dress code of most women in the community consisted of covering the entire body, leaving only the hands and feet exposed. Among the 78 mother-infant pairs for whom measurements were both available, hypovitaminosis D (25-OH-vitamin D <10 ng/mL) was detected in 61% of the mothers and 82% of babies. Infants with hypovitaminosis D had significantly higher median serum alkaline phosphatase, suggestive of early metabolic bone disease. The authors concluded that in this population of exclusively nursing infants and their mothers, vitamin D deficiency is *"almost the rule rather than the exception."* Moreover, in order to prevent nutritional rickets, they recommended that beginning in the first month of life, all breastfeeding infants receive vitamin D supplementation (Dawodu *et al.*, 2003).

The vitamin D status of the exclusively breastfed unsupplemented infant has also been documented via prospective longitudinal investigations. One of the earliest examples is a study from Otago, New Zealand (latitude 45° south), of 25-OH-vitamin D_3 levels over the first six months postpartum in full-term breastfeeding dyads. At birth, three weeks, and three and six months, maternal and infant sera were collected. Only 14 subjects were initially enrolled and three subjects completed the study. During this time, infants were not given any other foods and neither mothers nor infants received any vitamin D supplements. Season of birth was not specified and neither sunshine exposure nor maternal dietary vitamin D was assessed. At delivery, this small cohort had robust mean 25-OH-vitamin D_3 concentrations (maternal = 32.5°±13.2 ng/mL, neonatal = 27.8°±11.1 ng/mL). Although there was a significant drop in maternal and infant levels between birth and three weeks, through the entire six months, they remained comfortably above the classic deficiency threshold of 11 ng/mL. Based on finding vitamin D sufficiency through the first six months of life in three subjects, the authors contended that "in optimum circumstances human milk alone can provide sufficient dietary vitamin D for the needs of the term infant for up to the first six months of life." Furthermore, they stated that there is no justification for the routine administration of vitamin D supplements (Birkbeck & Scott, 1980).

In Rotterdam, The Netherlands (latitude 51° north), Hoogenboezem *et al.* prospectively followed the vitamin D status of 39 unsupplemented exclusively breastfed Caucasian infants through the first five months of life who were born at the end of summer. Being delivered at this time of year afforded the mother the opportunity for several months prior to delivery to benefit from exposure to solar radiation capable of initiating endogenous vitamin D synthesis. Presumably, this would ensure robust maternal and fetal vitamin D levels. As expected, at delivery the mean maternal and neonatal serum 25-OH-vitamin D concentrations were 32 and 25 ng/mL, respectively. However, by eight weeks of life, the mean 25-OH-vitamin D level fell to 10 ng/mL. For the remainder of the study period, no further significant change in vitamin D status was noted. The rapid decline of the cohort's vitamin D levels while receiving only breastmilk with presumably low amounts of vitamin D was thought to signify the depletion of prenatally acquired vitamin D stores. Since these summer-born exclusively nursing infants became deficient so quickly, the authors advised that, regardless of season of birth, vitamin D supplementation should be initiated in the first or second week of life (Hoogenboezem, 1989).

In Greece, with the exception of infant formulas, no foods are vitamin D fortified. Yet, it is a country with abundant sunshine. Its relatively moderate latitude (34 to 41° north) affords inhabitants the opportunity of nearly year-round exposure to levels of ultraviolet B radiation sufficient to effect cutaneous vitamin D production. Therefore, it would not be unreasonable to posit that few, if any, individuals would be vitamin D deficient. However, in a recent investigation of the vitamin D status in 178 healthy Greek children aged three to 18 years, Lapatsanis *et al.* observed during the winter months that 47% and 14% of subjects aged 15 to 18 and 13 to 14 years, respectively, were vitamin D deficient (25-OH-vitamin D concentration < 10 ng/mL). By contrast, children and adolescents tested in the summer months were all vitamin D sufficient (Lapatsanis *et al.*, 2005). In the same town (Ioannina, latitude 37° north), a prospective observational study of the vitamin D status of 66 full-term exclusively breastfeeding dyads through the first six months postpartum was also conducted. Approximately one half of the subjects delivered in the winter, while the remainder delivered in the summer. During the study, as well as prenatally, none of the subjects received vitamin D supplements. Utilizing the same definition of vitamin D deficiency, Challa *et al.* found 91% of the winter-born and 56% of the summer born neonates to be deficient, while in both seasons approximately 35% of mothers were deficient. By six months of life, the mean 25-OH-vitamin D level of both groups rose significantly from 6.7±0.7 to 19.4±2.8 and 10.1±0.9 to 13.3±1.6ng/mL, respectively. Despite these increases, at six months of life, 30% of summer and 21% of winter infants were still vitamin D deficient. They concluded that for the first six months of life, exclusive breastfeeding *"does not seem to provide an adequate vitamin D supply."* The considerable percentage of vitamin D deficiency observed despite the ample sunshine was theorized to be the result of several factors: the absence of vitamin D-fortified foods, widespread use of sunscreens, and deficient sunlight exposure. They recommended that, irrespective of season, in countries where foods are not vitamin D-fortified either the mother should be supplemented during pregnancy and lactation and/or the infant should be supplemented during the period of exclusive breastfeeding (Challa *et al.*, 2005).

Both retrospective and prospective investigations from throughout the world have documented that breastfeeding without supplemental vitamin D is associated with vitamin D deficient rickets and vitamin D deficiency. Their reports have been accompanied by recommendations to institute one or more of the following measures: infant vitamin D supplementation, maternal vitamin D supplementation, or vitamin D-fortification of foods. As explained by Greer and others: "Rickets itself is the end stage of vitamin D deficiency. Deficiency must be present for many months before clinical rickets becomes obvious (Greer, 2003)." Since rickets is the result of a long-term deficit, the reports of rickets and the prospective detection of high rates of hypovitaminosis D in small cohorts of breastfed children suggest that it is common throughout the world. The merit of this stance is also based upon the recognition of the limited endogenous and exogenous sources of vitamin D for infants, children, and adults. Endogenous vitamin D synthesis is limited by the many factors which interfere with sunlight exposure, i.e., environment, lifestyle, cultural and religious practices, as well as by national and international public health campaigns to prevent skin cancer. Because melanin blocks the penetration of UVB rays into the skin and decreases or even completely inhibits cutaneous vitamin D synthesis, those individuals with darker skin color are faced with an additional impediment. The exogenous supply of vitamin D is limited by the low vitamin D content of human milk and the scarcity of vitamin D-containing foods. Even though cow's milk, breakfast cereals, orange juice, and margarine are vitamin D-fortified in the United States, the high prevalence of vitamin D deficiency in the country's adolescents and adults suggests that current fortification strategies are inadequate (Calvo & Whiting, 2003; Looker *et al.*, 2002; Nesby-O'Dell *et al.*, 2002; Tangpricha, 2002). Currently, the two most promising means of ensuring vitamin D sufficiency while breastfeeding are infant and maternal vitamin D supplementation.

VITAMIN D SUPPLEMENTATION OF THE BREASTFEEDING INFANT

It is widely acknowledged that for nearly every infant, breastmilk is the optimal form of nutrition, conferring numerous and varied short and long term health benefits. Lactation is also associated with medical advantages for the mother including: decreased rates of breast and ovarian cancers, increased child spacing, and earlier return to pre-pregnancy weight (Gartner *et al.*, 2005). To maximize the benefit from breastfeeding, many experts and healthcare organizations recommend exclusive breastfeeding for approximately the first six months of life. Furthermore, the AAP advises that lactation "should be continued for at least the first year of life and beyond for as long as mutually desired by mother and child (Gartner *et al.*, 2005)." However, as documented above, breastfeeding without supplemental vitamin D is associated with hypovitaminosis D and the development of vitamin D deficient rickets in infancy and early childhood. It is the result of limited sunlight exposure, low antirachitic activity of human milk, and scarcity of dietary vitamin D (Hollis & Wagner, 2004). In other words, by being protected from the sun by staying indoors and/or being covered by clothing and sunscreen, receiving breastmilk containing only 20-70 IU per liter and, if no longer exclusively nursing, consuming foods with little or no vitamin D, the typical breastfeeding infant and toddler is deprived of both endogenous and exogenous vitamin D. Vitamin D is essential for calcium homeostasis and bone health, and has a role in a multitude of other physiologic processes. Additionally, preliminary studies suggest that vitamin D deficiency may increase the risk of certain cancers and autoimmune disorders. Given the multiple functions of vitamin D, ensuring its adequate supply will prevent the multiple advantages of breastfeeding from being attenuated and eliminate the established and potential risks of vitamin D deficiency.

Hypothetically, the vitamin D status of the nursing child can be supported in a direct or indirect fashion. Indirectly, one may provide sufficient vitamin D by maternal supplementation or increased exposure to UVB radiation. While both methods have been shown to significantly enhance the vitamin D content of breastmilk, only the former approach has been formally evaluated. Small, well-designed clinical trials have shown maternal vitamin D supplementation to be safe and effective (discussed below in the section "Vitamin D Supplementation of the Breastfeeding Mother"). Alternatively, one may enhance a child's vitamin D levels directly via increased exposure to UVB radiation, thereby raising the cutaneous production of vitamin D. In fair-skinned children, this approach has been shown to be effective. However, because of the long-term morbidities associated with sunlight exposure in childhood, this approach is not currently advocated (AAP, 1999). Additionally, the numerous biologic, geographic, environmental, and seasonal factors impacting upon the occurrence and quantity of endogenous vitamin D production make this a challenging and unreliable method of ensuring vitamin D sufficiency. The final and most widely advocated option is to provide the breastfeeding child with a daily oral dose of vitamin D.

One of the earliest investigations which suggested that vitamin D supplementation was advantageous for the nursing infant was a prospective case-control study conducted by Martha Eliot, MD. Beginning in August

1923, 116 infants in New Haven, Connecticut (latitude 41° north), received a daily "antirachitic treatment" of one teaspoon of cod liver oil and regular sunlight exposure. One teaspoon of cod liver oil contains approximately 400 IU of vitamin D_3. A group of 127 untreated infants born during the same months served as controls. Rickets was diagnosed via regular clinical and roentgenographic examinations. Although some degree of rickets was nearly universal in all infants, compared to the control subjects, the study infants had a much lower incidence of "moderate" or "marked" rickets (4.3 vs. 23%). It was also noted that, among infants diagnosed with rickets, daily cod liver oil and regular sunlight exposure was associated with a significantly higher proportion of improvement (Eliot, 1925). Unfortunately, neither sunlight exposure nor bone biochemistries (e.g., serum alkaline phosphatase, calcium, and phosphorous) were measured. Despite these design flaws, this was one of the first human studies to intimate the relative importance of vitamin D supplementation and sunlight on the development of rickets.

It was not until the 1980s that researchers in the United States began to utilize randomized trials to evaluate and compare bone mineralization, vitamin D status, and risk of nutritional rickets in formula-fed and vitamin D supplemented and unsupplemented breastfeeding Caucasian infants. In 1981, a randomized double-blind prospective trial of 18 healthy full-term exclusively breastfed Caucasian infants designed to determine "whether or not supplemental vitamin D affected bone mineralization" was published. From two weeks through 26 weeks of life, subjects from Cincinnati, Ohio (latitude 39° north), were given ergocalciferol (vitamin D_2) 400 IU per day or placebo. An additional 12 term exclusively formula fed infants served as a comparison group for bone mineralization only. They were fed a single production batch of Similac 20 with iron, containing an average of 427 IU of vitamin D_3 per liter. At the time of enrollment, both groups of breastfeeding infants had normal and similar 25-OH-vitamin D levels, and bone mineral content (BMC) at the ⅓ distal radius was similar in all infants. Throughout the study, daily sunshine exposure of mothers and infants as well as intake of vitamin D and calcium-containing foods were similar between the two breastfeeding groups. By 12 weeks of life, compared to the supplemented group, placebo subjects had significantly lower 25-OH-vitamin D values (20 vs. 38 ng/mL, $P < 0.01$). However, the two groups had similar mean serum parathyroid hormone levels. The difference in vitamin D status at 12 weeks was mirrored by a significantly lower BMC in the unsupplemented nursing infants. At 12 weeks of age, the formula and vitamin D supplemented infants had similar BMC. At 26 weeks, the serum 25-OH-vitamin D levels decreased further in the placebo group to 12.9 ng/mL (vs. 32.7 in the study infants). Although none of the placebo infants had clinical signs of rickets, two had 25-OH-vitamin D values below the limit of sensitivity for the assay (4ng/mL). In contrast to the disparity in vitamin D status at 26 weeks of age, BMC, alkaline phosphatase, and parathyroid hormone values of the supplemented and unsupplemented groups were not significantly different. The authors speculated that the vitamin D content of human milk "may not be adequate." Since mineralization occurs predominantly at the distal end of growing bones and BMC was measured at the distal 1/3 of the radius, they theorized that the discrepancy between the comparable BMC and the significantly lower 25-OH-vitamin D levels of the placebo subjects might be secondary to the failure to measure bone mineralization at the distal end of the radius (Greer *et al.*, 1981; Greer *et al.*, 1982).

In a second study published that year, Roberts *et al.* reported the findings of a trial of vitamin D supplementation among a small cohort of full-term Caucasian infants in Salt Lake City, Utah (latitude 40° north). At two weeks of life, 19 breastfeeding infants were randomized to receive a daily vitamin D supplement of 400 IU (type of vitamin D not specified), while another 22 breastfeeding subjects were randomized not to receive a supplement. Additionally, 32 exclusively formula-fed infants were enrolled (Similac containing 400 IU of vitamin D_3 per liter). BMC, bone biochemical measurements, and 25-OH-vitamin D levels were assessed at baseline and 16 weeks of age. Both groups of nursing women were taking a daily multivitamin with 400 IU of vitamin D and, at enrollment, had similar mean serum 25-OH-vitamin D values. Sunlight exposure was not monitored. Researchers found that whereas initially all groups had similar results in the three parameters, by 16 weeks, the unsupplemented breastfed group had a significantly lower 25-OH-vitamin D level (17±3 vs. 25±2 and 22±3 ng/mL). However, all three groups had vitamin D levels in the normal range and had similar BMC. In light of these results, it was inferred that "*during the first 16 weeks of life, human milk appears to provide sufficient nutrients for adequate bone mineralization.*" Nevertheless, researchers cautioned that, in the exclusively breastfed infants, bone mineralization may have occurred at the expense of vitamin D stores (Roberts, 1981).

In an accompanying editorial, Finberg raised important and insightful issues regarding Roberts *et al.* conclusions that: "*... when environmental and social conditions are favorable, routine vitamin D supplementation of breastfed infants during the first 16 weeks of life is not necessary.*" He posited that if this recommendation were to be followed throughout the United States in 1981, the following scenario would occur. Assuming that 20% of the 3.5 million babies born that year in the United States were to be breastfed for 16 weeks, in order to determine whether vitamin D supplementation should be initiated, practitioners would need to evaluate the potential impact of environmental and social conditions on the bone mineralization of 700,000 nursing infants. Given the absence of any data or guidelines defining 'favorable' and 'unfavorable' conditions for bone mineralization, the importance of infant skin color on vitamin D status, the occurrence of rickets among breastfed infants even in the warmest and sunniest regions of the Earth, as well as the small number of infants studied by Roberts *et al.*, an alternative approach was proposed. Finberg suggested that universal Vitamin D supplementation of nursing infants with 400 IU per day be implemented. In addition to preventing vitamin D deficient rickets, this approach would entail minimal expense and inconvenience and has (and still has) no known risks (Finberg, 1981). In light of our current knowledge of vitamin D's multitude of functions, the possible long-term effects of early vitamin D deficiency, and numerous case reports of rickets which have and to this day continue to emanate from throughout the world, the challenges of and approach to ensuring vitamin D sufficiency discussed in this 1981 editorial are still relevant today.

Using the same study design, the group from Salt Lake City enrolled a second cohort of 91 breast- and formula-fed infants, assessing their growth and bone mineralization through the first year of life. At two weeks, two months, four months, and six months of life, 25-OH-vitamin D levels were measured. As in their first study, sunlight exposure was not monitored. Throughout the study, the three groups had similar infant growth, BMC, and maternal 25OH-vitamin D levels. The only age at which a significantly lower vitamin D value was noted in the unsupplemented infants was four months of life. It was concluded that "human milk provides for adequate growth and bone mineralization for the first year of life." However, in light of prior reports which noted an association between exclusive breastfeeding and rickets in infants raised in "unfavorable environmental and social conditions," the authors urged healthcare providers to ascertain whether "proper maternal conditions prevailed" prior to foregoing the recommendation of vitamin D supplementation (Chan *et al.*, 1982).

Another vitamin D supplementation trial which found no evidence of vitamin D deficiency in unsupplemented breastfed infants was conducted in Madison, Wisconsin (latitude 43° north). Utilizing a randomized double-blind design, 46 term, Caucasian, exclusively breastfeeding infants were placed on vitamin D_2 400 IU/day or placebo. For comparison, 12 similar formula-fed (containing vitamin D_3 427 IU/L) infants were also followed. Throughout pregnancy and the study, all women took a daily multivitamin containing 400 IU of vitamin D. Total maternal vitamin D intake averaged 701 IU and 652 IU per day at 1.5 and six months, respectively, and was similar between the two groups. At 1.5, three, and six months of life, serum vitamin D, bone biochemistries, and BMC were assessed. In addition, at each interval, limited monitoring of infant UVB exposure was conducted with a personal dosimeter. Initially, the vitamin D status of the three groups was comparable and, by current standards, within normal limits (mean 25-OH-vitamin D levels: 19.2 vs. 23.9 ng/mL). However, by six months of age, although the placebo group with an estimated maternal vitamin D intake of 700 IU per day still had a normal 25-OH-vitamin D level, it was significantly lower than that of the vitamin D_2 and formula groups (23.5±9.9 vs. 37±11.9 and 37.6±8.5). Despite the disparity in vitamin D levels at six months, all three groups had similar BMC and bone biochemistries. It was concluded that for the first six months of life, Caucasian breastfeeding infants in Madison, Wisconsin, with normal neonatal vitamin D status do not require supplementation to maintain adequate vitamin D levels (Greer & Marshall, 1989).

In order to assess whether amounts of vitamin

D lower than the 'standard' dose of 400 IU per day would be effective in preventing rickets, Specker *et al.* conducted a prospective randomized trial in 256 term Chinese newborns. In the fall and the spring in the first week of life, subjects were recruited in two northern (latitudes 47° and 40° north) and two southern (latitudes 30° and 22° south) cities. They were randomly assigned to one of three groups to receive 100, 200, or 400 IU of vitamin D per day. (Note: The type of vitamin D given was not specified in the paper.) The investigators did not control the infants' diet. In this era, a Chinese infant's diet consisted of various combinations of human milk, powdered cow's milk, and rice porridge. Moreover, neither adult nor infant foods were vitamin D-fortified and multivitamins were not routinely administered during pregnancy. Investigators collected serum from the umbilical cord and at six months, and obtained a wrist radiograph in the first week and at six months of age. Vitamin D deficiency was defined as a 25-OH-vitamin D level of <11 ng/mL *"because concentrations less than this value are observed in infants with vitamin D-deficiency rickets."* At birth, 57% of all subjects were vitamin D deficient. Compared to infants born in the south, those born in the north had a significantly lower mean cord serum 25-OH-vitamin D concentration and were much less likely to have a radiographically detectable wrist ossification center. During the study period, adherence to the supplementation regimen, caloric intake of breastmilk, and mean ultraviolet exposure scores did not differ between dosage groups. According to dietary histories collected during the fifth month of life, 20% were not consuming any human milk and the remainder were receiving an average of 66% of their estimated caloric intake from human milk. At six months, 19% of the entire cohort were still vitamin D deficient and, as noted at birth, there was a significantly greater percentage of deficiency in the north. In the northern and southern infants, there was a significant relationship between vitamin D dose and 25-OH-vitamin D levels. Although no cases of rickets were found, it is disturbing that even when receiving 400 IU per day some of the northern and southern subjects still had undetectable (<3 ng/mL) 25-OH-vitamin D concentrations. In summary, regardless of latitude, even up to 400 IU per day of vitamin D did not eliminate vitamin D deficiency in this cohort of term Chinese combination-fed infants (Specker & Ho, 1992).

Maternal and infant serum 25-OH-vitamin D concentrations with maternal and infant supplementation

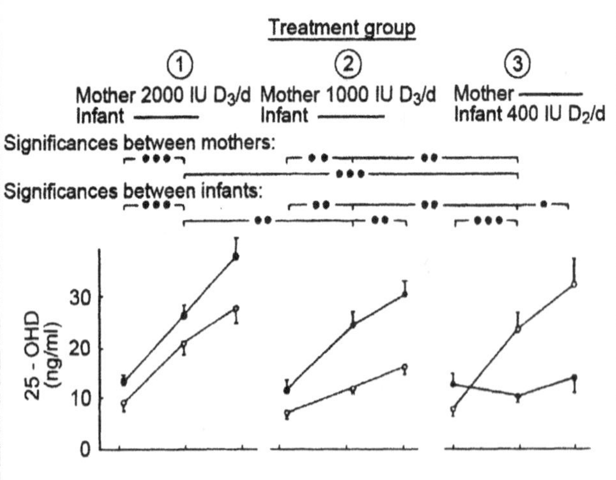

Figure 6. **Serum vitamin D metabolite concentrations (mean(SEM)) in winter of mothers (●) and infants (O) in different groups with vitamin D supplementation at delivery and 15 weeks later. Source: Ala-Houhala et al., 1986; reprinted with permission of BMJ Publishing Group.**

In summary, these four randomized clinical trials found that breastfeeding without supplemental vitamin D may expose the Caucasian American infant to a transient decrease in bone density and a risk of vitamin D deficiency, but will not lead to the development of nutritional rickets. However, further analysis of these studies and inclusion of additional data to evaluate the necessity of vitamin D supplementation for Caucasian breastfeeding infants reveals significant flaws in this position. Thus far, only four randomized controlled trials involving a total of 231 subjects have been published. While two of the studies followed the infants through the end of the first year of life, one trial concluded after six months and the fourth study ended after only four months of life (Chan *et al.*, 1982; Greer *et al.*, 1981; Greer *et al.*, 1982; Greer & Marshall, 1989; Roberts, 1981). It is also important to consider the extensive American literature of breastfed infants and toddlers diagnosed with vitamin D deficient rickets. Together, Cosgrove *et al.* and Weisberg *et al.* noted that between 1975 and 2003, 259 children from all regions of the country were diagnosed with the disorder. In nearly every instance, the child had been or was currently nursing and received little or no supplemental vitamin D. Additionally, almost ten percent of cases were Caucasian subjects (Cosgrove & Dietrich, 1985; Weisberg, 2004). Without a reporting system for vitamin D rickets, the numbers cited in the literature are presumed to represent a fraction of the actual total. The numerous cases of nutritional rickets in breastfed African-American and Caucasian children are in seeming contradiction to the absence of rickets among subjects enrolled in published vitamin D supplementation trials. The inconsistency between these two types of data may be explained in part by the low estimated incidence (five to nine per one million children) as well as by the prolonged time course of the disease (Weisberg, 2004). Even assuming that the actual incidence of nutritional rickets in the U.S. is much higher than described, enrolling 231 infants in studies lasting between four to 12 months is inadequate to assess the efficacy of and need for vitamin D supplementation in Caucasian breastfeeding infants. Given the low vitamin D content of human milk, current adequate intake (AI) for vitamin D of 200 IU per day, detection of vitamin D deficiency in breastfeeding infants, continued occurrence of vitamin D deficient rickets, as well as the limited data from prospective clinical trials, it appears that, in the U.S., Caucasian breastfeeding infants require additional vitamin D.

Does this requirement also apply to dark-skinned breastfeeding infants? Clinical trials of supplemental vitamin D for nursing infants have only enrolled Caucasian subjects. However, considering that approximately 90% of all reported cases of nutritional rickets have occurred in African-American children and that, compared to fair-skinned individuals, darker-skinned individuals require greater amounts of sunlight exposure to cutaneously generate a given amount of vitamin D_3, it is prudent to extend the recommendation of supplemental vitamin D to include all breastfeeding infants of color.

VITAMIN D SUPPLEMENTATION OF THE BREASTFEEDING MOTHER

Extensive research has established that human milk is species specific and "*uniquely superior for infant feeding* (Gartner *et al.*, 2005)." However, it is well known that human milk contains only small amounts of vitamin D. The most likely explanation for breastmilk's low antirachitic activity is the borderline or deficient vitamin D status of the typical modern-day lactating woman (Basile *et al.*, 2006). Because of the low vitamin D content of human milk, breastfeeding without vitamin D supplementation is associated with both hypovitaminosis D and vitamin D deficient rickets. Prevention of vitamin D deficiency and its complications in the exclusively nursing infant can be accomplished by several means. Increasing maternal UVB exposure (via natural or

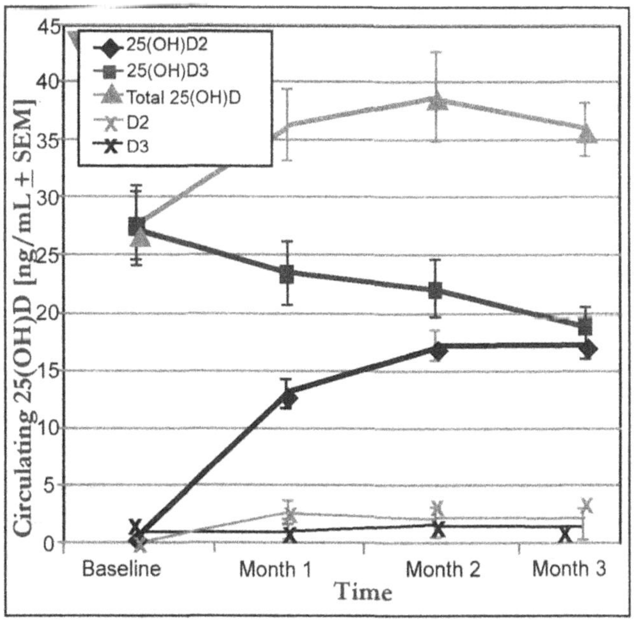

Figure 7. Circulating vitamin D concentrations (mean ±SEM) over time among lactating mothers receiving 1600 IU/day D_2 and 400 IU/day D_3. Source: Hollis & Wagner, 2004 (Figure 1); reprinted with permission from *The American Journal of Clinical Nutrition.*

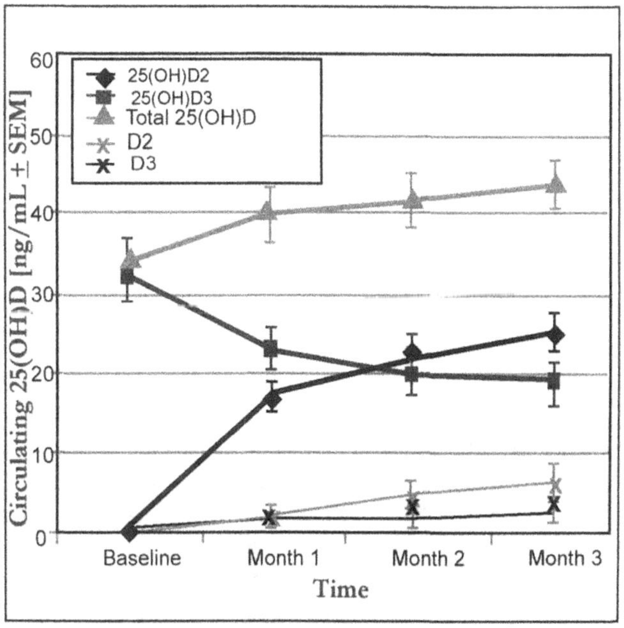

Figure 8. Circulating vitamin D concentrations (mean ±SEM) over time among lactating mothers receiving 3600 IU/day D_2 and 400 IU/day D_3. Source: Hollis & Wagner, 2004 (Figure 2); reprinted with permission from *The American Journal of Clinical Nutrition.*

artificial sources) elicits increased levels of cutaneous vitamin D synthesis, thereby enhancing both serum and milk vitamin D levels. Alternatively, increasing infant UVB exposure will directly boost the infant's vitamin D status. Due to the significant risks of sunburn for the baby and skin cancer for both mother and baby, neither of these options is currently advocated. As described in the preceding section, infant vitamin D supplementation has been shown to be both safe and effective. The one disadvantage of supplementing the child is its failure to impact maternal vitamin D levels. Studies of vitamin D status of lactating and non-lactating women of childbearing ages from throughout the world have found a high prevalence of vitamin D deficiency (Ala-Houhala, 1985; Carnevale *et al.*, 2001; Dawodu *et al.*, 2003; Lamberg-Allardt *et al.*, 2001; Meddeb *et al.*, 2005; Nesby-O'Dell *et al.*, 2002; Nowson & Margeison, 2002). Hypovitaminosis D in women is associated with osteoporosis and increased risk of fractures (Raisz, 2005). Studies also suggest vitamin D deficiency is associated with an increased risk of breast cancer and autoimmune disorders (Zittermann, 2003). Not only does maternal vitamin D supplementation address the needs of the woman, it also increases breastmilk vitamin D content to a level that maintains normal vitamin D concentrations in the exclusively nursing infant, thereby fulfilling the needs of the child as well.

During the 1980's, researchers began to examine the effects of maternal vitamin D supplementation on the vitamin D status of both the breastfeeding woman and her infant. In a prospective observational study of seven exclusively breastfed infants living in Tromso, Norway (latitude 70° north), serum vitamin D concentrations were measured at three, six, and 12 months of life. Throughout lactation, the mothers had "well balanced diets," but only three received approximately 400 IU of vitamin D per day. In all subjects, 25-OH-vitamin D levels decreased during winter. All but one infant were found to be vitamin D deficient on at least one occasion (study definition of vitamin D deficiency: <20 nanomoles/L or 8 ng/mL.) Therefore, in Tromso, Norway, maternal supplementation with 400 IU per day did not prevent the exclusively nursing infant from becoming vitamin D deficient. Although none of the babies had clinical or biochemical evidence of rickets, it was construed that the vitamin D content of their breastmilk was inadequate. For breastfed infants deprived of sunlight for a significant portion of the year, the authors recommended routine supplementation of the infant (Markestad *et al.*, 1984).

Table 5. Sociodemographic Data and Clinical Factors for Subjects as a Function of Study Group

Maternal and infant factors	2000 IU group	4000 IU group
Maternal	*n* = 9	*n* = 9
Age (y) (mean SD)	29.0 ± 6.0	30.8 ± 5.2
Race (no.)		
African American	3 (33.3%)	2 (22.2%)
White	6 (66.6%)	7 (77.8%)
Insurance status (no.)		
Private	5 (55.6%)	6 (66.7%)
Indigent/Medicaid	4 (44.4%)	3 (33.3%)
Parity (median)	0.5	0.1
Gravidity (median)	2.0	2.0
Compliance with vitamin D supplement (%) mean ± SD)		
Amount supplement returned month 1	10.3 ± 9.0	8.4 ± 8.9
Amount supplement returned month 2	12.1 ± 9.0	10.4 ± 14.4
Amount supplement returned month 3	10.2 ± 9.9	7.6 ± 7.94
Infant	*n* = 9	*n* = 8
Birth weight (g) (mean ± SD)	3526.6 ± 497.5	3368.8 ± 552.1
Gestational age (wk) (mean ± SD)	39.1 ± 1.5 (range: 37-41)	38.4 ± 1.7 (range: 36-41)

No significant differences were found between the two groups with respect to sociodemographic data and maternal/infant clinical factors.

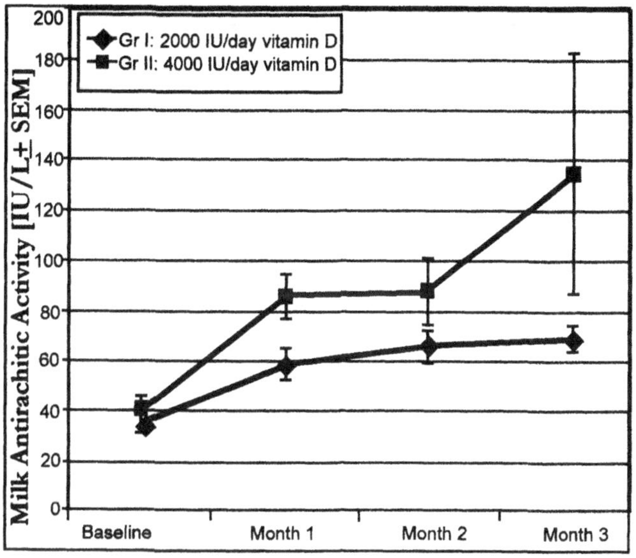

Figure 9. Milk antirachitic activity (mean±SEM) over time among 18 mothers receiving 2000 or 4000 IU/day of vitamin D. Source: Hollis & Wagner, 2004 (Figure 3); reprinted with permission from *The American Journal of Clinical Nutrition*.

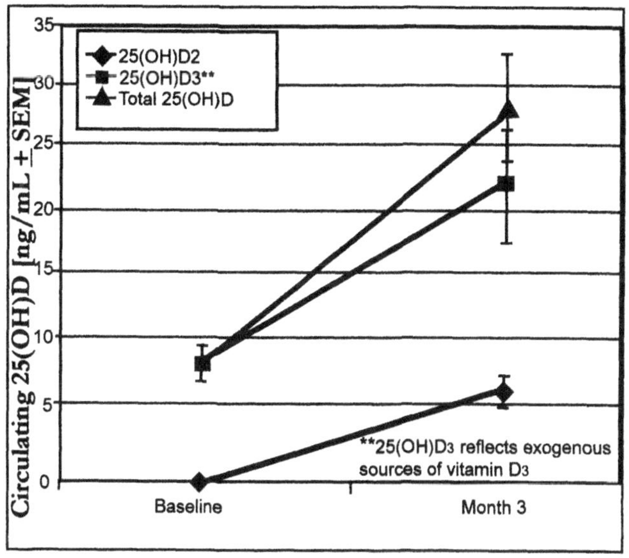

Figure 11. Circulating vitamin D concentrations (mean ±SEM) over time among lactating mothers receiving 1600 IU/day D_2 and 400 IU/day D_3. Source: Hollis & Wagner, 2004 (Figure 4); reprinted with permission from *The American Journal of Clinical Nutrition*.

In a sunny, southern climate, Rothberg *et al.* also noted the ineffectiveness of 'low' levels of maternal supplementation. Beginning on the fourth postpartum day, nursing women in Johannesburg, South Africa (latitude 26° south), were randomized in a double-blind fashion to receive either placebo, vitamin D 500 IU, or vitamin D 1000 IU per day for six weeks following delivery. (Note: the form of vitamin D was not specified in the paper.) A control group of nursing mothers did not receive vitamin D, but their infants were given 400 IU of vitamin D per day. At baseline, all four groups of mothers and newborns had similar serum 25-OH-vit-D values. At the conclusion of the study, placebo infants had the lowest vitamin D levels of any group and were severely vitamin D deficient (total 25-0H-vit-D 1.1 ± 1.4 ng/mL). By contrast, the control infants given 400 IU per day had the highest mean vitamin D levels (15.2±3.7). Additionally, all infant 25-OH-vitamin D levels were significantly and directly related to those of their mother. Surprisingly, compared to 500 IU per day, maternal supplementation with 1000 IU per day was not associated with higher maternal or infant vitamin D levels. Given the significantly lower vitamin D levels in the placebo infants living in proximity to the Equator and the superiority of administration of vitamin D directly to the infant as opposed to the mother, the authors recommended, even in the absence of biochemical rickets, routine supplementation of breastfed infants whose mothers have a low intake of vitamin D "irrespective of climate (Rothberg *et al.*, 1982)."

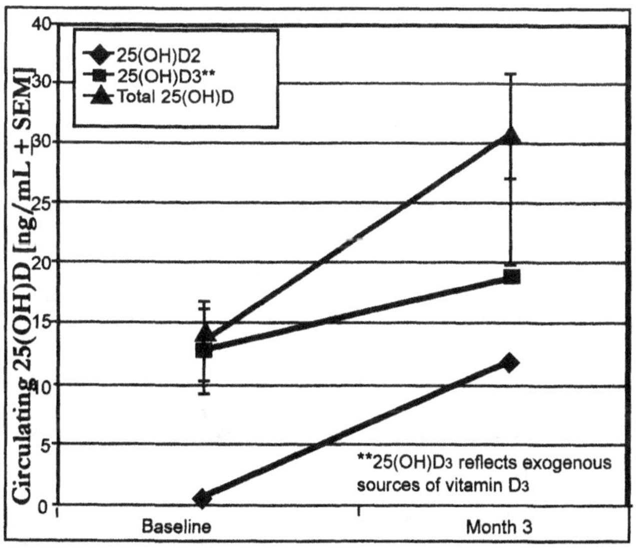

Figure 10. Circulating vitamin D concentrations (mean ±SEM) over time among lactating mothers receiving 3600 IU/day D_2 and 400 IU/day D_3. Source: Hollis & Wagner, 2004 (Figure 5); reprinted with permission from *The American Journal of Clinical Nutrition*.

A few years later, Ala-Houhala *et al.* compared the effects of a somewhat higher level of daily maternal supplementation to 'standard' infant and maternal vitamin D supplementation on infant vitamin D status. During January, in Tampere, Finland (latitude 61° north), 49 exclusively breastfeeding dyads were "divided in succession into three groups": Group 1, maternal supplementation with 2,000 IU of vitamin D_3, Group 2, maternal supplementation with 1,000 IU of vitamin D_3, and Group 3, mothers not supplemented and infants supplemented with 400 IU of vitamin D_3. At delivery and at eight and 15 weeks postpartum, maternal and infant serum was collected. Because of the increased solar zenith angle in this region throughout the study period, threshold levels of UVB radiation would not be reached. Therefore, exposure to sunlight would not result in cutaneous vitamin D synthesis. That is to say, for the duration of the study, vitamin D status was entirely dependent upon exogenous intake and body stores. At delivery, maternal and infant 25-OH-vitamin D values were comparable in all three groups. However, at both the mid-point and conclusion of the trial, infant 25-OH-vitamin D levels of Groups 1 and 3 increased significantly above baseline and were similar to each other. Additionally, compared to the vitamin D status of infants in groups 1 and 3, the vitamin D status of group 2 infants was significantly lower (**Figure 6**).

Presumably, the relatively inferior vitamin D status of the Group 2 infants at eight and 15 weeks postpartum was caused by the consumption of breastmilk with lower levels of antirachitic activity. The authors concluded that administering 400 IU of vitamin D_3 per day directly to the baby was sufficient to maintain vitamin D sufficiency. Their findings are comparable to those of Greer *et al.* and Rothberg *et al.* in which a daily maternal vitamin D intake of approximately 1000 IU was not associated with an increase in infant vitamin D levels (see above) (Greer & Marshall, 1989; Rothberg *et al.*, 1982). Although maternal supplementation with 2,000 IU and infant supplementation with only 400 IU of vitamin D_3 had similar efficacies, they cautioned against using this higher maternal dose until the safety of prolonged administration could be established (Ala-Houhala *et al.*, 1986).

An understanding of the types and proportions of vitamin D metabolites present in breastmilk can be obtained by examining published reports from the 1980's. From delivery until the 25th day postpartum, Greer *et al.* analyzed breastmilk and maternal, infant, and umbilical cord sera from an exclusively breastfeeding dyad whose mother, pre- and postnatally, was being treated for chronic hypoparathyroidism with 100,000 IU of vitamin D_2 per day. On postpartum day 14, her breastmilk was found to contain a total antirachitic activity of 6700 to 7660 IU/L. Over 95% of the antirachitic activity was derived solely from vitamin D_2 (ergocalciferol) and 25-OH-vitamin D_2. Of the two primary metabolites, which accounted for 95% of the activity, vitamin D_2 accounted for approximately 95% by weight and 80% of the breastmilk antirachitic activity of this fraction (Greer *et al.*, 1984a). In contrast to the use of pharmacologic doses of vitamin D_2, Takeuchi *et al.* assessed the effects of low-level supplementation on the concentrations of vitamin D compounds in human milk. At one week postpartum, 25 healthy lactating women

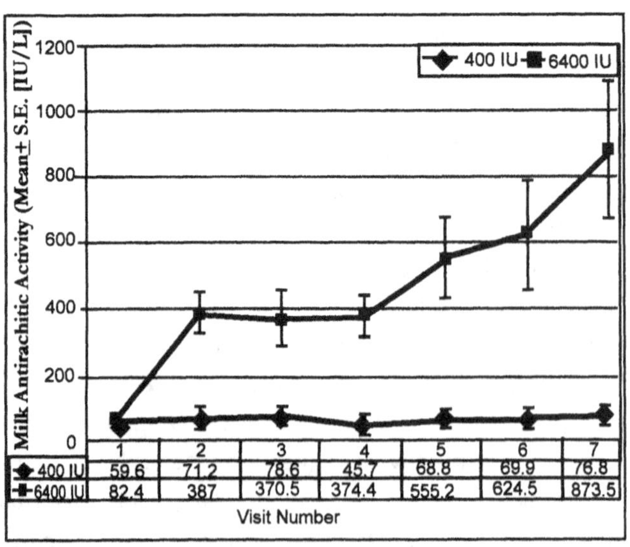

Figure 12. Milk antirachitic activity as a function of maternal vitamin D3 dose: 400 vs. 6400 IU/day. Source: Wagner *et al.*, 2006 (Figure 3); reprinted with permission of Liebert Publishing.

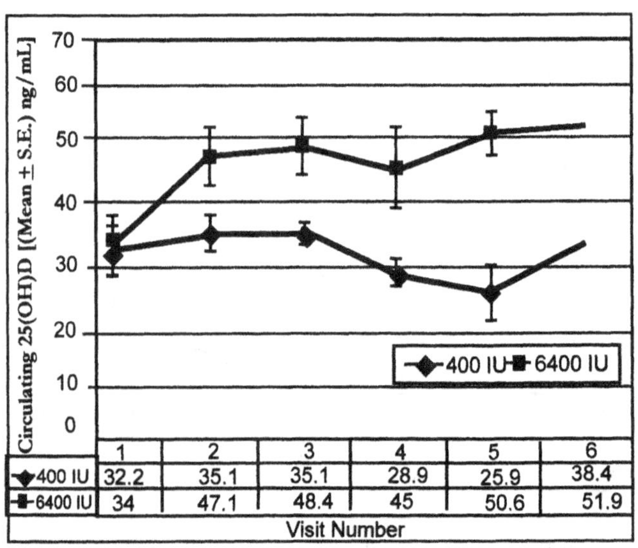

Figure 13. Maternal 25-OH-vitamin D status as a function of maternal vitamin D dose: 400 vs. 6400 IU/day. Source: Wagner *et al.*, 2006 (Figure 1); reprinted with permission of Liebert Publishing.

were given 1,200 IU of vitamin D_2 daily for four weeks. At baseline, over 90% of milk antirachitic activity was attributed to 25-OH-vitamin D_3. In addition, extremely low concentrations of vitamin D_2 and no 25-OH-vit-D_2 were detected. After four weeks of therapy, mean 25-OH-vitamin D_2 levels went from being undetectable to 32 ng/liter and vitamin D_2 increased from 11 to 125 ng/liter. Thus, after four weeks of supplementation with ergocalciferol, the parent compound (vitamin D) was the most abundant vitamin D metabolite in breastmilk (Takeuchi *et al.*, 1989).

In another case report, the impact of maternal exposure to brief, relatively intense doses of UVB radiation on vitamin D levels in breastmilk was described. In Madison, Wisconsin, USA, five Caucasian lactating women were exposed to 1.5 minimal erythemal doses (MED) of UVB via a walk-in irradiation chamber. For fair-skinned individuals, one MED of UVB is equivalent to the amount of UV radiation received from 30 minutes of sunshine exposure in the middle of a clear summer day at temperate latitudes (Diffey, 1982). At baseline, 24 and 48 hours, and one and two weeks after exposure, serum and milk vitamin D measurements were performed. During this period, subjects carefully limited their exposure to sunlight. This dose of UVB radiation was associated with a significant improvement in maternal vitamin D status. Serum 25-OH-vitamin D_3 levels increased from a mean of 13.9 to 20.5 ng/mL and, compared to pre-exposure measurements, remained

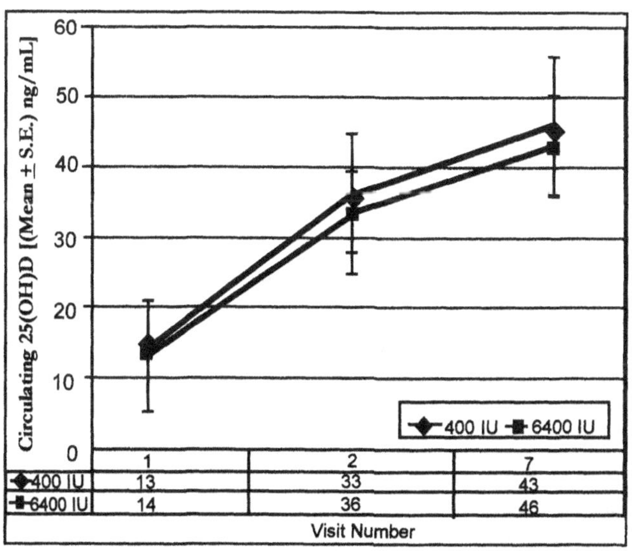

Figure 14. Infant 25-OH-vitamin D status as a function of maternal vitamin D dose: 400 vs. 6400 IU/day. Source: Wagner *et al.*, 2006 (Figure 4); reprinted with permission of Liebert Publishing.

elevated throughout. Analysis of their breastmilk revealed only a small increase in 25-OH-vitamin D_3, but a 2200% elevation in vitamin D_3 levels. They also noted a strong correlation between maternal serum and breastmilk vitamin D_3 levels (**Figures 7, 8**) (Greer *et al.*, 1984b). In summary, early studies found that both orally ingested vitamin D_2 and cutaneously synthesized vitamin D_3 appear to be the primary forms of vitamin D in milk. Additionally, at least a portion of both molecules (vitamin D and 25-OH-vit-D) are transferred to breastmilk. These human data are consistent with findings from a rat model in which high intraperitoneal doses of radiolabeled vitamin D_3 resulted in milk whose vitamin D content consisted primarily of the radiolabeled vitamin D_3 (Dostal *et al.*, 1983).

In an effort to better quantify the rate of transfer of vitamin D compounds from plasma to breastmilk, Hollis *et al.* conducted a detailed analysis of vitamin D compounds in plasma and milk of 51 lactating women who, according to dietary recall, were consuming approximately 400 IU of vitamin D per day. They noted the total antirachitic activity of human milk to be 68 IU/L. Although most of the vitamin D activity was due to 25-OH-vitamin D, vitamin D was the most abundant compound. A comparison of milk and plasma levels of these two metabolites revealed total breastmilk vitamin D and 25-OH-vitamin D concentrations were 30% and 1%, respectively, of that found in plasma. Utilizing a regression analysis, a significant positive correlation and regression slope was noted between concentrations of vitamin D_2 (vitamin D_2 and 25-OH-vitamin D_2) and vitamin D_3 metabolites (vitamin D_3 and 25-OH-vitamin D_3) in maternal milk and plasma. According to their calculations, approximately 10 to 20% of plasma ergocalciferol and cholecalciferol were transferred into milk (B. Hollis, personal communication, August 2006). These findings indicate that the concentration of the primary vitamin D compounds in the circulation (and indicative of overall maternal vitamin D status) "*has a direct bearing on that in the milk* (Hollis *et al.*, 1986)."

Within the first postpartum month, 18 "fully lactating" Caucasian and African-American mothers in Charleston, South Carolina (latitude 32° north), were randomly assigned to receive either an additional 1600 or 3600 IU of vitamin D_2 per day for three months (**Table 5**). Given the scarcity of dietary vitamin D_2 and that endogenous synthesis does not generate vitamin D_2, supplementing with D_2 enabled the accurate assessment of the effects of maternal D_2 supplementation on maternal and infant vitamin D status. Participants were instructed to limit sunshine exposure and intake of infant formula and all mothers received an additional daily multivitamin containing 400 IU of vitamin D_3. Therefore, for three months, subjects were consuming either 10 (2000 IU) or 20 times (4000 IU) the current Adequate Intake (AI) for vitamin D. For the duration of the study, maternal blood, breastmilk, and urine were collected at monthly intervals. At one and four months of life, infant blood was collected. Serum calcium concentrations remained within normal limits and no episodes of hypercalciuria were noted. Whereas, compared to baseline, both regimens resulted in a significant enhancement in maternal serum 25 OH-vitamin D_2 concentrations and breastmilk antirachitic activity, the increase observed in both body fluids was far superior in the higher dose group (**Figures 7, 8, 9**). These changes in maternal vitamin D status were paralleled by similar elevations in infant vitamin D levels (**Figures 10, 11**). In other words, whereas compared to baseline, both regimens resulted in a substantial elevation in infant serum vitamin D levels, those infants whose mothers were receiving the higher dose (4000 IU per day) had a significantly greater increase in their levels (32.9±2.4 to 44.5±3.9 vs. 27.6±3.3 to 36.1±2.3 ng/mL). In quantifying the alterations in both forms of vitamin D (D_2 and D_3), it was noted that over the three month trial while maternal total serum 25-OH-vitamin D concentrations were rising, maternal serum 25-OH-vitamin D_3 levels decreased significantly. Moreover, the elevation in milk antirachitic activity was only attributable to 25-OH-vitamin D_2 and vitamin D_2. This suggests that even in a warm and sunny climate, when sunlight exposure is limited, maternal supplementation during lactation with 400 IU of vitamin D_3 per day is inadequate. Based on the data, the authors concluded that "*the current DRI of 400 IU per day of vitamin D is irrelevant to the vitamin D nutritional status of mothers and nursing infants*" and that 4000 IU per day is safe and represents an adequate dose for the mother and her nursing infant (Hollis & Wagner, 2004).

In considering the maternal efficacy and safety of administering 4000 IU per day of a combination of vitamin D_2 and D_3 to a nursing mother, it is essential to point out that, prior to this study, other investigators had demonstrated that supplementation of vitamin D sufficient adult men and non-lactating women with up to 10,000 IU of vitamin D_3 for as long as five months was well tolerated. In Toronto, Canada (latitude 43° north), 61 middle-aged adults were closely monitored for as long as five months while daily receiving either 1000 or 4000 IU of vitamin D_3. They observed that a daily intake of 4000 IU was needed to achieve vitamin D levels in the low-normal range (Vieth *et al.*, 2001). In a second trial conducted in Omaha, Nebraska (latitude 41° north), a different group conducted a 20-week formal pharmacokinetic evaluation of oral vitamin D_3 therapy. During winter, they administered between zero to 10,000 IU of vitamin D_3 per day to 67 men. After three months on 10,000 IU of vitamin D_3, the mean serum 25-OH-vitamin D concentrations peaked in the high normal range (63.5±6.7 ng/mL). It was concluded that healthy men utilize 3000 to 5000 IU of vitamin D_3 per day (Heaney, 2003). Despite taking up to 10,000 IU of vitamin D_3 per day, no subject in either study developed hypervitaminosis D or hypercalcemia. Additionally, there was a similar incidence of hypercalciuria between the different dosage groups (Vieth *et al.*, 2001; Heaney, 2003). In 1998, the group out of Omaha also published results from an eight week open-label trial providing 1000 IU to 50,000 IU of vitamin D_3 per day to 37 vitamin D sufficient men. Once again, no episodes of hypercalcemia were detected (Barger-Lux *et al.*, 1998). These, as well as other data, have undermined the validity of the current adequate intake (AI) of 200 IU per day, the safe upper limit (2000 IU per day), and the Lowest Observed Adverse Effect Level (3800 IU per day) for vitamin D intake established in 1997 by the United States Food and Nutrition Board (Standing Committee, 1997). In estimating the vitamin D requirements of a lactating woman, one must also take into consideration Hollis *et al.*'s earlier finding that 10 to 20% of her serum cholecalciferol was transferred into the breastmilk (Hollis *et al.*, 1986).

In light of previous observations from lactating and non-lactating women, Wagner and Hollis recently completed another pilot trial in which "fully lactating" subjects received 400 or 6400 IU of vitamin D_3 per day for six months. In this investigation, vitamin D_2 was not used because the increase in maternal serum and breastmilk levels observed in their previous study was much lower than expected. The relatively poor response with vitamin D_2 administration was consistent with recent investigations. In comparing the ability of equal molar quantities of vitamin D_2 and D_3 to increase serum 25-OH-vitamin D concentrations, Trang *et al.* and Armas *et al.* found vitamin D_3 to be 1.7 and three times more effective, respectively (Trang *et al.*, 1998; Armas *et al.*, 2004). Therefore, at one month postpartum, 19 breastfeeding dyads (15 of whom were Caucasians) were enrolled in a randomized, double-blind, placebo-control study. In the experimental group, mothers were given 6400 IU of vitamin D_3 per day and infants were given placebo. In the control group, mothers were given 400 IU and the infants were given 300 IU of vitamin D_3 per day. The authors formulated two hypotheses. They posited that high dose maternal vitamin D alone would enhance the vitamin D status of the mother and her nursing infant. They also hypothesized that compared to the combination regimen (maternal of 400 IU and infant of 300 IU per day), the high dose maternal regimen (maternal of 6400 IU and infant placebo) would result in superior maternal vitamin D levels, but comparable infant levels. Participants were instructed to limit sunshine exposure or to use sunscreen. At monthly intervals, breastmilk and infant and maternal serum and urine were collected. Additionally, at each visit, maternal and infant changes in skin pigmentation (an indirect measure of UVB exposure) were assessed and dietary and outdoor activity questionnaires were completed. There were no group differences with respect to demographics, dietary profiles, outdoor activity, skin pigmentation changes, or compliance with therapy. According to the food frequency questionnaires, in both cohorts, mean maternal dietary vitamin D intake was approximately 270 IU per day (Wagner, 2006).

While receiving a daily supplement of 400 IU vitamin D_3, total maternal 25-OH-vitamin D levels were stable and ranged between 25.9 to 38.4 ng/mL. Many experts now define optimal adult vitamin D status as a 25-OH-vitamin D concentration of >32 ng/mL (Bischoff-Ferrari, 2004; Meier, 2004). Therefore, a total vitamin D intake of 670 IU per day (via the diet and supplement) in the control women was associated with low-normal vitamin D status. In the low dose subjects, breastmilk antirachitic activity did not increase and ranged between 45.7 to 76.3 IU per liter. Given this level of breastmilk antirachitic activity, in order to receive the current AI of 200 IU vitamin D per day, the exclusively nursing control infants would have needed to consume approximately three to four liters of breastmilk per day.

By comparison, high dose maternal vitamin D_3 supplementation significantly increased both milk antirachitic activity and maternal 25 OH-vitamin D levels (**Figures 12, 13**). Daily administration of 6400 IU of vitamin D_3 for six months was associated with mean maternal 25-OH-vitamin D concentration of 58.8 ng/mL and breastmilk antirachitic activity of 873.5 IU per liter. (Note: baseline breastmilk antirachitic activity was 82.4 IU.) Approximately 90% of the antirachitic activity was due to vitamin D_3 (B. Hollis, personal communication, March 2006). In contrast to the discrepant maternal vitamin D status, both regimens resulted in comparable infant 25-OH-vitamin D concentrations (**Figure 14**). No adverse events, including hypercalcemia, hypercalciuria, or hypervitaminosis D, were detected. The authors concluded that administering 6400 IU of vitamin D_3 per day to a nursing woman and none to her infant "eliminates hypovitaminosis D in both mother and infant." Moreover, because maternal supplementation with 400 IU per day was associated with low normal maternal 25-OH-vitamin D and low milk vitamin D levels, it was also concluded that this dose is "*irrelevant to the vitamin D nutritional status of the mother and her nursing infant.*" However, they advised that the safety of 6400 IU per day needs to be confirmed by larger, multi-site trials among a more diverse population of breastfeeding dyads. Additionally, it was acknowledged that further research is needed to determine the optimal 25-OH-vitamin D levels for lactating women and their infants.

In 2006, data derived from several small studies supports the contention that during lactation, maternal vitamin D supplementation alone with a minimum of 2000 IU of cholecalciferol (vitamin D_3) daily appears to be safe and will increase vitamin D levels of both the mother and her full-term nursing infant. The increase in infant levels appears to be directly related to the enhanced breastmilk antirachitic activity. Consistent with other trials involving non-lactating women of reproductive ages, investigators in Johannesburg, South Africa (latitude 26° south), and Tampere, Finland (latitude 61° north), found that for both members of the breastfeeding dyad, a maternal supplement of 1000 IU daily was associated with low-normal vitamin D concentrations (Ala-Houhala *et al.*, 1986; Rothberg *et al.*, 1982). Compared to subjects receiving only a maternal dose of 1000 IU of vitamin D_3 per day, a maternal dose of 2000 IU helped mothers and infants achieve robust and significantly greater circulating vitamin D levels. The vitamin D status of these infants was similar to those who were given vitamin D_3 400 IU per day but whose mothers were not supplemented (Rothberg *et al.*, 1982; Ala-Houhala *et al.*, 1986). Similarly, almost 20 years later, Hollis *et al.* observed that, for mother and baby, maternal supplementation with 2000 IU (1600 IU of which were vitamin D_2) was safe and efficacious (Hollis & Wagner, 2004). This dose is ten times the current AI for lactating women established by the U.S. Food and Nutrition Board in 1997. Several recent well-designed adult investigations in which subjects were given up to 50,000 IU of vitamin D_3 per day found normal vitamin D levels and no adverse effects. Utilizing safety data from their first study as well as from trials involving non-lactating adults, Wagner *et al.* have just completed a study which appears to have extended the 'safety zone' for maternal vitamin D consumption during lactation. While receiving a maternal supplement of 6400 IU of vitamin D_3 per day for six months, a high breastmilk antirachitic activity of 873.5 IU per liter, consisting primarily of vitamin D_3, was achieved. The nine fully lactating mothers and their infants developed robust serum 25-OH-vitamin D concentrations. Compared to infants in the high dose cohort, those in the low dose combination cohort (consisting of a daily maternal vitamin D_3 supplement of 400 IU and an infant vitamin D_3 supplement of 300 IU) had similar vitamin D levels. Over the six month study period, no adverse effects were noted (Wagner *et al.*, 2006). Confirmation of the efficacy and safety of this dose requires evaluation by larger, multicentered trials. More importantly, maternal supplementation alone is a feasible and safe means to simultaneously support the vitamin D status of the mother and her nursing infant. However, delineation of the 'correct' maternal dose during lactation is largely dependent on the determination of optimal circulating vitamin D levels for children and adults.

CONCLUSIONS AND IMPLICATIONS

Vitamin D is a nutrient with a wide range of functions throughout the body and whose deficiency, according to a rapidly growing body of knowledge, may play a role in a multitude of acute and chronic diseases. Breastfeeding and the use of human milk confer "*diverse and compelling advantages for infants, mothers, families, and society* (Gartner *et al.*, 2005)." Unfortunately, it has been well-documented that this preeminent form of nutrition is deficient in vitamin D. Throughout the world, breastfeeding without vitamin D supplementation has been associated with vitamin D deficiency and an increased risk of rickets. Rather than viewing this as a shortcoming of human milk, the low levels of antirachitic compounds contained therein are best understood as a consequence of modern civilization's severe curtailment of exposure to UVB light, along with a diet naturally lacking in vitamin D. Deprived of both exogenous and endogenous sources of vitamin D, many modern-day human beings are vitamin D deficient. Viewed in this context, providing supplemental vitamin D, either to the nursing mother or her child, compensates for present day lifestyles and a diet low in vitamin D and enhances the health and well-being of the breastfeeding dyad.

Traditionally, vitamin D deficiency has been equated with the occurrence of vitamin D deficient rickets and adult osteomalacia and, for all ages, has been defined as a 25-OH-vitamin D concentration of <11 ng/mL (27.5 nmol/L). This threshold is the basis of all current vitamin D intake guidelines. The realization that vitamin D is a substance with numerous and varied biological functions has prompted a reassessment of the definition of vitamin D deficiency. In light of recent findings derived from adult studies examining the association between serum 25-OH-vitamin D levels and several biomarkers and clinical outcomes (e.g., PTH, bone mineral density, insulin sensitivity, and cancer risk), several experts have recommended that 25-OH-vitamin D concentrations be maintained at or above 30-32 ng/mL (75-80 nmol/L). Because similar studies have not been performed in infants and children, Frank Greer, MD, chairman of the AAP's Committee on Nutrition has questioned the veracity of the current definition of pediatric vitamin D deficiency (Greer, 2004). Recent adult trials suggest that the level of intake needed to reach and maintain this significantly higher threshold far exceed current guidelines for vitamin D. If a similar upward revision of pediatric vitamin D deficiency were to be proposed, current pediatric intake guidelines would also need to be re-evaluated.

Despite the uncertainties pertaining to vitamin D deficiency and intake, in the face of on-going worldwide efforts of governments, healthcare agencies, and providers to enhance breastfeeding rates and duration, it is imperative that breastfeeding women and their children are provided up-to-date evidence-based guidelines. Ensuring vitamin D sufficiency of both members of the nursing dyad may be accomplished via separate and concurrent supplementation of mother and child or via supplementation of the mother alone. Extensive data from lactating and non-lactating subjects has revealed that maternal supplementation with 400 IU of vitamin D_3 per day will not support normal maternal vitamin D levels and is associated with low concentrations of vitamin D compounds in her milk. This regimen is also associated with vitamin D deficiency in the exclusively nursing infant. It is also well-documented that providing a nursing infant with 200-400 IU of vitamin D_3 per day is safe and effective. Alternatively, supporting a normal vitamin D status for both members of the breastfeeding dyad via maternal supplementation alone appears to be a promising approach. Based on two clinical trials (only one of which was randomized) involving a total of 67 subjects, daily intakes of 2,000 IU and 6,400 IU of vitamin D_3 were both well-tolerated and associated with robust infant and maternal vitamin D levels. (Ala-Houhala *et al.*, 1986; Wagner, 2006). Given the limited experience with this method, it would seem prudent to adopt the approach of separately supplementing mother and child.

References

Achinger SG, Ayus JC. The role of vitamin D in left ventricular hypertrophy and cardiac function. *Kidney Int Suppl.* 2005; 95:S37-42.

Ahmed I, Atiq M, Iqbal J, *et al.* Vitamin D deficiency rickets in breast-fed infants presenting with hypocalcemic seizures. *Acta Paediatr.* 1995; 84:941-42.

Ala-Houhala M, Koskinen T, Terho A, *et al.* Maternal compared with infant vitamin D supplementation. *Arch Dis Child.* 1986; 61:1159-63.

Ala-Houhala M. 25-hydroxyvitamin D levels during breast-feeding with or without maternal or infantile supplementation of vitamin D. *J Pediatr Gastroenterol Nutr.* 1985; 4:220-26.

American Academy of Pediatrics, Committee on Environmental Health. Ultraviolet light: a hazard to children. *Pediatrics.* 1999; 104:328-33.

Andiran N, Yordam N, Ozon A. Risk factors for vitamin D deficiency in breast-fed newborns and their mothers. *Nutrition.* 2002; 18:47-50.

Armas LAG, Hollis BW, Heaney RP. Vitamin D2 is much less effective than vitamin D3 in humans. *J Clin Endocrinol Metab.* 2004; 89:5387-91.

Arnaud CD. Parathyroid hormone and its role in the pathophysiology of the common forms of rickets and osteomalacia. In: Glorieux FH. *Rickets.* Nestec, Vevey: Raven Press; 1991.

Atiq M, Suria A, Nizami SQ, *et al.* Vitamin D status of breastfed Pakistani infants. *Acta Paediatr.* 1998; 87:737-40.

Bachrach S, Fisher J, Parks JS. An outbreak of vitamin D deficiency rickets in a susceptible population. *Pediatrics.* 1979; 64:871-77.

Bahijri SM. Serum 25-hydroxy cholecalciferol in infants and preschool children in the western region of Saudi Arabia. *Saudi Med J.* 2001; 22:973-79.

Barger-Lux MJ, Heaney RP, Dowell S, *et al.* Vitamin D and its major metabolites: serum levels after graded oral dosing in healthy men. *Osteopor Int.* 1998; 8:222-30.

Basile LA, Taylor SN, Wagner CL, *et al.* The effect of high-dose vitamin D supplementation on serum vitamin D levels and milk calcium concentration in lactating women and their infants. *Breastfeeding Medicine.* 2006; 1:27-35.

Beer TM, Myrthue A. Calcitriol in cancer treatment: from the lab to the clinic. *Mol Cancer Ther.* 2004; 3:373-81.

Birkbeck JA, Scott HF. 25-hydroxycholecalciferol serum levels in breast-fed infants. *Arch Dis Child.* 1980; 55:691-95.

Bischoff-Ferrari H, Dietrich T, Orav E, *et al.* Positive association between 25(OH)D levels and bone mineral density: A population-based study of younger and older adults. *Amer J Med.* 2004; 116:634-39.

Bischoff-Ferrari HA, Giovannucci E, Willett WC, *et al.* Estimation of optimal serum concentrations of 25-hydroxyvitamin D for multiple outcomes. *Am J Clin Nutr.* 2006; 84:18-28.

Bohnsack BL, Hirschi KK. Nutrient regulation of cell cycle progression. *Annu Rev Nutr.* 2004; 24:433-53.

Bouillon R. Vitamin D: from photosynthesis, metabolism, and action to clinical applications. In: DeGroot L, Jameson JL. *Endocrinology.* 5th Ed. Philadelphia, PA: Elsevier Saunders; 2006.

Brunvand L, Haga P, Tangsrud SE, *et al.* Congestive heart failure caused by vitamin D deficiency? *Acta Paediatr.* 1995; 84:106-8.

Butte N, Lopez-Alarcon MG, Garza C. Nutrient adequacy of exclusive breastfeeding for the term infant during the first six months of life. *World Health Organization.* 2002. p. 47.

Calikoglu AS, Davenport ML. Prophylactic vitamin D supplementation. *Endocr Dev.* 2003; 6:233-58.

Calvo MS, Whiting SJ, Barton CN. Vitamin D fortification in the United States and Canada: current status and needs. *Am J Clin Nutr.* 2004; 80(suppl):1710S-16S.

Calvo MS, Whiting SJ, Barton CN. Vitamin D intake: a global perspective of current status. *J Nutr.* 2005; 135:310-16.

Calvo MS, Whiting SJ. Prevalence of vitamin D deficiency in Canada and the United States: importance to health status and efficacy of current food fortification and dietary supplement use. *Nutrition Rev.* 2003; 61:107-13.

Calvo MS, Whiting SJ. Public health strategies to overcome barriers to optimal vitamin D status in populations with special needs. *J Nutr.* 2006; 136:1135-39.

Cantorna MT, Mahon BD. D-hormone and the immune system. *J Rheumatol.* 2005; 76:11-20.

Cantorna MT, Mahon BD. Mounting evidence for vitamin D as an environmental factor affecting autoimmune disease prevalence. *Exp Biol Med.* 2004; 229:1136-42.

Carnevale V, Modoni S, Pileri M, *et al.* Longitudinal evaluation of vitamin D status in healthy subjects from southern Italy: seasonal and gender differences. *Osteoporos.* 2001; 12:1026-30.

Challa A, Ntourntoufi A, Cholevas V, *et al.* Breastfeeding and vitamin D status in Greece during the first 6 months of life. Eur *J Pediatr.* 2005; 164:724-29.

Chan GM, Roberts CC, Folland D, *et al.* Growth and bone mineralization of normal breast-fed infants and the effects of lactation on maternal bone mineral status. *Am J Clin Nutr.* 1982; 36:438-43.

Chesney RW. Rickets: an old form in a new century. *Pediatr Int.* 2003; 45:509-11.

Cosgrove L, Dietrich A. Nutritional rickets in breast-fed infants. *J Fam Pract.* 1985; 21:205-9.

Dancaster CP, Jackson WPU. Studies in rickets in the Cape peninsula. II Aetiology. *South Afr Med J.* 1961; 35:890-94.

Dawodu A, Agarwal M, Hossain M, *et al.* Hypovitaminosis D and vitamin D deficiency in exclusively breast-feeding infants and their mothers in summer: a justification for vitamin D supplementation of breastfeeding infants. *J Pediatr.* 2003; 142:169-73.

Dawson-Hughes B, Heaney RP, Holick MF, *et al.* Estimates of optimal vitamin D status. *Osteoporos Int.* 2005; 16:713-16.

Diffey BL. *Ultraviolet radiation in medicine.* Bristol (Avon): Adam Hilger in collaboration with the Hospital Physicists' Association; 1982.

Dostal LA, Boass A, Toverud SU, *et al.* Effects of high doses of vitamin D3 and 1,25-dihydroxyvitamin D3 in lactating rats on milk composition and calcium homeostasis of the suckling pups. *Endocrinology.* 1983; 112:1631-38.

Dusso AS, Brown AJ, Slatpolsky E. Vitamin D. *Am J Renal Physiol Renal Physiol.* 2005; 289:F8-F28.

Eliot MM. The control of rickets: preliminary discussion of the demonstration in New Haven. *JAMA.* 1925; 85:656-63.

Endo I, Inoue D, Mitsui T, *et al.* Deletion of vitamin D receptor gene in mice results in abnormal skeletal muscle development with deregulated expression of myoregulatory transcription factors. *Endocrinology.* 2003; 144:5138-44.

EURODIAB. Vitamin D supplement in early childhood and risk for type I (insulin-dependent) diabetes mellitus. The EURODIAB substudy 2 study group. *Diabetologia.* 1999; 42:51-54.

Feron F, Burne TH, Brown J, *et al.* Developmental vitamin D deficiency alters the rat adult brain. *Brain Res Bull.* 2005; 65:141-48.

Feskanich D. Ma J, Fuchs CS, *et al.* Plasma vitamin D metabolites and risk of colorectal cancer in women. *Cancer Epidemiol Biomarkewr Prev.* 2004; 13:1502-8.

Finberg L. Human milk feeding and vitamin D supplementation - 1981. *J Pediatr.* 1981; 99:228-29.

Gannagé-Yared MH, Chemali R, Yaacoub N, *et al.* Hypovitaminosis D in a sunny country: relation to lifestyle and bone markers. *J Bone Miner Res.* 2000; 15:1856-62.

Garland CF, Comstock GW, Garland FC, *et al.* Serum 25-hydroxyvitamin and colon cancer: eight-year prospective study. *Lancet.* 1989; 18:2(8673):1176-78.

Garland CF, Garland FC. Do sunlight and vitamin D reduce the likelihood of colon cancer? *Int J Epidemiol.* 1980; 9:227-31.

Gartner LM, Greer FR, Section on Breastfeeding and Committee on Nutrition. Prevention of rickets and vitamin D deficiency: new guidelines for vitamin D intake. *Pediatrics.* 2003; 111:908-10.

Gartner LM, Morton J, Lawrence RA, *et al.* Breastfeeding and the use of human milk. *Pediatrics.* 2005; 115:496-506.

Ghannam NN, Hammami MM, Bakheet SM, *et al.* Bone mineral density of the spine and femur in healthy Saudi females: relation to vitamin D status, pregnancy and lactation. *Calcif Tissue Int.* 1999; 65:23-28.

Gies P, Roy C, Javorniczky J, *et al.* Global solar UV index: Australian measurements, forecasts and comparison with the UK. *Photocem Photobiol.* 2004; 79:32-39.

Giovannucci E. The epidemiology of vitamin D and cancer incidence and mortality: A review (United States). *Cancer Causes Control.* 2005; 16:83-95.

Goswami R, Gupta N, Goswami D, *et al.* Prevalence and significance of low 25-hydroxyvitamin D concentrations in healthy subjects in Delhi. *Am J Clin Nutr.* 2000; 72:472-75.

Grant WB, Holick MF. Benefits and requirements of vitamin D for optimal health: a review. *Altern Med Rev.* 2005; 10:94-111.

Grant WB. An estimate of premature cancer mortality in the U.S. due to inadequate doses of solar ultraviolet-B radiation. *Cancer.* 2002; 94:1867-75.

Grant WB. Health benefits of solar UV-B radiation through the production of vitamin D. *Photochem Photobiol Sci.* 2003; 2:1307-8.

Greer FR, Hollis BW, Cirpps DJ, *et al.* Effects of maternal ultraviolet B irradiation on vitamin D content of human milk. *J Pediatr.* 1984; 105:431-33.

Greer FR, Hollis BW, Napoli JL. High concentrations of vitamin D2 in human milk associated with pharmacologic doses of vitamin D2. *J Pediatr.* 1984; 105:61-64.

Greer FR, Marshall S. Bone mineral content, serum vitamin D metabolite concentrations, and ultraviolet B light exposure in infants fed human milk with and without vitamin D2 supplements. *J Pediatr.* 1989; 114:204-12.

Greer FR, Searcy JE, Levin RS, *et al.* Bone mineral content and serum 25-hydroxyvitamin D concentration in breast-fed infants with and without supplemental vitamin D. *J Pediatr.* 1981; 98:696-701.

Greer FR, Searcy JE, Levin RS, *et al.* Bone mineral content and serum 25-hydroxyvitamin D concentrations in breast-fed infants with and without supplemental vitamin D: one-year follow-up. *J Pediatr.* 1982; 100:919-22.

Greer FR. Issues in establishing vitamin D recommendations for infants and children. *Am J Clin Nutr.* 2004; 80(Suppl):1759S-62S.

Greer FR. Vitamin D deficiency- its more than just rickets. *J Pediatr.* 2003; 143:422-23.

Harkness L, Cromer B. Low levels of 25-hydroxy vitamin D are associated with elevated pararthyroid hormone in healthy adolescent females. *Osteoporos Int.* 2005; 16:109-13.

Harris RS, Bunker JWM. Vitamin D potency of human breast milk. *Am J Public Hlth.* 1939; 29:744-47.

Harris SS, Dawson-Hughes B. Seasonal changes in plasma 25-hydroxyvitamin D concentrations of young American black and white women. *Am J Clin Nutr.* 1998; 67:1232-36.

Hatun S, Islam O, Cizmecioglu F, *et al.* Subclinical vitamin D deficiency is increased in adolescent girls who wear concealing clothing. *J Nutr.* 2005; 135:218-22.

Heaney RP. Long-latency deficiency disease: insights from calcium and vitamin D. *Am J Clin Nutr.* 2003; 78:912-19.

Heaney RP. The vitamin D requirement in health and disease. *J Steroid Biochem Mol Biol.* 2005; 97:13-19.

Holick MF. McCollum award lecture, 1994: Vitamin D- new horizons for the 21st century. *Am J Clin Nutr.* 1994; 60:619-30.

Holick MF. Vitamin D: the underappreciated D-lightful hormone that is important for skeletal and cellular health. *Curr Opin Endocrinol Diabetes.* 2002; 9:87-98.

Holick MF. Vitamin D: photobiology, metabolism, mechanism of action and clinical applications. In: Favus MJ. *Primer on the metabolic bone diseases and disorders of mineral metabolism.* 5th Ed. Washington, DC: American Society of Bone and Mineral Metabolism; 2003.

Holick MF. Sunlight and vitamin D for bone health and prevention of autoimmune diseases, cancers, and cardiovascular disease. *Am J Clin Nutr.* 2004; 80(suppl):1678S-88S.

Holick MF. The vitamin D epidemic and its health consequences. *J Nutr.* 2005; 135:2739S-2748S.

Holick MF, Frommer JE, McNeill SC, *et al.* Photometabolism of 7-dehydrocholesterol to previtamin D3 in skin. *Biochem Biophys Res Commun.* 1977; 76:107-14.

Holick MF, MacLaughlin JA, Clark MB, *et al.* Photosynthesis of previtamin D3 in human skin and the physiologic consequences. *Science.* 1980; 210:203-5.

Holick MF, MacLaughlin JA, Doppelt SH. Regulation of cutaneous previtamin D3 photosynthesis in man: skin pigment is not an essential regulator. *Science.* 1981; 211:590-93.

Hollis BW. Circulating 25-hydroxyvitamin D levels indicative of vitamin D sufficiency: implications for establishing a new effective dietary intake recommendation for vitamin D. *J Nutr.* 2005; 135:317-22.

Hollis BW, Pittard WB, Reinhardt TA. Relationships among vitamin D, 25-hydroxyvitamin D, and vitamin D-binding protein concentrations in the plasma and milk of human subjects. *J Clin Endocrinol Metab.* 1986; 62:41-44.

Hollis BW, Roos BA, Draper HH, *et al.* Vitamin D and its metabolites in human and bovine milk. *J Nutr.* 1981; 111:1240-48.

Hollis BW, Wagner CL. Vitamin D requirements during lactation: high-dose maternal supplementation as therapy to prevent hypovitaminosis D for both the mother and the nursing infant. *Am J Clin Nutr.* 2004; 80(suppl):1752S-58S.

Hollis BW, Wagner CL. Normal serum vitamin D levels. *NEJM.* 2005; 352:515-16.

Hoogenboezem T, Degenhart HJ, De Muinck SMPF, *et al.* Vitamin D metabolism in breast-fed infants and their mothers. *Pediatr Res.* 1989; 25:623-28.

Horst RL, Reinhardt TA, Reddy GS. Vitamin D metabolism. In: Feldman D, Pike JW, Glorieux FH. *Vitamin D.* Elsevier; 2005.

Hypponen E. Micronutrients and the risk of type 1 diabetes: vitamin D, vitamin E, and nicotinamide. *Nutr Rev.* 2004; 62:340-47.

Hypponen E, Laara E, Reunanen A, *et al.* Intake of vitamin D and risk of type I diabetes: a birth-cohort study. *Lancet* 2001; 358:1500-3.

John EM, Schwartz GG, Dreon DM, *et al.* Vitamin D and breast cancer risk: the NHANES I epidemiologic follow-up study, 1971-1975 to 1992. *Cancer Epidemiol Biomarkers Prev.* 1999; 8:399-406.

Katz A, Sluss PM, Lewandrwsli KB. Normal serum vitamin D levels. *NEJM.* 2005; 352:515-16.

Kollias N. The physical basis of skin color. *Clinics in Dermatology.* 1995; 13:361-67.

Kreiter SR, Schwartz RP, Kirkman HN, *et al.* Nutritional rickets in African American breast-fed infants. *J Pediatr.* 2000; 137:153-57.

Kruse K. Pathophysiology of calcium metabolism in children with vitamin D-deficiency rickets. *J Pediatr.* 1995; 126:736-41.

Ladizesky M, Lu Z, Oliveri B, *et al.* Solar ultraviolet B radiation and photoproduction of vitamin D3 in central and southern areas of Argentina. *J Bone Miner Res.* 1995; 10:545-49.

Lamberg-Allardt C. Vitamin D in foods and as supplements. *Prog Biophys Mol Biol.* 2006; 92:33-38.

Lamberg-Allardt CJ, Outila TA, Karkkainien MU, *et al.* Vitamin D deficiency and bone health in healthy adults in Finland: could this be a concern in other parts of Europe? *J Bone Miner Res.* 2001; 16:2066-73.

Lapatsanis D, Moulas A, Cholevas V, *et al.* Vitamin D: a necessity for children and adolescents in Greece. *Calcif Tissue Int.* 2005; 77:348-55.

Lebrun JB, Moffatt MEK, Mundy RJT, *et al.* Vitamin D deficiency in a Manitoba community. *Can J Public Health.* 1993; 84:394-96.

Li YC, Qiao G, Uskokovic M, *et al.* Vitamin D: a negative endocrine regulator of the renin-angiotensin system and blood pressure. *J Steroid Biochem Mol Biol.* 2004; 89-90:387-92.

Lips P. How to define normal values for serum concentrations of 25-hydroxyvitamin D? An Overview. In: Feldman D, Pike JW, Glorieux FH. *Vitamin D.* Elsevier; 2005.

Liu PT, Stenger S, Li H, *et al.* Toll-like receptor triggering of a vitamin D-mediated human antimicrobial response. *Science.* 2006; 311:1770-73.

Looker AC, Dawson-Hughes B, Calvo MS, *et al.* Serum 25-hydroxyvitamin D status of adolescents and adults in two seasonal subpopulations from NHANES III. *Bone.* 2002; 30:771-77.

Maiya S, Allgrove J, Mok Q, *et al.* Vitamin D deficiency and mortality and serious morbidity in infancy: time for action. *Arch Dis Child.* 2006; 91(Suppl 1):A71.

Markestad T, Kolmannskog S, Arntzen L, *et al.* Serum concentrations of vitamin D metabolites in exclusively breast-fed infants at 70 degrees north. *Act Paediatr Scand.* 1984; 73:29-32.

Mathieu C, Badenhoop K. Vitamin D and type I diabetes mellitus: state of the art. *Trends Endocrinol Metab.* 2005; 16:261-66.

Matsuoka LY, Wortsman J, Haddad JG, *et al.* Racial pigmentation and the cutaneous synthesis of vitamin D. *Arch Dermatol.* 1991; 127:536-38.

Matsuoka LY, Wortsman J, Hollis BW. Use of topical sunscreen for the evaluation of regional synthesis of vitamin D3. *J Am Acad Dermatol.* 1990; 22:772-75.

McCollum EV, Simmonds N, Becket JE, *et al.* Studies on experimental rickets. XXI. An experimental demonstration of the existence of a vitamin, which promotes calcium deposition. *J Biol Chem.* 1922; 53:293-312.

Meddeb N, Sahli H, Chahed M, *et al.* Vitamin D deficiency in Tunisia. *Osteporos Int.* 2005; 16:180-83.

Meier C, Woitge H, Witte K, *et al.* Supplementation with oral vitamin D3 and calcium during winter prevents seasonal bone loss: A randomized controlled open-label prospective trial. *J Bone Mineral Res.* 2004; 19:1221-30.

Mylott BM, Kump T, Bolton ML, *et al.* Rickets in the dairy state. *Wisc Med J.* 2004; 103:84-87.

Namgung R, Tsang RC, Lee C, *et al.* Low total body mineral bone content and high bone resorption in Korean winter-born versus summer-born newborn infants. *J Pediatr.* 1998; 132:421-25.

National Public Health Institute, Nutrition Unit. Fineli. *Finnish food composition database. Release 6.* Helsinki 2006. Available from: http://www.ktl.fi/fineli/.

Nesby-O'Dell S, Scanlon KS, Cogswell ME, *et al.* Hypovitaminosis D prevalence and determinants among African American and white women of reproductive age: Third National Health and Nutrition Examination Survey, 1988-1994. *Am J Clin Nutr.* 2002; 76:187-92.

Nowson CA, Margeison C. Vitamin D intake and vitamin D status of Australians. *Med J Aust.* 2002; 177:149-52.

Park E. The etiology of rickets. *Physiol Rev.* 1923; 3:106-19.

Peller S, Stephenson CS. Skin irritation and cancer in the United States Navy. *Am J Med Sci.* 1937; 194:326-33.

Peterlik M, Cross HS. Vitamin D and calcium deficits predispose for multiple chronic diseases. *Eur J Clin Invest.* 2005; 35:290-304.

Pettifor JM. Rickets and vitamin D deficiency in children and adolescents. *Endocrinol Metab Clin North Am.* 2005; 34:537-53.

Pike RL, Reinhardt TA, Reddy GS. Vitamin D metabolism. In: Feldman D, Pike JW, Glorieux FH. *Vitamin D.* Elsevier; 2005.

Raisz LG. Pathogenesis of osteoporosis: concepts, conflicts and prospects. *J Clin Invest.* 2005; 115:3318-25.

Raiten DJ, Picciano MF. Vitamin D and health in the 21st century: bone and beyond. Executive summary. *Am J Clin Nutr.* 2004; 80(suppl):1673S-77S.

Roberts CC, Chan GM, Folland D, *et al.* Adequate bone mineralization in breast-fed infants. *J Pediatr.* 1981; 99:192-96.

Robinson PD, Hogler W, Craig ME, *et al.* The re-emerging burden of rickets: a decade of experience from Sydney. *Arch Dis Child.* 2006; 91:564-68.

Rothberg AD, Pettifor JM, Cohen DF, *et al.* Maternal-infant vitamin D relationships during breast-feeding. *J Pediatr.* 1982; 101:500-3.

Scientific Committee for Food (SCF). *Nutrient intakes for the European community.* Luxembourg: Office for Official Publications of the European Communitities; 1993.

Shaw NJ. Vitamin D deficiency rickets. *Endocr Dev.* 2003; 6:93-104.

Specker BL, Ho ML, Oestreich A, *et al.* Prospective study of vitamin D supplementation and rickets in China. *J Pediatr.* 1992; 120:733-39.

Specker BL, Tsang RC, Hollis BW. Effect of race and diet on human-milk vitamin D and 25-hydroxyvitamin D. *Am J Dis Child.* 1985; 139:1134-37.

Scientific Committee on Food. *Report of the Scientific Committee on Food on the revision of reference values for nutrition labelling.* European Commission. Health and Consumer Protection Directorate-General. 6 March 2003. Available from: http://europa.eu.int/comm/food/fs/sc/scf/index_en.html.

Standing Committee on the Scientific Evaluation of Dietary Reference Intakes, Food and Nutrition Board, Institute of Medicine. *Dietary reference intakes for calcium, phosphorus, magnesium, vitamin D and fluoride.* National Academy Press; 1997.

Stumpf WE, Sar M, Reid FA, *et al.* Target cells for 1,25-dihydroxyvitamin D3 in intestinal tract, stomach, kidney, skin, pituitary and parathyroid. *Science.* 1979; 206:1188-90.

Takeuchi A, Okano T, Tsugawa N, *et al.* Effects of ergocalciferol supplementation on the concentration of vitamin D and its metabolites in human milk. *J Nutr.* 1989; 119:1639-46.

Tangpricha V, Pearce EN, Chen TC. Vitamin D insufficiency among free-living healthy young adults. *Am J Med.* 2002; 112:659-62.

Trang HM, Cole DE, Rubin LA, *et al.* Evidence that vitamin D3 increases serum 25-hydroxyvitamin D more efficiently than does vitamin D2. *Am J Clin Nutr.* 1998; 68:854-58.

Trump DL, Hershberger PA, Bernardi RJ, *et al.* Anti-tumor activity of calcitriol: pre-clinical and clinical studies. *J Steroid Biochem Mol Biol.* 2004; 89-90:519-26.

U.S. Department of Agriculture, Agricultural Research Service. USDA *nutrient database for standard reference.* Release 18;

2005. Nutrient Data Laboratory Home Page. Available from: http://www.ars.usda.gov/ba/bhnrc/ndl.

van Etten E, Mathieu C. Immunoregulation by 1,25-dihydroxyvitamin D3: basic concepts. *J Steroid Biochem Mol Biol.* 2005; 97:93-101.

van Leeuwen JPTM, Pols HA. Vitamin D: Cancer and differentiation. In: Feldman D, Pike JW, Glorieux FH. *Vitamin D*. Elsevier; 2005.

Vieth R. Why the optimal requirement for vitamin D3 is probably much higher than what is officially recommended for adults. *J Steroid Biochem Mol Biol.* 2004; 89-90:575-79.

Vieth R. Chapter 61: The pharmacology of vitamin D, including fortification strategies. In: Feldman D, Pike JW, Glorieux FH. *Vitamin D*. Elsevier; 2005.

Vieth R. What is the optimal vitamin D status for health? *Prog Biophys Mol Biol.* 2006; 92:26-32.

Vieth R, Chan PC, Macfarlane GD. Efficacy and safety of vitamin D3 intake exceeding the lowest observed adverse effect level. *Am J Clin Nutr.* 2001; 73.288-94.

Wagner CL, Hulsey TC, Fanning D, *et al.* High dose vitamin D3 supplementation in a cohort of breastfeeding mothers and their infants: a 6-month follow-up study. *Breastfeeding Medicine.* 2006; 1:59-70.

Webb AR, DeCosta BR, Holick MF. Sunlight regulates the cutaneous production of vitamin D3 by causing its photodegradation. *J Clin Endocrinol Metab.* 1989; 68:882-87.

Webb AR, Kline L, Holick MF. Influence of season and latitude on the cutaneous synthesis of vitamin D3: exposure to winter sunlight in Boston and Edmonton will not promote vitamin D3 synthesis in human skin. J *Clin Endocrinol Metab.* 1988; 67:373-78.

Webb AR. Who, what, where and when- influences on cutaneous vitamin D synthesis. *Prog Biophys Mol Biol.* 2006; 92:17-25.

Weiler H, Fitzpatrick-Wong S, Veitch R, *et al.* Vitamin D deficiency and whole-body and femur bone mass relative to weight in healthy newborns. *CMAJ.* 2005; 172:757-61.

Weisberg P, Scanlon KS, Li R, *et al.* Nutritional rickets among children in the United States: review of cases reported between 1986 and 2003. *Am J Clin Nutr.* 2004; 80(suppl):1697S-705S.

Welch TR, Bergstrom WH, Tsang RC. Vitamin D-deficient rickets: the reemergence of a once-conquered disease. *J Pediatr.* 2000; 137:143-45.

Whiting SJ, Calvo MS. Dietary recommendations to meet both endocrine and autocrine needs of vitamin D. *J Steroid Biochem Mol Biol.* 2005; 97:7-12.

Zeitz U, Weber K, Soegiarto DW, *et al.* Impaired insulin secretory capacity in mice lacking a functional vitamin D receptor. *FASEB J.* 2003; 17:509-11.

Zinser GM, Packman K, Welsh J. Accelerated mammary gland development during pregnancy and delayed postlactational involution in vitamin D3 receptor null mice. *Mol Endocrinol.* 2004; 18:2208-23.

Zittermann A. Vitamin D in preventative medicine: are we ignoring the evidence? *Br J Nutr.* 2003; 89:552-72.

SECTION VI

MEDICATIONS

Chapter 24

The Transfer of Medications into Human Milk

Thomas W. Hale, Judith H. Kristensen, and Kenneth F. Ilett

ALVEOLAR SUBUNIT OF THE BREAST

Human milk is a complex mixture composed of thousands of substances including proteins, peptides, lipids, carbohydrates, cytokines, and living cells, such as macrophages, leukocytes, stem cells, and other cellular species. These substances exist in several compartments: an aqueous phase containing water-soluble components, colloidal dispersions of proteins (casein), oil-in-water emulsions of triglyceride-rich fat globules, and living cells (macrophages, lymphocytes, leukocytes, etc).

During pregnancy, the human breast undergoes a massive change which includes the migration of ductal tissues from the nipple through the naive breast thoracic fat pads and connective tissue to form a tree-like structure within the fatty tissue. The forming ducts canalize themselves through the fat pad during the first and second trimester of pregnancy, ultimately ending in extensive lobulo-alveolar clusters, lined by the alveolar epithelium which actually creates milk (Neville, 2001).

The terminal ends of the ductal tissues resemble a cluster of grapes. The marked proliferation of ductal and alveolar epithelium is largely dependent on elevated levels of prolactin, estrogen, and progesterone. Studies in knockout mice suggest that removal of the receptor sites for any of these hormones blocks development of milk-secreting alveolar tissues (Brisken *et al.*, 2000, Miyoshi *et al.*, 2002). Because only 10-15 ducts terminate at the nipple, the breast is therefore subdivided into numerous lobulo-alveolar clusters, each of which is drained by an individual ductal system.

The alveolus in each lobulo-alveolar cluster is lined with a single layer of polarized epithelial cells (now termed lactocytes) which are ultimately responsible for the creation of milk (McManaman *et al.*, 2003). Each alveolus is surrounded by a supporting connective tissue stroma. On top of this stroma is a basket-like layer of specialized smooth muscle or "myoepithelial" cells. The myoepithelial cells contain receptors for oxytocin, and on release of oxytocin from the mother's posterior pituitary,

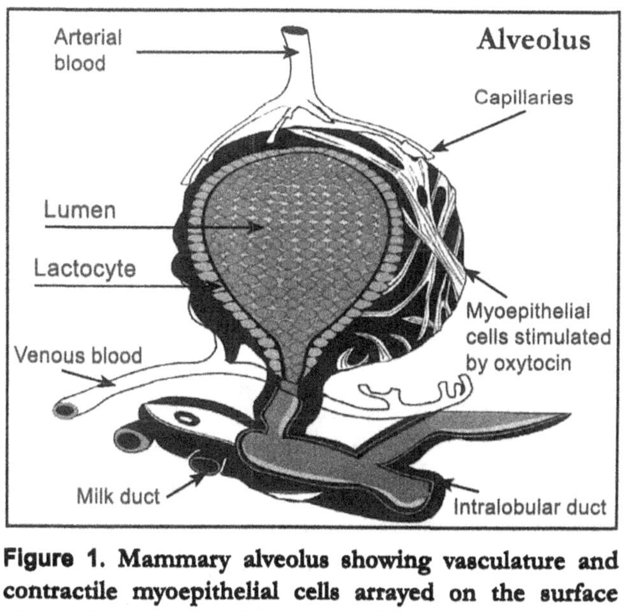

Figure 1. Mammary alveolus showing vasculature and contractile myoepithelial cells arrayed on the surface along with the intralobular duct. The secretory alveolar epithelia (lactocytes) line the interior of the alveolus.

the myoepithelial cell contracts thus forcing milk into the ductal system toward the nipple (milk ejection or letdown).

THE ALVEOLAR EPITHELIUM

Secretory differentiation of the breast tissue begins around mid-pregnancy. The initial phase is characterized by growth in number and size of the alveolar epithelium (**Figure 1**). At this time, alveolar cells start producing small amounts of secretions containing lactose and selected proteins, including α-lactalbumin (Arthur *et al.*, 1991; Cox *et al.*, 1999). The production of this *pre-milk* is limited, probably due to high circulating levels of progesterone.

From early gestation until parturition, the endocrine system coordinates development of the mammary gland. As levels of estrogen, progesterone, placental lactogen, oxytocin, and prolactin increase during gestation, they act directly on mammary tissue to stimulate ductal growth, alveolar cell proliferation, and development. During gestation, a significant amount of lactose is secreted from the alveolar cells, but having nowhere to go, diffuses back into the maternal plasma and is excreted in the urine. It is apparent that the primary inhibiting factor that prevents milk production is the high level of plasma progesterone. Once the placenta is delivered and progesterone/estrogen levels drop rapidly, milk production by the lactocyte ensues.

Each alveolus is lined with secretory epithelial lactocytes. The cytoplasm of each epithelial cell is filled with a large nucleus, numerous mitochondria and an extensive rough endoplasmic reticulum. A complete Golgi apparatus is located near the luminal (apical) surface of the cell (Clermont *et al.*, 1993, Mather *et al.*, 1998). Milk proteins such as casein and α-lactalbumin, triglycerides, and phospholipids are synthesized by the endoplasmic reticulum, and packaged and secreted by the Golgi apparatus. Lactose, the major carbohydrate in human milk, is also synthesized and secreted by the Golgi. During milk production, fat globules migrate toward the luminal surface and then by exocytosis are expelled from the interior of the cell into the alveolar lumen. Milk proteins are packaged into secretory vesicles by the Golgi and then passed across the luminal membrane into milk. Water and a range of ions (Na^+, K^+, Mg^{++}, Ca^{++}, Cl^-, phosphate, and citrate) pass readily in both directions across the luminal membrane. For a thorough review of milk synthesis, see Neville (2001), McManaman *et al.* (2003), and Chapter 7 in this textbook.

LACTOGENESIS

Stage I - Colostrum

This occurs during pregnancy when the lactocyte initiates the secretion of small quantities of milk components, such as casein and lactose. After this stage has begun, the gland is sufficiently differentiated to secrete small quantities of a unique milk called colostrum (Neville, 2001). Colostrum contains rather high concentrations of protein, Na^+, Cl^-, immunoglobulins such as IgG, IgM, IgA, and lactoferrin. Because the lactocytes are small in size and without tight cell to cell junctions, lymphocytes, macrophages, and other cellular components easily transfer into colostrum. Casein and lactose are low in concentration at this stage. Production of colostrum generally lasts for two to three days postpartum when the transitional period ensues. In this period, there is a gradual change in composition from that of colostrum to that of mature milk. Transitional milk production starts after about three to four days postpartum when maternal progesterone and estrogen levels have reached their lowest point in plasma. During the period in which colostrum is produced, there are open-junctions between the lateral cell walls of adjacent lactocytes. Thus, drugs may pass through these gaps, as well as through the lactocytes to enter into milk. There have been few longitudinal studies of drug transfer into milk in the first few days of lactation. For example, the mean amount of the analgesic methadone available to the infant changes gradually from 6 μg on postnatal day one through to 84 μg on day four (Jansson *et al.*, 2007). This finding suggests that despite having both transcellular and paracellular avenues for drugs to access milk, the small volumes of colostrum (30-60 mL/day) and intermediate volumes of transitional milk (400-600 mL/day) produced in the first few days of lactation limit the quantity of drug that is able to be transferred.

Stage II - Transitional/ Mature Milk

Lactogenesis II starts early in the postnatal period. This phase is characterized by a major increase in milk protein synthesis, migration of the Golgi apparatus to the apical surface, induction of all major protein and lipid biosynthetic processes, and closure of the tight-junction complexes between the cells. This process is dependent on the rapid elimination of progesterone from the maternal plasma. The secretory alveolar epithelium undergoes a rapid increase in function within 48-72 hours of birth. With delivery of the placenta and the rapid decrease in blood levels of progesterone and estrogens, prolactin-mediated cell growth occurs rapidly, leading to enlargement of the alveolar cell (lactocyte) and closure of the open-junctions between these cells. Ultimately, this leads to trapping of lactose within the alveolar lumen. Water follows lactose producing increasing volumes of milk. Transitional milk is produced starting a few days after birth and progressing gradually to mature milk after about two weeks (Lawrence *et al.*, 2005).

Passage of Drugs Across the Alveolar Epithelium

Unfortunately, our understanding of the transport of proteins, lipids, and drugs across the apical membrane is not well defined. However, it is clear that the transport of lipids, proteins, and electrolytes is controlled by the alveolar cell, yielding milk with a uniform day to day composition. Electrolyte composition of human milk is tightly controlled once closure of the open-junctions between adjacent lactocytes occurs, and the composition (electrolyte) of milk varies little during the course of lactation.

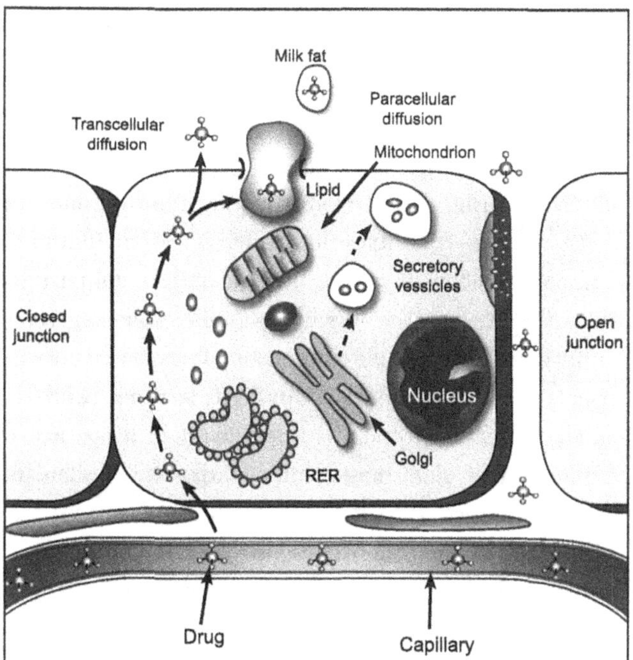

Figure 2. Diagrammatic representation of the pathways of milk secretion and the way in which drugs in plasma may traverse the lactocyte and enter milk.

The pathways for milk secretion and for drug transfer from plasma to milk are illustrated in **Figure 2.**

Drugs that are small and relatively lipid soluble, pass from the blood across the alveolar epithelium and into the alveolar ducts largely by passive diffusion. Drug transfer into the milk compartment is largely controlled by the physicochemical characteristics of the drug (its pKa, lipid solubility, molecular weight), patient characteristics (drug concentration in the maternal plasma, extent of protein binding, milk and plasma pH), and by the other constituents in milk (lipid content) (Hale *et al.*, 2002a). In the first one to two days after birth when colostrum is produced, the junctions between adjacent epithelial cells are still open, allowing diffusion of both small drug molecules and large proteins through the open cell junctions and into the milk (*paracellular* pathway). As the junctions between the epithelial cells close (day two onwards), passive diffusion (*transcellular* pathway) becomes the predominant method for transfer of small lipid soluble molecules such as drugs. In general, large molecular weight drugs and proteins do not penetrate through the epithelial cells in to milk in clinically relevant amounts.

PASSIVE DIFFUSION AS A PATHWAY FOR DRUG TRANSFER INTO MILK

The major factors influencing passive diffusion of drugs into milk are discussed below. It is important to remember that while individual factors are important for individual drugs, it is the combination of several factors that will ultimately determine the amount of drug transfer into milk.

Molecular Weight of the Drug

The passive diffusion of drugs across the lactocyte membranes is a function of the molecular weight of the drug. Basically, the smaller the drug, the more likely it is to diffuse into milk. A medication such as lithium with no protein binding and a very low molecular weight (6.94 daltons) readily transfers into milk (Sykes *et al.*, 1976). Small lipophilic drug molecules (200-400 daltons) also readily diffuse into milk, providing other factors, such as protein binding, pH, and pKa, are permissive. Conversely, large drug molecules with high molecular weights, such as heparin (12,000-15,000 daltons), do not passively diffuse into milk. However, this is not to say that all large molecules cannot penetrate into milk. Active transport systems and receptor-mediated endocytosis provide mechanisms of access for some large endogenous molecules. For example, insulin is normally transported into breastmilk (range 7-306 mU/L) from nondiabetic mothers (Koldovsky, 1995; Kulski *et al.*, 1983). The mechanism by which insulin transfers from the blood into milk is unclear. However it is probably transported into the lactocytes by receptor-mediated endocytosis, as has been demonstrated in some vascular endothelial cells (Wang *et al.*, 2006). Once inside the lactocyte, insulin may be packaged by the golgi and secreted with other components of milk. In addition, since insulin is administered as replacement therapy, its plasma levels after exogenous use are of similar magnitude to those resulting from normal endogenous insulin production (5-40 mU/L) (Verge, 2004). Hence, exogenous insulin can be expected to be subject to the same tightly controlled cellular regulation and disposition as endogenous insulin. Other large molecular weight proteins from the maternal plasma compartment are also transported or at least diffuse into milk to a limited degree. These include insulin growth factor, prolactin, and many others.

Drug Concentration in the Maternal Circulation and Protein Binding in Plasma

Both *passive* diffusion and *paracellular* diffusion processes are driven by the concentration of drug in the plasma. High concentrations favor passage from plasma into milk, while low concentrations do not. Many small drug molecules (e.g., 300 daltons) are able to reversibly associate with plasma proteins, such as albumin (67,000 daltons). This leads to an equilibrium between drug *bound* to protein (high molecular weight; e.g., 67,300 daltons) and drug that is not bound to protein (*free drug*) (molecular weight still 300 daltons) in the plasma. Only the low molecular weight *free* drug is able to passively diffuse across the lactocyte membrane into milk. Hence, drugs that are highly and/or avidly bound to plasma proteins are often largely retained in the plasma compartment, thus restricting the extent of their distribution into milk. The NSAID celecoxib is an example of a drug with high protein binding (97%), poor transfer into milk (milk/plasma ratio (M/P)=0.23), and a low relative infant dose (0.3%) (Hale *et al.*, 2004). By contrast, drugs which have low plasma protein binding will have higher free concentrations in plasma and an increased opportunity to distribute into milk. The antiepileptic, levetiracetam, is an example of a drug with low protein binding (<10%), where milk levels are similar to those in plasma (M/P =1.05), and the relative infant dose (8%) is larger (Tomson *et al.*, 2007). Thus, a drug with high protein binding (low *free* drug concentrations *in vivo*) is unlikely to transfer into milk in significant amounts.

Milk pH and Drug pKa

The pKa of a drug is a unique physicochemical property that controls its ionization state. When the pH of the environment in which the drug is placed (e.g., milk or plasma) is the same as its pKa, 50% of the drug exists with a positive or negative charge (*ionized*) and 50% is *unionized*. As the environmental pH moves away from the pKa, the ratio of *ionized* and *unionized* drug species changes. This is important because only the drug in the *unionized* state can passively diffuse from the plasma across the lactocyte membrane into the milk. The mean pH of milk is around 7.2, which is a little lower than that of plasma (7.4). The pKa for some basic drugs (e.g., those with ionizable NH_2 functional groups) is such that they tend to accumulate in milk where they are trapped in their *ionized* form at the slightly lower pH of milk. This phenomenon is called *ion trapping,* and it partly explains why many basic drugs accumulate in milk.

Lipid Solubility of the Drug and Co-transport into Milk

The lipid content of milk can vary significantly (1-20%) due to diet and other factors (Lawrence *et al.*, 2005). It is also well recognized that the lipid content of milk increases during a feed from a low level in foremilk (e.g. 2-3%) to two to three-fold higher levels in hindmilk. The lipophilicity of a drug is measured as its partition ratio (P) between the highly lipophilic solvent octanol and water. Because the numerical values for P can vary over several orders of magnitude, it is often expressed as $\log_{10}P$. Values of $\log_{10}P$ for individual drugs can be experimentally determined in the laboratory or calculated from theoretical considerations of the physicochemical properties of the drug of interest (ACD I Lab Software available at: http://www.acdlabs.com/download/logp.html).

Drugs with high lipophilicity tend to dissolve more readily in the lactocyte membranes and hence have increased opportunity to passively diffuse through the lactocyte into the milk. They can also accumulate in lipid droplets within the lactocyte and ultimately be co-transported into milk within the lipid secretions (Atkinson *et al.*, 1988). The antidepressant mirtazapine provides a good example of lipid-dependent transfer into milk. The concentration of mirtazapine in hindmilk was 2.3 times higher than in foremilk, corresponding to a mean creamatocrits of 13.7% and 6.2% in hind- and foremilk, respectively (Kristensen *et al.*, 2007). Its metabolite desmethylmirtazapine also showed a similar lipid-dependant distribution into milk. High lipid solubility ($\log_{10}P$ for mirtazapine=2.74) and co-transport in milk lipids provides an explanation for these observations.

Bioavailability of Drugs in Mother and Infant

The concentration of drug in maternal plasma is a function of the dose, its bioavailability, and the maternal clearance of the drug by the liver and kidneys. The bioavailability of a medication refers to the proportion of a dose that reaches the systemic circulation after its administration by a non IV route. This can vary somewhat with the route of administration (oral, IV, IM, SC, topically). Drugs administered orally are absorbed directly into the portal circulation and pass through the liver on their way into the general circulation. The liver often sequesters or metabolizes such medications, thus decreasing their bioavailability. Medications applied topically (e.g., to skin, eye) may have low bioavailability because their dose is low (intended for local effect only), and/or their absorption is limited. In addition, some drugs have low or no bioavailability because their physicochemical makeup does not allow them to be absorbed (e.g., large proteins), and/or because they are chemically unstable in the acid pH of the stomach (e.g., insulin). Hence, bioavailability in the mother is important since it is a major determinant of drug concentration in the plasma, which in turn is the driving force for drug transfer into milk.

Because infants receive drugs via the mother's milk, oral bioavailability in the infant is important for determining how much drug reaches the systemic circulation. The acidic pH in the infant's stomach can chemically degrade some drugs and thereby limit their bioavailability (e.g., omeprazole). In neonates, gastric emptying time is delayed and intestinal absorption irregular and in some cases limited (Besunder *et al.*, 1988a; Besunder *et al.*, 1988b). Slower intestinal absorption tends to be advantageous, as this would tend

Table 1. Maternal Medications that are Low Risk for the Breastfed Infant

Drug	Molecular weight (Daltons)	Oral bioavailability in adults (%)	Comment
Gentamicin (and related aminoglycosides)	478	Insignificant.	Inactivated by first-pass metabolism in the liver. Administered IM.
Omeprazole	345	60	Chemically unstable in stomach pH. Extensive metabolism by hepatic CYP's. Half-life is about 1-1.2 hours.
Lansoprazole	369	80	Chemically unstable in stomach pH. Extensive metabolism by hepatic CYP's. Half-life is about 1 hour.
Pantoprazole	405	77	Chemically unstable in stomach pH. Extensive metabolism by hepatic CYP's. Half-life is about 1 hour.
Salbutamol (and related inhaled b_2-agonists)	239	Insignificant.	Inactivated by first-pass metabolism in the gut and liver. Administered by metered aerosol inhalation.
Fluticasone (and related inhaled corticosteroids)	500	<0.5	Administered by metered aerosol inhalation to avoid systemic exposure.
Cefpirome (and other 3rd generation cephalosporins	482	Not absorbed.	Administered IV.
Insulin	5,808	Not absorbed.	Chemically unstable at pH of gut contents. Administered IV, SC mainly.
Etanercept (recombinant TNFα fusion protein)	51,235	Not absorbed.	Decomposed by gut pH and enzymes. Administered SC.
Heparin	12,000-15,000	Not absorbed.	Administered SC or IV.
Interferon-α and interferon-β	Approx 20,000	Not absorbed.	Decomposed by gut pH and enzymes. Administered SC.
Infliximab (TNFα neutralizing monoclonal antibody)	144,190	Not absorbed.	Decomposed by gut pH and enzymes. Administered IV.

to keep drug plasma concentrations lower in the infant.

Table 1 summarizes examples of medications that are unlikely to cause problems in a breastfed infant as a result of low or no bioavailability. In some instances, the drugs have low or no oral bioavailability in adults (mothers) because of their large molecular weight (e.g., infliximab) or because they are chemically degraded in the gastrointestinal tract (e.g., insulin). Low or no absorption in a mother means low or no transfer to milk and compatibility with breastfeeding. In other cases, drugs such as omeprazole, lansoprazole, and pantoprazole have low bioavailability in the infant because they are chemically degraded by the stomach acid. They have moderate to good bioavailability in adults because they are formulated as tablets that disintegrate and are absorbed only when they reach the intestine. In addition, these three drugs are also rapidly cleared from the maternal circulation by hepatic metabolism, leading to less opportunity for their transfer to milk. Quantitative examples for such drugs are sparse, but a mother who took 40 mg of pantoprazole daily had a M/P ratio of 0.02, and her breastfed infant received only 0.14% of her weight-adjusted dose (Plante *et al.*, 2004).

However, even low exposure to some medications may cause adverse effects in breastfed infants. For example, diarrhea and thrush are common complications following the maternal use of some antibiotics, even though the dose received via milk is small (Ilett *et al.*, 2006). (See also Chapter 28.)

ACTIVE TRANSPORT AS A MECHANISM FOR DRUG TRANSFER INTO MILK

Although most drug transport into milk can be explained by passive diffusion, a review of the literature shows that there are a few drugs where the measured milk transfer assessed as M/P ratio is significantly larger than would be predicted by passive diffusion. These observations suggest that active transport may enhance the passage of these drugs across the lactocytes.

For example, the predicted mean M/P for nitrofurantoin in human milk was 0.28, compared to an observed mean M/P of 6 (Gerk *et al.*, 2001a). Active transport has also been demonstrated for nitrofurantoin in lactating rats (Gerk *et al.*, 2001b; Kari *et al.*, 1997), and in cultured lactocytes (Gerk *et al.*, 2003; Toddywalla *et al.*, 1997). In addition, the M/P for cimetidine in human milk was 5.5 times higher than that predicted (Oo *et al.*, 1995). Alcorn and McNamara have shown that acyclovir accumulated in rat milk by active transport, whereas transport of ganciclovir and zidovudine into milk was consistent with a passive diffusion process (Alcorn *et al.*, 2002b). It has also been suggested that active transport may be involved in the distribution of acyclovir into human milk (Lau *et al.*, 1987), but *in vitro* experiments subsequently showed that passive diffusion provided an adequate explanation (Bork *et al.*, 2000). Thus, it seems that active transport probably functions for only a few selected drugs. Nevertheless, there may be a wider role for active transport as gene expression of numerous transport proteins in human lactocytes has been demonstrated (Alcorn *et al.*, 2002a; Ito *et al.*, 2003). Using real-time RT-PCR, these authors screened for gene transcripts expression in an epithelial cell-enriched fraction from human milk and in a similarly processed fraction from breast tissues from non-lactating women (representing non-lactating epithelial cells). Of 30 genes examined, 19 were detectable either in lactating mammary epithelia or both lactating and non-lactating mammary epithelia. The lactating human mammary gland epithelia expressed the transporters OCT1, OCT3/EMT, OCTN1, and OCTN2, but not OCT2. There was substantial up-regulation of OCT1 expression in the lactating mammary gland compared to the non-lactating epithelia. Messenger RNA transcripts of CNT1, CNT3, ENT1, and ENT3 were also detected in lactating mammary gland epithelia. Both PEPT1 and PEPT2 were expressed in the lactating human mammary gland. Lactating mammary epithelial cells also expressed transcripts for MRP1, MRP2, and MRP5, but not for MRP3 and MRP4. Finally, MDR1 mRNA, the gene encoding for the drug transporter P-glycoprotein (P-gP), was also detected, but lactation appeared to down-regulate its expression.

It is also possible that active transport could be involved in limiting the entry of drugs into breastmilk, for example, P-gP codes for an efflux transporter located in either apical or basolateral epithelial membranes (Raub, 2006). Passage of some drugs across the blood-brain epithelial barrier is limited by P-gP, while in the gut P-gP functions to limit absorption of other drugs across the intestinal epithelial barrier. A possible role for P-gP in the transport of the antiviral drug, nelfinavir, into milk has been investigated in lactating rats (Edwards *et al.*, 2005) because the observed M/P (0.56) was lower than anticipated from its high lipid solubility ($\log_{10}P=4.1$). Their study showed that P-gP was expressed in mammary epithelium, but nelfinavir transport into milk was not blocked by the specific inhibitor GF120981, indicating that P-gP did not have a significant role in nelfinavir transport in this model. In addition, studies (Briggs *et al.*, 2005a; Gardiner *et al.*, 2003a; Hale *et al.*, 2002b) of the antidiabetic drug, metformin, have reported low mean M/P values (0.63, 0.35, and 0.46, respectively) and a flat milk concentration-time profile. Assuming a passive diffusion model (Begg *et al.*, 1992), the theoretical M/P for metformin was 2.93 (Hale *et al.*, 2002b). The lower observed M/P may indicate the effects of an active "efflux" transporter pumping metformin out of milk and back into the blood (Gardiner *et al.*, 2003a). Support for this hypothesis comes from the observation that metformin is a substrate for the OCT1 and OCT2 organic cation transporters in human kidney (Kimura *et al.*, 2005) and that OCT1 is expressed in human mammary gland epithelium (Alcorn *et al.*, 2002a).

In summary, active transport is a novel and interesting mechanism that may play a role in drug transport across the lactocyte membrane. Presently, only a few drugs are transported into human milk by active transport and the significance of such transport for infant exposure has not been determined.

MILK/PLASMA (M/P) RATIO

The ratio of the concentration of drug in milk to that in plasma is known as the milk:plasma (M/P) ratio. The primary use of M/P is in quantifying the extent of drug transfer into milk and giving some indication of the underlying mechanisms. M/P has no role in assessing drug safety in breastfeeding. The concentration of a drug in milk (C_{milk}) is the determinant of infant exposure, which in turn can be used to assess safety. M/P can be used to calculate milk drug concentration when only maternal plasma concentration is known. However, given that modern analytical methods can measure drugs in milk easily, there is little justification for using this indirect calculation of C_{milk}.

$$C_{milk} = C_{plasma} \times M/P$$

A detailed discussion of the measurement of M/P and factors that can influence the reliability of such measurement is given in Chapter 33.

INFANT DOSE: CONTROLLING FACTORS AND INTERPRETATION

Drug Disposition in Mother and Infant

Figure 3 shows how the concentration in the mother's and infant's drug levels interact to influence the infant's exposure to drugs.

Drug concentrations in the maternal plasma are controlled by the balance of the maternal daily drug dose and the maternal elimination rate constant ($k_{el\text{-}maternal}$). The ratio of the rate constants for drug transfer from maternal plasma into milk and from milk back to plasma (k_{pm}/k_{mp}) controls the equilibrium M/P for the drug and the concentration of drug in milk.

The drug concentration in the infant's plasma is the balance of intake and output over time. Intake by the infant comes entirely from mother's milk and is

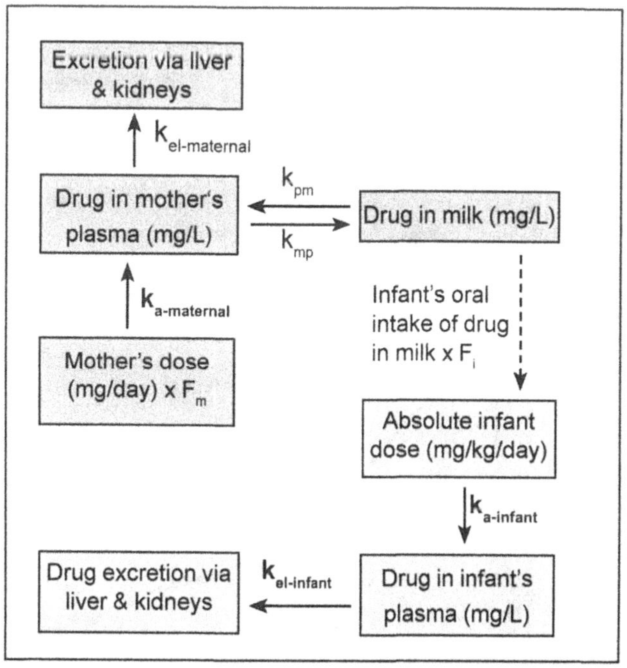

Figure 3. Drug transfer from mother to infant via milk and its disposition in the infant. $k_{a\text{-}maternal}$ = mother's oral absorption rate constant, k_{pm} and k_{mp} = transfer rate constants between plasma and milk, $k_{el\text{-}maternal}$ = elimination rate constant for drug from maternal plasma, F_m = drug bioavailability in mother, F_i = drug bioavailability in infant, $k_{a\text{-}infant}$ = oral absorption rate constant in the infant, and $k_{el\text{-}infant}$ = rate constant for drug elimination from infant plasma.

calculated as concentration in milk multiplied by volume of milk ingested. Output from the infant's plasma is controlled by hepatic and renal elimination processes. The elimination of drug from the infant's plasma is controlled by the capacity of hepatic and renal excretion pathways. The latter is age-dependent and starts from around 33% of maternal drug elimination capacity at birth (full-term infant), rising to adult levels at about seven months of age (Begg, 2003). Thus, increasing age gives the infant increased drug clearance capacity and therefore decreased exposure to drugs absorbed from milk. In considering the infant's exposure to drugs, the health of the liver and kidney should also be considered as intercurrent illness may independently decrease drug clearance and thereby alter exposure.

Calculation of Infant Dose and Its Interpretation

Absolute Infant Dose

Absolute infant dose (AID) can be calculated as follows:

$$AID = \text{Drug concentration in milk } (C_{max} \text{ or } C_{average}) \times \text{Volume of milk ingested/day}$$

Where C_{max} = maximum concentration of drug in milk and $C_{average}$ = average concentration of drug in milk. In the calculation, concentration of drug in milk has units of mg/L, and the average estimate of the volume of milk ingested/day is 0.15 L/kg (Bennett, 1996), so that AID has units of mg/kg/day. Most investigators use the $C_{average}$ drug concentration in milk over a dose interval in the calculation. Using C_{max} gives a higher, more conservative estimate of dose. This calculation should be modified appropriately where breastfeeding is not exclusive. Note also that C_{max} in milk does not necessarily occur at the same time as C_{max} in mother's plasma. The concentration-time profiles in milk and plasma are often different as illustrated in **Figure 4** for an individual patient taking olanzapine (Gardiner *et al.*, 2003b). The median time for C_{max} in a group of six patients in the study was 2.5 hours in plasma compared to 5.2 hours in milk. A similar but more marked delay in the milk C_{max} time has been reported for sumatriptan (Wojnar-Horton *et al.*, 1996). However, data for escitalopram shows a similar time of C_{max} in milk and plasma (Rampono *et al.*, 2006).

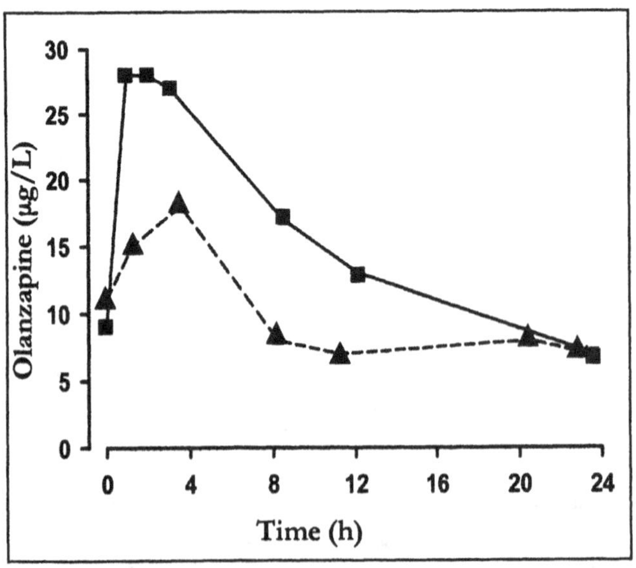

Figure 4. Steady-state olanzapine concentration-time data from a patient described in a study by Gardiner *et al.* (2003b). The concentration in milk (▲---▲) occurs at a later time after dose than that in plasma (■–■).

AID is best interpreted by direct comparison with known safe doses of the drug in neonates or infants. Thus, the direct application of AID comparison is limited to those drugs that have therapeutic applications in neonatology or pediatrics. An arbitrary limit of no more than 10% of the infant therapeutic dose has been suggested as an acceptable level of exposure (Ito, 2000).

Relative Infant Dose

Relative infant dose (RID) is the most useful parameter for assessing drug safety in breastfeeding. It is calculated as follows:

$$RID\ (\%) = \frac{\text{Absolute infant dose (mg/kg/day)}}{\text{Maternal dose (mg/kg/day)}} \times 100$$

RID thus provides a standardized means of referencing infant exposure to maternal exposure on a dose/weight basis. Note that the RID calculation assumes that the maternal dose lies within the "usual range" of therapeutic doses. Hence, maternal doses that are unusually high may result in increased infant exposure (in AID terms), and therefore require additional consideration.

Interpretation of RID is by reference to a notional safe "level of concern." In 1966, Bennett suggested that a cut-off value of 10% for RID can be used to indicate drug compatibility during breastfeeding, and this has been widely accepted in the literature (Bennett, 1996). This generally works well for full-term infants (38-40 weeks post-conceptual age) whose clearance capacity is around 33% of maternal values (Begg, 2003). As discussed above, the comparison becomes more conservative as the infant ages and drug clearance capacity increases to adult levels (at about seven months of age). Similarly the 10% level of concern should be decreased in pre-term infants whose clearance capacities are lower (5% at 24-28 weeks and 10% at 28-34 weeks post-conceptual age).

When considering early neonatal exposure to drugs in milk, one should also ascertain whether the neonate may have been exposed to drugs *in utero*. The level of exposure in pregnancy is usually five to 10-fold greater than that received via breastmilk, and drugs with long $t_{1/2}$ values may continue to contribute to postnatal exposure for one to two weeks after birth.

Risk-Benefit Analysis

The breastfed infant has nothing to gain from exposure to drugs via his mother's milk and is but an "innocent bystander" (Begg, 2000). Reducing or avoiding infant exposure should therefore be a desired outcome. Careful consideration of non-drug therapies must be given before embarking on a course of drug treatment. Postponing treatment should also be considered as an option. Topical application of the drug may be an alternative to systemic drug therapy. For example, an oxymetazoline nasal spray could replace the oral decongestant pseudoephedrine and avoid any effects that the latter might have on milk production.

If maternal drug treatment is necessary, then the decision to breastfeed should be made following an individual *risk-benefit analysis* carried out by or on instruction from the prescriber. Following this assessment, involvement of the mother and her partner is essential in agreeing on a therapeutic plan. Indirectly, the infant can be expected to benefit from drug-related improvements in mother's health and wellbeing. The algorithm shown in **Figure 5** summarizes the steps in the risk-benefit assessment. Recommended sources of information on drugs and breastfeeding include textbooks (Bennett *et al.*, 1996; Briggs *et al.*, 2005b; Hale, 2006), the US National Library of Medicine TOXNET LactMed data base (available online at http://toxnet.nlm.nih.gov/), as well as reviews and individual published papers from the scientific literature.

In the First Stage, the Information Collected Should Include:

1. Any already published/known information about the absolute and/or relative infant dose for the drug and/or active metabolites, the plasma levels in exposed infants, and reported adverse effects in exposed infants.
2. The relative toxicity of the medication. Radioisotopes, antimetabolites, anticancer agents may be extremely dangerous, even in miniscule doses. Breastfeeding may need to cease temporarily.
3. The maternal dose to be used.
4. The duration of maternal therapy.
5. The infant's post-conceptual age.
6. Any inter-current illness or other pathology in the infant that might compromise drug clearance.
7. Whether breastfeeding is exclusive or the infant is supplemented with a bottle or solid foods.

In the next stage, infant absorption of drugs in milk is considered. Some drugs (e.g., large proteins or those that are chemically unstable in the stomach) may not be bioavailable and can thus be classified as being compatible with breastfeeding. For all other drugs, the published data on absolute and relative infant doses, levels in plasma of exposed infants, and adverse effects in exposed infants should be evaluated. Where possible, the dose calculation should be individualized for the mother's intended dose.

In the Final Stage, from the Published and Individualized Information Available, The Drug is Classified as Having or not Having:

1. An acceptable AID and/or RID.
2. Acceptable plasma levels (usually compared as a % of levels in the maternal plasma).
3. An acceptable adverse effect profile in exposed infants.

On the basis of the above evaluation, it can then be decided if the drug is compatible with breastfeeding. In our experience, the AID is infrequently used in the assessment of drug safety, as few of the drugs that mothers consume have neonatal or pediatric applications. Hence, a RID with a 10% cut-off is usually the primary measure used in the risk-benefit analysis (Bennett, 1996).

There are no firm guidelines for assessing the infant's plasma drug levels as a percentage of those in mother's plasma. Obviously, the lower the value, the less likely it becomes that there will be significant effects in the infant. However, it is interesting to note that quite high values are sometimes considered acceptable for drugs like lithium (up to 30%) (Moretti *et al.*, 2003) and lamotrigine (23-50%) (Ohman *et al.*, 2000). In such cases,

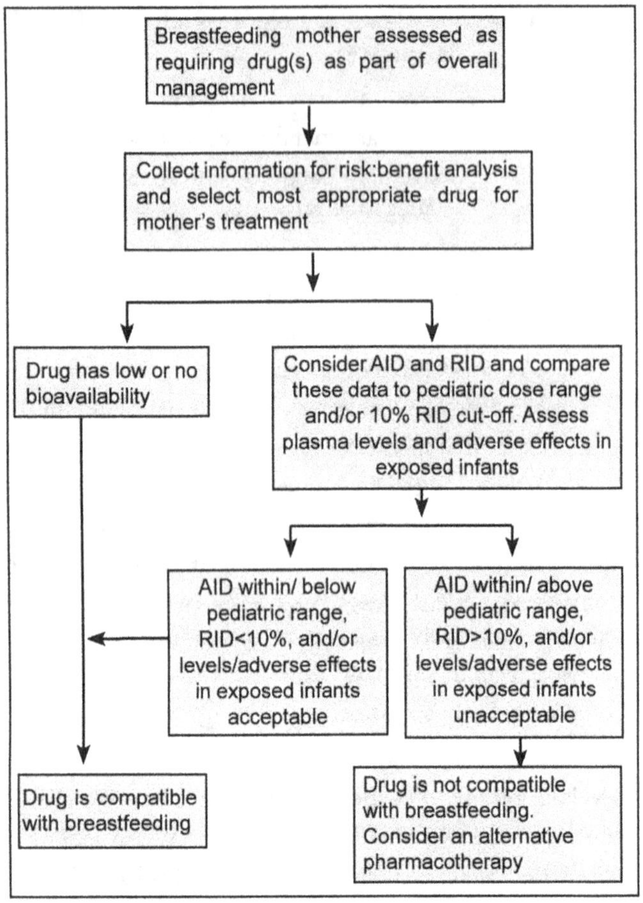

Figure 5. Risk-benefit analysis algorithm for assessment of drug use in breastfeeding, where AID=absolute infant dose and RID=relative infant dose

it is recommended that the infant's progress is monitored at appropriate intervals and that occasional drug levels in plasma are also measured.

Published information on adverse effects in infants exposed to drugs needs to be evaluated critically, preferably using a validated assessment tool. In one study of the published literature on adverse effects in breastfed infants, none of 100 reports were considered to be "definite" using a standard ranking scale; 47% were "probable" and 53% were "possible" (Anderson *et al.*, 2003).

Once drug treatment starts, the infant should be assessed at appropriate intervals to confirm that there are no significant adverse effects. The degree and type of assessment needs to be matched to the drug class and to likely adverse effects. Where there is any doubt or the mother needs reassurance, it can sometimes be helpful to measure drug levels in milk, in the infant, and in maternal plasma. These data can then be fed back through the second and third stages of the algorithm to produce individualized estimates of infant dose and exposure.

Minimizing infant exposure to drug in milk

Withholding breastfeeding temporarily is a useful strategy where the drug regimen to be used is single dose or intermittent (e.g., some radioisotopes or anticancer drugs). Milk produced during the withholding period should be pumped and discarded.

If maternal drug therapy is justifiable, then choosing a drug that has a lower relative infant dose is also a way of minimizing exposure. For example, with the SSRI antidepressants, one might prefer sertraline (RID = 0.3-0.9%) over fluoxetine (RID = 2.6-6.5%). However, such a choice should not preclude using a drug with a higher relative infant dose, where it has been efficacious in a previous treatment cycle for the patient.

It is often suggested that feeding immediately before mother's next drug dose is due (i.e., at the time of trough milk concentration) is helpful in minimizing infant exposure to drug. This strategy may offer significant benefit when the drug has a short half-life and there is minimal accumulation after repeated doses, as well as for drugs that are given once a day immediately before the infant's longest sleep period. It is unlikely to be of great benefit for drugs with long half-lives, where the magnitude of the differences between peak and trough concentrations at steady-state is small. Others have suggested that taking the drug immediately after a feed may reduce drug exposure (Anonymous, 2007). However, since infants can be expected to feed at intervals of three to five hours, there is no guarantee that this strategy would avoid peak concentrations in milk. Alternating bottle- and breastfeeding can also assist in limiting exposure.

Beneficial Effects of Maternal Drug Therapy in the Breastfed Infant

Occasionally, maternal drug therapy can directly benefit the infant. For example, 60-90% of neonates whose mothers took methadone for an opioid dependency during pregnancy suffer a neonatal abstinence syndrome in the first one to two weeks of life (Newman *et al.*, 1975; Ostrea *et al.*, 1976; Strauss *et al.*, 1974). These infants are exposed to high levels of methadone via the placenta during pregnancy. Postnatally, they experience a marked decrease in exposure and essentially undergo an opiate withdrawal. The amount of drug delivered via breastmilk is much smaller (Begg *et al.*, 2001;

Jansson *et al.*, 2007; Wojnar-Horton *et al.*, 1997), but can partially alleviate withdrawal symptoms in some infants (Abdel-Latif *et al.*, 2006; Malpas *et al.*, 1995), although this depends on the maternal dose. As the dose rises, virtually all infants exposed in utero will to some degree require exogenous opiates to suppress withdrawal symptoms. Indirect benefits can also be expected to flow to the breastfed infant from improvements in mother's health as a result of pharmacotherapy. For example, if mothers with significant postnatal depression are not treated, their infants show increased behavioral problems and delayed language development (Lee *et al.*, 1991; Murray *et al.*, 1996; Sinclair *et al.*, 1998; Zekoski *et al.*, 1987).

In summary, the following chapters in this section provide extensive detail on the transfer of specific classes of medications to the breastfed infant. In reality, we do have rather an extensive database on drugs and their transfer into human milk. Most drugs transfer into human milk, but most do so in subclinical amounts and it is often quite safe to breastfeed while using a medication. However, the choice of medication is extremely important. Physicians and patients are advised to carefully choose those with lower RIDs and limited side effect profiles. But this might not always be possible, and each physician and mother must as a team, determine the best choice for their individual case. Almost always, with the proper choice of medication, the mother can continue to breastfeed while undergoing drug therapy.

References

Abdel-Latif ME, Pinner J, Clews S, Cooke F, Lui K, Oei J. Effects of breast milk on the severity and outcome of neonatal abstinence syndrome among infants of drug-dependent mothers. *Pediatrics.* 2006; 117:e1163-e1169.

Alcorn J, Lu X, Moscow JA, McNamara PJ. Transporter gene expression in lactating and nonlactating human mammary epithelial cells using real-time reverse transcription-polymerase chain reaction. *J Pharmacol Exp Ther.* 2002a; 303:487-96.

Alcorn J, McNamara PJ. Acyclovir, ganciclovir, and zidovudine transfer into rat milk. *Antimicrob Agents Chemother.* 2002b; 46:1831-6.

Anderson PO, Pochop SL, Manoguerra AS. Adverse drug reactions in breastfed infants: less than imagined. *Clin Pediat (Phila).* 2003; 42:325-40.

Anonymous. Prescribing for breastfeeding women. In: Bochner F (ed.). *Australian medicines handbook.* Adelaide, Australia: RACGP, ASCEPT & PSA; 2007. p. xv.

Arthur PG, Kent JC, Potter JM, Hartmann PE. Lactose in blood in nonpregnant, pregnant, and lactating women. *J Pediatr Gastroenterol Nutr.* 1991; 13:254-59.

Atkinson HC, Begg EJ, Darlow BA. Drugs in human milk. Clinical pharmacokinetic considerations. *Clin Pharmacokinet.* 1988; 14:217-40.

Begg EJ. Clinical Pharmacology Essentials. *The principles behind the prescribing process.* Auckland: Adis International; 2000.

Begg EJ. *Instant clinical pharmacology.* 1st Ed. Oxford, UK: Blackwell Publishing Ltd; 2003.

Begg EJ, Atkinson HC, Duffull SB. Prospective evaluation of a model for the prediction of milk:plasma drug concentrations from physicochemical characteristics. *Br J Clin Pharmacol.* 1992; 33:501-5.

Begg EJ, Malpas TJ, Hackett LP, Ilett KF. Distribution of *R*- and *S*-methadone into human milk at steady state during ingestion of medium to high doses. *Br J Clin Pharmacol.* 2001; 52:681-85.

Bennett PN. Use of the monographs on drugs. In: Bennett PN (ed.). *Drugs and human lactation.* 2nd Ed. Amsterdam: Elsevier; 1996. p. 67-74.

Bennett PN, Astrup-Jensen A, Bates CJ, Begg EJ, Edwards S, Lazarus CR, *et al. Drugs and human lactation.* 2nd Ed. Amsterdam: Elsevier Science B.V.; 1996.

Besunder JB, Reed MD, Blumer JL. Principles of drug biodisposition in the neonate. A critical evaluation of the pharmacokinetic-pharmacodynamic interface (Part I). *Clin Pharmacokinet.* 1988a; 14:189-216.

Besunder JB, Reed MD, Blumer JL. Principles of drug biodisposition in the neonate. A critical evaluation of the pharmacokinetic-pharmacodynamic interface (Part II). *Clin Pharmacokinet.* 1988b; 14:261-86.

Bork K, Kaiser T, Benes P. Transfer of aciclovir from plasma to human breast milk. *Arzneimittelforschung* .2000; 50:656-58.

Briggs GG, Ambrose PJ, Nageotte MP, Padilla G, Wan S. Excretion of metformin into breast milk and the effect on nursing infants. *Obstet Gynecol.* 2005a; 105:1437-41.

Briggs GG, Freeman RK, Yaffe SJ. *Drugs in pregnancy and lactation.* 7th Ed. Philadelphia: Lippincott Williams and Wilkins; 2005b.

Brisken C, Heineman A, Chavarria T, Elenbaas B, Tan J, Dey SK, *et al.* Essential function of Wnt-4 in mammary gland development downstream of progesterone signaling. *Genes Dev.* 2000; 14:650-54.

Clermont Y, Xia L, Rambourg A, Turner JD, Hermo L. Transport of casein submicelles and formation of secretion granules in the Golgi apparatus of epithelial cells of the lactating mammary gland of the rat. *Anat Rec.* 1993; 235:363-73.

Cox DB, Kent JC, Casey TM, Owens RA, Hartmann PE. Breast growth and the urinary excretion of lactose during human pregnancy and early lactation: endocrine relationships. *Exp Physiol.* 1999; 84:421-34.

Edwards JE, Alcorn J, Savolainen J, Anderson BD, McNamara PJ. Role of P-glycoprotein in distribution of nelfinavir across the blood-mammary tissue barrier and blood-brain barrier. *Antimicrob Agents Chemother.* 2005; 49:1626-28.

Gardiner SJ, Kirkpatrick CMJ, Begg EJ, Zhang M, Moore MP, Saville DJ. Transfer of metformin into human milk. *Clin Pharmacol Ther.* 2003a; 73:71-77.

Gardiner SJ, Kristensen JH, Begg EJ, Hackett LP, Wilson DA, Ilett KF, *et al.* Transfer of olanzapine into breast milk, calculation of infant drug dose, and effect on breast-fed infants. *Am J Psychiatry.* 2003b; 160:1428-31.

Gerk PM, Kuhn RJ, Desai NS, McNamara PJ. Active transport of nitrofurantoin into human milk. *Pharmacotherapy.* 2001a; 21:669-75.

Gerk PM, Moscow JA, McNamara PJ. Basolateral active uptake of nitrofurantoin in the CIT3 cell culture model of lactation. *Drug Metab Dispos.* 2003; 31:691-93.

Gerk PM, Oo CY, Paxton EW, Moscow JA, McNamara PJ. Interactions between cimetidine, nitrofurantoin, and probenecid active transport into rat milk. *J Pharmacol Exp Ther.* 2001b; 296:175-80.

Hale TW. *Medications and mothers' milk.* 11th Ed. Amarillo, TX, USA: Pharmasoft Publishing; 2006.

Hale TW, Ilett KF. *Drug therapy and breastfeeding. From theory to clinical practice.* 1st Ed. London: The Parthenon Publishing Group; 2002a.

Hale TW, Kristensen JH, Hackett LP, Kohan R, Ilett KF. Transfer of metformin into human milk. *Diabetologia.* 2002b; 45:1509-14.

Hale TW, McDonald R, Boger J. Transfer of celecoxib into human milk. *J Hum Lact.* 2004; 20:397-403.

Ilett KF, Hackett LP, Ingle B, Bretz PJ. Transfer of probenecid and cephalexin into breast milk. *Ann Pharmacother.* 2006; 40:986-89.

Ito S. Drug therapy for breast-feeding women. N Engl J Med 2000;343:118-126.

Ito S, Alcorn J. Xenobiotic transporter expression and function in the human mammary gland. *Adv Drug Deliv Rev.* 2003; 55:653-65.

Jansson LM, Choo RE, Harrow C, Velez M, Schroeder JR, Lowe R, *et al.* Concentrations of methadone in breast milk and plasma in the immediate perinatal period. *J Hum Lact.* 2007; 23:184-90.

Kari FW, Weaver R, Neville MC. Active transport of nitrofurantoin across the mammary epithelium in vivo. *J Pharmacol Exp Ther.* 1997; 280:664-68.

Kimura N, Masuda S, Tanihara Y, Ueo H, Okuda M, Katsura T et al. Metformin is a superior substrate for renal organic cation transporter OCT2 rather than hepatic OCT1. *Drug Metab Pharmacokin.* 2005; 20:379-86.

Koldovsky O. Hormones in milk. *Vitam Horm.* 1995; 50:77-149.

Kristensen JH, Ilett KF, Rampono J, Kohan R, Hackett LP. Transfer of the antidepressant mirtazapine into breast milk. *Br J Clin Pharmacol.* 2007; 63:322-27.

Kulski JK, Hartmann PE. Milk insulin, GH and TSH: relationship to changes in milk lactose, glucose and protein during lactogenesis in women. *Endocrinol Exp.* 1983; 17:317-26.

Lau RJ, Emery MG, Galinsky RE. Unexpected accumulation of acyclovir in breast milk with estimation of infant exposure. *Obstet Gynecol.* 1987; 69:468-71.

Lawrence RA, Lawrence RM. Biochemistry of human milk. In: Lawrence RA, Lawrence RM (eds.). *Breastfeeding; a guide for the medical profession.* 6th Ed. St Louis USA: Mosby; 2005. p. 105-70.

Lee CM, Gotlib IH. Adjustment of children of depressed mothers: a 10-month follow-up. *J Abnorm Psychol.* 1991; 100:473-77.

Malpas TJ, Darlow BA, Lennox R, Horwood LJ. Maternal methadone dosage and neonatal withdrawal. *Aust N Z J Obstet Gynaecol.* 1995; 35:175-77.

Mather IH, Keenan TW. Origin and secretion of milk lipids. *J Mammary Gland Biol Neoplasia.* 1998; 3:259-73.

McManaman JL, Neville MC. Mammary physiology and milk secretion. *Adv Drug Deliv Rev.* 2003; 55:629-41.

Miyoshi K, Meyer B, Gruss P, Cui Y, Renou JP, Morgan FV, *et al.* Mammary epithelial cells are not able to undergo pregnancy-dependent differentiation in the absence of the helix-loop-helix inhibitor Id2. *Mol Endocrinol.* 2002; 16:2892-901.

Moretti ME, Koren G, Verjee Z, Ito S. Monitoring lithium in breast milk: An individualized approach for breast-feeding mothers. *Ther Drug Monit.* 2003; 25:364-66.

Murray L, Fiori-Cowley A, Hooper R, Cooper P. The impact of postnatal depression and associated adversity on early mother-infant interactions and later infant outcome. *Child Dev.* 1996; 67:2512-26.

Neville MC. Anatomy and physiology of lactation. *Periatr Clin North Am.* 2001; 48:13-34.

Newman RG, Bashkow S, Calko D. Results of 313 consecutive live births of infants delivered to patients in the New York City Methadone Maintenance Treatment Program. *Am J Obstet Gynecol.* 1975; 121:233-37.

Ohman I, Vitols S, Tomson T. Lamotrigine in pregnancy: pharmacokinetics during delivery, in the neonate, and during lactation. *Epilepsia.* 2000; 41:709-13.

Oo CY, Kuhn RJ, Desai N, McNamara PJ. Active transport of cimetidine into human milk. *Clin Pharmacol Ther.* 1995; 58:548-55.

Ostrea EM, Chavez CJ, Strauss ME. A study of factors that influence the severity of neonatal narcotic withdrawal. *J Pediatr.* 1976; 88:642-45.

Plante L, Ferron GM, Unruh M, Mayer PR. Excretion of pantoprazole in human breast. *J Reprod Med.* 2004; 49:825-7.

Rampono J, Hackett LP, Kristensen JH, Kohan R, Page-Sharp M, Ilett KF. Transfer of escitalopram and its metabolite demethylescitalopram into breastmilk. *Br J Clin Pharmacol.* 2006; 62:316-22.

Raub TJ. P-glycoprotein recognition of substrates and circumvention through rational drug design. *Mol Pharmacol.* 2006; 3:3-25.

Sinclair D, Murray L. Effects of postnatal depression on children's adjustment to school. Teacher's reports. *Brit J Psychiatry.* 1998; 172:58-63.

Strauss ME, Andresko M, Stryker JC, Wardell JN, Dunkel LD.

Methadone maintenance during pregnancy: pregnancy, birth, and neonate characteristics. *Am J Obstet Gynecol.* 1974; 120:895-900.

Sykes PA, Quarrie J, Alexander FW. Lithium carbonate and breast-feeding. *Br Med J.* 1976; 2:1299.

Toddywalla VS, Kari FW, Neville MC. Active transport of nitrofurantoin across a mouse mammary epithelial monolayer. *J Pharmacol Exp Ther.* 1997; 280:669-76.

Tomson T, Palm R, Kallen K, Ben-Menachem E, Soderfeldt B, Danielsson B, *et al.* Pharmacokinetics of levetiracetam during pregnancy, delivery, in the neonatal period, and lactation. *Epilepsia.* 2007; 48:1111-16.

Verge D. Biotechnological and administration innovations in insulin therapy. *Med Sci (Paris).* 2004; 20:986-98.

Wang H, Liu Z, Li G, Barrett EJ. The vascular endothelial cell mediates insulin transport into skeletal muscle. *Am J Physiol Endocrinol Metab.* 2006; 291:E323-E332.

Wojnar-Horton RE, Hackett LP, Yapp P, Dusci LJ, Paech M, Ilett KF. Distribution and excretion of sumatriptan in human milk. *Br J Clin Pharmacol.* 1996; 41:217-21.

Wojnar-Horton RE, Kristensen JH, Yapp P, Ilett KF, Dusci LJ, Hackett LP. Methadone distribution and excretion into breast milk of clients in a methadone maintenance programme. *Br J Clin Pharmacol.* 1997; 44:543-47.

Zekoski EM, O'Hara MW, Wills KE. The effects of maternal mood on mother-infant interaction. *J Abnorm Child Psychol.* 1987; 15:361-78.

Chapter 25

Medications that Alter Milk Production

Thomas W. Hale

HORMONAL REGULATION OF MILK PRODUCTION

The production of human milk is a complex task requiring the interaction of many hormones, the most important of which are prolactin and oxytocin. While this is thoroughly reviewed in Chapter 9, for the purposes of discussing drugs that affect milk production, some review of the hormonal control of milk synthesis is in order.

During gestation, milk production is largely inhibited due to high circulating levels of progesterone and estrogen. Although it is not exactly clear how elevated circulating levels of progesterone/estrogen inhibit lactation, it is probably by down regulating the activity of prolactin and/or the homogeneous expression of milk protein genes by alveolar cells (secretory activation)(Robinson *et al.*, 1995).

We now know that progesterone has a profound effect on milk production, but it is dependent on timing. Early postnatally, progesterone may still suppress milk production as is evident in cases of retained placenta. Exogenous progesterone has also been shown to inhibit lactose and lipid synthesis by mammary glands in pregnant rats (Kuhn, 1969). But, at about 40 hours or later, the lactocyte apparently becomes less sensitive to exogenous progesterone, and milk production is no longer affected. This is evident by the fact that many mothers use progestin-only birth control pills without problems.

With parturition and delivery of the intact placenta, progesterone and estrogen levels fall rapidly to trough levels within about 40 hours in most mothers. The fall in progesterone is now well recognized as the initiating factor that activates the biosynthetic process for the production of milk (Kuhn, 1969; Neville *et al.*, 2002). Thus, prior to parturition, the lactocyte is exceedingly sensitive to elevated levels of progesterone; later, it is much less sensitive.

Prolactin is the primary hormone responsible for the biosynthesis of milk, and in its absence, milk production ceases. Elevated levels of maternal prolactin first appear at about eight weeks gestation and continue to increase to a mean level of approximately 200 ng/mL or greater at term (Jacobs, 1977), then decline progressively by six months postpartum to 80 ng/mL (Cox *et al.*, 1996). At term, prolactin levels are 10-20 times higher than non-pregnant levels. Thus, prolactin attains its highest concentration in the last trimester and actually falls significantly after delivery and during lactation. Prolactin release is dependent on the sucking stimulus and peaks at about 45 minutes following stimulus (Tyson *et al.*, 1975). It then returns to pre-feed levels within three hours of feeding. This is termed the prolactin surge, which is evident in virtually all breastfeeding mothers.

It is now well known that no relationship exists between prolactin blood levels and the short-term rate of milk synthesis (Cox *et al.*, 1996). Mothers can produce just as much milk at 70 ng/mL as they can at

200 ng/mL (Cox *et al.*, 1996). While this is true when prolactin levels are elevated above baseline, it may not be true when maternal prolactin levels fall into the baseline ranges of 10-20 ng/mL or lower. This appears to be supported by the fact that the drugs discussed below all increase baseline levels of prolactin to some degree and also increase milk production in those mothers whose levels were initially low. The drugs apparently do not function well as galactagogues when maternal levels of prolactin are higher.

PROLACTIN AND ITS RELEASE

Prolactin is a polypeptide hormone that is synthesized and released by specialized cells in the anterior pituitary, the lactotrophs. Although mammals differ enormously in the type and hormonal requirements for milk production, the common requisite hormone is without doubt prolactin. While its presence in the plasma has always been associated with milk production, prolactin actually has over 300 separate biological activities and homeostatic roles all over the body (Bole-Feysot *et al.*, 1998). Prolactin is synthesized in many tissues other than the pituitary, including the breast. Prolactin receptors are found in peripheral tissues, such as heart, lung, thymus, spleen, liver, pancreas, kidney, adrenal gland, uterus, skeletal muscle, and skin, although their functions in those organs are unknown (Bole-Feysot *et al.*, 1998; Nagano *et al.*, 1994).

Prolactin has numerous effects on the mammary gland, including its growth and development (mammogenesis), synthesis of milk (lactogenesis), and maintenance of milk synthesis (galactopoiesis) (Freeman *et al.*, 2000). While prolactin is a common requisite hormone for galactopoiesis, it is still only a single member in an ensemble of hormones required for milk production, which include corticosteroids, growth hormone, and others. Even though we know they are required, the interplay of all these hormones in milk production is still somewhat obscure.

In the pituitary, there is obvious functional heterogeneity among lactotrophs with regard to their distribution in the anterior lobe and even their responsiveness to various secretagogues (dopamine, etc). Certain lactotrophs on the outer zone respond greater to thyrotrophin releasing hormone (TRH) than those on the inner zone. Dopamine-responsive lactotrophs are located in the inner zone of the pituitary (Arita *et al.*, 1991).

In humans, prolactin release is highest during sleep and lowest during waking hours, which is considered true circadian rhythm (Parker *et al.*, 1974). It is now well known that dopamine tone exerts inhibitory effect over prolactin secretion (Ben-Jonathan *et al.*, 2001) and that this tone apparently varies during the day, creating the diurnal rhythm. Thus, the release of dopamine into the long portal vessels reaching the anterior lobe of the pituitary is lowest prior to the peak of prolactin.

The well known prolactin surge seen during lactation is a physiologic response affected by the suckling stimulus applied by the infant and is classified as a neuroendocrine reflex. Somewhat enigmatic, the sucking-induced release of prolactin is in part due to a reduced secretion of the inhibiting dopamine into the portal circulation. However, the plasma levels of prolactin rise so high, that it exceeds the amount commonly stored in the lactotrophs of the pituitary. Thus, it is theorized that some change in 'production' of prolactin is induced by a prolactin releasing factor that is responsible for the exceedingly high prolactin levels released during this phase. Under the influence of this releasing factor, the lactotrophs are capable of much greater production and release of prolactin during the 'surge' phase.

At this juncture, it is thought that the typical galactagogues (dopamine antagonists) in use today increase circulating levels of prolactin by inhibiting the release of dopamine from the hypothalamus. In almost all cases, they increase the circulating levels of prolactin. It is also apparent that in those individuals whose plasma prolactin levels are already elevated, these drugs are unable to induce a higher level of galactopoiesis. In addition, the use of postlactational dopamine antagonists apparently stimulates prolactin release maximally, thus the prolactin 'surge' upon suckling disappears.

DRUGS THAT MAY INHIBIT MILK PRODUCTION

Some medications are well known to inhibit galactopoiesis, particularly those that are dopamine agonists at the D_2 receptor site. Almost invariably, most of the medications in use today do so by inhibiting the release of prolactin from the pituitary (ergot alkaloids),

Table 1. Drugs that may Reduce Milk Production
• Progestins • Estrogens • Ethanol • Bromocriptine • Ergotamine • Cabergoline • Pseudoephedrine • Testosterone • Antiestrogens • Clomiphene

although others may have alternate or unknown mechanisms. Some drugs may inhibit oxytocin release (ethanol) or even have direct effects on the lactocyte (prostaglandins, estrogens). Further, it is not even known if dopamine is the sole prolactin inhibitory factor (PIF). Other inhibitors have been theorized, but their role is unclear - GABA, somatostatin (Freeman *et al.*, 2000), and pseudoephedrine (Aljazaf *et al.*, 2003)(**Table 1**).

Dopamine receptors located on the lactotroph membranes belong to the D_2 subclass of dopamine receptors (Caron *et al.*, 1978). Agonists at this receptor site reduce the release of prolactin from the lactotroph, similar to that of dopamine from the hypothalamus via the portal circulation. Drugs that inhibit milk production by reducing maternal plasma prolactin levels classically include the ergot alkaloids and potentially some of the new dopamine agonist drugs used for Parkinsonian syndromes. Ergot alkaloids inhibit prolactin release in all vertebrate species tested so far, including man. Drugs, such as bromocriptine, metergoline, cabergoline, pergolide, and pramipexole, are potent dopamine D_2 receptor agonists, and therefore are potent inhibitors of prolactin release.

Bromocriptine has been used in the past to reduce engorgement and inhibit milk production, although it was associated with numerous cases of cardiac dysrhythmias, stroke, intracranial bleeding, cerebral edema, convulsions, and myocardial infarction (Dutt *et al.*, 1998; Iffy *et al.*, 1998; Pop *et al.*, 1998; Webster, 1996). A newer analog, cabergoline, has proven much safer and is now recommended for both hyperprolactinemia and inhibition of lactation (Bravo-Topete *et al.*, 2004; Ferrari *et al.*, 1995; Webster *et al.*, 1992). Doses of 1 mg administered early postpartum will completely inhibit lactation. For established lactation, 0.25 mg twice daily for two days has been found to completely inhibit lactation (Anonymous, 1991; Caballero-Gordo *et al.*, 1991).

While bromocriptine is a strong agonist of D_2 and partial agonist of D_1, pergolide is an agonist of both classes of receptors. Ropinirole and pramipexole are specific agonists for the D_2 receptor site. All of the dopamine receptor agonists listed above probably suppress prolactin release, although we do not have studies in lactating women with these newer antiparkinsonian agents.

Methylergonovine and ergonovine have been used in the past as oxytocic agents to prevent uterine hemorrhage, and they have been used during lactation. They are potent agonists at the α-receptor; however, several reports suggest that their D_2 agonist activity is enough to suppress prolactin levels and milk production (Peters *et al.*, 1979; Weiss *et al.*, 1975). Their effect on prolactin appears limited when used briefly and in minimal doses. They are probably suitable but not ideal agents to use to prevent uterine hemorrhage in breastfeeding mothers.

Clomiphene is an agent that stimulates the release of the pituitary gonadotropins, follicle-stimulating hormone (FSH), and luteinizing hormone (LH), which results in development and maturation of the ovarian follicle, ovulation, and subsequent development and function of the corpus luteum. It has both estrogenic and anti-estrogenic effects, but ultimately leads to increased follicle formation.

In a study of 60 postpartum women (one to four days postpartum), clomiphene was effective in totally inhibiting lactation early postnatally and in suppressing established lactation on day four postpartum (Masala *et al.*, 1978). Only seven of 40 women receiving clomiphene to inhibit lactation had signs of congestion or discomfort, suggesting it suppresses milk production. In the 20 women who received clomiphene to suppress established lactation (on day four), a rapid amelioration of breast engorgement and discomfort was produced. After five days of treatment, no signs of lactation were present. In another study of 177 postpartum women, clomiphene was very effective at inhibiting lactation (Zuckerman *et al.*, 1973). Other studies also suggest suppression of lactation following the use of clomiphene

(Peters *et al.*, 1979; Weinstein *et al.*, 1976; Weiss *et al.*, 1975). While clomiphene appears to suppress lactation in women, particularly in early postpartum, there is still some question as to its ability to suppress lactation after lactation is firmly established (months later).

Both estrogens (Tankeyoon *et al.*, 1984; Treffers, 1999) and antiestrogens (Shaaban, 1975) are known to have profound effects on lactation. Estrogens have a long but poorly documented history of suppressing milk production in patients (Booker *et al.*, 1967; Booker *et al.*, 1970; Gambrell, 1970; Tankeyoon *et al.*, 1984; Treffers, 1999). In contrast in animal models, estrogens are known to actually increase the release and synthesis of prolactin. Most of this work has been done in rats, and we do not know with certainty that the same occurs in humans. In rats, estradiol is antidopaminergic at the lactotroph (Raymond *et al.*, 1978), and reduces dopamine's potency to inhibit prolactin release in vivo. Apparently, estradiol exerts this effect by decreasing the number of prolactin receptors on the lactotroph membranes (Raymond *et al.*, 1978). We do not know if estradiol in the human ultimately reduces prolactin and milk synthesis. However, clinically we know that estrogens have a high likelihood of ultimately suppressing milk production, although data supporting this in the literature is suggestive but limited. The effect of estrogens from contraceptives and other forms seems inconsistent, as estrogens are known to increase prolactin production in the pituitary. While estrogens may have no effect whatsoever in some mothers, others seem to be exceedingly sensitive to them. The onset may be rapid or slow, and the change in milk volume may not be readily noticed by many mothers.

Regardless, all mothers who take estrogen-containing birth control preparations should be forewarned of its possible effect on milk production. When required, low-dose progestin-only oral contraceptives should be used. Even low-dose progestins may suppress milk production in some mothers if used too early postpartum. The most sensitive time for suppression is early postpartum before the mothers' milk supply is firmly established. Waiting as long as possible (weeks to months) prior to use is recommended. All mothers should be warned that in some cases a reduction in their milk supply may result, and they should be observant for such changes.

There are recent suggestions that the nasal decongestant pseudoephedrine may suppress milk production. In one study, milk production in mothers in late-stage lactation was significantly reduced (>63 weeks postpartum) (Aljazaf *et al.*, 2003). The mechanism by which pseudoephedrine could affect prolactin levels or milk production directly, is unknown.

The use of alcohol in breastfeeding mothers is somewhat controversial. Numerous studies in rodents suggest that the use of alcohol dramatically increases prolactin release (Sawagado *et al.*, 1988; Schrauzer *et al.*, 1982), but reduces milk production and lowers mammary gland weight and pup weight, suggesting that ethanol interrupts development of the mammary or production of milk (Heil *et al.*, 1999; Jones *et al.*, 1984; Vilaro *et al.*, 1987). Studies in humans suggest that alcohol may alter the taste and smell of milk. Infants suckle quickly at first, but ultimately consume less milk (Mennella *et al.*, 1991). Older studies have suggested that at high levels, alcohol may suppress oxytocin release and hence let down (Cobo, 1973). At this time, it is apparent that alcohol may suppress letdown.

DRUGS THAT STIMULATE MILK PRODUCTION

Many studies in the literature have demonstrated that antidopaminergic agents, such as metoclopramide (Booker *et al.*, 1967; Booker *et al.*, 1970; Budd *et al.*, 1993; Ehrenkranz *et al.*, 1986; Gambrell, 1970; Kauppila *et al.*, 1981; Kauppila *et al.*, 1983), domperidone (Motilium®) (Hofmeyr *et al.*, 1983; Hofmeyr *et al.*, 1985; Petraglia *et al.*, 1985), sulpiride (Aono *et al.*, 1979a; Aono *et al.*, 1982b; Ehrenkranz *et al.*, 1986; McMurdo *et al.*, 1987; Ylikorkala *et al.*, 1982) and many others are potentially useful in raising plasma prolactin levels and improving milk production in mothers. Although there are dozens of dopamine antagonists, including most of the antipsychotics (sulpiride, chlorpromazine, risperidone, etc.), most are far too toxic to use clinically to stimulate milk production in mothers. Thus, the only two commonly used clinically are domperidone (Motilium®) and metoclopramide (Reglan®)(**Table 2**).

Table 2. Drugs Known to Increase Milk Synthesis
• Domperidone • Metoclopramide • Sulpiride • Chlorpromazine • Haloperidol • Pimozide

Dopamine from the hypothalamus maintains a constant inhibitory tone on the lactotroph, preventing the release of stored prolactin. Dopamine D_2 receptor blockers block the 'inhibitory' tone of dopamine and free the lactotroph to release prolactin from the pituitary. As the pituitary is outside the blood-brain barrier, hyperprolactinemia is a typical side-effect occurring with all antidopaminergic prokinetics.

Galactagogues in this category clearly block or impede the D_2 receptor site in the lactotroph, and prolactin is therefore released at greater levels. However, intrinsic prolactin 'synthesis' may or may not be increased with continued release from the pituitary, as dopamine blockers only 'release' prolactin previously synthesized and stored in the lactotroph storage granules. Further, it is apparent from several studies that the prolactin 'surge' which normally occurs following nipple stimulation disappears, and prolactin levels, while higher, are level and do not increase dramatically following each suckling.

With respect to milk production, baseline maternal prolactin levels are critical. It is important to remember that these drugs work by initiating the release of additional prolactin, thus elevating maternal plasma levels of prolactin. In those mothers whose baseline prolactin levels are low, these drugs are known to stimulate milk synthesis significantly. In those mothers whose plasma prolactin levels are already elevated (probably > 50 ng/mL), additional milk synthesis may not occur.

Metoclopramide

Metoclopramide (Reglan®) is the most commonly used agent for increasing milk synthesis, and in some cases, profoundly stimulates milk production as much as 100%. Metoclopramide is an antidopaminergic gastrointestinal prokinetic drug, and its affect on milk synthesis has been known and used for more than 25 years. Early brief reports that metoclopramide could be used to increase milk production appeared in papers in 1975. Kauppila *et al.* were perhaps the first group to study the transfer of metoclopramide, maternal prolactin levels, and levels of metoclopramide attained in human milk (Kauppila *et al.*, 1981). In this study, they found that both prolactin levels and milk synthesis increased significantly following the use of 10-15 mg doses three times daily. Milk production increased by 42-50 mL per feed, while prolactin levels increased from 77 to 175 ng/mL. In another more thorough study, Ehrenkranz *et al.* found that daily milk production increased from 93.3 to 197 mL between the first and seventh day of therapy with 10 mg three times daily. This increase was associated with a significantly increased basal serum prolactin level from 18.1 ng/mL (pretreatment) to 121.8 ng/mL following treatment. This study was perhaps the first to demonstrate that the post-lactational 'surge' of prolactin is blocked following therapy with a dopamine blocker. In treated mothers, basal prolactin levels were identical to post-expression levels. This suggests that the release of prolactin from the pituitary lactotroph is maximized and extra prolactin to produce a surge is no longer available for release. Their data also clearly suggests that in patients with already elevated prolactin levels (> 100 ng/mL) the baseline levels of prolactin do not necessarily increase with metoclopramide treatment. Only when baseline levels are low (20-30 ng/mL) do they subsequently increase with treatment. This correlates well with clinical experience. Mothers with elevated prolactin levels do not necessarily respond with increased milk synthesis following the use of metoclopramide. Those with exceedingly low prolactin levels (20-30 ng/mL) respond rapidly.

In another study by Kauppila *et al.*, the unique effect of metoclopramide on prolactin levels was confirmed (Kauppila *et al.*, 1983). In this study, three mothers with the lowest prolactin levels responded to metoclopramide treatment with major baseline increases of prolactin. Those with elevated baseline levels of prolactin before treatment (>300ng/mL) failed to respond to treatment.

The transfer of metoclopramide into human milk and to the infant was perhaps first studied by Lewis. In ten patients who received a single oral dose of 10 mg, the mean maternal plasma and milk levels at two hours was 68.5 ng/mL and 125.7 μg/L, respectively (Lewis *et al.*, 1980).

In a study by Kauppila *et al.*, the concentration of metoclopramide in milk was consistently higher than the maternal serum levels (Kauppila *et al.*, 1983). The peak occurred at two to three hours after administration of the medication. During the late puerperium, the concentration of metoclopramide in milk varied from 20 to 125 μg/L which was less than the 28 to 157 μg/L noted during the early puerperium. The authors estimated the daily dose to the infant varied from 6 to 24 μg/kg/day during the early puerperium and from 1 to 13 μg/kg/day during the late phase. These doses are minimal compared to those used for therapy of reflux in pediatric patients (0.1 to 0.5 mg/kg/day). In these studies, only one of five infants studied had detectable blood levels of metoclopramide; hence, no accumulation or side effects were observed. While plasma prolactin levels in the newborns were comparable to those in the mothers prior to treatment, Kaupilla found slight increases in prolactin levels in four of seven newborns following treatment with metoclopramide; although, a more recent study did not find such changes. However, prolactin levels are highly variable and subject to diurnal rhythm, thus timing is essential in measuring prolactin levels and could account for this inconsistency.

In another study of 23 women with premature infants, milk production increased from 93 mL/day to 197 mL/day between the first and seventh day of therapy with 30 mg/day (Ehrenkranz *et al.*, 1986). Prolactin levels, although varied, increased from 18.1 to 121.8 ng/mL.

In a study of five breastfeeding women who were receiving 30 mg/day, daily milk production increased significantly from 150.9 mL/day to 276.4 mL/day (Ertl *et al.*, 1991). However, the plasma prolactin levels in their breastfed infants were determined on the fifth postnatal day and no changes were noted; thus, the amount of metoclopramide transferred in milk was not enough to change the infant's prolactin levels.

In a group of 17 women receiving 10 mg orally three times daily, metoclopramide levels in the milk of three mothers was undetectable. In the remaining mothers, levels of metoclopramide averaged 45 µg/L. The authors estimated that an infant would receive approximately 11 µg/kg/day (Hansen *et al.*, 2001).

In summary, it is well documented that metoclopramide may significantly increase a mothers' milk supply, but it is exceedingly dose dependent, and some mothers simply do not respond. In those mothers who do not respond, Kaupila's work suggests that they may already have elevated prolactin levels. In his study, three of the five mothers who did not respond with increased milk production had the highest basal prolactin levels (300-400 ng/mL) (Kauppila *et al.*, 1981). Thus it may be advisable to obtain plasma prolactin levels on under-producing mothers prior to instituting metoclopramide therapy. If the maternal plasma levels are high (>100 ng/mL), metoclopramide therapy may not work. If prolactin levels are in the low (nonlactational) range of 20, then this medication may proved highly effective. Prolactin levels should be drawn approximately three hours after nursing, so that trough prolactin levels are obtained.

Side Effects

Metoclopramide is not without significant side effects in some patients, including gastric cramping, diarrhea, extrapyramidal symptoms, and major depression. GI symptoms are normal and are a result of the gastrokinetic activity of this medication. Although extrapyramidal symptoms are rare, they are a concern, but fortunately, are rarely seen. Major depression is often seen, although we do not have data on its frequency. Appearing after three to four weeks of therapy, many women complain of severe and prolonged depressive symptoms. Therefore, the long-term use of this medication is not advised. Tapering of the dose is generally recommended once lactation is firmly established (three weeks). One possible regimen is to decrease the dose by 10 mg per week while observing for changes in milk production. Rapid discontinuation of the medication may lead to rapid failure of lactation, so mothers should be carefully withdrawn.

Two recent cases of serotonin-like reactions (agitation, dysarthria, diaphoresis, and extrapyramidal movement disorder) have been reported when metoclopramide was used in patients receiving sertraline or venlafaxine (Fisher *et al.*, 2002).

Domperidone

Domperidone (Motilium ®) is a benzimidazole derivative that is a potent dopamine D2 receptor antagonist. It has been marketed in Europe and 88 other countries as a prokinetic and antiemetic since 1978. A popular, but off-label use for domperidone has been the stimulation of breastmilk production. With the removal of cisapride from the market due to pro-arrhythmic side effects, relatively few prokinetic drugs have become available for the treatment of gastrointestinal motility disorders. For this reason, domperidone and metoclopramide have become quite popular in the treatment of milk production disorders.

The pharmacokinetics of domperidone is somewhat unique. Domperidone penetrates the blood-brain barrier very poorly and rarely causes the extrapyramidal side-effects that limit the use of metoclopramide, particularly in the elderly and pediatric populations (Barone, 1999; Brogden *et al.*, 1982). Because of extensive first-pass uptake in the liver and metabolism in the gut wall, its oral bioavailability is only 13-17% (Barone, 1999). For these two reasons alone, published plasma levels and milk levels are extraordinarily low.

In a study of 16 women, seven of whom received domperidone (10 mg three times daily), the baseline production of milk was 112.8 mL in the domperidone group and 48.2 mL in the placebo group. The mean daily volume of milk collected in the domperidone group following treatment was 162.2 mL and 65.1 mL in the placebo group (da Silva *et al.*, 2001). This was a 44.5% increase in milk synthesis in the domperidone group. Prolactin levels increased from 12.9 to 119.3 μg/L in the domperidone group and 15.6 to 18.1 μg/L in the placebo group. Note that the levels of prolactin were in the normal, non-lactating range for females. On day five, the mean domperidone concentration was 6.6 ng/mL in plasma and 1.2 μg/L in the breastmilk of the treated group (n=6). No adverse effects were reported in infants or mothers.

In another study of five patients who received a single 20 mg dose, plasma prolactin levels rose from a mean of 150 ng/mL to 255 ng/mL within two hours (Hofmeyr *et al.*, 1985). Plasma and milk domperidone levels taken between 1.75 and three hours were 10.3 ng/mL and 2.6 ng/mL, respectively. Thus the plasma prolactin levels rose approximately 70%. Unfortunately, no milk volumes were reported in this study.

Domperidone has no established dose as a galactagogue. The usual oral dose for controlling GI motility problems is 10-20 mg three to four times daily; although, for nausea and vomiting the dose can be higher (up to 40 mg). The doses used as a galactagogue in the available studies were 10 mg three times daily or a single 20 mg dose (da Silva *et al.*, 2001; Hofmeyr *et al.*, 1985). These studies clearly show that doses of 10-20 mg three to four times daily elevate prolactin levels to levels more than adequate to produce milk. Doses higher than this should be avoided in breastfeeding mothers. There is simply no evidence available that using doses higher than listed above provide higher plasma prolactin levels. Indeed, the pituitary seems to have a ceiling, above which it cannot go. For instance, in mothers using metoclopramide or domperidone, the prolactin surge which occurs upon attachment of the infant to the nipple disappears. This clearly suggests that the release of prolactin from the pituitary has reached its maximum and can no longer respond. Thus, extraordinarily high doses may not lead to higher levels of prolactin.

Recently, the U.S. FDA issued a warning on domperidone stating that it could induce cardiac arrhythmias in patients. This warning against the use of domperidone in breastfeeding mothers was based on the increased risk of cardia arrhythmias in patients undergoing high dose intravenous therapy for nausea and vomiting associated with chemotherapy (Osborne *et al.*, 1985; Roussak *et al.*, 1984). In one of these studies, four patients were receiving platinum-containing chemotherapy and were given 20 mg IV (Osborne *et al.*, 1985). All four of these patients were hypokalemic (2.0-3.3 mmol/L) prior to injection.

Domperidone is one of many HERG potassium channel blockers (ziprasidone, quetiapine, risperidone, olanzapine, and numerous antihistamines). The HERG receptor (human ether-a-go-go subunit) is the primary pore-forming and voltage-sensing component of potassium channels in cardiac tissue. HERG channel dysfunction ultimately leads to cardiac arrhythmias typified by prolonged QT syndrome. Many drugs still on the market affect this receptor to varying degrees, so in reality, domperidone is just one of many such drugs.

Fortunately, the pharmacokinetics of domperidone is ideal for breastfeeding mothers. Because of its poor oral bioavailability, the use of domperidone orally produces plasma levels far less than when it is used intravenously. Heykants *et al.* reported peak blood levels of 23 ng/mL following an oral dose of 10 mg, and plasma levels approximately 30 times higher following the same dose intravenously (Heykants *et al.*, 1981). Thus, it is questionable whether one can induce arrhythmias in normal non-hypokalemic mothers with normal doses of domperidone used orally. However, patients with severe cardiac disease, those with prolonged QT intervals, or those using higher than normal doses should be warned of the risk of cardiac arrhythmias associated with domperidone. Thus far, we do not have any recent published data suggesting that domperidone used orally in breastfeeding mothers is arrhythmogenic. We do have a wealth of clinical experience with this product suggesting it is not arrhythmogenic in this population.

Sulpiride

Sulpiride is an antipsychotic drug that is a substituted benzamide with selective dopaminergic blocking activity. Sulpiride not only blocks the dopamine (D_2) receptor site, but also the D_3 and D_4 sites. It has poor oral bioavailability (35%) and has many of the same complications as other antipsychotics including: sedation, extrapyramidal effects, tardive dyskinesia, and neuroleptic malignant syndrome.

In the initial study by Ylikorkala *et al.*, 26 women completed a study with 14 consuming sulpiride (50 mg TID) and 12 placebo (Ylikorkala *et al.*, 1982). In the sulpiride-treated group, prolactin levels rose from 49 ng/mL to 402 ng/mL at two weeks; in the placebo group, prolactin levels actually fell from 84.7 to 24 ng/mL. In 13 of the 14 women given sulpiride, the daily milk production increased by 90-730 mL. One patient had a decreased milk production. Average milk production increased by 212-265 mL in the sulpiride-treated group and fell in the placebo group.

In a subsequent study by these authors of 36 puerperal women, prolactin levels increased dramatically at one week (380 ng/mL versus 23 ng/mL in placebo groups), and milk production per day increased (628 mL/day versus 440 mL/day in placebo group) (Ylikorkala *et al.*, 1984).

In another interesting study of prolactin's dose-response to sulpiride, doses as low as 3 mg produced similar plasma prolactin levels to 50 mg doses (McMurdo *et al.*, 1987). However with chronic dosing, prolactin response was attenuated to 50% of the peak levels attained with acute dosing.

In other studies, sulpiride was found to dramatically increase milk production and prolactin levels in primiparous women at day four and five (Aono *et al.*, 1982a), and to dramatically increase milk production in 66 women when given daily (50 mg BID) over seven days postpartum (1211 mL/day versus 916 mL/day in placebo group) (Aono *et al.*, 1979b). Interestingly, sulpiride apparently does not work as well on multiparous women, as milk volumes were not increased with sulpiride (Aono *et al.*, 1982a).

HERBAL GALACTAGOGUES

The use of herbal products to stimulate milk production is quite common today. However, good supporting data suggesting that these agents stimulate milk production/synthesis is minimal to nil. Fenugreek is the most commonly used herbal for this purpose. In a recent abstract of ten women who ingested three capsules three times daily, the average milk production during the week increased significantly from 207 mL/day (range 57-1057 mL) to 464 mL/day (range 63-1140 mL) (Swafford & Berens, 2000). No untoward effects were reported; however, this was not a blinded or controlled study. Other herbal galactagogues have been reported, but again, we have no real scientific data that confirms the efficacy of these agents. For a complete description of these herbal drugs, see Chapter 35.

Table 3. Steps in Evaluating the Use of Galactagogues

1. Evaluate baseline plasma prolactin levels if possible. Levels near baseline indicate these medications will probably work. High levels of prolactin indicate that galactagogues will probably fail to work.
2. If levels of prolactin are low, use domperidone or metoclopramide at the proper dose. Do not overdose or under dose.
3. Monitor milk synthesis. If significantly increased within one week, then continue medication for up to three to four weeks if necessary.
4. If no significant change within one week, discontinue medication.
5. There is no evidence that prolactin levels are dose related when higher and higher doses are used. Do not presume that doubling or tripling the dose of these drugs leads to higher prolactin levels.
6. Slowly discontinue medication over two to three weeks.

SUMMARY

The use of drugs or herbals to suppress or stimulate milk synthesis is widespread and has been for thousands of years. Almost without exception, all of the medications listed above produce changes in the release of prolactin from the pituitary. All of the medications known to suppress breastmilk production do so by preventing the release of prolactin from the pituitary (ergot alkaloids, cabergoline) and are generally considered to be dopamine agonists. Those medications known to increase milk synthesis do so by increasing the release of prolactin from the pituitary (domperidone, metoclopramide, sulpiride, etc.) and are dopamine antagonists.

While dopamine stimulants work consistently to suppress prolactin release and milk synthesis, dopamine antagonists may or may not elevate the release of prolactin, and may or may not always increase milk synthesis. Thus, the clinical response to the use of dopamine antagonists, such as domperidone and metoclopramide, is highly variable among patients (**Table 3**).

For milk production to be sustained, it requires a prolonged and elevated level of prolactin that is above baseline non-lactational levels (>20 ng/mL). But milk synthesis also requires the presence of sensitive and active lactocytes in the breast. There are numerous examples of insufficient milk production, even in women with high prolactin levels. Thus, dopamine antagonists don't always work, and the most predictive factor in this case is perhaps the presence of sufficient lactational tissue in the breast or enlargement of the breasts during gestation. Unfortunately, we can't test for the presence of active lactocytes other than simply administering domperidone or metoclopramide and waiting to see if milk synthesis ensues in the next 24-48 hours.

Testing for baseline plasma prolactin levels is useful as long as the levels are drawn at the proper time. Levels drawn when prolactin is peaking at 45 minutes following breastfeeding would be useless. Baseline levels should be drawn at least two to four hours following a breastfeeding or just before the next feeding. These levels should be higher than the normal non-lactational baseline levels (>30-50 ng/mL) for milk production to persist. In mothers whose baseline levels drop to the non-lactational range (20 ng/mL), milk synthesis will probably suffer. These mothers will probably respond rapidly and effectively to a dopamine antagonist.

To effectively treat mothers with insufficient milk syndrome, clinicians must be cognizant of the side effects of these medications. In general, the amount of medication (domperidone and metoclopramide) transferred to the infant is subclinical and is of limited consequence. Secondly, while domperidone may induce arrhythmias in the rare proarrhythmic patient, it is considered to be the safest in this family of drugs with virtually no side effects in the average patient other than minor headache and GI cramping. On the other hand, metoclopramide's propensity to induce depression is troublesome and mothers should be monitored for this complication. Nevertheless, it is still quite useful short term (<1 month) for stimulating milk synthesis in most mothers.

Lastly, if medications are used to stimulate milk synthesis, all patients should be carefully withdrawn from these medications over several weeks to prevent rapid loss of milk production. We do not have an adequate understanding of this mechanism, but, apparently, rapid withdrawal frequently leads to a rapid loss of milk synthesis. However, we do know that many thousands of women have alternatively been slowly withdrawn from the drugs and have managed to maintain adequate milk production for long periods.

References

Aljazaf K, Hale TW, Ilett KF, Hartmann PE, Mitoulas LR, Kristensen JH, *et al.* Pseudoephedrine: effects on milk production in women and estimation of infant exposure via breastmilk. *Br J Clin Pharmacol.* 2003; 56:18-24.

Anonymous. Single dose cabergoline versus bromocriptine in inhibition of puerperal lactation: randomised, double blind, multicentre study. European Multicentre Study Group for Cabergoline in Lactation Inhibition [see comments]. *BMJ.* 1991; 302:1367-71.

Arita J, Kojima Y, Kimura F. Identification by the sequential cell immunoblot assay of a subpopulation of rat dopamine-unresponsive lactotrophs. *Endocrinology.* 1991; 128:1887-94.

Barone JA. Domperidone: a peripherally acting dopamine2-receptor antagonist. *Ann Pharmacother.* 1999; 33:429-40.

Ben-Jonathan N, Hnasko R. Dopamine as a prolactin (PRL) inhibitor. *Endocr Rev.* 2001; 22:724-63.

Bole-Feysot C, Goffin V, Edery M, Binart N, Kelly PA. Prolactin (PRL) and its receptor: actions, signal transduction pathways and phenotypes observed in PRL receptor knockout mice. *Endocr Rev.* 1998; 19:225-68.

Booker DE, Pahl IR. Control of postpartum breast engorgement with oral contraceptives. *Am J Obstet Gynecol.* 1967; 98:1099-101.

Booker DE, Pahl IR, Forbes DA. Control of postpartum breast engorgement with oral contraceptives. II. *Am J Obstet Gynecol.* 1970; 108:240-42.

Bravo-Topete EG, Mendoza-Hernandez F, Cejudo-Alvarez J, Briones-Garduno C. [Cabergoline for inhibition of lactation]. *Cir Cir.* 2004; 72:5-9.

Brogden RN, Carmine AA, Heel RC, Speight TM, Avery GS. Domperidone. A review of its pharmacological activity, pharmacokinetics and therapeutic efficacy in the symptomatic treatment of chronic dyspepsia and as an antiemetic. *Drugs.* 1982; 24:360-400.

Budd SC, Erdman SH, Long DM, Trombley SK, Udall JNJ. Improved lactation with metoclopramide. A case report. *Clin Pediatr (Phila).* 1993; 32:53-57.

Caballero-Gordo A, Lopez-Nazareno N, Calderay M, Caballero JL, Mancheno E, Sghedoni D. Oral cabergoline. Single-dose inhibition of puerperal lactation. *J Reprod Med.* 1991; 36:717-21.

Caron MG, Beaulieu M, Raymond V, Gagne B, Drouin J, Lefkowitz RJ, *et al.* Dopaminergic receptors in the anterior pituitary gland. Correlation of [3H]dihydroergocryptine binding with the dopaminergic control of prolactin release. *J Biol Chem.* 1978; 253:2244-53.

Cobo E. Effect of different doses of ethanol on the milk-ejecting reflex in lactating women. *Am J Obstet Gynecol.* 1973; 115:817-21.

Cox DB, Owens RA, Hartmann PE. Blood and milk prolactin and the rate of milk synthesis in women. *Exp Physiol.* 1996; 81:1007-20.

da Silva OP, Knoppert DC, Angelini MM, Forret PA. Effect of domperidone on milk production in mothers of premature newborns: a randomized, double-blind, placebo-controlled trial. *CMAJ.* 2001; 164:17-21.

Dutt S, Wong F, Spurway JH. Fatal myocardial infarction associated with bromocriptine for postpartum lactation suppression. *Aust N Z J Obstet Gynaecol.* 1998; 38:116-17.

Ehrenkranz RA, Ackerman BA. Metoclopramide effect on faltering milk production by mothers of premature infants. *Pediatrics.* 1986; 78:614-20.

Ertl T, Sulyok E, Ezer E, Sarkany I, Thurzo V, Csaba IF. The influence of metoclopramide on the composition of human breast milk. *Acta Paediatr Hung.* 1991; 31:415-22.

Ferrari C, Piscitelli G, Crosignani PG. Cabergoline: a new drug for the treatment of hyperprolactinaemia. *Hum Reprod.* 1995; 10:1647-52.

Fisher AA, Davis MW. Serotonin syndrome caused by selective serotonin reuptake-inhibitors-metoclopramide interaction. *Ann Pharmacother.* 2002; 36:67-71.

Freeman ME, Kanyicska B, Lerant A, Nagy G. Prolactin: structure, function, and regulation of secretion. *Physiol Rev.* 2000; 80:1523-1631.

Gambrell RDJ. Immediate postpartum oral contraception. *Obstet Gynecol.* 1970; 36:101-6.

Hansen W, Hunter S. Metoclopramide concentration in breast milk of women delivering between 23-34 weeks gestation. *Am J Obstet Gynecol.* 2001; 185:S116.

Heil SH, Hungund BL, Zheng ZH, Jen KL, Subramanian MG. Ethanol and lactation: effects of milk lipids and serum constituents. *Alcohol.* 1999; 18:43-48.

Heykants J, Hendriks R, Meuldermans W, Michiels M, Scheygrond H, Reyntjens H. On the pharmacokinetics of domperidone in animals and man. IV. The pharmacokinetics of intravenous domperidone and its bioavailability in man following intramuscular, oral and rectal administration. *Eur J Drug Metab Pharmacokinet.* 1981; 6:61-70.

Hofmeyr GJ, Van Iddekinge B. Domperidone and lactation [letter]. *Lancet.* 1983; 1:647.

Hofmeyr GJ, Van Iddekinge B, Blott JA. Domperidone: secretion in breast milk and effect on puerperal prolactin levels. *Br J Obstet Gynaecol.* 1985; 92:141-44.

Iffy L, O'Donnell J, Correia J, Hopp L. Severe cardiac dysrhythmia in patients using bromocriptine postpartum. *Am J Ther.* 1998; 5:111-15.

Jacobs LS. The role of prolactin in mammogenesis and lactogenesis. *Adv Exp Med Biol* 1977; 80:173-91.

Jones WL, Stewart DB. Effects of orally-administered ethanol on mammary gland morphology and functional efficiency in lactating rats. *Exp Pathol.* 1984; 25:205-13.

Kauppila A, Arvela P, Koivisto M, Kivinen S, Ylikorkala O, Pelkonen O. Metoclopramide and breast feeding: transfer into milk and the newborn. *Eur J Clin Pharmacol.* 1983; 25:819-23.

Kauppila A, Kivinen S, Ylikorkala O. A dose response relation between improved lactation and metoclopramide. *Lancet.* 1981; 1:1175-77.

Kuhn NJ. Progesterone withdrawal as the lactogenic trigger in the rat. *J Endocrinol.* 1969; 44:39-54.

Lewis PJ, Devenish C, Kahn C. Controlled trial of metoclopramide in the initiation of breast feeding. *Br J Clin Pharmacol.* 1980; 9:217-19.

Masala A, Delitala G, Alagna S, Devilla L, Stoppelli I, Lo DG. Clomiphene and puerperal lactation. *Panminerva Med.* 1978; 20:161-63.

McMurdo ME, Howie PW, Lewis M, Marnie M, McEwen J, McNeilly AS. Prolactin response to low dose sulpiride. *Br J Clin Pharmacol.* 1987; 24:133-37.

Mennella JA, Beauchamp GK. The transfer of alcohol to human milk. Effects on flavor and the infant's behavior. *N Engl J Med.* 1991; 325:981-85.

Nagano M, Kelly PA. Tissue distribution and regulation of rat prolactin receptor gene expression. Quantitative analysis by polymerase chain reaction. *J Biol Chem.* 1994; 269:13337-45.

Neville MC, McFadden TB, Forsyth I. Hormonal regulation of mammary differentiation and milk secretion. *J Mammary Gland Biol Neoplasia.* 2002; 7:49-66.

Osborne RJ, Slevin ML, Hunter RW, Hamer J. Cardiac arrhythmias during cytotoxic chemotherapy: role of domperidone. *Hum Toxicol.* 1985; 4:617-26.

Parker DC, Rossman LG, Vanderlaan EF. Relation of sleep-entrained human prolactin release to REM-nonREM cycles. *J Clin Endocrinol Metab.* 1974; 38:646-51.

Peters F, Lummerich M, Breckwoldt M. Inhibition of prolactin and lactation by methylergometrine hydrogenmaleate. *Acta Endocrinol (Copenh.)* 1979; 91:213-16.

Petraglia F, De L, V, Sardelli S, Pieroni ML, D'Antona N, Genazzani AR. Domperidone in defective and insufficient lactation. *Eur J Obstet Gynecol Reprod Biol.* 1985; 19:281-87.

Pop C, Metz D, Matei M, Wagner E, Tassan S, Elaerts J. [Postpartum myocardial infarction induced by Parlodel]. *Arch Mal Coeur Vaiss.* 1998; 91:1171-74.

Raymond V, Beaulieu M, Labrie F, Boissier J. Potent antidopaminergic activity of estradiol at the pituitary level on prolactin release. *Science.* 1978; 200:1173-75.

Robinson GW, McKnight RA, Smith GH, Hennighausen L. Mammary epithelial cells undergo secretory differentiation in cycling virgins but require pregnancy for the establishment of terminal differentiation. *Development.* 1995; 121:2079-90.

Roussak JB, Carey P, Parry H. Cardiac arrest after treatment with intravenous domperidone. *Br Med J (Clin Res Ed).* 1984; 289:1579.

Sawagado L, Houdebine LM. Identification of the lactogenic compound present in beer. *Ann Biol Clin (Paris).* 1988; 46:129-34.

Schrauzer GN, Hamm D, Kuehn K, Nakonecny G. Effects of long term exposure to beer on the genesis and development of spontaneous mammary adenocarcinoma and prolactin levels in female virgin C3H/St mice. *J Am Coll Nutr.* 1982; 1:285-91.

Shaaban MM. Suppression of lactation by an antiestrogen, tamoxifen. *Eur J Obstet Gynecol Reprod Biol.* 1975; 4:167-69.

Swafford S, Berens P. Effect of fenugreek on breast milk production. [Abstract]. *BM News and Views.* 2000; 6(3):2000. Annual meeting abstracts Sept. 11-13, 2000.

Tankeyoon M, Dusitsin N, Chalapati S, Koetsawang S, Saibiang S, Sas M *et al.* Effects of hormonal contraceptives on milk volume and infant growth. WHO Special Programme of Research, Development and Research Training in Human Reproduction Task force on oral contraceptives. *Contraception.* 1984; 30:505-22.

Treffers PE. [Breastfeeding and contraception]. *Ned Tijdschr Geneeskd.* 1999; 143:1900-4.

Tyson JE, Khojandi M, Huth J, Andreassen B. The influence of prolactin secretion on human lactation. *J Clin Endocrinol Metab.* 1975; 40:764-73.

Vilaro S, Vinas O, Remesar X, Herrera E. Effects of chronic ethanol consumption on lactational performance in rat: mammary gland and milk composition and pups' growth and metabolism. *Pharmacol Biochem Behav.* 1987; 27:333-39.

Webster J. A comparative review of the tolerability profiles of dopamine agonists in the treatment of hyperprolactinaemia and inhibition of lactation [published erratum appears in Drug Saf 1996 May;14(5):342]. *Drug Saf.* 1996; 14:228-38.

Webster J, Piscitelli G, Polli A, D'Alberton A, Falsetti L, Ferrari C *et al.* Dose-dependent suppression of serum prolactin by cabergoline in hyperprolactinaemia: a placebo controlled, double blind, multicentre study. European Multicentre Cabergoline Dose-finding Study Group. *Clin Endocrinol (Oxf).* 1992; 37:534-41.

Weinstein D, Ben David M, Polishuk WZ. Serum prolactin and the suppression of lactation. *Br J Obstet Gynaecol.* 1976; 83:679-82.

Weiss G, Klein S, Shenkman L, Kataoka K, Hollander CS. Effect of methylergonovine on puerperal prolactin secretion. *Obstet Gynecol.* 1975; 46:209-10.

Ylikorkala O, Kauppila A, Kivinen S, Viinikka L. Sulpiride improves inadequate lactation. *Br Med J (Clin Res Ed).* 1982; 285:249-51.

Ylikorkala O, Kauppila A, Kivinen S, Viinikka L. Treatment of inadequate lactation with oral sulpiride and buccal oxytocin. *Obstet Gynecol.* 1984; 63:57-60.

Zuckerman H, Carmel S. The inhibition of lactation by clomiphene. *J Obstet Gynaecol Br Commonw.* 1973; 80:822-23.

Chapter 26

Analgesic and Anti-Inflammatory Drugs

Kenneth F. Ilett and Judith H. Kristensen

INTRODUCTION

Analgesics are commonly used in breastfeeding mothers early postpartum, particularly when cesarean section has been necessary for the delivery of their newborn. In this situation, post-operative pain often requires repeated administration of moderate to strong analgesics for up to several days. Since lactation does not commence until one to two days after birth and when colostrum is produced in modest volumes (30-60 mL/day) (Neville *et al.*, 1988), the opportunity for transfer of analgesics into early milk is generally low. Nevertheless by day three, the volume of transitional milk has increased to a mean of around 400 mL/day, and by day 7-14 to a mean of 650 mL/day of mature milk (Neville *et al.*, 1988), and drug transfer may become significant. Analgesics and antipyretics may also be needed for pain control in a variety of other situations/conditions during mature milk production. Short-term pain control (e.g., headache) is often limited to one or two doses and obviously exposes the breastfed infant to a much lower level of risk than when long-term pain control is required (e.g., osteoarthritis).

The general area of analgesics and breastfeeding was most recently reviewed by Spigset and colleagues (Spigset *et al.*, 2000). In this chapter, we have chosen to address the comparative safety of drugs in breastfeeding by looking primarily at their relative infant dose. For the most part, this strategy works reasonably well and provides information that can assist in providing a risk/benefit analysis. However, for some drugs that are used as single doses, it is perhaps easier to step back to consideration of the absolute infant dose, particularly when the drug also has a pediatric indication that can provide a comparative yardstick in the assessment of safety (e.g., fentanyl). Whatever primary yardstick one chooses, it needs to be coupled with careful consideration of associated data that can indicate safety or otherwise of breastfeeding. Such data may include validated reports of adverse effects in breastfed infants and reports that indicate that cohorts of infants have achieved expected developmental milestones and normal cognitive abilities in comparison with matched controls. In addition, the use of analgesics (particularly opiates) in infants who are weak or apneic following delivery should be approached with great caution. Indeed, the frequent repeated use of such drugs has been reported to produce extreme sedation in breastfed infants (Koren *et al.*, 2006).

Table 1 summarizes the relative infant dose data and our recommendations for a range of analgesics that may be commonly encountered. Some antagonists related to the opiate analgesics are also included in this section. Selected examples are discussed in more detail in the sections that follow.

COMMON ANALGESICS

Acetaminophen ± Codeine

Acetaminophen (paracetamol) or acetaminophen/

Table 1. Analgesic and Anti-Inflammatory Drugs in Breastfeeding

Drug	Relative infant dose (%)	Comment	References
Common analgesics			
Aspirin	<0.1, 9.4, 10	Compatible in low doses. Prolonged use could be problematic. Others preferred.	Bailey *et al.*, 1982; Findlay *et al.*, 1981; Putter *et al.*, 1974
Acetaminophen (paracetamol)	1 - 2.8	Compatible.	Berlin Jr. *et al.*, 1980; Bitzen *et al.*, 1981; Notarianni *et al.*, 1987
Nonsteroidal anti-inflammatory drugs			
Celecoxib	0.2, 0.3	Compatible.	Gardiner *et al.*, 2006; Hale *et al.*, 2004
Diclofenac	1.4 or less	Compatible.	Sioufi *et al.*, 1982; Todd *et al.*, 1988
Ibuprofen	0.001	Compatible.	Townsend *et al.*, 1984; Weibert *et al.*, 1982
Indomethacin	0.3, 0.5	Compatible.	Beaulac-Baillargeon *et al.*, 1993; Lebedevs *et al.*, 1991
Ketoprofen		No data available.	
Ketorolac	0.2	Compatible.	Wischnik *et al.*, 1989
Meloxicam		No data available.	
Mefenamic acid		No data available, low transfer anticipated.	Buchanan *et al.*, 1968
Naproxen	2.0, 2.8	Low transfer to milk, but drug has long half-life. One report of bleeding and anemia in an exposed infant. Compatible for short term use.	Figalgo, 1989; Jamali *et al.*, 1983
Parecoxib		No data available.	
Piroxicam	3.5	Average exposure estimate.	Ostensen, 1983; Ostensen *et al.*, 1988
Opioids and related drugs			
Buprenorphine	<1 – 2.4	Single study only indicates low transfer. Variable dose ranges. Use with caution. May affect milk production.	Grimm *et al.*, 2005; Hirose *et al.*, 1997; Jernite *et al.*, 1999; Marquet *et al.*, 1997
Buprenorphine + naloxone		No data for the combination or for naloxone alone.	
Butorphanol	0.3 - 0.4	Single study. Compatible.	Pittman *et al.*, 1980
Codeine	0.6, 1.2	Compatible; others preferred because of (a) possible association with apnea or bradycardia and (b) one report of an infant death where the mother had the UM CYP2D6 genotype.	Findlay *et al.*, 1981; Koren *et al.*, 2006; Meny *et al.*, 1993
Fentanyl	0.6, 3	Compatible, but some concerns about successfully establishing lactation.	Leuschen *et al.*, 1990; Steer *et al.*, 1992
Hydrocodone		Compatible; some sedation in infants has been associated with higher doses and for longer periods; caution recommended.	Bodley *et al.*, 1997
Hydromorphone	0.7	Single 2 mg maternal intranasal dose. Compatible.	Edwards *et al.*, 2003
Meperidine (pethidine)	0.6 - 3.5	Low transfer, but adverse neurobehavioral side-effects reported. Safer alternatives available.	Freeborn *et al.*, 1980; Peiker *et al.*, 1980; Quinn *et al.*, 1986; Wittels *et al.*, 1990; Wittels *et al.*, 1997
Methadone	1 - 5.6	Low transfer to milk; levels generally insufficient to prevent withdrawal. Compatible.	Begg *et al.*, 2001; Geraghty *et al.*, 1997; Jansson *et al.*, 2007; Wojnar-Horton *et al.*, 1997
Morphine	0.4 - 3.4	Compatible in usual analgesic doses used in the perinatal period. Caution with high dose extended-release preparations as there are no data.	Baka *et al.*, 2002; Feilberg *et al.*, 1989; Kim *et al.*, 2006; Robieux *et al.*, 1990; Wittels *et al.*, 1990
Naltrexone	1	Compatible. Single case report only.	Chan *et al.*, 2004
Oxycodone	1-3.5, 8	Dose calculated on maximum levels in milk. Low or single doses compatible, but caution suggested with higher dose extended-release preparations.	Seaton *et al.*, 2007; Marx *et al.*, 1986
Propoxyphene	2	Compatible.	Kunka *et al.*, 1984; Kunka *et al.*, 1985
Tramadol	2.4	Compatible for short-term use.	Ilett *et al.*, 2007, submitted

codeine combinations are considered safe to use within the usual recommended daily dose ranges and have been approved by the American Academy of Pediatrics for use in breastfeeding mothers. Two studies reported apnea, bradycardia, or cyanosis in breastfed infants after repeated four to six hourly maternal doses of 60 mg codeine (Davis *et al.*, 2005; Naumburg *et al.*, 1987), but a third found no such effects (Meny *et al.*, 1993).

Typically, infants exposed to codeine-containing products have morphine serum concentrations of 0.5-2.2 μg/L (Meny *et al.*, 1993). One infant death has been reported following the maternal use of codeine (60 mg every 12 hours, reduced to 30 mg every 12 hours from day two to two weeks because of maternal somnolence and constipation) (Koren *et al.*, 2006). Morphine concentration in milk was 87 μg/L, corresponding to a relative infant dose of only 1.5%. CYP2D6 genotyping of the mother indicated that she had the ultra-rapid (UM) genotype [UM frequency range: 1% in Caucasians, 10% in Greeks and Portuguese, and 29% in Ethiopians (Cascorbi, 2003)] which results in a marked increase in the formation of morphine from codeine. However, the low relative infant dose is inconsistent with the apparent safety of morphine when used at the lower end of its usual dose range (see Opiates section below and **Table 1**). In addition, although a postmortem showed no anatomical defects that might explain a respiratory death, the investigation of alternative causes, such as infection, was not mentioned. CYP2D6 genotyping is available in many laboratories, and although expensive, its diagnostic use could be contemplated for mothers who need to take high doses of codeine chronically. Ultimately, each breastfed infant's response to codeine exposure should be determined by frequent careful observation. Adverse effects, such as overt somnolence, apnea, or poor feeding, should be investigated promptly. In most mothers, codeine taken in short courses and at low doses should be safe for the breastfed infant. Nevertheless, until further evidence emerges, it would seem prudent to rank codeine as a third line analgesic choice, after NSAIDs or paracetamol.

Aspirin

The available data for aspirin relate to the excretion of salicylic acid and/or some related metabolites of aspirin (Bailey *et al.*, 1982; Findlay *et al.*, 1981; Putter *et al.*, 1974). Given the very short (31 minute) half-life of aspirin in man (Kershaw *et al.*, 1987), transfer of aspirin itself into milk is probably low. However, given that aspirin is strongly associated with Reye's syndrome (Calvani, 2000; Glasgow, 2006), its use in breastfeeding mothers should be discouraged, but not necessarily contraindicated.

NONSTEROIDAL ANTI-INFLAMMATORY DRUGS (NSAIDS)

In reviewing this area, the authors of LactMed (US National Library of Medicine, 2006) express the view that the earlier NSAIDs (usually inhibitors of both COX-1 and COX-2) with short half-lives (e.g., diclofenac, ibuprofen) should be preferred over those with longer half-lives (e.g., naproxen, piroxicam). While this is a sensible evaluation, the relative infant doses for all of these drugs are low and the American Academy of Pediatrics considers most to be compatible in breastfeeding (American Academy of Pediatrics Committee on Drugs, 2001).

Naproxen

Naproxen used for periods less than two weeks is probably compatible, although one case of prolonged bleeding, hemorrhage, and acute anemia in a seven-day-old infant has been reported (Figalgo, 1989). The relative infant dose would probably be less than three percent.

Indomethacin

Seizures have been reported in an infant exposed to indomethacin via breastmilk, despite low transfer (Eeg-Olofsson *et al.*, 1978). However, the relative infant dose of indomethacin is low (Lebedevs *et al.*, 1991), and the link between the seizures and indomethacin exposure has not been proven (Paech *et al.*, 1998). Unfortunately, there are no data available for ketoprofen or meloxicam.

Celecoxib, Rofecoxib and Parecoxib

Of the more selective COX-2 NSAIDs, celecoxib has low transfer into milk, with a relative infant dose of only 0.3%, as does the closely related rofecoxib (0.25%) (Gardiner *et al.*, 2005), which was withdrawn from the market because of adverse cardiovascular effects in adults. There are presently no data available for parecoxib or its active metabolite valdecoxib.

Ketorolac

One of the more popular NSAIDs used orally, IV, and IM postoperatively, is ketorolac, which has mixed COX-1/COX-2 NSAID activity in animal models (Waterbury *et al.*, 2006). It is a highly effective analgesic, but has inhibitory effects on platelet function that may limit its use in postpartum women due to risk of hemorrhage (Anonymous, 2006). However, its transfer into milk is negligible (Wischnik *et al.*, 1989). In ten lactating women who received 10 mg orally four times daily, ketorolac was not detected in milk from four of the subjects, while in the remainder the concentration was <5μg/L. A maximum relative infant dose of <0.2% can be calculated from these data.

OPIOIDS AND ANTAGONISTS

Fentanyl

For fentanyl (**Table 1**), we calculated relative infant doses of 0.6% or 3% based on the average maternal dose per time and highest milk fentanyl concentration reported in two separate studies of fentanyl administration for cesarian section, postpartum tubal ligation, or labor (Leuschen *et al.*, 1990; Steer *et al.*, 1992). The absolute infant doses used in the above calculation (0.02 μg/kg/day and 0.06 μg/kg/day) can also be put into risk perspective by comparing them to the usual infant IV infusion dose of 1-3 μg/kg/hour for fentanyl (Hirshfeld *et al.*, 2000). Both methods of evaluation suggest a low infant exposure with an acceptable low level of risk. However, there is conflicting evidence that fentanyl administration during labor might be associated with difficulty in establishing breastfeeding (Beilin *et al.*, 2005; Halpern *et al.*, 2005). There is also one study indicating an association between fentanyl administration and an increased incidence of bottle feeding at discharge from the hospital. Nevertheless, establishing a clear cause and effect in such studies is difficult (Jordan *et al.*, 2005).

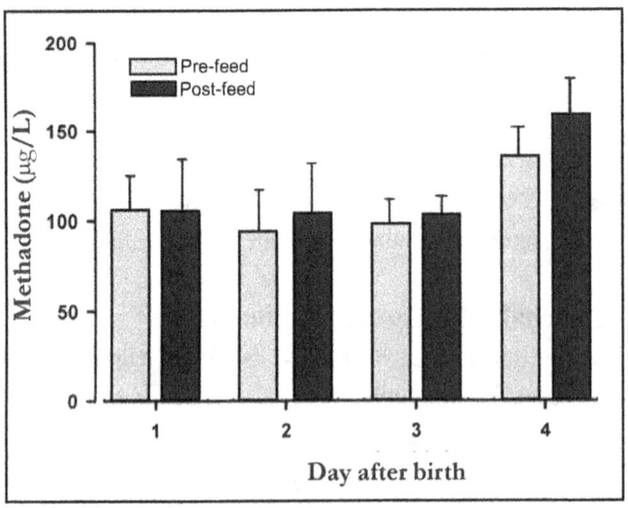

Figure 1. Pre- and post-feed methadone concentrations in colostrum/early milk in the immediate perinatal period. Data as mean ± SEM of peak and trough concentrations. Source: Jansson *et al.*, 2007.

Methadone

Because of its wide use as a maintenance treatment for opiate addiction, methadone has been extensively studied. For many years, The American Academy of Pediatrics recommended breastfeeding only for maternal methadone doses of <20 mg/day (Philipp *et al.*, 2003). However, as shown in **Table 1**, relative infant doses of between 1-5.6% have been reported in maternal doses ranging from 20-180 mg daily, and hence it is considered safe for use in breastfeeding (Begg *et al.*, 2001; Geraghty *et al.*, 1997; Wojnar-Horton *et al.*, 1997). This recommendation is now supported by the American Academy of Pediatrics (American Academy of Pediatrics Committee on Drugs, 2001). There is also published information on the levels of methadone in colostrum/transitional milk in the first four days after birth (Jansson *et al.*, 2007) (**Figure 1**). These women received a mean methadone dose of 76 mg daily (approximately 1086 μg/kg/day assuming a weight of 70 kg). Although pre- and post-feed concentrations of methadone in milk were statistically different overall, the differences were small. The authors calculated that the mean doses received by the infants were 6, 18, 39, and 84 μg on days one, two, three, and four, respectively. At day four, assuming an average infant weight of 3.1 kg, the mean absolute infant dose is 27 μg/kg/day and the estimated mean relative infant dose is 2.5%, which is in agreement with earlier studies in older infants (Begg *et al.*, 2001; Geraghty *et al.*, 1997; Wojnar-Horton *et al.*, 1997).

Starting one to two days after birth, up to 80% of newborns of mothers receiving methadone suffer from a neonatal abstinence syndrome (NAS) (Brown *et al.*, 1991; Rosen *et al.*, 1975). Newborns of methadone maintenance patients will have been exposed to high concentrations of methadone throughout pregnancy. At birth, they have significant concentrations of the drug in their blood and are essentially dependent on the drug. Withdrawal symptoms, such as tremor, hypotonia, irritability, fever, vomiting, diarrhea, and respiratory distress occur, and the degree of distress is measured using an instrument called the Finnegan Scale (Finnegan *et al.*, 1975). Treatment consists of general supportive measures and administration of sedatives and/or opiates (Carin *et al.*, 1983). The half-life of methadone in neonates varies from 16-25 hours (Rosen *et al.*, 1975; Rosen *et al.*, 1976), which is shorter than the population mean of 39 hours for adults in a methadone maintenance program (Foster *et al.*, 2004). Ingestion of methadone via breastmilk is only sufficient to ameliorate the symptoms of NAS in some cases (Malpas *et al.*, 1995; Malpas *et al.*, 1999; Ostrea *et al.*, 1976; Strauss *et al.*, 1974). Nevertheless, a recent study (Abdel-Latif *et al.*, 2006) showed that mean Finnegan scores over the first nine days of life were significantly lower in breastfed neonates compared to matched controls who received formula. The breastfed infants were also significantly less likely to require pharmacologic treatment for withdrawal. Hence, we conclude that breastfeeding is to be encouraged in mothers on methadone maintenance.

Buprenorphine

Buprenorphine, a partial μ-opioid receptor agonist is widely used at doses of 4-32 mg/day for treatment of opioid dependency (Robinson, 2002). A relative infant dose ranging from <1% to 2.4% can be calculated (Grimm *et al.*, 2005; Jernite *et al.*, 1999; Marquet *et al.*, 1997). However, some caution is suggested from the observation that buprenorphine may suppress oxytocin release and thus interfere with milk letdown (Hirose *et al.*, 1997).

Tramadol

Tramadol, a synthetic analgesic with agonist effects at μ-opioid receptors and an ability to block both 5-hydroxytryptamine and noradrenaline reuptake in central synapses has recently been studied in our laboratory. The drug was administered orally (100 mg 6-hourly for 4 doses prior to sampling) to a group of 75 women who had undergone cesarian sections and samples of transitional milk taken on day three to four after delivery showed low transfer into milk. At steady-state, the mean relative infant dose was 2.24% for tramadol, with an additional 0.64% for its *O*-desmethylmetabolite which is also a μ-opioid receptor agonist (Ilett *et al.*, 2007, submitted). The exposed infants had similar Neurologic and Adaptive Capacity Scores to a matched control group of infants whose mothers received alternative analgesics.

Meperidine

Calculations for meperidine (pethidine) give relative infant doses of <0.6-3.5% (Freeborn *et al.*, 1980; Peiker *et al.*, 1980; Quinn *et al.*, 1986; Wittels *et al.*, 1990). While this dose range is low, there could also be a similar contribution from its major metabolite normeperidine (Quinn *et al.*, 1986). One study has looked at saliva concentrations of meperidine in infants whose mothers received 100 mg meperidine during labor. In a sub-group of breastfed infants, salivary meperidine was higher at 24 hours than at two to three hours after birth, and remained elevated at 48 hours. By contrast, a sub-group of newborns who were bottle fed showed slowly decreasing meperidine concentrations over the first 48 hours after birth. Given the observation of adverse neurobehavioral effects in three to four day old infants whose mothers received patient-controlled meperidine analgesia after cesarian section (Wittels *et al.*, 1990; Wittels *et al.*, 1997), together with the long half-life of normeperidine in adults, the drug is probably best avoided during lactation.

Morphine

The available data on morphine transfer into milk arise mostly from its intravenous, intramuscular, or epidural use for post-operative analgesia following cesarian section (Feilberg *et al.*, 1989; Oberlander *et al.*, 2000; Robieux *et al.*, 1990; Wittels *et al.*, 1990). Only one study has measured the highly active metabolite, morphine-6-glucuronide, as well as morphine in colostrum (Baka *et al.*, 2002). Using the median concentrations of morphine and morphine-6-glucuronide reported over the first 48 hours of an intravenous infusion in four patients, relative infant doses of 0.6% and 17% can be calculated for parent drug and metabolite respectively. Based on its low relative infant dose, morphine appears safe to use in the standard doses administered in patient-controlled analgesic pumps, epidural injections, or repeated intramuscular or intravenous doses. If the absorption of morphine from the infant's gastrointestinal tract is low as in adults (30%) because of conversion to inactive morphine-3-glucuronide, then poor bioavailability may give the infant added protection. The significance of the presence of a high relative infant dose of morphine-6-glucuronide in colostrum (Baka *et al.*, 2002) has not been satisfactorily addressed. The glucuronide itself would presumably have low bioavailability, but there could be bacterial (β-glucuronidase-mediated) hydrolysis to release morphine in the distal small intestine and colon. Given the generally low morphine exposure and in the absence of adverse events being reported in breastfed infants (Wittels *et al.*, 1990; Wittels *et al.*, 1997) whose mothers received patient controlled analgesia with morphine after cesarian section, we conclude that morphine is compatible with breastfeeding. Since there are no data for high dose controlled-release oral morphine preparations, there should be careful observation of the breastfed infant if use of these dose forms is required during breastfeeding.

Hydrocodone

Hydrocodone, a semisynthetic derivative of codeine is metabolized to a number of active metabolites, and is considered to have approximately six times the potency of codeine. While it is commonly used as an analgesic in breastfeeding mothers, there are no published data on its transfer in milk. Anecdotally, when used in 5-10 mg doses every six hours, it has not been reported to sedate breastfeeding infants. Prolonged use has led to some reports of infant sedation (Bodley *et al.*, 1997). In the absence of data, we conclude that it is preferable to use other agents.

Butorphanol and Nalbuphine

Butorphanol and nalbuphine are narcotic analgesics with a partial agonist mechanism of action (i.e., they can both simulate and block opioid receptors). They are commonly used during delivery and postpartum because they are less likely to cause respiratory sedation. No data are available on their transfer into milk. In addition, they have been reported to cause psychotomimetic effects at higher doses (Zola *et al.*, 1983). Again, in the absence of data, we conclude that it is preferable to use other agents.

Oxycodone

Oxycodone is a semisynthetic narcotic analgesic derived from thebaine that is metabolized to the active metabolites oxymorphone and noroxycodone. It is commonly used as an analgesic in postpartum and other breastfeeding mothers. Like hydrocodone, it is an analgesic which is somewhat stronger than codeine. Following doses of 5-10 mg every four to seven hours, milk concentrations ranged from <5 to 226 μg/L (Marx *et al.*, 1986). Corresponding maternal plasma levels were 14-35 μg/L, giving a M/P of around 3.4. Using mid-range data from this study, a relative infant dose of around 3.2% can be calculated. A study of oxycodone use in 50 breastfeeding women post-cesarian section indicates a relative infant dose ranging from 1-3.5% in the first 72 hours after delivery (Seaton *et al.*, 2007). Oxycodone levels in milk ranged from 0-168 μg/L, and the authors calculated that a breastfed infant might receive more than 10% of an infant therapeutic dose. However, oxycodone was only detected in plasma (at a level of 6.6-7.4 μg/L) in one out of forty-one infants tested. While there are no reports of untoward effects in infants, sedation of the breastfed infant is a likely adverse effect and higher doses should be avoided.

Naltrexone

Transfer of the narcotic antagonist naltrexone into milk is low, with a relative infant dose of 0.86% (naltrexone + 6,β-naltrexol metabolite) for a 50 mg maternal oral dose regimen at steady-state (Chan *et al.*, 2004). Plasma concentrations of naltrexone in this patient ranged from 1.5-4 μg/L in the four to eight hours after the morning dose. While the transfer resulting from the use of naltrexone implants has not been studied, the plasma concentrations of around 3-5 μg/L typically achieved with these devices over months (Foster *et al.*, 2003; Hulse *et al.*, 2004) strongly suggests that breastfeeding should also be safe.

CONCLUSIONS

On balance, the data suggest that there are no absolute contraindications to breastfeeding for mothers who need to take the various analgesics, antipyretics, and some related drugs listed in **Table 1**.

Opiate analgesics that suppress the respiratory centers should be used with great caution where the breastfed infant has breathing difficulties, apnea, or other respiratory syndromes. Where their use is unavoidable, the dose, frequency, and duration of therapy should be minimized. NSAIDs and paracetamol should be preferred when analgesics are needed.

While the absolute and/or relative infant doses are useful guides to assessing safety of drug use in lactation, consideration should also be given to reports of adverse effects, the lack of adverse effects in breastfed infants, reports of blood levels of drugs in exposed infants, and the duration for which the mother needs to take the medication. As with all drug use in breastfeeding, an individual risk/benefit analysis should be conducted before starting therapy.

References

Abdel-Latif ME, Pinner J, Clews S, Cooke F, Lui K, Oei J. Effects of breast milk on the severity and outcome of neonatal abstinence syndrome among infants of drug-dependent mothers. *Pediatrics.* 2006; 117:e1163-69.

American Academy of Pediatrics Committee on Drugs. Transfer of drugs and other chemicals into human milk. *Pediatrics.* 2001; 108:776-89.

Anonymous. Toradol, MIMS Abbreviated prescribing information. *E-MIMS 2006.* 2006; Version 5.00.0270

Bailey DN, Weibert RT, Naylor AJ, Shaw RF. A study of salicylate and caffeine excretion in the breast milk of two nursing mothers. *J Anal Toxicol.* 1982; 6:64-68.

Baka NE, Bayoumeu F, Boutroy MJ, Laxenaire MC. Colostrum morphine concentrations during postcesarean intravenous patient-controlled analgesia. *Anesth Analgesia.* 2002; 94:184-87, table.

Beaulac-Baillargeon L, Allard G. Distribution of indomethacin in human milk and estimation of its milk to plasma ratio in vitro. *Br J Clin Pharmacol.* 1993; 36:413-16.

Begg EJ, Malpas TJ, Hackett LP, Ilett KF. Distribution of R- and S-methadone into human milk at steady state during ingestion of medium to high doses. *Br J Clin Pharmacol.* 2001; 52:681-85.

Beilin Y, Bodian CA, Weiser J, Hossain S, Arnold I, Feierman DE, *et al.* Effect of labor epidural analgesia with and without fentanyl on infant breast-feeding: a prospective, randomized, double-blind study. *Anesthesiology.* 2005; 103:1211-17.

Berlin CM Jr., Yaffe SJ, Ragni M. Disposition of acetaminophen in milk, saliva, and plasma of lactating women. *Pediatr Pharmacol* (NY). 1980; 1:135-41.

Bitzen PO, Gustafsson B, Jostell KG, Melander A, Wahlin-Boll E. Excretion of paracetamol in human breast milk. *Eur J Clin Pharmacol.* 1981; 20:123-25.

Bodley V, Powers D. Long-term treatment of a breastfeeding mother with fluconazole-resolved nipple pain caused by yeast: a case study. *J Hum Lact.* 1997; 13:307-11.

Brown ER, Zuckerman B. The infant of the drug-abusing mother. *Pediatr Ann.* 1991; 20:555-63.

Buchanan RA, Eaton CJ, Koeff ST, Kinkel AW. The breast milk excretion of mefenamic acid. *Curr Ther Res Clin Exp.* 1968; 10:592-97.

Calvani M. Reye's syndrome: the death of a syndrome? (Or death by a syndrome?). *Recenti Prog Med.* 2000; 91:675-80.

Carin I, Glass L, Parekh A, Solomon N, Steigman J, Wong S. Neonatal methadone withdrawal. Effect of two treatment regimens. *Am J Dis Child.* 1983; 137:1166-69.

Cascorbi I. Pharmacogenetics of cytochrome p4502D6: genetic background and clinical implication. *Eur J Clin Invest.* 2003; 33 Suppl 2:17-22.

Chan CF, Page-Sharp M, Kristensen JH, O'Neil G, Ilett KF. Transfer of naltrexone and its metabolite 6,beta-naltrexol into human milk. *J Hum Lact.* 2004; 20:322-26.

Davis JM, Bhutari VK. Neonatal apnea and maternal codeine use. *Pediatr Res.* 2005; 19:170A.

Edwards JE, Rudy AC, Wermeling DP, Desai N, McNamara PJ. Hydromorphone transfer into breast milk after intranasal administration. *Pharmacotherapy.* 2003; 23:153-58.

Eeg-Olofsson O, Malmros I, Elwin CE, Steen B. Convulsions in a breast-fed infant after maternal indomethacin [letter]. *Lancet.* 1978; 2:215.

Feilberg VL, Rosenborg D, Broen CC, Mogensen JV. Excretion of morphine in human breast milk. *Acta Anaesthesiol Scand.* 1989; 33:426-28.

Figalgo I. Anemia aguda, rectaorragia y hematuria asociadas a la ingestion de naproxen. *An Esp Pediatr.* 1989; 30:317-19.

Findlay JW, DeAngelis RL, Kearney MF, Welch RM, Findlay JM. Analgesic drugs in breast milk and plasma. *Clin Pharmacol Ther.* 1981; 29:625-33.

Finnegan LP, Connaughton JF Jr, Kron RE, Emich JP. Neonatal abstinence syndrome: assessment and management. *Addictive Dis.* 1975; 2:141-58.

Foster DJ, Somogyi AA, White JM, Bochner F. Population pharmacokinetics of (R)-, (S)- and rac-methadone in methadone maintenance patients. *Br J Clin Pharmacol.* 2004; 57:742-55.

Foster J, Brewer C, Steele T. Naltrexone implants can completely prevent early (1-month) relapse after opiate detoxification: a pilot study of two cohorts totalling 101 patients with a note on naltrexone blood levels. *Addict Biol.* 2003; 8:211-17.

Freeborn SF, Calvert RT, Black P, Macfarlane T, D'Souza SW. Saliva and blood pethidine concentrations in the mother and the newborn baby. *Br J Obstet Gynaecol.* 1980; 87:966-69.

Gardiner SJ, Begg EJ, Zhang M, Hughes RC. Transfer of rofecoxib into human milk. *Eur J Clin Pharmacol.* 2005; 61:405-8.

Gardiner SJ, Doogue MP, Zhang M, Begg EJ. Quantification of infant exposure to celecoxib through breast milk. *Br J Clin Pharmacol.* 2006; 61:101-4.

Geraghty B, Graham EA, Logan B, Weiss EL. Methadone levels in breast milk. *J Hum Lact.* 1997; 13:227-30.

Glasgow JF. Reye's syndrome: the case for a causal link with aspirin. *Drug Saf.* 2006; 29:1111-21.

Grimm D, Pauly E, Poschl J, Linderkamp O, Skopp G. Buprenorphine and norbuprenorphine concentrations in human breast milk samples determined by liquid chromatography-tandem mass spectrometry. *Ther Drug Monit.* 2005; 27:526-30.

Hale TW, McDonald R, Boger J. Transfer of celecoxib into human milk. *J Hum Lact.* 2004; 20:397-403.

Halpern SH, Ioscovich A. Epidural analgesia and breast-feeding. *Anesthesiology.* 2005; 103:1111-12.

Hirose M, Hosokawa T, Tanaka Y. Extradural buprenorphine suppresses breast feeding after caesarean section. *Br J Anaesth.* 1997; 79:120-21.

Hirshfeld AB, Getachew A, Sessions J. Drug doses. In: Siberry GK, Iannone R (eds.). *The Harriet Lane handbook. A manual for pediatric house officers.* 15th Ed. St Louis, USA: Mosby; 2000. p. 599-892.

Hulse GK, Arnold-Reed DE, O'Neil G, Chan CT, Hansson R, O'Neil P. Blood naltrexone and 6-beta-naltrexol levels following naltrexone implant: comparing two naltrexone implants. *Addict Biol.* 2004; 9:59-65.

Jamali F, Stevens DR. Naproxen excretion in milk and its uptake by the infant. *Drug Intell Clin Pharm.* 1983; 17:910-11.

Jansson LM, Choo RE, Harrow C, Velez M, Schroeder JR, Lowe R, *et al.* Concentrations of methadone in breast milk and plasma in the immediate perinatal period. *J Hum Lact.* 2007; 23:184-90.

Jernite M, Diemumunsch P, Kibtz P. Buprenorphine excretion in breast milk. *Anesthesiology.* 1999; 91:A1095.

Jordan S, Emery S, Bradshaw C, Watkins A, Friswell W. The impact of intrapartum analgesia on infant feeding. *Br J Obstet Gynaecol.* 2005; 112:927-34.

Kershaw RA, Mays DC, Bianchine JR, Gerber N. Disposition of aspirin and its metabolites in the semen of man. *J Clin Pharmacol.* 1987; 27:304-9.

Kim J, Riggs KW, Misri S, Kent N, Oberlander TF, Grunau RE, *et al.* Stereoselective disposition of fluoxetine and norfluoxetine during pregnancy and breast-feeding. *Br J Clin Pharmacol.* 2006; 61:155-63.

Koren G, Cairns J, Chitayat D, Gaedigk A, Leeder SJ. Pharmacogenetics of morphine poisoning in a breastfed neonate of a codeine-prescribed mother. *Lancet.* 2006; 368:704.

Kunka RL, Venkataramanan R, Stern RM, Ladik CF. Excretion of propoxyphene and norpropoxyphene in breast milk. *Clin Pharmacol Ther.* 1984; 35:675-80.

Kunka RL, Yong CL, Ladik CF, Bates TR. Liquid chromatographic determination of propoxyphene and norpropoxyphene in plasma and breast milk. *J Pharm Sci.* 1985; 74:103-4.

Lebedevs TH, Wojnar-Horton RE, Yapp P, Roberts MJ, Dusci LJ, Hackett LP, *et al.* Excretion of indomethacin in breast milk. *Br J Clin Pharmacol.* 1991; 32:751-54.

Leuschen MP, Wolf LJ, Rayburn WF. Fentanyl excretion in breast milk [letter]. *Clin Pharm.* 1990; 9:336-37.

Malpas TJ, Darlow BA. Neonatal abstinence syndrome following abrupt cessation of breastfeeding. *NZ Med J.* 1999; 112:12-13.

Malpas TJ, Darlow BA, Lennox R, Horwood LJ. Maternal methadone dosage and neonatal withdrawal. *Aust NZ J Obstet Gynaecol.* 1995; 35:175-77.

Marquet P, Chevrel J, Lavignasse P, Merle L, Lachatre G. Buprenorphine withdrawal syndrome in a newborn. *Clin Pharmacol Ther.* 1997; 62:569-71.

Marx CM, Pucino F, Carlson JD. Oxycodone excretion in human milk in the puerperium. *Drug Intell Clin Pharm.* 1986; 20:474.

Meny RG, Naumburg EG, Alger LS, Brill-Miller JL, Brown S. Codeine and the breastfed neonate. *J Hum Lact.* 1993; 9:237-40.

Naumburg EG, Meny RG, Alger LS. Codeine and morphine levels in breast milk and neonatal plasma. *Pediatr Res.* 1987; 21:240A.

Neville MC, Keller R, Seacat J, Lutes V, Neifert M, Casey C, *et al.* Studies in human lactation: milk volumes in lactating women during the onset of lactation and full lactation. *Am J Clin Nutr.* 1988; 48:1375-86.

Notarianni LJ, Oldham HG, Bennett PN. Passage of paracetamol into breast milk and its subsequent metabolism by the neonate. *Br J Clin Pharmacol.* 1987; 24:63-67.

Oberlander TF, Robeson P, Ward V, Huckin RS, Kamani A, Harpur A, *et al.* Prenatal and breast milk morphine exposure following maternal intrathecal morphine treatment. *J Hum Lact.* 2000; 16:137-42.

Ostensen M. Piroxicam in human breast milk. *Eur J Clin Pharmacol.* 1983; 25:829-30.

Ostensen M, Matheson I, Laufen H. Piroxicam in breast milk after long-term treatment. *Eur J Clin Pharmacol.* 1988; 35:567-69.

Ostrea EM, Chavez CJ, Strauss ME. A study of factors that influence the severity of neonatal narcotic withdrawal. *J Pediatr.* 1976; 88:642-45.

Paech M, Kristensen J, Ilett KF. Nonsteroidal antiinflammatory drugs during lactation [letter; comment]. *Anesth Analgesia.* 1998; 87:977.

Peiker G, Muller B, Ihn W, Noschel H. Excretion of pethidine in mother's milk (author's transl). *Zentralbl Gynakol.* 1980; 102:537-41.

Philipp BL, Merewood A, O'Brien S. Methadone and breastfeeding: new horizons. *Pediatrics.* 2003; 111:1429-30.

Pittman KA, Smyth RD, Losada M, Zighelboim I, Maduska AL, Sunshine A. Human perinatal distribution of butorphanol. *Am J Obstet Gynecol.* 1980; 138:797-800.

Putter J, Satravaha P, Stockhausen H. Quantitative analysis of the main metabolites of acetylsalicylic acid. Comparative analysis in the blood and milk of lactating women (author's transl). *Z Geburtshilfe Perinatol.* 1974; 178:135-38.

Quinn PG, Kuhnert BR, Kaine CJ, Syracuse CD. Measurement of meperidine and normeperidine in human breast milk by selected ion monitoring. *Biomed Environ Mass Spectrometry.* 1986; 13:133-35.

Robieux I, Koren G, Vandenbergh H, Schneiderman J. Morphine excretion in breast milk and resultant exposure of a nursing infant. *J Toxicol Clin Toxicol.* 1990; 28:365-70.

Robinson SE. Buprenorphine: an analgesic with an expanding role in the treatment of opioid addiction. *CNS Drug Rev.* 2002; 8:377-90.

Rosen TS, Pippenger CE. Disposition of methadone and its relationship to severity of withdrawal in the newborn. *Addictive Dis.* 1975; 2:169-78.

Rosen TS, Pippenger CE. Pharmacologic observations on the neonatal withdrawal syndrome. *J Pediatr.* 1976; 88:1044-48.

Seaton S, Reeves M, McLean S. Oxycodone as a component of multimodal analgesia for lactating mothers after Caesarian section: relationships between maternal plasma, breast milk and neonatal plasma levels. *Aust NZ J Obstet Gynaecol.* 2007; 47:181-85.

Sioufi A, Stierlin H, Schweizer A. Recent findings concerning clinically relevant pharmacokinetics of diclofenac sodium. In: Kass E (Ed.). *Voltaren-new findings.* Bern, Switzerland: Hans Huber Publishers; 1982. p. 19-30.

Spigset O, Hagg S. Analgesics and breast-feeding: safety considerations. *Paediatr Drugs.* 2000; 2:223-38.

Steer PL, Biddle CJ, Marley WS, Lantz RK, Sulik PL. Concentration of fentanyl in colostrum after an analgesic dose. *Can J Anaesth.* 1992; 39:231-35.

Strauss ME, Andresko M, Stryker JC, Wardell JN, Dunkel LD. Methadone maintenance during pregnancy: pregnancy, birth, and neonate characteristics. *Am J Obstet Gynecol.* 1974; 120:895-900.

Todd PA, Sorkin EM. Diclofenac sodium. A reappraisal of its pharmacodynamic and pharmacokinetic properties, and therapeutic efficacy. *Drugs.* 1988; 35:244-85.

Townsend RJ, Benedetti TJ, Erickson SH, Cengiz C, Gillespie WR, Gschwend J, *et al.* Excretion of ibuprofen into breast milk. *Am J Obstet Gynecol.* 1984; 149:184-86.

US National Library of Medicine. *Drugs and lactation database (LactMed).* TOXNET Toxicology Data Network. 2006. Available from: http://toxnet.nlm.nih.gov/cgi-bin/sis/htmlgen?LACT.

Waterbury LD, Silliman D, Jolas T. Comparison of cyclooxygenase inhibitory activity and ocular anti-inflammatory effects of ketorolac tromethamine and bromfenac sodium. *Curr Med Res Opin.* 2006; 22:1133-40.

Weibert RT, Townsend RJ, Kaiser DG, Naylor AJ. Lack of ibuprofen secretion into human milk. *Clin Pharm.* 1982; 1:457-58.

Wischnik A, Manth SM, Lloyd J, Bullingham R, Thompson JS. The excretion of ketorolac tromethamine into breast milk after multiple oral dosing. *Eur J Clin Pharmacol.* 1989; 36:521-24.

Wittels B, Glosten B, Faure EA, Moawad AH, Ismail M, Hibbard J, *et al.* Postcesarean analgesia with both epidural morphine and intravenous patient-controlled analgesia: neurobehavioral outcomes among nursing neonates. *Anesth Analgesia.* 1997; 85:600-6.

Wittels B, Scott DT, Sinatra RS. Exogenous opioids in human breast milk and acute neonatal neurobehavior: a preliminary study. *Anesthesiology.* 1990; 73:864-69.

Wojnar-Horton RE, Kristensen JH, Yapp P, Ilett KF, Dusci LJ, Hackett LP. Methadone distribution and excretion into breast milk of clients in a methadone maintenance programme. *Br J Clin Pharmacol.* 1997; 44:543-47.

Chapter 27

Anesthetic and Analgesic Medications: Implications for Breastfeeding

Thomas W. Hale

INTRODUCTION

The use of anesthetic and analgesic medications during delivery and other surgical procedures is commonplace in breastfeeding mothers. Unfortunately, we still know little about the transfer of these medications to the fetus or to the mother's breastmilk. While analgesics have been covered in another chapter, the use of specific analgesics during anesthetic procedures will be covered again in this chapter. Labor and birth, while a normal process, is still a painful undertaking. In recent years, more and more mothers have requested suitable pain management by their physicians, and it has now become almost standard practice to provide mothers with various anesthetic procedures to make labor more comfortable. While systemic and regional anesthesia has become less common, the newer neuroaxial techniques with minimal neuromotor blockade have become incredibly popular. Low dose epidurals, spinal anesthesia, and combined spinal-epidural analgesia have replaced the older epidural for labor. Now the mother can more completely participate in the delivery of her infant without the depressing effects of systemic analgesics. The introduction of new techniques such as the combined spinal epidural analgesia (CSE), newer anesthetic drugs, and the use of opiate drugs combined with local anesthetics has transformed obstetrical analgesia.

However, opiates and local anesthetics are still used in neuroaxial anesthesia and may sedate the infant and produce profound effects on the breastfeeding experience several days later. This chapter will provide a review of the current systemic analgesics, regional and neuroaxial analgesic techniques, and how they are used for pain management in labor, birth, early postpartum and postpartum anesthesia, and their possible implication in breastfeeding outcomes.

DESCRIPTIONS

The pharmacologic control of pain in obstetrical anesthesia, labor and birth require numerous agents and, more importantly, different methods/sites of administration. Numerous terms are commonplace in this field and are herewith described:

Analgesia: Control of pain using various analgesic medications, including opiates, opioids, nonsteroidal analgesics (NSAIDs), or other medications.

Anesthesia: The use of medications to induce analgesia and in some cases complete loss of sensation and consciousness.

Arachnoid Mater: The arachnoid mater is a thin, filmy membrane closely attached to the inner surface of the dura mater. It is penetrated by subdural penetration, hence the term subarachnoid. Its cells are metabolically active in transporting CSF and debris out of the subarachnoid space.

Combined spinal-epidural: This procedure consists of the placement of an analgesic in the subarachnoid space, followed by the use of a local anesthetic/analgesic in the epidural space. Sometimes it is called a "Walking Epidural."

Dura mater: A tough fibroelastic sheath that encloses the spinal cord and runs from the foramen magnum to the S2 vertebral level. It is very impervious and holds the CSF (cerebrospinal fluid) within the spinal cord.

Intrathecal: Injection of drugs into the subdural space and directly on top of the pia mater.

Local Anesthetic: Agent that induces complete loss of sensation by blocking pain transmission via local application of medications directly to the nerve, nerve trunk, or ganglion.

Neuroaxial Analgesia: Analgesia produced by local injection of analgesics and local anesthetics directly into the epidural or intrathecal space.

Opiate: Drugs derived from opium, such as heroin, morphine, codeine, and hydrocodone.

Opioid: Generally describes drugs that act at the opiate receptor site. This can include an opiate, but also a non-opiate drug, such as meperidine. Meperidine, fentanyl, sufentanil are considered opioids, but not opiates.

Patient-controlled Analgesia: Technique which permits the patient to directly control the application of analgesics with an infusion pump directly into the epidural (PCEA) or intravenous spaces (PCA).

Pia Mater: Thin membrane that covers the surface of the brain, spinal cord, and nerves. The space between the pia and the arachnoid is called the subarachnoid space. This is where most medications are injected.

Regional Anesthesia: Technique involving the injection of local anesthetics, with or without opiates, directly into the epidural or subarachnoid space producing complete analgesia below the block.

Subdural Space: Because the arachnoid mater is attached so closely to the inner surface of the dura, puncturing the dura is considered synonymous with entering the subarachnoid or "subdural" space. It is also referred to as an 'intrathecal' injection.

ANESTHETIC TECHNIQUES

No description of anesthesia is complete without a suitable description of the injection sites and techniques where drugs are injected. In reality, the site where the medication is injected largely controls the transfer of the specific medication to the fetus and has a major impact on the fetal outcome. All medications injected peripherally, ultimately end up in the plasma and are distributed to the fetus to some degree.

Systemic Analgesia

Despite the popularity of regional anesthesia, systemic medications are still commonly used in some procedures. They are generally administered intravenously (IV), subcutaneously, or intramuscularly. Because these agents have a greater potential to transfer to the fetus, some problems, such as neonatal sedation, are encountered and must be understood. Ideal systemic medications should have certain unique characteristics, such as rapid onset and clearance, rapid metabolism and elimination, and minimal transfer to the fetus. Most of the medications currently used lack these characteristics, but instead tend to have high volumes of distribution and slow clearance from the body. Systemic analgesia has been used in managing obstetrical pain for more than 100 years. While the goal is pain control, this method suffers from the fact that plasma levels of these medications are higher, and transfer to the fetus is higher still. Because of their lipophilicity and low molecular weights, all opioids can easily cross the placenta by diffusion and may produce neonatal respiratory depression. Use of parenteral opioids during delivery also results in decreased beat-to-beat variability in the fetal heart rate which fails to indicate the status of fetal oxygenation or acid-base balance (Visalyaputra, 2000). Conversely, epidural opioids (morphine 3 mg, fentanyl 75 ug, sufentanil 50 ug) administered to the mother seldom produces a depressant effect on the fetus (Celleno *et al.*, 1991), although these doses are somewhat lower than commonly used.

Induction Agents

Induction agents are commonly used in cesarean sections and other major surgical procedures. Induction agents are commonly used to rapidly transport the patient past the second, or excitatory stage of surgery into the third stage of surgery. The most common agents are now propofol, ketamine, and thiopental sodium.

Ketamine

Ketamine is a potent and effective anesthetic agent for rapid induction. Used less frequently in the USA, it is probably the most commonly used agent in other parts of the world. Ketamine is most frequently chosen for parturients with significant hemorrhage or those with possible allergies and asthma. Doses of ketamine in excess of 2 mg/kg have been reported to increase the risk of neonatal depression (Lindblad *et al.*, 1987). While many of these agents may affect uteroplacental perfusion, ketamine in lower doses ($\leq$ 1 mg/kg) has not. Ketamine is well known for inducing a 'dysphoric reaction' upon withdrawal, although this is seldom observed in neonates.

Propofol

Propofol is a widely used drug of induction and is becoming increasingly popular because of its rapid onset, short duration of action, and rapid recovery with a low incidence of postoperative side-effects. While it has been used extensively in emergency cesarean sections, some reports suggest it is associated with a slightly higher risk of hypotension when compared to thiopental (Celleno *et al.*, 1989), although these reports are highly controversial and are probably dose-related.

Thiopental

Thiopental (thiopentone) is the most commonly used drug of induction for cesarean section in the United States. Although it rapidly distributes to the fetus, neonatal outcome is generally good due to its rapid redistribution out of the fetal circulation and back to the mother. This drug, like no other, rapidly redistributes from the plasma compartment to muscle and adipose almost instantly following injection. Thiopental is a barbiturate. It induces rapid hypnosis and protects against seizures.

Sedatives/Hypnotics

Various medications from sedatives to analgesics are sometimes used. During the early stage of labor, they (promethazine, hydroxyzine) are primarily used to suppress nausea and vomiting sometimes associated with the use of opioids. While they have little effect on the progress of labor, they may depress fetal respiration and impair fetal platelet function. They may also block the vasopressor effects of adrenergic drugs (phenylephrine, epinephrine). Benzodiazepines, particularly midazolam or lorazepam, may occasionally be used to control seizures or to sedate an agitated patient. Midazolam is commonly used as an adjunct to anesthesia (induction) and for its amnesic qualities. Its primary benefit over others in this class is its brief half-life and limited transfer to the fetus. Diazepam is seldom used today because it has a prolonged half-life in the fetus, produces profound fetal sedation, hypotonia, and impaired thermogenesis.

Opiates/Opioids

The use of systemic opioids is somewhat problematic. While they are well known to reduce shivering, they can also produce nausea, vomiting, pruritus, dysphoria, drowsiness, hypoventilation, neonatal depression, and reduction of uterine contractures (Mattingly *et al.*, 2003). Therefore, they are not always used systemically during delivery.

Meperidine

Meperidine is still one of the most popular analgesics used in obstetrical delivery even though it readily crosses the placenta and produces prolonged fetal depression. Administered in doses of 25-50 mg intravenously and 50-100 mg intramuscularly, it has a rather brief duration of action (3-4 hours) in adults. Pharmacologically, it is considered a weak analgesic, but a strong sedative. The most common maternal complaint following its use is somnolence. Following intravenous administration, it rapidly enters the fetal circulation. The umbilical vein/maternal vein ratio is 1 within 6 minutes of its administration (Belfrage *et al.*, 1981; Kuhnert *et al.*, 1985). Meperidine is rapidly metabolized to normeperidine and a significant accumulation occurs in the fetus (Kuhnert *et al.*, 1985). The half-life of meperidine in the fetus is long, approximately 20 hours. However, the half-life of normeperidine is much longer, 60-73 hours.

Meperidine and its metabolite suppress fetal respiration, and normeperidine is believed to lower the seizure threshold in some patients (Marinella, 1997). Together in the neonate, they cause lower Apgar scores, prolonged time to sustain respiration (Belfrage *et al.*, 1981), and approximately a 3 fold increase in apneic episodes (Hamza *et al.*, 1992). Most important is the time interval between administration of meperidine and delivery (Belfrage *et al.*, 1981). If delivery occurs within 1 hour of maternal administration of intramuscular meperidine, neonatal respiratory depression is unlikely. If, however, delivery ensues 2-3 hours following administration of meperidine, significant neonatal respiratory difficulties have been reported. Because of its documented neonatal complications, the use of meperidine in obstetrical anesthesia has decreased with good reason. Many have suggested that meperidine should probably be abandoned due to prolonged neonatal respiratory depression (Bruyere *et al.*, 2005; Kanto, 1991).

Morphine

The use of morphine systemically is controversial and is seldom used because of its delayed onset time, prolonged duration of action, severe maternal and fetal respiratory depression, nausea, vomiting, and pruritus, although recent data seems to suggest that neonatal sedation may not be as severe as once thought. More recently, morphine has become popular when administered in the subarachnoid space as a part of regional anesthesia, where doses of 0.25 mg produce long-term analgesia with minimal fetal effects (Mattingly *et al.*, 2003). This dose is significantly less than the 3-5mg used epidurally or the 5-10mg used intramuscularly.

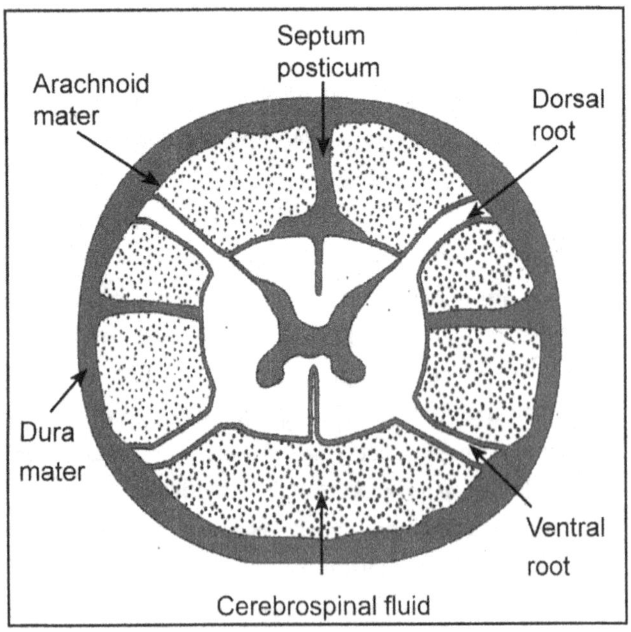

Figure 1. Anatomy of the spinal cord, including dura and arachnoid mater.

Fentanyl

Fentanyl and sufentanil are sometimes used systemically, generally for acute short-term needs, such as in patient-controlled analgesia. However, the use of fentanyl intravenously has been associated with a 44% incidence of moderately depressed neonates with an Apgar score ≤ 6 at 1 minute (Morley-Forster *et al.*, 1998). Nevertheless, fentanyl is still the most commonly used epidural anesthetic in this field.

Remifentanil

Remifentanil is a new ultra-short-acting opioid similar to fentanyl. Because of an ester linkage, it is rapidly metabolized by all tissue and plasma esterases and is completely independent of liver function. Its half-life is extremely short (<3 minutes). While it would seem that this agent is ideal for systemic use in delivery, its use has shown inconsistent results. In some studies, it has been found to provide suitable analgesia with minimal side effects in the fetus.

NEURAXIAL ANALGESIA AND ANESTHESIA

In the past decade, epidural, spinal, and the newer combined spinal-epidural anesthetic techniques have become the methods of choice for analgesia of labor and anesthesia for cesarean delivery. Unlike intravenous anesthesia/analgesia (systemic) where the doses are significantly higher, regional anesthesia generally reduces (but does not eliminate) the risk of maternal or neonatal respiratory depression.

Regional analgesia techniques have changed dramatically over the past decade to allow for more effective pain relief while reducing the density of the block, the risk of maternal hypotension, and reducing neonatal depression. The use of localized injections into the epidural and subarachnoid spaces of the spinal cord, combined with much lower doses of these analgesics, provides significant pain relief to patients without the corresponding neonatal sedation induced following systemic administration of these same agents.

Spina/Intrathecal

Spinal analgesic/anesthesia permits the injection of small anesthetic doses of opioids, with or without local anesthetics, into the subarachnoid space **(Figure 1)**. Because the doses used are substantially less than those used epidurally or systemically, the clinical effects on the mother and fetus are generally significantly less. While single injections may provide suitable analgesia for short procedures, the introduction of the new microcatheter now allows for the continuous infusion of small doses of analgesics into the subarachnoid space, and thus analgesia for prolonged procedures (Visalyaputra, 2000). However, numerous cases of transient radicular irritation (TRI) were initially reported and the microcatheter was removed from the market by the FDA. Many of these problems have been solved in the last few years, and these catheters may ultimately gain approval again. Continuous spinal (subarachnoid) anesthesia uses less local anesthetic and/or analgesic, thus reducing the risk of systemic toxicity and neonatal sedation, although it may have any number of other problems. While postdural puncture headaches may occur, they are less likely with the new microcatheter.

The use of opioids via continuous spinal infusion has become increasingly appealing. The infusion of opioids produces a dose-dependent analgesia without significant motor block which can also be reversed by naloxone. While morphine was perhaps the first used, its use is less appealing because it is slow in onset (45 or more minutes) and produces significant pruritus and nausea (Hurley, 2000). Alternate opioids, such as fentanyl and sufentanil, have rapid onset and are commonly used, but may produce some tachyphylaxis.

The use of subarachnoid local anesthetics is subject to some controversy due to the risk of TRI. Bupivacaine and, more recently, ropivacaine appear to be the safest. Numerous new reports suggest this technique may offer significant benefits in certain surgical procedures (Forster *et al.*, 2006; Okutomi *et al.*, 2006).

Epidural

The epidural space consists of the spinal canal exterior to the dura mater and extends from the foramen magnum to the S2 vertebral level. The epidural space contains connective and adipose tissue, lymphatics, arteries, an extensive plexus of veins, and the spinal nerve roots as they exit the dural sac and pass through the intervertebral foramina. When anesthetic agents are injected into the epidural space, some analgesic enters the adipose tissue, some penetrates through the dura mater into the spinal cord, and the remaining (probably most) is absorbed into the veins and capillaries and enters the plasma compartment for peripheral distribution to the mother and, unfortunately, the fetus. Thus, for drugs to traverse the dura mater, they must be highly lipophilic, small in molecular weight, and highly potent, as only limited quantities are capable of entering the subarachnoid levels of the spinal cord. Epidural analgesia has evolved from producing total loss of sensation to analgesia with minimal block. These changes have occurred with newer drugs and better dosing regimens. This change has been particularly advantageous to parturients as they can now be more mobile and can participate in delivery.

Complications of epidural and spinal analgesia include hypotension, accidental intravascular injection, dural puncture headache, inadequate block or pain relief, and perhaps fetal sedation (Paull, 2000; Visalyaputra, 2000). Hypotension is primarily associated with the use of local anesthetics due to the sympathectomy and vasodilation that occurs. Because hypotension is dose-related, the co-administration of opioids with local anesthetics has dramatically reduced the concentration of local anesthetics required, so the risks of hypotension have been significantly reduced in the past decade. Dura puncture occurs in approximately 0.2% to 4% of all epidural insertions (Zakowski, 2002). If the injection occurs in the subarachnoid space, severe complications may arise, although infrequently, and may include motor blockade caudally with rapidly increasing motor blockade, progressive respiratory paralysis, and loss of consciousness (Zakowski, 2002).

Numerous medications have been used epidurally, but the more popular seems to include fentanyl, sufentanil, morphine, meperidine, bupivacaine, and ropivacaine. Opioids were added some years ago to epidural procedures to reduce the dose of bupivacaine required and also the incidence of shivering. After defining the epidural space by loss of resistance, a test dose of lidocaine may sometimes be administered to determine if the needle is in the subarachnoid space or a capillary. A rapid, dense, ensuing block would suggest entry into the subarachnoid space, while tachycardia, hypotension, or tingling of the lips would suggest entry into the vascular system rather than the epidural

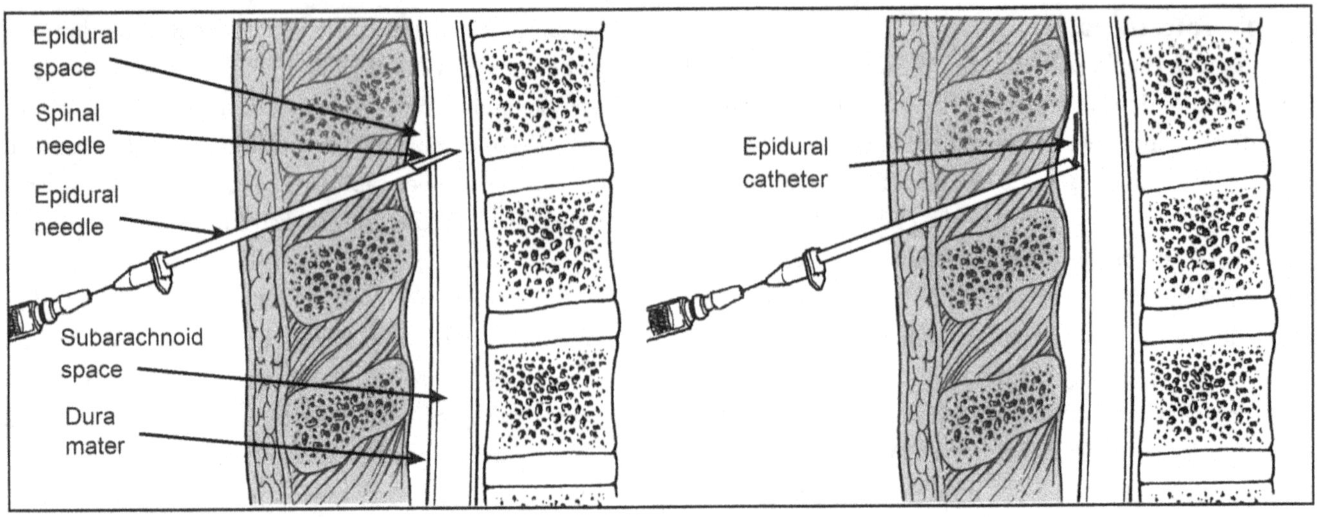

Figure 2. Combined Spinal-Epidural (CSE) injection into the spine. The first needle (epidural) is passed into the epidural space. The second needle is then passed through the epidural needle into the subarachnoid space. A small amount of anesthetic or opioid is injected, and the needle is removed. A soft catheter is then threaded into the epidural space for subsequent injections.

space. Test doses are, however, often considered optional. Some anesthesiologists use a stepwise method of simply injecting small amounts to start with while monitoring the patient, followed by additional amounts later. Ultimately, the mother's blood pressure should be continuously checked during the first 5-10 minutes and at frequent intervals thereafter until her hemodynamic status has stabilized. At present, fentanyl and bupivacaine are the most frequently used epidural drugs.

Combined Spinal-Epidural (CSE)

A combined spinal-epidural procedure (walking epidural) was first described in 1937 by a New York surgeon (Soresi, 1937) who described the use of a combined epidural and subarachnoid injection (then termed "episubdural block"). Since then, this procedure has undergone numerous changes. The many techniques currently involved in this procedure are beyond the scope of this chapter, but the needle-through-needle technique is generally used today with the use of flexible catheters left remaining in the epidural space.

In this procedure (**Figure 2**), an epidural or Tuohy needle is inserted in the epidural (below L2) space as a guide. After locating the epidural space, a long, small gauge spinal needle (24-27 gauge) is inserted through the epidural needle into the subarachnoid space. Fentanyl or sufentanil alone, or with local anesthetic is then administered into the subarachnoid space. After removal, a flexible catheter is then placed in the epidural space and left for administering drugs for later pain control.

The CSE technique has been used for many procedures including general surgery, orthopedic surgery, trauma surgery, urologic surgery, and many gynecologic procedures. Currently, CSE is most often used in cesarean section, assisted vaginal delivery, and major orthopedic surgeries requiring treatment for severe postoperative pain.

The use of the CSE technique for cesarean delivery has gained wide popularity around the world. CSE provides rapid onset of analgesia and, at the same time, prolonged analgesia postoperatively. Even small doses of morphine (0.1-0.3 mg) can provide adequate analgesia for more than 24 hours. Because the doses of analgesics are quite low, fetal sedation is generally minimal. However, sensory block from T4 to S5 required for cesarean section may also be associated with a higher risk of hypotension and some fetal risk (Rawal *et al.*, 2000). Because the intrathecal dose is a one-time injection, failure of an adequate block is problematic. But in general, CSE has several benefits. Fewer patients experience motor blockade, patient satisfaction is higher than with the standard epidural technique (Collis *et al.*, 1995), and cervical dilation may be accelerated. Disadvantages of CSE include maternal hypotension with the extensive block (T4-S5), occasional failures due to misplaced subarachnoid medications, and the typical postdural puncture headache.

In a large retrospective review, no difference was found in the incidence of emergency cesarean delivery in women who received CSE (n=1217) versus women (n=1140) who did not receive neuraxial analgesia (Albright *et al.*, 1997). However, the impact of epidural/CSE on the rate of cesarean is still somewhat controversial because of the numerous variables, and the reader is referred to other major reviews in this field (Beilin *et al.*, 1999). For a complete review of the CSE technique, the reader is referred to the following thorough review (Rawal *et al.*, 2000).

The intrathecal injection of fentanyl (10-20 ug) or sufentanil (2.5-5 ug), alone or in combination with isobaric bupivacaine (0.25%-0.75%), produces profound

Table 1. Drugs of Induction, Local Anesthetics, and Analgesic Drugs in Obstetrical Anesthesia

Drug	Relative infant dose (%)	Comment	References
Drugs of Induction			
Propofol	4.4	Levels reported in milk are minimal. Probably safe. Commonly used in infants.	Dailland *et al.*, 1989
Thiopental sodium	2.5	Levels in milk range from 0.34 mg/L in colostrum to 0.9 mg/L in mature milk. Probably safe. Rapidly cleared.	Andersen *et al.*, 1987
Ketamine	Not reported	Data is limited, but is commonly used in many parts of the world without problem.	
Local Anesthetics			
Bupivacaine	< 1.15	Levels are low (<0.02 to 0.09 mg/L) in two studies. Compatible.	Naulty, 1983; Ortega *et al.*, 1999
Lidocaine	2.8-4.9	Levels are low and range according to dose. Generally 0.5 to 0.86 mg/L. Compatible.	Dryden *et al.*, 2000; Ortega *et al.*, 1999
Ropivacaine	Not reported	No data available, but probably compatible. Commonly used to replace bupivacaine.	
Opioids and related drugs			
Buprenorphine	<1 – 2.4	Single study only indicates low transfer. Variable dose ranges. Use with caution. May affect milk production.	Grimm *et al.*, 2005; Hirose *et al.*, 1997; Jernite *et al.*, 1999; Marquet *et al.*, 1997
Butorphanol	0.3-0.4	Single study. Compatible.	Pittman *et al.*, 1980
Fentanyl	0.6, 3	Compatible, but some concerns about successfully establishing lactation.	Leuschen *et al.*, 1990; Steer *et al.*, 1992
Hydrocodone		Compatible; some sedation in infants has been associated with higher doses and for longer periods; caution recommended.	Bodley *et al.*, 1997
Meperidine (pethidine)	0.6-3.5	Low transfer, but adverse neurobehavioral side-effects reported. Safer alternatives available.	Freeborn *et al.*, 1980; Peiker *et al.*, 1980; Quinn *et al.*, 1986; Wittels *et al.*, 1990; Wittels *et al.*, 1997
Morphine	0.4-3.4	Compatible in usual analgesic doses used in the perinatal period. Caution with high dose extended-release preparations as there are no data.	Baka *et al.*, 2002; Feilberg *et al.*, 1989; Kim *et al.*, 2006; Robieux *et al.*, 1990; Wittels *et al.*, 1990
Naltrexone	1	Compatible. Single case report only.	Chan *et al.*, 2004
Oxycodone	8	Dose calculated on maximum levels in milk. Low or single doses compatible, but caution suggested with higher dose extended-release preparations.	Marx *et al.*, 1986
Propoxyphene	2	Compatible.	Kunka *et al.*, 1984; Kunka *et al.*, 1985

analgesia lasting for 90-120 minutes with minimal motor blockade. The use of opioid alone during the early latent phase may control pain, but ultimately, the use of bupivacaine is required to control heavy labor pain. The most common complication of intrathecal opioids, such as fentanyl, is pruritus, nausea, vomiting, and urinary retention.

Patient-Controlled Epidural Analgesia (PCEA)

Patient controlled epidural analgesia is the newest of these techniques and is becoming increasingly popular for management of acute pain in labor and delivery. PCEA has been suggested to offer many advantages over continuous epidural infusions, particularly fewer physician interventions, improved analgesia, and patient satisfaction. Described first in 1988 by Gambling *et al.* in 27 patients (Gambling *et al.*, 1988), PCEA has been found in a meta analysis of nine studies to produce significant analgesia with lower doses of analgesics and fewer unscheduled clinician top-ups (Van *et al.*, 2002). While somewhat controversial, this technique allows the patient to control the dose of epidural medication as labor and pain patterns change. However, the equipment required for PCEA is more expensive than that used for continuous epidural infusion, and more time is ultimately required to educate the patient on its use. Patient hemodynamic status is more stable with this technique, and hypotension is rare.

The choice of analgesics and local anesthetics is large and too numerous to review here. Fentanyl and bupivacaine 0.125% are generally the drugs of choice and are infused at varying rates. Currently, there is no consensus on the choice of medications used, their basal infusion rates, or almost any aspect of this technique. It is largely up to the preference of the individual anesthesiologist.

TRANSPORT OF MEDICATIONS INTO HUMAN MILK

Virtually all medications used during anesthetic procedures will pass to some degree into human milk (Table 1). Fortunately, the transport is generally subclinical due to the rapid redistribution and clearance of the medications by the mother. Thus far, few medications other than some of the opiates have been correlated with neonatal sedation via milk. For a review of the transfer of the opiates and other analgesics, please see Chapter 26 on analgesics. Other anesthetic agents are included below.

Propofol

In one study of 4 women who received a bolus propofol of 2.5 mg/kg IV, milk levels ranged from 0.089 to 0.24 µg/mL (Dailland *et al.*, 1989). In a second group of 3 who received a bolus and continuous infusions of propofol (5 mg/kg/h), milk levels ranged from 0.33 to 0.74 µg/mL. The second breastmilk level obtained 24 hours after delivery contained only 6% of the 4-hour sample. Similar levels (0.12-0.97 mg/L) were noted by Schmitt in colostrum samples obtained 4-8 hours after induction with propofol (Schmitt *et al.*, 1987).

In a study of 5 women who received a single dose of 2.5 mg/kg propofol, the amount of propofol measured in milk collected at 5, 7, 9, 11, and 24 hours ranged from 0.004% - 0.082% of the maternal dose. Following a single dose, the authors estimated an infant would receive only 0.0052 mg/kg/24 hours (Nitsun *et al.*, 2006).

From these data, it is apparent that only minimal amounts of propofol are transferred to human milk. No data are available on the oral absorption of propofol.

Midazolam

After oral administration of 15 mg for up to 6 days postnatally in 22 women, midazolam was below the limit of detection (<3 µg/L) in 11 mothers. In the additional 11 mothers, the mean milk/plasma ratio was 0.15 in six paired samples. The average maximum level of midazolam in breastmilk was 9 nanogram/mL and occurred 1-2 hours after administration. Midazolam and its hydroxy-metabolite were undetectable 4 hours after administration. Therefore, the amount of midazolam transferred to an infant via early milk is minimal, particularly if the baby is breastfed more than 4 hours after administration. After repeated evening dosing, none was detectable in milk in the morning.

In a further study of 5 women who received 2 mg midazolam intravenously, the authors estimated the infants would receive via milk an estimated 0.016 µg/kg/d. The relative infant dose was estimated to be 0.06% (Nitsun *et al.*, 2006).

Thiopental Sodium

In a study of two groups of 8 women who received from 5.0 to 5.4 mg/kg thiopental sodium, the maximum concentration in breastmilk occurred immediately after anesthesia and was 0.9 mg/L in mature milk and 0.34 mg/L in colostrum. The milk/plasma ratio was 0.3 for colostrum and 0.4 for mature milk. The maximum daily dose to the infant would be 0.135 mg/kg or approximately 2.5% of the adult dose (Andersen *et al.*, 1987). Most authors agree that the dose received by the infant would be subclinical.

Bupivacaine/Lidocaine

In one study of five patients, levels of bupivacaine in breastmilk were below the limits of detection (< 0.02 mg/L) at 2 to 48 hours postpartum (Naulty, 1983). These authors concluded that bupivacaine is a safe drug for perinatal use in mothers who plan to breastfeed.

In another study of 27 parturients who received an average of 183.3 mg lidocaine and 82.1 mg bupivacaine via an epidural catheter, lidocaine milk levels at 2, 6, and 12 hours post administration were 0.86, 0.46, and 0.22 mg/L respectively (Ortega *et al.*, 1999). Levels of bupivacaine in milk at 2, 6, and 12 hours were 0.09, 0.06, and 0.04 mg/L, respectively. The milk/serum ratio bases upon area under the curve values (AUC) were 1.07 and 0.34 for lidocaine and bupivacaine, respectively. Based on AUC data of lidocaine and bupivacaine milk levels, the average milk concentration of these agents over 12 hours was 0.5 and 0.07 mg/L. Most of the infants had a maximal APGAR score.

Magnesium

In one study of 10 preeclamptic patients who received a 4 gm IV loading dose followed by 1 gm per hour IV for more than 24 hours, the average milk magnesium levels in treated subjects were 6.4 mg/dl. This was only slightly higher than controls (untreated), which were 4.77 mg/dl (Cruikshank *et al.*, 1982). On day 2, the average milk magnesium levels in treated groups were 3.83 mg/dl, which was not significantly different from untreated controls, 3.19 mg/dl. By day 3, the treated and control groups breastmilk levels were identical (3.54 vs. 3.52 mg/dl). The mean maternal serum magnesium level on day 1 in treated groups was 3.55 mg/dl, which was significantly higher than untreated controls, 1.82 mg/dl. In both treated and control subjects, levels of milk magnesium were approximately twice those of maternal serum magnesium levels, with the milk-to-serum ratio being 1.9 in treated subjects and 2.1 in control subjects. This study clearly indicates a normal concentrating mechanism for magnesium in human milk. It is well known that oral magnesium absorption is very poor, averaging only 4% following large oral doses (Morris *et al.*, 1987). Further, this study indicates that in treated groups, infants would only receive about 1.5 mg of oral magnesium more than the untreated controls. It is very unlikely that the amount of magnesium in breastmilk would be clinically relevant to an infant.

EFFECTS ON BREASTFEEDING AND NEWBORNS

The secondary effects of anesthetic agents on breastfeeding and infant neurobehavioral outcome are highly controversial. Perhaps more important is the method of administration. Numerous new neuraxial techniques have been introduced in recent years with the aim of increasing the comfort level in laboring women while reducing the dose and side effects of the anesthetic agents on the fetus. Almost invariably, they have reduced the overall dose administered to the parturient and the dose transferred to the fetus.

Three things seem clear about the use of anesthetic agents in breastfeeding infants. One - the transfer to the fetus depends on the total dose administered, its timing, and route (IV, IM, epidurally, intrathecally). At present in the literature, it is all but impossible to distinguish the effect of a prolonged or difficult labor from the use of anesthetic agents. This makes interpretation of the overall effects of labor medications on breastfeeding infinitely difficult. Two - the infant stands a much higher probability of being sedated if the duration of exposure is longer, and the dose of anesthetic medication (particularly with meperidine or fentanyl) is higher. This seems logical. Sedated infants simply don't breastfeed as soon or as well and, therefore, are at higher risk for hyperbilirubinemia and slower weight gain. Three - virtually all of these agents redistribute rapidly out of the maternal plasma compartment to peripheral compartments, and therefore, milk levels of these agents are almost invariably low and subclinical. Almost all of our current published data concerning these drugs, with exception of meperidine, suggests that milk levels of these agents in milk do not affect the newborn infant clinically.

Some literature suggests that the effects of anesthetic agents, particularly those administered intrathecally or epidurally, are of minimal concern to a breastfeeding mother (Beilin *et al.*, 2005; Radzyminski, 2003). On the other hand, there are numerous reports that suggest that the use of opiates and local anesthetics may produce suboptimal breastfeeding due to sedation in the neonate (Anonymous, 1980; Baumgarder *et al.*, 2003; Dewey *et al.*, 2003). While it is rather clear that the transfer of these agents into colostrum and milk is negligible, most of the concern about the use of general anesthesia, epidural, or systemic analgesics involves the direct sedation of the neonate via transplacental passage of these drugs, which results in sedated infants that feed poorly. The possibility that intrapartum analgesia with opiates and local anesthetics may be affecting breastfeeding has been poorly studied, often in studies with inadequate numbers and poor inclusion criteria. Breastfeeding as an outcome is all but never determined in the outcome variables of most obstetrical studies. However, there are some studies which show a dose-response relationship between opioid use and the rate of breastfeeding. One such study showed that higher doses of neuroaxial fentanyl in 425 parturients actually reduced the rate of breastfeeding (Jordan *et al.*, 2005). However, this was an observational study. In contrast, other studies detected no newborn abnormalities in neonatal behavior or Apgar scores following the use of fentanyl (Bader *et al.*, 1995; Fernando *et al.*, 1997). Mothers who receive epidural or intrathecal injections often have a higher risk of elevated body temperatures (Lieberman *et al.*, 1999). While this may cause extra interventions, such as antibiotic use, it is not believed to affect breastfeeding itself.

It is not a stretch of logic to assume that any anesthetic medication used during delivery may ultimately end up in the fetus. Whether this is sufficient to affect a newborn, neurobehaviorally is yet to be answered, although it seems rather obvious to assume some sedation is likely. Ultimately, the neurobehavioral affect of these drugs really depends on the type and dose of medications used, their site of administration, the duration of labor, and the difficulty of labor. Until we can adequately control for all of these study parameters, the answer to the neurobehavioral effects of these drugs on newborns is yet to be determined.

References

Albright GA, Forster RM. Does combined spinal-epidural analgesia with subarachnoid sufentanil increase the incidence of emergency cesarean delivery? *Reg Anesth.* 1997; 22:400-5.

Andersen LW, Qvist T, Hertz J, Mogensen F. Concentrations of thiopentone in mature breast milk and colostrum following an induction dose. *Acta Anaesthesiol Scand.* 1987; 31:30-32.

Anonymous. Levels of free amino acids in lactating women following ingestion of the sweetener aspartame. *Nutr Rev.* 1980; 38:183-84.

Bader AM, Fragneto R, Terui K, Arthur GR, Loferski B, Datta S. Maternal and neonatal fentanyl and bupivacaine concentrations after epidural infusion during labor. *Anesth Analg.* 1995; 81:829-32.

Baka NE, Bayoumeu F, Boutroy MJ, Laxenaire MC. Colostrum morphine concentrations during postcesarean intravenous patient-controlled analgesia. *Anesth Analgesia.* 2002; 94:184-87.

Baumgarder DJ, Muehl P, Fischer M, Pribbenow B. Effect of labor epidural anesthesia on breast-feeding of healthy full-term newborns delivered vaginally. *J Am Board Fam Pract.* 2003; 16:7-13.

Beilin Y, Bodian CA, Weiser J, Hossain S, Arnold I, Feierman DE, *et al.* Effect of labor epidural analgesia with and without fentanyl on infant breast-feeding: a prospective, randomized, double-blind study. *Anesthesiology.* 2005; 103:1211-17.

Beilin Y, Leibowitz AB, Bernstein HH, Abramovitz SE. Controversies of labor epidural analgesia. *Anesth Analg.* 1999; 89:969-78.

Belfrage P, Boreus LO, Hartvig P, Irestedt L, Raabe N. Neonatal depression after obstetrical analgesia with pethidine. The role of the injection-delivery time interval and of the plasma concentrations of pethidine and norpethidine. *Acta Obstet Gynecol Scand.* 1981; 60:43-49.

Bodley V, Powers D. Long-term treatment of a breastfeeding mother with fluconazole-resolved nipple pain caused by yeast: a case study. *J Hum Lact.* 1997; 13:307-11.

Bruyere M, Mercier FJ. Alternative techniques to labour epidural analgesia. *Ann Fr Anesth Reanim.* 2005; 24:1375-82.

Celleno D, Capogna G, Sebastiani M, Costantino P, Muratori F, Cipriani G, *et al.* Epidural analgesia during and after cesarean delivery. Comparison of five opioids. *Reg Anesth.* 1991; 16:79-83.

Celleno D, Capogna G, Tomassetti M, Costantino P, Di FG, Nisini R. Neurobehavioural effects of propofol on the neonate following elective caesarean section. *Br J Anaesth.* 1989; 62:649-54.

Chan CF, Page-Sharp M, Kristensen JH, O'Neil G, Ilett KF. Transfer of naltrexone and its metabolite 6,beta-naltrexol into human milk. *J Hum Lact.* 2004; 20:322-26.

Collis RE, Davies DW, Aveling W. Randomised comparison of combined spinal-epidural and standard epidural analgesia in labour. *Lancet.* 1995; 345:1413-16.

Cruikshank DP, Varner MW, Pitkin RM. Breast milk magnesium and calcium concentrations following magnesium sulfate treatment. *Am J Obstet Gynecol.* 1982; 143:685-88.

Dailland P, Cockshott ID, Lirzin JD, Jacquinot P, Jorrot JC, Devery J, *et al.* Intravenous propofol during cesarean section: placental transfer, concentrations in breast milk, and neonatal effects. A preliminary study. *Anesthesiology.* 1989; 71:827-34.

Dewey KG, Nommsen-Rivers LA, Heinig MJ, Cohen RJ. Risk factors for suboptimal infant breastfeeding behavior, delayed onset of lactation, and excess neonatal weight loss. *Pediatrics.* 2003; 112:607-19.

Dryden RM, Lo MW. Breast milk lidocaine levels in tumescent liposuction. *Plast Reconstr Surg.* 2000; 105:2267-68.

Feilberg VL, Rosenborg D, Broen CC, Mogensen JV. Excretion of morphine in human breast milk. *Acta Anaesthesiol Scand.* 1989; 33:426-28.

Fernando R, Bonello E, Gill P, Urquhart J, Reynolds F, Morgan B. Neonatal welfare and placental transfer of fentanyl and bupivacaine during ambulatory combined spinal epidural analgesia for labour. *Anaesthesia.* 1997; 52:517-24.

Forster JG, Rosenberg PH, Niemi TT. Continuous spinal microcatheter (28 gauge) technique for arterial bypass surgery of the lower extremities and comparison of ropivacaine with or without morphine for postoperative analgesia. *Br J Anaesth.* 2006; 97:393-400.

Freeborn SF, Calvert RT, Black P, Macfarlane T, D'Souza SW. Saliva and blood pethidine concentrations in the mother and the newborn baby. *Br J Obstet Gynaecol.* 1980; 87:966-69.

Gambling DR, Yu P, Cole C, McMorland GH, Palmer L. A comparative study of patient controlled epidural analgesia (PCEA) and continuous infusion epidural analgesia (CIEA) during labour. *Can J Anaesth.* 1988; 35:249-54.

Grimm D, Pauly E, Poschl J, Linderkamp O, Skopp G. Buprenorphine and norbuprenorphine concentrations in human breast milk samples determined by liquid chromatography-tandem mass spectrometry. *Ther Drug Monit.* 2005; 27:526-30.

Hamza J, Benlabed M, Orhant E, Escourrou P, Curzi-Dascalova L, Gaultier C. Neonatal pattern of breathing during active and quiet sleep after maternal administration of meperidine. *Pediatr Res.* 1992; 32:412-16.

Hirose M, Hosokawa T, Tanaka Y. Extradural buprenorphine suppresses breastfeeding after caesarean section. *Br J Anaesth.* 1997; 79:120-21.

Hurley RJ. Continuous spinal anesthesia techniques for labor and delivery. In: Birnbach DJ, Gatt SP, Datta S (eds.). *Textbook of obstetric anesthesia.* New York: Churchill Livingston; 2000. p. 183-202.

Jernite M, Diemumunsch P, Kibtz P. Buprenorphine excretion in breast milk. *Anesthesiology.* 1999; 91.

Jordan S, Emery S, Bradshaw C, Watkins A, Friswell W. The impact of intrapartum analgesia on infant feeding. *BJOG.* 2005; 112:927-34.

Kanto J. Risk-benefit assessment of anaesthetic agents in the puerperium. *Drug Saf.* 1991; 6:285-301.

Kim J, Riggs KW, Misri S, Kent N, Oberlander TF, Grunau RE, *et al.* Stereoselective disposition of fluoxetine and norfluoxetine during pregnancy and breast-feeding. *Br J Clin Pharmacol.* 2006; 61:155-63.

Kuhnert BR, Kuhnert PM, Philipson EH, Syracuse CD. Disposition of meperidine and normeperidine following multiple doses during labor. II. Fetus and neonate. *Am J Obstet Gynecol.* 1985; 151:410-15.

Kunka RL, Venkataramanan R, Stern RM, Ladik CF. Excretion of propoxyphene and norpropoxyphene in breast milk. *Clin Pharmacol Ther.* 1984; 35:675-80.

Kunka RL, Yong CL, Ladik CF, Bates TR. Liquid chromatographic determination of propoxyphene and norpropoxyphene in plasma and breast milk. *J Pharm Sci.* 1985; 74:103-4.

Leuschen MP, Wolf LJ, Rayburn WF. Fentanyl excretion in breast milk [letter]. Clin Pharm. 1990; 9:336-37.

Lieberman E, Cohen A, Lang J, Frigoletto F, Goetzl L. Maternal intrapartum temperature elevation as a risk factor for cesarean delivery and assisted vaginal delivery. *Am J Public Health.* 1999; 89:506-10.

Lindblad A, Bernow J, Marsal K. Obstetric analgesia and fetal aortic blood flow during labour. *Br J Obstet Gynaecol.* 1987; 94:306-11.

Marinella MA. Meperidine-induced generalized seizures with normal renal function. *South Med J.* 1997; 90:556-58.

Marquet P, Chevrel J, Lavignasse P, Merle L, Lachatre G. Buprenorphine withdrawal syndrome in a newborn. *Clin Pharmacol Ther.* 1997; 62:569-71.

Marx CM, Pucino F, Carlson JD. Oxycodone excretion in human milk in the puerperium. *Drug Intell Clin Pharm.* 1986; 20:474.

Mattingly JE, D'Alessio J, Ramanathan J. Effects of obstetric analgesics and anesthetics on the neonate: a review. *Paediatr Drugs.* 2003; 5:615-27.

Morley-Forster PK, Weberpals J. Neonatal effects of patient-controlled analgesia using fentanyl in labor. *Int J Obstet Anesth.* 1998; 7:103-7.

Morris ME, LeRoy S, Sutton SC. Absorption of magnesium from orally administered magnesium sulfate in man. *J Toxicol Clin Toxicol.* 1987; 25:371-82.

Naulty JS. Bupivacaine in breast milk following epidural anesthesia for vaginal delivery. *Regional Anesthesia.* 1983; 8:44-45.

Nitsun M, Szokol JW, Saleh HJ, Murphy GS, Vender JS, Luong L, *et al.* Pharmacokinetics of midazolam, propofol, and fentanyl transfer to human breast milk. *Clin Pharmacol Ther.* 2006; 79:549-57.

Okutomi T, Saito M, Koura M, Hoka S. Spinal anesthesia using a continuous spinal catheter for cesarean section in a parturient with prior surgical correction of scoliosis. *J Anesth.* 2006; 20:223-26.

Ortega D, Viviand X, Lorec AM, Gamerre M, Martin C, Bruguerolle B. Excretion of lidocaine and bupivacaine in breast milk following epidural anesthesia for cesarean delivery. *Acta Anaesthesiol Scand.* 1999; 43:394-97.

Paull J. Epidural analgesia for labor. In: Birnbach DJ, Gatt SP, Datta S (eds.). *Textbook of obstetric anesthesia.* 1st Ed. New York: Churchill Livingstone; 2000. p. 145-56.

Peiker G, Muller B, Ihn W, Noschel H. Excretion of pethidine in mother's milk (author's transl). *Zentralbl Gynakol.* 1980; 102:537-41.

Pittman KA, Smyth RD, Losada M, Zighelboim I, Maduska AL, Sunshine A. Human perinatal distribution of butorphanol. *Am J Obstet Gynecol.* 1980; 138:797-800.

Quinn PG, Kuhnert BR, Kaine CJ, Syracuse CD. Measurement of meperidine and normeperidine in human breast milk by selected ion monitoring. *Biomed Environ Mass Spectrom.* 1986; 13:133-35.

Radzyminski S. The effect of ultra low dose epidural analgesia on newborn breastfeeding behaviors. *J Obstet Gynecol Neonatal Nurs.* 2003; 32:322-31.

Rawal N, Holmstrom B, Van Zundert A, Crowhurst JA. The combined spinal-epidural technique. In: Birnbach DJ, Gatt SP, Datta S (eds.). *Textbook of obstetric anesthesia.* 1st Ed. New York: Churchill Livingstone; 2000. p. 157-82.

Robieux I, Koren G, Vandenbergh H, Schneiderman J. Morphine excretion in breast milk and resultant exposure of a nursing infant. *J Toxicol Clin Toxicol.* 1990; 28:365-70.

Schmitt JP, Schwoerer D, Diemunsch P, Gauthier-Lafaye J. [Passage of propofol in the colostrum. Preliminary data]. *Ann Fr Anesth Reanim.* 1987; 6:267-68.

Soresi A. Episubdural anesthesia. *Anesth Analg.* 1937; 16:306-10.

Steer PL, Biddle CJ, Marley WS, Lantz RK, Sulik PL. Concentration of fentanyl in colostrum after an analgesic dose. *Can J Anaesth.* 1992; 39:231-35.

Van D, V, Halpern S, Joseph G. Patient-controlled epidural analgesia versus continuous infusion for labour analgesia: a meta-analysis. *Br J Anaesth.* 2002; 89:459-65.

Visalyaputra S. Systemic analgesia for labor. In: Birnbach DJ, Gatt SP, Datta S (eds.). *Textbook of obstetric anesthesia.* 1st Ed. New York: Churchill Livingstone; 2000. p. 209-27.

Wittels B, Glosten B, Faure EA, Moawad AH, Ismail M, Hibbard J, *et al.* Postcesarean analgesia with both epidural morphine and intravenous patient-controlled analgesia: neurobehavioral outcomes among nursing neonates. *Anesth Analgesia.* 1997; 85:600-6.

Wittels B, Scott DT, Sinatra RS. Exogenous opioids in human breast milk and acute neonatal neurobehavior: a preliminary study. *Anesthesiology.* 1990; 73:864-69.

Zakowski M. Complications associated with regional anesthesia in the obstetric patient. *Semin Perinatol.* 2002; 26:154-68.

Chapter 28

Antibiotic, Antifungal, Antiviral, and Antiretroviral Drugs

Judith H. Kristensen and Kenneth F. Ilett

INTRODUCTION

Antimicrobial drugs are used in breastfeeding mothers, often in the immediate postpartum period, to treat conditions such as wound infection post surgery, endometritis, mastitis, or other acute infections.

The transfer of maternal antibiotics into breastmilk has been reviewed several times in recent years (Bar-Oz *et al.*, 2003; Chung *et al.*, 2002; Mathew, 2004; Nahum *et al.*, 2006). These reviews have concentrated on the potential for antibiotics to cause acute toxicity in the breastfed infant. In addition, a recent review documents how individual gut flora species specifically induce gene activation within the host and thus modulate mucosal and systemic immune function and also impact metabolic programming (Bedford Russell *et al.*, 2006). This raises the possibility that alteration in the infant's gastrointestinal flora could have long-term effects and highlights the need for studies in breastfed infants exposed to antimicrobials. Antifungal, antiviral, anthelmintic, and antimalarial drug use during breastfeeding has also been reviewed (Mathew, 2004). A critical review of the published literature on infant adverse reactions claimed to be associated with breastmilk found only 100 case reports, with the majority in infants under two month of age (Anderson *et al.*, 2003). Of these, 43% were "probable" and 57% "possible" using the Naranjo scale (Naranjo *et al.*, 1981). Moreover, antimicrobials were the most frequently implicated class, comprising 17% of all reports.

As with all maternal drug use during lactation, the questions that need to be asked are (a) is there significant drug transfer into milk, (b) is drug exposure likely to cause any short-term toxicity in the infant, and (c) is drug exposure likely to cause any long-term adverse effects in the infant? In this chapter, we summarize the safety of representative antimicrobials in **Tables 1-3** and discuss selected antibiotics, antifungals, antivirals, and antiretrovirals in more detail.

ANTIBIOTICS

Penicillins and Cephalosporins

The penicillins and cephalosporins have been studied extensively in breastfeeding mothers. Only trace amounts have been detected in milk. With relative infant doses of <1% of the weight-adjusted maternal dose, they are compatible with breastfeeding (Bar-Oz *et al.*, 2003; Briggs *et al.*, 2005; Hale, 2006; Mathew, 2004). The addition of β−lactamase enzymes inhibitor clavulanic acid to amoxicillin to extend its spectrum has also been studied (Benyamini *et al.*, 2005). These authors compared reports of adverse effects in breastfed infants whose mothers had taken amoxicillin (n=40) or amoxicillin/clavulanic acid (n=67). While there was a higher percentage of reactions in the latter group (22.3% versus 7.5%), the odds ratio (95% CI) of 2.99 (0.95-9.68) showed that the difference was not significant.

Probenecid is occasionally used to enhance plasma levels of penicillins and cephalosporins when high tissue penetration is required. A single case involving maternal prescription of cephalexin and probenecid for a breast infection was recently reported (Ilett *et al.*, 2006). The average concentrations of probenecid and cephalexin in milk were 964 and 745 μg/L, respectively, corresponding to absolute and relative infant doses of 145 μg/kg/day and 0.7% for probenecid and 112 μg/kg/day and 0.5% for cephalexin. During the course of treatment, the infant developed diarrhea and related adverse effects which, based on the Naranjo Probability Scale (Naranjo *et al.*, 1981), were rated as "possible" for probenecid and "probable" for cephalexin. The case also illustrates that even at very low infant doses, antibiotics can alter the infant's gut flora and cause problems, such as diarrhea, dehydration, or candidiasis.

Macrolides

Erythromycin, with a low transfer to milk and relative infant doses ranging from 1.4-2.3, is considered compatible in breastfeeding mothers (Knowles, 1972; Matsuda, 1984; Stang, 1986), although hypertrophic pyloric stenosis in infants has been linked to exposure to the drug via milk (Sorensen *et al.*, 2003). In the latter study, infantile hypertrophic pyloric stenosis was 2.3 to 3 times more prevalent when the mother had taken a macrolide antibiotic (93% erythromycin, 7% clarithromycin) during the three months after delivery. Clarithromycin has absolute and relative infant doses of 0.15 mg/kg/day and 2% respectively (Sedlmayr *et al.*, 1993). There were no adverse effects in the 12 breastfed infants studied, and given that the usual pediatric dose of clarithromycin is 15 mg/kg/day (Anonymous, 2006), it can be concluded that clarithromycin is also compatible with breastfeeding. Azithromycin, a newer macrolide with a long half-life, has a somewhat higher relative infant dose (5.8%) (Kelsey *et al.*, 1994), but the absolute infant dose of 0.42 mg/kg/day is still well below the pediatric therapeutic dose range (10 mg/kg/day) (Young *et al.*, 2006). In addition, ten infants exposed to azithromycin for three days via breastmilk showed no vomiting, diarrhea, rash, or other adverse effects (Bar-Oz *et al.*, 2003). There are presently no data for roxithromycin use in breastfeeding. However, given its similarity to the other macrolides discussed above, it is also compatible (American Academy of Pediatrics Committee on Drugs, 2001).

Fluoroquinolones

Fluoroquinolone use in breastfeeding has often been prohibited because of reports of arthropathy in immature animals. There is also one reported case of pseudomembranous colitis in a breastfed infant exposed to ciprofloxacin for six days (Harmon *et al.*, 1992). However, ciprofloxacin use in pediatrics has increased in recent years (Ghaffer *et al.*, 2003), and there are now several studies indicating that there is little risk from ciprofloxacin exposure (Belet *et al.*, 2004; Drossou-Agakidou *et al.*, 2004; Gurpinar *et al.*, 1997; van den Oever *et al.*, 1998). The manufacturer's product information indicates that ionized calcium (Ca^{++}) may compromise the bioavailability of ciprofloxacin in adults (Product Information Ciproxin, 2006), and hence milk may be expected to limit its absorption by the breastfed infant. Using the maximum milk ciprofloxacin data from one study (Giamarellou *et al.*, 1989), the absolute infant dose is around 0.57 mg/kg/day. This is well below the pediatric therapeutic dose of 10-30 mg/kg/day (Anonymous, 2006).

The American Academy of Pediatrics considers ciprofloxacin to be safe during breastfeeding (American Academy of Pediatrics Committee on Drugs, 2001). The data available for norfloxacin comprise one case where the drug was not detected in milk for up to six hours after a single 200 mg oral dose (Takase *et al.*, 1981).

Metronidazole and Tinidazole

The safety of metronidazole use during breastfeeding has been questioned in the past (American Academy of Pediatrics Committee on Drugs, 2001) because of its known genotoxicity and mutagenicity in bacteria, genotoxicity in human cell lines, and carcinogenicity in animals (Bendesky *et al.*, 2002; Dobias *et al.*, 1994). However, the relevance of *in vitro* and animal studies is uncertain, and there are no definitive studies of its mutagenicity in humans (Bendesky *et al.*, 2002). It is frequently used postpartum to treat intra-uterine infections, and both the parent drug and its active hydroxyl metabolite are transferred to milk in significant amounts (Erickson *et al.*, 1981; Heisterberg *et al.*, 1983; Passmore *et al.*, 1988). The relative infant doses for metronidazole (10.5-13%) and hydroxymetronidazole (around 5%) are also a cause for concern. The absolute infant dose for a 1.2 g/day dose is calculated to be 2.3 mg/kg/day (Astrup-Jensen *et al.*, 1996; Hale,

Table 1. Antibiotics in Breastfeeding

Drug	Relative infant dose (%)	Comment	References
Penicillins and cephalosporins			
Amoxicillin (± clavulanic acid)	0.9	Compatible. Observe infant for diarrhea or thrush. Addition of clavulanic acid did not alter the percent of adverse reactions in infants.	Benyamini *et al.*, 2005; Kafetzis *et al.*, 1981; Matsuda, 1984
Cephalexin	0.5	Compatible. Observe infant for diarrhea or thrush.	Ilett *et al.*, 2006; Kafetzis *et al.*, 1981; Matsuda, 1984
Cefotaxime	0.17	Compatible. Observe infant for diarrhea or thrush.	Harms *et al.*, 1980; Kafetzis *et al.*, 1980
Dicloxacillin	1	Compatible. Observe infant for diarrhea or thrush.	Matsuda, 1984
Macrolides			
Azithromycin	5.8	Compatible. Observe infant for diarrhea or thrush.	Kelsey *et al.*, 1994
Clarithromycin	2	Compatible. One study showed an absolute infant dose of around 0.15 mg/kg/day that can be compared with the usual pediatric dose of 7.5 mg/kg twice daily. Observe infant for diarrhea or thrush.	Sedlmayr *et al.*, 1993; Young *et al.*, 2003
Erythromycin	1.4, 2.3	Compatible. Association between exposure via milk and infantile hypertrophic pyloric stenosis reported. Observe infant for diarrhea or thrush.	Knowles, 1972; Matsuda, 1984; Sorensen *et al.*, 2003; Stang, 1986
Roxithromycin	ND	No specific information, but related drugs in same class are compatible.	American Academy of Pediatrics Committee on Drugs, 2001
Quinolones			
Ciprofloxacin	2.1, 2.6	Compatible. Theoretical risk of arthropathy. One case of pseudomembranous colitis reported. Observe infant for diarrhea or thrush.	Gardner *et al.*, 1992; Giamarellou *et al.*, 1989; Harmon *et al.*, 1992
Norfloxacin	ND	Compatible. Not detected in breastmilk after a single 200 mg maternal dose.	Takase *et al.*, 1981
Ofloxacin	3.1	Compatible. Observe infant for diarrhea or thrush.	Giamarellou, 1989
Tetracyclines			
Doxycycline	4, 6	Compatible for short term use (<3 weeks). Avoid chronic dosing. Observe infant for diarrhea or thrush.	Lutziger, 1969; Morganti *et al.*, 1968
Tetracycline	0.8, 1.3	Compatible for short-term use. Absorption from milk may be limited by chelation to Ca^{++}. Observe infant for diarrhea or thrush.	Gruner, 1955; Matsuda, 1984; Posner *et al.*, 1955
Others			
Clindamycin	1.4-2.8	Compatible. One case of bloody stools and diarrhea reported. Observe infant for diarrhea or thrush.	Mann, 1980; Matsuda, 1984; Smith *et al.*, 1975; Steen *et al.*, 1982; Zhang *et al.*, 1997
Gentamicin	0.7, 1.9	Compatible. Poor oral absorption from milk also anticipated on molecular weight considerations.	Celiloglu *et al.*, 1994; Ito, 1970
Nitrofurantoin	6.8	Compatible. Avoid in infants with glucose-6-phosphate dehydrogenase deficiency or jaundice.	Gerk *et al.*, 2001
Metronidazole	10.5-13	Moderate transfer to milk, but no adverse effects reported in exposed infants. Dose significantly less than therapeutic dose. May impose bitter taste to milk. For 2 g single oral dose, express and discard milk for 12-24 hours.	Erickson *et al.*, 1981; Heisterberg *et al.*, 1983; Passmore *et al.*, 1988
Sulfamethoxazole (± trimethoprim)	2.3, 3, 6	Compatible. Avoid in infants with glucose-6-phosphate dehydrogenase deficiency or jaundice.	Chung *et al.*, 2002; Ito *et al.*, 1993; Miller *et al.*, 1974
Tinidazole	≈15	After large single doses, express and discard milk for up to 72 hours.	Evaldson *et al.*, 1985; Mannisto *et al.*, 1983
Trimethoprim	5.5, 5.9, 9.8	Compatible. Absolute infant dose is 6-11% of pediatric dose.	Anonymous, 2006; Arnauld *et al.*, 1972; Borderon *et al.*, 1975; Ito *et al.*, 1993
Vancomycin	6.6	Compatible. Minimal oral bioavailability anticipated on molecular weight considerations. Absolute infant dose is about 5% of infant dose for pseudomembranous colitis. Observe infant for diarrhea or thrush.	Reyes *et al.*, 1989; Young *et al.*, 2006

Table 2. Antifungal Drugs in Breastfeeding

Drug	Relative infant dose (%)	Comment	References
Nystatin	ND	Undetectable in maternal plasma after oral administration and therefore transfer into milk likely to be negligible.	Rothermel *et al.*, 1975
Amphotericin	ND	Minimal oral bioavailability anticipated on molecular weight considerations; unlikely to be present in milk in clinically significant quantities.	Hale, 2006
Fluconazole	16	Relatively high transfer into milk. However, absolute infant dose is only 6-12% of the therapeutic infant dose (3-6 mg/kg) administered to preterm infants for treatment of systemic fungal infections.	Force, 1995; Kaufman *et al.*, 2001; Schilling *et al.*, 1993; Young *et al.*, 2006

Table 3. Antiviral and Antiretroviral Drugs in Breastfeeding

Drug	Relative infant dose (%)	Comment	References
Antivirals			
Acyclovir	1.4, 1.9, 1, 8.5	Compatible.	Bork *et al.*, 1995; Lau *et al.*, 1987; Meyer *et al.*, 1988; Taddio *et al.*, 1994
Famciclovir	1.5	Greater bioavailability than acyclovir. Consider acyclovir or valacyclovir as alternatives.	Hale, 2006
Valacyclovir	2.4	Metabolized to acyclovir in blood, prior to transfer into milk. Compatible.	Sheffield *et al.*, 2002
Antiretrovirals			
Lamivudine	4.3, 6.4	Compatible. Median infant plasma concentrations were only 5% of the therapeutic IC_{50} for HIV-1.	Moodley *et al.*, 1998; Shapiro *et al.*, 2005
Nevirapine	17.8	Compatible. Median infant plasma concentrations are 40-times the therapeutic IC_{50} for HIV-1.	Shapiro *et al.*, 2005
Zidovudine	0.4	Compatible. In combination with a daily dose of zidovudine 4-6 mg/kg/day, median infant plasma concentrations were 25-times the therapeutic IC_{50} for HIV-1.	Shapiro *et al.*, 2005

2006). Metronidazole is commonly used orally to treat infections in infants at doses of 7.5-22.5 mg/kg/day (Young *et al.*, 2006). Nevertheless, the metronidazole in milk is absorbed by the breastfed infant. In one study, infant plasma metronidazole concentrations ranged from 4 to 32% of those in maternal plasma, while hydroxymetronidazole plasma concentrations ranged from 8 to 96% of those in maternal plasma. Thus, by whatever yardstick we choose, the breastfed infant is exposed to significant amounts of unwanted drug. Nevertheless, overt adverse effects in exposed infants do not appear to be a frequent problem. There is one report of diarrhea and secondary lactose intolerance (Clements, 1980) balanced by others where no adverse effects were noted in 16 exposed infants (Heisterberg *et al.*, 1983) and where diaper rash, feeding, and weight gain at discharge were similar for 35 exposed infants and controls whose mothers received either amoxicillin or no drug (Passmore *et al.*, 1988). Thus, we conclude that short courses of metronidazole at common therapeutic oral doses (600-1200 mg/day) are compatible with breastfeeding when no other alternative drug is acceptable. When larger single doses are needed (e.g., 2 g for trichonomiasis), expressing and discarding milk for 12-24 hours is recommended (American Academy of Pediatrics Committee on Drugs, 2001).

Tinidazole, which is closely related to metronidazole, is also a drug where there may be concern about use during breastfeeding. Usually a single 2 g dose is used for trichomoniasis or giardiasis in adults (Product Information Fasigyn, 2006). Literature data on its concentrations in breastmilk give relative infant doses of up to 15% in the first 24 hours after a single dose, and this exposure falls to about two percent at 72 hours. Hence, it is recommended that milk should be pumped and discarded for up to three days after such doses (American Academy of Pediatrics Committee on Drugs, 2001).

Tetracyclines

Tetracyclines are another drug group where there has been controversy over their use during breastfeeding. Issues of staining of the infant's developing teeth and interference with bone growth have been cited. However, the relative infant dose is moderate (4%, 6%) for doxycycline (Lutziger, 1969; Morganti *et al.*, 1968) and low (0.8%,1.3%) for tetracycline (Gruner, 1955; Matsuda, 1984; Posner *et al.*, 1955). Tetracyclines are well known to have their bioavailability compromised by divalent metal ions, such as Ca^{++}, and one can surmise that human milk would therefore limit its absorption in the infant. Moreover no adverse effects in breastfed infants were reported (Gruner, 1955; Posner *et al.*, 1955). Being conservative, it seems reasonable to advise against chronic dosing with tetracyclines during lactation and to observe the infant for diarrhea or candidiasis which may indicate an adverse local effect on gut flora. Therapy for up to three weeks is considered safe (Hale, 2006). Alternative drugs with a comparable activity spectrum could be considered when chronic therapy is necessary.

Sulfamethoxazole and Trimethoprim

Although quite an old drug, sulfamethoxazole is still widely used, often in a combination formulation with trimethoprim. The relative infant dose of sulfamethoxazole is low (range 2.3-6) (Chung *et al.*, 2002; Miller *et al.*, 1974), and no adverse effects were found in infants from 12 women who took the drug while breastfeeding (Ito *et al.*, 1993). It is therefore compatible with breastfeeding (American Academy of Pediatrics Committee on Drugs, 2001). However, it is suggested that sulfonamides should be avoided if the infant has glucose-6-phosphate dehydrogenase deficiency or is jaundiced, as they may exacerbate symptoms (American Academy of Pediatrics Committee on Drugs, 2001; Chung *et al.*, 2002). Trimethoprim has a somewhat higher range of relative infant doses (5.6-9.8%) (Arnauld *et al.*, 1972; Borderon *et al.*, 1975), but this is only 6-11% of the pediatric dose of 4-8 mg/kg/day (Anonymous, 2006), and it should be considered compatible. In healthy infants, the combination of sulfamethoxazole and trimethoprim should also be compatible with breastfeeding as no adverse effects were found in infants from 12 women who took the drug while breastfeeding (Ito *et al.*, 1993).

Aminoglycosides

The aminoglycosides, gentamicin and tobramycin, which are usually administered IM or IV, are compatible with breastfeeding. They both have low relative infant doses (ranging from undetectable to 2.6%) together with poor oral bioavailability, so significant infant exposure is unlikely (Celiloglu *et al.*, 1994; Festini *et al.*, 2006; Ito, 1970; Takase, 1975; Uwaydah *et al.*, 1975).

ANTIFUNGALS

Of the antifungals, amphotericin and nystatin are both considered compatible for breastfeeding mothers based on their poor oral bioavailability (Hale, 2006; Rothermel *et al.*, 1975). Fluconazole has a higher transfer to milk with an absolute infant dose of 0.34 mg/kg/day and a relative infant dose of 16% (Force, 1995; Kaufman *et al.*, 2001; Schilling *et al.*, 1993). While this is higher than the notional 10% limit of safety (Bennett, 1996), it is only about 6-12% of the intravenous dose (3-6 mg/kg/day) suggested for prophylaxis against fungal infection in preterm infants (Young *et al.*, 2006). Amphotericin, nystatin, and miconazole are often used topically for fungal infections of the nipple. Infant exposure from this use is considered minimal, provided that minimal amounts are placed on the nipple and that the area is washed before feeding. Nystatin oral drops (100,000 U, four times daily) (Product Information Nilstat Oral Drops, 2006) and miconazole oral gel (5 mg, four times daily) (Product Information Daktarin Oral Gel, 2006) also have a therapeutic use in the local treatment of oral thrush in infants, but again exposure is not considered to be significant.

ANTIVIRALS

Acyclovir

Acyclovir, with a low (1%, 1.9%, 8.5%) relative infant dose (Bork *et al.*, 1995; Lau *et al.*, 1987; Meyer *et al.*, 1988; Taddio *et al.*, 1994) is considered safe for use in breastfeeding mothers, as is valacyclovir (relative infant dose 2.4%) because it is a pro-drug that is rapidly converted to acyclovir (Sheffield *et al.*, 2002). These are probably safer alternatives than famciclovir which has a higher bioavailability than acyclovir and for which there are currently no available data on its transfer into milk. Topical application of acyclovir is not considered to be a risk for the breastfed infant.

ANTIRETROVIRALS

Lamiduvine, Nevirapine and Zidovudine

Antiretroviral drugs are used widely in the developing world in the treatment of HIV-1 infections. If these drugs are not administered to mothers with HIV-1 and/or their infants, mother-to-child transmission of HIV-1 from breastfeeding occurs in 9-16% of breastfed infants (The Breastfeeding and HIV-1 International Transmission Study Group, 2004). In western countries, we generally choose to advise mothers positive for HIV-1 not to breastfeed in order to limit horizontal transmission. However, in developing countries, formula feeding is associated with increased infant morbidity and mortality from a variety of infectious diseases (World Health Organization (WHO) Collaborative Study Team, 2000), and breastfeeding is often preferred even when the mother is HIV-1 positive. The focus on antiretroviral drugs and breastfeeding concerns whether the concentration of drug transferred via milk is sufficient to contribute to the prevention of infection in the infant, rather than on possible adverse effects. Some small studies have suggested that the concentration in milk might be sufficient to contribute to antiviral actions in the infant (Colebunders *et al.*, 2005; Moodley *et al.*, 1998; Musoke *et al.*, 1999). In a study of 20 women who received highly active antiretroviral treatment (HAART) with lamivudine (300 mg/day), nevirapine (400 mg/day), and zidovudine (600 mg/day), infant plasma concentrations achieved during breastfeeding were 40-times IC_{50} values (concentration for 50% inhibition of virus growth) for nevirapine, but only 5% of the IC_{50} values for lamivudine (Shapiro *et al.*, 2005). For zidovudine, infant plasma concentrations during breastfeeding were 25-times the IC_{50} value, but the interpretation of these data was complicated by ongoing treatment of the infants with therapeutic doses of zidovudine. Hence, it appears that, at least for some of its individual constituents, maternal HAART may have the potential to minimize the transmission of HIV-1 to the breastfed infant. The possibility of drug-related adverse effects in the infants as a result of this exposure remains to be investigated. In addition, the lowering of plasma viral titers with HAART treatment should also reduce the maternal-infant transfer of the virus.

CONCLUSIONS

On balance, the data suggest that there are few absolute contraindications to breastfeeding for mothers who need to take antimicrobials. Local application of these drugs to the nipples (e.g., neomycin, clotrimazole, miconazole, nystatin) or in the ears or eyes (e.g., chloramphenicol, framycetin) of the mother is unlikely to be a risk for the breastfed infant. Although most antimicrobials discussed above transfer into milk in small amounts, many have the potential to modify bowel flora, causing short-term adverse effects in the form of gastrointestinal symptoms, such as diarrhea or thrush (diaper rash). They could also interfere with interpretation of culture results. Notable exceptions are metronidazole and tinidazole where a withholding period is required after high doses.

Some reviewers have recommended strategies of minimizing infant exposure to antimicrobials in milk by feeding at a time in the dose interval when drug concentrations in milk will be lowest (Mathew, 2004). While the latter is a laudable aim, it is usually impractical. In addition, peak to trough variation in maternal drug concentration for many drugs is small, thus making it difficult to achieve a significant decrease in exposure. Using drugs with high maternal clearance has also been suggested, and could perhaps work best when single or intermittent dosing is appropriate.

While the relative infant doses for these drugs are useful guides to assessing safety of drug use in lactation, absolute infant dose is often a robust comparator for evaluating safety as these drugs often have a pediatric application. Consideration should also be given to reports of adverse effects, the lack of adverse effects in breastfed infants, reports of blood levels of drugs in exposed infants, and the duration for which mother needs to take the medication. When weighing up the information from any report, due consideration should be given to the number of subjects studied and the quality of the data, particularly if they are related to adverse events. With regard to the latter, it is worth remembering that a review of the literature found only 100 adverse event reports up to 2003 (Anderson *et al.*, 2003). Of these, 17% were associated with maternal antibiotic use, but overall the study found that only 47% of the adverse events were "probably" attributable to the suspected drug. As with all drug use in breastfeeding, an individual risk/benefit analysis should be conducted before starting therapy.

References

American Academy of Pediatrics Committee on Drugs. Transfer of drugs and other chemicals into human milk. *Pediatrics.* 2001; 108:776-89.

Anderson PO, Pochop SL, Manoguerra AS. Adverse drug reactions in breastfed infants: less than imagined. *Clin Pediat (Phila).* 2003; 42:325-40.

Anonymous. *BNF for children.* 2nd Ed. London, UK: MBJ Publishing Group Ltd; 2006.

Arnauld R, Soutoul JH, Gallier J. Etude du passage de la trimethoprim dans le lait maternel. *Ouest Med.* 1972; 25:959-64.

Astrup-Jensen A, Bates CJ, Begg EJ, Edwards S, Lazarus CR, Matheson I, *et al. Drugs and human lactation.* 2nd Ed. Amsterdam: Elsevier; 1996.

Bar-Oz B, Bulkowstein M, Benyamini L, Greenberg R, Soriano I, Zimmerman D, *et al.* Use of antibiotic and analgesic drugs during lactation. *Drug Saf.* 2003; 26:925-35.

Bedford Russell AR, Murch SH. Could peripartum antibiotics have delayed health consequences for the infant? *BJOG.* 2006; 113:758-65.

Belet N, Haciomeroglu P, Kucukoduk S. Ciprofloxacin treatment in newborns with multi-drug-resistant nosocomial Pseudomonas infections. *Biol Neonate.* 2004; 85:263-68.

Bendesky A, Menendez D, Ostrosky-Wegman P. Is metronidazole carcinogenic? *Mutat Res.* 2002; 511:133-44.

Bennett PN. Use of the monographs on drugs. In: Bennett PN (ed.). *Drugs and human lactation.* 2nd Ed. Amsterdam: Elsevier; 1996. p. 67-74.

Benyamini L, Merlob P, Stahl B, Braunstein R, Bortnik O, Bulkowstein M, *et al.* The safety of amoxicillin/clavulanic acid and cefuroxime during lactation. *Ther Drug Monit.* 2005; 27:499-502.

Borderon E, Soutoul JH. Excretion of antibiotics in human milk. *Med Mal Infect.* 1975; 5:373-76.

Bork K, Benes P. Concentration and kinetic studies of intravenous acyclovir in serum and breast milk of a patient with eczema herpeticum. *J Am Acad Dermatol.* 1995; 32:1053-55.

Briggs GG, Freeman RK, Yaffe SJ. *Drugs in pregnancy and lactation.* 7th Ed. Philadelphia: Lippincott Williams and Wilkins; 2005.

Celiloglu M, Celiker S, Guven H, Tuncok Y, Demir N, Erten O. Gentamicin excretion and uptake from breast milk by nursing infants. *Obstet Gynecol.* 1994; 84:263-65.

Chung AM, Reed MD, Blumer JL. Antibiotics and breast-feeding: a critical review of the literature. *Paediatr Drugs.* 2002; 4:817-37.

Clements CJ. Metronidazole and breast feeding. *NZ Med J.* 1980; 92:329.

Colebunders R, Hodossy B, Burger D, Daems T, Roelens K, Coppens M, *et al.* The effect of highly active antiretroviral treatment on viral load and antiretroviral drug levels in breast milk. *AIDS.* 2005; 19:1912-15.

Dobias L, Cerna M, Rossner P, Sram R. Genotoxicity and carcinogenicity of metronidazole. *Mutat Res.* 1994; 317:177-94.

Drossou-Agakidou V, Roilides E, Papakyriakidou-Koliouska P, Agakidis C, Nikolaides N, Sarafidis K, *et al.* Use of ciprofloxacin in neonatal sepsis: lack of adverse effects up to one year. *Pediatr Infect Dis J.* 2004; 23:346-49.

Erickson SH, Oppenheim GL, Smith GH. Metronidazole in breast milk. *Obstet Gynecol.* 1981; 57:48-50.

Evaldson GR, Lindgren S, Nord CE, Rane AT. Tinidazole milk excretion and pharmacokinetics in lactating women. *Br J Clin Pharmacol.* 1985; 19:503-7.

Festini F, Ciuti R, Taccetti G, Repetto T, Campana S, De MM. Breast-feeding in a woman with cystic fibrosis undergoing antibiotic intravenous treatment. *J Maternal Fetal Neonatal Med.* 2006; 19:375-76.

Force RW. Fluconazole concentrations in breast milk. *Pediatr Infect Dis J.* 1995; 14:235-36.

Gardner DK, Gabbe SG, Harter C. Simultaneous concentrations of ciprofloxacin in breast milk and in serum in mother and breast-fed infant. *Clin Pharm.* 1992; 11:352-54.

Gerk PM, Kuhn RJ, Desai NS, McNamara PJ. Active transport of nitrofurantoin into human milk. *Pharmacotherapy.* 2001; 21:669-75.

Ghaffer F, McCraken GH. Quinolones in pediatrics. In: Hoper DC, Rubenstein E (eds). *Quinolone antimicrobial agents.* Washington DC, USA: ASM Press; 2003. p. 343-54.

Giamarellou H, Kolokythas E, Petrikkos G, Gazis J, Aravantinos D, Sfikakis P. Pharmacokinetics of three newer quinolones in pregnant and lactating women. *Am J Med.* 1989; 87:49S-51S.

Gruner JM. The excretion of terramycin and tetracycline in human milk. *Geburtshilfe Frauenheilkd.* 1955; 15:354-60.

Gurpinar AN, Balkan E, Kilic N, Kiristioglu I, Dogruyol H. The effects of a fluoroquinolone on the growth and development of infants. *J Int Med Res.* 1997; 25:302-6.

Hale TW. *Medications and mothers' milk.* 11th Ed. Amarillo, TX, USA: Pharmasoft Publishing; 2006.

Harmon T, Burkhart G, Applebaum H. Perforated pseudomembranous colitis in the breast-fed infant. *J Pediatr Surg.* 1992; 27:744-46.

Harms K, Gerke G, Zaloudek D. Konzentrationsbestimmungen von cetotaxim aus der muttermilch. *Infection.* 1980; 8 (Suppl 4):S451-S453.

Heisterberg L, Branebjerg PE. Blood and milk concentrations of metronidazole in mothers and infants. *J Perinat Med.* 1983; 11:114-20.

Ilett KF, Hackett LP, Ingle B, Bretz PJ. Transfer of probenecid and cephalexin into breast milk. *Ann Pharmacother.* 2006; 40:986-89.

Ito S, Blajchman A, Stephenson M, Eliopoulos C, Koren G. Prospective follow-up of adverse reactions in breast-fed infants exposed to maternal medication. *Am J Obstet Gynecol.* 1993; 168:1393-99.

Ito T. Absorption, excretion and effects of gentamicin in newborn infants. *Jap J Antibiotics.* 1970; 23:298-311.

Kafetzis DA, Lazarides CV, Siafas CA, Georgakopoulos PA, Papadatos CJ. Transfer of cefotaxime in human milk and from mother to foetus. *J Antimicrob Chemother.* 1980; 6 Suppl A:135-41.

Kafetzis DA, Siafas CA, Georgakopoulos PA, Papadatos CJ. Passage of cephalosporins and amoxicillin into the breast milk. *Acta Paediatr Scand.* 1981; 70:285-88.

Kaufman D, Boyle R, Hazen KC, Patrie JT, Robinson M, Donowitz LG. Fluconazole prophylaxis against fungal colonization and infection in preterm infants. *N Engl J Med.* 2001; 345:1660-66.

Kelsey JJ, Moser LR, Jennings JC, Munger MA. Presence of azithromycin breast milk concentrations: a case report. *Am J Obstet Gynecol.* 1994; 170:1375-76.

Knowles JA. Drugs in milk. *Pediatric Currents.* 1972; 21:28-32.

Lau RJ, Emery MG, Galinsky RE. Unexpected accumulation of acyclovir in breast milk with estimation of infant exposure. *Obstet Gynecol.* 1987; 69:468-71.

Lutziger H. Concentration determinations and clinical effectiveness of doxycycline (Vibramycin) in the uterus, adnexa and maternal milk. *Ther Umsch.* 1969; 26:476-80.

Mann CF. Clindamycin and breast-feeding [letter]. *Pediatrics.* 1980; 66:1030-31.

Mannisto PT, Karhunen M, Koskela O, Suikkari AM, Mattila J, Haataja H. Concentrations of tinidazole in breast milk. *Acta Pharmacol Toxicol (Copenh).* 1983; 53:254-56.

Mathew JL. Effect of maternal antibiotics on breast feeding infants. *Postgrad Med J.* 2004; 80:196-200.

Matsuda S. Transfer of antibiotics into maternal milk. *Biol Res Pregnancy Perinatol.* 1984; 5:57-60.

Meyer LJ, de Miranda P, Sheth N, Spruance S. Acyclovir in human breast milk. *Am J Obstet Gynecol.* 1988; 158:586-88.

Miller RD, Salter AJ. *The passage of trimethoprim/sulfamethoxazole into breast milk and its significance.* Athens: Hellenic Society for Chemotherapy; 1974. p. 687-91.

Moodley J, Moodley D, Pillay K, Coovadia H, Saba J, van LR, *et al.* Pharmacokinetics and antiretroviral activity of lamivudine alone or when coadministered with zidovudine in human immunodeficiency virus type 1-infected pregnant women and their offspring. *J Infect Dis.* 1998; 178:1327-33.

Morganti G, Ceccarelli G, Ciaffi G. Comparative concentrations of a tetracycline antibiotic in serum and maternal milk. *Antibiotica.* 1968; 6:216-23.

Musoke P, Guay LA, Bagenda D, Mirochnick M, Nakabiito C, Fleming T, *et al.* A phase I/II study of the safety and pharmacokinetics of nevirapine in HIV-1-infected pregnant Ugandan women and their neonates (HIVNET 006). *AIDS.* 1999; 13:479-86.

Nahum GG, Uhl K, Kennedy DL. Antibiotic use in pregnancy and lactation: what is and is not known about teratogenic and toxic risks. *Obstet Gynecol.* 2006; 107:1120-38.

Naranjo CA, Busto U, Sellers EM, Sandor P, Ruiz I, Roberts EA, *et al.* A method for estimating the probability of adverse drug reactions. *Clin Pharmacol Ther.* 1981; 30:239-45.

Passmore CM, McElnay JC, Rainey EA, D'Arcy PF. Metronidazole excretion in human milk and its effect on the suckling neonate. *Br J Clin Pharmacol.* 1988; 26:45-51.

Posner AC, Prigot A, Konicoff NG. Further observations on the use of tetracycline hydrochloride in prophylaxis and treatment of obstetric infections. *Antibiotics Annual 1955.* 1954-1955:594-95.

Product Information Ciproxin. MIMS Abbreviated product information. E-MIMS 2006; Version 5.00.0270.

Product Information Daktarin Oral Gel. MIMS Abbreviated Product Information. E-MIMS 2006; Version 5.00.0270.

Product Information Fasigyn. MIMS Abbreviated product information. E-MIMS 2006; Version 5.00.0270.

Product Information Nilstat Oral Drops. MIMS Abbreviated product information. E-MIMS 2006; Version 5.00.0270.

Reyes MP, Ostrea EMJ, Cabinian AE, Schmitt C, Rintelmann W. Vancomycin during pregnancy: does it cause hearing loss or nephrotoxicity in the infant? [see comments]. *Am J Obstet Gynecol.* 1989; 161:977-81.

Rothermel P, Faber M. Drugs in breastmilk: a consumer's guide. *Birth Fam J.* 1975; 2:76-78.

Schilling CG, Seay RE, Larson TA. Excretion of fluconazole in human breast milk. *Pharmacotherapy.* 1993; 13:287.

Sedlmayr T, Peters F, Raasch W, Kees F. Clarithromycin, a new macrolide antibiotic. Effectiveness in puerperal infections and pharmacokinetics in breast milk. *Geburtshilfe Frauenheilkd.* 1993; 53:488-91.

Shapiro RL, Holland DT, Capparelli E, Lockman S, Thior I, Wester C, *et al.* Antiretroviral concentrations in breast-feeding infants of women in Botswana receiving antiretroviral treatment. *J Infect Dis.* 2005; 192:720-27.

Sheffield JS, Fish DN, Hollier LM, Cadematori S, Nobles BJ, Wendel GD. Acyclovir concentrations in human breast milk after valaciclovir administration. *Am J Obstet Gynecol.* 2002; 186:100-2.

Smith JA, Morgan JR. Clindamycin in human breast milk. *Can Med Assoc J.* 1975; 112:806.

Sorensen HT, Skriver MV, Pedersen L, Larsen H, Ebbesen F, Schonheyder HC. Risk of infantile hypertrophic pyloric stenosis after maternal postnatal use of macrolides. *Scand J Infect Dis.* 2003; 35:104-6.

Stang H. Pyloric stenosis associated with erythromycin ingested through breastmilk. *Minn Med.* 1986; 69:669-70.

Steen B, Rane A. Clindamycin passage into human milk. *Br J Clin Pharmacol.* 1982; 13:661-64.

Taddio A, Klein J, Koren G. Acyclovir excretion in human breast milk. *Ann Pharmacother.* 1994; 28:585-87.

Takase Z. Laboratory and clinical studies on tobramycin in the field of obstetrics and gynecology. *Chemotherapy (Tokyo).* 1975; 23:1402.

Takase Z, Shirafuji H, Uchida M. Basic and clinical studies on AM-715 in the field of obstetrics and gynecology. *Chemotherapy (Tokyo).* 1981; 29 (Suppl 4):697-704.

The Breastfeeding and HIV-1 International Transmission Study Group. Late postnatal transmission of HIV-1 in breast-fed children: an individual patient data meta-analysis. *J Infect Dis.* 2004; 189:2154-66.

Uwaydah M, Bibi S, Salman S. Therapeutic efficacy of tobramycin-a clinical and laboratory evaluation. *J Antimicrob Chemother.* 1975; 1:429-37.

van den Oever HL, Versteegh FG, Thewessen EA, van den Anker JN, Mouton JW, Neijens HJ. Ciprofloxacin in preterm neonates: case report and review of the literature. *Eur J Pediatr.* 1998; 157:843-45.

World Health Organisation (WHO) Collaborative Study Team. Effect of breastfeeding on infant and child mortality due to infectious diseases in less developed countries: a pooled analysis. *Lancet.* 2000; 355:451-55.

Young TE, Mangum B. *Neofax; A manual of drugs used in neonatal care.* 18th Ed. Raleigh, NC, USA: Acorn Publishing Inc; 2003.

Young TE, Mangum B. *Neofax.* 19th Ed. Raleigh, NC, USA: Acorn Publishing, Inc; 2006.

Zhang Y, Zhang Q, Xu Z. Tissue and body fluid distribution of antibacterial agents in pregnant and lactating women. *Zhonghua Fu Chan Ke Za Zhi.* 1997; 32:288-92.

Chapter 29

Anthelmintics and Antiprotozoals; Scabicides and Pediculicides; Antimalarials and Antimycobacterials

Kenneth F. Ilett and Judith H. Kristensen

INTRODUCTION

These are drugs with restricted but important applications in breastfeeding women. The antiprotozoals, anthelmintics, pediculicides, and scabicides are widely used both in tropical countries where transmission is high, as well as in western countries where such infections are more sporadic. The antimalarials and antimycobacterials are more likely to be needed in tropical countries where such infections are prevalent, and use may be both for prophylaxis and/or acute treatment. Prophylactic use of antimalarial drugs may also be necessary in lactating mothers who need to travel to malarious areas.

There have been few published reviews for these drug groups. Anthelmintics, pediculicides, and scabicides were reviewed in 2003 (Porto, 2003), antimalarials in 1992 and 1993 (Fulton *et al.*, 1992; Parke, 1993) and antimycobacterials in 1998 (Tran *et al.*, 1998). Anthelmintic drug use during breastfeeding has also been reviewed in 2004 (Mathew, 2004). Detailed monographs for many individual drugs are also available in reference texts (Bennett *et al.*, 1996; Briggs *et al.*, 2005; Hale, 2006) and from LactMed (US National Library of Medicine, 2006).

As with all maternal drug use during lactation, the questions that need to be asked are (a) is there significant drug transfer into milk, (b) is drug exposure likely to cause any short-term toxicity in the infant and, (c) is drug exposure likely to cause any long-term adverse effects in the infant? In this chapter, we summarize the safety of representative antiprotzoals, anthelmintics, pediculicides, and scabicides in **Table 1**, antimalarials in **Table 2**, and antimycobacterials in **Table 3**, and also discuss selected drugs in detail in the text.

ANTHELMINTICS AND ANTIPROTOZOALS

Mebendazole

Mebendazole has a low oral absorption of 2-10% and high protein binding (95%). In a single case, mebendazole was undetected in breastmilk after a maternal dose of 100 mg twice a day for three days (Kurzel *et al.*, 1994). In the same study, no change in milk production was noted in four mothers after a course of mebendazole. This contrasts with a report of significantly decreased milk supply in a mother who had taken the same dose (Rao, 1983).

Albendazole

There are no reports quantifying albendazole transfer to milk. The drug has low oral absorption <5% (Hale, 2006) and is unlikely to be present in milk in clinically relevant quantities. It has been suggested that a single dose of albendazole may be given to a breastfeeding mother (Allen *et al.*, 2002), and that in order to minimize infant exposure, the dose should be given prior to the infant's longest sleep period.

Thiabendazole

Thiabendazole is rapidly absorbed orally and is commonly associated with central nervous system side effects. There are no data on the transfer of thiabendazole to breastmilk, but as the drug is completely eliminated from the plasma in 24 to 48 hours, expressing and discarding the milk for this period of time may provide an alternative to feeding if use of the drug is essential (Porto, 2003).

Ivermectin

Ivermectin is considered compatible with breastfeeding by the American Academy of Pediatrics (American Academy of Pediatrics Committee on Drugs, 2001). In a study of four subjects given a single dose of 150 μg/kg, it was estimated that a breastfeeding infant would receive 1.47 μg/kg, with a relative infant dose of 0.98% (Ogbuokiri *et al.*, 1993; Ogbuokiri *et al.*, 1994). No adverse effects attributable to the drug were observed in infants exposed to ivermectin through breastmilk in a population of lactating women living in an endemic area (Ogbuokiri *et al.*, 1993; Ogbuokiri *et al.*, 1994; Porto, 2003).

Praziquantal

Very small amounts of praziquantal are transferred to breastmilk. Relative infant doses of 0.44% and 0.56% were reported in women ingesting either a single dose of 50 mg/kg or three doses of 20 mg at four hourly intervals. Based on the low transfer to milk, it is suggested that praziquantal is not contraindicated in breastfeeding mothers (Allen *et al.*, 2002; Olds, 2003). Again, it is recommended that a single dose is given prior to the infant's longest sleep period, or the milk may be expressed and discarded for 24 to 36 hours after the praziquantal dosing is completed (Porto, 2003).

Pyrantel

Although there is no data on the transfer of pyrantel to breastmilk, the low oral absorption and correspondingly low plasma levels would suggest low breastmilk concentrations of the drug (Hale, 2006).

Metronidazole

Metronidazole and tinidazole have a spectrum of activity that includes anaerobic protozoa, such as *Giardia lamblia,* as well as anaerobic bacteria. The safety of metronidazole use during breastfeeding has been questioned in the past (American Academy of Pediatrics Committee on Drugs, 2001) because of its known genotoxicity and mutagenicity in bacteria, genotoxicity in human cell lines, and carcinogenicity in animals (Dobias *et al.*, 1994; Bendesky *et al.*, 2002). However, the relevance of *in vitro* and animal studies is uncertain, and there are no definitive studies of its mutagenicity in humans (Bendesky *et al.*, 2002). It is frequently used postpartum to treat intra-uterine infections and both the parent drug and its active hydroxyl metabolite are transferred to milk in significant amounts (Erickson *et al.*, 1981; Heisterberg *et al.*, 1983; Passmore *et al.*, 1988). The relative infant doses for metronidazole (10.5-13%) and hydroxymetronidazole (around 5%) are also a cause for concern. The absolute infant dose for a 1.2 g/day maternal dose is calculated to be 2.3 mg/kg/day (Astrup-Jensen *et al.*, 1996; Hale, 2006). Metronidazole is commonly used orally to treat infections in infants at doses of 7.5-22.5 mg/kg/day (Young *et al.*, 2006). Nevertheless, the metronidazole in milk is absorbed by the breastfed infant and in one study, infant plasma metronidazole concentrations ranged from 4-32% of those in maternal plasma, while hydroxymetronidazole plasma concentrations ranged from 8-96% of those in maternal plasma. Thus, by whatever yardstick we choose, the breastfed infant is exposed to significant amounts of unwanted drug. Nevertheless, overt adverse effects in exposed infants do not appear to be a frequent problem. There is one report of diarrhea and secondary lactose intolerance (Clements, 1980), balanced by others where no adverse effects were noted in 16 exposed infants (Heisterberg *et al.*, 1983), and where diaper rash, feeding, and weight gain at discharge were similar for 35 exposed infants and controls whose mother's received either amoxicillin or no drug (Passmore *et al.*, 1988). Thus, we conclude that short courses of metronidazole at common therapeutic oral doses (600-1200 mg/day) are compatible with breastfeeding when no other alternative drug is acceptable. When larger single doses are needed (e.g., 2 grams for bacterial vaginosis), expressing and discarding milk for 12-24 hours is recommended (American Academy of Pediatrics Committee on Drugs, 2001). Metronidazole is reported to impart a metallic taste to milk which may be offensive to some infants (Hale, 2006).

Table 1. Selected Drugs for the Treatment of Protozoal and Helminth Parasitic Infections and Ectoparasitic Infections

Drug	Relative infant dose (%)	Comment	References
Anthelmintics and antiprotozoals			
Albendazole	ND	Low oral absorption. A single dose is safe. Take before infant's longest sleep period to reduce exposure.	Allen *et al.*, 2002; Porto, 2003
Bithional	ND		
Diloxanide	ND		
Furazolidine	ND	Caution. Low oral absorption and mostly inactivated in gut.	Hale, 2006
Iodoquinol	ND		
Ivermectin	0.98	Compatible.	Ogbuokiri *et al.*, 1993; Ogbuokiri *et al.*, 1994
Mebendazole	0.06, less than analytical limit of detection	Compatible. Low transfer to breastmilk. Reduced milk production reported in single case.	Rao, 1983; Stoukides, 1994; Kurzel *et al.*, 1994
Metronidazole	10.5-13	Moderate transfer to milk, but no adverse effects reported in exposed infants. Dose significantly less than therapeutic dose. May impose bitter (metallic) taste to milk. For 2 gram single oral dose, express and discard milk for 12-24 hours.	Erickson *et al.*, 1981; Heisterberg *et al.*, 1983; Passmore *et al.*, 1988
Nitazoxanide	ND		
Paromomycin	ND		
Praziquantel	0.44[1], 0.56[1]	Compatible. Low transfer to milk. Take before infant's longest sleep period to reduce exposure.	Putter *et al.*, 1979; Olds, 2003
Pyrantel	ND	Probably compatible. Low oral absorption and minimal plasma levels.	Hale, 2006
Quinacrine	ND	Caution, probably compatible. Low transfer to milk. Potential to accumulate in infant because of low rate of excretion. Avoid in babies with G6PD.	Briggs *et al.*, 2005; Hale, 2006
Thiabendazole	ND		
Tinidazole	≈15	After large single doses, express and discard milk for up to 72 hours.	Mannisto *et al.*, 1983; Evaldson *et al.*, 1985
Pediculicides and scabicides			
Benzyl benzoate	ND	Not recommended during breastfeeding. Use has been associated with severe neurological adverse effects.	Roos *et al.*, 2001
Crotamiton	ND	Minimally absorbed from topical preparations.	
Gamma-benzene hexachloride (Lindane®)	ND	Well absorbed after topical application and has been detected in breastmilk. Use has been associated with severe neurological adverse effects, and, therefore, is not recommended in breastfeeding.	Angel *et al.*, 2000; Roos *et al.*, 2001
Malathion (Maldison®)	ND	Levels less than 5 μg/l in milk from women living in areas where malathion used in agricultural spraying. Less than 10% of topically applied malathion is absorbed. There is significant first-pass metabolism. Occasional use for head lice is considered safe.	Nash, 2003; Taylor, 2006; Anonymous, 2006a
Permethrin	ND	Compatible. Low absorption from cream. Preferred agent in lactation.	Centers for Disease Control and Prevention (CDC), 1998; Hale, 2006
Pyrethrins (with piperonyl butoxide)	ND	Minimally absorbed from topical preparations. Preferred agents in lactation.	Centers for Disease Control and Prevention (CDC), 1998

ND = no data; [1] infant dose as % total maternal dose

Tinidazole

Tinidazole, which is closely related to metronidazole, is also a drug where there may be concern about use during breastfeeding. Usually a single 2 gram dose is used for trichomoniasis or giardiasis in adults (Product Information Fasigyn, 2006). Data on its concentrations in breastmilk report relative infant doses of up to 15% in the first 24 hours after a single dose, and this exposure falls to about 2% at 72 hours. Hence, it is recommended that milk should be pumped and discarded for up to three days after such doses (American Academy of Pediatrics Committee on Drugs, 2001).

SCABICIDES AND PEDICULICIDES

Despite a comprehensive review of the general therapeutic uses and toxicity of scabicides and pediculcides (Roos *et al.*, 2001), there is little information on their transfer into breastmilk. Both gamma-benzene hexachloride (Lindane®) and benzyl benzoate are unsuitable for use in breastfeeding mothers (Centers for Disease Control and Prevention (CDC), 1998). These chemicals are significantly absorbed transcutaneously from topical preparations, and both have been implicated in severe neurological side effects in children (Angel *et al.*, 2000; Roos *et al.*, 2001; Porto, 2003). Gamma-benzene hexachloride breastmilk concentrations have been reported to be 60 times higher after topical application, compared with those in milk from untreated women (Roos *et al.*, 2001).

Crotamiton

Crotamiton is both a pediculicide and antipruritic. It is minimally absorbed after topical application and is not associated with severe side effects (Roos *et al.*, 2001). However, there are no data on breastmilk transfer.

Malathion

The transfer of malathion (Maldison®) into breastmilk is also unknown, but less than 10% of topically applied malathion is systemically absorbed. There is high first-pass clearance (Taylor, 2006), and occasional use for the treatment of head lice is considered safe (Nash, 2003).

Permethrin and Pyrethrins

Permethrin and pyrethrins (including piperonyl butoxide) are minimally absorbed topically. Although the amount transferred to breastmilk is unknown, it is thought to be negligible, and thus these are the preferred agents to be used in lactating women (Centers for Disease Control and Prevention (CDC), 1998). Permethrin shampoos and creams have been used clinically in infants greater than two months of age with no adverse effects reported (Roos *et al.*, 2001). For the treatment of scabies, the topical cream containing 1% permethrin is preferred.

Herbal preparations containing ingredients such as tea tree oil have also been used for the treatment of pediculosis, but thc efficacy and safety of these products has not been determined in breastfeeding. A safe alternative treatment in breastfeeding mothers is the application of hair conditioner to the hair, followed by combing it through with a fine tooth comb, daily for ten days (Kmietowicz, 2003).

ANTIMALARIALS

As can be seen from **Table 2**, our knowledge of the transfer of these drugs into breastmilk and the safety of infant exposure is far from complete. In considering the antimalarials, many of which have long half-lives and are administered either as short treatment courses (e.g., daily for three days for chloroquine) or less frequently for prophylaxis (e.g., once weekly for chloroquine), where appropriate some authors have estimated infant exposure (as relative infant dose) for the approximate maintenance dose interval (e.g., one week for chloroquine). The basis of the calculation of infant exposure is, however, quite variable for antimalarials and the usual calculation method for relative infant dose (from C_{avg} or C_{max} in milk and daily average milk intake) has been used in some cases (e.g., azithromycin, doxycycline, isoniazid, and mefloquine).

Doxycycline

Doxycycline belongs to the tetracycline class where there has been some controversy over use during breastfeeding, with issues of staining of the infant's developing teeth and interference with bone growth being cited. However, the relative infant dose is moderate (4%, 6%) for doxycycline (Morganti *et al.*, 1968; Lutziger, 1969). Interestingly, unlike some tetracyclines, the bioavailability of doxycycline is not significantly altered by food or milk (Anonymous, 2007a), and it is well known to produce the least amount of dental staining. The American Academy of Pediatrics considers doxycycline to be safe during breastfeeding (American Academy of

Pediatrics Committee on Drugs, 2001). Nevertheless, it seems reasonable to advise against long-term use during lactation (>3 weeks), and if used short-term, to observe the infant for diarrhea or candidiasis which may indicate an adverse local effect on gut flora. Therapy for up to three weeks is considered safe (Hale, 2006). The chemoprophylactic dose of doxycycline for malaria is 100 mg daily for two days before entering and while in a malarious area, and for two weeks after leaving the area (Anonymous, 2007a). Hence, if the duration of stay in a malarious area is expected to be more than one week, it would be preferable to use alternative antimalarials and/or general protective measures, such as repellants, protective clothing, and bed nets.

Chloroquine

Chloroquine is still very widely used for intermittent preventative treatment of malaria in pregnancy (Anonymous, 2007d), despite increasing parasite resistance in many parts of the tropics (Edwards *et al.*, 2002). Prophylactic use of chloroquine is also common during lactation (Ette *et al.*, 1987; Ogunbona *et al.*, 1987; Akintonwa *et al.*, 1988). As summarized in **Table 2**, the relative infant dose of chloroquine in the first two weeks of a prophylactic dose regimen ranges from 1.8 to 6.6% of the maternal dose (Deturmeny *et al.*, 1984; Edstein *et al.*, 1986; Ette *et al.*, 1987; Ogunbona *et al.*, 1987; Witte *et al.*, 1990), and the American Academy of Pediatrics considers chloroquine to be safe during breastfeeding (American Academy of Pediatrics Committee on Drugs, 2001). During this time, the breastmilk concentrations of the major metabolite of chloroquine range from about 20-50% of those of chloroquine (Edstein *et al.*, 1986; I. Law, personal communication, January 2007), and this would be an additional infant exposure. Chloroquine also has some activity against HIV, and a potential benefit of its use during lactation is its ability to accumulate in mammary epithelial cells (Boelaert *et al.*, 2001), which in turn can decrease viral load in breastmilk (Semrau *et al.*, 2006).

Piperaquine

Piperaquine, which is structurally related to chloroquine and currently enjoying a resurgence of use as artemisinin combination therapy (with dihydroartemisinin or artemisinin) (Davis *et al.*, 2005), has not been studied in breastmilk. Its high lipid solubility would be expected to facilitate transfer into milk. In addition, while its plasma concentrations (on a molar basis) after standard therapeutic doses are lower than those for chloroquine, it also has a long terminal half-life in adults (23 days) (Hung *et al.*, 2004) and would be expected to result in a level of infant exposure similar to that of chloroquine.

The transfer into milk of the artemisinin group of antimalarials, which are the mainstay of artemisinin combination therapy for acute malaria infections (Ashley *et al.*, 2005), also has not been studied. Given that these drugs have an excellent safety profile, short half-lives, and are used in treatment courses administered over two to four days (Ilett *et al.*, 2005), they probably represent a low risk to the breastfed infant.

Azithromycin

Azithromycin is a macrolide antibiotic that has been shown to have additive or synergistic actions *in vitro* with other antimalarials (Nakornchai *et al.*, 2006; Noedl *et al.*, 2007). When used in combination with either artesunate or quinine, azithromycin has been demonstrated to be safe and effective for treatment of uncomplicated *P. falciparum* infections (Noedl *et al.*, 2006). The author of a 1994 case report (Kelsey *et al.*, 1994) used the maximum concentration (2.8 mg/L) measured 30 hours after three x 500 mg daily doses for cellulitis to calculate an absolute infant dose of 155 μg/kg/day (assuming a bioavailability of 37% in the infant). When compared to the mother's daily dose adjusted for bioavailability (1532 μg/kg/day), a relative infant dose of 10.1% can be calculated. Although the American Academy of Pediatrics classifies azithromycin as being compatible with breastfeeding (American Academy of Pediatrics Committee on Drugs, 2001), caution is appropriate if the drug is used long-term for two reasons. First, azithromycin has quite a long half-life (two to four days), and accumulation (approximately three-fold at trough) occurs during a treatment course (Anonymous, 2007h). Second, a study of breastfed infants with hypertrophic pyloric stenosis reported an association with mothers who were taking macrolide antibiotics (Sorensen *et al.*, 2003). While it is clear that erythromycin may induce hypertrophic pyloric stenosis even in breastfed infants, most infectious disease experts believe this does not occur with azithromycin.

Mefloquine

Mefloquine has been the subject of only one breastmilk study (Edstein *et al.*, 1988). From the concentrations measured in milk, the authors calculated an absolute

Table 2. Selected Antimalarial Drugs and Breastfeeding

Drug	Relative infant dose (%)	Comment	References
Amodiaquine	ND	Probably compatible. The desethyl- metabolite would also make a 30-50% additional contribution to infant exposure to pharmacologically active drug. Disposition and activity reviewed in Li *et al.*, 2002.	
Atovaquone	ND	Has high lipid solubility which would favor transfer into milk. The manufacturer's PI says that milk concentrations in rats were 30% of those in plasma and advises against its use in breastfeeding.	Anonymous, 2007e
Artesunate, dihydroartemisinin, artemether, arteether or artelinic acid	ND	Probably compatible. The parent artemisinins or their active metabolites often have high lipid solubility, which would favor transfer into milk. Nevertheless, infant exposure may be low as these agents generally have both short half-lives and poor oral bioavailabilities that would limit absorption by the infant.	
Azithromycin	10.1	Compatible. Caution with long-term use. Observe infant for diarrhea or thrush.	Kelsey *et al.*, 1994; American Academy of Pediatrics Committee on Drugs, 2001
Chloroquine	4.2, 1.8, 4.2, 6.6[1], 2.3[1]	Compatible. Unless otherwise specified, dose calculated from milk C_{avg} first week following a treatment dose. An additional contribution to infant dose can also be expected from desethylchloroquine, which has milk concentrations of 20-50% of those for chloroquine.	Deturmeny *et al.*, 1984; Edstein *et al.*, 1986; Ette *et al.*, 1987; Ogunbona *et al.*, 1987; Witte *et al.*, 1990
Doxycycline	4, 6	Compatible for short term use (3 weeks). Avoid chronic dosing. Observe infant for diarrhea or thrush.	Morganti *et al.*, 1968; Lutziger, 1969
Mefloquine	3.8[2]	Compatible.	Edstein *et al.*, 1988; Anonymous, 2007c
Naphthoquine	ND		
Piperaquine	ND	Probably compatible, despite having a high lipid solubility that would favor transfer into milk.	
Primaquine	ND	Short half-life (4.3-7.1 h). Its carboxy metabolite has longer half-life and accumulates during the usual 14 day treatment course for P. vivax. The pediatric dose is 0.5 mg/kg base up to adult dose orally, once/day for 14 days after departure from the malarious area. Avoid use in infants with hyperbilirubinemia or glucose-6-phosphate dehydrogenase deficiency.	Anonymous, 2007c; Anonymous, 2007g
Pyrimethamine	45, 17, 28, 46[3]	Compatible. Studies show significant infant exposure over 9-10 days after maternal dosing. The amount received by the infant may be therapeutic in some cases.	Clyde *et al.*, 1956; Edstein *et al.*, 1986
Proguanil	ND	Compatible. The manufacturer's information and other sources indicate that small quantities of proguanil are excreted in human milk. Pediatric dose of proguanil is 25 mg for infants < 1 year and up to 4 years indicates safety of full treatment doses in infants and, therefore, indirectly of dose via milk.	Anonymous, 1990; Anonymous, 2007f
Pyronaridine	ND	Avoid. Has high lipid solubility which would favor transfer into milk.	
Quinine	2.2-4.8	Compatible.	Phillips *et al.*, 1986; Bennett *et al.*, 1996
Sulfadoxine	ND	Compatible. Long half-life may increase likelihood of infant exposure, but no data for milk transfer available. Avoid use in infants with hyperbilirubinemia or glucose-6-phosphate dehydrogenase deficiency.	

ND = no data; [1] Dose calculated from C_{max} in milk for a total period of 9.1 to 9.5 days after the maternal dose; [2] Infant dose calculated for a total period of 56 days after the maternal dose; [3] Infant dose calculated for a total period of 9.1 to 9.5 days after the maternal dose.

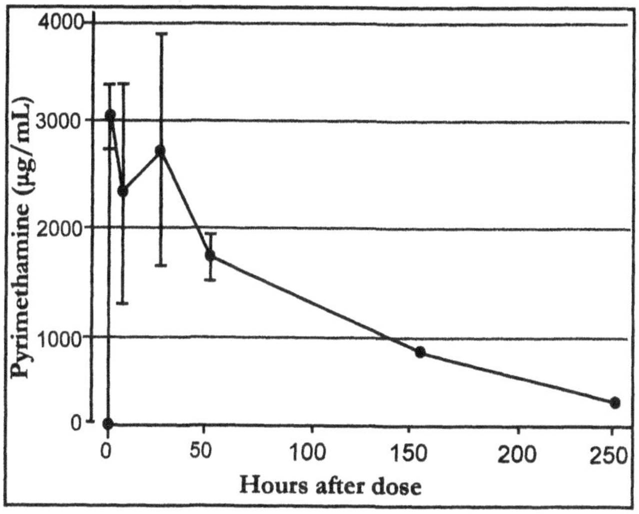

Figure 1. Pyrimethamine concentration in milk (normalized to a 50 mg dose at time zero) as mean ± SEM up to 48 h after dose (Clyde *et al.*, 1956). Extrapolation from 50 to 248 hours (10.3 days) was achieved by assuming a mean maternal half-life of 100 hours (Anonymous, 2007b).

infant dose of around 136 µg/kg/day and a relative infant dose of 3.8% of the weight-adjusted maternal dose (estimated from milk C_{max}). Since the recommended dose for infants ≤9 kg is 4.6 mg/kg/day, the absolute infant dose is only about 2.9% of the therapeutic dose and, therefore, considered safe (Anonymous, 2007c). The low dose received via milk also highlights the requirement for independent pharmacologically adequate prophylaxis in the breastfed infant.

Proguanil

Proguanil can be deduced to be safe in breastfeeding as the dose via milk is reported to be very small (Anonymous, 1990; Anonymous, 2007f), and the drug is recommended in doses of 25 mg/day for infants less than one year and up to four years of age (Anonymous, 2007f). The amount received via milk is also unlikely to be sufficient to be therapeutic for malaria in the infant.

Pyrimethamine

Pyrimethamine excretion in milk has been documented in four studies (Clyde *et al.*, 1956; Clyde, 1957; Clyde, 1960; Edstein *et al.*, 1986). Mean milk concentrations from six volunteers who received a single dose of pyrimethamine (25-75 mg) are shown in **Figure 1** (Clyde *et al.*, 1956). From the milk C_{avg} from 0 to 248 hours (14,923 µg/L), a relative infant dose of 45% of the maternal weight adjusted dose can be calculated. Similar milk C_{avg} data extracted from Edstein's study (Edstein *et al.*, 1986) give relative infant doses of 17, 28, and 46%, respectively, of the weight adjusted maternal dose (12.5 mg single dose) over a period of 10.1-10.3 days. Hence, pyrimethamine illustrates an unusual situation where the infant dose exposure via milk is quite large. Indeed, Clyde goes on to describe an experiment where the mothers in mother/baby dyads (three separate groups of 17, 10, and 5) infected with *P. falciparum* were treated with two sequential doses of pyrimethamine (75 mg and 50 mg). The number of infants remaining infected decreased after both the first and second doses. In the first group, all 17 infants were parasite negative after the second dose, while in the other two groups 10% and 40%, respectively, remained infected after two doses. Cure was ascribed to the amount of pyrimethamine received via milk. The treatment failures were investigated and found in part to be explained by less than exclusive breastfeeding or resistant parasite strains. They concluded that while treating malaria infected infants in this way was successful in a percentage of cases, it was not reliable and that infants should receive individual pharmacotherapy whenever possible.

Quinine

Quinine transfer into milk has been reported in several studies (Terwilliger *et al.*, 1934; White, 1985; Phillips *et al.*, 1986; Looareesuwan *et al.*, 1987). The most informative of these reported a mean milk concentration of 2.6 mg/L (range 0.5-3.6 mg/L) in five breastfeeding women who received between two and seven IV doses of quinine (8.3 mg/kg as base given eight hourly). Using the maximum observed concentration, the calculated relative infant dose was 2.6% (Bennett *et al.*, 1996). Similarly, in 25 patients in the same study who received oral quinine therapy for one to ten days, mean milk concentration was 3.4 mg/L (range 0.5-8 mg/L), and relative infant dose was calculated to be 4.8% (Bennett *et al.*, 1996). The American Academy of Pediatrics classifies quinine as compatible with breastfeeding (American Academy of Pediatrics Committee on Drugs, 2001).

Sulfadoxine

Sulfadoxine is administered with pyrimethamine as combination pharmacotherapy for malaria (Fansidar®). The half-life of sulfadoxine in adults is around 200 hours (Anonymous, 2007b). Unfortunately, we were unable to locate any milk transfer data for sulfadoxine.

Table 3. Selected Antimycobacterial Drugs and Breastfeeding

Drug	Relative infant dose (%)	Comment	References
p-Aminosalicylic acid	0.3	Probably compatible. Single case report only.	Holdiness, 1984
Clarithromycin	2	Compatible. One study showed an absolute infant dose of around 0.15 mg/kg/day that can be compared with the usual pediatric dose of 7.5 mg/kg twice daily. Observe infant for diarrhea or thrush.	Sedlmayr *et al.*, 1993; Young *et al.*, 2006
Clofazimine	22.1	Avoid. Colors maternal skin and milk, pink to red. One report of skin coloration in a breastfed infant.	Browne *et al.*, 1962; Waters, 1969; Freerksen *et al.*, 1992; Venkatesan *et al.*, 1997
Cycloserine	14	Probably compatible. Report of use in 5 mother/infant dyads. No adverse effects reported in the infants.	Charles *et al.*, 1955
Dapsone	9.6[1]	Probably compatible. One case report of mild hemolytic anemia in a breastfed infant. Avoid use in infants with hyperbilirubinemia or glucose-6-phosphate dehydrogenase deficiency. AAP OK.	Dreisbach, 1952; Sanders *et al.*, 1982; Edstein *et al.*, 1986
Ethambutol	ND	Probably compatible. Two cases reported in literature, with infant dose calculated as 3.4-4.7% of the pediatric dose.	Snider *et al.*, 1984; Toddywalla *et al.*, 1995
Ethionamide	ND	Transfer into milk probable. Avoid until data available.	
Isoniazid	11[2], 13.7 and 0[3], 2.3[4]	Probably compatible. Both isoniazid and its acetyl metabolite found in milk.	Lass *et al.*, 1953; Ricci *et al.*, 1954; Berlin *et al.*, 1979; Toddywalla *et al.*, 1995
Levofloxacin	17.2	Probably compatible. Observe infant for diarrhea or thrush.	Giamarellou *et al.*, 1989; Cahill, Jr. *et al.*, 2005
Minocycline	4.2[4]	Other tetracyclines preferred. Single case report. Black discoloration of milk reported.	Mizuno *et al.*, 1969; Basler *et al.*, 1985; Hunt *et al.*, 1996
Ofloxacin	3.1	Compatible. Observe infant for diarrhea, overgrowth of *C. difficle*, or candida.	Giamarellou, 1989
Pyrazinimide	0.3	Single case report.	Holdiness, 1984; Bennett *et al.*, 1996
Rifampin (Rifampicin)	<1%	Compatible. Calculated from peak milk concentrations in one case, assuming usual daily maternal dose of 10 mg/kg.	Lenzi *et al.*, 1969

ND = no data; [1] Dose calculated for percent of maternal drug recovered in milk for a mean period of 3.9 days after a single oral dose; [2] calculated from average peak concentrations in milk at 2 hours after dose; [3] mean of 11% at peak 2 hours after dose and essentially undetected at 12 hours; [4] as % of dose in milk over 24 hours after dose. [4] Calculated peak concentrations in milk 6 hours after dose.

However, a relative infant dose of 2-2.5% has been calculated for the related antibacterial, sulfamethoxazole, which has a much shorter half-life (11 hours) (Bennett *et al.*, 1996). If transfer across the mammary epithelium is similar for sulfadoxine, its longer half-life could well result in higher infant exposure. Nevertheless, the American Academy of Pediatrics classifies related sulfonamides (sulfapyridine, sulfisoxazole, and sulfamethoxazole) as compatible with breastfeeding (American Academy of Pediatrics Committee on Drugs, 2001), and we expect that sulfadoxine should also be compatible. One suggested precaution is to avoid exposure to sulfonamides in infants with hyperbilirubinemia or glucose-6-phosphate dehydrogenase deficiency.

ANTIMYCOBACTERIALS

Clarithromycin

Clarithromycin has absolute and relative infant doses of 0.15 mg/kg/day and 2%, respectively (Sedlmayr *et al.*, 1993). There were no adverse effects in the 12 breastfed infants studied, and given that the usual pediatric dose of clarithromycin is 15 mg/kg/day (Anonymous, 2006b), it can be concluded that clarithromycin also is compatible with breastfeeding.

Clofazimine

Clofazimine is used in the treatment of leprosy and causes a pink to red coloration of both maternal skin and milk (Waters, 1969; Freerksen *et al.*, 1992). Coloration (ruddy and slightly hypermelanotic) of a breastfed infant's skin, which slowly returned to normal five months after cessation of maternal therapy, has also been documented (Browne *et al.*, 1962). The mean relative infant dose in five exposed infants at maternal steady-state was 22.1% (range 13.5-30%) (Venkatesan *et al.*, 1997). Given that the relative infant dose is high and that there is a possibility of skin discoloration in the infant, use of clofazimine in breastfeeding should be avoided.

Isoniazid

Isoniazid is metabolized to *N*-acetylisoniazid by *N*-acetyltransferase 2 and both compounds appear in milk (Berlin *et al.*, 1979). The relative infant dose at the time of peak concentrations for isoniazid in milk (about two hours after dose) are high and variable (11-50%) (Lass *et al.*, 1953; Ricci *et al.*, 1954; Berlin *et al.*, 1979). However, the half-life of isoniazid in milk is only about six hours, while that of *N*-acetylisoniazid is around 13.5 hours (Berlin *et al.*, 1979). Hence, 7-12 hours after dose, the relative infant dose falls rapidly to between 0 and 2.4%. Concentrations of *N*-acetylisoniazid in milk were some 23% of those for isoniazid (Berlin *et al.*, 1979), suggesting that it makes a lesser contribution to total drug exposure. Urinary recovery of isoniazid in two of three breastfed infants studied by Ricci and Copaitch was some 2.3% of the 600 mg maternal dose (Ricci *et al.*, 1954). Infant exposure to isoniazid and its metabolite over a dose interval is likely to be in the 1-3% range and, hence, the American Academy of Pediatrics classifies isoniazid as compatible with breastfeeding (American Academy of Pediatrics Committee on Drugs, 2001).

Ofloxacin and Levofloxacin

Ofloxacin and levofloxacin are compatible or probably compatible with breastfeeding, respectively (Giamarellou *et al.*, 1989; Cahill Jr. *et al.*, 2005). Early animal data that raised the possibility of interference with joint development in infants (arthropathy) from the fluoroquinolones are no longer considered valid (Gurpinar *et al.*, 1997; van den Oever *et al.*, 1998).

p-Aminosalicylic Acid, Pyrizinimide, and Rifampicin

There are only limited data for the use of *p*-aminosalicylic acid (Holdiness, 1984), cycloserine (Charles *et al.*, 1955), dapsone (Dreisbach, 1952; Sanders *et al.*, 1982; Edstein *et al.*, 1986), ethambutol (Snider *et al.*, 1984; Toddywalla *et al.*, 1995), pyrizinimide (Holdiness, 1984), and rifampicin (Lenzi *et al.*, 1969) in breastfeeding, but all are considered to be reasonably compatible.

Minocycline

Although the relative infant dose of minocycline is low (4.2%) (Mizuno *et al.*, 1969), the black discoloration of milk (Basler *et al.*, 1985; Hunt *et al.*, 1996) that is apparently due to iron chelation by the drug suggests that other agents should be preferred.

References

Akintonwa A, Gbajumo SA, Mabadeje AF. Placental and milk transfer of chloroquine in humans. *Ther Drug Monit.* 1988; 10:147-49.

Allen HE, Crompton DW, deSilva SN, LoVerde PT, Olds GR. New policies for using anthelmintics in high risk groups. *Trends Parasitol.* 2002; 18:381-82.

American Academy of Pediatrics Committee on Drugs. Transfer of drugs and other chemicals into human milk. *Pediatrics.* 2001; 108:776-89.

Angel TA, Nigro J, Levy ML. Infestations in the pediatric patient. *Pediatr Clin North Am.* 2000; 47:921-35, viii.

Anonymous. Recommendations for the prevention of malaria among travelers. *MMWR Recommendations and Reports. MMWR Morb Mortal Wkly Rep.* 1990; 39:1-10.

Anonymous. In: Mehta DK (ed.). *BNF for children.* 2nd Ed. London, UK: MBJ Publishing Group Ltd; 2006b. p. 343.

Anonymous. In: McEvoy GK (ed.). *AHFS drug information.* Bethesda, MD, USA: American Society of Health-System Pharmacists; 2006a. p. 3441-44.

Anonymous. *Doryx, MIMS abbreviated prescribing information.* Version 5.01. 2005 Ed. St Leonards, Australia: CMP Medica Australia Pty Ltd.; 2007a.

Anonymous. *Fansidar, MIMS abbreviated prescribing information.* Version 5.01. 2005 Ed. St Leonards, Australia: CMP Medica Australia Pty Ltd.; 2007b.

Anonymous. *Information for health care providers: preventing malaria in infants and children.* Atlanta, GA: Centers for Disease Control and Prevention; 2007c.

Anonymous. *Malaria in pregnancy.* World Health Organisation; 2007d; Available from: URL: http://www.rbm.who.int/cmc_upload/0/000/015/369/RBMInfosheet_4.htm 23-2-2007d.

Anonymous. *Malarone, MIMS abbreviated prescribing information.* Version 5.01. 2005 Ed. St Leonards, Australia: CMP Medica Australia Pty Ltd.; 2007e.

Anonymous. *Paludrine, MIMS abbreviated prescribing information.* Version 5.01. 2005 Ed. St Leonards, Australia: CMP Medica Australia Pty Ltd.; 2007f.

Anonymous. *Primacin, MIMS abbreviated prescribing information.* Version 5.01. 2005 Ed. St Leonards, Australia: CMP Medica Australia Pty Ltd.; 2007g.

Anonymous. *Zithromax, MIMS abbreviated prescribing information.* Version 5.01. 2005 Ed. St Leonards, Australia: CMP Medica Australia Pty Ltd.; 2007h.

Ashley EA, White NJ. Artemisinin-based combinations. *Curr Opin Infect Dis.* 2005; 18:531-36.

Astrup-Jensen A, Bates CJ, Begg EJ, Edwards S, Lazarus CR, Matheson I, *et al. Drugs and human lactation.* 2nd Ed. Amsterdam: Elsevier; 1996.

Basler RS, Lynch PJ. Black galactorrhea as a consequence of minocycline and phenothiazine therapy. *Arch Dermatol.* 1985; 121:417-18.

Bendesky A, Menendez D, Ostrosky-Wegman P. Is metronidazole carcinogenic? *Mutat Res.* 2002; 511:133-44.

Bennett PN, Astrup-Jensen A, Bates CJ, Begg EJ, Edwards S, Lazarus CR, *et al. Drugs and human lactation.* 2nd Ed. Amsterdam: Elsevier Science B.V.; 1996.

Berlin CMJ, Lee C. Isoniazid and acetylisoniazid disposition in human milk, saliva and plasma. *Fed Proc.* 1979; 38 (Part 1):426.

Boelaert JR, Yaro S, Augustijns P, Meda N, Schneider YJ, Schols D, *et al.* Chloroquine accumulates in breast-milk cells: potential impact in the prophylaxis of postnatal mother-to-child transmission of HIV-1. *AIDS.* 2001;15:2205-7.

Briggs GG, Freeman RK, Yaffe SJ. *Drugs in pregnancy and lactation.* 7th Ed. Philadelphia: Lippincott Williams and Wilkins; 2005.

Browne SG, Hogerzeil LM. "B 663" in the treatment of leprosy. Preliminary report of a pilot trial. *Lepr Rev.* 1962; 33:6-10.

Cahill Jr JB, Bailey EM, Chien S, Johnson GM. Levofloxacin secretion in breast milk: a case report. *Pharmacotherapy.* 2005; 25:116-18.

Centers for Disease Control and Prevention (CDC). 1998 Guidelines for treatment of sexually transmitted diseases. *MMWR Recomm Rep.* 1998; 47:1-118.

Charles E, McKenna MH, Morton RF. Studies on the absorption, diffusion, and excretion of cycloserine. *Antibiot Annu.* 1955; 3:169-72.

Clements CJ. Metronidazole and breast feeding. *NZ Med J.* 1980; 92:329.

Clyde DF. An examination of factors involved in the transfer of pyrimethamine in human milk. *East Afr Med J.* 1957; 34:81-85.

Clyde DF. Prolonged malaria prophylaxis through pyrimethamine in mothers' milk. *East Afr Med J.* 1960; 37:659-60.

Clyde DF, Press J, Shute GT. Transfer of pyrimethamine in human milk. *J Trop Med Hyg.* 1956; 59:277-84.

Davis TM, Hung TY, Sim IK, Karunajeewa HA, Ilett KF. Piperaquine: a resurgent antimalarial drug. *Drugs.* 2005; 65:75-87.

Deturmeny E, Viala A, Durand A, Nosny Y. [Chloroquine transfer to milk. A case]. *Therapie.* 1984; 39:438-40.

Dobias L, Cerna M, Rossner P, Sram R. Genotoxicity and carcinogenicity of metronidazole. *Mutat Res.* 1994; 317:177-94.

Dreisbach JA. Sulphone levels in breast milk of mothers on sulphone therapy. *Lepr Rev.* 1952; 23:101-6.

Edstein MD, Veenendaal JR, Hyslop R. Excretion of mefloquine in human breast milk. *Chemotherapy.* 1988; 34:165-9.

Edstein MD, Veenendaal JR, Newman K, Hyslop R. Excretion of chloroquine, dapsone and pyrimethamine in human milk. *Br J Clin Pharmacol.* 1986; 22:733-35.

Edwards G, Bray P, Ward SA. 4-Aminoquinolines (Amodiaquine, Chloroquine). In: Yu VL, Edwards G, McKinnon PS, Peloquin CA, Morse G (eds.). *Antimicrobial therapy and vaccines,* Volume II. 2nd Ed. Pittsburgh, PA, USA: ESun Technologies, LLC; 2002. p. 961-72.

Erickson SH, Oppenheim GL, Smith GH. Metronidazole in breast milk. *Obstet Gynecol.* 1981; 57:48-50.

Ette EI, Essien EE, Ogonor JI, Brown-Awala EA. Chloroquine in human milk. *J Clin Pharmacol.* 1987; 27:499-502.

Evaldson GR, Lindgren S, Nord CE, Rane AT. Tinidazole milk excretion and pharmacokinetics in lactating women. *Br J Clin Pharmacol.* 1985; 19:503-7.

Freerksen E, Seydel JK. Critical comments on the treatment of leprosy and other mycobacterial infections with clofazimine. *Arzneimittelforschung.* 1992; 42:1243-45.

Fulton B, Moore LL. Antiinfectives in breastmilk. Part II: Sulfonamides, tetracyclines, macrolides, aminoglycosides and antimalarials. *J Hum Lact.* 1992; 8:221-23.

Giamarellou H, Kolokythas E, Petrikkos G, Gazis J, Aravantinos D, Sfikakis P. Pharmacokinetics of three newer quinolones in pregnant and lactating women. *Am J Med.* 1989; 87:49S-51S.

Gurpinar AN, Balkan E, Kilic N, Kiristioglu I, Dogruyol H. The effects of a fluoroquinolone on the growth and development of infants. *J Int Med Res.* 1997; 25:302-6.

Hale TW. *Medications and mothers' milk.* 11th Ed. Amarillo, TX, USA: Pharmasoft Publishing; 2006.

Heisterberg L, Branebjerg PE. Blood and milk concentrations of metronidazole in mothers and infants. *J Perinat Med.* 1983; 11:114-20.

Holdiness MR. Antituberculosis drugs and breast-feeding. *Arch Intern Med.* 1984; 144:1888.

Hung TY, Davis TM, Ilett KF, Karunajeewa H, Hewitt S, Denis MB, *et al.* Population pharmacokinetics of piperaquine in adults and children with uncomplicated falciparum or vivax malaria. *Br J Clin Pharmacol.* 2004; 57:253-62.

Hunt MJ, Salisbury EL, Grace J, Armati R. Black breast milk due to minocycline therapy. *Br J Dermatol.* 1996; 134:943-44.

Ilett KF, Batty KT. Artemisinin and its derivatives. In: Yu VL, Edwards G, McKinnon PS, Peloquin CA, Morse G (eds). *Antimicrobial therapy and vaccines. Volume II: Antimicrobial agents.* 2nd Ed. Pittsburgh, PA, USA: ESun Technologies LLC; 2005. p. 981-1002.

Kelsey JJ, Moser LR, Jennings JC, Munger MA. Presence of azithromycin breast milk concentrations: a case report. *Am J Obstet Gynecol.* 1994; 170:1375-76.

Kmietowicz Z. Information for patients: removal of lice and eggs by combing. *BMJ.* 2003; 326:1258.

Kurzel RB, Toot PJ, Lambert LV, Mihelcic AS. Mebendazole and postpartum lactation. *NZ Med J.* 1994; 107:439.

Lass A, Bunger P. Studies on the diffusion of isoniazid in the fetal circulation, the amniotic fluid and human milk. *Klin Wochenschr.* 1953; 31:606-8.

Lenzi E, Santuari S. Preliminary observations on the use of a new semi-synthetic rifamycin derivative in gynecology and obstetrics. *Atti Accad Lancisiana Roma.* 1969; 13:87-94.

Li XQ, Bjorkman A, Andersson TB, Ridderstrom M, Masimirembwa CM. Amodiaquine clearance and its metabolism to N-desethylamodiaquine is mediated by CYP2C8: a new high affinity and turnover enzyme-specific probe substrate. *J Pharmacol Exp Ther.* 2002; 300:399-407.

Looareesuwan S, White NJ, Silamut K, Phillips RE, Warrell DA. Quinine and severe falciparum malaria in late pregnancy. *Acta Leiden.* 1987; 55:115-20.

Lutziger H. Concentration determinations and clinical effectiveness of doxycycline (Vibramycin) in the uterus, adnexa and maternal milk. *Ther Umsch.* 1969; 26:476-80.

Mannisto PT, Karhunen M, Koskela O, Suikkari AM, Mattila J, Haataja H. Concentrations of tinidazole in breast milk. *Acta Pharmacol Toxicol (Copenh).* 1983; 53:254-56.

Mathew JL. Effect of maternal antibiotics on breast feeding infants. *Postgrad Med J.* 2004; 80:196-200.

Mizuno S, Takata M, Sano S, Ueyama T. Minocycline. *Jpn J Antibiot.* 1969; 22:473-79.

Morganti G, Ceccarelli G, Ciaffi G. [Comparative concentrations of a tetracycline antibiotic in serum and maternal milk. *Antibiotica.* 1968; 6:216-23.

Nakornchai S, Konthiang P. Activity of azithromycin or erythromycin in combination with antimalarial drugs against multidrug-resistant Plasmodium falciparum in vitro. *Acta Tropica.* 2006; 100:185-91.

Nash B. Treating head lice. *BMJ.* 2003; 326:1256-57.

Noedl H, Krudsood S, Chalermratana K, Silachamroon U, Leowattana W, Tangpukdee N, *et al.* Azithromycin combination therapy with artesunate or quinine for the treatment of uncomplicated Plasmodium falciparum malaria in adults: a randomized, phase 2 clinical trial in Thailand. *Clin Infect Dis.* 2006; 43:1264-71.

Noedl H, Krudsood S, Leowattana W, Tangpukdee N, Thanachartwet W, Looareesuwan S, *et al.* In vitro antimalarial activity of azithromycin, artesunate, and quinine in combination and correlation with clinical outcome. *Antimicrob Agents Chemother.* 2007; 51:651-56.

Ogbuokiri JE, Ozumba BC, Okonkwo PO. Ivermectin levels in human breastmilk. *Eur J Clin Pharmacol.* 1993; 45:389-90.

Ogbuokiri JE, Ozumba BC, Okonkwo PO. Ivermectin levels in human breast milk. *Eur J Clin Pharmacol.* 1994; 46:89-90.

Ogunbona FA, Onyeji CO, Bolaji OO, Torimiro SE. Excretion of chloroquine and desethylchloroquine in human milk. *Br J Clin Pharmacol.* 1987; 23:473-76.

Olds GR. Administration of praziquantel to pregnant and lactating women. *Acta Tropica.* 2003; 86:185-95.

Parke AL. Antimalarial drugs, pregnancy and lactation. *Lupus.* 1993; 2 Suppl 1:S21-S23.

Passmore CM, McElnay JC, Rainey EA, D'Arcy PF. Metronidazole excretion in human milk and its effect on the suckling neonate. *Br J Clin Pharmacol.* 1988; 26:45-51.

Phillips RE, Looareesuwan S, White NJ, Silamut K, Kietinun S, Warrell DA. Quinine pharmacokinetics and toxicity in pregnant and lactating women with falciparum malaria. *Br J Clin Pharmacol.* 1986; 21:677-83.

Porto I. Antiparasitic drugs and lactation: focus on anthelmintics, scabicides, and pediculicides. *J Hum Lact.* 2003; 19:421-25.

Product Information *Fasigyn. MIMS abbreviated product information.* E-MIMS 2006; Version 5.00.0270.

Putter J, Held F. Quantitative studies on the occurrence of praziquantel in milk and plasma of lactating women. *Eur J Drug Metab Pharmacokin.* 1979; 4:193-98.

Rao TS. Does mebendazole inhibit lactation? *NZ Med J.* 1983; 96:589-90.

Ricci G, Copaitich T. Elimination of orally administered isoniazid in human milk. *Rass Clin Ter.* 1954; 53:209-14.

Roos TC, Alam M, Roos S, Merk HF, Bickers DR. Pharmacotherapy of ectoparasitic infections. *Drugs.* 2001; 61:1067-88.

Sanders SW, Zone JJ, Foltz RL, Tolman KG, Rollins DE. Hemolytic anemia induced by dapsone transmitted through breast milk. *Annals Intern Med.* 1982; 96:465-66.

Sedlmayr T, Peters F, Raasch W, Kees F. Clarithromycin, a new macrolide antibiotic. Effectiveness in puerperal infections and pharmacokinetics in breast milk. *Geburtshilfe Frauenheilkd.* 1993; 53:488-91.

Semrau K, Kuhn L, Kasonde P, Sinkala M, Kankasa C, Shutes E, *et al.* Impact of chloroquine on viral load in breast milk. *Trop Med Int Health.* 2006; 11:800-3.

Snider DEJ, Powell KE. Should women taking antituberculosis drugs breast-feed? *Arch Intern Med.* 1984; 144:589-90.

Sorensen HT, Skriver MV, Pedersen L, Larsen H, Ebbesen F, Schonheyder HC. Risk of infantile hypertrophic pyloric stenosis after maternal postnatal use of macrolides. *Scand J Infect Dis.* 2003; 35:104-6.

Stoukides C. Can a mother safely breastfeed while on mebendazole (Vermox)? *J Hum Lact.* 1994; 10:269.

Taylor P. Anticholinesterase agents. In: Brunton LL, Lazo JS, Parker KL (eds). *Goodman and Gilman's The pharmacological basis of therapeutics.* 11th Ed. New York: McGraw Hill Medical Publishing Division; 2006. p. 201-16.

Terwilliger WG, Hatcher RA. The elimination of morphine and quinine in human milk. *Surg Gynecol Obstet.* 1934; 58:823-6.

Toddywalla VS, Patel SB, Betrabet SS, Kulkarni RD, Kombo I, Saxena BN. Can chronic maternal drug therapy alter the nursing infant's hepatic drug metabolizing enzyme pattern? *J Clin Pharmacol.* 1995; 35:1025-29.

Tran JH, Montakantikul P. The safety of antituberculosis medications during breastfeeding. [Review] [18 refs]. *J Hum Lact.* 1998; 14:337-40.

van den Oever HL, Versteegh FG, Thewessen EA, Van den Anker JN, Mouton JW, Neijens HJ. Ciprofloxacin in preterm neonates: case report and review of the literature. *Eur J Pediat.* 1998; 157:843-45.

US National Library of Medicine. *Drugs and lactation database (LactMed).* TOXNET Toxicology Data Network. 2006. Available from: http://toxnet.nlm.nih.gov/cgi-bin/sis/htmlgen?LACT.

Venkatesan K, Mathur A, Girdhar A, Girdhar BK. Excretion of clofazimine in human milk in leprosy patients. *Lepr Rev.* 1997; 68:242-46.

Waters MF. G 30 320 or B 663--Lampren (Geigy). *Lepr Rev.* 1969; 40:21-47.

White NJ. Clinical pharmacokinetics of antimalarial drugs. *Clin Pharmacokinet.* 1985; 10:187-215.

Witte AM, Klever HJ, Brabin BJ, Eggelte TA, Van der Kaay HJ, Alpers MP. Field evaluation of the use of an ELISA to detect chloroquine and its metabolites in blood, urine and breast-milk. *Trans R Soc Trop Med Hyg.* 1990; 84:521-25.

Young TE, Mangum B. *Neofax.* 19th Ed. Raleigh, NC, USA: Acorn Publishing, Inc; 2006.

Chapter 30

Antidepressants and Antipsychotics

Jonathan Rampono, Judith H. Kristensen, and Kenneth F. Ilett

INTRODUCTION

The postnatal period is, regrettably, often accompanied by significant psychiatric disorders. These include depressive, anxiety spectrum, and psychotic disorders.

The frequency of depression in women in the postnatal period is around 10–15% (O'Hara *et al.*, 1990). The clinical symptoms of depressive disorder include: disturbances of mood, sleep, motivation, and irritability; impairment in cognitive function; reduction in energy; and despair, and are sometimes accompanied by suicidal ideation. There are also consequences for the neonate of depressed mothers in terms of increased behavioral problems and delayed language development (Zekoski *et al.*, 1987; Lee *et al.*, 1991; Murray *et al.*, 1996; Sinclair *et al.*, 1998). Depression can also interfere in the relationship of the mother with her partner and other children.

The incidence and impact of anxiety spectrum disorders is potentially as potent as those of the depressive disorders. Women with generalized anxiety disorder, social phobia, panic disorder, and post traumatic stress disorder can be quite disabled by the impact of these disorders in the postnatal period. Obsessive compulsive disorder often accompanies anxiety disorders and the obsessional thoughts and fears, rituals, and other behaviors associated with obsessive compulsive disorder can be quite overwhelming for new mothers. Antidepressant medication (in conjunction with psychological therapy and psychosocial adjustments) has been shown to be very effective in the management of the above disorders.

The consequences of psychotic disorders in the postpartum period may be significant and may be associated with suicide and/or infanticide. The incidence of schizophrenia is around one percent. In the past, the use of some of the original "typical" antipsychotics in the management of schizophrenia was associated with significant hyperprolactinemia (leading to galactorrhea) and secondary sub-fertility in women. Hyperprolactinemia is infrequent with the newer "atypical" antipsychotic agents. Some of the reduction in hyperprolactinemia with the newer antipsychotic medication may be associated with increasing rates of conception in women with schizophrenia. Some authors have suggested that estrogens may have a protective effect in women with schizophrenia (Kulkarni *et al.*, 2002). The significant fall in estrogen levels postpartum and with breastfeeding may be linked to an increase in the symptoms and severity of schizophrenia in the postpartum period.

The presentation of bipolar mood disorder in the postpartum period may sometimes be quite florid, and the rate of progression of mania is often greater in the postpartum period compared to other periods in a woman's life (Brockington, 1996). The grandiose and paranoid delusions associated with mania may pose a grave threat to the mother and/or baby. Following a manic phase, there is an increased risk of a profound morbid depressive phase (Llewellyn *et al.*, 1998). For these reasons, drug treatment is highly desirable and the benefits and risks of using antipsychotic and mood stabilizer medication during breastfeeding need to be carefully weighed for the individual case (Gentile, 2004).

Use of antidepressants and/or antipsychotics in lactation has been reviewed in recent years (Hale *et al.*, 2002; Weissman *et al.*, 2004; Gentile, 2004; Rubin *et al.*, 2004; Gentile, 2005; Ilett *et al.*, 2005; Hatzopoulos *et al.*, 2006; Gentile, 2007). Detailed monographs for many individual drugs are also available in reference texts (Bennett *et al.*, 1996; Briggs *et al.*, 2005; Hale, 2007) and from LactMed (US National Library of Medicine, 2006). As with all maternal drug use during lactation, the questions that need to be asked are (a) is there significant drug transfer into milk, (b) is drug exposure likely to cause any short-term toxicity in the infant, and (c) is drug exposure likely to cause long-term adverse effects in the infant? For some antidepressants, there is clear evidence that placental exposure can result in adverse effects in the early neonatal period, and these must be distinguished from effects that occur postpartum due to exposure via the drug present in milk.

In this chapter, we summarize the data for infant exposure to selective serotonin reuptake inhibitor (SSRI), serotonin norepinephrine reuptake inhibitor (SNRI), norepinephrine reuptake inhibitor (NRI), and related antidepressants in **Table 1**, tricyclic, tetracyclic, and related antidepressants in **Table 2,** and typical and atypical antipsychotics in **Table 3**. In considering the effects of exposure to these drugs, many have active metabolites that should be considered in the risk-benefit analysis. A summary of the pharmacological activity of metabolites for many antidepressants is available (Weissman *et al.*, 2004).

Since antidepressants have no direct therapeutic application in neonates, consideration of absolute infant dose *per se* is not helpful. Therefore, in considering the exposure of infants to these drugs via milk, we will confine our evaluation to relative infant dose, plasma levels and effects of the drugs in exposed infants, and effects of the drugs on maternal serum prolactin. The latter is largely of academic interest as many antipsychotics occasionally cause increased prolactin levels (via blockade of central dopaminergic pathways) which would not be expected to alter milk production. Selected drugs are discussed in detail in the text that follows.

ANTIDEPRESSANTS

The American Academy of Pediatrics classifies all antianxiety, antidepressant, and neuroleptic drugs as having unknown effects in the breastfed infant and therefore as drugs where concern is appropriate if they need to be used in breastfeeding (American Academy of Pediatrics Committee on Drugs, 2001). While at first sight, this appears to be justifiable, their most recent review of the literature was done some years ago and much more information is now at hand for many of these drugs.

SSRI's and SNRI's and Related Drugs

Some of the new information in the area of SSRI's relates to drug-related adverse effects in the neonate that result in overexposure to 5-hydroxytryptamine (5-HT) during both pregnancy and/or lactation. For example, Oberlander and colleagues reported that infants exposed to an SSRI, either during pregnancy and/or lactation, had blunted responses to pain compared to controls (Oberlander *et al.*, 2005). They concluded that the mechanisms that may have altered 5-HT-mediated pain modulation in infants after SSRI exposure were unclear. They recommended maternal use of antidepressants during and after pregnancy where indicated. They also recommended promotion of breastfeeding in this setting as a key goal for all clinicians. In addition, a recent study by Chambers and colleagues in 377 women whose infants had persistent pulmonary hypertension of the newborn and 836 matched control women and their infants found that 14 infants had been exposed to an SSRI after the 20th week of gestation compared to six of the control infants (Chambers *et al.*, 2006). The significance of this association is unclear, but the low frequency of the syndrome (1.9-1000) and well defined supportive treatment procedures mitigate against restrictions on the maternal use of SSRI's where these are necessary treatments. Patients should be fully informed about this possible adverse effect, and the option of reducing the antidepressant dose in the weeks prior to delivery should be discussed with them.

Citalopram and Escitalopram

The peer-reviewed published data for the transfer of these SSRI's into milk consist of around 27 cases for citalopram and 10 for escitalopram (Spigset *et al.*, 1997; Jensen *et al.*, 1997; Ohman *et al.*, 1997; Rampono

Table 1. Selective Serotonin (SSRI), Serotonin Norepinephrine (SNRI), and Norepinephrine (NRI) Reuptake Blockers, and Related Antidepressants and Breastfeeding

	Relative infant dose (%)	Comment	References
Citalopram (*N*-desmethylcitalopram)	0.7-7.3 (0.9-1.9)	Compatible. Most studies report few adverse events.	Spigset *et al.*, 1997; Jensen *et al.*, 1997; Ohman *et al.*, 1997; Rampono *et al.*, 2000; Schmidt *et al.*, 2000; Nordeng *et al.*, 2001; Heikkinen *et al.*, 2002; Berle *et al.*, 2004; Franssen *et al.*, 2006
Duloxetine	0.14	Unpublished data from 6 lactating volunteers available from the manufacturer. Probably compatible but others preferred.	Data on file, Lilly Research Laboratories, July 7, 2007.
Escitalopram (*N*-desmethylescitalopram)	3.9, 7.7 (1.7)	Compatible. Preferred over citalopram as absolute infant dose of *S*-enantiomer is lower.	Rampono *et al.*, 2006; Castberg *et al.*, 2006
Fluoxetine (norfluoxetine)	2.6-6.5 (2.6-3.4)	Compatible despite reports of colic, irritability, and seizures in some infants.	Isenberg, 1990; Burch *et al.*, 1992; Lester *et al.*, 1993; Taddio *et al.*, 1996; Brent *et al.*, 1998; Yoshida *et al.*, 1998b; Kristensen *et al.*, 1999; Hendrick *et al.*, 2001c; Fish *et al.*, 2003; Kim *et al.*, 2006
Fluvoxamine	0.5-1.6	Compatible. Six cases reported for infant dose. No adverse events. Undetectable in infant plasma in nine cases. Detected at >10% of mother's level in one case.	Wright *et al.*, 1991; Yoshida *et al.*, 1997a; Arnold *et al.*, 2000; Hagg *et al.*, 2000; Nordeng *et al.*, 2001; Piontek *et al.*, 2001; Hendrick *et al.*, 2001b; Kristensen *et al.*, 2002
Mirtazapine (*N*-desmethylmirtazapine)	2.8-6.8 (0.4)	Compatible. Ten cases reported with no adverse events.	Aichhorn *et al.*, 2004; Kristensen *et al.*, 2007; Klier *et al.*, 2007
Paroxetine	1.1-1.4	Compatible. No adverse events reported.	Spigset *et al.*, 1996; Begg *et al.*, 1999; Ohman *et al.*, 1999; Stowe *et al.*, 2000; Misri *et al.*, 2000; Hendrick *et al.*, 2001b; Berle *et al.*, 2004
Reboxetine	2.1	Compatible, but only four cases reported.	Hackett *et al.*, 2006
Sertraline (*N*-demethylsertraline)	0.3-0.9 (0.3-1.4)	Compatible. No adverse events reported.	Altshuler *et al.*, 1995; Stowe *et al.*, 1997; Mammen *et al.*, 1997b; Kristensen *et al.*, 1998; Wisner *et al.*, 1998; Dodd *et al.*, 2000; Hendrick *et al.*, 2001b
St John's Wort	ND	Observational study with matched control group. No significant difference in adverse events. Compatible	Lee *et al.*, 2003
Trazodone	0.7, 0.6	Probably compatible.	Verbeeck *et al.*, 1986; Misri *et al.*, 1991
Venlafaxine (including *O*-desmethylvenlafaxine)	5, 6.4	Probably compatible. Exposure is moderate, but can be managed with careful observation of the infant.	Ilett *et al.*, 1998; Hendrick *et al.*, 2001a; Ilett *et al.*, 2002; Berle *et al.*, 2004

ND = no data

et al., 2000; Schmidt *et al.*, 2000; Nordeng *et al.*, 2001; Heikkinen *et al.*, 2002; Berle *et al.*, 2004; Rampono *et al.*, 2006). Both the racemate and its *S*-enantiomer have intermediate relative infant doses of around 1-6% with a lesser contribution of up to 2% from their respective *N*-desmethyl metabolites (Rampono *et al.*, 2000; Rampono *et al.*, 2006).

Both citalopram and escitalopram are well tolerated by breastfed infants exposed via milk, with infrequent reports of adverse events in a total of about 50 breastfed infants studied (Rampono *et al.*, 2000; Heikkinen *et al.*, 2002; Berle *et al.*, 2004; Lee *et al.*, 2004b; Rampono *et al.*, 2006; Castberg *et al.*, 2006). Symptoms such as irregular breathing, sleep disorders, hypotonia, hypertonia, restlessness, or irritability have been reported in three cases where citalopram was taken. In one, symptoms were considered to be due to prior exposure during pregnancy (Franssen *et al.*, 2006), and in the other two, symptoms resolved after maternal dose reduction and a reduction to partial breastfeeding (Schmidt *et al.*, 2000) or after cessation of breastfeeding (Lee *et al.*, 2004b).

Escitalopram is preferred over citalopram in treating lactating women. It offers similar maternal therapeutic benefit to citalopram, but absolute maternal doses are about 50% of those for citalopram. Although the relative infant dose is similar for escitalopram and citalopram, the absolute infant dose of escitalopram delivered via milk is only about 50% of that for citalopram (Rampono *et al.*, 2006).

Citalopram is one of a small number of antidepressants for which long-term neurodevelopment of exposed infants has been studied (Heikkinen *et al.*, 2002). Infants from 11 women who had taken citalopram (average dose 20 mg/day) both during pregnancy and lactation were followed up to one year of age. Compared with a matched control group, there were no differences in neurodevelopment in the exposed infants.

Fluoxetine and Norfluoxetine

The SSRI fluoxetine has an active metabolite, norfluoxetine, that has similar pharmacological activity and a longer half-life (Weissman *et al.*, 2004). Using the data from a pooled analysis of 20 published (Isenberg, 1990; Burch *et al.*, 1992; Lester *et al.*, 1993; Taddio *et al.*, 1996; Brent *et al.*, 1998; Yoshida *et al.*, 1998b; Kristensen *et al.*, 1999) and unpublished cases for the SSRI fluoxetine (Weissman *et al.*, 2004), a mean relative infant dose of 2.8% can be calculated. However, the contribution of norfluoxetine to infant dose needs to be considered as it has a much longer half-life (eight to nine days) than the parent drug (one to two days) and is a contributor to adverse effects in exposed infants. One study in 14 breastfed infants reported a mean relative infant dose of 6.8% (range 2-12%) for fluoxetine and norfluoxetine combined (Kristensen *et al.*, 1999), while another with 10 cases reported a combined dose of 3.8% when the exposed infants were three-months-old (Heikkinen *et al.*, 2003). Finally a third study calculated a combined relative infant dose of 1.02% in a group of 30 breastfeeding mothers (Kim *et al.*, 2006). Although the total dose differs considerably between these three studies, they all show an approximately equal individual contribution to dose from fluoxetine and norfluoxetine.

Levels of fluoxetine and norfluoxetine in infant serum have been investigated in a number of studies (Kristensen *et al.*, 1999; Epperson *et al.*, 2001; Heikkinen *et al.*, 2003; Oberlander *et al.*, 2005; Kim *et al.*, 2006). The absolute concentrations in infant serum vary widely between studies, depending on maternal dose, exclusivity of breastfeeding, and the extent of contribution from placental exposure. In these studies, the range for fluoxetine was 3-250 μg/L and for norfluoxetine 2-187 μg/L. Typically, fluoxetine was only detected in 20-50% of cases, while norfluoxetine was seen in all cases. This indicates that while infants may be exposed to both drugs in milk, they have the capacity to demethylate ingested fluoxetine. For fluoxetine alone, it has been calculated that the average concentration in plasma of exposed infants is a mean of 7% (range 3-12%) of that in maternal plasma (Weissman *et al.*, 2004). However, norfluoxetine will also be present in the infant's plasma and will contribute significantly to exposure.

Given the level of exposure to both fluoxetine and norfluoxetine via milk, it is not surprising that there are a significant number of reports of adverse effects, such as sleepiness, colic, seizure-like activity, irritability, hyperglycemia, and glycosuria (Epperson *et al.*, 2001), in exposed breastfed infants (Lester *et al.*, 1993; Mhanna *et al.*, 1997; Rohan, 1997; Brent *et al.*, 1998; Kristensen *et al.*, 1999; Mohan *et al.*, 2000; Hale *et al.*, 2001). Some of these reports are complicated by recent exposure to the drug during pregnancy and the subsequent emergence of a neonatal serotonin toxicity syndrome. Nevertheless, there is no doubt that exposure via breastmilk makes a contribution to infant exposure in many cases.

However, the degree of exposure varies widely between cases. Symptoms of serotonin excess arising from exposure in pregnancy are most likely to arise in the first week after birth (Hostetter *et al.*, 2000; Laine *et al.*, 2003; Rampono *et al.*, 2004) and can be controlled by conservative management without the need to withdraw breastfeeding.

Because fluoxetine has been on the market for a long period of time and has been used in a large number of pregnant/breastfeeding women, there are also data on other effects in exposed infants. A full discussion of the topic is available online via the LactMed database (Anonymous, 2007a). For example, 26 infants exposed to fluoxetine via milk showed decreased weight gain (compared to a retrospective control group) at six months of age (Chambers *et al.*, 1999). However, the weights were still in the expected range and the investigators suggested that the effect should only be a problem in cases where there was also weight loss from other causes as well. A prospective study of women who took either tricyclic antidepressants (N=46) or fluoxetine (40) and controls (36) found that neither tricyclic antidepressants nor fluoxetine adversely affected the child's global IQ, language development, or behavior over the period of 15 to 71 months of age. By contrast, IQ was significantly and negatively associated with duration of depression, whereas language was negatively associated with the number of depression episodes after delivery (Nulman *et al.*, 2002).

In summary, the research summarized above does not support a prohibition of the use of fluoxetine in breastfeeding mothers. If it is the drug of choice for the individual patient, it may be used during breastfeeding provided the infant is routinely monitored for expected milestones and side effects, such as colic, fussiness, or sedation.

Fluvoxamine

Relative infant dose has been estimated for the SSRI fluvoxamine in a total of six cases and ranges from 0.5-1.6% (Wright *et al.*, 1991; Yoshida *et al.*, 1997a; Arnold *et al.*, 2000; Hagg *et al.*, 2000; Kristensen *et al.*, 2002). Four investigations (nine cases) have also reported that fluvoxamine was undetected in the plasma of exposed infants (Piontek *et al.*, 2001; Kristensen *et al.*, 2002; Hendrick *et al.*, 2001b) , while one case was reported where infant plasma level was >10% of the maternal level (Weissman *et al.*, 2004). Importantly, none of the above studies reported any adverse effects in the exposed infants.

Paroxetine

Paroxetine is an SSRI, but it has no metabolites of interest. A pooled analysis of the published literature (N=50) on levels in breastmilk (Spigset *et al.*, 1996; Begg *et al.*, 1999; Ohman *et al.*, 1999; Stowe *et al.*, 2000; Hendrick *et al.*, 2000; Misri *et al.*, 2000) enables us to calculate a mean relative infant dose of 1.4% (Weissman *et al.*, 2004). The same pooled analysis reported that paroxetine was undetected in plasma of 40 exposed infants (usual analytical limit of detection 1-2 μg/L). Two other studies reported undetectable levels in infant serum (N=16) (Hendrick *et al.*, 2001b), or levels (0.9 μg/L) that were 5% of the corresponding maternal serum concentration (N=19) (Oberlander *et al.*, 2005). All of the latter cases had maternal doses in the usual 10-50 mg/day range.

There are several studies containing information on the possibility of adverse effects in breastfed infants exposed to paroxetine at doses ranging from 20-40 mg/day. In most of these, the infants (N=26) did not show any adverse effects and achieved age-related milestones (Hendrick *et al.*, 2003; Berle *et al.*, 2004; Misri *et al.*, 2006). In one infant exposed in both pregnancy and lactation, adverse effects (symptoms of serotonin toxicity) were noted at birth, but the infant was assessed as having no neurological problems and had achieved expected weight at four months of age (Laine *et al.*, 2004). There is also a report that a breastfed infant exposed to maternal paroxetine (40 mg daily for a year) developed metabolic abnormalities leading to inappropriate secretion of antidiuretic hormone syndrome (Abdul Aziz *et al.*, 2004). Although paroxetine was thought to be causative, alternative diagnoses were not excluded. Finally, there is a report of agitation and difficulty with feeding in an infant whose mother took paroxetine, but the detail is lacking and the outcome unknown (Rohan, 1997).

Hence, the low infant dose and levels in infant serum together with few adverse events reported for paroxetine (**Table 2**) has resulted in it being a preferred treatment for postnatal maternal depression (Wisner *et al.*, 2002; Weissman *et al.*, 2004; Berle *et al.*, 2004).

Sertraline and *N*-Desmethylsertraline

For the SSRI sertraline, the mean relative infant dose is very low (0.3, 0.2, 0.9, <2%) with a similar percentage

Table 2. Tricyclic, Tetracyclic, Monoamine Oxidase Inhibitor Antidepressants and Breastfeeding

Drug	Relative infant dose (%)	Comment	References
Tricyclics and tetracyclics			
Amitriptyline (nortriptyline)	0.1-2 (0.1-1)	Compatible.	Bader *et al.*, 1980; Brixen-Rasmussen *et al.*, 1982; Pittard III *et al.*, 1986; Breyer-Pfaff *et al.*, 1995; Yoshida *et al.*, 1999b
Amoxapine (8-hydroxyamoxapine)	0.08 (0.5-0.7)	Compatible.	Gelenberg, 1979
Bupropion (3-4 metabolites)	0.4, 0.14 (1.9, 2.0)	Compatible. One report of a possible bupropion-related seizure in an exposed infant.	Briggs *et al.*, 1993; Haas *et al.*, 2004; Chaudron *et al.*, 2004
Clomipramine	1.8-4.4, 1.5	Compatible.	Schimmell *et al.*, 1991; Yoshida *et al.*, 1997b
Desipramine	1.2	Compatible.	Stancer *et al.*, 1986
Dothiepin		Compatible.	Ilett *et al.*, 1993; Buist *et al.*, 1995
Doxepin (includes *N*-desmethyldoxepin)	0.35, 2.2, 2.6	Two cases showing significant adverse effects (sedation, hypotonia, etc). Consider alternative drugs.	Kemp *et al.*, 1985; Matheson *et al.*, 1985; Frey *et al.*, 1999; Weissman *et al.*, 2004
Imipramine	0.5, 2.9	Compatible.	Sovner *et al.*, 1979; Yoshida *et al.*, 1997b
Mianserin (N-desmethylmianserin)	0.5, 0.7, 1.4 (0.1, 0.2, 0.5)	Probably compatible. Data from three cases only.	Buist *et al.*, 1993; unpublished data Kay et al., 1998
Maprotiline	1.1, 1.8	Probably compatible.	Anonymous, 2007b
Nortriptyline	1.3	Compatible.	Brixen-Rasmussen *et al.*, 1982; Matheson *et al.*, 1988; Breyer-Pfaff *et al.*, 1995; Weissman *et al.*, 2004
Protriptyline		Probably compatible, but no data.	
Monoamine oxidase inhibitors			
Moclobemide (including metabolite)	1%	Compatible.	Pons *et al.*, 1990
Phenelzine	ND	Others preferred.	
Tranylcypromine	ND	Others preferred.	

ND = no data available

contribution from its metabolite demethylsertraline (0.2, 1.3%) (Altshuler *et al.*, 1995; Stowe *et al.*, 1997; Kristensen *et al.*, 1998; Dodd *et al.*, 2000). While *N*-desmethylsertraline apparently has low neurological activity (about 10% of the parent drug), both it and the parent drug have significant anti-platelet aggregation activity *in vitro* (Serebruany *et al.*, 2001). Using data from a 2004 review that considered the above published milk drug concentration data as well as some additional unpublished cases, a mean relative infant dose of 0.6% can be calculated for sertraline (Weissman *et al.*, 2004). There are also data showing that breastfed infants (56 cases; maternal dose range 25-200 mg/day) had undetectable (42 cases), or very low concentrations of sertraline (2-8 μg/L) and/or its metabolite (2-26 μg/L) in their blood (Altshuler *et al.*, 1995; Stowe *et al.*, 1997; Mammen *et al.*, 1997b; Kristensen *et al.*, 1998; Wisner *et al.*, 1998; Hendrick *et al.*, 2001b). No significant adverse events attributable to breastfeeding were reported in the above cases. Spontaneously resolving agitation or minor sleep disturbances have been reported in two exposed infants (Rohan, 1997; Mammen *et al.*, 1997b). In another study, there was no change in platelet reuptake of 5-hydroxytryptamine (a biomarker of SSRI effects) in breastfed infants whose mothers were taking therapeutic doses of sertraline, again confirming that significant drug concentrations do not occur as a result of infant exposure via milk (Epperson *et al.*, 2001). The American Academy of Pediatrics lists sertraline as a drug of concern in lactation (American Academy of Pediatrics Committee on Drugs, 2001). Nevertheless, given its low dose via milk and low frequency of adverse effects in exposed infants, sertraline is considered safe in lactation and is often preferred over related drugs (Wisner *et al.*, 2002; Weissman *et al.*, 2004; Berle *et al.*, 2004).

SNRI ANTIDEPRESSANTS

Venlafaxine and O-Desmethylvenlafaxine

The mean relative infant doses of venlafaxine and its *O*-desmethyl metabolite are 3.2% and 3.2%, respectively (i.e., a combined 6.4%) in a total of nine cases (Ilett *et al.*, 1998; Ilett *et al.*, 2002). Venlafaxine was not detected in plasma from any of the infants studied. However, *O*-desmethylvenlafaxine (mean 41 μg/L) was detected in the plasma of seven of eight infants studied. None of the infants showed any adverse effects at the time of study. *O*-desmethylvenlafaxine alone was also reported in plasma from two infants exposed to venlafaxine and its metabolite via milk (Hendrick *et al.*, 2001a). In these two cases, there were no acute adverse effects and the infants had made normal progress at one year of age. Three other cases of infants exposed to venlafaxine via milk also reported moderate levels of *O*-desmethylvenlafaxine (mean 24 μg/L) in serum of all three infants and venlafaxine in one (Berle *et al.*, 2004). The amount of drug in the infant serum was 10.2% of that in the mother's serum. As in the other studies, no adverse effects were seen. A relative infant dose of 5% (venlafaxine plus *O*-desmethylvenlafaxine) can be calculated from their data.

Overall, these data indicate that venlafaxine and *O*-desmethylvenlafaxine in milk are absorbed by the infants, and that most infants can efficiently *O*-demethylate the parent drug. While no adverse events were seen in the 14 cases reported to date, venlafaxine should only be used where it is the preferred prescription for the mother with careful observation of the breastfed infant. It is also interesting that one case report suggested that the amount of venlafaxine and its metabolite in milk may have been sufficient to ameliorate symptoms of serotonin excess from exposure during pregnancy (Koren *et al.*, 2006).

Duloxetine

In six lactating women given 40 mg duloxetine twice daily for 3.5 days, the M/P was 0.25 and the relative infant dose was approximately 0.14% of the weight-adjusted maternal dose (Data on file, Lilly Research Laboratories, July 7, 2007).

NRI ANTIDEPRESSANTS

Reboxetine

Presently, there is only one study of the NRI reboxetine (Hackett *et al.*, 2006). Because of its selective action on norepinephrine uptake, reboxetine is usually used as an add-on to SSRI pharmacotherapy. Its distribution into milk and effects in exposed infants have been studied in only four mother-baby dyads. Maternal dose ranged between 2-10 mg/day and two were also taking either escitalopram or sertraline, respectively. The transfer of reboxetine from plasma into milk was very low (mean M/P=0.06) and combined with average plasma reboxetine levels of 245 μg/L, this resulted in a mean relative infant dose of 2% (95% CI=1.3-2.7%). Plasma reboxetine in the breastfed infants was undetectable in one infant, with levels of 2.6, 2.3, and 5 μg/L, respectively, in the other three. Three of the infants showed normal development for age, while the fourth was lower than predicted for age, but this was considered to be unrelated to reboxetine exposure. In summary, despite there being only one small study, the very low levels in milk and low infant exposure, combined with a lack of adverse effects in the infants, suggests that this drug is compatible with breastfeeding. Since it is often used as an add-on therapy, consideration also needs to be given to its partner drug in the assessment of the risks and benefits of breastfeeding for an individual patient.

OTHER RELATED ANTIDEPRESSANTS

Mirtazapine

Mirtazapine is an antagonist of central alpha$_2$-auto and hetero-adrenoceptors, and it increases both norepinephrine and serotonin release that, in turn, stimulates $5HT_1$ receptors. It also blocks $5HT_2$, $5HT_3$, and histamine receptors. Desmethylmirtazapine, formed by CYP3A4, is also of interest because it has steady-state plasma concentrations that are about 33% of those of mirtazapine and a similar but less active (five- to 10-fold lower) pharmacological profile (Timmer *et al.*, 2000). There are two studies of the transfer of mirtazapine into breastmilk and effects in exposed infants. The first is a single case report of a woman taking 30 mg mirtazapine daily and fully breastfeeding her four-month-old infant (Aichhorn *et al.*, 2004). The average concentration of mirtazapine in milk was 31 μg/L, from which a relative infant dose of 1.1% can be estimated. The concentration of mirtazapine in the infant's plasma was 0.2 μg/L and no adverse effects (e.g., sedation) were seen. The second study was larger with eight breastfeeding women and their infants participating (Kristensen *et al.*, 2007). Median mirtazapine daily dose (maternal) was 38 mg (range 30-120 mg). Both mirtazapine and its active metabolite desmethylmirtazapine (plasma levels 33%, activity 5-10%, compared to parent) were measured in milk and plasma at steady-state. The mean M/P was 1.1 for mirtazapine and 0.6 for the metabolite, indicating a moderate to low transfer capacity. Mean relative infant dose was 1.5% (95% CI=0.8-2.2%) for mirtazapine and 0.4% (95% CI=0.2-0.6%) for desmethylmirtazapine. Plasma samples were available for only four of the eight infants. Mirtazapine (1.5 μg/L) was detected in plasma from one infant, and both parent and metabolite were undetected in the other three infants. A Denver developmental assessment done on seven of the infants (one unavailable) showed normal development for age, and no adverse effects were noted in any of the eight infants. On the basis of the findings in these investigations, we conclude that mirtazapine treatment is probably compatible with breastfeeding.

St John's Wort

The antidepressant herb St John's Wort has been studied in an observational study in 101 breastfeeding women taking the drug and a matched disease-free control group of breastfeeding women (Lee *et al.*, 2003). There were no differences in milk production, adverse events in mother or infant, or infant weight gain in the first year of life. Nevertheless, the antidepressant efficacy of the herb has not been clearly demonstrated (Linde *et al.*, 2005), and other antidepressants should be preferred during lactation.

Trazodone

Trazodone is a serotonin reuptake inhibitor as well as a 5-HT_2 receptor antagonist. In six women taking 50 mg/day, peak trazodone levels in milk averaged 100 μg/L at two hours after dose (Verbeeck *et al.*, 1986). Using these data, a relative infant dose of around 0.7% can be calculated. A second study reported 40 μg/L in milk for a 75 mg daily dose (Misri *et al.*, 2006), corresponding to a relative infant dose of 0.6%. In two cases, infants were followed up after 12 and 52 weeks exposure via milk and no adverse effects of development were noted (Misri *et al.*, 1991; Misri *et al.*, 2006), but no measurements of the drug in infant plasma have been reported.

Tricyclic,Tetracyclic, and Related Antidepressants

The American Academy of Pediatrics lists the tricyclic antidepressants as drugs of concern when used during lactation (American Academy of Pediatrics Committee on Drugs, 2001). They generally have low relative infant doses and a low incidence of adverse effects in the breastfed infant. The only exception is doxepin, where significant toxicity was observed in two exposed infants. The quantity and quality of the data varies widely for the different drugs in the group, and this can help in guiding drug selection.

Amitriptyline

Milk concentrations of amitriptyline (maternal dose range 75-175 mg daily) are available from six patients (Bader *et al.*, 1980; Brixen-Rasmussen *et al.*, 1982; Pittard III *et al.*, 1986; Breyer-Pfaff *et al.*, 1995; Yoshida *et al.*, 1997b). The mean relative infant dose for amitriptyline in these studies ranged from 0.1-2% and for nortriptyline from 0.1-1%. The metabolite *E*-10-hydroxynortriptyline has also been calculated to have a relative infant dose of 0.5%, following amitriptyline administration (Breyer-Pfaff *et al.*, 1995). A recent pooled analysis of these data can be used to calculate a mean relative infant dose of 0.7% for amitriptyline (Weissman *et al.*, 2004).

With one exception where amitriptyline was detected in plasma (7.5 μg/L) from an infant whose mother was taking 100 mg daily (Yoshida *et al.*, 1997b), amitriptyline and/or nortriptyline have not been detected in infant serum after therapeutic (75-175 mg daily) doses of amitriptyline (Erickson *et al.*, 1979; Bader *et al.*, 1980; Brixen-Rasmussen *et al.*, 1982; Breyer-Pfaff *et al.*, 1995).

However, poor analytical sensitivity is likely to explain the latter finding. No adverse effects or developmental delays have been found in infants exposed to amitriptyline and its metabolites via milk (Misri *et al.*, 1991; Yoshida *et al.*, 1997b; Nulman *et al.*, 2002).

Despite a relatively small number of studies, the low relative infant dose, lack of adverse effects, and large number of breastfeeding patients treated with amitriptyline suggest that this drug is compatible with breastfeeding.

Clomipramine

Data for clomipramine and breastfeeding are limited. In one case report of a mother taking 125-150 mg daily (Schimmell *et al.*, 1991), levels in milk indicated a relative infant dose ranging from 1.8-4.4% of the weight-adjusted maternal dose. Clomipramine was detected in the infant's blood at birth (267 μg/L) and at 4-35 days after birth (slowly decreasing from 128 to 10 μg/L, with a half-life of 93 hours). The infant had Apgar scores of six at birth, as well as respiratory distress, hypotonia, and jitteriness that resolved spontaneously by day six. Breastfeeding started on day 10, and the infant remained asymptomatic despite an estimated relative infant dose ranging from 1.8-4.4%. The second study reports two patients taking 100 or 125 mg daily (Yoshida *et al.*, 1997b) and an average relative infant dose of 1.5% can be calculated. Clomipramine was present in the serum from one of these infants at levels varying from undetectable to 5.5 μg/L. The drug was not detected in the other infant's serum. No adverse effects were noted. Clomipramine was undetected (limit of detection 10 μg/L) in serum from four exposed infants whose mothers took 75-150 mg daily (Wisner *et al.*, 1995). Again, there were no adverse effects in these infants. There are other reports of pregnancy-related exposure to clomipramine resulting in adverse effects, such as respiratory distress and jitteriness in the early neonatal period and the presence of metabolites in the infant's serum at birth (Musa *et al.*, 1979; Pedersen *et al.*, 1981; Ostergaard *et al.*, 1982). These are clearly attributable to placental transfer of clomipramine causing direct short-lived toxicity.

Desipramine

Milk levels of desipramine and its pharmacologically equally active 2-hydroxy metabolite (Weissman *et al.*, 2004) after 300 mg daily averaged a combined 338 μg/L at nine hours after a dose at steady-state. This translates to a relative infant dose of 1.2%. Birnbaum and colleagues reported that desipramine was undetectable in serum from four infants exposed via breastmilk, but their assay sensitivity was relatively high (10-25 μg/L) (Birnbaum *et al.*, 1999). No adverse effects on infant growth and development were reported in a case where the mother took 100 mg daily for eight weeks while breastfeeding (Misri *et al.*, 1991).

Dothiepin

The original study on dothiepin in milk describes the excretion of dothiepin, nordothiepin, dothiepin-*S*-oxide, and nordothiepin-*S*-oxide into breastmilk in eight women taking 25-225 mg daily (Ilett *et al.*, 1993). The metabolites all have significant pharmacological activity (Fulton *et al.*, 1982). The mean relative infant daily doses (in dothiepin equivalents) were 0.58% for dothiepin, 0.23% for nordothiepin, 2.47% for dothiepin-S-oxide, and 1.17% for nordothiepin-*S*-oxide. Interestingly, this study also presented clear evidence for cotransport of the lipid soluble dothiepin and its metabolite nordothiepin in milk fat, with M/P increasing from means of 0.8 or 0.9 in foremilk to 1.6 or 1.4, respectively, in hindmilk. By contrast, this effect was not seen with the more water soluble *S*-oxide metabolites of dothiepin. Plasma samples were obtained from five infants; in one, both dothiepin and nordothiepin were below their minimum quantifiable levels (2 μg/L), while in four others both dothiepin-*S*-oxide and nordothiepin-S-oxide were below their minimum quantifiable levels (10 μg/L). No adverse effects were found in any of the eight infants. A single case report also enables the calculation of a relative infant dose of 0.2% for dothiepin at a maternal dose of 75 mg/day (Rees *et al.*, 1976).

A study in infants from 30 depressed women taking dothiepin (only 15 breastfed) and 36 non-depressed controls used the McCarthy Scale to examine the children's progress three to five years postpartum (Buist *et al.*, 1995). Overall cognitive scores for the children did not differ between the groups. Higher levels of dothiepin and nordothiepin were associated with higher cognitive scores on subscales.

Doxepin

Doxepin also has an active *N*-desmethyl metabolite. Levels in milk in a mother taking 150 mg at night were 35-68 μg/L for doxepin and 65-131 μg/L for *N*-desmethyldoxepin (Kemp *et al.*, 1985). This corresponds to a combined relative infant dose of around 2.2%. A second case, where the maternal dose was 75 mg/day reported milk doxepin of 7-29 μg/L and *N*-desmethyldoxepin up to 11 μg/L, corresponding to a combined relative infant dose of about 0.4% (Matheson *et al.*, 1985). In a third case with a maternal dose of 35 mg/day, combined levels for doxepin and *N*-desmethyldoxepin averaged 87 μg/L, corresponding to a relative infant dose of 2.6% (Frey *et al.*, 1999). Adverse effects have been reported in two breastfed infants exposed to doxepin via milk (Matheson *et al.*, 1985; Frey *et al.*, 1999), although there were no problems in a third case (Kemp *et al.*, 1985). One nine-day-old boy was admitted because of drowsiness and poor sucking and swallowing, with muscle hypotonia and vomiting. However, his mother had taken doxepin through pregnancy (35 mg/day) and placental exposure may have been a contributing factor to his symptoms (Frey *et al.*, 1999). In the second case, an eight-week-old infant was found pale, limp, somnolent, and breathing poorly after the maternal dose was increased from 10 to 25 mg/day. His condition resolved within 24 hours of discontinuing breastfeeding (Matheson *et al.*, 1985).

Imipramine

One published case of imipramine in breastmilk gave a relative infant dose of 0.5% for the sum of imipramine and its active metabolite desipramine (Sovner *et al.*, 1979), while in another four breastfeeding mothers (75-150 mg/day) gave a relative infant dose of 2.9% (Yoshida *et al.*, 1999b). Imipramine and/or desipramine have been detected at low levels (0.6, 5.5 μg/L) in serum of two exposed infants (Birnbaum *et al.*, 1999), but were undetected in serum from two others (Misri *et al.*, 1991). Adverse effects and/or failure to achieve normal development were not seen in a total of 31 infants exposed to maternal imipramine (25-200 mg/day) (Sovner *et al.*, 1979; Misri *et al.*, 1991; Yoshida *et al.*, 1997b; Nulman *et al.*, 2002).

Maprotiline

Maprotiline is a tetracyclic antidepressant with strong norepinephrine reuptake and only weak effects on serotonin and dopamine reuptake properties. Two studies give limited details of maprotiline transfer into milk. In the first, peak levels of 110 μg/L occurred after a single oral dose of 100 mg (Lloyd, 1977), while in the second, a dose of 50 mg thrice daily gave levels between 180 and 200 μg/L (Reiss, 1975). These data allow the calculation of a relative infant dose ranging from 1.1-1.8%. There are no data for serum levels in infants. In the course of a larger study, no adverse effects were noted in the infant of one mother who was taking maprotiline (Nulman *et al.*, 2002). The lack of adverse effects in infants receiving other tricyclics might be used as an additional guide to breastfeeding safety for maprotiline (Buist *et al.*, 1995; Yoshida *et al.*, 1997b; Nulman *et al.*, 2002).

Mianserin

Mianserin is a tetracyclic antidepressant that blocks inhibitory α_2-autoreceptors and blocks neuronal norepinephrine reuptake. It also has some effect at the histamine and 5HT receptors. The only published data come from two single case reports (Buist *et al.*, 1993), where the mothers took 60 and 40 mg daily. The relative infant doses were 1.4 and 0.5%, respectively, for mianserin and 0.2 and 0.5%, respectively, for its metabolite, *N*-desmethylmianserin. The two exposed infants showed no adverse effects. We can also contribute one unpublished case (Kay O, Rampono J, Hackett LP, Ilett KF, 06/03/1998). The maternal dose was 100 mg daily, and relative infant dose at steady-state (14 hours after dose) was calculated as 0.7% for mianserin and 0.1% for *N*-desmethylmianserin. Information on the infant was not available.

Nortriptyline

As well as being a metabolite of amitriptyline, nortriptyline is also marketed as an antidepressant. The drug is metabolized to *E*-10-hydroxynortriptyline and *Z*-10-hydroxynortriptyline by CYP2D6 and 3A4 (Venkatakrishnan *et al.*, 1999). The metabolites have about 50% of the potency of nortriptyline on neuronal reuptake of norepinephrine (Bertilsson *et al.*, 1979) and 5% of its anticholinergic activity (Nordin *et al.*, 1987). Its relative infant dose after amitriptyline administration is discussed earlier. There is only a single case where nortriptyline alone was administered at a dose of 125 mg/day (Matheson *et al.*, 1988); a relative infant dose of 1.3% was reported. The authors noted that milk levels were much higher in fore- than in hindmilk, a finding that was suggested to be related to milk-fat content. Nortriptyline and its active metabolites in serum from exposed infants are low and not present in all cases (Wisner *et al.*, 1991; Altshuler *et al.*, 1995; Wisner *et al.*, 1997; Mammen *et al.*, 1997a). Out of 13 exposed infants, nortriptyline was only detected in the serum from one, *E*-10-hydroxynortriptyline in four, and *Z*-10-hydroxynortriptyline in six infants. Nortriptyline was not detected in infant serum in another case where it was co-administered with sertraline (Altshuler *et al.*, 1995). While in another two cases, only *Z*-10-hydroxynortriptyline was detected (Mammen *et al.*, 1997a). None of the infants in the above studies had adverse effects from their exposure to nortriptyline or its metabolites alone. As noted in the amitriptyline paragraph, there are also additional cases where exposure to nortriptyline after maternal amitriptyline treatment did not result in adverse effects.

OTHERS

Bupropion

Although bupropion is not a tricyclic, it is mechanistically related as it inhibits neuronal reuptake of norepinephrine and dopamine. While bupropion was originally marketed as an antidepressant, it is usually encountered in its alternative pharmacotherapeutic use as a treatment for smoking cessation (Holm *et al.*, 2000). Its transfer into milk has been the subject of two studies. The first was a case report and measured the drug and two of its major metabolites in the first six hours after 100 mg thrice daily dosing (Briggs *et al.*, 1993). Relative infant doses were 0.13, 0.3, 0.2, and 1.4% for bupropion, hydroxybupropion, erythrohydroxybupropion, and threohydroxybupropion, respectively. Similar transfer data were also reported in the second study in 10 women taking 300 mg/day (Haas *et al.*, 2004). Relative infant doses were 0.4, 0.35, and 1.5% for bupropion, hydroxybupropion, and threohydroxybupropion, respectively. Consideration of the total dose including metabolites is appropriately conservative as the various metabolites have some pharmacological activity in rodent studies (Schroeder, 1983). Levels of bupropion and its metabolites in the serum of three breastfed infants were below assay limits of detection at steady-state maternal doses of 150-300 mg/day, and no adverse effects were observed in these infants. However, there is one case report possibly linking an infant seizure with breastfeeding while using bupropion (Chaudron *et al.*, 2004). Given that the infant was only partially breastfed and that the mother had taken only two doses (150 mg) at the time of the event, the link to the seizure symptoms seems tenuous. The American Academy of Pediatrics recommendation of caution in the use of the drug predates most of the information that is now available (The American Academy of Pediatrics Committee on Drugs, 2001). Overall, the available data on milk transfer, limited levels in infant serum, and infant well being suggest that bupropion is probably compatible with breastfeeding. However, it should be noted that the manufacturer's product information lists a 0.1% prevalence of seizures in routine use of the drug, and, therefore, has a contraindication on its use in patients (including breastfeeding mothers), with risk factors that may predispose them to seizures.

Amoxapine and Protriptyline

The data for amoxapine (a tetracyclic inhibitor of neuronal norepinephrine reuptake) arise as a result of development of galactorrhea in a non-breastfeeding woman treated with amoxapine 250 mg daily (Gelenberg, 1979). At 0.75 and 11.5 hours after dose, amoxapine was detected (limit of detection 20 μg/L), while the pharmacologically active 8-hydroxyamoxapine was quantified at 113 and 168 μg/L, respectively, at the same times. No data are available for protriptyline.

Monoamine Oxidase Inhibitors

Like the tricyclics, monoamine oxidase inhibitor drugs are now infrequently used in psychiatry. There are no published data for phenelzine and tranylcypromine, but there is one study on moclobemide (Pons *et al.*, 1990). Both moclobemide and its major metabolite (Ro 12-8095) were quantified in milk and plasma. Milk levels of both compounds were highest three hours after dose, and the metabolite was undetectable after 12 hours. The percentages of the dose excreted as moclobemide and RO 12-8095 in milk were 0.06% and 0.03%, respectively, over 24 hours, and the relative infant dose of moclobemide was calculated to be approximately one percent.

ANTIPSYCHOTICS

In general (except for lithium), as shown in **Table 3**, the relative infant doses for the various antipsychotics are usually low. However, because of the nature of the illness in patients taking these drugs and their

Table 3. Typical and Atypical Antipsychotics and Breastfeeding

Drug	Relative infant dose (%)	Comment	References
Amisulpride	ND	Probably compatible. Others preferred until data are available.	
Aripiprazole	0.95	Low transfer into milk. Single case report.	Schlotterbeck *et al.*, 2007
Chlorpromazine	0.14, 0.25, 0.73	Low transfer to milk. Drowsiness and lethargy reported in some infants. May cause galactorrhea.	Blacker, 1962; Wiles *et al.*, 1978; Ohkubo *et al.*, 1993
Clozapine	1.2%	Low transfer to milk. Adverse effects reported in exposed infants. Alternatives recommended.	Barnas *et al.*, 1994
Haloperidol	0.2 -11.2	Probably compatible with careful observation. Infant development delayed in combination with chlorpromazine.	Stewart *et al.*, 1980; Whalley *et al.*, 1981; Ohkubo *et al.*, 1992; Yoshida *et al.*, 1998a
Lithium	0-30	Exposure can be high. May be compatible only if managed by monitoring infant progress, including serum lithium.	Tunnessen *et al.*, 1972; Schou *et al.*, 1973; Sykes *et al.*, 1976; Skausig *et al.*, 1977; Llewellyn *et al.*, 1998; Koren *et al.*, 1999; Viguera *et al.*, 2000; Moretti *et al.*, 2003
Olanzapine	0.9, 1.6, 1.12	Probably compatible. Drowsiness reported in some infants.	Kirchheiner *et al.*, 2000; Croke *et al.*, 2002; Gardiner *et al.*, 2003; Ambresin *et al.*, 2004
Quetiapine	0.09-0.27	A total of eight cases now available documenting very low infant exposure. Probably compatible with careful observation.	Lee *et al.*, 2004a; Misri *et al.*, 2006; Rampono *et al.*, 2007
Risperidone (including 9-hydroxyrisperidone)	0.62-6.5	Only five cases studied. Probably compatible, with careful observation.	Hill *et al.*, 2000; Ilett *et al.*, 2004; Aichhorn *et al.*, 2005
Ziprasidone	ND	Others preferred until data are available.	

ND – no data available

circumstances, accumulating a series of breastfeeding case reports is difficult, as is often reflected in the sparse data on their transfer into milk and effects in exposed infants.

Typical Antipsychotics

Chlorpromazine

Several small studies (Blacker, 1962; Citterio, 1964; Uhlir *et al.*, 1973; Wiles *et al.*, 1978; Ohkubo *et al.*, 1993) have described the transfer of chlorpromazine into breastmilk in a total of 25 cases. Relative infant doses of 0.25% and 0.14% were calculated after single doses of 1200 mg and 40 mg, respectively (Blacker, 1962; Ohkubo *et al.*, 1993). Chlorpromazine or its metabolites have been detected in breastmilk in varying quantities that do not appear to be dose related (Blacker, 1962; Citterio, 1964; Uhlir *et al.*, 1973; Ohkubo *et al.*, 1993), and the drug has been detected in infant serum at 7 and 92 μg/L, although the relative milk concentrations and maternal doses were not stated (Wiles *et al.*, 1978). A lack of side effects and the achievement of normal developmental milestones have been reported in several babies exposed to chlorpromazine via milk (Kris *et al.*, 1957; Ayd, 1973), but drowsiness and lethargy was reported in one infant who ingested milk containing 92 μg/L of chlorpromazine (Wiles *et al.*, 1978). However, another study reports that occasionally breastfed infants of mothers taking chlorpromazine exhibit drowsiness (Bonello, 1956), while three infants exposed to both chlorpromazine and haloperidol via breastmilk showed developmental delay, and an infant exposed only to chlorpromazine was unaffected (Yoshida *et al.*, 1998a). Finally, chlorpromazine has been used to increase milk supply, as galactorrhea is a reported side effect of phenothiazines (Bonello, 1956; Nemba, 1994). The American Academy of Pediatrics recommends the exercise of concern in the use of chlorpromazine in breastfeeding (American Academy of Pediatrics Committee on Drugs, 2001).

Haloperidol

Haloperidol transfers into breastmilk in low concentrations and reported relative infant doses range from 0.2-11.2% (Stewart *et al.*, 1980; Whalley *et al.*, 1981; Ohkubo *et al.*, 1992; Sugawara *et al.*, 1999). Haloperidol has been detected in the urine from exposed infants (Whalley *et al.*, 1981; Sugawara *et al.*, 1999) and in the plasma of two exposed infants at 6.8 and 8 μg/L, respectively (Sugawara *et al.*, 1999). The latter levels are within the adult therapeutic concentration range (6-17 μg/L) (Ulrich *et al.*, 1998). Adverse effects in exposed infants were not seen in two cases (Whalley *et al.*, 1981; Yoshida *et al.*, 1998a), while in three others, where there was exposure to both haloperidol and chlorpromazine via milk, developmental milestones were not met (Yoshida *et al.*, 1998a). The American Academy of Pediatrics recommends the exercise of concern in the use of haloperidol in breastfeeding (American Academy of Pediatrics Committee on Drugs, 2001).

Lithium

Lithium use during breastfeeding is controversial, as the concentration in milk is around 50% of that in mother's serum (Viguera *et al.*, 2007) and the concentration in the infant's serum ranges from 10 to 50% of that in maternal serum (Tunnessen *et al.*, 1972; Sykes *et al.*, 1976; Skausig *et al.*, 1977; Moretti *et al.*, 2000). Hence, the relative infant dose can be very high (around 20%) (Moretti *et al.*, 2000; Viguera *et al.*, 2007), and at least two cases with adverse lithium-related effects have been reported (Chaudron *et al.*, 2000). An unpublished case where a mother took 675-1125 mg lithium carbonate/day has shown a relative infant dose of 21-49% and infant serum lithium levels of around 0.2 mmol/L, compared to 0.59-0.71 mmol/L in the mother's serum (Rampono J, Kristensen JH, Ilett KF, Hackett LP, 07/19/2000). The latter can be compared to the usual therapeutic range of 0.5-1 mmol/L. No adverse effects were seen in the exposed infant. The published literature also describes some 21 cases where infants were exposed to maternal lithium via milk for several months without adverse effects (Weinstein *et al.*, 1969; Sykes *et al.*, 1976; Wise *et al.*, 1990; Moretti *et al.*, 2000; Viguera *et al.*, 2007). Reports of adverse effects in exposed infants comprise three cases with a range of symptoms (cyanosis, lethargy, ECG T-wave inversion, and elevated TSH) (Tunnessen *et al.*, 1972; Skausig *et al.*, 1977; Viguera *et al.*, 2007). The American Academy of Pediatrics suggests prohibition of breastfeeding when lithium therapy is necessary (American Academy of Pediatrics Committee on Drugs, 2001). However, some have expressed the opinion that breastfeeding is acceptable provided there is careful observation of the infant and regular monitoring of the infant's serum lithium levels (Koren *et al.*, 1999; Moretti *et al.*, 2003).

OTHERS

There are no published studies of the use of fluphenazine, molindone, or thiothixene in breastfeeding and other agents, such as haloperidol, olanzapine, or risperidone, may be preferred.

Atypical Antipsychotics

Amisulpride

There are presently no data available for this selective dopamine D_2 and D_3 antagonist drug.

Aripiprazole

Aripiprazole appears to mediate its antipsychotic effects primarily by partial agonist action at D_2 and $5HT_{1A}$ receptors, as well as having moderate affinity at H_1 and α-adrenoceptors. There is only one published case report for aripiprazole (Schlotterbeck *et al.*, 2007). A lactating mother taking 15 mg aripiprazole daily for formal thought disorder and delusions of persecution had 71 μg/L in plasma and 13-14 μg/L in milk at steady-state, giving a M/P ratio of 0.2. Assuming a body weight of 70 kg, the calculated relative infant dose is 0.95% of the maternal weight-adjusted dose.

Clozapine

Experience with clozapine (an antagonist at D_1, D_2, D_3, and D_5 receptors, as well as at selected adrenergic, cholinergic, histaminergic, and serotonergic receptors) during breastfeeding, comprises a single case where milk levels were 64-116 μg/L in a woman taking 50-100 mg/day (Barnas *et al.*, 1994). Her infant was not breastfed, but a relative infant dose of around 1.2% can be calculated. Adverse effects (drowsiness or agranulocytosis) were seen in two of four exposed infants in one report (Dev *et al.*, 1995). In view of the small but important potential for agranulocytosis, other antipsychotics would be preferred over clozapine. The American Academy of Pediatrics lists clozapine as a drug to be treated with concern in breastfeeding (American Academy of Pediatrics Committee on Drugs, 2001). Clozapine has minimal effects on serum prolactin (Maguire, 2002).

Olanzapine

Olanzapine (an antagonist at $5HT_2$, D_2, and H_1 receptors) transfer into milk has been studied in a total of 14 cases, with relative infant doses ranging from 0.9-1.6% for maternal doses of 2.5-20 mg daily (Kirchheiner *et al.*, 2000; Croke *et al.*, 2002; Gardiner *et al.*, 2003; Ambresin *et al.*, 2004). These studies also reported that olanzapine was undetectable in serum from seven of the breastfed infants from whom samples were obtained (Kirchheiner *et al.*, 2000; Croke *et al.*, 2002; Gardiner *et al.*, 2003). Adverse effects in exposed infants have been reported infrequently in the above studies. Drowsiness was reported in one of seven exposed infants (Gardiner *et al.*, 2003) and resolved when the mother's dose (originally 10 mg/day) was halved. In addition, drowsiness, diarrhea, diaper rash, lethargy, and poor suckling were considered to be associated with olanzapine use in two of 23 cases reported in a conference proceeding (Goldstein *et al.*, 2002). Olanzapine is generally considered to have minimal effects on serum prolactin, although there is one report of galactorrhea (Miller *et al.*, 2005). The American Academy of Pediatrics lists olanzapine as a drug to be treated with concern in breastfeeding (American Academy of Pediatrics Committee on Drugs, 2001).

Quetiapine

The effects of the antipsychotic quetiapine are mediated through antagonist activity mainly at D_1, D_2, $5\text{-}HT_{1A}$, and $5\text{-}HT_2$ receptor subtypes. Again, the data on breastmilk transfer for quetiapine are sparse, with a total of eight cases documenting a very low relative infant dose, ranging from 0.09-0.27% (Lee *et al.*, 2004a; Misri *et al.*, 2006; Rampono *et al.*, 2007). In one case, despite the low intake and no adverse effects in the infant, infant plasma levels were 6% of those in the maternal circulation (Rampono *et al.*, 2007). In another single case (Lee *et al.*, 2004a), no adverse effects were seen. In a third study of six cases, there were also no adverse effects attributable to quetiapine (Misri *et al.*, 2006). A fourth case reported no adverse effects in a breastfed infant exposed to maternal quetiapine (200 mg/day) for two months (Ritz, 2005).

Although the relative infant dose of quetiapine is low and adverse effects are infrequent, the small database suggests that this drug should only be used with careful monitoring of the infant's progress. Occasional measurement of plasma quetiapine in the infant could also be used to confirm the expected minimal exposure. The American Academy of Pediatrics lists quetiapine as a drug to be treated with concern in breastfeeding (American Academy of Pediatrics Committee on Drugs, 2001). Quetiapine can occasionally increase serum prolactin and cause galactorrhea (Pae *et al.*, 2004), but this would be unlikely to affect an established lactation.

Risperidone

Transfer of risperidone (an antagonist at D_1, D_2, and $5HT_{2A}$ receptors subtypes) and its major metabolite 9-hydroxyrisperidone into milk has been described in only five women, four mother-baby pairs and one patient with galactorrhea (Hill *et al.*, 2000; Ilett *et al.*, 2004; Aichhorn *et al.*, 2005). The metabolite was detected in infant plasma in one case (Aichhorn *et al.*, 2005), and both risperidone and its metabolite were below the analytical limit of detection in another case (Ilett *et al.*, 2004). No adverse effects have been detected in the four exposed infants studied (Ratnayake *et al.*, 2002; Ilett *et al.*, 2004; Aichhorn *et al.*, 2005).

Ziprasidone

There are presently no published studies of the atypical antipsychotic, ziprasidone, in breastfeeding, and other agents, such as haloperidol, olanzapine, or risperidone, are preferred.

CONCLUSIONS

Most of the data for antidepressants pertain to the potential for acute adverse effects arising subsequent to the drug's transport into milk and its oral absorption by the breastfeeding infant. Since maternal use of these drugs is often necessary during pregnancy as well as during lactation, it should not be surprising that there is a well described syndrome of short-term, self-limiting adverse effects in neonates exposed to SSRI or SNRI antidepressants during pregnancy (Zeskind *et al.*, 2004; Oberlander *et al.*, 2005; Levinson-Castiel *et al.*, 2006; Agut-Quijano *et al.*, 2006; Ferreira *et al.*, 2007). The syndrome has sometimes been described as a "Neonatal Abstinence Syndrome," assuming similarity to the withdrawal symptoms seen in neonates born to mothers taking methadone as an opiate substitute. However, in the case of the SSRI's and SNRI's, the symptoms seen in exposed infants are more akin to those of serotonin overdose in adults and are more appropriately described as a "Serotonin Toxicity Syndrome" (Isbister *et al.*, 2001). Several studies show that there is significant infant drug exposure via the placenta (Hostetter *et al.*, 2000; Laine *et al.*, 2003; Rampono *et al.*, 2004). Exposure via the placenta is usually quantified from the concentration of drug in the infant's circulation at birth (cord blood at delivery), and varies from 50-100% of that in the mother's circulation. It is also reported that placental exposure to tricyclics that have significant 5-HT reuptake blocking activity (e.g., doxepin and clomipramine) can cause the same serotonin toxicity syndrome in the early neonatal period (Musa *et al.*, 1979; Pedersen *et al.*, 1981; Ostergaard *et al.*, 1982; Schimmell *et al.*, 1991; Frey *et al.*, 1999). By contrast, infant exposure to maternal drugs via milk is generally less than 10% of the maternal daily intake. Hence, when adverse effects are noted in the neonate, it is extremely important to discriminate between placental transport of a drug, its transfer via milk, or even a withdrawal syndrome in determining causality.

The effects of long-term exposure of infants to antidepressant drugs in breastmilk have received only limited attention. Nevertheless, there are some useful data for tricyclic antidepressants, fluoxetine, and citalopram administered during pregnancy and/or lactation that show no differences in measures of cognitive development at one to five years of age (Buist *et al.*, 1995; Nulman *et al.*, 1997; Nulman *et al.*, 2002; Heikkinen *et al.*, 2002; Heikkinen *et al.*, 2003). These studies are very reassuring, and it is to be hoped that future studies will extend our knowledge in this important area.

Maternal psychosis itself correlates negatively with cognitive development for infants at seven months of age (Yoshida *et al.*, 1999a), mainly as a result of lifestyle factors. As illustrated above, short-term adverse effects in infants whose mothers received antipsychotic medications during breastfeeding do not appear to be a significant problem for some drugs. Nevertheless, the potential for long-term effects following infant exposure to these drugs is an important consideration for which there are presently no data.

For the antidepressants and antipsychotics which have no therapeutic application in infants, relative infant dose is the most useful primary measure for assessing safety of their use in lactation. However, this needs to be interpreted together with evidence of levels of these drugs in infant serum and case reports/studies of adverse effects (or lack thereof) in exposed infants. When evaluating the information from any report, due consideration should be given to the number of subjects studied and the quality of the data, particularly with respect to adverse events that are claimed to be due to the drug in question. With regard to the latter, it is worth remembering that a review of the literature found only 100 adverse event reports up to 2003 (Anderson *et al.*, 2003). Only 47% of adverse events were "probably" attributable to the suspected drug. As with all drug use in breastfeeding, an individual risk/benefit analysis should be conducted before initiating therapy with an antidepressant or antipsychotic medication.

References

Abdul Aziz A, Agab WA, Kalis NN. Severe paroxetine induced hyponatremia in a breast fed infant. *J Bahrain Med Soc.* 2004; 16:195-98.

Agut-Quijano T, Martinez-Nadal S, Elizari-Saco MJ, Sala-Castellvi P, Vila-Ceren C, Raspall-Torrent F. Neonatal withdrawal syndrome to selective serotonin reuptake inhibitors: case report and literature review. *Rev Neurol.* 2006; 42:660-62.

Aichhorn W, Stuppaeck C, Whitworth AB. Risperidone and breast-feeding. *J Psychopharmacol.* 2005; 19:211-13.

Aichhorn W, Whitworth AB, Weiss U, Stuppaeck C. Mirtazapine and breast-feeding. *Am J Psychiatry.* 2004; 161:2325.

Altshuler LL, Burt VK, McMullen M, Hendrick V. Breastfeeding and sertraline: a 24-hour analysis. *J Clin Psychiatry.* 1995; 56:243-45.

Ambresin G, Berney P, Schulz P, Bryois C. Olanzapine excretion into breast milk: a case report. *J Clin Psychopharmacol.* 2004; 24:93-95.

American Academy of Pediatrics Committee on Drugs. Transfer of drugs and other chemicals into human milk. *Pediatrics.* 2001; 108:776-89.

Anderson PO, Pochop SL, Manoguerra AS. Adverse drug reactions in breastfed infants: less than imagined. *Clin Pediat (Phila).* 2003; 42:325-40.

Anonymous. Fluoxetine. Toxnet drugs and lactation (Lactmed) database 2007a. Available from: http://toxnet.nlm.nih.gov/cgi-bin/sis/htmlgen?LACT.

Anonymous. Maprotiline. Toxnet drugs and lactation (Lactmed) database 2007b. Available from: http://toxnet.nlm.nih.gov/cgi-bin/sis/htmlgen?LACT.

Arnold LM, Suckow RF, Lichtenstein PK. Fluvoxamine concentrations in breast milk and in maternal and infant sera. *J Clin Psychopharmacol.* 2000; 20:491-93.

Ayd FJ Jr. Excretion of psychotropic drugs in human breast milk. *Int Drug Ther News Bull.* 1973; 8:33-40.

Bader TF, Newman K. Amitriptyline in human breast milk and the nursing infant's serum. *Am J Psychiatry.* 1980; 137:855-56.

Barnas C, Bergant A, Hummer M, Saria A, Fleischhacker WW. Clozapine concentrations in maternal and fetal plasma, amniotic fluid, and breast milk. *Am J Psychiatry.* 1994; 151:945.

Begg EJ, Duffull SB, Saunders DA, Buttimore RC, Ilett KF, Hackett LP, *et al.* Paroxetine in human milk. *Br J Clin Pharmacol.* 1999; 48:142-47.

Bennett PN, Astrup-Jensen A, Bates CJ, Begg EJ, Edwards S, Lazarus CR, *et al. Drugs and human lactation.* 2nd Ed. Amsterdam: Elsevier Science B.V.; 1996.

Berle JO, Steen VM, Aamo TO, Breilid H, Zahlsen K, Spigset O. Breastfeeding during maternal antidepressant treatment with serotonin reuptake inhibitors: infant exposure, clinical symptoms, and cytochrome p450 genotypes. *J Clin Psychiatry.* 2004; 65:1228-34.

Bertilsson L, Mellstrom B, Sjoqvist F. Pronounced inhibition of noradrenaline uptake by 10-hydroxymetabolites of nortriptyline. *Life Sciences.* 1979; 25:1285-92.

Birnbaum CS, Cohen LS, Bailey JW, Grush LR, Robertson LM, Stowe ZN. Serum concentrations of antidepressants and benzodiazepines in nursing infants: A case series. *Pediatrics.* 1999; 104:e11.

Blacker KH. Mothers milk and chlorpromazine. *Am J Psychiatry.* 1962; 114:178-79.

Bonello FJ. Chlorpromazine in general practice. *Int Rec Med Gen Pract Clin.* 1956; 169:197-212.

Brent NB, Wisner KL. Fluoxetine and carbamazepine concentrations in a nursing mother/infant pair. *Clin Pediat (Phila).* 1998; 37:41-44.

Breyer-Pfaff U, Nill K, Entenmann KN, Gaertner HJ. Secretion of amitriptyline and metabolites into breast milk. *Am J Psychiatry.* 1995; 152:812-13.

Briggs GG, Freeman RK, Yaffe SJ. *Drugs in pregnancy and lactation.* 7th Ed. Philadelphia: Lippincott Williams and Wilkins; 2005.

Briggs GG, Samson JH, Ambrose PJ, Schroeder DH. Excretion of bupropion in breast milk. *Ann Pharmacother.* 1993; 27:431-33.

Brixen-Rasmussen L, Halgrener J, Jorgensen A. Amitriptyline and nortriptyline excretion in human breast milk. *Psychopharmacology (Berl).* 1982; 76:94-95.

Brockington IF. *Motherhood and mental illness.* Oxford, UK: Oxford University Press; 1996.

Buist A, Janson H. Effect of exposure to dothiepin and northiaden in breast milk on child development. *Brit J Psychiatry.* 1995; 167:370-73.

Buist A, Norman TR, Dennerstein L. Mianserin in breast milk [letter]. *Br J Clin Pharmacol.* 1993; 36:133-34.

Burch KJ, Wells BG. Fluoxetine/norfluoxetine concentrations in human milk. *Pediatrics.* 1992; 89:676-77.

Castberg I, Spigset O. Excretion of escitalopram in breast milk. *J Clin Psychopharmacol.* 2006; 26:536-38.

Chambers CD, Anderson PO, Thomas RG, Dick LM, Felix RJ, Johnson KA, *et al.* Weight gain in infants breastfed by mothers who take fluoxetine. *Pediatrics.* 1999; 104:1120-21.

Chambers CD, Hernandez-Diaz S, Van Marter LJ, Werler MM, Louik C, Jones KL, *et al.* Selective serotonin-reuptake inhibitors and risk of persistent pulmonary hypertension of the newborn. *New Engl J Med.* 2006; 354:579-87.

Chaudron LH, Jefferson JW. Mood stabilizers during breastfeeding: A review. *J Clin Psychiatry.* 2000; 61:79-90.

Chaudron LH, Schoenecker CJ. Bupropion and breastfeeding: a case of a possible infant seizure. *J Clin Psychiatry.* 2004; 65:881-82.

Citterio C. Riconoscimento e dosaggio di derivati fenotiazinici nella secrezione lattea. *Neuropsichiatria.* 1964; 20:141-46 (quoted by Toxnet/LactMed NLM Database).

Croke S, Buist A, Hackett LP, Ilett KF, Norman T, Burrows GD. Olanzapine excretion in human breast milk: estimation of infant exposure. *Int J Neuropsychopharmacol.* 2002; 5:243-47.

Dev VJ, Krupp P. Adverse event profile and safety of clozapine. *Rev Contemp Pharmacother.* 1995; 6:197-208.

Dodd S, Stocky A, Buist A, Burrows GD, Maguire K, Norman TR. Sertraline in paired blood plasma and breast-milk samples from nursing mothers. *Hum Psychopharmacol.* 2000; 15:161-264.

Epperson N, Czarkowski KA, Ward-O'Brien D, Weiss E, Gueorguieva R, Jatlow P, *et al.* Maternal sertraline treatment and serotonin transport in breast-feeding mother-infant pairs. *Am J Psychiatry.* 2001; 158:1631-37.

Erickson SH, Smith GH, Heidrich F. Tricyclics and breast feeding. *Am J Psychiatry.* 1979; 136:1483-84.

Ferreira E, Carceller AM, Agogue C, Martin BZ, St-Andre M, Francoeur D, *et al.* Effects of selective serotonin reuptake inhibitors and venlafaxine during pregnancy in term and preterm neonates. *Pediatrics.* 2007; 119:52-59.

Fish EW, Faccidomo S, Gupta S, Miczek KA. Anxiolytic-like effects of escitalopram, citalopram and R-citalopram in maternally separated mouse pups. *J Pharmacol Exp Ther.* 2004; 308(2):474-80. Epub 2003 Oct 30.

Franssen EJ, Meijs V, Ettaher F, Valerio PG, Keessen M, Lameijer W. Citalopram serum and milk levels in mother and infant during lactation. *Ther Drug Monit.* 2006; 28:2-4.

Frey OR, Scheidt P, von Brenndorff AI. Adverse effects in a newborn infant breast-fed by a mother treated with doxepin. *Ann Pharmacother.* 1999; 33:690-93.

Fulton A, Norman TR, Cheng H, Burrows GD. Assessment of the antidepressant activity of dothiepin and its metabolites by preclinical tests. *J Affect Disord.* 1982; 4:261-69.

Gardiner SJ, Kristensen JH, Begg EJ, Hackett LP, Wilson DA, Ilett KF, *et al.* Transfer of olanzapine into breast milk, calculation of infant drug dose, and effect on breast-fed infants. *Am J Psychiatry.* 2003; 160:1428-31.

Gelenberg AJ. Single case study. Amoxapine, a new antidepressant, appears in human milk. *J Nerv Ment Dis.* 1979; 167:635-36.

Gentile S. Clinical utilization of atypical antipsychotics in pregnancy and lactation. *Ann Pharmacother.* 2004; 38:1265-71.

Gentile S. The safety of newer antidepressants in pregnancy and breastfeeding. *Drug Saf.* 2005; 28:137-52.

Gentile S. Use of contemporary antidepressants during breastfeeding: a proposal for a specific safety index. *Drug Saf.* 2007; 30:107-21.

Goldstein DJ, Corbin LA, Wohlreich MM, Kwong K. Olanzapine use during breast-feeding. *Schizophrenia Res.* 2002; 53:185.

Haas JS, Kaplan CP, Barenboim D, Jacob P III, Benowitz NL. Bupropion in breast milk: an exposure assessment for potential treatment to prevent post-partum tobacco uses. *Tobacco Control.* 2004; 13:52-56.

Hackett LP, Ilett KF, Rampono J, Kristensen JH, Kohan R. Transfer of reboxetine into breastmilk, its plasma concentrations and lack of adverse effects in the breastfed infant. *Eur J Clin Pharmacol.* 2006; 62:633-68.

Hagg S, Granberg K, Carleborg L. Excretion of fluvoxamine into breast milk. *Br J Clin Pharmacol.* 2000; 49:286-88.

Hale TW. *Medications and mothers' milk.* 12th Ed. Amarillo, TX, USA: Pharmasoft Publishing; 2006.

Hale TW, Ilett KF. *Drug therapy and breastfeeding. From theory to clinical practice.* 1st Ed. London: The Parthenon Publishing Group; 2002.

Hale TW, Shum S, Grossberg M. Fluoxetine toxicity in a breastfed infant. *Clin Pediat (Phila).* 2001; 40:681-84.

Hatzopoulos FK, Albrecht LM. Antidepressant use during breastfeeding. *J Hum Lact.* 2006; 12:139-41.

Heikkinen T, Ekblad U, Kero P, Ekblad S, Laine K. Citalopram in pregnancy and lactation. *Clin Pharmacol Ther.* 2002; 72:184-91.

Heikkinen T, Ekblad U, Palo P, Laine K. Pharmacokinetics of fluoxetine and norfluoxetine in pregnancy and lactation. *Clin Pharmacol Ther.* 2003; 73:330-37.

Hendrick V, Altshuler L, Wertheimer A, Dunn WA. Venlafaxine and breast-feeding. *Am J Psychiatry.* 2001a; 158:2089-90.

Hendrick V, Fukuchi A, Altshuler L, Widawski M, Wertheimer A, Brunhuber MV. Use of sertraline, paroxetine and fluvoxamine by nursing women. *Brit J Psychiatry.* 2001b; 179:163-66.

Hendrick V, Smith LM, Hwang S, Altshuler LL, Haynes D. Weight gain in breastfed infants of mothers taking antidepressant medications. *J Clin Psychiatry.* 2003; 64:410-12.

Hendrick V, Stowe ZN, Altshuler LL, Hostetter A, Fukuchi A. Paroxetine use during breast-feeding. *J Clin Psychopharmacol.* 2000; 20:587-89.

Hendrick V, Stowe ZN, Altshuler LL, Mintz J, Hwang S, Hostetter A, *et al.* Fluoxetine and norfluoxetine concentrations in nursing infants and breast milk. *Biol Psychiatry.* 2001c; 50:775-82.

Hill RC, McIvor RJ, Wojnar-Horton RE, Hackett LP, Ilett KF. Risperidone distribution and excretion into human milk: case report and estimated infant exposure during breast-feeding [letter]. *J Clin Psychopharmacol.* 2000; 20:285-86.

Holm KJ, Spencer CM. Bupropion: a review of its use in the management of smoking cessation. *Drugs.* 2000; 59:1007-24.

Hostetter A, Ritchie JC, Stowe ZN. Amniotic fluid and umbilical cord blood concentrations of antidepressants in three women. *Biol Psychiatry.* 2000; 48:1032-34.

Ilett KF, Hackett LP, Dusci LJ, Roberts MJ, Kristensen JH, Paech M, *et al.* Distribution and excretion of venlafaxine and O-desmethylvenlafaxine in human milk. *Br J Clin Pharmacol.* 1998; 45:459-62.

Ilett KF, Hackett LP, Kristensen JH, Vaddadi KS, Gardiner SJ, Begg EJ. Transfer of risperidone and 9-hydroxyrisperidone into human milk. *Ann Pharmacother.* 2004; 38:273-76.

Ilett KF, Kristensen JH. Drug use and breastfeeding. *Expert Opin Drug Saf.* 2005; 4:745-68.

Ilett KF, Kristensen JH, Hackett LP, Paech M, Kohan R, Rampono J. Distribution of venlafaxine and its O-desmethyl metabolite in human milk and their effects in breastfed infants. *Br J Clin Pharmacol.* 2002; 53:17-22.

Ilett KF, Lebedevs TH, Wojnar-Horton RE, Yapp P, Roberts MJ, Dusci LJ, *et al.* The excretion of dothiepin and its primary metabolites in breast milk. *Br J Clin Pharmacol.* 1993; 33:635-39.

Isbister GK, Dawson A, Whyte IM, Prior FH, Clancy C, Smith AJ. Neonatal paroxetine withdrawal syndrome or actually serotonin syndrome? *Arch Dis Child Fetal Neonatal Ed.* 2001; 85:F147-48.

Isenberg KE. Excretion of fluoxetine in human breast milk [letter]. *J Clin Psychiatry.* 1990; 51:169.

Jensen PN, Olesen OV, Bertelsen A, Linnet K. Citalopram and desmethylcitalopram concentrations in breast milk and in serum of mother and infant. *Ther Drug Monit.* 1997; 19:236-39.

Kemp J, Ilett KF, Booth J, Hackett LP. Excretion of doxepin and N-desmethyldoxepin in human milk. *Br J Clin Pharmacol.* 1985; 20:497-99.

Kim J, Riggs KW, Misri S, Kent N, Oberlander TF, Grunau RE, *et al.* Stereoselective disposition of fluoxetine and norfluoxetine during pregnancy and breast-feeding. *Br J Clin Pharmacol.* 2006; 61:155-63.

Kirchheiner J, Berghöfer A, Bolk-Weischedel D. Healthy outcome under olanzapine treatment in a pregnant woman. *Pharmacopsychiatry.* 2000; 33:78-80.

Klier CM, Mossaheb N, Lee A, Zernig G. Mirtazapine and breastfeeding: maternal and infant plasma levels. *Am J Psychiatry.* 2007; 164:348-49.

Koren G, Moretti M, Ito S. Continuing drug therapy while breastfeeding. Part 2. Common misconceptions of physicians. *Can Fam Physician.* 1999; 45:1173-75.

Koren G, Moretti M, Kapur B. Can venlafaxine in breast milk attenuate the norepinephrine and serotonin reuptake neonatal withdrawal syndrome. *J Obstet Gynaecol Can.* 2006; 28:299-302.

Kris EB, Carmichael DM. Chlorpromazine maintenance therapy during pregnancy and confinement. *Psychiatr Q.* 1957; 31:690-95.

Kristensen JH, Hackett LP, Kohan R, Paech MJ, Ilett KF. The amount of fluvoxamine in milk is unlikely to be a cause of adverse effects in breastfed infants. *J Hum Lact.* 2002; 18:139-43.

Kristensen JH, Ilett KF, Dusci LJ, Hackett LP, Yapp P, Wojnar-Horton RE, *et al.* Distribution and excretion of sertraline and N-desmethylsertraline in human milk. *Br J Clin Pharmacol.* 1998; 45:453-57.

Kristensen JH, Ilett KF, Hackett LP, Yapp P, Paech M, Begg EJ. Distribution and excretion of fluoxetine and norfluoxetine in human milk. *Br J Clin Pharmacol.* 1999; 48:521-27.

Kristensen JH, Ilett KF, Rampono J, Kohan R, Hackett LP. Transfer of the antidepressant mirtazapine into breast milk. *Br J Clin Pharmacol.* 2007; 63:322-27.

Kulkarni J, Riedel A, de Castella AR, Fitzgerald PB, Rolfe TJ, Taffe J, *et al.* A clinical trial of adjunctive oestrogen treatment in women with schizophrenia. *Arch Womens Ment Health.* 2002; 5:99-104.

Laine K, Heikkinen T, Ekblad U, Kero P. Effects of exposure to selective serotonin reuptake inhibitors during pregnancy on serotonergic symptoms in newborns and cord blood monoamine and prolactin concentrations. *Arch Gen Psychiatry.* 2003; 60:720-26.

Laine K, Kytola J, Bertilsson L. Severe adverse effects in a newborn with two defective CYP2D6 alleles after exposure to paroxetine during late pregnancy. *Ther Drug Monit.* 2004; 26:685-87.

Lee A, Giesbrecht E, Dunn E, Ito S. Excretion of quetiapine in breast milk. *Am J Psychiatry.* 2004a; 161:1715-16.

Lee A, Minhas R, Matsuda N, Lam M, Ito S. The safety of St. John's wort (Hypericum perforatum) during breastfeeding. *J Clin Psychiatry.* 2003; 64:966-68.

Lee A, Woo J, Ito S. Frequency of infant adverse events that are associated with citalopram use during breast-feeding. *Am J Obstet Gynecol.* 2004b; 190:218-21.

Lee CM, Gotlib IH. Adjustment of children of depressed mothers: a 10-month follow-up. *J Abnorm Psychol.* 1991; 100:473-77.

Lester BM, Cucca J, Andreozzi L, Flanagan P, Oh W. Possible association between fluoxetine hydrochloride and colic in an infant. *J Am Acad Child Adolesc Psychiatry.* 1993; 32:1253-55.

Levinson-Castiel R, Merlob P, Linder N, Sirota L, Klinger G. Neonatal abstinence syndrome after in utero exposure to selective serotonin reuptake inhibitors in term infants. *Arch Pediatr Adolesc Med.* 2006; 160:173-76.

Linde K, Mulrow CD, Berner M, Egger M. St John's wort for depression. *Cochrane Database Syst Rev.* 2005; CD000448.

Llewellyn A, Stowe ZN, Strader JRJ. The use of lithium and management of women with bipolar disorder during pregnancy and lactation. *J Clin Psychiatry.* 1998; 59 (Suppl 6):57-64.

Lloyd AH. Practical considerations in the use of maprotiline (Ludiomil) in general practice. *J Int Med Res.* 1977; 5 (Suppl 4):122-38.

Maguire GA. Prolactin elevation with antipsychotic medications: mechanisms of action and clinical consequences. *J Clin Psychiatry.* 2002; 63 (Suppl 4):56-62.

Mammen O, Perel JM, Wheeler S. Antidepressants and breast-feeding. *Am J Psychiatry.* 1997a; 154:1174-75.

Mammen OK, Perel JM, Rudolph G, Foglia JP, Wheeler SB. Sertraline and norsertraline levels in three breastfed infants. *J Clin Psychiatry.* 1997b; 58:100-3.

Matheson I, Pande H, Alertsen AR. Respiratory depression caused by N-desmethyldoxepin in breast milk. *Lancet.* 1985; 2:1124.

Matheson I, Skjaeraasen J. Milk concentrations of flupenthixol, nortriptyline and zuclopenthixol and between-breast differences in two patients. *Eur J Clin Pharmacol.* 1988; 35:217-20.

Mhanna MJ, Bennet JB, Izatt SD. Potential fluoxetine chloride (Prozac) toxicity in a newborn. *Pediatrics.* 1997; 100:158-59.

Miller DE, Sebastian CS. Olanzapine-induced hyperprolactinemia and galactorrhea reversed with addition of bromocriptine: a case report. *J Clin Psychiatry.* 2005; 66:269-70.

Misri S, Corral M, Wardrop AA, Kendrick K. Quetiapine augmentation in lactation: a series of case reports. *J Clin Psychopharmacol.* 2006; 26:508-11.

Misri S, Kim J, Riggs KW, Kostaras X. Paroxetine levels in postpartum depressed women, breast milk, and infant serum. *J Clin Psychiatry.* 2000; 61:828-32.

Misri S, Sivertz K. Tricyclic drugs in pregnancy and lactation: a preliminary report. *Int J Psychiatry Med.* 1991; 21:157-71.

Mohan CG, Moore JJ. Fluoxetine toxicity in a preterm infant. *J Perinatol.* 2000; 20:445-46.

Moretti ME, Koren G, Verjee Z, Ito S. Monitoring lithium in breast milk: An individualized approach for breast-feeding mothers. *Ther Drug Monit.* 2003; 25:364-66.

Moretti ME, Lee A, Ito S. Which drugs are contraindicated during breastfeeding? Practice guidelines. *Can Fam Physician.* 2000; 46:1753-57.

Murray L, Fiori-Cowley A, Hooper R, Cooper P. The impact of postnatal depression and associated adversity on early mother-infant interactions and later infant outcome. *Child Dev.* 1996; 67:2512-26.

Musa AB, Smith CS. Neonatal effects of maternal clomipramine therapy. *Archives of Diseases in Childhood.* 1979; 54:405.

Nemba K. Induced lactation: a study of 37 non-puerperal mothers. *J Trop Pediatr.* 1994; 40:240-42.

Nordeng H, Bergsholm YK, Bohler E, Spigset O. Excretion of selective serotonin reuptake inhibitors in breast milk. *Tidsskr Nor Laegeforen.* 2001; 121:199-203.

Nordin C, Bertilsson L, Otani K, Widmark A. Little anticholinergic effect of E-10-hydroxynortriptyline compared with nortriptyline in healthy subjects. *Clin Pharmacol Ther.* 1987; 41:97-102.

Nulman I, Rovet J, Stewart DE, Wolpin J, Gardner HA, Theis JG, *et al.* Neurodevelopment of children exposed in utero to antidepressant drugs. *New Engl J Med.* 1997; 336:258-62.

Nulman I, Rovet J, Stewart DE, Wolpin J, Pace-Asciak P, Shuhaiber S, *et al.* Child development following exposure to tricyclic antidepressants or fluoxetine throughout fetal life: a prospective, controlled study. *Am J Psychiatry.* 2002; 159:1889-95.

O'Hara MW, Zekoski EM, Philipps LH, Wright EJ. Controlled prospective study of postpartum mood disorders: comparison of childbearing and nonchildbearing women. *J Abnorm Psychol.* 1990; 99:3-15.

Oberlander TF, Grunau RE, Fitzgerald C, Papsdorf M, Rurak D, Riggs W. Pain reactivity in 2-month-old infants after prenatal and postnatal serotonin reuptake inhibitor medication exposure. *Pediatrics.* 2005; 115:411-25.

Ohkubo T, Shimoyama R, Sugawara K. Measurement of haloperidol in human breast milk by high-performance liquid chromatography. *J Pharm Sci.* 1992; 81:947-49.

Ohkubo T, Shimoyama R, Sugawara K. Determination of chlorpromazine in human breast milk and serum by high-performance liquid chromatography. *J Chromatogr.* 1993; 614:328-32.

Ohman R, Hagg S, Carleborg L, Spigset O. Excretion of paroxetine into breast milk. *J Clin Psychiatry.* 1999; 60:519-23.

Ohman R, Norstedt B, Vitols WS. Citalopram and metabolite levels in plasma and breast milk in two nursing women. *Br J Clin Pharmacol.* 1997; A179.

Ostergaard GZ, Pedersen SE. Neonatal effects of maternal clomipramine treatment. *Pediatrics.* 1982; 69:233-34.

Pae CU, Kim JJ, Lee CU, Chae JH, Lee SJ, Lee C, *et al.* Very low dose quetiapine-induced galactorrhea in combination with venlafaxine. *Hum Psychopharmacol.* 2004; 19:433-34.

Pedersen S, Ostergaard GZ. Neonatal complications caused by maternal clomipramine treatment. *Ugeskr Laeger.* 1981; 143:417-18.

Piontek CM, Wisner KL, Perel JM, Peindl KS. Serum fluvoxamine levels in breastfed infants. *J Clin Psychiatry.* 2001; 62:111-13.

Pittard WB III, O'Neal W Jr. Amitriptyline excretion in human milk. *J Clin Psychopharmacol.* 1986; 6:383-84.

Pons G, Schoerlin MP, Tam YK, Moran C, Pfefen JP, Francoual C, *et al.* Moclobemide excretion in human breast milk. *Br J Clin Pharmacol.* 1990; 29:27-31.

Rampono J, Hackett LP, Kristensen JH, Kohan R, Page-Sharp M, Ilett KF. Transfer of escitalopram and its metabolite demethylescitalopram into breastmilk. *Br J Clin Pharmacol.* 2006; 62:316-22.

Rampono J, Kristensen JH, Hackett LP, Paech M, Kohan R, Ilett KF. Citalopram and demethylcitalopram in human milk; distribution, excretion and effects in breast fed infants. *Br J Clin Pharmacol.* 2000; 50:263-68.

Rampono J, Kristensen JH, Ilett KF, Hackett LP, Kohan R. Quetiapine and breastfeeding. *Ann Pharmacother.* 2007; 41:711-14.

Rampono J, Proud S, Hackett LP, Kristensen JH, Ilett KF. A pilot study of newer antidepressant concentrations in cord and maternal serum and possible effects in the neonate. *Int J Neuropsychopharmacol.* 2004; 7:329-34.

Ratnayake T, Libretto SE. No complications with risperidone treatment before and throughout pregnancy and during the nursing period. *J Clin Psychiatry.* 2002; 63:76-77.

Rees JA, Glass RC, Sporne GA. Seum and breastmilk concentrations of dothiepin. *Practitioner.* 1976; 217:686.

Riess W. The relevance of blood level determinations during the evaluation of maprotiline in man. In: Murphy JE (ed.). *Research and Clinical Investigation in Depression.* Northampton, England: Cambridge Medical Publications; 1976. p.19-38.

Ritz S. Quetiapine monotherapy in post-partum onset bipolar disorder with a mixed affective state. *Eur Neuropsychopharmacol.* 2005; 15 (Suppl 3):S407.

Rohan A. Drug distribution in milk. *Aust Prescriber.* 1997; 20:84.

Rubin ET, Lee A, Ito S. When breastfeeding mothers need CNS-acting drugs. *Can J Clin Pharmacol.* 2004; 11:e257-66.

Schimmell MS, Katz EZ, Shaag Y, Pastuszak A, Koren G. Toxic neonatal effects following maternal clomipramine therapy. *J Toxicol Clin Toxicol.* 1991; 29:479-84.

Schlotterbeck P, Leube D, Kircher T, Hiemke C, Grunder G. Aripiprazole in human milk. *Int J Neuropsychopharmacol.* 2007; 10:433.

Schmidt K, Olesen OV, Jensen PN. Citalopram and breast-feeding: serum concentration and side effects in the infant. *Biol Psychiatry.* 2000; 47:164-65.

Schou M, Amdisen A. Lithium and pregnancy. 3. Lithium ingestion by children breast-fed by women on lithium treatment. *Br Med J.* 1973; 2:138.

Schroeder DH. Metabolism and kinetics of bupropion. *Journal of Clinical Psychiatry.* 1983; 44:79-81.

Serebruany VL, Gurbel PA, O'Connor CM. Platelet inhibition by sertraline and N-desmethylsertraline: a possible missing link between depression, coronary events, and mortality benefits of selective serotonin reuptake inhibitors. *Pharmacol Res.* 2001; 43:453-62.

Sinclair D, Murray L. Effects of postnatal depression on children's adjustment to school. Teacher's reports. *Brit J Psychiatry.* 1998; 172:58-63.

Skausig OB, Schou M. Breast feeding during lithium therapy. *Ugeskr Laeger.* 1977; 139:400-1.

Sovner R, Orsulak PJ. Excretion of imipramine and desipramine in human breast milk. *Am J Psychiatry.* 1979; 136:451-52.

Spigset O, Carieborg L, Ohman R, Norstrom A. Excretion of citalopram in breast milk. *Br J Clin Pharmacol.* 1997; 44:295-98.

Spigset O, Carleborg L, Norstrom A, Sandlund M. Paroxetine level in breast milk [letter]. *J Clin Psychiatry.* 1996; 57:39.

Stancer HC, Reed KL. Desipramine and 2-hydroxydesipramine in human breast milk and the nursing infant's serum. *Am J Psychiatry.* 1986; 143:1597-600.

Stewart RB, Karas B, Springer PK. Haloperidol excretion in human milk. *Am J Psychiatry.* 1980; 137:849-50.

Stowe ZN, Cohen LS, Hostetter A, Ritchie JC, Owens MJ, Nemeroff CB. Paroxetine in human breast milk and nursing infants. *Am J Psychiatry.* 2000;157:185-89.

Stowe ZN, Owens MJ, Landry JC, Kilts CD, Ely T, Llewellyn A, *et al.* Sertraline and desmethylsertraline in human breast milk and nursing infants. *Am J Psychiatry.* 1997; 154:1255-60.

Sugawara K, Shimoyama R, Ohkubo T. Determinations of psychotropic drugs and antiepileptic drugs by high-performance liquid chromatogaphy and its monitoring in human breast milk. *Hirosaki Med J.* 1999; 51 (Suppl):S81-86.

Sykes PA, Quarrie J, Alexander FW. Lithium carbonate and breast-feeding. *Br Med J.* 1976; 2:1299.

Taddio A, Ito S, Koren G. Excretion of fluoxetine and its metabolite, norfluoxetine, in human breast milk. *J Clin Pharmacol.* 1996; 36:42-47.

The American Academy of Pediatrics Committee on Drugs. Transfer of drugs and other chemicals into human milk. *Pediatrics.* 2001; 108:776-89.

Timmer CJ, Sitsen JM, Delbressine LP. Clinical pharmacokinetics of mirtazapine. *Clin Pharmacokinet.* 2000; 38:461-74.

Tunnessen WW Jr, Hertz CG. Toxic effects of lithium in newborn infants: a commentary. *J Pediatr.* 1972; 81:804-7.

Uhlir F, Ryznar J. Appearance of chlorpromazine in the mother's milk. *Act Nerv Super (Praha).* 1973; 15:106.

Ulrich S, Neuhof S, Braun V, Meyer FP. Therapeutic window of serum haloperidol concentration in acute schizophrenia and schizoaffective disorder. *Pharmacopsychiatry.* 1998; 31:163-69.

US National Library of Medicine. *Drugs and lactation database (LactMed).* TOXNET Toxicology Data Network. 2007. Available from: http://toxnet.nlm.nih.gov/cgi-bin/sis/htmlgen?LACT.

Venkatakrishnan K, von Moltke LL, Greenblatt DJ. Nortriptyline E-10-hydroxylation in vitro is mediated by human CYP2D6 (high affinity) and CYP3A4 (low affinity): implications for interactions with enzyme-inducing drugs. *J Clin Pharmacol.* 1999; 39:567-77.

Verbeeck RK, Ross SG, McKenna EA. Excretion of trazodone in breast milk. *Br J Pharmacol.* 1986; 22:367-70.

Viguera AC, Newport DJ, Ritchie J, Stowe Z, Whitfield T, Mogielnicki J, *et al.* Lithium in breast milk and nursing infants: clinical implications. *Am J Psychiatry.* 2007; 164:342-45.

Viguera AC, Nonacs R, Cohen LS, Tondo L, Murray A, Baldessarini RJ. Risk of recurrence of bipolar disorder in pregnant and nonpregnant women after discontinuing lithium maintenance. *Am J Psychiatry.* 2000; 157:179-84.

Weinstein MR, Goldfield M. Lithium carbonate treatment during pregnancy; report of a case. *Dis Nerv Syst.* 1969; 30:828-32.

Weissman AM, Levy BT, Hartz AJ, Bentler S, Donohue M, Ellingrod VL, *et al.* Pooled analysis of antidepressant levels in lactating mothers, breast milk, and nursing infants. *Am J Psychiatry.* 2004; 161:1066-78.

Whalley LJ, Blain PG, Prime JK. Haloperidol secreted in breast milk. *Br Med J (Clin Res Ed).* 1981; 282:1746-47.

Wiles DH, Orr MW, Kolakowska T. Chlorpromazine levels in plasma and milk of nursing mothers. *Br J Clin Pharmacol.* 1978; 5:272-73.

Wise MG, Javors MA, Funderburg LG. Lithium levels in bodily fluids of a nursing mother and infant. *Lithium.* 1990; 1:189-91 (cited by Toxnet/LactMed Database, accessed 04-30/2007).

Wisner KL, Parry BL, Piontek CM. Clinical practice. Postpartum depression. *New Engl J Med.* 2002; 347:194-99.

Wisner KL, Perel JM. Serum nortriptyline levels in nursing mothers and their infants. *Am J Psychiatry.* 1991; 148:1234-36.

Wisner KL, Perel JM, Blumer J. Serum sertraline and N-desmethylsertraline levels in breast-feeding mother-infant pairs. *Am J Psychiatry.* 1998; 155:690-92.

Wisner KL, Perel JM, Findling RL, Hinnes RL. Nortriptyline and its hydroxymetabolites in breastfeeding mothers and newborns. *Psychopharmacol Bull.* 1997; 33:249-51.

Wisner KL, Perel JM, Foglia JP. Serum clomipramine and metabolite levels in four nursing mother-infant pairs. *J Clin Psychiatry.* 1995; 56:17-20.

Wright S, Dawling S, Ashford JJ. Excretion of fluvoxamine in breast milk. *Br J Clin Pharmacol.* 1991; 31:209.

Yoshida K, Marks MN, Craggs M, Smith B, Kumar R. Sensorimotor and cognitive development of infants of mothers with schizophrenia. *Brit J Psychiatry.* 1999a; 175:380-87.

Yoshida K, Smith B, Channikumar R. Fluvoxamine in breast-milk and infant development. *Br J Clin Pharmacol.* 1997a; 44:210-11.

Yoshida K, Smith B, Craggs M, Kumar R. Neuroleptic drugs in breast-milk: a study of pharmacokinetics and of possible adverse effects in breast-fed infants. *Psychol Med.* 1998a; 28:81-91.

Yoshida K, Smith B, Craggs M, Kumar RC. Investigation of pharmacokinetics and of possible adverse effects in infants exposed to tricyclic antidepressants in breast-milk. *J Affect Disord.* 1997b; 43:225-37.

Yoshida K, Smith B, Craggs M, Kumar RC. Fluoxetine in breast-milk and developmental outcome of breast-fed infants. *Brit J Psychiatry.* 1998b; 172:175-78.

Yoshida K, Smith B, Kumar R. Psychotropic drugs in mothers' milk: a comprehensive review of assay methods, pharmacokinetics and of safety of breast-feeding. *J Psychopharmacol.* 1999b; 13:64-80.

Zekoski EM, O'Hara MW, Wills KE. The effects of maternal mood on mother-infant interaction. *J Abnorm Child Psychol.* 1987; 15:361-78.

Zeskind PS, Stephens LE. Maternal selective serotonin reuptake inhibitor use during pregnancy and newborn neurobehavior. *Pediatrics.* 2004; 113:368-75.

Chapter 31

Antihypertensives, Diuretics, and Anticoagulants

Judith H. Kristensen and Kenneth F. Ilett

INTRODUCTION

Breastfeeding women frequently require prescribed drugs for hypertension. The drugs used in this area have the potential to cause bradycardia and hypotension that might be recognized in the infant as cyanosis. There have been two reviews of these classes of drugs in recent years (Beardmore *et al.*, 2002; Qasqas *et al.*, 2004), and detailed monographs for many individual drugs are also available (Hale, 2006).

As with all maternal drug use during lactation, the questions that need to be asked are (a) is there significant drug transfer into milk, (b) is drug exposure likely to cause any short-term toxicity in the infant, and (c) is drug exposure likely to cause any long-term adverse effects in the infant? In this chapter, we summarize the safety of representative antihypertensives, diuretics and anticoagulants in **Tables 1 and 2** and also discuss selected drugs in detail in the text.

ANTIHYPERTENSIVES

β-Adrenoceptor Blockers

Low plasma protein binding has been suggested to be an important factor in drug transfer from plasma to milk (Atkinson *et al.*, 1988) and has been suggested as a means of selecting "safe" β-blockers for use in lactation (Anderson, 2006; Riant *et al.*, 1986). This latter concept has also been endorsed by the authors of LactMed, who have additionally drawn attention to the half-life of the drug and to the extent of its renal excretion as additional indicators of infant exposure (http://toxnet.nlm.nih.gov). We previously suggested that lipophilicity of the β-blocker could be inversely related to its relative infant dose (Hale *et al.*, 2002). Nevertheless, neither protein binding nor lipophilicity are robust predictors of the potential for adverse effects in the breastfed infant. In addition, for protein binding, the primary outcome variable in the correlation between infant exposure and protein binding for β-blockers was M/P (Riant *et al.*, 1986), which we now know to be a flawed predictor of drug safety in lactation. Indeed, as suggested specifically for β-blockers (Atkinson *et al.*, 1990), and as is the case with all drugs (Atkinson *et al.*, 1988), it is more appropriate to consider the potential for adverse events in the breastfed infant in terms of the relative infant dose. It is interesting that a recent review also recommended the use of protein binding as a marker for high infant exposure when experimental data are unavailable (Anderson, 2006).

The various physicochemical and pharmacokinetic properties of a range of β-adrenoceptor blockers as well as their relative infant doses are summarized in **Table 1.** More detailed data on relative infant dose for common orally administered β-adrenoceptor blockers are also summarized in **Table 2.**

Acebutolol and atenolol have been associated with adverse events, such as hypotension, bradycardia, and transient tachypnea in breastfed infants (Boutroy *et al.*, 1986; Schimmel *et al.*, 1989). Measurable serum or urine levels of atenolol have also been found in exposed breastfed infants, some of whom showed symptoms of β-blockade (Bhamra *et al.*, 1983; Kulas *et al.*, 1984; Liedholm *et al.*, 1981; Liedholm, 1983; Schimmel *et al.*, 1989). No adverse effects have been reported in infants exposed to metoprolol (Ho *et al.*, 1999; Schimmel *et al.*, 1989), or labetalol (Michael, 1979), and there is no published information for propranolol.

The comments on compatibility of the β-blockers with breastfeeding (**Table 1**) are our distillation of published relative infant dose data, route of administration (dose after ocular administration likely to be very low), and expert opinion (The American Academy of Pediatrics Committee on Drugs, 2001). Drugs, such as propranolol (Smith *et al.*, 1983), metoprolol (Sandstrom *et al.*, 1980), and labetalol, with a low relative infant dose and minimal reports of adverse effects in breastfed infants, are preferred over atenolol, sotalol, and acebutolol, which generally have a higher relative infant dose and for which there are reports of adverse effects in breastfed infants.

As discussed above, although values for either plasma protein binding or log D_{pH7} [logarithm of the octanol/water partition coefficient at pH7, for the mixture of the neutral and ionic forms of the drug (Chemical Abstract Services, 2006)] superficially appear to predict the extent to which β-blockers may cause problems in breastfeeding, it is our view that this association can be predictive only in a general way. In the final analysis, reports of relative infant dose, plasma concentrations, and/or effects (or lack thereof) in exposed infants are the best data on which decisions about the safety of breastfeeding can be made. Second, the likelihood of accumulation of a β-blocker by the exposed breastfed infant (and hence of toxicity) may be refined by looking at adult data for drug half-life and the extent to which the kidney excretes the drug unchanged. This consideration could be particularly important for neonates where renal function is not fully developed.

Some β-blockers are used primarily as eye drops in the treatment of glaucoma (e.g., timolol, betaxolol, levobunolol). While there is measurable but variable

Table 1. Physicochemical and Pharmacokinetic Descriptors and Relative Infant Doses of Representative β-blockers (oral administration unless otherwise specified)

Drug	log D_{pH7}[1]	Plasma protein binding (%)[2]	Half-life (h)[2]	Renal excretion parent drug[2] (%)	Relative infant dose (%)[9]	Comments for use in breastfeeding
Atenolol	-2.02	3	7-9	90	4.9-33.6	Compatible but not preferred.
Sotalol	-1.82	5	12.7	75	18	Compatible but not preferred.
Timolol	-1.77	10	2.6[5]	ND	0.96-1.2	Compatible. Predominant ocular use. Exposure likely to be low.
Nadolol	-0.83	25[14]	22[13]	70[14]	4.8[13]	Compatible.
Metoprolol	-0.33	12	3-5	3	2-4.4	Compatible.
Pindolol	-0.18	40	3.3	40	ND	Compatible but not preferred.
Acebutolol	-0.11	15	4[6]		3.9[3]	Compatible but not preferred.
Bisprolol	0.03	35	10-12	50	ND	Compatible but not preferred.
Oxprenolol	0.17	80	1-2	2-5	ND	Compatible but not preferred.
Labetalol	0.33	52	6-8	5	0.06-0.57	Compatible.
Dilevalol (R,R'-labetalol)	0.33	ND	8.3[7]	ND	0.007[8]	Compatible.
Betaxolol	0.56	50	14.7[4]	15[10]	ND	Compatible. Predominant ocular use. Exposure likely to be low.
Levobunolol	0.77	ND	6.1[11]	14.7[12]	ND	Compatible. Predominant ocular use. Exposure likely to be low.
Propranolol	1	93	3-6	0-5	0.03-0.7	Compatible.
Carvedilol	2.93	98	6-10	Very low	ND	Compatible but not preferred.

[1] Logarithm of octanol/water partition coefficient at pH7 for the mixture of the neutral and ionic forms of the drug (Chemical Abstract Services, 2006); [2] Manufacturer's Product Information (eMIMS, 2006) unless otherwise specified; [3] Boutroy *et al.*, 1986; [4] Stagni *et al.*, 1991; [5] Kaila *et al.*, 1993; [6] Lilja *et al.*, 2005; [7] Kramer *et al.*, 1988; [8] Radwanski *et al.*, 1988; [9] From **Table 2** unless otherwise specified; [10] http://products.sanofi-aventis.us/kerlone/kerlone.html ; [11] Di Carlo *et al.*, 1977; [12] Leinweber *et al.*, 1978; [13] Devlin *et al.*, 1981a; [14] LactMed (http://toxnet.nlm.nih.gov); ND=no data available

systemic absorption (and effects) following conjunctival application of these drugs (Salminen, 1990), the dose is small (usually 1-2 drops of a 0.25-0.5% solution administered once or twice daily), and significant transfer to the breastfed infant is unlikely. There is one report of no adverse effects in a breastfed infant whose mother was using 0.5% timolol eye drops twice daily in the right eye (Lustgarten *et al.*, 1983).

Angiotensin Converting Enzyme Inhibitors and Angiotensin II Receptor Blockers

Fetal mortality and morbidity have been reported when angiotensin converting enzyme inhibitor drugs or angiotensin II receptor blockers were used to treat hypertension during the second half of pregnancy (Quan, 2006). Adverse effects reported include oligohydramnios, fetal growth restriction, stillbirth, and neonatal renal failure. Caution has therefore been recommended in their use in lactation when the infant is preterm or very young (Hale, 2004).

Nevertheless, the angiotensin converting enzyme inhibitors captopril, enalapril, and quinapril have low to very low relative infant doses (0.01%, 0.3%, and 1.6%, respectively), and there are no reports of adverse events from their use during breastfeeding (Begg *et al.*, 2001; Devlin *et al.*, 1981b; Huttunen *et al.*, 1989; Redman *et al.*, 1990). Presently, there are no studies of the use of fosinopril, lisinopril perindopril, ramipril, or trandolapril during lactation.

There is one report of low milk production in one of 12 lactating women studied while taking 100 mg captopril thrice daily (Devlin *et al.*, 1981b). However, in controlled studies, neither captopril or enalapril altered prolactin levels in normal or hyperprolactinemic subjects (Anderson *et al.*, 1989). Hence, the low milk production in the one woman in Devlin's 1981 study seems unlikely to have been related to captopril. The American Academy of Pediatrics lists these agents as being usually compatible with breastfeeding (American Academy of Pediatrics Committee on Drugs, 2001). There are presently no data on milk concentrations, infant dose, or adverse effects for the angiotensin II receptor blockers, such as candesartan, eprosartan, irbesartan, losartan, or telmisartan. Until relevant data are available, it would seem prudent to use alternative antihypertensives during lactation.

Calcium Channel Blockers

Relative infant doses reported for these agents are low (nifedipine 1-2.4%) (Ehrenkranz *et al.*, 1989; Manninen *et al.*, 1991; Penny *et al.*, 1989), verapamil (0.1-1%) (Anderson *et al.*, 1987; Inoue *et al.*, 1984; Miller *et al.*, 1986), and diltiazem (1%) (Okada *et al.*, 1985). Low serum levels of verapamil (2 μg/L) were reported in one neonate where the mother was taking 80 mg verapamil thrice daily, but transplacental transfer may have been involved (Andersen, 1983). Two older infants had no detectable plasma levels of verapamil or its nor-metabolite following maternal doses of 100 mg and 80 mg thrice daily (Anderson *et al.*, 1987; Miller *et al.*, 1986). As well as its use as an antihypertensive agent, nifedipine (usual dose 30 mg/day) is also used as a treatment for the pain associated with nipple vasospasm (Anderson *et al.*, 2004; Page *et al.*, 2006). The calcium channel blockers are usually compatible with breastfeeding (American Academy of Pediatrics Committee on Drugs, 2001).

Diuretics

Some of these compounds have been used early after birth to prevent the establishment of lactation and may therefore be expected to inhibit milk production (Cominos *et al.*, 1976; Healy, 1961; Miller *et al.*, 1982; Reiher, 1963; Stout, 1962). At least for furosemide, this effect is not mediated through a decrease in prolactin levels (Kalk *et al.*, 1977). Nevertheless, suppression of established lactation does not appear to be a significant problem with diuretics, and they are generally compatible with breastfeeding (American Academy of Pediatrics Committee on Drugs, 2001).

Other Antihypertensive Agents

In this area, we have chosen to consider hydralazine (direct smooth muscle vasodilator), methyldopa (a dopa decarboxylase inhibitor), and prazosin (α_2-adrenoceptor blocker) which are used in the treatment of pregnancy-induced hypertension, and where treatment may extend into the early part of lactation (**Table 1**). In addition, we have reviewed clonidine (central α_2-adrenoceptor agonist) because of its use in hypertension, migraine, and recurrent vascular headache prophylaxis (**Table 1**).

Hydralazine has a low relative infant dose of 0.9%, and no adverse effects were seen in one infant who was breastfed for eight weeks (Liedholm *et al.*, 1982).

Table 2. Antihypertensives, Diuretics, and Anticoagulants in Breastfeeding

Drug	Relative infant dose (%)	Comment	References
Antihypertensives			
Beta blockers			
Atenolol	4.9- 33.6	Compatible. Other agents preferred. Detected in infant plasma, and adverse effects reported in some infants.	Atkinson *et al.*, 1988a; Bhamra *et al.*, 1983; Kulas *et al.*, 1984; Thorley *et al.*, 1983; White *et al.*, 1984
Labetolol	0.06-0.57	Compatible. No adverse effects.	Leitz *et al.*, 1983; Lunell *et al.*, 1985; Michael, 1979
Metoprolol	2– 4.4	Compatible.	Kulas *et al.*, 1984; Liedholm *et al.*, 1981; Lindeberg *et al.*, 1984; Sandstrom *et al.*, 1980
Propranolol	0.03-0.7	Compatible.	Bauer *et al.*, 1979; Karlberg *et al.*, 1974; Lewis *et al.*, 1981; Smith *et al.*, 1983; Thorley *et al.*, 1983
Sotalol	20-23	Compatible. Other agents preferred.	Hackett *et al.*, 1990
ACE Inhibitors			
Captopril	0.02	Compatible. No adverse effects reported in infants, but caution with preterm infants due to possible renal toxicity of ACE inhibitors.	Devlin *et al.*, 1981b
Enalapril	0.17, 0.2, 0.27	Compatible.	Redman *et al.*, 1990; Rush *et al.*, 1991
Quinapril	1.6	Compatible.	Begg *et al.*, 2001
Other ACE inhibitors	ND	Probably compatible, but consider alternative agents where data are available.	
Calcium channel blockers			
Diltiazem	1	Compatible.	Okada *et al.*, 1985
Nifedipine	0.1, 1.2,1.8	Compatible.	Ehrenkranz *et al.*, 1989; Manninen *et al.*, 1991; Penny *et al.*, 1989; Taddio *et al.*, 1996
Verapamil	0.1, 0.2, 0.3, 1.0	Compatible.	Andersen, 1983; Anderson *et al.*, 1987; Inoue *et al.*, 1984; Miller *et al.*, 1986
Others			
Clonidine	4.8 – 9.9	Moderate transfer to milk. Significant infant plasma levels obtained. Consider alternative.	Boutroy *et al.*, 1988; Bunjes *et al.*, 1993;, Hartikainen-Sorri *et al.*, 1987; Heim *et al.*, 1979
Hydralazine	0.9	Compatible. Low transfer to milk. Infant dose low compared with clinical infant dose 0.25-1mg/kg/dose 6-8 hourly.	Liedholm *et al.*, 1982; Young *et al.*, 2003
Methyldopa	0.7, 0.84	Compatible.	Jones *et al.*, 1978; White *et al.*, 1985
Prazosin	ND	No data. Others preferred.	
Diuretics			
Chlorothiazide	ND	Less than 1 μg/L in milk after a 500 mg single dose. Can decrease milk supply.	Healy, 1961; Reiher, 1963; Stout, 1962; Werthmann, Jr. *et al.*, 1972
Chlorthalidone	3.8	Has been used to suppress lactation. Low transfer to milk. No effect in established lactation.	Mulley *et al.*, 1978; Reiher, 1963; Vercruysse, 1966
Furosemide	ND	Amount in milk unknown.	Cominos *et al.*, 1976; Healy, 1961
Hydrochlorothiazide	5.8 (calculated from peak)	Low transfer to milk. Not detectable in infant plasma. Can decrease milk supply at higher doses.	Healy, 1961; Miller *et al.*, 1982; Reiher, 1963; Stout, 1962
Indapamide	ND	Can decrease milk supply. No data on milk transfer or infant effects, and others therefore preferred.	Healy, 1961; Reiher, 1963; Stout, 1962
Spironolactone	0.8 (as active metabolite)	Low transfer to milk. Unlikely to suppress lactation.	Phelps *et al.*, 1977

Anticoagulants			
Warfarin	ND	No drug detected in milk or drug activity in infant plasma. No adverse effects in infants. Compatible.	Ito *et al.*, 1993; McKenna *et al.*, 1983; Orme *et al.*, 1977
Heparin	ND	Compatible.	Not studied.
Dalteparin	ND	Compatible.	Harenberg *et al.*, 1987; Richter *et al.*, 2001
Enoxaparin	ND	Approximate molecular weight 4,500 daltons. Not detected in milk. Anticoagulant activity undetected in milk. No bleeding in infants. Compatible.	Guillonneau *et al.*, 1996
Lepirudin	ND	Not detectable in milk (<0.1 mg/L) in one patient. No bleeding in exposed infant.	Lindhoff-Last *et al.*, 2000
Nadroparin	ND	Expected to behave similarly to dalteparin and enoxaparin.	Not studied.
ND= no data available			

Methyldopa also has a low relative infant dose (0.7% and 0.84%) at usual therapeutic doses (250 mg 3-4 times daily) (Jones *et al.*, 1978; White *et al.*, 1985). Methyldopa was not measurable in the infant's plasma, but was detected in urine (Hauser *et al.*, 1985). Nevertheless, several studies show no adverse effects in the breastfed infant (Hauser *et al.*, 1985; Hoskins *et al.*, 1982; Jones *et al.*, 1978; White *et al.*, 1985). There are no data for prazosin, and it is therefore best avoided. Despite small maternal dose rates for clonidine (usually 150 μg twice daily), the relative infant dose ranges from 4.8-9.9% (Boutroy *et al.*, 1988; Bunjes *et al.*, 1993; Hartikainen-Sorri *et al.*, 1987). Although infant serum levels of clonidine were <96 μg/L in one exposed infant (Bunjes *et al.*, 1993), levels ranging from 350-690 μg/L were consistently detected in nine exposed infants across the first 60 days of lactation (Hartikainen-Sorri *et al.*, 1987). These levels were about 66% of those measured simultaneously in the mother's serum. Typical adult clonidine side-effects (sedation) were not seen in these exposed infants (Hartikainen-Sorri *et al.*, 1987). Three breastfed infants whose mothers took usual therapeutic doses of clonidine also showed normal growth and psychomotor development at 12 months of age (Boutroy *et al.*, 1988). Although clonidine has been reported to cause postpartum hyperprolactinemia and galactorrhea (Heim *et al.*, 1979), it is unlikely to alter an established lactation. In summary, although clonidine use may be compatible in lactation, the high levels of infant exposure suggest that alternative medications should be explored first.

Anticoagulants

Warfarin is highly protein bound and on theoretical grounds would be expected to transfer poorly into milk. This indeed is the case, with no drug detected in milk (McKenna *et al.*, 1983; Orme *et al.*, 1977) or adverse effects in breastfed infants (Ito *et al.*, 1993). Hence, warfarin is considered compatible during lactation (American Academy of Pediatrics Committee on Drugs, 2001; Clark *et al.*, 2000).

Heparin and the newer low molecular weight heparins (dalteparin, enoxaparin, and nadroparin) are all acidic mucopolysaccharides. Heparin is composed of a mixture of polysaccharides with molecular weights from 6,000 to 26,000 daltons (commercial production material usually 12,000 to 15,000 daltons). The other three are produced from heparin by controlled depolymerization to yield dalteparin (molecular weight 4,000-6,000), enoxaparin (mean molecular weight 4,500), and nadroparin (mean molecular weight 4,500). The final drug in this area is lepirudin, a single-chain polypeptide of about 65 amino acids (7000 daltons) that is derived from leeches. It has a neutral hydrophobic N terminus, an acidic hydrophilic C terminus, and a compact, hydrophobic core region.

On theoretical grounds, such large molecules are unlikely to transfer into milk or to be absorbed across the infant's gastrointestinal cell barriers. Moreover, they are acid labile and would be expected to breakdown in the infant's gastrointestinal tract and have very low bioavailability. Heparin itself has not been studied, but given its much larger molecular weight range, it is predicted to be less likely to transfer into milk than its depolymerized derivatives. There are limited studies for enoxaparin and lepirudin that broadly support the proposition of low milk transfer (Guillonneau *et al.*, 1996; Lindhoff-Last *et al.*, 2000). Dalteparin has conflicting data with one study showing no drug in milk

(Harenberg *et al.*, 1987) and a second demonstrating anticoagulant activity in milk ranging from 2.5-22.4% of that in maternal plasma (Richter *et al.*, 2001). The reason for the discrepancy is unclear.

CONCLUSION

The relative infant dose for these drugs is perhaps the most useful primary guide to assessing safety of drug use in lactation, but needs to be interpreted together with evidence of levels of these drugs in infant serum and case reports/studies of adverse effects (or lack thereof) in exposed infants. When weighing the information from any report, due consideration should be given to the number of subjects studied and the quality of the data, particularly if they are related to adverse events. With regard to the latter, it is worth remembering that a review of the literature found only 100 adverse event reports up to 2003 (Anderson *et al.*, 2003). Only 47% of adverse events were "probably" attributable to the suspected drug. As with all drug use in breastfeeding, an individual risk/benefit analysis should be conducted before starting therapy.

On balance, the data suggest that there are few contraindications to breastfeeding for mothers who need to take antihypertensives or anticoagulants. Some β-blockers are clearly better avoided because of high relative infant doses and reports of adverse effects. Clonidine is probably best avoided on the basis of its high levels in infant serum compared to those in paired maternal serum samples.

References

American Academy of Pediatrics Committee on Drugs. Transfer of drugs and other chemicals into human milk. *Pediatrics.* 2001; 108:776-89.

Andersen HJ. Excretion of verapamil in human milk. *Eur J Clin Pharmacol.* 1983; 25:279-80.

Anderson GD. Using pharmacokinetics to predict the effects of pregnancy and maternal-infant transfer of drugs during lactation. *Expert Opinion on Drug Metabolism and Toxicology.* 2006; 2:947-60.

Anderson JE, Held N, Wright K. Raynaud's phenomenon of the nipple: a treatable cause of painful breastfeeding. *Pediatrics.* 2004; 113:360-64.

Anderson P, Bondesson U, Mattiasson I, Johansson BW. Verapamil and norverapamil in plasma and breastmilk during breastfeeding. *Eur J Clin Pharmacol.* 1987; 31:625-27.

Anderson PO, Pochop SL, Manoguerra AS. Adverse drug reactions in breastfed infants: less than imagined. *Clin Pediatr (Phila).* 2003; 42:325-40.

Anderson PW, Malarkey WB, Salk J, Kletsky OA, Hsueh WA. The effect of angiotensin-converting enzyme inhibition on prolactin responses in normal and hyperprolactinemic subjects. *J Clin Endocrinol Metab.* 1989; 69:518-22.

Atkinson H, Begg EJ. Concentrations of beta-blocking drugs in human milk. *J Pediatr.* 1990; 116:156.

Atkinson HC, Begg EJ, Darlow BA. Drugs in human milk. Clinical pharmacokinetic considerations. *Clin Pharmacokinet.* 1988; 14:217-40.

Bauer JH, Pape B, Zajicek J, Groshong T. Propranolol in human plasma and breast milk. *Am J Cardiol.* 1979; 43:860-62.

Beardmore KS, Morris JM, Gallery ED. Excretion of antihypertensive medication into human breast milk: a systematic review. *Hypertens Pregnancy.* 2002; 21:85-95.

Begg EJ, Robson RA, Gardiner SJ, Hudson LJ, Reece PA, Olson SC, *et al.* Quinapril and its metabolite quinaprilat in human milk. *Br J Clin Pharmacol.* 2001; 51:478-81.

Bhamra RK, Thorley KJ, Vale JA, Holt DW. High-performance liquid chromatographic measurement of atenolol: methodology and clinical applications. *Ther Drug Monit.* 1983; 5:313-18.

Boutroy MJ, Bianchetti G, Dubruc C, Vert P, Morselli PL. To nurse when receiving acebutolol: is it dangerous for the neonate? *Eur J Clin Pharmacol.* 1986; 30:737-39.

Boutroy MJ, Gisonna CR, Legagneur M. Clonidine: placental transfer and neonatal adaption. *Early Hum Dev.* 1988; 17:275-86.

Bunjes R, Schaefer C, Holzinger D. Clonidine and breast-feeding [letter]. *Clin Pharm.* 1993; 12:178-79.

Chemical Abstract Services. SciFinder Scholar. American Chemical Society, Washington DC, USA. 2006; Available from: http://cas.org./SCIFINDER/SCHOLAR/.

Clark SL, Porter TF, West FG. Coumarin derivatives and breast-feeding. *Obstet Gynecol.* 2000; 95:938-40.

Cominos DC, van der WA, van Rooyen AJ. Suppression of postpartum lactation with furosemide. *S Afr Med J.* 1976; 50:251-52.

Devlin RG, Duchin KL, Fleiss PM. Nadolol in human serum and breast milk. *Br J Clin Pharmacol.* 1981a; 12:393-96.

Devlin RG, Fleiss PM. Captopril in human blood and breast milk. *J Clin Pharmacol.* 1981b; 21:110-13.

Di Carlo FJ, Leinweber FJ, Szpiech JM, Davidson IW. Metabolism of l-bunolol. *Clin Pharmacol Ther.* 1977; 22:858-63.

Ehrenkranz RA, Ackerman BA, Hulse JD. Nifedipine transfer into human milk. *J Pediatr.* 1989; 114:478-80.

eMIMS. *MIMS Abbreviated prescribing information.* St Leonards, Australia: CMPMedica Australia Pty Ltd.; 2006. Version 5.00.0270

Guillonneau M, de CA, Aufrant C, Hurtaud-Roux MF, Jacqz-Aigrain E. Breast-feeding is possible in case of maternal treatment with enoxaparin. *Arch Pediatr.* 1996; 3:513-14.

Hackett LP, Wojnar-Horton RE, Dusci LJ, Ilett KF, Roberts MJ. Excretion of sotalol in breast milk. *Br J Clin Pharmacol.* 1990; 29:277-78.

Hale TW. Maternal medications during breastfeeding. *Clin Obstet Gynecol.* 2004; 47:696-711.

Hale TW. *Medications and mothers' milk.* 12th Ed. Amarillo, TX, USA: Pharmasoft Publishing; 2006.

Hale TW, Ilett KF. *Drug therapy and breastfeeding. From theory to clinical practice.* 1st Ed. London: The Parthenon Publishing Group; 2002.

Harenberg J, Leber G, Zimmermann R, Schmidt W. Prevention of thromboembolism with low-molecular weight heparin in pregnancy. *Geburtshilfe Frauenheilkd.* 1987; 47:15-18.

Hartikainen-Sorri AL, Heikkinen JE, Koivisto M. Pharmacokinetics of clonidine during pregnancy and nursing. *Obstet Gynecol.* 1987; 69:598-600.

Hauser GJ, Almog S, Tirosh M, Spirer Z. Effect of alpha-methyldopa excreted in human milk on the breast-fed infant. *Helv Paediatr Acta.* 1985; 40:83-86.

Healy M. Suppressing lactation with oral diuretics. *Lancet.* 1961;1:1353-54.

Heim J, Massart C, Auvray E, Allannic H. Post-partum galactorrhea with hyperprolactinaemia persistent during a clonidine treatment (author's transl). *Sem Hop.* 1979; 55:1933-34.

Ho TK, Moretti ME, Shaeffer IJ, Ito S, Koren G. Maternal beta-blocker usage and breast feeding in the neonate. *Pediatr Res.* 1999; 45:67A.

Hoskins JA, Holliday SB. Determination of alpha-methyldopa and methyldopate in human breast milk and plasma by ion-exchange chromatography using electrochemical detection. *J Chromatogr Biomed Appl.* 1982; 230:162-67.

Huttunen K, Gronhagen-Riska C, Fyhrquist F. Enalapril treatment of a nursing mother with slightly impaired renal function. *Clin Nephrol.* 1989; 31:278.

Inoue H, Unno N, Ou MC, Iwama Y, Sugimoto T. Level of verapamil in human milk [letter]. *Eur J Clin Pharmacol.* 1984; 26:657-58.

Ito S, Blajchman A, Stephenson M, Eliopoulos C, Koren G. Prospective follow-up of adverse reactions in breast-fed infants exposed to maternal medication. *Am J Obstet Gynecol.* 1993; 168:1393-99.

Jones HM, Cummings AJ. A study of the transfer of alpha-methyldopa to the human foetus and newborn infant. *Br J Clin Pharmacol.* 1978; 6:432-34.

Kaila T, Karhuvaara S, Huupponen R, Iisalo E. The analysis of plasma kinetics and beta-receptor binding and -blocking activity of timolol following its small intravenous dose. *Int J Clin Pharmacol.* 1993; 31:351-57.

Kalk WJ, Cominos DC, van der WA, van Rooyen AJ. The effect of furosemide on serum prolactin levels in the postpartum period. *S Afr Med J.* 1977; 52:485-86.

Karlberg B, Lundberg D, Aberg H. Letter: Excretion of propranolol in human breast milk. *Acta Pharmacol Toxicol (Copenh).* 1974; 34:222-24.

Kramer WG, Nagabhushan N, Affrime MB, Perentesis GP, Symchowicz S, Patrick JE. Pharmacokinetics and bioavailability of dilevalol in normotensive volunteers. *J Clin Pharmacol.* 1988; 28:644-48.

Kulas J, Lunell NO, Rosing U, Steen B, Rane A. Atenolol and metoprolol. A comparison of their excretion into human breast milk. *Acta Obstet Gynecol Scand Suppl.* 1984; 118:65-69.

Leinweber FJ, Szpiech JM, Di Carlo FJ. l-Bunolol metabolites in human urine. *Pharmacology.* 1978; 16:70-77.

Leitz F, Bariletto S, Gural R, Jaworsky L, Patrick J, Symchowicz S. Secretion of labetalol in breast-milk of lactating women. *Fed Proc.* 1983; 42:378.

Lewis AM, Patel L, Johnston A, Turner P. Mexiletine in human blood and breast milk. *Postgrad Med J.* 1981; 57:546-47.

Liedholm H. Transplacental passage and breast milk accumulation of atenolol in humans. *Drugs.* 1983; 25 (Suppl 2):217-18.

Liedholm H, Melander A, Bitzen PO, Helm G, Lonnerholm G, Mattiasson I, *et al.* Accumulation of atenolol and metoprolol in human breast milk. *Eur J Clin Pharmacol.* 1981; 20:229-31.

Liedholm H, Wahlin-Boll E, Hanson A, Ingemarsson I, Melander A. Transplacental passage and breast milk concentrations of hydralazine. *Eur J Clin Pharmacol.* 1982; 21:417-19.

Lilja JJ, Raaska K, Neuvonen PJ. Effects of grapefruit juice on the pharmacokinetics of acebutolol. *Br J Clin Pharmacol.* 2005; 60:659-63.

Lindeberg S, Sandstrom B, Lundborg P, Regardh CG. Disposition of the adrenergic blocker metoprolol in the late-pregnant woman, the amniotic fluid, the cord blood and the neonate. *Acta Obstet Gynecol Scand Suppl.* 1984; 118:61-64.

Lindhoff-Last E, Willeke A, Thalhammer C, Nowak G, Bauersachs R. Hirudin treatment in a breastfeeding woman. *Lancet.* 2000; 355:467-68.

Lunell NO, Kulas J, Rane A. Transfer of labetalol into amniotic fluid and breast milk in lactating women. *Eur J Clin Pharmacol.* 1985; 28:597-99.

Lustgarten JS, Podos SM. Topical timolol and the nursing mother. *Arch Ophthal.* 1983; 101:1381-82.

Manninen AK, Juhakoski A. Nifedipine concentrations in maternal and umbilical serum, amniotic fluid, breast milk and urine of mothers and offspring. *Int J Clin Pharmacol Res.* 1991; 11:231-36.

McKenna R, Cole ER, Vasan U. Is warfarin sodium contraindicated in the lactating mother? *J Pediatr.* 1983; 103:325-27.

Michael CA. Use of labetalol in the treatment of severe hypertension during pregnancy. *Br J Clin Pharmacol.* 1979; 8:211S-15S.

Miller ME, Cohn RD, Burghart PH. Hydrochlorothiazide disposition in a mother and her breast-fed infant. *J Pediatr.* 1982; 101:789-91.

Miller MR, Withers R, Bhamra R, Holt DW. Verapamil and breast-feeding. *Eur J Clin Pharmacol.* 1986; 30:125-26.

Mulley BA, Parr GD, Pau WK, Rye RM, Mould JJ, Siddle NC. Placental transfer of chlorthalidone and its elimination in maternal milk. *Eur J Clin Pharmacol.* 1978; 13:129-31.

Okada M, Inoue H, Nakamura Y, Kishimoto M, Suzuki T. Excretion of diltiazem in human milk [letter]. *New Engl J Med.* 1985; 312:992-93.

Orme ML, Lewis PJ, de SM, Serlin MJ, Sibeon R, Baty JD, *et al.* May mothers given warfarin breast-feed their infants? *Br Med J.* 1977; 1:1564-65.

Page SM, McKenna DS. Vasospasm of the nipple presenting as painful lactation. *Obstet Gynecol.* 2006; 108:806-8.

Penny WJ, Lewis MJ. Nifedipine is excreted in human milk. *Eur J Clin Pharmacol.* 1989; 36:427-28.

Phelps DL, Karim Z. Spironolactone: relationship between concentrations of dethioacetylated metabolite in human serum and milk. *J Pharm Sci.* 1977; 66:1203.

Qasqas SA, McPherson C, Frishman WH, Elkayam U. Cardiovascular pharmacotherapeutic considerations during pregnancy and lactation. *Cardiol Rev.* 2004; 12:201-21.

Quan A. Fetopathy associated with exposure to angiotensin converting enzyme inhibitors and angiotensin receptor antagonists. *Early Hum Dev.* 2006; 82:23-28.

Radwanski E, Nagabhushan N, Affrime MB, Perentesis G, Symchowicz S, Patrick JE. Secretion of dilevalol in breast milk. *J Clin Pharmacol.* 1988; 28:448-53.

Redman CW, Kelly JG, Cooper WD. The excretion of enalapril and enalaprilat in human breast milk. *Eur J Clin Pharmacol.* 1990; 38:99.

Reiher KH. Suppression of lactation by stimulation of diuresis. *Zentralbl Gynakol.* 1963; 85:188-90.

Riant P, Urien S, Albengres E, Duche JC, Tillement JP. High plasma protein binding as a parameter in the selection of betablockers for lactating women. *Biochem Pharmacol.* 1986; 35:4579-81.

Richter C, Sitzmann J, Lang P, Weitzel H, Huch A, Huch R. Excretion of low molecular weight heparin in human milk. *Br J Clin Pharmacol.* 2001; 52:708-10.

Rush JE, Snyder DL, Barrish A, Hichens M. Comment on Huttunen K, Gronhagen-Riska C and Fyhrquist F, 1989. Enalapril treatment of a nursing mother with slightly impaired renal function. Clin Nephrol. 31: 278. *Clin Nephrol.* 1991; 35:234.

Salminen L. Review: systemic absorption of topically applied ocular drugs in humans. *J Ocul Pharmacol.* 1990; 6:243-49.

Sandstrom B, Regardh CG. Metoprolol excretion into breast milk. *Br J Clin Pharmacol.* 1980; 9:518-19.

Schimmel MS, Eidelman AI, Wilschanski MA, Shaw DJ, Ogilvie RJ, Koren G, *et al.* Toxic effects of atenolol consumed during breast feeding. *J Pediatr.* 1989; 114:476-78.

Smith MT, Livingstone I, Hooper WD, Eadie MJ, Triggs EJ. Propranolol, propranolol glucuronide, and naphthoxylactic acid in breast milk and plasma. *Ther Drug Monit.* 1983; 5:87-93.

Stagni G, Davis PJ, Ludden TM. Human pharmacokinetics of betaxolol enantiomers. *J Pharm Sci.* 1991; 80:321-24.

Stout G. Suppression of lactation. *Br Med J.* 1962; 1150.

Taddio A, Oskamp M, Ito S, Bryan H, Farine D, Ryan D, *et al.* Is nifedipine use during labour and breast-feeding safe for the neonate? *Pediatr Res.* 1996; 39:1471.

The American Academy of Pediatrics Committee on Drugs. Transfer of drugs and other chemicals into human milk. *Pediatrics.* 2001; 108:776-89.

Thorley KJ, McAinsh J. Levels of the beta-blockers atenolol and propranolol in the breast milk of women treated for hypertension in pregnancy. *Biopharm Drug Dispos.* 1983; 4:299-301.

US National Library of Medicine. *Drugs and lactation database (LactMed).* TOXNET Toxicology Data Network. 2006. Available from: http://toxnet.nlm.nih.gov/cgi-bin/sis/htmlgen?LACT.

Vercruysse J. Inhibition of lactation. Comparative study of an estro-androgen and of a diuretic. *Brux Med.* 1966; 46:1258-66.

Werthmann MW, Jr., Krees SV. Excretion of chlorothiazide in human breast milk. *J Pediatr.* 1972; 81:781-83.

White WB, Andreoli JW, Cohn RD. Alpha-methyldopa disposition in mothers with hypertension and in their breast-fed infants. *Clin Pharmacol Ther.* 1985; 37:387-90.

White WB, Andreoli JW, Wong SH, Cohn RD. Atenolol in human plasma and breast milk. *Obstet Gynecol.* 1984; 63:42S-44S.

Young TE, Mangum B. *Neofax: A manual of drugs used in neonatal care.* 18th Ed. Raleigh, NC, USA: Acorn Publishing Inc; 2003.

Chapter 32

Antihistamines, Anticholinergics, and Endocrine Drugs

Kenneth F. Ilett and Judith H. Kristensen

INTRODUCTION

Antihistamines are predominantly available over the counter in pharmacies and are widely used in their own right and as components in many cough and cold remedies. One previous review specifically covered the topic, while in another, it was a small part of a larger article (Mitchell, 1999; Spencer *et al.*, 2001). Probably the only anticholinergic agent that breastfeeding mothers may occasionally need to use is hyoscine (scopolamine), either in its role as an anti-nauseant for travel sickness or as an anti-spasmodic for gut pain. The use of endocrine drugs in breastfeeding is also relatively infrequent, but can cover replacement therapy (e.g., insulin, thyroid hormone), corticosteroid use for asthma and other diseases with an inflammatory component, and increasingly, the need for oral antidiabetic drugs in the treatment of type 2 diabetes. Use of endocrine drugs by breastfeeding women was last reviewed as part of a broader article on drugs and breastfeeding (Ilett *et al.*, 2005), and there has also been a review of endocrine-active substances of environmental origin and breastfeeding (Dorea, 2006). When looking for additional or new information on any drugs in these categories, we recommend articles in current journals, as well as textbooks (Briggs *et al.*, 2005b; Hale, 2006), and the US National Library of Medicine TOXNET LactMed data base, available online at http://toxnet.nlm.nih.gov/.

ANTIHISTAMINES

The generic term "antihistamines" conventionally refers to drugs that block histamine H_1 receptors. These drugs are widely used in the community, mainly for their effects in suppressing the inflammatory and allergic effects of histamine on mucous membranes in the eyes, nose, and ears. While some are available only by prescription, most are readily available "over the counter" in pharmacies and hence self-medication is common.

Many of the older "sedating" or "first generation" antihistamines, such as brompheniramine, chlorpheniramine, cyproheptadine, diphenhydramine, doxylamine, promethazine, and triprolidine, readily cross the blood-brain barrier and have significant side-effects (mainly sedation) by blocking H_1 receptors (Skidgel *et al.*, 2006). Diphenhydramine, doxylamine, and promethazine are used for their H_1-blocking central nervous system sedative properties, as well as for their effects on H_1 receptors at mucous membrane surfaces. Many of the first generation antihistamines also have anticholinergic activity. For example, promethazine has strong anticholinergic activity and also is used as an antiemetic in preventing motion sickness, as well as nausea, arising from disorders of the labyrinthine system. The newer "non-sedating" or "second generation" anthistamines, such as cetirizine, fexofenadine (the active metabolite of terfenadine), and loratidine, have negligible or poor penetration across the blood-brain barrier and hence their effects are predominantly at H_1 receptors in the periphery (Skidgel *et al.*, 2006). Nevertheless, the manufacturer's product information for cetirizine notes that the drug may cause mild sedation. The incidence of somnolesence was 14.7% in patients taking the drug, compared to 7.6% for a matched placebo group (Anonymous, 2007b). Cyproheptadine also blocks 5-HT_2 receptors and therefore finds use in the treatment of migraine, while levocabastine is a selective second-generation H_1-receptor antagonist used for allergic conjunctivitis.

The major but largely theoretical concern with breastfeeding and the maternal use of older sedating antihistamines is the possibility of irritability, drowsiness, and poor feeding in exposed infants (Simons, 2003). Nevertheless, the data for first generation antihistamines (**Table 1**) clearly indicate that breastmilk transfer and effects in exposed infants have received only very limited study. In the absence of published data, the conservative view is to recommend that antihistamines should be restricted to short-term use during breastfeeding, that exposed infants should be monitored for any signs of irritability and drowsiness, and that the non-sedating antihistamines should be preferentially used. Although there are no data for levocabastine, it is only used topically for allergic conjunctivitis and infant exposure is therefore not likely to be a problem.

There has also been concern that the sedating antihistamines may decrease prolactin secretion in the anterior pituitary and thereby decrease milk supply. Histamine and 5-HT (5-hydroxytryptamine) are two neurotransmitters that can negatively regulate the secretion of dopamine in the neurons of the tuberoinfundibular system (Freeman *et al.*, 2000). This system connects directly with the anterior pituitary where prolactin is synthesized and secreted, and a decrease in dopamine leads to an increase in prolactin secretion. Conversely, in non-pregnant women, the antihistamines promethazine and dexchlorpheniramine block H_1 receptors in the tuberoinfundibular neurones and have been shown to increase dopamine, and thus to decrease prolactin secretion by the anterior pituitary (Pontiroli *et al.*, 1981; Messinis *et al.*, 1985). However, in breastfeeding women, these two antihistamines did not alter the normal suckling-induced increase in prolactin secretion (Messinis *et al.*, 1985). Overall, as a group, the sedating antihistamines are therefore unlikely to affect milk production. Nevertheless, some authorities recommend that cyproheptadine should be avoided as it may decrease milk production (Anonymous, 2007a). There is no direct evidence for this claim, but the dual effects of the drug on blocking both H_1 and $5HT_2$ receptors in the tuberoinfundibular system may provide an explanation for the suggestion.

Our understanding of the newer non-sedating antihistamines (**Table 1**) is slightly better. Studies of fexofenadine (deduced from a 60 mg dose of parent terfenadine) (Lucas Jr. *et al.*, 1995) and loratadine (40 mg dose) (Hilbert, 1988) suggest low transfer into milk (relative infant doses of <0.1% and 1.1%, respectively). There are presently no data for cetirizine in its own right or for hydroxyzine from which it is metabolically derived. Effects in the infant are unlikely, but exposed infants should be observed if its use is necessary.

Moreover, a large prospective study of 838 breastfed infants whose mothers took various drugs, including antihistamines [terfenadine (n=25), diphenhydramine (n=12), astemizole (n=10), dimenhydrinate (n=7), and chlorpheniramine (n=5)] found no major adverse reactions requiring medical intervention (Ito *et al.*, 1993). They also reported that irritability and occasionally drowsiness were minor adverse effects associated with antihistamines, and they concluded that short-term effects, if any, on breastfed infants were mild and posed little risk to the infants.

The American Academy of Pediatrics lists brompheniramine, fexofenadine, loratadine, and triprolidine as usually compatible with breastfeeding, promethazine as having unknown effects but may be of concern, and does not list other drugs in this class. In summary, our review of the literature suggests that the antihistamines are generally compatible with breastfeeding. However, the possible sedative effects associated particularly with the first generation antihistamines can be completely avoided by using either loratadine or fexofenadine, both of which have acceptably low relative infant doses.

ANTICHOLINERGICS

Hyoscine finds application both as an antispasmodic for reducing gut pain (e.g., 10-20 mg of the butylbromide salt four times daily) and as an antiemetic/antinauseant for prevention of travel sickness (e.g., 0.3-0.6 mg of the hydrobromide salt four times daily). Another

Table 1. Selected Antihistamine and Anticholinergic Drugs and Breastfeeding

Drug	Relative infant dose (%)	Comment	References
Sedating antihistamines			
Chlorpheniramine	ND	Suitable for occasional use. Observe infant for sedation.	
Cyproheptadine	ND	Avoid. May reduce milk supply.	Wortsman *et al.*, 1979
Dexbrompheniramine	ND	Suitable for occasional use. Observe infant for sedation.	
Dexchlorpheniramine	ND	Suitable for occasional use. Observe infant for sedation. Excreted into human milk.	O'Brien, 1974
Diphenhydramine	ND	Suitable for occasional use. Observe infant for sedation.	
Doxylamine	ND	Suitable for occasional use. Observe infant for sedation.	
Levocabastine	ND	Compatible. Used topically thus insignificant milk concentrations.	
Promethazine	ND	Suitable for occasional use. Observe infant for sedation.	
Triprolidine	<1.8	Suitable for occasional use. Observe infant for sedation.	Findlay *et al.*, 1984
Non-sedating antihistamines			
Cetirizine	ND	Suitable for occasional use. Observe infant for sedation, as mild sedation noted in manufacturer's product information.	
Fexofenadine	<0.1	Compatible. Low milk concentrations. Lack of sedation in infants but observe infant for irritability.	Ito *et al.*, 1993
Loratadine	1.1	Compatible. Low transfer to milk.	Hilbert, 1988
Anticholinergics			
Hyoscine	ND	Human milk transfer unknown. Caution as children are susceptible to anticholinergic side effects.	Hale, 2006
ND = no data			

antispasmodic formulation contains atropine sulphate (0.195 mg), hyoscine hydrobromide (0.065 mg), and hyoscyamine sulfate (0.104 mg) with a recommended dose of 1-2 tablets four times daily. The doses of these preparations are modest, but the duration of use could vary from 1-2 doses for travel sickness to multiple doses over several days for gut pain. A practical approach would be to allow short-term use with careful observation of the infant (**Table 1**). Previously, many authors have anecdotally suggested that anticholinergics might suppress milk production due to their "drying" effect. There is no evidence to support this effect.

ENDOCRINE DRUGS

In this section, we have summarized information about insulin, oral antidiabetics, thyroid hormone and antithyroid drugs, and corticosteroids, which are sometimes needed in lactating women (**Table 2**).

Insulin and Oral Antidiabetic Agents

Insulin

Insulin has a molecular weight of around 5808 daltons and is synthesized from preproinsulin in the pancreas within the endoplasmic reticulum of the β-cells in the islets of Langerhans. Within these cells, it is transported to the golgi where it is cleaved to insulin and packaged into vesicles that are secreted into the blood. Because of its molecular size, exogenously administered insulin would not be expected to transfer from maternal plasma into milk by passive diffusion. In addition, since insulin is administered as replacement therapy, plasma levels after exogenous use are of similar magnitude to those resulting from normal endogenous production (5-40 mu/L) (Verge, 2004). Hence, exogenous insulin can be expected to be subject to the same cellular regulation and disposition as endogenous insulin. There are no reports of significant insulin levels in breastmilk in lactating women using exogenous insulin for type 1 diabetes. In addition, no adverse effects have been reported in breastfed infants of diabetic mothers using insulin. Hence, insulin use is completely compatible with breastfeeding.

Insulin appears to be permissive for lactation. Controlling blood glucose tightly increases maternal serum and milk prolactin levels and decreases the delay in establishing lactation that can occur in diabetes (Neubauer *et al.*, 1993; Ostrom *et al.*, 1993). Interestingly, insulin is normally present in breastmilk (range 7-306 mU/L) from nondiabetic mothers (Kulski *et al.*, 1983; Koldovsky, 1995). It is thought to be necessary for intestinal maturation and may also assist in decreasing the risk of developing type 1 diabetes in breastfed infants (Shehadeh *et al.*, 2001a; Shehadeh *et al.*, 2001b). The way in which insulin gets from the maternal circulation into milk is unclear. However, as shown in cell culture systems, it is likely to traverse the vascular endothelium by a mix of paracellular diffusion and receptor-mediated endocytosis (Wang *et al.*, 2006). Transport into the lactocytes might also be by receptor-mediated endocytosis, and once inside the cell, it may be packaged by the golgi apparatus and secreted with other components of milk.

Oral Antidiabetic Agents

The prevalence of type 2 diabetes in the general population and in pregnant women has increased in recent years (Feig *et al.*, 2006). Women with pregestational diabetes are usually treated with oral antidiabetic agents. During pregnancy, they are generally switched to insulin to avoid adverse effects, such as increased perinatal mortality and neonatal hyperglycemia, that have been encountered with some drugs in this group. However, after delivery, they are keen to return to their usual and more convenient oral therapy. The commonly available oral antidiabetic agents consist of the biguanides (metformin), sulphonylureas (glipizide, gliclazide, glyburide, glimepiride, and tolbutamide), the thiazolidinediones or glitazones (pioglitazone, rosiglitazone), alpha-glucosidase inhibitors (acarbose), and meglitinides (repaglinide). The use of the biguanides and sulphonylureas in pregnancy and lactation has been reviewed recently (Feig *et al.*, 2007).

Acarbose

Acarbose inhibits intestinal enzymes (α-glucosidases) involved in the degradation of ingested disaccharides, oligosaccharides, and polysaccharides, and reduces the postprandial rise in blood glucose. It has a molecular weight of 646, and only 1 to 2% of an oral dose of acarbose is absorbed from the gastrointestinal tract as unchanged drug. Although there are no data for its use during breastfeeding, its minimal oral bioavailability clearly indicates that it will not be significantly transferred to the infant and therefore poses no risk. Metformin reduces hepatic glucose production and promotes glucose uptake and utilization in skeletal muscle. Most importantly, it does not reduce plasma glucose levels in nondiabetic individuals (including breastfeeding infants). It has a short $t_{1/2}$, and there are now four studies (n=20) where maternal doses ranged from a single 500 mg dose through to 1500 mg daily. Collectively, these studies suggest that the relative infant dose of metformin is low (range 0.11-0.65%) and that effects in the exposed infant were not problematic (Hale *et al.*, 2002b; Gardiner *et al.*, 2003; Briggs *et al.*, 2005a; Glueck *et al.*, 2006). In another study comparing outcomes in 61 breastfed and 50 formula-fed infants from 92 mothers taking a mean of 2.55 g metformin daily, no differences in weight, height, and motor-social development were found at three and six months of age (Briggs *et al.*, 2005a). Intercurrent illnesses also did not differ between the groups. The authors concluded that metformin use during lactation was safe for the exposed infant. The effects of metformin on success in lactation has also been investigated (Thatcher *et al.*, 2006). Of the 250 women taking between 0.5 and 2 g daily, 124 attempted to breastfeed and 78% were successful. Failures were attributed to poor milk production, demands of multiple births, infant prematurity, cleft palate, and mastitis.

Sulfonylureas

Tolbutamide is a first generation oral antidiabetic that acts by stimulating insulin production by β-cells. It has a $t_{1/2}$ of 6-12 hours. One study of two patients who took a single 500 mg dose found relative infant doses of 6 and 38%, using milk concentration data measured four hours after dose (Moiel *et al.*, 1967). These values represent peak exposure calculated from milk data collected at the time of peak levels in plasma. Tolbutamine use is considered compatible with breastfeeding in conjunction with occasional monitoring of infant blood glucose (Everett, 1997, Berlin *et al.*, 2005). Glipizide, gliclazide, glimepiride, and glyburide are all second generation sulfonylureas with the same mechanism of action as the earlier drugs in this series. Glyburide has been studied in eight women taking either 5 or 10 mg daily (Feig *et al.*, 2005). Milk levels were less than the 5 μg/L limit of detection of their assay, and they calculated relative infant doses of <1.5% or <0.7% of the weight-adjusted maternal dose, respectively. Blood glucose was normal in one exposed infant. The same authors also studied two mother/baby pairs where the mother was taking 5 mg of glipizide daily (Feig *et al.*, 2005). Trough drug concentrations in milk were below the limit of detection (<80 μg/L), and they calculated that the relative infant dose was <27%. While this seems high, it must be borne in mind that the high dose is directly related to the high analytical detection limit. Blood glucose was normal in both exposed infants. Presently, there are no data on either transfer into milk or effects in infants for the drugs gliclazide and glimepiride. In summary, the experience with these second generation sulfonylureas is very limited. For the ones where there are data, transfer into milk appears to be low, and adverse effects in exposed infants have not been reported. We suggest they be used with caution and with appropriate monitoring of plasma glucose in exposed infants (Everett, 1997; Berlin *et al.*, 2005).

Thiazolidinediones

The thiazolidinediones are selective agonists for nuclear peroxisome proliferator-activated receptor-γ and thereby activate insulin-responsive gene regulation of carbohydrate and lipid metabolism. Their activity depend on the presence of some insulin, and they exert their effects by lowering glucose production in the liver and increasing insulin sensitivity in peripheral tissues. Currently, there are no data on milk transfer or effects in exposed infants for the commonly used antidiabetics pioglitazone and rosiglitazone. Given their broad spectrum of pharmacological activity and range of adverse effects, their use in breastfeeding should be discouraged until relevant data become available. If used, infants should be closely observed, including monitoring of plasma glucose (Everett, 1997; Berlin *et al.*, 2005).

Meglitinides

Repaglinide, representative of the meglitinide class of antidiabetics, lowers blood glucose by stimulating the release of insulin from the pancreas. Currently, there are no breastfeeding or infant exposure data for this drug and other agents are therefore preferred. If used, infants should be closely observed, including monitoring of plasma glucose (Everett, 1997; Berlin *et al.*, 2005).

Thyroid and Anti-Thyroid Drugs

Levothyroxine and Liothyronine

Replacement therapy for hypothyroidism is undertaken using either levothyroxine (*l*-thyroxine; T4) or liothyronine (triiodothyronine; T3). Levels of these two closely related hormones in milk following exogenous administration have not been measured. However, they are both present in human milk with transfer of liothyronine said to be greater than that of levothyroxine (Oberkotter, 1983; Koldovsky, 1995). However, the amounts present in milk are insufficient to influence thyroid hormone levels in the preterm breastfed infant's plasma (van Wassenaer *et al.*, 2002). There are two reports (six exposed infants) suggesting that levothyroxine caused some adverse effects in breastfed infants (Ito *et al.*, 1993; Caplan *et al.*, 1993), but effects in infants after liothyronine use have not been studied. The American Academy of Pediatrics regards thyroxine as being compatible with breastfeeding (American Academy of Pediatrics Committee on Drugs, 2001).

Carbimazole and Methimazole

Carbimazole is quantitatively converted to its active metabolite methimazole in the body and both drugs are marketed in different countries. After administration of either carbimazole or methimazole, ranging from 5-40 mg daily, the relative infant dose varied from 1.5-5.8% (Tegler *et al.*, 1980; Johansen *et al.*, 1982; Cooper *et al.*, 1984; Abe *et al.*, 1995). After maternal doses of methimazole (5-30 mg daily), 18 exposed infants all had normal thyroid function, and serum levels in a subgroup of exposed infants were undetectable (n=6) or low (30 and 35 μg/L; n=2) (Azizi, 2003). This group also reported normal infant thyroid function (n=88; age 1 year) and no deficits in physical or intellectual

Table 2. Selected Endocrine Drugs and Breastfeeding

Drug	Relative infant dose (%)	Comment	References
Insulin and oral antidiabetics			
Acarbose	ND	Compatible. No transfer to milk expected because oral bioavailability is only 1-2%.	
Glipizide	<27	Compatible. Calculated dose is from trough milk assay, with a high limit of detection (<80 μg/L). Infant blood glucose levels were normal (n=2).	Feig *et al.*, 2005
Glyburide	<0.7, <1.5	Compatible. Blood glucose levels were normal in an infant exposed to a 5 mg daily maternal dose.	Ito, 2000; Feig *et al.*, 2005
Gliclazide	ND	Probably compatible. Use with caution and monitor infant's plasma glucose.	
Glimepiride	ND	Probably compatible. Use with caution and monitor infant's plasma glucose.	
Insulin	ND	Compatible.	
Metformin	0.28, 0.11-0.25, 0.65	Compatible. No adverse effects in exposed infants.	Hale *et al.*, 2002b; Gardiner *et al.*, 2003; Briggs *et al.*, 2005a; Glueck *et al.*, 2006
Pioglitazone	ND	Others preferred until data are available. Use with caution and monitor infant's plasma glucose.	
Repaglinide	ND	Others preferred until data are available. Use with caution and monitor infant's plasma glucose.	
Rosiglitazone	ND	Others preferred until data are available. Use with caution and monitor infant's plasma glucose.	
Tolbutamide	6, 38	Compatible. Monitor infant blood glucose. Only two patients studied. Dose corresponds to C_{max} in plasma.	Moiel *et al.*, 1967
Thyroid and anti-thyroid drugs			
Carbimazole (Methimazole; active metabolite)	0.14-5.8	No adverse infant effects at usual maternal therapeutic doses. Compatible. Monitor infant thyroid function if high doses used.	Johansen *et al.*, 1982; Rylance *et al.*, 1987; Azizi, 1996; Azizi *et al.*, 2000; Azizi, 2003
Levothyroxine and liothyronine	ND	Very low concentrations in milk. Compatible.	Oberkotter, 1983; Ito *et al.*, 1993; Caplan *et al.*, 1993; Koldovsky, 1995; van Wassenaer *et al.*, 2002
Propylthiouracil	0.3, 0.8	Compatible.	Kampmann *et al.*, 1980; Cooper, 1987
Corticosteroids			
Budesonide, fluticasone, and mometasone (asthma)	ND	Compatible.	Ellsworth, 1994; Spencer *et al.*, 2001
Beclomethasone, hydrocortisone, mometasone and triamcinolone (topical)	ND	Compatible.	
Hydrocortisone		Low levels normally present in milk. Compatible.	Kulski *et al.*, 1981
Prednisone	3-5.5	Compatible.	Katz *et al.*, 1975; Sagraves *et al.*, 1981
Prednisolone	0.02-0.14[1]		
Methylprednisolone	1.2	Compatible. Withholding breastfeeding for several hours has been suggested for very large single doses.	Coulam *et al.*, 1982

ND = no data, [1] infant dose as percent exposure of total maternal dose (single dose only).

development (n=14) in infants exposed to maternal doses of up to 20 mg methimazole daily (Azizi *et al.*, 2000). Some of the same infants (n=42) were studied again at four years of age; all showed normal intellectual development (Azizi *et al.*, 2003). Overall, these data suggest that methimazole use is compatible with breastfeeding.

Propylthiouracil

The relative infant dose of propylthiouracil can be calculated to be 0.3% (Kampmann *et al.*, 1980) and 0.8% (Cooper, 1987). While there are no data for levels in plasma of exposed infants, some 24 breastfed infants exposed to maternal doses of 50-300 mg daily showed no adverse effects or changes in their thyroid function (Kampmann *et al.*, 1980; Lamberg *et al.*, 1984; McDougall *et al.*, 1986; Momotani *et al.*, 1989; Momotani *et al.*, 2000; Lee *et al.*, 2000). Like methimazole, the American Academy of Pediatrics classifies propylthiouracil as compatible with breastfeeding (American Academy of Pediatrics Committee on Drugs, 2001), but others have expressed a preference for propylthiouracil (Cooper, 1987; Mandel *et al.*, 2001) presumably because of the lower relative infant dose and perhaps the lower adverse effects profile in adults.

Corticosteroids

The glucocorticoids have a broad range of applications that may require their use during breastfeeding.

Budesonide, Fluticasone and Mometasone (Asthma)

These corticosteroids have important applications in long-term prevention of asthma. They are most commonly administered in small doses by metered-dose aerosol or dry powder inhaler. The dose is intended to have local actions in the lung with low absorption via the gut. Drug entering the systemic circulation via the lung is pharmacologically active, while that entering via the gut is largely inactivated by first-pass metabolism. Oral bioavailability for these drugs ranges from 1-26% (Hubner *et al.*, 2005). While systemic adverse effects can occur in the persons inhaling these drugs (Lipworth, 1999), the small doses used and their low oral bioavailability suggest that amounts transferred into milk and subsequently absorbed by the infant will be minimal. There are no data on their transfer into breastmilk, or on plasma levels or adverse effects in exposed infants, but reviews of pharmacotherapy of asthma and allergic rhinitis have suggested that they are compatible with breastfeeding (Greenberger *et al.*, 1987; Ellsworth, 1994; Leimgruber, 2007).

Betamethasone, Hydrocortisone, Mometasone, Triamcinolone (Topical)

These corticosteroids find wide application in dermatology (e.g., psoriasis, atopic dermatitis, seborrheic dermatitis) and are applied locally to the skin. There are no data on their transfer into breastmilk or on plasma levels or adverse effects in exposed infants. However, given that systemic absorption via skin is generally <10% and their use is generally short-term and intermittent, they pose a very low risk to the breastfed infant. If direct application to the breast is necessary, formulations with an aqueous base should be used. Only minimal quantities should be applied to the nipple, or the cream should be washed off prior to breastfeeding to prevent oral absorption by the infant. There is a reported case of severe adverse effects (prolonged QT interval, cushingoid appearance, severe hypertension, decreased growth, and electrolyte abnormalities) in an infant exposed to use (on the nipples) of the corticosteroid 9-α-isofluprednisolone acetate, a drug with relatively high mineralocorticoid activity (De *et al.*, 1983). Additional caution should be exercised in the use of these drugs during breastfeeding when high concentration, high potency topical corticosteroids are used on large areas of the skin or for prolonged periods. In addition, high potency topical steroids should never be applied to the nipples of breastfeeding mothers.

Hydrocortisone

Hydrocortisone (cortisol) is a normal constituent of human milk. Kulski and Hartmann reported that average levels in plasma during pregnancy were 25 μg/L, and this decreased within two days postpartum, establishing low levels by day ten (Kulski *et al.*, 1981). The mean concentration in mature milk averaged 7 μg/L (range <1-32 μg/L). There are no reports of adverse effects or serum levels of hydrocortisone in exposed infants. Given that hydrocortisone is a normal secretion of the adrenal glands in both adults and children and that the American Academy of Pediatrics considers the closely related prednisone and prednisolone to be compatible with breastfeeding (American Academy of Pediatrics

Committee on Drugs, 2001), hydrocortisone should be classified similarly. Again, topical application to the nipples should be limited to prevent the absorption of higher doses by the infant.

Methylprednisolone

A relative infant dose of 1.2% can be calculated from data for a single case of a woman taking 6 mg of methyprednisolone daily (Coulam *et al.*, 1982). There are no reports of levels in serum of exposed infants, and no adverse effects were reported in three infants exposed to maternal methylprednisolone (6-8 mg daily) (Coulam *et al.*, 1982; Grekas *et al.*, 1984). For very large doses (e.g., 1-2 g) in treatment of multiple sclerosis, it has been suggested that withholding breastfeeding for 12 hours after the daily dose would substantially avoid infant exposure (Hale *et al.*, 2002a).

Prednisone and Prednisolone

Prednisone is quantitatively metabolized to prednisolone in the body, and both compounds have similar pharmacological potency and actions. Using peak levels of prednisone plus its metabolite in milk after single doses of 10, 20, or 120 mg prednisone, relative infant doses of 3, 5.3, and 5.5%, respectively, can be calculated (Katz *et al.*, 1975; Sagraves *et al.*, 1981). Following administration of a single 5 mg dose of prednisolone in seven women, the total infant exposure over the subsequent 2-2.5 days was 0.14% of the maternal dose (McKenzie *et al.*, 1975). Similarly, in six women taking 10-80 mg prednisolone daily, it can be calculated that total infant dose is about 0.02% of the maternal dose (Ost *et al.*, 1985). Finally, following a single 50 mg IV dose. Greenberger *et al.* estimated that the nursing infant would be exposed to 0.074% of the maternal dose (Greenberger *et al.*, 1993). Note that the percentage exposures in the three studies of prednisolone have calculated the infant dose as a percent of the mother's total dose.

Serum levels of these two corticosteroids have not been reported in exposed infants. In addition, there are no reports of adverse effects in exposed infants following usual therapeutic doses of either prednisone (unspecified or 5-7.5 mg daily; n=8) (Ito *et al.*, 1993; Munoz-Flores-Thiagarajan *et al.*, 2001; Moretti *et al.*, 2003), or prednisolone (5-10 mg daily; n=14) (Nyberg *et al.*, 1998). These exposures were mostly in an organ transplant situation where long-term immunosuppression was required.

In summary, a variety of corticosteroids with oral, parenteral, inhalational, or topical routes of administration are compatible with breastfeeding. The American Academy of Pediatrics has a usually compatible recommendation only for prednisone and prednisolone (American Academy of Pediatrics Committee on Drugs, 2001). Withholding breastfeeding for 12 hours or so after very large doses of methylprednisolone may be a conservative maneuver to limit infant exposure.

References

Abe Y, Sato H, Sakai H. Antithyroid treatment of maternal hyperthyroidism during lactation. *Thyroid.* 1995; 5 (Suppl 1):S108.

American Academy of Pediatrics Committee on Drugs. Transfer of drugs and other chemicals into human milk. *Pediatrics.* 2001; 108:776-89.

Anonymous. *Cyproheptadine. Toxnet drugs and lactation (Lactmed) database.* 2007a. Available from: URL: http://toxnet.nlm.nih.gov/cgi-bin/sis/htmlgen?LACT.

Anonymous. *Zyrtec. MIMS abbreviated prescribing information.* Version 5.01.2005 Ed. St. Leonards, Australia: CMP Medica Australia Pty Ltd.; 2007b.

Azizi F. Effect of methimazole treatment of maternal thyrotoxicosis on thyroid function in breast-feeding infants. *J Pediatr.* 1996; 128:855-58.

Azizi F. Thyroid function in breast-fed infants is not affected by methimazole-induced maternal hypothyroidism: results of a retrospective study. *J Endocrinol Invest.* 2003; 26:301-4.

Azizi F, Bahrainian M, Khamseh ME, Khoshniat M. Intellectual development and thyroid function in children who were breast-fed by thyrotoxic mothers taking methimazole. *J Pediatr Endocrinol Metab.* 2003; 16:1239-43.

Azizi F, Khoshniat M, Bahrainian M, Hedayati M. Thyroid function and intellectual development of infants nursed by mothers taking methimazole. *J Clin Endocrinol Metab.* 2000; 85:3233-38.

Berlin CM, Briggs GG. Drugs and chemicals in human milk. *Semin Fetal Neonatal Med.* 2005; 10:149-59.

Briggs GG, Ambrose PJ, Nageotte MP, Padilla G, Wan S. Excretion of metformin into breast milk and the effect on nursing infants. *Obstet Gynecol.* 2005a; 105:1437-41.

Briggs GG, Freeman RK, Yaffe SJ. *Drugs in pregnancy and lactation.* 7th Ed. Philadelphia: Lippincott Williams and Wilkins; 2005b.

Caplan RH, Wickus GG. Reduced calcitriol requirements for treating hypoparathyroidism during lactation. A case report. *J Reprod Med.* 1993; 38:914-18.

Cooper DS. Antithyroid drugs: to breast-feed or not to breast-feed. *Am J Obstet Gynecol.* 1987; 157:234-35.

Cooper DS, Bode HH, Nath B, Saxe V, Maloof F, Ridgway EC. Methimazole pharmacology in man: studies using a newly developed radioimmunoassay for methimazole. *J Clin Endocrinol Metab.* 1984; 58:473-79.

Coulam CB, Moyer TP, Jiang NS, Zincke H. Breast-feeding after renal transplantation. *Transplant Proc.* 1982; 14:605-9.

De SP, Bongo IG, Borgna-Pignatti C, Severi F. Factitious hypertension with mineralocorticoid excess in an infant. *Helv Paediatr Acta.* 1983; 38:185-89.

Dorea JG. Maternal exposure to endocrine-active substances and breastfeeding. *Am J Perinatol.* 2006; 23:305-12.

Ellsworth A. Pharmacotherapy of asthma while breastfeeding. *J Hum Lact.* 1994; 10:39-41.

Everett JA. Use of oral antidiabetic agents during breastfeeding. *J Hum Lact.* 1997; 13:319-21.

Feig DS, Briggs GG, Koren G. Oral antidiabetic agents in pregnancy and lactation: a paradigm shift? *Ann Pharmacother.* 2007; 41:xx-yy.

Feig DS, Briggs GG, Kraemer JM, Ambrose PJ, Moskovitz DN, Nageotte M, *et al.* Transfer of glyburide and glipizide into breast milk. *Diabetes Care.* 2005; 28:1851-55.

Feig DS, Cleave B, Tomlinson G. Long-term effects of a diabetes and pregnancy program: does the education last? *Diabetes Care.* 2006; 29:526-30.

Findlay JW, Butz RF, Sailstad JM, Warren JT, Welch RM. Pseudoephedrine and triprolidine in plasma and breast milk of nursing mothers. *Br J Clin Pharmacol.* 1984; 18:901-6.

Freeman ME, Kanyicska B, Lerant A, Nagy G. Prolactin: structure, function, and regulation of secretion. *Physiol Rev.* 2000; 80:1523-631.

Gardiner SJ, Kirkpatrick CMJ, Begg EJ, Zhang M, Moore MP, Saville DJ. Transfer of metformin into human milk. *Clin Pharmacol Ther.* 2003; 73:71-77.

Glueck CJ, Salehi M, Sieve L, Wang P. Growth, motor, and social development in breast- and formula-fed infants of metformin-treated women with polycystic ovary syndrome. *J Pediatr.* 2006; 148:628-32.

Greenberger PA, Odeh YK, Frederiksen MC, Atkinson AJ. Pharmacokinetics of prednisolone transfer to breast milk. *Clin Pharmacol Ther.* 1993; 53:324-28.

Greenberger PA, Patterson R. The management of asthma during pregnancy and lactation. *Clin Rev Allergy.* 1987; 5:317-24.

Grekas DM, Vasiliou SS, Lazarides AN. Immunosuppressive therapy and breast-feeding after renal transplantation. *Nephron.* 1984; 37:68.

Hale TW. *Medications and mothers' milk.* 11th Ed. Amarillo, TX, USA: Pharmasoft Publishing; 2006.

Hale TW, Ilett KF. *Drug therapy and breastfeeding. From theory to clinical practice.* 1st Ed. London: The Parthenon Publishing Group; 2002a.

Hale TW, Kristensen JH, Hackett LP, Kohan R, Ilett KF. Transfer of metformin into human milk. *Diabetologia.* 2002b; 45:1509-14.

Hilbert J. Excretion of loratadine in human breast milk. *J Clin Pharmacol.* 1988; 28:234-39.

Hubner M, Hochhaus G, Derendorf H. Comparative pharmacology, bioavailability, pharmacokinetics, and pharmacodynamics of inhaled glucocorticosteroids. *Immunol Allergy Clin North Am.* 2005; 25:469-88.

Ilett KF, Kristensen JH. Drug use and breastfeeding. *Expert Opin Drug Saf.* 2005; 4:745-68.

Ito S. Drug therapy: Drug therapy for breast-feeding women. *New Engl J Med.* 2000; 343:118-26.

Ito S, Blajchman A, Stephenson M, Eliopoulos C, Koren G. Prospective follow-up of adverse reactions in breast-fed infants exposed to maternal medication. *Am J Obstet Gynecol.* 1993; 168:1393-99.

Johansen K, Andersen AN, Kampmann JP, Molholm HJ, Mortensen HB. Excretion of methimazole in human milk. *Eur J Clin Pharmacol.* 1982; 23:339-41.

Kampmann JP, Johansen K, Hansen JM, Helweg J. Propylthiouracil in human milk. Revision of a dogma. *Lancet.* 1980; 1:736-7.

Katz FH, Duncan BR. Entry of prednisone into human milk [letter]. *New Engl J Med.* 1975; 293:1154.

Koldovsky O. Hormones in milk. *Vitam Horm.* 1995; 50:77-149.

Kulski JK, Hartmann PE. Changes in the concentration of cortisol in milk during different stages of human lactation. *Aust J Exp Biol Med Sci.* 1981; 59:769-78.

Kulski JK, Hartmann PE. Milk insulin, GH and TSH: relationship to changes in milk lactose, glucose and protein during lactogenesis in women. *Endocrinol Exp.* 1983; 17:317-26.

Lamberg BA, Ikonen E, Osterlund K, Teramo K, Pekonen F, Peltola J, *et al.* Antithyroid treatment of maternal hyperthyroidism during lactation. *Clin Endocrinol (Oxf).* 1984; 21:81-87.

Lee A, Moretti ME, Collantes A, Chong D, Mazzotta P, Koren G, *et al.* Choice of breastfeeding and physicians' advice: A cohort study of women receiving propylthiouracil. *Pediatrics.* 2000; 106:27-30.

Leimgruber A. Treatment of asthma and rhinitis during pregnancy and breast feeding. *Rev Med Suisse.* 2007; 3:1044-49.

Lipworth BJ. Systemic adverse effects of inhaled corticosteroid therapy: A systematic review and meta-analysis. *Arch Intern Med.* 1999; 159:941-55.

Lucas BD, Jr., Purdy CY, Scarim SK, Benjamin S, Abel SR, Hilleman DE. Terfenadine pharmacokinetics in breast milk in lactating women. *Clin Pharmacol Ther.* 1995; 57:398-402.

Mandel SJ, Cooper DS. The use of antithyroid drugs in pregnancy and lactation. *J Clin Endocrinol Metab.* 2001; 86:2354-9.

McDougall IR, Bayer MF. Should a woman taking propylthiouracil breast-feed? *Clin Nucl Med.* 1986; 11:249-50.

McKenzie SA, Selley JA, Agnew JE. Secretion of prednisolone into breast milk. *Arch Dis Child.* 1975; 50:894-96.

Messinis IE, Souvatzoglou A, Fais N, Lolis D. Histamine H1 receptor participation in the control of prolactin secretion in postpartum. *J Endocrinol Invest.* 1985; 8:143-6.

Mitchell JL. Use of cough and cold preparations during breastfeeding. *J Hum Lact.* 1999; 15:347-49.

Moiel RH, Ryan JR. Tolbutamide orinase in human breast milk. *Clin Pediatr (Phila).* 1967; 6:480.

Momotani N, Yamashita R, Makino F, Noh JY, Ishikawa N, Ito K. Thyroid function in wholly breast-feeding infants whose mothers take high doses of propylthiouracil. *Clin Endocrinol (Oxf).* 2000; 53:177-81.

Momotani N, Yamashita R, Yoshimoto M, Noh J, Ishikawa N, Ito K. Recovery from foetal hypothyroidism: evidence for the safety of breast-feeding while taking propylthiouracil. *Clin Endocrinol (Oxf).* 1989; 31:591-5.

Moretti ME, Sgro M, Johnson DW, Sauve RS, Woolgar MJ, Taddio A, *et al.* Cyclosporine excretion into breast milk. *Transplantation.* 2003; 75:2144-46.

Munoz-Flores-Thiagarajan KD, Easterling T, Davis C, Bond EF. Breast-feeding by a cyclosporine-treated mother. *Obstet Gynecol.* 2001; 97:816-18.

Neubauer SH, Ferris AM, Chase CG, Fanelli J, Thompson CA, Lammi-Keefe CJ, *et al.* Delayed lactogenesis in women with insulin-dependent diabetes mellitus. *Am J Clin Nutr.* 1993; 58:54-60.

Nyberg G, Haljamae U, Frisenette-Fich C, Wennergren M, Kjellmer I. Breast-feeding during treatment with cyclosporine. *Transplantation.* 1998; 65:253-55.

O'Brien TE. Excretion of drugs in human milk. *Am J Hosp Pharm.* 1974; 31:844-54.

Oberkotter LV. Thyroid function and human breast milk [letter]. *Am J Dis Child.* 1983; 137:1131.

Ost L, Wettrell G, Bjorkhem I, Rane A. Prednisolone excretion in human milk. *J Pediatr.* 1985; 106:1008-11.

Ostrom KM, Ferris AM. Prolactin concentrations in serum and milk of mothers with and without insulin-dependent diabetes mellitus. *Am J Clin Nutr.* 1993; 58:49-53.

Pontiroli AE, De Castro e Silva E, Mazzoleni F, Alberetto M, Baio G, Pellicciotta G, *et al.* The effect of histamine and H1 and H2 receptors on prolactin and luteinizing hormone release in humans: sex differences and the role of stress. *J Clin Endocrinol Metab.* 1981; 52:924-28.

Rylance GW, Woods CG, Donnelly MC, Oliver JS, Alexander WD. Carbimazole and breastfeeding. *Lancet.* 1987; 1:928.

Sagraves R, Kaiser D, Sharpe GL. Prednisone and prednisolone concentrations in milk of a lactating mother. *Drug Intell Clin Pharm.* 1981; 15:484.

Shehadeh N, Gelertner L, Blazer S, Perlman R, Solovachik L, Etzioni A. Importance of insulin content in infant diet: suggestion for a new infant formula. *Acta Paediatr.* 2001a; 90:93-95.

Shehadeh N, Shamir R, Berant M, Etzioni A. Insulin in human milk and the prevention of type 1 diabetes. *Pediatr Diabetes.* 2001b; 2:175-77.

Simons SER. Antihistamines. In: Adkinson J, Franklin N, Yunginger JW, Busse WW, Bochner BS, Simons FER, *et al.* (eds.). *Middelton's allergy: principles and practice.* 6th Ed. Philadelphia, PA: Mosby; 2003. p. 834-69.

Skidgel RA, Erdos EG. Histamine, bradykinin and their antagonists. In: Brunton LL, Lazo JS, Parker KL (eds.). *Goodman & Gilman's the pharmacological basis of therapeutics.* 11th Ed. New York: McGraw Hill Medical Publishing Division; 2006. p. 629-51.

Spencer JP, Gonzalez LS, III, Barnhart DJ. Medications in the breast-feeding mother. *Am Fam Physician.* 2001; 64:119-26.

Tegler L, Lindstrom B. Antithyroid drugs in milk. *Lancet.* 1980; 2:591.

Thatcher SS, Jackson EM. Pregnancy outcome in infertile patients with polycystic ovary syndrome who were treated with metformin. *Fertil Steril.* 2006; 85:1002-9.

van Wassenaer AG, Stulp MR, Valianpour F, Tamminga P, Ris SC, de Randamie JS, *et al.* The quantity of thyroid hormone in human milk is too low to influence plasma thyroid hormone levels in the very preterm infant. *Clin Endocrinol (Oxf).* 2002; 56:621-27.

Verge D. Biotechnological and administration innovations in insulin therapy. *Med Sci (Paris).* 2004; 20:986-98.

Wang H, Liu Z, Li G, Barrett EJ. The vascular endothelial cell mediates insulin transport into skeletal muscle. *Am J Physiol Endocrinol Metab.* 2006; 291:E323-32.

Wortsman J, Soler NG, Hirschowitz J. Cyproheptadine in the management of the galactorrhea-amenorrhea syndrome. *Ann Intern Med.* 1979; 90:923-25.

Chapter 33

Drugs of Abuse and Breastfeeding

Ghia McAfee

INTRODUCTION

Drug abuse causes extreme burden, not only on the drug user and his/her family, but also on the country as a whole. It was estimated that in the United States of America (USA), the economical cost of drug abuse in 1992 was approximately $245.7 billion (illicit drugs, legal drugs taken for non-medical purposes, excluding nicotine and alcohol abuse) (National Institute on Drug Abuse InfoFacts, 1995).

Survey results from 1991-1993 indicated that 1.2% of the USA population aged twelve or older were dependent on or had abused illicit drugs in the past year (Substance Abuse and Mental Health Services Administration, 1996), compared to approximately three percent reported in 2002-2003 (**Figure 1**).

There is a large body of literature available pertaining to the physical and psychological consequences of drug abuse, the pharmacological properties of the substances, and their mechanisms of action. This particular chapter will, however, largely focus on the effects of maternal drug abuse and its affect on the breastfed infant.

Abusing drugs to try and cope with stress is a common phenomenon in today's society, and it is no different for women during the early postpartum period. Since drug abuse during pregnancy is a probable proxy for abusing drugs postpartum, some reference is made in this chapter to significant studies where the infant was affected by drug abuse during gestation and subsequent breastfeeding.

Although some drugs that are abused are considered illegal to possess, sell, or manufacture, others are available with a physicians prescription (opioids and benzodiazepines), over the counter (pseudoephedrine), or in grocery stores (various inhalants, alcohol, and tobacco products). The focus of this chapter will mainly be on the effect that illicit drug use, but also alcohol and cigarette smoke, has on the breastfed infant.

Although virtually all drugs of abuse enter the milk compartment, the level at which it appears in breastmilk is dependent on various factors including, but not limited to the physiochemical properties of the compound, maternal blood levels, and frequency of drug abuse. Therefore, reference is made to the milk to plasma (M/P) ratio of some of the drugs discussed in this chapter. The M/P ratio is calculated by taking the concentration of the drug in the breastmilk and maternal plasma into account. A M/P ratio of less than 1 generally indicates that only a minimal amount of the drug is transferred into breastmilk. Regardless, in general the M/P ratio is a poor estimate of the amount of drug that a breastfed infant is exposed to. Note that the absolute dose of a drug that reaches the breastfed infant is partially dependent on the drug concentration in maternal plasma.

Another important point is that of polydrug use, where drug users abuse multiple drugs concomitantly. One well-known example of a polydrug combination is that of cigarette smoke and alcohol. Various other drug abuse combinations exist, such as cocaine and heroin

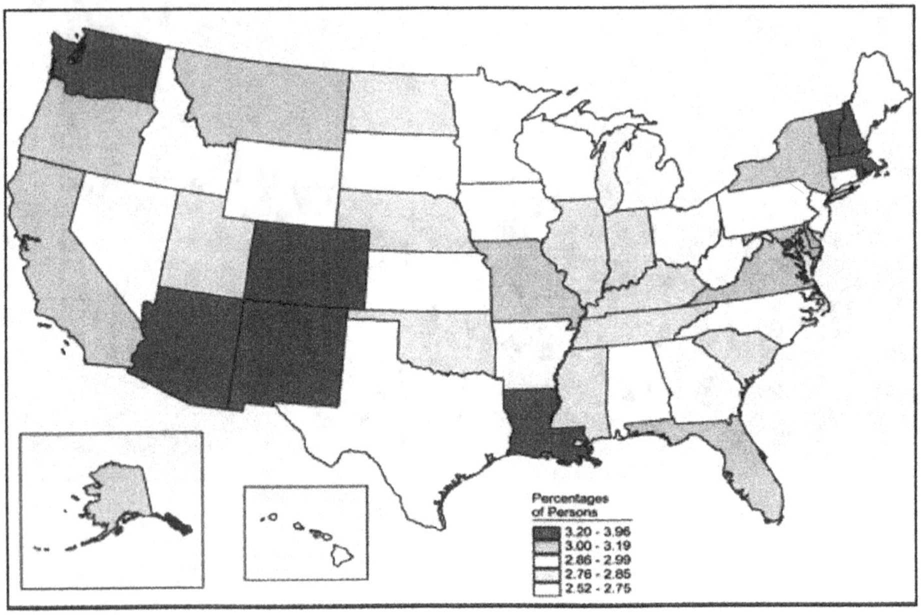

Figure 1. Any illicit drug abuse or dependence in the past year among persons who are 12 years or older (annual averages based on 2002 and 2003 data) (National Surveys on Drug Use and Health, 2002–2003).

or cocaine and alcohol. Although limited information is available on the effect of these various drug combinations on the breastfed infant, some information will be supplied and discussed in this chapter.

AMPHETAMINE, DEXTROAMPHETAMINE, AND METHAMPHETAMINE

In the USA, amphetamine is used in the treatment of attention-deficit hyperactivity disorder (ADHD), and narcolepsy. However, amphetamine is widely abused due to the likelihood of severe psychological and physiological dependency. Amphetamine concentrates in breastmilk and ultimately attains levels of between 55 and 138 ng/mL. In one study, its M/P ratio was reported to be between 2.8 and 7.5, following a 20 mg daily dose. Small amounts of amphetamine were present in the urine of the breastfed infant. In addition, the infant presented with irritability and poor sleeping patterns (Steiner *et al.*, 1984). In another study of four mothers who received 15-45 mg/day dextroamphetamine, the dextrorotary stereoisomer of amphetamine, the average absolute infant dose was 21 (11-39) μg/kg/day. The relative infant dose was 5.7% (4-10.6%). Plasma levels in the infants ranged from undetectable to 18 μg/L. No untoward effects were noted in any of the four infants (Ilett *et al.*, 2007).

According to the Drug Enforcement Administration, 80% of the methamphetamine in the United States originate from Mexico, where "super labs" can produce more than ten pounds of methamphetamine in one production cycle. The second source of methamphetamine is small toxic labs in the USA itself and account for 20% of the methamphetamine consumed in the USA (Tandy, 2006).

Methamphetamine is structurally related to amphetamine (**Figure 2**), but in comparable doses methamphetamine has a longer half-life, is more potent, and has the potential of leading to reversible schizoid side effects. Methamphetamine is a highly addictive substance that can be snorted, smoked, injected or taken orally. The half-life of methamphetamine ranges between 10.7 and 11.4 hours regardless of its route of administration (Harris *et al.*, 2003a). The

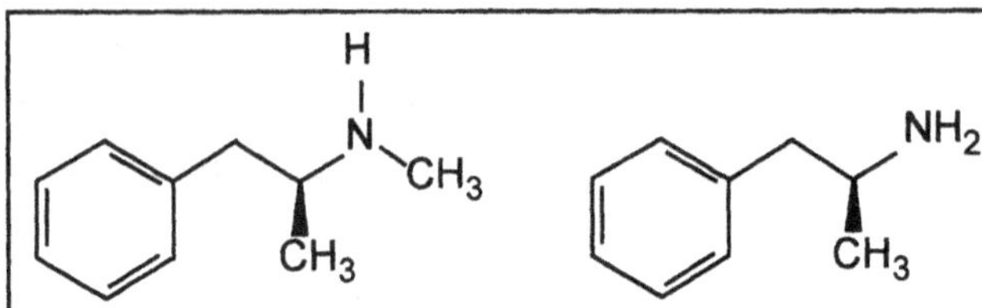

Methamphetamine **Amphetamine**

Figure 2. Chemical structure of methamphetamine and amphetamine.

physical appearance of the hydrochloride salt form of methamphetamine resembles that of ice, hence its street names - ice, crystal, and glass.

Only one case report of exposure of an infant to methamphetamine is available. In this case of an infant fatality, the mother abused methamphetamine and reportedly breastfed her infant. Postmortem methamphetamine blood levels were reported to be 39 ng/mL (Ariagno *et al.*, 1995). However, according to the authors, blood levels in amphetamine-related deaths are associated with much higher levels, such as 300 ng/mL to 40 μg/mL. Therefore, it is more likely that the infant died of sudden infant death syndrome (SIDS) than methamphetamine-related intoxication (Ariagno *et al.*, 1995).

In a lay report in a newspaper, methamphetamine was detected in the mother's breastmilk, but no levels were reported. According to this report, the infant presented with trace amounts of methamphetamine in his stomach contents and system. No cause of death was listed (Hall, 2005).

Experimental Animal Studies

Animal studies clearly suggest that methamphetamine is both addictive and alters maternal behavior. Slamberova and coworkers (2005) suggested that methamphetamine administration to rats during the pre-mating, gestational, and lactational periods impaired maternal behavior toward their pups.

Conclusion

Amphetamine and dextroamphetamine transfer into breastmilk, but apparently at less than therapeutic levels when maternal doses are within normal limits. At these doses present in milk, side affects in the breastfed infant are apparently minimal. However, each infant should be closely monitored for side effects, such as poor feeding, insomnia, and excitement.

Methamphetamine, on the other hand, is a highly addictive compound with a long half-life and numerous risks. Although limited data are available on the effects of methamphetamine on the breastfeeding infant, it has been reported that methamphetamine is excreted in breastmilk and that it is responsible for impaired maternal behavior. Methamphetamine is not listed in the American Academy of Pediatrics (AAP) Committee on Drugs' review of drugs. According to the AAP, amphetamine (or dextroamphetamine) is contraindicated for use during breastfeeding (American Academy of Pediatrics, 2001), although there are reports of its safe use in mothers with ADHD (Hale, 2006). Therefore, based on methamphetamine's extreme potency and significant hazards to the breastfeeding infant, its use during nursing is strongly contraindicated.

ALCOHOL

In 2005, 55.4% of females, aged 18 to 25 in the USA were current alcohol (ethanol) users (National Survey on Drug Use and Health, 2005). Although this data indicates the prevalence of alcohol use among women of child-bearing age, the Substance Abuse and Mental Health Services Administration (SAMHSA) do not have any specific data on the prevalence of alcohol use during breastfeeding. Nonetheless, according to the AAP, alcohol is usually compatible with breastfeeding (American Academy of Pediatrics, 1989). In addition, if the amount and duration of alcohol exposure is limited, it is not considered harmful to the breastfeeding infant (Hale, 2004; Liston, 1998).

However, more recent studies have indicated that modest amounts of alcohol intake by a nursing mother may have long-term effects on the breastfed infant (Little *et al.*, 1989; Schulte, 1995).

Transfer of Alcohol into Breastmilk

When lactating women ingest alcohol, as is the case with caffeine, less than 2% of the dose reaches the bloodstream and breastmilk (Mennella, 2001). Alcohol is not stored in breastmilk, rather it readily diffuses back and forth between the blood and breastmilk. Thus, it maintains a close equilibrium with the plasma compartment during elimination (Lawton, 1985). Alcohol's rate of transfer between blood and breastmilk is independent of pH, since it is a non-polar compound. In addition, alcohol is highly water soluble and therefore able to pass easily through biological membranes where it can distribute throughout the water compartments of the body (Lawton, 1985).

Alcohol
M/P concentration ratio = 1.0
Relative infant dose = 16%
Adult half-life = 0.24 hours

Since breastmilk has a higher water content than blood (87.5% vs. 85%), alcohol levels in breastmilk will be equal or slightly higher than of that in plasma (Lawton, 1985; Mennella, 2001). In addition, the distribution of alcohol in fore- and hind-milk, relative to blood samples, is similar since the water content of fore- and hind-milk is virtually constant. Conversely, in a study by Kesäniemi (1974), alcohol levels in breastmilk were marginally lower than that in maternal blood. Differences in reported levels in these two compartments may be due to the timing of measurement. Regardless, levels of alcohol in breastmilk ranges between 80 and 90 mg/100 mL after the consumption of 30 to 50 grams of alcohol by a breastfeeding mother (Kesäniemi, 1974).

While alcohol is metabolized through oxidation to acetaldehyde, no acetaldehyde has been detected in breastmilk, irrespective of high blood alcohol levels (Kesäniemi, 1974; Liston, 1998).

The Effect of Alcohol on Breastmilk Composition and the Mammary Gland

The teratogenic effects of alcohol are well recognized. Fetal alcohol syndrome (FAS) is characterized by distinctive facial anomalies, including a smooth philtrum, epicanthal folds, flat nasal bridge and midface, small palpebral fissures, "railroad track" ears, small head circumference, upturned nose and thinner upper lip. In addition, FAS is characterized by structural or functional central nervous system abnormalities, as well as prenatal and postnatal growth retardation (Wattendorf & Muenke, 2005). Infants born with FAS present with severe feeding dysfunction. The infant tires quickly, suckles poorly, and is easily distracted while breastfeeding (Van Dyke *et al.*, 1982). This is important because suckling stimulates prolactin and oxytocin release, which is critical for the initiation of lactation and milk ejection.

However, the effect of alcohol on the pregnant mammary gland and the composition of breastmilk postnatally is not as well understood. Only one animal study is available, and it suggested that animals who received 5% alcohol during the second half of pregnancy had mammary glands that weighed less and milk that was less efficiently secreted from the mammary glands (Jones & Stewart, 1984).

In addition, other animal studies indicate that chronic alcohol consumption during pregnancy changes the composition of milk. These studies suggest that chronic alcohol exposure before mating, and/or during pregnancy, and/or during lactation, resulted in:

- impaired casein production and secretion in milk (Vilaro *et al.*, 1989),
- increased lipid and decreased lactose content, as well as increased alkalinity of milk (Sanchis & Guerri, 1986),
- impaired amino acid uptake by mammary gland (Viñas *et al.*, 1987),
- incomplete alveolar development of the mammary glands, increased lipoprotein lipase activity with correlating increased lipoprotein levels (Vilaro *et al.*, 1987),
- increased phosphatidyl-serine levels in milk (Heil *et al.*, 1999).

Another syndrome that is of importance is SIDS, which can be defined as the *"sudden death of an infant under one year of age which remains unexplained after a thorough case investigation, including performance of a complete autopsy, examination of the death scene, and review of the clinical history"* (Willinger *et al.*, 1991). The etiology of SIDS is still unclear, although neurological, pulmonary, endocrine, and cardiac causes have been considered (Makielski, 2006). However, any drug that can cause drowsiness, such as alcohol, can be associated with SIDS (Liston, 1998), contrary to the weak scientific evidence linking maternal alcohol intake to SIDS in those breastfed infants.

Alcohol's Effect on the Breastfeeding Process

Lactation Performance

It has been shown that chronic alcohol exposure in rats significantly impairs lactation performance, as indicated by the decline in milk production, altered amino acid uptake pattern, and milk composition (Vilaro *et al.*, 1987; Viñas *et al.*, 1987).

Let-down Reflex

Although there is significant variation between individual nursing mothers, it has been found that maternal doses of alcohol greater than 1-2 g/kg can interfere with the let-down reflex (Cobo, 1973). The effect of alcohol on let-down is apparently a direct pharmacologic effect, as low doses of alcohol did not significantly reduce the response (Cobo, 1973). This finding was evident in mothers who often consume alcohol and experience delayed let-down and a reported reduced milk supply (Liston, 1998). Conversely, in another study, nursing mothers who consumed one alcoholic drink reported an improved let-down reflex (Liston, 1998).

Prolactin and Oxytocin

Moderate alcohol consumption reportedly disrupts the two pituitary gland hormones, prolactin and oxytocin, that are of critical importance to lactation performance (Mennella *et al.*, 2005). The posterior pituitary hormone, oxytocin, is released as a conditioned response, stimulated by a variety of sensory inputs, including hearing the infant cry or seeing the infant, as well as suckling (Chatterton *et al.*, 2000; Cowley, 2005; Gimpl & Fahrenholz, 2001; McNeilly *et al.*, 1983). Oxytocin is responsible for the contraction of the myoepithelial cells surrounding the alveoli and interlobular ducts in the breasts, or milk ejection (Chatterton *et al.*, 2000; Liston 1998; Subramanian, 1999; Wakerley *et al.*, 1973). In turn, milk is forced into the larger ducts which makes the milk available for the infant to retrieve (Liston 1998; Subramanian, 1999). Oxytocin thus "facilitates emptying of the breast and thereby the continuation of milk secretion" (Chatterton *et al.*, 2000; Newton, 1992a, 1992b).

During pregnancy, prolactin is required for the lobuloalveolar development in the mammary gland. In addition, prolactin is required for lactogenesis at parturition and the maintenance of breastmilk secretion during lactation (Grattan, 2002). Prolactin is secreted by lactotrophs located in the adenohypophysis (anterior pituitary gland). Dopamine secreted by the tuberoinfundibular dopamine (TIDA) neurons, located in the arcuate nucleus of the hypothalamus, stimulate D2 receptors on the pituitary lactotrophs which subsequently inhibit prolactin secretion (Freeman *et al.*, 2000). Prolactin regulates its own secretion by stimulating the TIDA neurons (Freeman *et al.*, 2000).

With the onset of lactation, the suckling of the infant at the nipple provides a powerful prolactin stimulus called the prolactin surge (Selmanoff & Gregerson, 1985). According to Grattan (2002), these adaptations are essential for mammary gland functional development and maintenance during pregnancy and lactation. The basal serum prolactin level varies widely among women after the early postpartum period, during which acceptable breastmilk production is maintained (Howie *et al.*, 1980). However, it is reported that a number of women breastfeed successfully at basal prolactin levels that are equivalent to that of non-lactating women (Akre, 1989; Minchin, 1991).

Under normal conditions, prolactin and oxytocin levels increase in response to infant suckling (Johnston & Amico, 1986; Leake *et al.*, 1983; McNeilly *et al.*, 1983; Mennella *et al.*, 2005). Various studies have been performed in animals and humans to examine the effect of alcohol on prolactin release, with inconsistent results. This can be partially attributed to differences in species, sex, age, amount, and the dose of alcohol consumed.

However, a recent study suggests that during the hours immediately following alcohol consumption, prolactin levels increased while oxytocin levels decreased during and after breast stimulation in lactating women (Mennella *et al.*, 2005). Mennella and coworkers (2005) proposed that alcohol acts at the central nervous system level by inhibiting synaptic transmission of afferent impulses to the hypothalamus or through a general depression. According to Mennella and coworkers (2005), this inhibition or depression will result in decreased oxytocin levels (Gimpl & Fahrenholz, 2001), and an increase in prolactin levels since the projections from the hypothalamus exert an inhibitory control on prolactin (Freeman *et al.*, 2000). However, animal studies suggest that chronic alcohol exposure increases prolactin levels by increasing the number of lactotropes in the anterior pituitary gland and by increasing prolactin release from lactotropes (De *et al.*, 2002).

In addition, there is a strong correlation between prolactin levels and the degree of fullness of the breasts of nursing mothers (Cox *et al.*, 1996). Conversely, there is no correlation between prolactin levels and the amount of milk that is produced (Bohnet & Kato, 1985; Chatterton *et al.*, 2000; Howie *et al.*, 1980; Mennella *et al.*, 2005). Since alcohol may increase breast fullness, nursing mothers erroneously believe that their milk production increased. In addition, since alcohol inhibits oxytocin release (Fuchs, 1969; Fuchs & Wagner, 1963; Gibbens & Chard, 1976; Mennella *et al.*, 2005; Subramanian, 1999; Wagner & Fuchs, 1968), the reduced milk ejection and yield (Mennella *et al.*, 2005) may result in a disruption of milk delivery to the infant (Mennella & Beauchamp, 1991, 1993a, 1993b).

Milk Ingestion by Infant

Thirty minutes after a nursing mother ingests one drink, it reportedly produces a mild sedative effect in the breastfed infant (Liston, 1998), but also changes the odor of her breastmilk (Liston, 1998; Mennella & Beauchamp, 1991). This may result in the refusal of the infant to breastfeed due to taste, with subsequent less breastmilk intake (Mennella & Beauchamp, 1993b).

In fact, three to four hours after a nursing mother had an alcoholic beverage (0.3 g/kg), the infant consumed approximately 20% less breastmilk (Ito, 2000; Mennella & Beauchamp, 1991, 1993b). This finding correlates with a study performed in rats where milk consumption by rat pups was significantly reduced after acute alcohol administration to lactating rats (Subramanian & Abel, 1988).

Conversely, other studies found that infants exposed to alcohol through breastmilk, consume less milk, although it was not because of the change in the flavor of the breastmilk (Mennella, 1997) or because the infant nursed for shorter periods of time (Mennella & Beauchamp, 1991, 1993b).

Alcohol's Effect on the Breastfed Infant

It is known that alcohol is poorly metabolized by infants. In addition, there are reports that serial doses of alcohol delivered through breastmilk can cause alcohol accumulation in the breastfed infant (Little *et al.*, 1989), which is probably due to the slower metabolism and/or excretion of alcohol (Le Guennec & Billon, 1987; Little *et al.*, 1989). During the first weeks of life, infants metabolize alcohol at about half the rate of adults. Alcohol exposure in younger infants may have a greater effect when compared to older infants. In 1987 however, Le Guennec and Billon suggested that breastmilk contains a component that temporarily inhibits the postnatal maturation of hepatic cytochrome P450. This finding is critical since alcohol as well as caffeine are metabolized by cytochrome P450 2E1 (CYP2E1) (Mennella, 2001; Terelius *et al.*, 1991).

Alcohol ingested orally is subject to gastric first pass metabolism, largely by class I and IV isoforms of alcohol dehydrogenase (ADH), but also to a minor extent by the class III isoform of ADH (Moreno & Parés, 1991; Moreno *et al.*, 1994; Parés *et al.*, 1992). ADH activity is dependent on age (Harada & Okubo, 1993; Moreno *et al.*, 1994; Seitz *et al.*, 1993), gender (Frezza *et al.*, 1990; Seitz & Oneta, 1998; Seitz *et al.*, 1993), ethnicity (Baraona *et al.*, 1991; Yin *et al.*, 1997), concentration of alcohol ingested (Koivusalo *et al.*, 1989), gastric mucosal injury (DiPadova *et al.*, 1987; Pedrosa *et al.*, 1996; Thuluvath *et al.*, 1994), gastric emptying of alcohol (Oneta *et al.*, 1998), and co-administration of alcohol with drugs that might inhibit ADH activity, such as cimetidine and ranitidine (DiPadova *et al.*, 1992; Hernandez-Munoz *et al.*, 1990; Roine *et al.*, 1990). Pikkarainen and Räihä (1967) found that infants between the age of ten days and seven months presented with liver ADH activity of approximately 20% when compared to that of adults between the ages of 20 to 50 years. Interestingly, the ADH activity of two month old infants approximately doubles when they reach the age of seven months, but their ADH activity will still be <50% of that of adults during the first year of life (Pikkarainen & Räihä, 1967). Thus, neonates/infants who breastfeed from mothers that ingest alcohol may have a lower capacity to metabolize alcohol, which may predispose these infants to higher levels of alcohol.

Excessive intake of alcohol by mothers who breastfed their infants may lead to drowsy, fussy, weak, and sleepy babies (Liston, 1998) that may not suck well, which in turn may lead to reduced milk supply (Hale, 1998). In another study (Binkiewicz *et al.*, 1978), a four month old breastfeeding infant presented with Pseudo-Cushing syndrome. The mother reportedly consumed more than fifty 12 ounce beers and other alcoholic beverages per week. The infant was considered obese, short statured, and had a "balloon-shaped" or "moon-shaped" facial appearance. The appearance and growth of the infant gradually returned to normal when the mother discontinued consuming alcohol (Binkiewicz *et al.*, 1978).

Acute exposure to alcohol through breastmilk can also result in altered sleep-wake patterns of the infant. These infants tend to fall asleep faster, but will be asleep for significantly shorter periods of time (Mennella & Gerrish, 1998). In addition, one study indicated that breastfed infants at one year of age presented with slightly, though statistically insignificant, decreased motor development when the mothers had one alcoholic drink per day during the first three months postpartum (Little *et al.*, 1989). Conversely, these results could not be duplicated in a subsequent study (Little *et al.*, 2002).

Another study (Backstrand *et al.*, 2004) concluded that heavy intake of "pulque" by nursing mothers was associated with poorer child growth. Pulque is a mild beverage that contains approximately 4-6% alcohol.

Lastly, breastfed infants exposed to alcohol have been reported to exhibit impaired neurological development as evident by lower Psychomotor Development Index scores (Ito, 2000; Little *et al.*, 1989).

Conclusion

Alcohol follows zero-order metabolism (Ito *et al.*, 2000), and it should take approximately two hours for one drink to be eliminated in adults. Its elimination cannot be accelerated by resting, drinking water, or "pumping and dumping" breastmilk (Anderson, 1995). In addition, the time needed for alcohol to be eliminated from breastmilk is dependent on various factors, including a person's weight and height (Koren, 2002).

Koren (2002) produced an algorithm through pharmacokinetic modeling that determines the time needed for alcohol to be eliminated from breastmilk. According to this report, it requires approximately two to three hours for one alcoholic drink to be totally eliminated from breastmilk in women weighing between 90 to 210 pounds with an average height of 5'4" (Koren, 2002). Although the calculations yield theoretical values, one shortcoming of this study is that the values are based on patients with a specific height of 5'4". Furthermore, Koren does not provide a supporting mathematical formula, without which it is difficult to customize the calculation to suit a specific patient of a different height.

Breastfeeding women who chronically ingest alcohol or who are heavy consumers of alcohol should avoid breastfeeding their infants (Hale, 2004; Hale & McAfee, 2005). It is advised that nursing women do not consume more than one alcoholic beverage between each breastfeeding session (Ito, 2000).

The effects of alcohol on the breastfed infant are concentration and exposure dependent (Dillon *et al.*, 1997). Social drinking is thought to only have a mild sedative effect (Lindmark, 1990), whereas greater alcohol intake is linked to drowsy, fussy, weak, and sleepy babies (Hale & McAfee, 2005). Heavy alcohol use may have profound neurobehavioral effects on the nursing mother, including fatigue and increased susceptibility to depression, thereby reducing her ability to function as a caregiver. Heavy exposure to alcohol may also reduce appetite and could reduce the nutritional components in milk.

The goal of all nursing mothers should be to limit the exposure of their infants to alcohol. This can be accomplished by eating before and during alcohol consumption, waiting for at least two hours after consuming alcohol to breastfeed the infant, choosing low-alcoholic drinks, and expressing and storing alcohol-free breastmilk for use after moderate to heavy alcohol consumption, particularly during the first three months of the infant's life (Liston, 1998).

COCAINE

The *Erythroxylon* coca bush grows primarily in Bolivia and Peru where pure cocaine was first extracted from the leaf of the plant in the mid 19th century (National Institute on Drug Abuse, 1999). Today, cocaine is one of the oldest drugs known to be abused with its popularity soaring during the 1980's and 1990's. Two chemical forms of cocaine exists: the "freebase" which can be smoked and the hydrochloride salt, a powder form of cocaine that can be snorted or taken intravenously when dissolved in water. On the street, cocaine is known as 'C,' snow, coke, flake, or blow, among other names (**Figure 3**). Most often, drug dealers dilute cocaine with inert substances or with active drugs, such as procaine or amphetamines (National Institute on Drug Abuse, 1999).

Gestational Cocaine Use and Its Effects on the Infant Postnatally

Studies show that infants born of mothers abusing cocaine during pregnancy presented with:

- lower gestational age at delivery (MacGregor *et al.*, 1987),

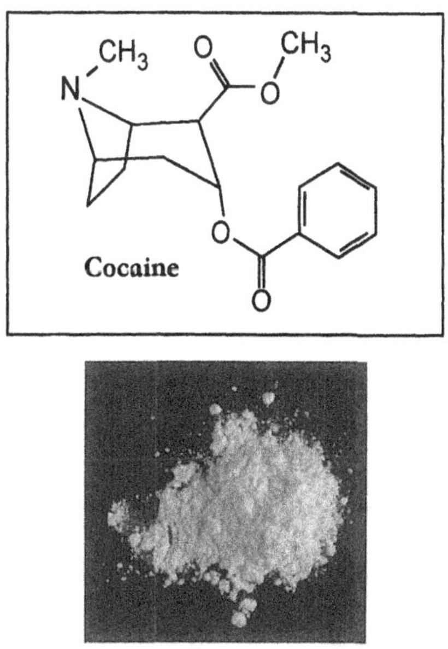

Figure 3. Chemical structure (top) and photograph of cocaine (photo image courtesy of the Drug Enforcement Administration).

- lower birth weight (Bendersky & Lewis, 1999; MacGregor *et al.*, 1987, Zuckerman *et al.*, 1989),
- prematurity (Chasnoff, 1989; MacGregor *et al.*, 1987),
- intrauterine growth retardation (Chasnoff, 1989),
- delivery of an infant who is small for its gestational age (MacGregor *et al.*, 1987),
- high incidence of pregnancy complications,
- microcephaly,
- perinatal morbidity (Chasnoff, 1989),
- a 15% increased risk of SIDS compared to methadone exposed infants (Chasnoff *et al.*, 1987a),
- abnormal sleeping ventilatory patterns that may be related to the increased SIDS risk among those infants (Ward *et al.*, 1986), and
- increased risk of congenital cardiovascular malformations (Lipshultz *et al.*, 1991).

Chronic Exposure of Cocaine in Rats During Gestation

Experiments in rodents suggest that cocaine decreases oxytocin levels in certain brain areas. **Table 1** offers a summary of the specific brain areas and the effects induced by cocaine.

Table 1. Neurologic Effects Subsequent to Cocaine-induced Reduction of Oxytocin Levels as a Function of Brain Area

Brain area	Cocaine induced effects
Medial preoptic area (MPOA) of the hypothalamus, Ventral tegmental area (VTA) and Hippocampus (Johns *et al.*, 1997)	Disruptions in the onset of maternal behavior (Heyser *et al.*, 1992; Johns *et al.*, 1994; Kinsley *et al.*, 1994; Vernotica *et al.*, 1996; Zimmerberg & Gray, 1992)
Amygdala (Johns *et al.*, 1995)	Heightened postpartum aggression (Johns *et al.*, 1995)

Cocaine Pharmacokinetics And Its Effect on Breastfed Infants

During the 1990's, it was believed that concurrent cocaine abuse and breastfeeding was a common phenomenon (Dickson *et al.*, 1994), however, its prevalence in the 21st century is not known. Unfortunately, the physiochemistry of cocaine is ideal for producing toxic concentrations in breastmilk and the plasma compartment of the breastfed infant (Bailey, 1993). The M/P ratio in rats has been reported as 7.8 (Wiggins *et al.*, 1989), and it is likely to have a high value in humans as well. Cocaine concentrations in breastmilk of mothers who abuse cocaine can reach up to 12 µg/mL (Winecker *et al.*, 2001). With a pKa of 8.6, it is likely to be trapped in the milk compartment of most species (Winecker *et al.*, 2001).

Polydrug Abuse of Cocaine and Alcohol

Two carboxylesterase enzymes, human liver carboxylesterases form 1 and 2 (hCE-1 and hCE-2) have been identified to take part in the metabolism of cocaine. hCE-1 and hCE-2 are more abundant in liver, but also present in the heart, colon, kidney, stomach, and other tissues. Cocaine is normally metabolized by hydrolysis to benzoylecgonine via hCE-1 and to ecgonine methyl ester via hCE-2 (Brzezinski *et al.*, 1994; Dean *et al.*, 1991) and pseudocholinesterase (Stewart *et al.*, 1977, 1979) with subsequent elimination by the kidneys. Both benzoylecgonine and ecgonine methyl ester are pharmacologically inactive (Sun & Lau, 2001).

Cocaine abuse is often complicated by the concurrent intake of alcohol, probably since the users experience a prolonged and more pronounced euphoric effect as opposed to when the drugs are taken separately (Harris *et al.*, 2003b; McCance-Katz *et al.*, 1993). Cocaine does not undergo hydrolysis in the presence of alcohol, but rather transesterification via hCE-1, producing the active metabolite cocaethylene (**Figure 4**).

Both the behavioral and psychomotor stimulant effects of cocaethylene are similar to those of cocaine. Cocaethylene inhibits dopamine uptake into synaptosomes by binding to the dopamine transporter (Bailey, 1997). However, the toxicity of cocaethylene is greater as is evident by its lower LD50 value (Hearn *et al.*, 1991). Cocaethylene had a significantly longer plasma half-life (mean = 3.5 hours) when compared to cocaine (1 hour) in a study performed by Bailey (1993). In addition, cocaethylene to cocaine plasma concentration ratios ranged between 0.1 and 4.7 (mean = 1.3), with mean plasma levels of 353 nmol/L and 386 nmol/L, respectively (Bailey, 1996).

Cocaethylene has been detected in the breastmilk of mothers following ingestion of cocaine (Bailey, 1998; Dickson *et al.*, 1994). A study by Bailey (1998) suggests that cocaethylene binds to breastmilk to a higher degree than cocaine (61% vs. 55%). In addition, the lower pH of breastmilk provides an "ion trap" for both cocaine

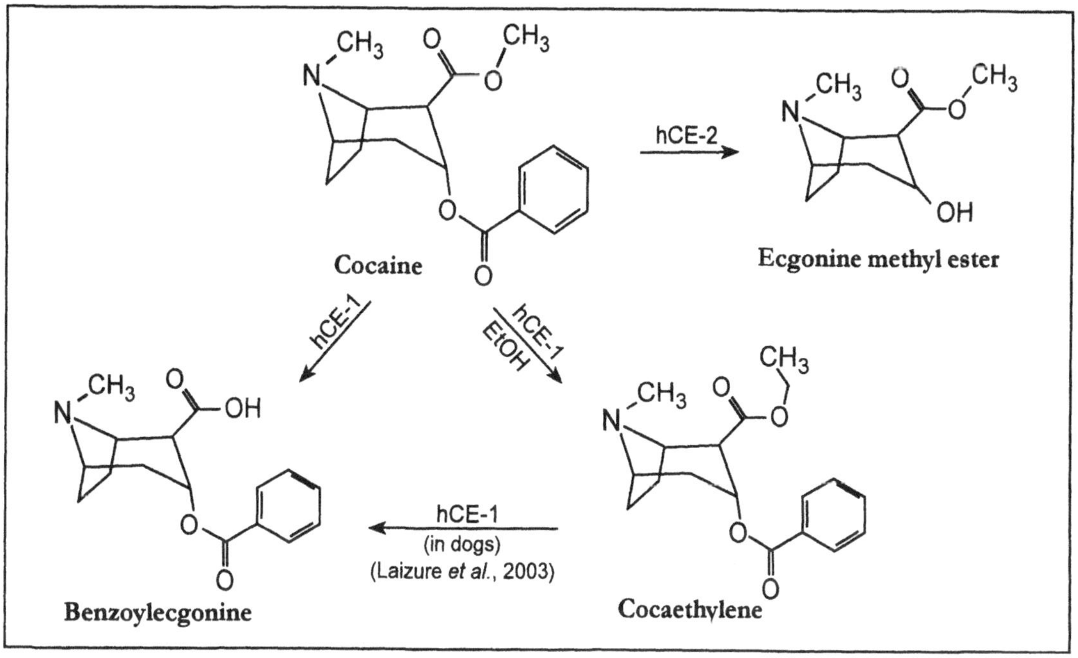

Figure 4. Metabolism of cocaine by hCE-1 or hCE-2, producing ecgonine methyl ester and benzoylecgonine. In the presence of ethanol, cocaine is metabolized to cocaethylene via hCE-1 (Laizure *et al.*, 2003).

and cocaethylene, with pKa values of 8.60 and 8.23, respectively. Cocaethylene is therefore of toxicological importance not only to the drug users but also to the breastfeeding infant.

Cocaine is not only concomitantly taken with alcohol, but also with heroin. For more information, refer to "Polydrug use" under the heroin section.

Case Studies

As noted before, drug abuse will likely continue throughout pregnancy and the postpartum period. However, in a case where cocaine was solely abused during the postpartum period, the breastfed infant presented with tachycardia, hypertension, and irritability three hours after nursing at two weeks postpartum (Chasnoff *et al.*, 1987b). Symptoms were transient and subsided 48 hours after nursing ceased. Cocaine and its major metabolite, benzoylecgonine, were detected in the mother's breastmilk for 36 hours after the last reported cocaine use and was present in the infant's urine for 60 hours after nursing was ceased (Chasnoff *et al.*, 1987b).

In case studies by Winecker and coworkers (2001), only trace amounts of cocaine were present in breastmilk. However, breastmilk samples may test positive for cocaine up to 60 hours after exposure to the drug (Chaney *et al.*, 1988). Furthermore, maternal history is not a reliable indicator of prenatal cocaine exposure (Schutzman *et al.*, 1991). In cases of suspected maternal cocaine abuse, infant urine screens and even breastmilk are good sources for determining exposure to cocaine.

In another case, an 11 week old breastfed infant was admitted to the hospital, following symptoms of gasping, choking, and hypoxia. The breastmilk of the mother was negative for cocaine and metabolites, but the infants' urine tested positive. Further investigation revealed that the mother applied cocaine to her nipples as treatment for nipple soreness. The infant presented with symptoms of acute cocaine ingestion, including seizures. The infant was discharged after five days, had no further seizures, and the physical examination was normal. At six months of age, the findings of the neurological and physical examinations were normal (Chaney *et al.*, 1988).

Miscellaneous

Since the hydrochloride salt of cocaine can be injected, there is a severe risk of contracting human immunodeficiency virus (HIV) when using non-sterile syringes and needles (National Institute on Drug Abuse, 1999). It is important to note that the infant will be exposed to HIV at birth and when breastfed (Jeffery & Mercer, 2000).

Conclusion

Lifetime cocaine prevalence rates among youths, twelve years and older, peaked at an all time high of 2.7% in

2002 compared to that of 0.1% in 1967 and 2.2% in 1987 (National Institute on Drug Abuse, 1999). Various health risks are associated with cocaine abuse, including heart attacks, strokes, respiratory failure, seizures, and violent and bizarre behavior. Sadly, more is known about the social and behavioral complications of cocaine abuse than what is known about the levels present in breastmilk and its effects on the breastfed infant.

Cocaine abuse by a mother who is breastfeeding her infant is without a doubt a major health risk to the infant. The combination of high maternal cocaine blood concentrations with a high M/P ratio could easily produce toxic blood concentrations in the infant. Furthermore, since the infant's metabolic pathways are still immature, higher plasma levels could result (Dickson *et al.*, 1994), with detrimental effects. Unfortunately, limited data are available on the effects of cocaine on a breastfeeding infant. Conversely though, this does not prevent the AAP's Committee on Drugs to contraindicate cocaine use during breastfeeding (American Academy of Pediatrics Committee on Drugs, 2001).

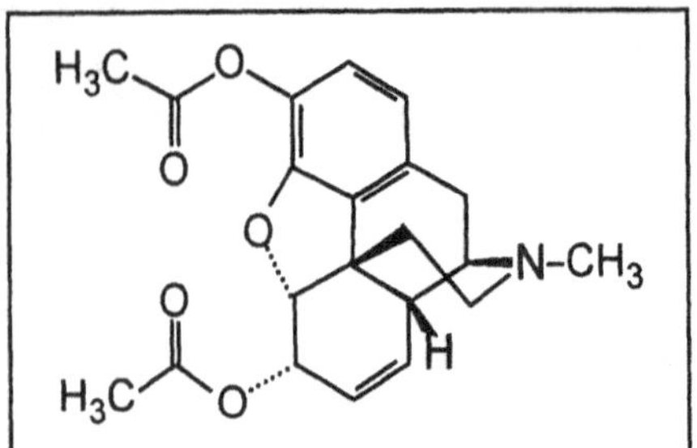

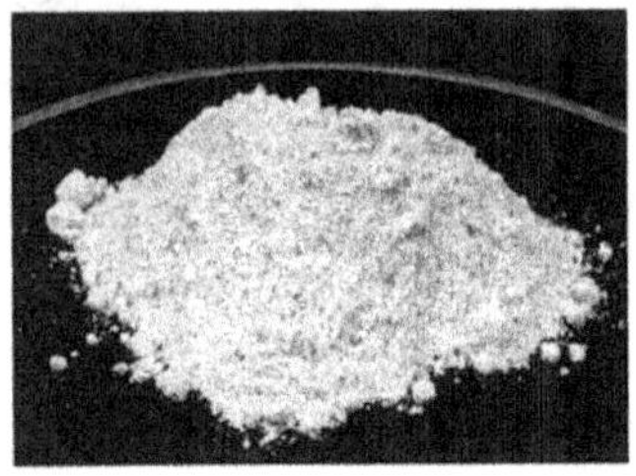

Figure 5. Chemical structure of heroin (top) and photo of heroin powder (photo image courtesy of the Drug Enforcement Administration).

HEROIN

A British chemist, C.R. Wright, first synthesized diacetylmorphine (heroin) (**Figure 5**) in 1874 by boiling anhydrous morphine alkaloid with acetic anhydride for several hours. It was not until 23 years later that its commercial potential was realized when it was resynthesized at Bayer Pharmaceutical in Germany by Felix Hoffman in 1897. Sales skyrocketed when it was marketed as a non-addictive cough remedy and shipped to over 20 countries worldwide as an ingredient in elixirs, lozenges, tablets, and water soluble salts. By 1902, American and French researchers reported on the "addictive" properties of heroin and in 1913 Bayer stopped its manufacture of the drug (Anon, 1998).

Today, heroin is a legal drug in some countries and in the United Kingdom it is available under the trade name diamorphine hydrochloride, which is prescribed for acute pulmonary edema, myocardial infarction, as well as for acute and chronic pain. In the USA on the other hand, it is illegal to possess, sell, or manufacture heroin.

Metabolism of Heroin

The pharmacological activity of heroin stems from its metabolites, 6-monoacetylmorphine and morphine (**Figure 6**) (Hosztafi, 2003; Reisine & Pasternak, 1996). However, heroin and 6-monoacetylmorphine are more lipid soluble than morphine and therefore are likely to enter the central nervous system and breastmilk in greater concentrations.

The 3-acetyl group of heroin undergoes hydrolysis by hCE-1 and hCE-2 (Brzezinski *et al.*, 1994; Kamendulis *et al.*, 1996) as well as pseudocholinesterase (Lockridge *et al.*, 1980) (serum cholinesterase found primarily in the liver) to form 6-monoacetylmorphine. Subsequent hydrolysis of 6-monoacetylmorphine to morphine is catalyzed mainly by hCE-2 (Kamendulis *et al.*, 1996; Pindel *et al.*, 1997).

Heroin and the Breastfed Infant

Since illicit heroin is most often "cut" (mixed) with other substances, such as powdered milk, sugar, starch, quinine, strychnine, or other substances, it is virtually impossible to determine the actual dose of heroin administered under these circumstances.

To date there are no published data on the transfer of heroin into human milk. However, taking into account that the half-life of heroin is only three minutes after an intravenous injection (Sawynok, 1986) and the fact that only the metabolites of heroin are active, one should rather consider the transfer of 6-monoacetylmorphine and morphine (M/P ratio of morphine = 2.45) as opposed to heroin (Feilberg *et al.*, 1989). In addition,

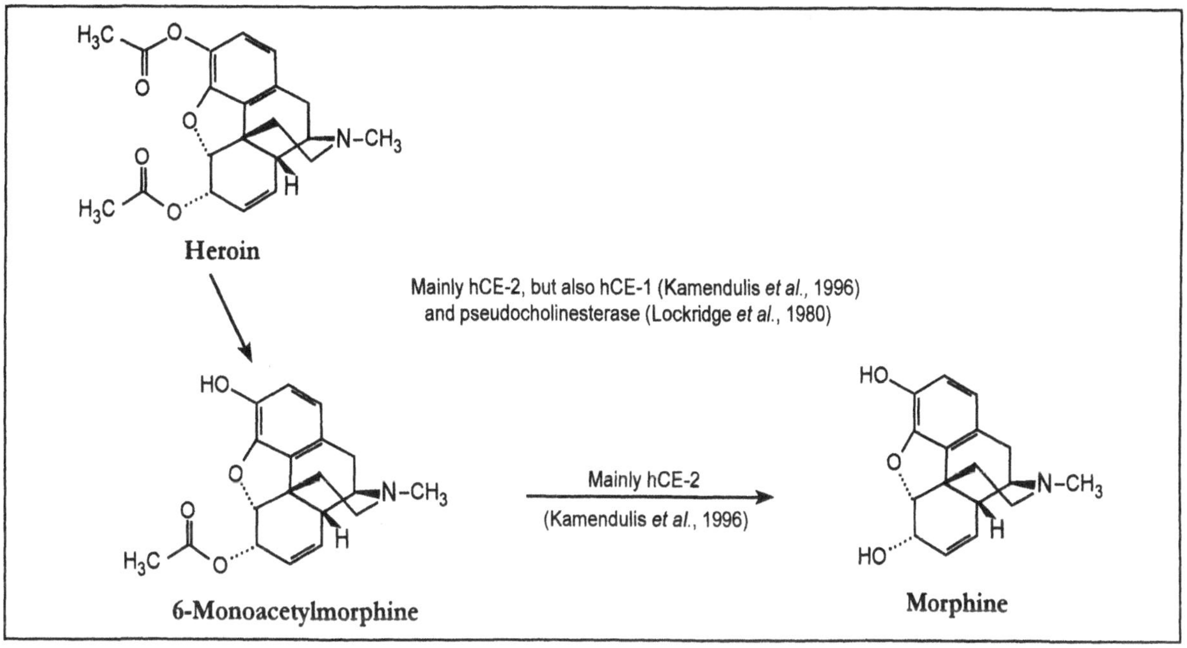

Figure 6. Hydrolysis of heroin (diacetylmorphine) to 6-monoacetylmorphine and subsequently to morphine.

morphine bioavailability following oral administration (<30%) is limited by first pass sequestration in the liver. With the exception of morphine, the milk levels of all of the above mentioned compounds are still unknown.

A study by Girardin and coworkers (2003) in heroin addicts suggests that although heroin is absorbed orally it yields negligible systemic heroin and 6-monoacetylmorphine levels. To date, there are no data on the actual presence of heroin in breastmilk and its subsequent bioavailability in breastfed infants from heroin abusing mothers. Only one case study has been reported on the oral use of heroin. In this case, a breastfed infant whose mother was abusing heroin postnatally, presented with withdrawal symptoms when feeding was withheld or when the mother was deprived of the drug (Catz & Giacoia, 1972).

Polydrug Use

Many drug users often prefer abusing multiple drugs to increase the level of neurobehavorial effects. This is especially true in the case of heroin and cocaine, also called 'speedballing' or 'snowballing', which may result in an increased risk of lethal drug overdose. When used concomitantly, cocaine competitively inhibits the metabolism of heroin (Kamendulis *et al.*, 1996). There are no data available to date on the effects of speedballing on the breastfed infant.

Heroin is also abused concomitantly with marijuana. However, no data are available on the effect of this polydrug use on breastfed infants.

Miscellaneous

Traditionally heroin is injected intravenously, but it can also be snorted or 'smoked' (inhaling the vapors of heated heroin is also known as 'chasing the dragon'). According to the National Institute on Drug Abuse, injecting heroin is still the most common method of heroin abuse (National Institute on Drug Abuse, 2005b).

Intravenous heroin abusers have an increased risk of contracting blood-borne pathogens, such as HIV, hepatitis B, and hepatitis C, and may ultimately transfer HIV and hepatitis B to the breastfed infant. Mothers with hepatitis B may continue to breastfeed following immunization with the hepatitis B vaccine and treatment with the hepatitis immune globulin. Thus far, no cases of hepatitis C transmission to breastfed infants have been reported. The Centers for Disease Control and Prevention (2006) endorses breastfeeding if the mother is infected with hepatitis C; however, the nursing mother should temporarily cease breastfeeding and pump and discard her milk if her nipples are cracked and bleeding. The HIV virus on the other hand, has been isolated from breastmilk and nursing therefore poses a great risk to the infant (Goldfarb, 1993). Nursing women living in the USA who are infected with HIV are advised not to breastfeed their infants.

Conclusion

At present, we do not have data on the transfer of heroin into human milk. It is known that heroin, an inactive compound, undergoes hydrolysis to active metabolites, including 6-monoacetylmorphine and morphine. Morphine subsequently undergoes conjugation to morphine-6-glucuronide. With a half-life of only three minutes, the transfer of heroin into breastmilk is unlikely. Rather, morphine, the active metabolite of heroin, is well known to be excreted in breastmilk.

Potential effects on the breastfed infant exposed to opiates (Hosztafi, 2003) include respiratory depression, drowsiness, bradycardia, and apnea (Chrisholm & Kuller, 1997). The ability of the mother to assume care of the infant is also compromised while under the influence of opiates. The AAP contraindicates heroin use during breastfeeding (American Academy of Pediatrics, 1989).

LYSERGIC ACID DIETHYLAMIDE (LSD)

LSD, more commonly known as acid, blotter, dots, microdot, pane, sugar cubes, trip, and window pane among numerous other names, is a hallucinogen that causes extreme distortions in a user's perception of reality (National Institute on Drug Abuse InfoFacts, 2006b). The most common form of LSD that is sold is blotter paper (**Figure 7**), where sheets of paper are soaked in LSD and perforated into small squares of individual dosage units (National Institute on Drug Abuse, 2001).

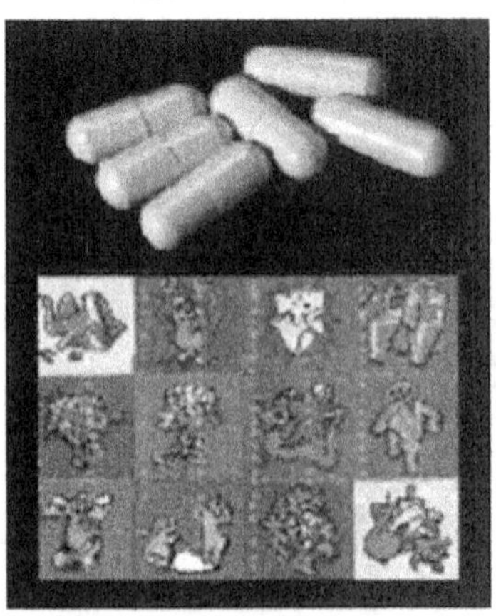

Figure 7. LSD capsules and blotter paper (photo images courtesy of the Drug Enforcement Administration).

Unfortunately, no data are available on the transfer of LSD into human milk. However, LSD is an enormously potent hallucinogen, and microscopic amounts present in breastmilk could potentially harm an infant. While we do not have specific data concerning the levels of LSD present in breastmilk, its physiochemistry is ideal for the transfer into breastmilk. Combined with its enormous potency, LSD poses an enhanced risk to breastfed infants.

It has been confirmed through radioactive studies on rats and mice that LSD crosses the placenta and enters the fetus during different stages of gestation. The half-life of LSD in rats is seven minutes and within 15 to 20 minutes after an intravenous injection, LSD accumulates in the brain of the rat. Receptor bound LSD localizes in the midbrain, medulla, and cortex where LSD distributes to the hippocampus choroidal plexus, cerebellum, pituitary and pineal glands (Tuchmann-Duplessis, 1983).

In man, the half-life of LSD has been reported as 175 minutes. An increased risk of spontaneous abortion has been identified in human LSD users (Tuchmann-Duplessis, 1983). Older *in vitro* studies suggests that LSD use leads to chromosomal damage. However, it seems that LSD use is not realistically linked to chromosomal damage in humans (Dishotsky *et al.*, 1971; Long, 1972). Thus, there is insufficient evidence to suggest that LSD is indeed teratogenic (Cohen & Shiloh, 1977-1978; Tuchmann-Duplessis, 1983).

Although the chemical structure (**Figure 8**) of a compound does not provide an indication of its possible teratogenetic effects (Tuchmann-Duplessis, 1983), it does provide clues to whether it will appear in the breastmilk of the lactating mother. Having a small molecular weight

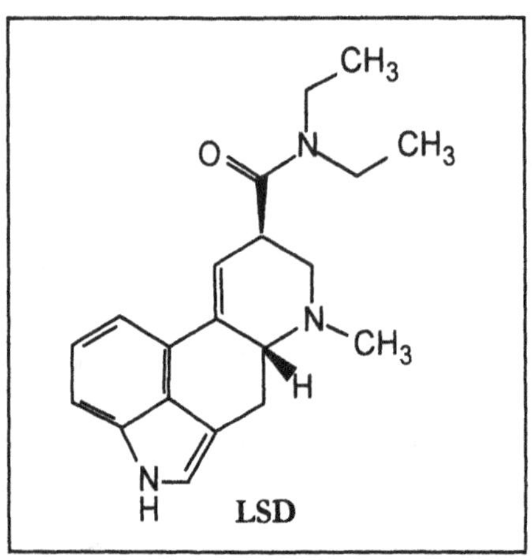

Figure 8. Chemical structure of lysergic acid diethylamide (LSD).

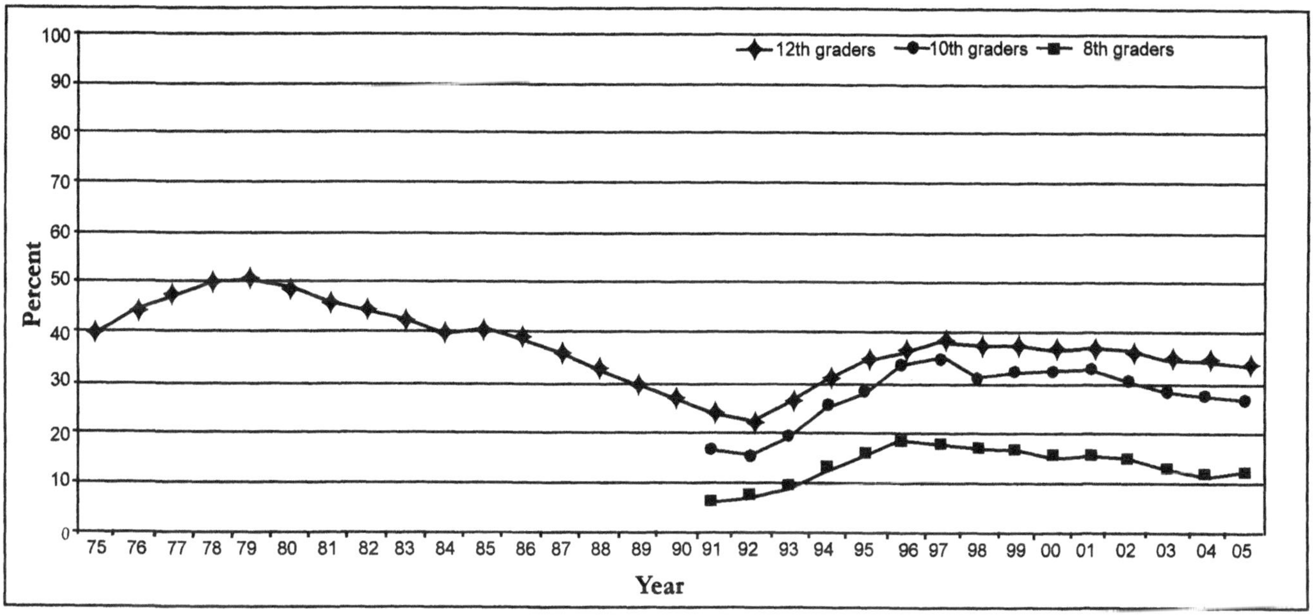

Figure 9: Trends in annual marijuana use for 8th, 10th, and 12th graders from 1975 to 2005 (Johnston *et al.*, 2006).

(323.44 g/mol) and enormous lipophilicity, it is probable that LSD would significantly enter into breastmilk and produce psychomimetic effects in the breastfeeding infant (Dillon *et al.*, 1997).

In a study performed by Meltzer and coworkers (1977) in rodents, LSD was reported to directly or indirectly inhibit prolactin release because of its significant dopamine receptor agonistic properties in the pituitary. In addition, a study performed in rats by Quadri and Meites (1971) showed that LSD is a potent inhibitor of prolactin release by the pituitary gland. These findings are supported by an *in vitro* study performed by Giacomelli and coworkers (1998) on pituitary cell cultures, which indicated that LSD inhibits prolactin release in a concentration-dependent manner. While performed in a rodent and *in vitro* model system, these studies suggest that prolactin release may be affected in lactating women who abuse LSD. Considering the importance of prolactin in the synthesis of breastmilk (Selmanoff & Gregerson, 1985), it can be concluded that LSD could potentially affect milk production.

However, the psychotomimetic effects of LSD are profound, and the ability of the mother to tend to her infant's needs is highly questionable. A study in lactating rats showed that LSD severely disrupted maternal behavior, indicated by a delay in the onset of nursing and significantly shorter nursing time (Uyeno, 1970).

Conclusion

Unfortunately, no data are available on the effects of LSD on the breastfed infant. However, taking into consideration that LSD is extremely potent at low doses, has a molecular weight of 323.43 g/mol, and a high degree of lipophilicity (XLogP = 2.1), its use is definitely contraindicated during breastfeeding.

MARIJUANA

Marijuana, known by its various street names as pot, weed, mj, reefer, grass, mary jane or herb was the most commonly used illicit drug across the USA in 2005 (National Survey on Drug Use and Health, 2005). The annual trend between 1975 and 2005 of 8th, 10th and 12th graders who used marijuana is shown in **Figure 9**.

The psychological effects associated with the use of marijuana include euphoria, slowed reaction time and thinking, impaired motor performance and coordination, altered perception, poor short memory, impaired judgment and attention, anxiety, panic attacks, and dizziness. The adverse effects of marijuana (physiological) include increased heart rate, redness of eyes, dry mouth, nausea, increased appetite, immune system dysfunction, and respiratory disorder (Djulus *et al.*, 2005; Heyman *et al.*, 1999; Thomas, 1993).

Active Ingredient of Marijuana

Marijuana smoke contains more than 150 compounds (Djulus *et al.*, 2005). Δ^9-Tetrahydrocannabinol (THC), the main ingredient in the marijuana plant, *Cannabis sativa*, produces psychotic-like symptoms and anxiety (Zuardi, 2006). The amount of THC in the preparation that is smoked, eaten (mixed with foods), or drank (tea) determines the potency and, therefore, the effects of the marijuana (National Institute on Drug Abuse, 2005a). Today's marijuana plant is much more potent when compared to those of 30 years ago since the content of THC increased from less than 1% in the mid-1970's to more than 6% in 2002 (Office of National Drug Control Policy, 2003).

Excretion of THC in Breastmilk

After using marijuana, THC is absorbed from the lungs or gastrointestinal tract and rapidly distributes throughout the body, accumulating in the brain and fatty tissues. It subsequently redistributes from the central nervous system (CNS) to adipose tissue, where it is slowly released over prolonged periods. THC is extensively bound to plasma protein (97%). Ten minutes after marijuana is smoked, THC reaches its peak plasma levels (7-18 ng/mL) (Huestis *et al.*, 1992). Fifteen to 20% of the smoked THC is ultimately excreted in the urine as acidic metabolites, whereas 30 to 35% is excreted in the feces as 11-hydroxy-Δ^9-tetrahydrocannabinol (11-OH-THC) and 11-nor-9-carboxy-Δ^9-tetrahydrocannabinol (9-carboxy-THC). The metabolism of THC is shown in **Figure 10**, here 11-OH-THC, the active metabolite of THC, is formed via hydroxylation by cytochrome P450 followed by oxidation to yield the inactive metabolite, 9-carboxy-THC (Huestis, 2002).

To determine the elimination half-life of THC (between three to five days) in heavy smokers, Johansson and coworkers (1988) used deuterium-labeled THC and a sensitive analytical procedure (gas chromatography/mass spectrometry with selected ion monitoring). Care should be taken when a less sensitive assay is used to determine the half-life of THC, since it can result in a much lower estimate of its half-life.

After marijuana is ingested by the lactating mother, THC and its metabolites, 11-OH-THC and 9-carboxy-THC, are secreted in the breastmilk and absorbed by the nursing infant (Perez-Reyes & Wall, 1982). The levels of THC in the blood and breastmilk of a marijuana user is dependent on the amount of marijuana ingested, the content of THC in the marijuana that is used, and the length of time between drug use and sample collection

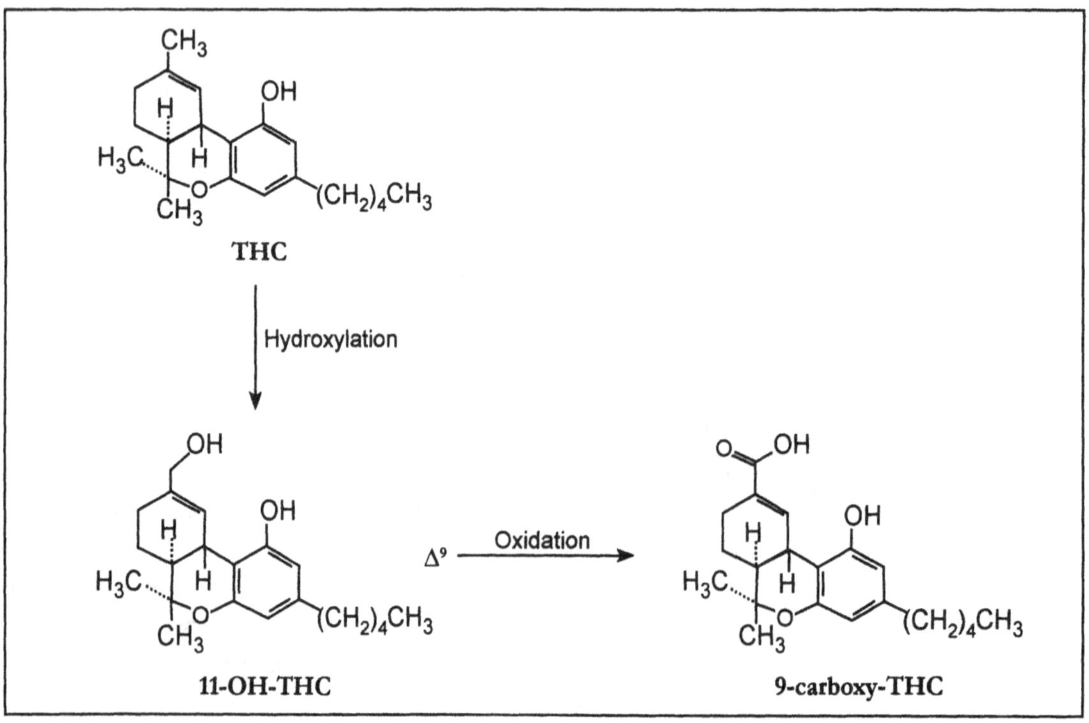

Figure 10. Metabolic fate of Δ^9 tetrahydrocannabinol (THC) to form 11-hydroxy-Δ^9-tetrahydrocannabinol (11-OH-THC) and, subsequently, 11-nor-9-carboxy-Δ^9-tetrahydrocannabinol (9-carboxy-THC) (Huestis, 2002).

(blood or breastmilk) (Perez-Reyes & Wall, 1982). A breastfed infant exposed to marijuana will test positive for a urine screen test for up to two to three weeks (Hale, 1998).

A study performed by Perez-Reyes & Wall (1982) indicate that one hour after the last drug use there is an eightfold accumulation of THC in breastmilk versus that in maternal plasma (M/P ratio = 8). Such accumulation does not occur in the case of the metabolites, 11-OH-THC and 9-carboxy-THC, most likely because of their lower lipophilicity when compared to THC. Maternal plasma levels reported in this study for the various compounds are as follows: THC 7.2 ng/mL; 11-OH-THC 2.5 ng/mL; 9-carboxy-THC 19 ng/mL, with respective breastmilk levels as: THC 60.3 ng/mL; 11-OH-THC 1.1 ng/mL; 9-carboxy-THC 1.6 ng/mL. The nursing infant excreted THC, 11-OH-THC, and 9-carboxy-THC in its stool. The proportion of the metabolites to THC was higher in the feces when compared to that of the breastmilk, suggesting that the infant's body metabolizes THC to 11-OH-THC and 9-carboxy-THC.

Marijuana's Effect on Lactation (Animal Studies) and the Breastfed Infant

Some animal studies suggest that marijuana reduces milk production (Borgen, 1971), possibly due to reduced prolactin levels and/or decreased mammary gland growth caused by THC after chronic use (Asch *et al.*, 1979; Hughes *et al.*, 1981; Kramer & Ben-David, 1978; Raine *et al.*, 1978; Rettori *et al.*, 1988). Unfortunately, there are no data in humans to confirm these results.

Taking into account that an infant's brain is still developing postnatally, THC could theoretically affect the normal brain development of breastfed infants exposed to marijuana (Djulus *et al.*, 2005), although there is conflicting evidence that this occurs. In one study of 27 women who smoked marijuana routinely during breastfeeding, no differences were noted in outcomes on growth, mental, and motor development (Tennes *et al.*, 1985). In another study performed by Astley and Little (1990), exposure to marijuana during lactation was associated with decreased motor development in one year old infants.

Lethargy and shorter, less frequent feedings have been observed after infants were exposed to THC through breastmilk (Djulus *et al.*, 2005). In addition, use of marijuana can compromise the ability of a nursing mother to adequately care for the infant, since it can affect her judgment and mood.

The Effect of Prenatal and Postnatal Marijuana Exposure on the Fetus, Infant, and Findings of Animal Studies

Effects of Marijuana on the Fetus and Infant Exposed Prenatally

Prenatal marijuana use is associated with decreased maternal weight gain and a shorter gestation period, but has no effect on the length of labor (Fried, 1982). Recent data suggest that early maternal marijuana use is linked to a reduction in foot length and body weight in mid-gestation fetuses (Hurd *et al.*, 2005). Moreover, the reduced fetal foot length was inversely correlated with the frequency and amount of marijuana that was used during the early gestation period (Hurd *et al.*, 2005).

Studies in mice indicate that marijuana exposure during gestation was not associated with fetal anomalies (Harbison *et al.*, 1977), but that the pups were less active and had lower birth weights (Fried & Charlebois, 1979).

In humans, heavy marijuana use prenatally was significantly linked to a smaller head circumference observed in the offspring when early adolescence was reached (Fried *et al.*, 1999). However, no effect on the birth weight (Fried, 1982; Fried *et al.*, 1999) of the infant was observed.

Marijuana proved to be teratogenic (cleft palate, exencephaly) in extremely large doses in mice but not in macaque monkeys. In humans, however, marijuana has not been linked to teratogenic effects (Bennett, 1999), although some researchers do not deem the current available data as sufficient to make such a conclusion (Briggs *et al.*, 1998).

Motor Development of Infants Exposed to Marijuana Prenatally or Postnatally

Data are limited concerning the effect of prenatal and postnatal marijuana use on the motor development of the infant. Therefore, the results of the following studies need to be interpreted with caution.

Neonates of mothers who smoked five marijuana joints per week during pregnancy presented with marked tremors, startles, and altered visual responsiveness at two to four days of age. These symptoms were attenuated by 30 days (Fried, 1982). Fried and Watkinson (1988) conducted a follow-up study and showed no association between marijuana exposure prenatally and the motor development of infants at one and two years of age. In addition, a study by Astley and Little (1990) showed no association between prenatal marijuana exposure and the motor development of infants at one year of age. A subsequent study in 1990 performed by Fried and Watkinson suggested that at 48 months of age, maternal marijuana use was associated with significantly lower scores in memory and verbal domains. However, observations at 60 and 72 months of age did not parallel those at 48 months of age (Fried *et al.*, 1992).

Data are conflicting regarding the effect of postnatal marijuana use and its effect on the motor development of infants assessed at one year of age. Tennes and coworkers (1985) found no effects of postnatal marijuana exposure on the motor and mental skills of one year old infants. However, a study performed in 1990 by Astley and Little showed that exposure to marijuana during lactation is associated with decreased motor development in one year old infants.

Brain Development Studies in Experimental Animals

Marijuana use during gestation may result in a variety of disturbances in the development of the offspring by affecting the ontogeny of various neurotransmitter systems, leading to changes in different behavioral patterns. The transmission of serotonin, glutamate, gamma-aminobutyric acid (GABA), and endocannabinoid is effected by perinatal cannabinoid use.

However, upon maturing, animals present with changes in various processes, including social interaction, motor activity, neuroendocrine control, stress response, drug seeking behavior, and nociception. It is evident that the neurotransmitters, dopamine and endogenous opioids, are effected to a greater degree by the perinatal use of marijuana (Fernández-Ruiz *et al.*, 2004). The disturbances likely originate from cannabinoid that influence the expression of essential genes for both dopamine and endogenous opioids, in particular, tyrosine hydroxylase and opioid precursor proenkephalin. In addition, cannabinoids might be involved in apoptotic death (Bcl-2/Bax system) occurring during brain development and modulating the gene expression of neuron-glia cell adhesion molecules (Fernández-Ruiz *et al.*, 2004).

Conclusion

The prevalence of marijuana abuse among women of childbearing age is high, yet there is little known about the effect of marijuana on the breastfeeding infant and/or lactation as a whole. According to Perez-Reyes and Wall (1982), only small to moderate amounts of THC, 11-OH-THC, and 9-carboxy-THC are excreted in the breastmilk of mothers who abuse marijuana. Regardless, this could have an effect on the breastfeeding infant, including symptoms such as lethargy and shorter, less frequent feedings. Also, it is important to avoid smoking in the presence of infants to reduce the risk of SIDS (Klonoff-Cohen & Lam-Kruglick, 2001). Mothers should be strongly advised that marijuana is present in plasma and adipose tissue for an extended period of time, and that breastmilk may contain residues of marijuana for long periods (up to weeks). These residues when passed via milk may be evident in drug screens done on their breastfed infants. While the levels may not be pharmacologically active, they are enough to indicate to authorities that the mother is ingesting marijuana. The AAP's Committee on Drugs contraindicates the use of marijuana during breastfeeding (American Academy of Pediatrics, 1989).

NICOTINE

Cigarette smoking is of great importance from a societal and medico-ethical perspective since it has been described as the leading preventable cause of morbidity and mortality in developed countries (Peto *et al.*, 1992).

> Despite the well-known health dangers of using tobacco, almost **1.3 billion adults worldwide** continue to do so, a number that will climb to 1.9 billion users by the year 2025 if cigarette consumption remains unchanged (Guindon & Boisclair, 2003).

There are almost 4,000 chemicals in tobacco products, such as cigarettes, cigars, and pipe tobacco, of which nicotine (**Figure 11**) is the best known and the most studied (National Institute on Drug Abuse, 2002).

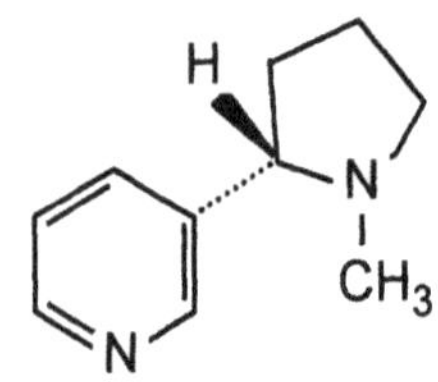

(*S*)-Nicotine

Figure 11. Chemical structure of (*S*)-nicotine.

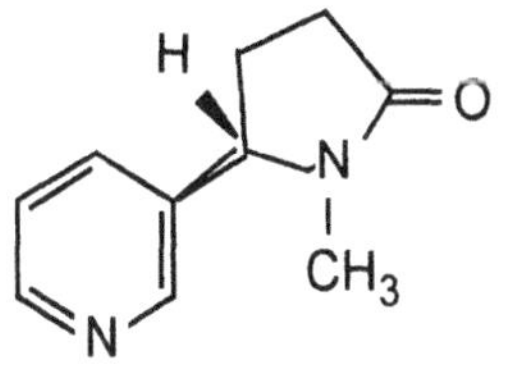

(*S*)-Cotinine

Figure 12. Chemical structure of (*S*)-cotinine.

Pharmacokinetics and the Transfer of Nicotine into Breastmilk and the Infant

Various studies have confirmed nicotine excretion in breastmilk of mothers who smoke cigarettes, where levels range from 13 to 114 μg/L (median = 51 μg/L) (Minchin, 1991; Woodward *et al.*, 1984), although some studies have reported higher values (Dahlström *et al.*, 2004; Ferguson *et al.*, 1976; Perlman *et al.*, 1942).

Nicotine, a naturally occurring alkaloid and basic compound, reaches higher concentrations in breastmilk, which is a slightly acidic compartment (pH 7.2), as opposed to serum (M/P ratio = 2.9 ± 1.1) (Dahlström *et al.*, 1990; Luck & Nau, 1984; Steldinger *et al.*, 1988). One small study found that the half-life of nicotine in breastmilk was 97 (± 20) minutes, which was slightly longer than the half-life in serum (81 ± 9 min) (Luck & Nau, 1984).

Once absorbed, nicotine is extensively metabolized by the liver to a number of major and minor metabolites (Snyder *et al.*, 1993). Metabolism of nicotine and its metabolites in living organisms involves phase I (microsomal oxidation) and phase II metabolism (N-glucuronidation and O-glucuronidation) (Yildiz, 2004). Cytochrome P450 2A6 (CYP2A6), present in human liver, nasal mucosa, and lung (Crawford *et al.*, 1998; Maurice *et al.*, 1991; Su *et al.*, 1996), and aldehyde oxidation metabolizes nicotine to its major metabolite, cotinine (**Figure 12**) (Yildiz, 2004).

Levels of cotinine reported in breastmilk range between 50 and 300 μg/L, which is substantially higher than that of nicotine in breastmilk (Ilett *et al.*, 2003; Minchin, 1991). In addition, there is a linear correlation between the levels of cotinine in breastmilk and in the serum of smoking mothers, although the cotinine concentrations in milk were lower than of that in serum (M/P ratio = 0.78 ± 0.19) (Luck & Nau, 1984).

Cigarette smoke contains other chemical by-products, namely nitrates and nitrites, which are found in breastmilk. However, the carcinogenic nitrosamines are not detectable in breastmilk (Minchin, 1991).

Factors Influencing Nicotine Concentrations in Breastmilk

The actual concentration of nicotine in breastmilk is dependent on the number of cigarettes smoked per day, but more so on the time lapse between nursing and the last cigarette smoked (Steldinger *et al.*, 1988). We will examine each factor in light of studies that were performed.

1. Number of cigarettes smoked:
   Mothers who smoke one to four cigarettes over a twelve hour period are regarded as occasional smokers and had an average nicotine concentration of between 120 and 160 μg/L in their breastmilk (Perlman *et al.*, 1942). Dahlström and coworkers (2004) report the mean nicotine concentration in breastmilk to be 440 μg/L in mothers who smoke between 10 and 20 cigarettes per day. The average concentration of nicotine in breastmilk ranged between 445 μg/L and 500 μg/L in a group of heavy smokers who smoked 11 to 20 and more cigarettes over a twelve hour period (Perlman *et al.*, 1942).
2. Time lapse between nursing and the last cigarette smoked:
   The body rapidly eliminates nicotine, which explains the low plasma and breastmilk concentrations after refraining from smoking (for example, overnight abstinence). In the study performed by Dahlström and coworkers (1990), the amount of nicotine transferred to the breastfed infant increased from 0.09 to 1.03 μg/kg infant body weight when mothers smoked before nursing their infants. Correspondingly, the cotinine concentrations transferred to the breastfed infant also increased from 2.0 to 2.6 μg/kg infant body weight (Dahlström *et al.*, 1990). The daily dose of nicotine that a breastfed infant received was 6 μg/kg infant body weight (Dahlström *et al.*, 1990).

Nicotine and Cotinine in the Serum and Urine of Breastfed Infants

Luck and Nau (1985) quantified nicotine (5-110 ng/mg creatinine; median = 14 ng/mg creatinine) in the urine of infants after nicotine exposure from breastmilk alone where the mothers smoked in separate rooms from the infants. Both nicotine and cotinine have been detected in the serum and urine of breastfed infants from smoking mothers (Dahlström *et al.*, 1990; Luck & Nau; 1985). However, there was no correlation between the amount of nicotine received through breastfeeding and the nicotine and cotinine concentrations in the infant's urine (Dahlström *et al.*, 1990).

Furthermore, cotinine elimination is considerably slower in infants as opposed to adults (Dahlström *et al.*, 1990). In fact, the elimination half-life of cotinine in neonates (68 hours) (Labrecque *et al.*, 1989) is two to three times that of adults (Etzel *et al.*, 1985). Therefore, single samples of urine cannot be used to quantify nicotine exposure in infants.

Passive Smoke, Nicotine, and Cotinine

It has long been known that non-smokers exposed to passive smoke have measurable amounts of nicotine in their blood and urine (Kyerematen *et al.*, 1982; Russell & Feverabend, 1975). Similarly, Luck and Nau (1985) found that nicotine concentrations ranged between 4.7 to 218 ng/mg creatinine (median = 35 ng/mg creatinine) in infants exposed to passive smoke.

A study by Hardee and coworkers (1983) found that non-smoking mothers exposed to passive smoke at work during the day presented with detectable levels of nicotine and cotinine in their breastmilk. In addition, a few studies found that breastmilk is a more important source of cotinine found in the urine of infants than inhaled nicotine from exposure to passive smoke (Mascola *et al.*, 1998; Schulte-Hobein *et al.*, 1992; Schwartz-Bickenbach *et al.*, 1987; Woodward *et al.*, 1986). Mascola and coworkers (1998) found that breastfed infants from mothers who smoked in the same room as their infant presented with a ten-fold higher median cotinine concentration in their urine (4667 ng/mg creatinine) than bottle-fed infants whose mothers smoked in the same room as the infant (413 ng/mg creatinine). Conversely, Luck and Nau (1985) also found that the median urine cotinine concentrations are higher in non-breastfed infants exposed to only passive smoke from parents (parents smoked 15-40 cigarettes per day; median = 327 ng/mg creatinine) as opposed to breastfeeding infants who are not exposed to passive smoke but only to nicotine from smoking mothers who nursed (10-30 cigarettes smoked per day by mother; 110 ng/mg creatinine).

Thus, cotinine levels are higher in the urine of infants exposed to passive smoke versus cotinine levels in adults that are exposed to passive smoke. Breastfed infants from smoking mothers excrete cotinine in their urine in the range of that of adult smokers (Schulte-Hobein *et al.*, 1992).

Previously, cotinine was believed to be pharmacologically inactive and therefore posed no risk to the infant. However, a study performed by Dwoskin and coworkers (1999) showed that (*S*)-(-)-cotinine does evoke the release of dopamine in rat striatal slices in a calcium- and concentration-dependent manner which resulted in the desensitization of the nicotinic receptors. The (*S*)-(-)-cotinine concentrations that caused dopamine release were not in the concentration range of that found in smokers. However, because cotinine has a very long half-life (68 hours), one can propose that it could accumulate after chronic exposure to nicotine to ultimately produce neuropharmacological effects (Dwoskin *et al.*, 1999). This issue needs to be further investigated to understand the role that cotinine plays in the addiction process and the effects that cotinine might have on the breastfeeding infant and/or on infants exposed to passive smoke.

Nicotine Patch and Smokeless Tobacco

Ilett and coworkers (2003) studied the use of three different strengths of nicotine patches and smoking in breastfeeding mothers. They showed that the absolute infant dose of nicotine and cotinine decreased by approximately 70% when subjects were using the 7 mg nicotine patch as opposed to smoking or using the 21 mg nicotine patch. The fact that mothers can stop smoking by using a nicotine patch regime is of critical importance to their breastfeeding infants. In addition, mothers using nicotine patches will avoid exposing their breastfeeding infants to other potentially harmful chemicals.

Smoking bans are public policies to prohibit people from smoking in public places in order to protect citizens from cancer, heart diseases, respiratory illnesses, as well as other acute and chronic diseases caused, at least partly, by prolonged exposure to passive smoke (Directgov, 2005). One pitfall of a smoking ban is that it does not, in general, include smokeless tobacco (snuff). Instead, it is probable that smokers will smoke less because of the ban, but will subsequently compensate by using snuff. This is of particular concern in women who are using smokeless tobacco and nursing their infants.

A small 2004 study by Dahlström and coworkers indicated that nursing women who use snuff are exposing their infants to higher nicotine concentrations when compared to the majority of women who smoke cigarettes. This can be partly due to the more frequent intake of nicotine by snuffing (Dahlström *et al.*, 2004).

Nicotine's Effect on Mammary Glands, Breastmilk Yield and Constituents, as well as the Motivation to Breastfeed

Nicotine has been reported to reduce milk production, although this is somewhat controversial (Perlman *et al.*, 1942). The effect of nicotine on mammary glands, breastmilk production, and the motivation of smoking mothers to breastfeed follows.

Mammary Gland Abscesses

Smoking cigarettes plays a significant role in non-lactation breast abscesses and may predispose women to anaerobic breast infections and the development of mammillary fistulae (Bundred *et al.*, 1992). According to Schäfer and coworkers (1988), smoking cigarettes might have an indirect toxic effect through hormonal stimulation of breast secretion or a direct toxic effect on the retroareolar lactiferous ducts. Fifty-three out of sixty patients that presented with recurrent subareolar breast abscesses were smokers. This condition is apparently more prevalent in younger women who smoke, (Boeckxstaens *et al.*, 1984; Schäfer *et al.*, 1988).

Low Prevalence Of Breastfeeding Among Nursing Mothers Who Smoke

At three months postpartum, 86% of non-smokers were still breastfeeding compared to only 51% of mothers who smoked (Woodward, 1988). The study by Hopkinson and coworkers (1992) might shed light on the etiology of these statistics, but at first the focus will fall on the general role of prolactin in lactation.

Role of Prolactin

Prolactin, as mentioned before (see section on alcohol and its effect on prolactin), is essential for successful lactation (Grattan, 2002; Uynas-Moberg *et al.*, 1990). Previous studies have indicated that smoking mothers have lower prolactin levels during the first weeks (Andersen *et al.*, 1982) and later months of lactation (Andersen & Schioler, 1982).

Other studies have provided either controversial or supporting results with regards to the prevalence of reduced prolactin levels in smoking mothers. Shieh and Pan (1997) conducted a study in rats and showed that nicotine inhibits TIDA neuronal activity, which resulted in increased prolactin serum levels. On the other hand, Coleman and Bancroft (1995) showed that nicotine directly affects the pituitary prolactin-secreting cells (GH3 cell-line) by decreasing the transcription of the prolactin gene, which subsequently reduces prolactin levels.

However, recently a controversial but interesting study in men investigated the effect of cigarette smoke on plasma prolactin levels (Mendelson *et al.*, 2003). Although the study was not performed in lactating women, it is of relevance to nicotine's effect on prolactin. In this study the subjects smoked low- or high-yield cigarettes, during which plasma nicotine and prolactin levels were determined. Before the results of this study are discussed, some background information will be supplied.

Nicotine yield should not be confused with the nicotine content of a cigarette (amount of nicotine contained in the cigarette before it is lit and smoked). Nicotine yield is rather a measurement of the amount of nicotine present in the smoke that a smoker inhales (The Massachusetts Tobacco Control Program, 1998-2004) and is dependent on the following factors:

- puff interval: time interval between puffs,
- puff volume: the length of time and depth of inhalation of each puff, and the
- percent filter ventilation of the smoke breathed in: amount of pure air drawn in during smoking through the vent holes that are present in the filter tip. The simultaneous breathing of air and smoke during the smoking process, decreases the air concentration in the smoke/air mixture that is breathed (The Massachusetts Tobacco Control Program, 1998-2004).

The Massachusetts Tobacco Control Program (1998-2004) classifies cigarettes as high-, moderate-, or low-yield nicotine cigarettes if the nicotine yield is >1.2 mg, between 0.2-1.2 mg, or 0.01-0.2 mg, respectively. However, a cigarette with a higher nicotine content can potentially deliver a higher nicotine yield (The Massachusetts Tobacco Control Program, 1998-2004).

In a study of men who smoked (Mendelson *et al.*, 2003), high-yield nicotine cigarettes (Marlboro Red) yielded 15.48 mg of nicotine based on the Massachusetts Department of Public Health analysis. The low-yield nicotine cigarette yielded 0.1 mg nicotine based on the manufacturer's analyses.

In the case of the low-yield cigarette, plasma nicotine levels increased significantly (mean peak = 3.9 ± 0.77 ng/mL) above pre-smoking baseline levels; however, no increase in plasma prolactin levels were evident. After a high-yield cigarette was smoked, a mean peak plasma nicotine concentration of 22.6 ± 3.4 ng/mL was reached and remained above baseline throughout the sampling period of 120 minutes. Yet, plasma prolactin levels increased to levels above the baseline for approximately 40 minutes after the cigarette smoking period ended (at approximately 12 minutes) (Mendelson *et al.*, 2003).

Interestingly, chronic smoking has been associated with low prolactin levels (Fuxe *et al.*, 1989), while prolactin levels were increased acutely after smoking a cigarette (Kirschbaum *et al.*, 1994; Seyler *et al.*, 1986; Wilkins *et al.*, 1982). Benowitz (1991) and Matheson & Rivrud (1989) suggested that nicotine decreases basal prolactin production. However, the exact mechanism of the effect of cigarette smoke on prolactin levels is yet to be understood.

Breastmilk Constituents and Yield

Hopkinson and coworkers (1992) found that mothers who smoke have a significantly lower milk yield when compared to those mothers who do not smoke (514 mL/day in non-smokers compared to 406 mL/day in smokers three days postpartum). Furthermore, Hopkinson and coworkers (1992) found that total protein, lactose, nitrogen, calcium, and phosphorous concentrations in breastmilk do not differ between mothers who smoke cigarettes and those who do not. However, the fat concentration of breastmilk was lower in mothers who smoked cigarettes (Hopkinson *et al.*, 1992).

Various studies found that infants from smoking mothers weaned earlier compared to the infants from non-smoking mothers (Counsilman & Mackay, 1985; Håkansson & Carlsson, 1992; Hopkinson *et al.*, 1992; Klinnert *et al.*, 2001; Schwartz-Bickenbach *et al.*, 1987). This might be attributed to the lower fat content in their breastmilk and reduced milk volume as induced by nicotine (Hopkinson *et al.*, 1992).

The effect of nicotine and smoking on milk production is somewhat controversial. A study performed by Ilett and coworkers (2003) found that no change in breastmilk intake by the infants was evident in mothers who smoked and who were later placed on a smoking cessation protocol with the aid of nicotine patches. This study extended over a period of 11 weeks when the mothers were totally weaned off the patch. The median milk intake by the infants from smoking mothers was 585 mL/day prior to the study and 717 mL/day when the mothers were using the 21 mg nicotine patch, 731 mL/day during the use of the 14 mg nicotine patch, and 619 mL/day during the use of the 7 mg nicotine patch. Interestingly, milk production did not increase with a decrease in nicotine (patch) content, which suggests that nicotine may not affect breastmilk production (Ilett *et al.*, 2003).

Lack of Motivation to Breastfeed?

It should be noted that the desire of a smoking mother to breastfeed is a variable that is not always taken into account in studies that determine the prevalence of breastfeeding among smoking and non-smoking women. One review found that women who smoke have significantly less intent to breastfeed and subsequently initiate breastfeeding less frequently (Amir & Donath, 2003). Apart from being less motivated to breastfeed (Amir & Donath, 2003), they are also less likely to seek help with breastfeeding difficulties as opposed to non-smoking mothers (Amir, 1999).

Donath and coworkers (2004), Amir (2001), and Amir & Donath (2003) found that smoking mothers are less likely to breastfeed their infants due to lower motivation, rather than the physiological effect smoking has on milk supply.

One should thus be careful to conclude that earlier weaning in mothers who smoke is due to their inability to do so, but rather take these variables into account when performing studies into the prevalence of early weaning among smoking mothers.

Nicotine's Effect on the Breastfed Infant

Poor Bodyweight, Colic, and Infant Development

The mean birth weight of neonates exposed to cigarette smoke during gestation is significantly lower when compared to controls (Schulte-Hobein *et al.*, 1992; Steyn *et al.*, 2006). However, postnatally, their weight was not significantly different from unexposed infants at twelve months of age (Schulte-Hobein *et al.*, 1992).

Breastfeeding infants from smoking mothers apparently show poorer growth, which might be attributed to the anorexic effect of nicotine or, in extreme cases, it can induce nausea and vomiting (Minchin, 1991). Breastfed infants of mothers who stopped smoking have similar outcomes in regards to birth weight (Andrews & McGarry, 1972; Counsilman & Mackay, 1985) and duration of breastfeeding (Mills, 1950).

The effect of passive smoking on neonatal birth weight is still controversial. Steyn and coworkers (2006) could not find a correlation between reduced birth weight and exposure to passive smoke. Misra & Nguyen (1999), however, clearly established a link and reported that infants who are born of mothers exposed to environmental tobacco smoke are generally two to four times more likely to be born small for gestational age.

Ninety percent of infants exposed to passive smoke from fathers presented with postprandial colic, compared to 57% where only the mother smoked (Said *et al.*, 1984). Infant irritability due to exposure to passive smoke may lead to postprandial colic. Distress in the infant may subsequently lead to more maternal stress and more smoking.

In addition, an infant's irritability may have many etiologies, including inadequate milk transfer which can be caused by poor positioning and subsequent nipple trauma (Minchin, 1989) or abdominal discomfort ("oversupply colic") caused by inappropriate breastfeeding management (Woolridge & Fisher, 1988).

According to a study by Schulte-Hobein and coworkers (1992), neither psychomotor nor mental development was affected in infants exposed to cigarette smoke during pregnancy and early lactation. However, long-term studies performed by Fried and Watkinson (1988, 1990) showed that prenatal exposure to cigarette smoke is significantly associated with lower cognitive scores and poorer language development at 12, 24, 36, 48, 60, and 72 months after birth (Fried & Watkinson, 1988, 1990; Fried *et al.*, 1992).

Taste of Breastmilk, Maternal Nutrient Deficiencies, and SIDS

An infant will probably tolerate the constant low level of tobacco intake from his mother's breastmilk if the infant has only had her milk as food. However, if a mother's cigarette consumption increases, the infant might refuse feeding to express their distaste for the milk. In addition, when the mother significantly reduces her tobacco use, the infant may suffer from withdrawal symptoms, such as sleep disturbances, irritability, and headaches (Minchin, 1991). It is therefore advised that mothers consider using nicotine patches to cut back or quit smoking (Ilett *et al.*, 2003). See the sections: *"Nicotine's effect on breastmilk constituents and yield"* and *"Nicotine patch and smokeless tobacco"* for more information with regards to the nicotine patch.

It is known that smokers present with lower blood levels of ascorbic acid (Keith & Mossholder, 1986), carotene, and folate (Witter *et al.*, 1982). Therefore, in severe cases, nutrient deficiencies may occur in breastfeeding infants, since women who smoke are more likely to present with nutrient depletion (Minchin, 1991). Smoking also depresses the immune system, which puts the breastfeeding infant in jeopardy of acquiring infections more easily (Minchin, 1991).

Maternal and antenatal smoking are associated with an increased risk of SIDS (Hunt & Hauck, 2006; Williams *et al.*, 2002). Prior belief was that breastfeeding had a protective effect in regards to SIDS, but a recent study found that breastfeeding is not associated with a decreased risk of SIDS, but rather of post-neonatal deaths overall. Currently, the data are inadequate to recommend breastfeeding as a strategy to reduce the risk of SIDS (Hunt & Hauck, 2006).

Respiratory Tract Infections

Nicotine was removed from the list of drugs contraindicated during breastfeeding by the AAP's Committee on Drugs in 2001. Part of their reasoning lies in the fact that there is no evidence documenting that nicotine excreted in breastmilk at 1.5-3.0 times the maternal plasma concentration (Steldinger *et al.*, 1988) with a half-life of 60-90 minutes (Luck & Nau, 1984) poses a health risk to the nursing infant (American Academy of Pediatrics Committee on Drugs, 2001).

Although the AAP Committee on Drugs (2001) finds that there is no clear evidence that nicotine might cause an increase in respiratory illnesses (including otitis media) in the nursing infant, various studies did find that parental (including maternal) smoking causes an increase in respiratory tract infections (including asthma) in their infants and children (Chen *et al.*, 1986; Colley *et al.*, 1974; Dezateux *et al.*, 2001; Dutau *et al.*, 1981; Fergusson *et al.*, 1980; Håkansson & Carlsson, 1992; Harlap & Davies, 1974; Klinnert *et al.*, 2001; Ogston *et al.*, 1987; Pedreira *et al.*, 1985; Rantakallio, 1978; Strachan & Cook, 1997; Taylor & Wadsworth, 1987; Young *et al.*, 2000).

Further investigation is therefore necessary to elucidate at what concentrations nicotine in maternal plasma attribute to the increased risk of respiratory tract infections.

On the other hand, Woodward and coworkers (1990) found that breastfeeding infants from mothers who smoke had a lower incidence of acute respiratory illness compared with bottle-fed infants from smoking mothers. Therefore, this might indicate that the outcomes are more detrimental for infants that are exposed to maternal smoke and bottle-fed as opposed to those who are breastfed and exposed to maternal smoke.

New Findings

Postnatal Obesity, Hypertension, and Diabetes Mellitus

Gao and coworkers (2005) showed that nicotine exposure in rats during gestation and lactation resulted in increased visceral adiposity with increased amounts of fat surrounding the vasculature, as well as accelerated postnatal weight gain (obesity). Of great interest is that Gao and coworkers (2005) found that fetal and neonatal nicotine exposure in the rat results in an attenuation of vessel relaxation in adult life, due to a change in the modulatory function of perivascular adipose tissue (PVAT). Further research needs to be performed to determine whether the role of PVAT in rats and humans is similar. Nevertheless, this is the first study to implicate nicotine's role in the increased prevalence of hypertension among children (Blake *et al.*, 2000; Morley *et al.*, 1995) who were exposed to cigarette smoke as a fetus and during breastfeeding (Gao *et al.*, 2005).

A recent epidemiological study has shown that offspring of smoking mothers present with an increased risk of developing diabetes mellitus type II (Montgomery & Ekbom, 2002). Progress in this field was made when Holloway and coworkers (2005) found that exposure to nicotine at levels relevant for human exposure during gestation and lactation in rats resulted in impaired glucose homeostasis. In addition, fetal nicotine exposure resulted in reduced serum insulin concentrations and an increase in the number of apoptotic islet cells on the first day postnatally. It is evident that further investigation is necessary into the effect of nicotine exposure to the fetus in association with long-term postnatal health.

Neuronal Nicotinic Receptor Upregulation

Previous studies have indicated that chronic nicotine exposure causes an upregulation in neuronal nicotinergic acetylcholine receptors (nAChRs) in humans, rats, and mice (Benwell *et al.*, 1988; Breese *et al.*, 1997; Marks *et al.*, 1983, 1985, 1992; Schwartz & Kellar, 1983, 1985; Wonnacott, 1990). Interestingly, the levels of tyrosine hydroxylase and dopamine transporter were upregulated in response to chronic administration of nicotine and nicotine containing smoke extract in a rat study in vivo. However, cotinine and nicotine-free smoke extract did not affect tyrosine hydroxylase and dopamine transporter regulation (McAfee, 2004).

In further support of these studies, results from a study performed in rat pups showed that nicotine exposure through breastmilk also induced an upregulation in nAChRs (Narayanan *et al.*, 2002). This is of significance since brain development continues postnatally, which impacts normal cognitive and synaptic development (Casey *et al.*, 2000). Nicotine exposure during the postnatal period can, therefore, result in permanent or long-term changes in synaptic structure and activity, which may become evident later in life as behavioral problems or cognitive deficits, including long-term behavioral, learning, and memory deficits (Narayanan *et al.*, 2002). Additional investigations are necessary in this exciting field to determine the true effect of nicotine found in breastmilk on the regulation of nAChRs in the nursing infant and subsequent long-term epidemiological studies are needed to determine the consequences.

Risk for Pulmonary Emphysema

It is well known that cigarette smoke is a significant risk factor for pulmonary emphysema, the abnormal enlargement of airspaces distal to the terminal bronchiole without fibrosis (American Thoracic Society, 1962; Snider, 1989; Snider *et al.*, 1985, 1986).

A study performed by Maritz and Dennis (1998) exposed rats to nicotine (1 mg/kg/day) subcutaneously during gestation and lactation. The results of this study indicated that the offspring presented with suppressed alveolarisation (increased alveolar volume, reduced internal surface area, and decreased alveolar number) in their lungs which reduced the effectiveness of the lungs to exchange gases. More importantly, the adverse effects of nicotine exposure during gestation and lactation on lung development in the offspring appeared to be irreversible (Maritz & Dennis, 1998). Maritz (2002) concluded that maternal nicotine exposure during gestation and lactation induces microscopic emphysema in the offspring.

In a follow-up study, Maritz and coworkers (2000) found that copper supplementation during gestation and lactation prevented the adverse effects of maternal nicotine exposure on the development and growth of the lung in rat pups. Lysyl oxidase, a copper-dependent enzyme, plays an essential role in cross-linking collagen and elastin (O'Dell *et al.,* 1978). It is therefore argued that nicotine interferes with the alveolarisation process by reducing the copper content and thus the lysyl oxidase activity (Maritz *et al.,* 2000).

In a 2003 rat study, Kordom and coworkers demonstrated that maternal nicotine exposure during gestation and lactation resulted in a reduced rate of glucose flux through the glycolic pathway which can be due to an inhibition of 6-phosphofructo-1-kinase, a rate-limiting enzyme for glycolysis. This finding is significant since glucose uptake and metabolism are essential for the survival and proliferation of cells (Kordom *et al.,* 2003).

Polydrug Use

Cigarette smokers are not exempt from being vulnerable to polydrug use, as is the case with other drug users. Cigarette smokers tend to smoke more when consuming alcohol, whereas marijuana users tend to smoke tobacco and marijuana concomitantly (Mello *et al.,* 1980). No data are available on the effect of concomitant use of marijuana and tobacco or increased tobacco use with alcohol consumption on the breastfed infant.

Conclusion

There is cause of concern for the well-being of infants when they are exposed to nicotine, cotinine, and various other harmful chemicals from passive smoke as well as through breastmilk from a mother who smokes. Infant exposure to nicotine and cotinine through breastmilk is dependent on various factors, including the number of cigarettes smoked per day, frequency of smoking, time of smoking, and the time interval between smoking the last cigarette and nursing (Luck & Nau, 1987), as well as nicotine yield. **Table 2** gives a brief overview of some of the variables covered in this particular section.

It has not yet been proven without a doubt that cotinine has pharmacological properties in the breastfeeding infant. Yet, it should still be of concern, considering the high levels of cotinine that is present in the infant who is exposed to passive smoke and/or breastmilk from a smoking mother.

It is expected that nicotine concentrations are lower during the night and early morning, when asleep, or waking up from a night's rest. Mothers are therefore encouraged to pump their breastmilk in the mornings, approximately eight to ten hours after their last cigarette, to ensure that their infants' exposure to nicotine through breastmilk is as low as possible (Hale & McAfee, 2005).

Table 2. A Comparison of Nicotine and Cotinine Variables in Infants

Nicotine	Variable	Cotinine
13-114 μg/L	Breastmilk concentration	50-300 μg/L
2.9 ± 1.1	M/P ratio	0.78 ± 0.19
0.09-1.03 μg/kg infant body weight	Amount transferred to breastfed infant	2.0-2.6 μg/kg infant body weight
35 ng/mg creatinine (median)	Urine concentrations in infants exposed to passive smoke alone	413 ng/mg creatinine (median)

It is advised that mothers refrain from smoking during the nursing period or, if that is not feasible, to extend the time between nursing and when the last cigarette was smoked (Steldinger *et al.,* 1988). For instance, it is recommended that a mother smoke after a feeding and then wait until after the next feeding before smoking another cigarette (Myr, 2004).

Finally, it is certainly not ideal for a mother who smokes to breastfeed or to expose her infant to passive smoke. However, it is clear that it is more beneficial for infants to receive breastmilk from smoking mothers than to be exposed to passive smoke and formula.

PHENCYCLIDINE (PCP)

Thirty years after its first synthesis in 1950, 1-(1-phenyl cyclohexyl)piperidine (also known as phencyclidine or PCP) was considered for human use as an anesthetic although it was never approved due to problems patients experienced when emerging from anesthesia that arose during clinical trials, including delirium and extreme agitation. PCP, a white crystalline powder, can be taken orally, snorted, or smoked and produces its effects by blocking N-methyl-D-aspartic acid (NMDA) type glutamate receptors in the cortex and limbic structures of the brain (O'Brien, 1996).

Pharmacokinetics of PCP

PCP is highly lipophilic (**Figure 13**), has a distribution half-life of one to four hours, and distributes into the brain and other fatty tissues (Martin & Freeman, 1983; Pradhan, 1984; Sioris & Krenzelok, 1978). The plasma

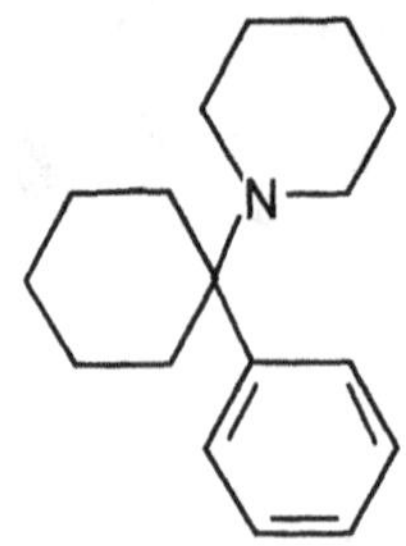

Figure 13. Chemical structure of phencyclidine (PCP).

elimination half-life is dependent on the dosage of PCP. For example, the elimination half-life ranges between 11 and 89 hours in patients that received an overdose. However, in patients that received a low dose of PCP, the elimination half-life ranged between 7 and 50 hours (mean = 17.6 hours) (Cook *et al.*, 1983; Sioris & Krenzelok, 1978).

Frequent PCP drug abusers present with a two compartment elimination model where PCP is slowly released from tissue compartments over a long period (Domino *et al.*, 1982). Interestingly, the brain to plasma ratio in rats for PCP is approximately seven to one after a single dose, while the fat to plasma ratio can be as high as 100:1 (Misra *et al.*, 1979). The volume of distribution is between 5.4 and 7.5 L/kg where the plasma clearance is between 0.25 and 0.30 L/kg/h (Martin & Freeman, 1983; Pradhan, 1984; Sioris & Krenzelok, 1978).

PCP undergoes hydroxylation on the cyclohexane ring (20%), piperidine ring (8%), or both (3%) to produce more polar compounds. Eighty-five percent of these compounds undergo conjugation with glucuronide or sulfate and are subsequently eliminated from the body in the urine. The 4-hydroxylated piperidine metabolite undergoes further metabolism to an open ring product, 5-(1-phenylcyclohexylamino)valeric acid, which is deposited in the meconium of the infant when PCP is used during gestation (Kuhnert *et al.*, 1983).

Contrary to earlier studies where it was suggested that none of the metabolites of PCP are active, recent data suggest that the major metabolite of PCP, 4-phenyl-4-(1-piperidinyl)cyclohexanol (trans isomer) may contribute to the psychotomimetic effects (Baba *et al.*, 1994a;1994b).

PCP's effect on prolactin and oxytocin

Data are limited with regards to PCP's effect on prolactin and oxytocin. However, a study performed in rats found that PCP reduced basal prolactin release (Hyde, 1992). This is of significance because reduced prolactin levels can result in reduced milk production (Hyde, 1992). It also appeared that PCP might inhibit oxytocin secretion during suckling (Hyde, 1992).

Transfer of PCP into Breastmilk

PCP is excreted into breastmilk with levels greater than that in maternal blood. In the only study available, the mother gave birth to a healthy infant 36 days after the last reported use of PCP. At the time of birth, maternal blood (0.77 ng/mL) and urine (0.16 ng/mL, pH 6.13) sample analyses showed the presence of PCP in low concentrations. Five days after the infant was born, PCP was detected in the breastmilk at 3.9 ng/mL (Kaufman *et al.*, 1983).

These results were supported by a mouse study performed by Nicholas and coworkers (1982) where the milk PCP concentrations were ten times higher than that in the maternal plasma. In this study, it appeared that the milk contained mainly PCP and not its metabolites, indicating that breastfed infants will be exposed to orally bioavailable PCP.

Conclusion

PCP is highly lipophilic and stored in adipose tissue for long periods of time. Therefore, PCP appears in much higher concentrations in breastmilk than in maternal plasma. In addition, since PCP is orally bioavailable, it poses a great risk to the breastfed infant. Taking the effects of PCP into account, as well as the doses the breastfed infant is exposed to, it is without a doubt that the use of PCP during breastfeeding is an absolute contraindication.

MISCELLANEOUS DRUGS

Mescaline

As a naturally occurring psychedelic, mescaline is found in several cactus species, but most notably the San Pedro, Peyote, and Peruvian Torch cactus. The "button" of the Peyote cactus is swallowed with subsequent absorption of mescaline from the stomach and intestine. A high percent (99.3%) of mescaline is ionized at physiological pH, and the un-ionized mescaline has a low lipid solubility (Taska & Schoolar, 1972). With a molecular weight of 211.26 g/mol, mescaline is small enough to pass into breastmilk, but with a XLogP value of 0.6 one can almost assume, that it will not readily pass into breastmilk. However, mescaline crosses the blood brain barrier and is therefore likely to enter breastmilk as well. In addition, it is the degree to which mescaline will pass into breastmilk that is not yet clear. It is subsequently advised that mothers who take mescaline refrain from breastfeeding.

Psilocybin

The fungi of genera Conocybe, Panaeolus, Gymnopilus, and Psilocybe, among others, are well-known as "magic" mushrooms, which contain the ingredient, psilocybin. The pro-drug, psilocybin, is converted by dephosphorylation to psilocin. The effect of psilocybin (psilocin) is similar to that of LSD (Reingardiene *et al.*, 2005). Psilocybin has a molecular mass of 284.25 g/mol and a XLogP value of 0.2, indicating low lipophilicity. However, the active ingredient, psilocin has a XLogP value of 1.6 indicating a higher probability of transfer into breastmilk. It's pharmacokinetics are comparable to nicotine, which has a molecular weight of 162.23 g/mol and a XLogP value of 1.1. Therefore, breastfeeding is certainly not advised while using "magic" mushrooms.

Club Drugs

Under this class defined by the National Institute on Drug Abuse are the following drugs: Ecstasy (MDMA), gamma hydroxybutyrate (GHB), Rohypnol, methamphetamine, ketamine, and LSD.

Methamphetamine and LSD have been discussed previously in the chapter. GHB is available under the trade name Xyrem in the USA for treatment of cataplexy with narcolepsy. Flunitrazepam is a benzodiazepine and is the active ingredient in Rohypnol, a drug not yet approved by the FDA for medicinal use. Ketamine is a general anesthetic used in veterinary and human medicine. GHB, flunitrazepam, and ketamine are not discussed in this chapter since, they are either indicated for medicinal use or belong to a class of drugs that is discussed elsewhere in the textbook.

3,4-Methylenedioxy-N-methylamphetamine (MDMA)

MDMA, commonly known as Ecstasy, E, X or XTC, is a chiral compound used as a racemate. The *S*-(+)-enantiomer is more active in terms of disruptiveness and degree of intoxication when compared to the R-(-)-enantiomer (Anderson *et al.*, 1978). One study indicated that the plasma half-life of the R-(-)-enantiomer is significantly longer (5.8 ± 2.2 h) than that of the *S*-(+)-enantiomer (3.6 ± 0.9 h) and that the plasma concentrations of the R-(-)-enantiomer exceeded that of the *S*-(+)-enantiomer (*R:S* AUC ratio = 2.4 ± 0.3) (Fallon *et al.*, 1999).

An average dose is one or two tablets of MDMA, where each tablet contains between 60 and 120 mg of MDMA. In one study, after a dose of 40 mg MDMA, most of the material was excreted in the urine within 24 hours after dose administration (Fallon *et al.*, 1999).

Considering the structure of MDMA (**Figure 14**), its relation to amphetamine (XLogP = 1.8) and methamphetamine (XLogP = 2.2), and it's XLogP value of 1.9, it is clear that MDMA will easily transfer into breastmilk. Refer to the section on methamphetamine in this chapter for further information about its transfer into breastmilk.

Breastfeeding following the use of MDMA is not advised and a waiting period of 32 to 48 hours before nursing is recommended.

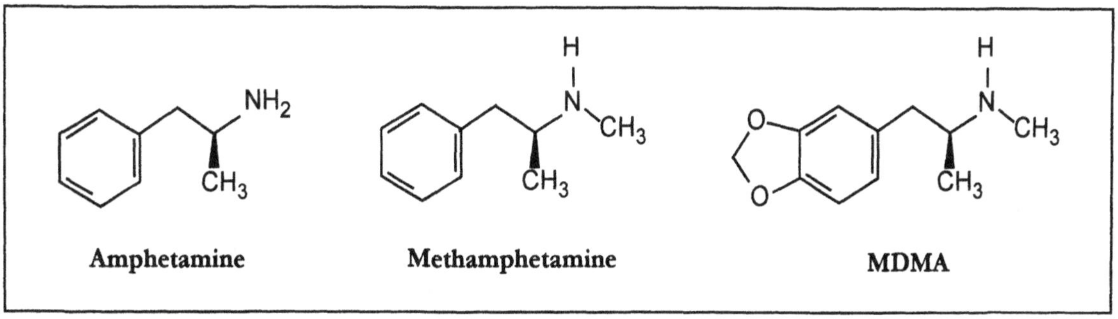

Figure 14. Chemical structures of amphetamine, methamphetamine and 3,4-methylenedioxy-N-methylamphetamine (MDMA).

Inhalants

An inhalant is a volatile chemical at room temperature that is ingested via inhalation. This category includes the following (National Institute on Drug Abuse Infofacts, 2006a):

- nitrites, such as cyclohexyl, butyl, and amyl nitrites (commonly sold as video head cleaners or room deodorizers, leather cleaner, or liquid aroma)
- volatile solvents, such as nail polish remover, paint thinners, degreasers, dry-cleaning fluids, gasoline, glue, correction fluid, and felt-tip marker fluid,
- aerosols, such as spray paints, hair or deodorant sprays, vegetable oil sprays, and aerosol computer cleaning products, and
- gases, such as propane tanks, whipping cream aerosols or dispensers, refrigerant gases, butane lighters, ether, chloroform, halothane, and nitrous oxide (laughing gas).

Nursing women are advised to avoid exposure to these substances. Exposure to inhalants needs to be minimized by using such household products only in well ventilated areas and avoiding skin contact. If it is possible, replace solvent-containing products with water-based products.

Unfortunately, no data are available on the transfer of these agents into breastmilk nor their effect on the breastfed infant. Although taking in consideration that most volatile substances have extremely short half-lives, it is advised that breastfeeding should be avoided while the mother is abusing the inhalant and/or feels intoxicated.

CHAPTER SUMMARY

The drugs discussed in this chapter range from mildly toxic to extremely hazardous for the breastfed infant. The list of contraindicated drugs during breastfeeding includes: cocaine, heroin, LSD, PCP, marijuana, and amphetamines. Other drugs, such as alcohol and tobacco smoke, are not contraindicated, but mothers are encouraged to refrain from using these products while in the presence of their infant and/or during breastfeeding. As in the case of alcohol, Binkiewicz and coworkers (1978) states it quite elegantly, *"We remain advocates of breastfeeding and would not prescribe alcohol. It is the combination that is undesirable."*

Another combination that is undesirable is that of the concomitant use of various drugs of abuse, also known as polydrug use. Although polydrug use is not a new trend among drug abusers, it is in the scientific community, as much needed research is necessary on the interactive effects of various drug combinations, not only on the drug abuser but also on the breastfed infant.

The aim of clinicians is to limit the exposure of the breastfed infant to maternal drugs of abuse. The famous aphorism of Sir Francis Bacon, "*knowledge is power,*" rings especially true when considering this topic. However, for clinicians and mothers to know and to act upon this knowledge is priceless.

References

Akre J. Infant feeding: the physiological basis. *Bull World Health Organ.* 1989; 67:Suppl 1-108.

American Academy of Pediatrics Committee on Drugs. The transfer of drugs and other chemicals into breastmilk. *Pediatrics.* 1989, 84:924-36.

American Academy of Pediatrics Committee on Drugs. Transfer of drugs and other chemicals into human milk. *Pediatrics.* 2001; 108:776-89.

American Thoracic Society. Statement on definitions and classification of emphysema. *Ann Rev Respir Dis.* 1962; 85:762-68.

Amir LH, Donath SM. Does maternal smoking have a negative physiological effect on breastfeeding? The epidemiological evidence. *Breastfeed Rev.* 2003; 11:19-29.

Amir LH. Maternal smoking and reduced duration of breastfeeding: a review of possible mechanisms. *Early Hum Dev.* 2001; 64:45-67.

Amir LH. Smoking status of breastfeeding women. *Acta Paediatr.* 1999; 88:1412-13.

Andersen AN, Schioler V. Influence of breastfeeding pattern on pituitary-ovarian axis of women in an industrialized community. *Am J Obstet Gynaecol.* 1982; 143:673-67.

Andersen AN, Lund-Andersen C, Larsen JF, Christensen NJ, Legros JJ, Louis F, *et al.* Suppressed prolactin but normal neurophysin levels in cigarette-smoking breastfeeding women. *Clin Endocrinol.* 1982; 17:363-68.

Anderson GM III, Braun G, Braun U, Nichols DE, Shulgin AT. Absolute configuration and psychotomimetic activity. *NIDA Res Monogr.* 1978; 22:8-15.

Anderson PO. Alcohol and breastfeeding. *J Hum Lact.* 1995; 11:321-23.

Andrews J, McGarry JM. A community study of smoking in pregnancy. *J Obstet Gynaecol Br.* 1972; 79:1057-73.

Anon. How aspirin turned hero. 1998. *Sunday Times.* Available from: http://opioids.com/heroin/heroinhistory.html [Date of access: 1 December 2006].

Ariagno R, Karch SB, Middleberg R, Stephens BG, Valdes-Dapena M. Methamphetamine ingestion by a breast-feeding mother and her infant's death: People v Henderson. *JAMA.* 1995; 274:215.

Asch RH, Smith CG, Siler-Kohdr TM, Pauerstein C. Acute decreases in serum prolactin concentrations caused by delta-9-tetrahydrocannabinol in nonhuman primates. *Fertil Steril.* 1979; 32:571-74.

Astley SJ, Little RE. Maternal marijuana use during lactation and infant development at one year. *Neurotoxicol Teratol.* 1990; 12:161-68.

Baba A, Yamamoto T, Kawai N, Yamamoto H, Suzuki T, Moroji T. Behavioral effects of phencyclidine and its major metabolite, (trans)4-phenyl-4-(1-piperidinyl)cycloh exanol, in mice. *Behav Brain Res.* 1994a; 65:75-81.

Baba A, Yamamoto T, Yamamoto H, Suzuki T, Moroji T. Effects of the major metabolite of phencyclidine, the trans isomer of 4-phenyl-4-(1-piperidinyl)cyclohexan ol, on [3H]N-(1-[2-thienyl] cyclohexyl)-3,4-piperidine ([3H]TCP) binding and [3H]dopamine uptake in the rat brain. *Neurosci Lett.* 1994b; 182:119-21.

Backstrand JR, Goodman AH, Allen LH, Pelto GH. Pulque intake during pregnancy and lactation in rural Mexico: alcohol and child growth from 1 to 57 months. *Eur J Clin Nutr.* 2004; 58:1626-34.

Bailey DN. Cocaethylene: a novel cocaine homolog. *West J Med.* 1997; 167:38-39.

Bailey DN. Cocaine and cocaethylene binding to human milk. *Am J Clin Pathol.* 1998; 110:491-94.

Bailey DN. Comprehensive review of cocaethylene and cocaine concentrations in patients. *Am J Clin Pathol.* 1996; 106:701-4.

Bailey DN. Serial plasma concentrations of cocoethylene, cocaine, and ethanol in trauma victims. *J Anal Toxicol.* 1993; 17:79-83.

Baraona E, Yokoyama A, Ishii H, Hernandez-Munoz R, Takagi T, Tsuchiya M, *et al.* Lack of alcohol dehydrogenase in enzyme activities in the stomach of Japanese. *Life Sci.* 1991; 52:2071.

Bendersky M, Lewis M. Prenatal cocaine exposure and neonatal condition. *Infant Behav Dev.* 1999; 22:353-66.

Bennett AD. Perinatal substance abuse and the drug-exposed neonate. *Adv Nurse Pract.* 1999; 7:32-36.

Benowitz NL. Nicotine replacement therapy during pregnancy. *JAMA.* 1991; 266:3174-77.

Benwell ME, Balfour DJ, Anderson JM. Evidence that tobacco smoking increases the density of (-)-[3H]nicotine binding sites in human brain. *J Neurochem.* 1988; 50:1243-47.

Binkiewicz A, Robinson MJ, Senior B. Pseudo-Cushing syndrome caused by alcohol in breastmilk. *J Pediatr.* 1978; 93:965-67.

Blake KV, Gurrin LC, Evans SF, Beilin LJ, Landau LI, Stanley FJ, *et al.* Maternal cigarette smoking during pregnancy, low birth weight and subsequent blood pressure in early childhood. *Early Hum Dev.* 2000; 57:137-47.

Boeckxstaens C, Gruwez J, Depauw AM. Chronic recurrent subareolar abscess formation. *Acta Chir Belg.* 1984; 84:233-38.

Bohnet HG, Kato K. Prolactin secretion during pregnancy and puerperium: response to metoclopromide and interactions with placental hormones. *Obstet Gynecol.* 1985; 65:789-92.

Borgen LA, Davis WM, Pace HB. Effects of synthetic 9-tetrahydrocannabinol on pregnancy and offspring in the rat. *Toxicol Appl Pharmacol.* 1971; 20:480-86.

Breese CR, Marks MJ, Logel J, Adams CE, Sullivan B, Collins AC, *et al.* Effect of smoking history on [3H]nicotine binding in human postmortem brain. *J Pharmacol Exp Ther.* 1997; 282:7-13.

Briggs GG, Freeman RK, Yaffe SJ. *Drugs in pregnancy and lactation.* 5th Ed. Baltimore: Williams & Wilkins; 1998.

Brzezinski MR, Abraham TL, Stone CL, Dean RA, Bosron WF. Purification and characterization of a human liver cocine carboxylesterase that catalyzes the purification of benzoylecgonine and the formation of cocaethylene from alcohol and cocaine. *Biochem Pharmacol.* 1994; 48:1747-55.

Bundred NJ, Dover MS, Coley S, Morrison JM. Breast abscesses and cigarette smoking. *Br J Surg.* 1992; 79:58-59.

Casey BJ, Giedd JN, Thomas KM. Structural and functional brain development and its relation to cognitive development. *Biol Psychol.* 2000; 54:241-57.

Catz CS, Giacoia, GP. Drugs and breast milk. *Pediatr Clin North Am.* 1972; 19:151-66.

Centers for Disease Control and Prevention. Frequently asked questions about hepatitis C. 2006. Available from: http://www.cdc.gov/ncidod/diseases/hepatitis/c/faq.htm#3c [Date of access: 28 January 2007]

Chaney NE, Frank J, Wadlington WB. Cocaine convulsions in a breast-feeding baby. *J Pediatr.* 1988; 112:134-35.

Chasnoff IJ, Burns KA, Burns WJ. Cocaine use in pregnancy: perinatal morbidity and mortality. *Neurotoxicol Teratol.* 1987a; 9:291-93.

Chasnoff IJ, Lewis DE, Squires L. Cocaine intoxication in a breast-fed infant. *Pediatrics.* 1987b; 80:836-38.

Chasnoff IJ. Cocaine, pregnancy, and the neonate. *Women Health.* 1989; 15:23-35.

Chatterton RT Jr, Hill PD, Aldag JC, Hodges KR, Belknap SM, Zinaman MJ. Relation of plasma oxytocin and prolactin concentrations to milk production in mothers of preterm infants: influence of stress. *J Clin Endocrinol Metab.* 2000; 85:3661-68.

Chen Y, Li W, Yu S. Influence of passive smoking on admissions for respiratory illness in early childhood. *Br Med J (Clin Res Ed).* 1986; 293:303-6.

Chrisholm CA, Kuller JA. A guide to the safety of CNS-active agents during breastfeeding. *Drug Saf.* 1997; 17:127-42.

Cobo E. Effect of different doses of ethanol on the milk ejecting reflex in lactating women. *Am J Obstet Gynecol.* 1973; 115:817-21.

Cohen MM, Shiloh Y. Genetic toxicology of lysergic acid diethylamide (LSD-25). *Mutat Res.* 1977-1978; 47:183-209.

Coleman DT, Bancroft C. Nicotine acts directly on pituitary GH3 cells to inhibit prolactin promoter activity. *J Neuroendocrinol.* 1995; 7:785-89.

Colley JR, Holland WW, Corkhill RT. Influence of passive smoking and parental phlegm on pneumonia and bronchitis in early childhood. *Lancet.* 1974; ii:1031-34.

Cook CE, Perez-Reyes M, Jeffcoat AR, Brine DR. Phencyclidine disposition in humans after small doses of radiolabelled drug. *Fed Proc.* 1983; 42:2566-69.

Counsilman JJ, Mackay EV. Cigarette smoking by pregnant women with particular reference to their past and subsequent breast feeding behaviour. *Aust NZ J Obstet Gynaecol.* 1985; 25:101-7.

Cowley KC. Psychogenic and pharmacologic induction of the let-down reflex can facilitate breastfeeding by tetraplegic women: a report of 3 cases. *Arch Phys Med Rehabil.* 2005; 86:1261-64.

Cox DB, Owens RA, Hartmann PE. Blood and milk prolactin and the rate of milk synthesis in women. *Exp Physiol.* 1996; 81:1007-20.

Crawford EL, Weaver DA, Demuth JP, Jackson CM, Khuder SA, Frampton MW, *et al.* Measurement of cytochrome P450 2A6 and 2E1 gene expression in primary human bronchial epithelial cells. *Carcinogenesis.* 1998; 19:1867-71.

Dahlström A, Ebersjo C, Lundell B. Nicotine exposure in breastfed infants. *Acta Paediatr.* 2004; 93:810-16.

Dahlström A, Lundell B, Curvall M, Thapper L. Nicotine and cotinine concentrations in the nursing mother and her infant. *Acta Paediatr Scand.* 1990; 79:142-47.

De A, Boyadjieva N, Oomizu S, Sarkar DK. Ethanol induces hyperprolactinemia by increasing prolactin release and lactotropes growth in female rats. *Alcohol Clin Exp Res.* 2002; 26:1420-29.

Dean RA, Christian CD, Sample RH, Bosron WF. Human liver cocaine esterases: ethanol-mediated formation of ethylcocaine. *FASEB J.* 1991; 5:2735-39.

Dezateux C, Stocks J, Wade AM, Dundas I, Fletcher ME. Airway function at one year: Association with premorbid airway function, wheezing, and maternal smoking. *Thorax.* 2001; 56:680-86.

Dickson PH, Lind A, Studts P, Nipper HC, Makoid M, Therkildsen D. The routine analysis of breast milk for drugs of abuse in a clinical toxicology laboratory. *J Forensic Sci.* 1994; 39:207-14.

Dillon AE, Wagner CL, Wiest D, Newman RB. Drug therapy in the nursing mother. *Obstet Gynecol Clin North Am.* 1997; 24:675-96.

DiPadova C, Roine R, Frezza M, Gentry RT, Baraona E, Lieber CS. Effects of ranitidine on blood alcohol levels after ethanol ingestion. Comparison with other H2-receptor antagonists. *JAMA.* 1992; 267:83-86.

DiPadova C, Worner TM, Julkunen RJ, Lieber CS. Effects of fasting and chronic alcohol consumption on the first pass metabolism of ethanol. *Gastroenterology.* 1987; 92:1169-73.

Directgov. New Health bill will ban smoking in majority of workplaces. 2005. Available from: http://www.direct.gov.uk/Nl1/Newsroom/NewsroomArticles/fs/en?CONTENT_ID=10027079&chk=5r8ic9 [Date of access: 7 November 2006].

Dishotsky NI, Loughman WD, Mogar RE, Lipscomb WR. LSD and genetic damage. *Science.* 1971; 172:431-40.

Djulus J, Moretti M, Koren G. Marijuana use and breastfeeding. *Can Fam Physician.* 2005; 51:349-50.

Domino SE, Domino LE, Domino EF. Comparison of two and three compartment models of phencyclidine in man. *Subst Alcohol Actions Misuse.* 1982; 3:205-11.

Donath SM, Amir LH, ALSPAC Study Team. The relationship between maternal smoking and breastfeeding duration after adjustment for maternal infant feeding intention. *Acta Paediatr.* 2004; 93:1514-18.

Dutau G, Enjaume C, Petrus M, Darcos P, Demenrisse P, Rochiccioli P. Epidemiology of passive smoking of children from 0 to 6 years. *Arch Fr Pediatr.* 1981; 38:721-25.

Dwoskin LP, Teng L, Buxton ST, Crooks PA. (*S*)-(-)-Cotinine, the major brain metabolite of nicotine, stimulates nicotinic receptors to evoke [3H]dopamine release from rat striatal slices in a calcium-dependent manner. *J Pharmacol Exp Ther.* 1999; 288:905-11.

Etzel RA, Greenberg RA, Haley NJ, Loda FA. Urine cotinine excretion in neonates exposed to tobacco smoke products in utero. *J Pediatr.* 1985; 107:146-48.

Fallon JK, Kicman AT, Henry JA, Milligan PJ, Cowan DA, Hutt AJ. Stereospecific analysis and enantiomeric disposition of 3,4-methylenedioxymethamphetamine (Ecstasy) in humans. *Clin Chem.* 1999; 45:1058-69.

Feilberg VL, Rosenborg D, Broen Christensen C, Mogensen JV. Excretion of morphine in human breast milk. *Acta Anaesthesiol Scand.* 1989; 33:426-28.

Ferguson BB, Wilson DJ, Schaffner W. Determination of nicotine concentrations in human milk. *Am J Dis Child.* 1976; 130:837-39.

Fergusson DM, Horwood LJ, Shannon FT. Parental smoking and respiratory illness in infancy. *Arch Dis Child.* 1980; 55:358-61.

Fernández-Ruiz J, Gomez M, Hernandez M, de Miguel R, Ramos JA. Cannabinoids and gene expression during brain development. *Neurotox Res.* 2004; 6:389-401.

Freeman ME, Kanyicska B, Lerant A, Nagy G. Prolactin: structure, function, and regulation of secretion. *Physiol Rev.* 2000; 80:1523-1631.

Frezza M, di Padova C, Pozzato G, Terpin M, Baraona E, Lieber CS. High blood alcohol levels in women. The role of decreased gastric alcohol dehydrogenase activity and first-pass metabolism. *N Engl J Med.* 1990; 322:95-99.

Fried PA. Marihuana use by pregnant women and effects on offspring: an update. *Neurobehav Toxicol Teratol.* 1982; 4:451-54.

Fried PA, Charlebois AT. Effects upon rat offspring following Cannabis inhalation before and/or after mating. *Can J Psychol.* 1979; 33:125-32.

Fried PA, O'Connell CM, Watkinson B. 60- and 72-month follow-up of children prenatally exposed to marijuana, cigarettes, and alcohol: cognitive and language assessment. *J Dev Behav Pediatr.* 1992; 13:383-91.

Fried PA, Watkinson B. 12- and 24-month neurobehavioural follow-up of children prenatally exposed to marijuana, cigarettes and alcohol. *Neurotoxicol Teratol.* 1988; 10:305-13.

Fried PA, Watkinson B. 36- and 48-month neurobehavioral follow-up of children prenatally exposed to marijuana, cigarettes, and alcohol. *J Dev Behav Pediatr.* 1990; 11:49-58.

Fried PA, Watkinson B, Gray R. Growth from birth to early adolescence in offspring prenatally exposed to cigarettes and marijuana. *Neurotoxicol Teratol.* 1999; 21:513-25.

Fuchs AR. Ethanol and the inhibition of oxytocin release in lactating rats. *Acta Endocrinol (Copenh).* 1969; 62:546-54.

Fuchs A, Wagner G. The effect of ethyl alcohol on the release of oxytocin in rabbits. *Acta Endocrinol (Copenh).* 1963; 44:593-605.

Fuxe K, Andersson K, Eneroth P, Harfstrand A, Agnati LF. Neuroendocrine actions of nicotine and of exposure to cigarette smoke: medical implications. *Psychoneuroendocrinology.* 1989; 14:19-41.

Gao YJ, Holloway AC, Zeng ZH, Lim GE, Petrik JJ, Foster WG, *et al.* Prenatal exposure to nicotine causes postnatal obesity and altered perivascular adipose tissue function. *Obes Res.* 2005; 13:687-92.

Giacomelli S, Palmery M, Romanelli L, Cheng CY, Silvestrini B. Lysergic acid diethylamide (LSD) is a partial agonist of D2 dopaminergic receptors and it potentates dopamine-mediated prolactin secretion in lactotrophs *in vitro*. *Life Sci.* 1998; 63:215-22.

Gibbens GL, Chard T. Observations on maternal oxytocin release during human labor and the effect of intravenous alcohol administration. *Am J Obstet Gynecol.* 1976; 126:243-46.

Gimpl G, Fahrenholz F. The oxytocin receptor system: structure, function and regulation. *Physiol Rev.* 2001; 81:629-83.

Girardin F, Rentsch KM, Schwab MA, Maggiorini M, Pauli-Magnus C, Kullak-Ublick GA, *et al.* Pharmacokinetics of high doses of intramuscular and oral heroin in narcotic addicts. *Clin Pharmacol Ther.* 2003; 74:341-52.

Goldfarb J. Breastfeeding. AIDS and other infectious diseases. *Clin Perinatol.* 1993; 20:225-43.

Grattan DR. Behavioural significance of prolactin signaling in the central nervous system during pregnancy and lactation. *Reproduction.* 2002; 123:497-506.

Guindon GE, Boisclair D. Past, current, and future trends in tobacco use. Vol 2003: The World Bank. Available from: http://www1.worldbank.org/tobacco/publications.asp [Date of access: 7 November 2006].

Håkansson A, Carlsson B. Maternal cigarette smoking, breast-feeding, and respiratory tract infections in infancy. *Scand J Prim Health Care.* 1992; 10:62-65.

Hale TW. *Medications and mothers' milk.* 7th Ed. Amarillo, TX: Pharmasoft Publishing; 1998.

Hale TW. *Medications and mothers' milk.* 11th Ed. Amarillo, TX: Pharmasoft Publishing; 2004.

Hale, TW. *Medications and mothers' milk.* 12th Ed. Amarillo, TX: Pharmasoft Publishing; 2006.

Hale TW, McAfee G. *A medication guide for breastfeeding moms.* Amarillo, TX: Pharmasoft Publishing; 2005.

Hall J. Woman sentenced in infant's death. 2005. Available from: http://www.nctimes.com/articles/2005/04/09/news/californian/23_24_174_8_05.txt [Date of access: 8 December 2006].

Harada S, Okubo T. Investigation of alcohol dehydrogenase isozymes of biopsy gastric mucosa in Japanese. *Alcohol Alcohol Suppl.* 1993; 1B:59-62.

Harbison RD, Mantilla-Plata B, Lubin DJ. Alteration of delta-9-tetrahydrocannabinol-induced teratogenicity by stimulation and inhibition of its metabolites. *J Pharmacol Exp Ther.* 1977; 202:455-65.

Hardee GE, Stewart T, Capomacchia AC. Tobacco smoke xenophobic compound appearance in mother's milk after involuntary smoke exposures I. Nicotine and cotinine. *Toxicol Lett.* 1983; 15:109-12.

Harlap S, Davies AM. Infant admissions to hospital and maternal smoking. *Lancet.* 1974; i:529-32.

Harris DS, Boxenbaum H, Everhart ET, Sequeria G, Mendelson JE, Jones RT. The bioavailability of intranasal and smoked methamphetamine. *Clin Pharmacol Ther.* 2003a; 74:475-86.

Harris DS, Everhart ET, Mendelson J, Jones RT. The pharmacology of cocaethylene in humans following cocaine and ethanol administration. *Drug Alcohol Depend.* 2003b; 72:169-82.

Hearn WL, Rose S, Wagner J, Ciarleglio A, Mash DC. Cocoethylene is more potent than cocaine in mediating lethality. *Pharmacol Biochem Behav.* 1991; 39:531-33.

Heil SH, Hungund BL, Zheng ZH, Jen KL, Subramanian MG. Ethanol and lactation: effects of milk lipids and serum constituents. *Alcohol.* 1999; 18:43-48.

Hernandez-Munoz R, Caballeria J, Baraona E, Uppal R, Greenstein R, Lieber CS. Human gastric alcohol dehydrogenase: its inhibition by H2-receptor antagonists, and its effect on the bioavailability of ethanol. *Alcohol Clin Exp Res.* 1990; 14:946-50.

Heyman RB, Anglin TM, Copperman SM, Joffe A, McDonald CA, Rogers PD, *et al.* American Academy of Pediatrics. Committee on substance abuse. Marijuana: A continuing concern for pediatricians. *Pediatrics.* 1999; 104:982-85.

Heyser CJ, Molina VA, Spear LP. A fostering study of the effects of prenatal cocaine exposure: I. Maternal behaviors. *Neurotoxicol Teratol.* 1992; 14:415-21.

Holloway AC, Lim GE, Petrik JJ, Foster WG, Morrison KM, Gerstein HC. Fetal and neonatal exposure to nicotine in Wistar rats results in increased beta cell apoptosis at birth and postnatal endocrine and metabolic changes associated with type 2 diabetes. *Diabetologia.* 2005; 48:2661-66.

Hopkinson JM, Schanler RJ, Fraley JK. Milk production by mothers of premature infants: influence of cigarette smoking. *Pediatrics.* 1992; 90:934-38.

Hosztafi S. Heroin, part III: the pharmacology of heroin. *Acta Pharm Hung.* 2003; 73:197-205.

Howie PW, McNeilly AS, McArdle T, Smart L, Houston M. The relationship between suckling-induced prolactin response and lactogenesis. *J Clin Endocrinol Metab.* 1980; 50:670-73.

Huestis MA. Cannabis (marijuana) - Effects on human behavior and performance. *Forensic Sci Rev.* 2002; 14:15-60.

Huestis MA, Henningfield JE, Cone EJ. Blood cannabinoids. I. Absorption of THC and formation of 11-OH-THC and THCCOOH during and after smoking marijuana. *J Anal Toxicol.* 1992; 16:276-82.

Hughes CL, Everett JW, Tyrey L. Δ^9-Tetrahydrocannabinol suppression of prolactin secretion in the rat: lack of direct pituitary effect. *Endocrinology.* 1981; 109:876-80.

Hunt CE, Hauck FR. Sudden infant death syndrome. *CMAJ.* 2006; 20:1861-69.

Hurd YL, Wang X, Anderson V, Beck O, Minkoff H, Dow-Edwards, D. Marijuana impairs growth in mid-gestation fetuses. *Neurotoxicol Teratol.* 2005; 27:221-29.

Hyde JF. Effects of phencyclidine on 5-hydroxytryptophan- and suckling-induced prolactin release. *Brain Res.* 1992; 573:204-8.

Ilett K, Hale TW, Page-Sharp M, Kristensen JH, Kohan R, Hackett LP. Use of nicotine patches in breast-feeding mothers: Transfer of nicotine and cotinine into human milk. *Clin Pharmacol Ther.* 2003; 74:516-24.

Ilett KF, Hackett LP, Kristensen JH, Kohan R. Transfer of dexamphetamine into breast milk during treatment for attention deficit hyperactivity disorder. *Br J Clin Pharmacol.* 2007; 63:371-75.

Ito S. Drug therapy for breast-feeding women. *N Engl J Med.* 2000; 343:118-26.

Jeffery BS, Mercer KG. Pretoria pasteurisation: a potential method for the reduction of postnatal mother to child transmission of the human immunodeficiency virus. *J Trop Pediatr.* 2000; 46:219-23.

Johansson E, Agurell S, Hollister LE, Halldin MM. Prolonged apparent half-life of delta 1-tetrahydrocannabinol in plasma of chronic marijuana users. *J Pharm Pharmacol.* 1988; 40:374-75.

Johns JM, Faggin BM, Noonan LR, Li L, Zimmerman LI, Pedersen CA. Chronic cocaine treatment decreases oxytocin levels in the amygdala and increases maternal aggression in Sprague-Dawley rats. *Soc Neurosci.* 1995; 21:766-7.

Johns JM, Lubin DA, Walker CH, Meter KE, Mason GA. Chronic gestational cocaine treatment decreases oxytocin levels in the medial preoptic area, ventral tegmental area and hippocampus in Sprague-Dawley rats. *Neuropeptides.* 1997; 31:439-43.

Johns JM, Noonan LR, Zimmerman LI, Li L, Pedersen CA. Effects of chronic and acute cocaine treatment on the onset of maternal behavior and aggression in Sprague-Dawley rats. *Behav Neurosci.* 1994; 108:107-112.

Johnston JM, Amico JA. A prospective longitudinal study of the release of oxytocin and prolactin in response to infants suckling in long term lactation. *J Clin Endocrinol Metab.* 1986; 62:653-57.

Johnston LD, O'Malley PM, Bachman JG, Schulenberg JE. Monitoring the future national survey results on drug use, 1975-2005: Volume I, Secondary school students (NIH Publication No. 06-5883). Bethesda, MD: National Institute on Drug Abuse. 2006. Available from: http://www.monitoringthefuture.org/pubs/monographs/vol1_2005.pdf.

Jones WL, Stewart DB. Effects of orally-administered ethanol on mammary gland morphology and functional efficiency in lactating rats. *Exp Pathol.* 1984; 25:205-13.

Kamendulis LM, Brzezinski MR, Pindel EV, Bosron WF, Dean RA. Metabolism of cocaine and heroin is catalyzed by the same human liver carboxylesterases. *J Pharmacol Exp Ther.* 1996; 279:713-17.

Kaufman KR, Petrucha RA, Pitts FN, Weekes ME. PCP in amniotic fluid and breast milk: case report. *J Clin Psychiatry.* 1983; 44:269-70.

Keith RE, Mossholder SB. Ascorbic acid status of smoking and nonsmoking adolescent females. *Int J Vitam Nutr Res.* 1986; 56:363-66.

Kesäniemi YA. Ethanol and acetaldehyde in the milk and peripheral blood of lactating women after ethanol administration. *J Obstet Gynaecol Br Commonw.* 1974; 81:84-86.

Kinsley CH, Turco D, Bauer A, Beverly M, Wellman J, Graham AL. Cocaine alters the onset and maintenance of maternal behavior in lactating rats. *Pharmacol Biochem Behav.* 1994; 47:857-64.

Kirschbaum C, Scherer G, Strasburger CJ. Pituitary and adrenal hormone responses to pharmacological, physical and psychological stimulation in habitual smokers and non-smokers. *Clin Investig.* 1994; 72:804-10.

Klinnert MD, Nelson HS, Price MR, Adinoff AD, Leung DY, Mrazek DA. Onset of persistence of childhood asthma: predictors from infancy. *Pediatrics.* 2001; 108:E69.

Klonoff-Cohen H, Lam-Kruglick P. Maternal and paternal recreational drug use and sudden infant death syndrome. *Arch Pediatr Adolesc Med.* 2001; 155:765-70.

Koivusalo M, Baumann M, Uotila L. Evidence for the identity of glutathione-dependent formaldehyde dehydrogenase and class III alcohol dehydrogenase. *FEBS Lett.* 1989; 257:105-9.

Kordom C, Maritz GS, De Kock M. Maternal nicotine exposure during pregnancy and lactation: I. Effect on glycolysis in the lungs of the offspring. *Exp Lung Res.* 2003; 29:79-89.

Koren G. Drinking alcohol while breastfeeding. Will it harm my baby? *Can Fam Physician.* 2002; 48:39-41.

Kramer J, Ben-David M. Prolactin suppression by (-)-Δ^9-tetrahydrocannabinol: involvement of serotoninergic and dopaminergic pathways. *Endocrinology.* 1978; 103:452-58.

Kuhnert BR, Bagby BS, Golden NL. Measurement of phencyclidine and two hydroxylated metabolites by selected ion monitoring. *J Chromatogr.* 1983; 276:433-37.

Kyerematen GA, Damiano MD, Dvorchik BH, Vesell ES. Smoking-induced changes in nicotine disposition: application of a new HPLC assay for nicotine and its metabolites. *Clin Pharmacol Ther.* 1982; 32:769-80.

Labrecque M, Marcoux S, Weber JP, Fabia J, Ferron L. Feeding and urine cotinine values in babies whose mothers smoke. *Pediatrics.* 1989; 83:93-97.

Laizure SC, Mandrell T, Gades NM, Parker RB. Cocaethylene metabolism and interaction with cocaine and ethanol: role of carboxylesterases. *Drug Metabolism Dispos.* 2003; 31:16-20.

Lawton ME. Alcohol in breast milk. *Aust NZ J Obstet Gynaec.* 1985; 25:71-73.

Le Guennec JC, Billon B. Delay in caffeine elimination in breast-fed infants. *Pediatrics.* 1987; 79:264-68.

Leake RD, Waters CB, Rubin RT, Buster JE, Fisher DA. Oxytocin and prolactin responses in long-term breast-feeding. *Obstet Gynecol.* 1983; 62:565-68.

Lindmark B. Maternal use of alcohol and breast-fed infants. *N Engl J Med.* 1990; 322:338-39.

Lipshultz SE, Frassica JJ, Orav EJ. Cardiovascular abnormalities in infants prenatally exposed to cocaine. *J Pediatr.* 1991; 118:44-51.

Liston J. Breastfeeding and the use of recreational drugs - alcohol, caffeine, nicotine and marijuana. *Breastfeeding Rev.* 1998; 6:27-30.

Little RE, Anderson KW, Ervin CH, Worthington-Roberts B, Clarren SK. Maternal alcohol use during breast-feeding and infant mental and motor development at one year. *N Engl J Med.* 1989; 321:425-30.

Little RE, Northstone K, Golding J, ALSPAC Study Team. Alcohol, breastfeeding, and development at 18 months. *Pediatrics.* 2002; 109:E72.

Lockridge O, Mottershaw-Jackson N, Eckerson HW, La Du BN. Hydrolysis of diacetylmorphine (heroin) by human serum cholinesterase. *J Pharmacol Exp Ther.* 1980; 215:1-8.

Long SY. Does LSD induce chromosomal damage and malformations? A review of the literature. *Teratology.* 1972; 6:75-90.

Luck W, Nau H. Nicotine and cotinine concentrations in serum and milk of nursing smokers. *Br J Clin Pharmacol.* 1984; 18:9-15.

Luck W, Nau H. Nicotine and cotinine concentrations in serum and urine of infants exposed via passive smoking or milk from smoking mothers. *J Pediatr.* 1985; 107:816-20.

Luck W, Nau H. Nicotine and cotinine concentrations in the milk of smoking mothers: influence of cigarette consumption and diurnal variation. *Eur J Pediatr.* 1987; 146:21-26.

MacGregor SN, Keith LG, Chasnoff IJ, Rosner MA, Chisum GM, Shaw P, *et al.* Cocaine use during pregnancy: adverse perinatal outcome. *Am J Obstet Gynecol.* 1987; 157:686-90.

Makielski JC. SIDS: genetic and environmental influences may cause arrhythmia in this silent killer. *J Clin Invest.* 2006; 116:297-99.

Maritz GS. Maternal nicotine exposure during gestation and lactation of rats induce microscopic emphysema in the offspring. *Exp Lung Res.* 2002; 28:391-403.

Maritz GS, Dennis H. Maternal nicotine exposure during gestation and lactation interferes with alveolar development in the neonatal lung. *Reprod Fertil Dev.* 1998; 10:255-61.

Maritz GS, Matthews HL, Aalbers, J. Maternal supplementation protects the neonatal rat lung against the adverse effects of maternal nicotine exposure. *Reprod Fertil Dev.* 2000; 12:97-103.

Marks MJ, Burch JB, Collins AC. Effects of chronic nicotine infusion on tolerance development and nicotinic receptors. *J Pharmacol Exp Ther.* 1983; 226:817-25.

Marks MJ, Pauly JR, Gross SD, Deneris ES, Hermans-Borgmeyer I, Heinemann SF, *et al.* Nicotine binding and nicotinic receptor subunit RNA after chronic nicotine treatment. *J Neurosci.* 1992; 12:2765-84.

Marks MJ, Stitzel JA, Collins AC. Time course study of the effects of chronic nicotine infusion on drug response and brain receptors. *J Pharmacol Exp Ther.* 1985; 235:619-28.

Martin BR, Freeman AS. Disposition of phencyclidine and its pyrolitic products in mice exposed to smoke. *Fed Proc.* 1983; 42:2561-65.

Mascola MA, Van Vunakis H, Tager IB, Speizer FE, Hanrahan JP. Exposure of young infants to environmental tobacco smoke: breast-feeding among smoking mothers. *Am J Public Health.* 1998; 88:893-96.

Matheson I, Rivrud GN. The effect of smoking on lactation and infantile colic. *JAMA.* 1989; 261:42-43.

Maurice M, Emiliani S, Dalet-Beluche I, Derancourt J, Lange R. Isolation and characterization of a cytochrome P450 of the IIA subfamily from human liver microsomes. *Eur J Biochem.* 1991; 1:511-17.

McAfee G. Smoking and brain dopaminergic neurochemistry. 2004. Potchefstroom: North-West University. Thesis - Ph.D. p. 107.

McCance-Katz EF, Price LH, McDougle CJ, Kosten TR, Black JE, Jatlow PI. Concurrent cocaine-ethanol ingestion in humans: pharmacology, physiology, behavior, and the role of cocaethylene. *Psychopharmacology (Berl).* 1993; 111:39-46.

McNeilly AS, Robinson IC, Houston MJ, Howie PW. Release of oxytocin and prolactin in response to suckling. *Br Med J (Clin Res Ed).* 1983; 22:257-59.

Mello NK, Mendelson JH, Sellers ML, Kuehnle JC. Effect of alcohol and marihuana on tobacco smoking. *Clin Pharmacol Ther.* 1980; 27:202-9.

Meltzer HY, Fessler RG, Simonovic M, Doherty J, Fang VS. Lysergic acid diethylamide: evidence for stimulation of pituitary dopamine receptors. *Psychopharmacology (Berl).* 1977; 54:39-44.

Mendelson JH, Sholar MB, Mutschler NH, Jaszyna-Gasior M, Goletiani NV, Siegel AJ, *et al.* Effects of intravenous cocaine and cigarette smoking on luteinizing hormone, testosterone, and prolactin in men. *J Pharmacol Exp Ther.* 2003; 307:339-48.

Mennella J. Alcohol's effect on lactation. *Alcohol Res Health.* 2001; 25:230-34.

Mennella JA. Infants' suckling responses to the flavor of alcohol in mother's milk. *Alcohol Clin Exp Res.* 1997; 21:581-85.

Mennella JA, Beauchamp GK. Beer, breast feeding and folklore. *Dev Psychobiol.* 1993a; 26:459-66.

Mennella JA, Beauchamp GK. Effects of beer on breast-fed infants. *JAMA.* 1993b; 269:1637-38.

Mennella JA, Beauchamp GK. The transfer of alcohol to human milk: effects on flavor and the infant's behavior. *N Engl J Med.* 1991; 325:981-85.

Mennella JA, Gerrish CJ. Effects of exposure to alcohol in mother's milk on infant sleep. *Pediatrics.* 1998; 101:915.

Mennella JA, Pepino MY, Teff KL. Acute alcohol consumption disrupts the hormonal milieu of lactating women. *J Clin Endocrinol Metab.* 2005; 90:1979-85.

Mills CA. Tobacco smoking: some hints of its biologic hazards. *Ohio State Med J.* 1950; 46:1165-70.

Minchin MK. Positioning for breastfeeding. *Birth.* 1989; 16:67-80.

Minchin MK. Smoking and breastfeeding: An overview. *J Hum Lact.* 1991; 7:183-88.

Misra AL, Pontani RB, Bartolomeo J. Persistence of phencyclidine (PCP) and metabolites in brain and adipose tissue and implications for long-lasting behavioral effects. *Res Commun Chem Pathol Pharmacol.* 1979; 24:431-45.

Misra DP, Nguyen RH. Environmental tobacco smoke and low birth weight: a hazard in the workplace? *Environ Health Perspect.* 1999; 107 Suppl 6:897-904.

Montgomery SM, Ekbom A. Smoking during pregnancy and diabetes mellitus in a British longitudinal birth cohort. *BMJ.* 2002; 324:26-27.

Moreno A., Parés A, Ortiz J, Enriquez J, Parés X. Alcohol dehydrogenase from human stomach: variability in normal mucosa and effect of age, gender, ADH3 phenotype and gastric region. *Alcohol Alcohol.* 1994; 29:663-68.

Moreno A, Parés X. Purification and characterization of a new alcohol dehydrogenase from human stomach. *J Biol Chem.* 1991; 226:1128-33.

Morley R, Leeson Payne C, Lister G, Lucas A. Maternal smoking and blood pressure in 7.5 to 8 year old offspring. *Arch Dis Child.* 1995; 72:120-24.

Myr R. Promoting, protecting, and supporting breastfeeding in a community with a high rate of tobacco use. *J Hum Lact.* 2004; 20:415-16.

Narayanan U, Birru S, Vaglenova J, Breese CR. Nicotinic receptor expression following nicotine exposure via maternal milk. *Neuroreport.* 2002; 13:961-63.

National Institute on Drug Abuse InfoFacts. Costs to society. 1995. Available from: http://www.drugabuse.gov/infofacts/costs.html [Date of access: 4 January 2007].

National Institute on Drug Abuse InfoFacts. Inhalants. 2006a. Available from: http://www.drugabuse.gov/Infofacts/Inhalants.html [Date of access: 19 December 2006].

National Institute on Drug Abuse InfoFacts. LSD. 2006b. Available from: http://www.nida.nih.gov/infofacts/lsd.html [Date of access: 14 November 2006].

National Institute on Drug Abuse. Research report series - Cocaine abuse and addiction. 1999. Available from: http://www.nida.nih.gov/ResearchReports/Cocaine/Cocaine.html [Date of access: 14 November 2006].

National Institute on Drug Abuse. Research report series - Hallucinogens and dissociative drugs. Including LSD, PCP, Ketamine, Dextromethorphan. 2001. Available from: http://www.nida.nih.gov/ResearchReports/Hallucinogens/Hallucinogens.html [Date of access: 14 November 2006].

National Institute on Drug Abuse. Research report series - Nicotine addiction. 2002. Available from: http://www.nida.nih.gov/researchreports/nicotine/nicotine2.html#what [Date of access: 13 May 2004].

National Institute on Drug Abuse. Research report series - Marijuana abuse. 2005a. Available from: http://www.nida.nih.gov/ResearchReports/Marijuana/default.html [Date of access: 21 November 2006].

National Institute on Drug Abuse. Research report series - Heroin abuse and addiction. 2005b. Available from: http://www.nida.nih.gov/ResearchReports/Heroin/Heroin.html [Date of access: 8 December 2006].

National Survey on Drug Use and Health. National findings, results from 2005. Available from: http://www.oas.samhsa.gov/NSDUH/2k5NSDUH/2k5results.htm [Date of access: 20 November 2006].

National Surveys on Drug Use and Health. State estimates of substance use, 2002–2003. Available from: http://oas.samhsa.gov/2k3State/toc.htm#TopOfPage [Date of access: 7 January 2007].

Newton N. The relation of the milk-ejection reflex to the ability to breast feed. *Ann NY Acad Sci.* 1992a; 652:484-86.

Newton N. The quantitative effect of oxytocin (pitocin) on human milk yield. *Ann NY Acad Sci.* 1992b; 652:481-83.

Nicholas JM, Lipshitz J, Schreiber EC. Phencyclidine: its transfer across the placenta as well as into breast milk. *Am J Obstet Gynecol.* 1982; 143:143-46.

O'Brien CP. Drug addiction and drug abuse. In: Goodman Gilman A (*ed.*). *Goodman and Gilman's the pharmacological basis of therapeutics.* 9th Ed. New York: McGraw-Hill; 1996. p. 557-77.

O'Dell BL, Kilburn KH, McKenzie WN, Thurstone RJ. The lung of the copper-deficient rat. *Am J Pathol.* 1978; 91:413-32.

Office of National Drug Control Policy. *What Americans need to know about marijuana.* Annual Report. ONDCP; 2003.

Ogston, SA, Florey CD, Walker CH. Association of infant alimentary and respiratory illness with parental smoking and other environmental factors. *J Epidemiol Community Health.* 1987; 41:21-25.

Oneta CM, Simanowski UA, Martinez M, Allali-Hassani A, Parés X, Homann N, *et al.* First pass metabolism of ethanol is strikingly influenced by the speed of gastric emptying. *Gut.* 1998; 43:612-19.

Parés X, Cederlund E, Moreno A, Saubi N, Hoog JO, Jornvall H. Class IV alcohol dehydrogenase (the gastric enzyme). Structural analysis of human sigma sigma-ADH reveals class IV to be variable and confirms the presence of a fifth mammalian alcohol dehydrogenase class. *FEBS Lett.* 1992; 303:69-72.

Pedreira FA, Guandolo VL, Feroli EJ, Mella GW, Weiss IP. Involuntary smoking and incidence of respiratory illness during the first year of life. *Pediatrics.* 1985; 75:594-97.

Pedrosa MC, Russell RM, Saltzman JR, Golner BB, Dallal GE, Sepe TE, *et al.* Gastric emptying and first-pass metabolism of ethanol in elderly subjects with and without atrophic gastritis. *Scand J Gastroenterol.* 1996; 31:671-77.

Perez-Reyes M, Wall ME. Presence of Δ^9-tetrahydrocannibinol in human milk. *N Engl J Med.* 1982; 23:819-20.

Perlman HH, Dannenberg AM, Sokoloff N. The excretion of nicotine in breast milk and urine from cigarette smoking: its effect on lactation and the nursing. *J Am Med Assoc.* 1942; 120:1003-9.

Peto R, Lopez AD, Boreham J, Thun M, Heath C Jr. Mortality from tobacco in developed countries: indirect estimation from national vital statistics. *Lancet.* 1992; 339:1268-78.

Pikkarainen PH, Räihä NCR. Development of alcohol dehydrogenase activity in the human liver. *Pediatr Res.* 1967; 1:165-68.

Pindel EV, Kedishvilli NY, Abraham TL, Brzezinski MR, Zhang J, Dean RA, *et al.* Purification and cloning of a broad substrate specificity human liver carboxylesterase that catalyzes the hydrolysis of cocaine and heroin. *J Biol Chem.* 1997; 272:14769-75.

Pradhan SN. Phencyclidine (PCP): some human studies. *Neurosci Biobehav Rev.* 1984; 8:493-501.

Quadri SK, Meites J. LSD-induced decrease in serum prolactin in rats. *Proc Soc Exp Biol Med.* 1971; 137:1242-43.

Raine JM, Wing DR, Paton WDM. The effects of delta-1-tetrahydrocannabinol on mammary gland growth, enzyme activity and plasma prolactin levels in the mouse. *Bur J Pharmacol.* 1978; S1:11-17.

Rantakallio P. Relationship of maternal smoking to morbidity and mortality of the child up to the age of five. *Acta Paediatr Scand.* 1978; 67:621-31.

Reingardiene D, Vilcinskaite J, Lazauskas R. Hallucinogenic mushrooms. *Medicina (Kaunas).* 2005; 41:1067-70.

Reisine T, Pasternak G. Opioid analgesics and antagonists. In: Goodman Gilman A. (ed.). *Goodman and Gilman's the pharmacological basis of therapeutics.* 9th Ed. New York: McGraw-Hill; 1996. p. 521-55.

Rettori V, Wenger T, Snyder G, Dalterio S, McCann SM. Hypothalamic action of delta-9-tetrahydrocannabinol to inhibit the release of prolactin and growth hormone in the rat. *Neuroendocrinology.* 1988; 47:498-503.

Roine R, Gentry RT, Hernandez-Munoz R, Baraona E, Lieber CS. Aspirin increases blood alcohol dehydrogenase in humans after ingestion of ethanol. *JAMA.* 1990; 264:2406-8.

Russell MA, Feverabend C. Blood and urinary nicotine in non-smokers. *Lancet.* 1975; 25:179-81.

Said G, Patois E, Lellouch J. Infantile colic and parental smoking. *Br Med J (Clin Res Ed).* 1984; 289:660.

Sanchis R, Guerri C. Chronic ethanol intake in lactating rats: milk analysis. *Comp Biochem Physiol C.* 1986; 85:107-10.

Sawynok J. The therapeutic use of heroin: a review of the pharmacological literature. *Can J Physiol Pharmacol.* 1986; 64:1-6.

Schäfer P, Fürrer C, Mermillod B. An association of cigarette smoking with recurrent subareolar breast abscess. *Int J Epidemiol.* 1988; 17:810-13.

Schulte P. Minimizing alcohol exposure of the breastfed infant. *J Hum Lact.* 1995; 11:317-319.

Schulte-Hobein B, Schwartz-Bickenbach D, Abt S, Plum C, Nau H. Cigarette smoke exposure and development of infants throughout the first year of life: influence of passive smoking and nursing on cotinine levels in breast milk and infant's urine. *Acta Paediatr.* 1992; 81:550-57.

Schutzman DL, Frankenfield-Dhernicoff M, Clatterbaugh HE, Singer J. Incidence of intrauterine cocaine exposure in a suburban setting. *Pediatrics.* 1991; 88:825-27.

Schwartz RD, Kellar KJ. In vivo regulation of [3H]acetylcholine recognition sites in brain by nicotinic cholinergic drugs. *J Neurochem.* 1985; 45:427-33.

Schwartz RD, Kellar KJ. Nicotinic cholinergic receptor binding sites in the brain: regulation in vivo. *Science.* 1983; 220:214-16.

Schwartz-Bickenbach D, Schulte-Hobein B, Abt S, Plum C, Nau H. Smoking and passive smoking during pregnancy and early infancy: effects on birth weight, lactation period, and cotinine concentrations in mother's milk and infant's urine. *Toxicol Lett.* 1987; 35:73-81.

Seitz HK, Egerer G, Simanowski UA, Waldherr R, Eckey R, Agarwal DP, *et al.* Human gastric alcohol dehydrogenase activity: effect of age, sex, and alcoholism. *Gut.* 1993; 34:1433-37.

Seitz HK, Oneta CM. Gastrointestinal alcohol dehydrogenase. *Nutr Rev.* 1998; 56:52-60.

Selmanoff M, Gregerson KA. Suckling decreases dopamine turnover in both medial and lateral aspects of the median eminence in the rat. *Neurosci Lett.* 1985; 57:25-30.

Seyler LE Jr, Pomerlean OF, Fertig JB, Hunt D, Parker K. Pituitary hormone response to cigarette smoking. *Pharmacol Biochem Behav.* 1986; 24:159-62.

Shieh KR, Pan JT. Nicotinic control of tuberoinfundibular dopaminergic neuron activity and prolactin secretion: diurnal rhythm and involvement of endogenous opioidergic system. *Brain Res.* 1997; 756:266-72.

Sioris LJ, Krenzelok EP. Phencyclidine intoxication - literature review. *Am J Hosp Pharm.* 1978; 35:1362-67.

Slamberova R, Charousova P, Pometlova M. Maternal behavior is impaired by methamphetamine administered during pre-mating, gestation and lactation. *Reprod Toxicol.* 2005; 20:103-10.

Snider GL. Chronic obstructive pulmonary disease: risk factors, path physiology and pathogenesis. *Annu Rev Med.* 1989; 40:411-29.

Snider GL, Kleinerman J, Thurlbeck WM. The definition of emphysema. Report of a national heart, lung and blood institute, division of lung diseases, workshop. *Ann Rev Respir Dis.* 1985; 132:182-85.

Snider GL, Lucy EC, Stone PJ. Animal models of emphysema. *Ann Rev Respir Dis.* 1986; 133:149-69.

Snyder MJ, Hsu E, Feyereisen R. Induction of cytochrome P-450 activities by nicotine in the tobacco hornworm, manduca sexta. *J Chem Ecol.* 1993; 19:2903-10.

Steiner E, Villen T, Hallberg M, Rane A. Amphetamine secretion in breast milk. *Eur J Clin Pharmacol.* 1984; 27:123-24.

Steldinger R, Luck W, Nau H. Half lives of nicotine in milk of smoking mothers: implications for nursing. *J Perinat Med.* 1988; 16:261-62.

Stewart DJ, Inaba T, Lucassen M, Kalow W. Cocaine metabolism: cocaine and norcocaine hydrolysis by liver and serum esterases. *Clin Pharmacol Ther.* 1979; 25:464-68.

Stewart DJ, Inaba T, Tang BK, Kalow W. Hydrolysis of cocaine in human plasma by cholinesterase. *Life Sci.* 1977; 20:1557-63.

Steyn K, de Wet T, Saloojee Y, Nel H, Yach, D. The influence of maternal cigarette smoking, snuff use and passive smoking on pregnancy outcomes: The birth to ten study. *Paediatr Perinat Epidemiol.* 2006; 20:90-99.

Strachan DP, Cook DG. Health effects of passive smoking. 1. Parental smoking and lower respiratory illness in infancy and early childhood. *Thorax.* 1997; 52:905-14.

Su T, Sheng JJ, Lipinskas TW, Ding X. Expression of CYP2A genes in rodent and human nasal mucosa. *Drug Metab Dispos.* 1996; 24:884-90.

Substance Abuse and Mental Health Services Administration, Office of Applied Studies (1996) Substance Abuse in States and Metropolitan Areas: Model based estimates from the 1991-1993 national household surveys on Drug Abuse. OAS Analytic Paper, DHHS Publication No. (SMA) 96-3095, Rockville, MD., September 1996. Available from: http://oas.samhsa.gov/96state/toc.htm [Date of access: 1 June 2007].

Subramanian MG. Alcohol inhibits suckling-induced oxytocin release. *Alcohol.* 1999; 19:51-55.

Subramanian MG, Abel EL. Alcohol inhibits suckling-induced prolactin release and milk yield. *Alcohol.* 1988; 5:95-98.

Sun L, Lau CE. Simultaneous pharmacokinetic modeling of cocaine and its metabolites, norcocaine and benzoylecgonine, after intravenous and oral administration in rats. *Drug Metab Dispos.* 2001; 29:1183-89.

Taska RJ, Schoolar JC. Placental transfer and fetal distribution of mescaline-^{14}C in monkeys. *J Pharmacol Exp Ther.* 1972; 183:427-32.

Tandy, KP. 2006. Drug Enforcement Administration. International meth trafficking. 2006. Available from: http://www.usdoj.gov/dea/speeches_meth.html [Date of access: 8 December 2006].

Taylor B, Wadsworth J. Maternal smoking during pregnancy and lower respiratory tract illness in early life. *Arch Dis Child.* 1987; 62:786-91.

Tennes K, Avitable N, Blackard C, Boyles C, Hassoun B, Holmes L, *et al.* Marijuana: prenatal and postnatal exposure in the human. *NIDA Res Monogr.* 1985; 59:48-60.

Terelius Y, Norsten-Hoog C, Cronholm T, Ingelman-Sundberg M. Acetaldehyde as a substrate for ethanol-inducible cytochrome P450 (CYP2E1). *Biochem Biophys Res Commun.* 1991; 179:689-94.

The Massachusetts Tobacco Control Program, Massachusetts Department of Public Health. Change in nicotine yields 1998 - 2004. Available from: http://www.mass.gov/Eeohhs2/docs/dph/tobacco_control/nicotine_yields_1998_2004_report.pdf. [Date of access: 7 November 2006].

Thomas H. Psychiatric symptoms in cannabis users. *Br J Psychiatry.* 1993; 163:141-49.

Thuluvath P, Wojno KJ, Yardley JH, Mezey E. Effects of Helicobacter pylori infection and gastritis on gastric alcohol dehydrogenase activity. *Alcohol Clin Exp Res.* 1994; 18:795-98.

Tuchmann-Duplessis H. The teratogenic risk. *Am J Ind Med.* 1983; 4:245-58.

Uyeno ET. Effects of lysergic acid diethylamide on the maternal behavior of the rat. *J Psychol.* 1970; 75:271-73.

Uynas-Moberg K, Widstrom AM, Werner S, Matthiesen AS, Winberg J. Oxytocin and prolactin levels in breast-feeding women. Correlation with milk yield and duration of breastfeeding. *Acta Obstet Gynecol Scand.* 1990; 69:310-16.

Van Dyke DC, Mackay L, Ziaylek EN. Management of severe feeding dysfunction in children with fetal alcohol syndrome. *Clin Pediatr (Phila).* 1982; 21:336-39.

Vernotica EM, Lisciotto CA, Rosenblatt JS, Morrell JI. Cocaine transiently impairs maternal behavior in the rat. *Behav Neurosci.* 1996; 110:315-23.

Vilaro S, Viñas O, Remesar X. Altered ultra structure of lactating rat mammary epithelial cells induced by chronic ethanol ingestion. *Alcohol Clin Exp Res.* 1989; 13:128-36.

Vilaro S, Viñas O, Remesar X, Herrera E. Effects of chronic ethanol consumption on lactational performance in rat: mammary gland and milk composition and pups' growth and metabolism. *Pharmacol Biochem Behav.* 1987; 27:333-39.

Viñas O, Vilaro S, Herrera E, Remesar X. Effects of chronic ethanol treatment on amino acid uptake and enzyme activities in the lactating rat mammary gland. *Life Sci.* 1987; 40:1745-49.

Wagner G, Fuchs AR. Effect of ethanol on uterine activity during suckling in post partum women. *Acta Endocrinol (Copenh).* 1968; 58:133-41.

Wakerley JB, Dyball RE, Lincoln DW. Milk ejection in the rat: the result of a selective release of oxytocin. *J Endocrinol.* 1973; 57:557-58.

Ward SL Schuetz S, Kirshna V, Bean X, Wingert W, Wachsman L, *et al.* Abnormal sleeping ventilatory pattern in infants of substance-abusing mothers. *Am J Dis Child.* 1986; 140:1015-20.

Wattendorf DJ, Muenke M. Fetal alcohol spectrum disorders. *Am Fam Physician.* 2005; 72:279-85.

Wiggins RC, Rolsten C, Ruiz B, Davis CM. Pharmacokinetics of cocaine: basic studies of route, dosage, pregnancy and lactation. *Neurotoxicology.* 1989; 10:367-81.

Wilkins JN, Carlson HE, Van Vunakis H, Hill MA, Gritz E, Jarvik ME. Nicotine from cigarette smoking increases circulating levels of cortical, growth hormone, and prolactin in male chronic smokers. *Psychopharmacology (Berl).* 1982; 305-308.

Williams SM, Mitchell EA, Taylor BJ. Are risk factors for sudden infant death syndrome different at night? *Arch Dis Child.* 2002; 87:274-78.

Willinger M, James LS, Catz C. Defining the sudden infant death syndrome (SIDS): deliberations of an expert panel convened by the National Institute of Child Health and Human Development. *Pediatr Pathol.* 1991; 11:667-84.

Winecker RE, Goldberger BA, Tebbett IR, Behnke M, Eyler FD, Karlix JL, *et al.* Detection of cocaine and its metabolites in breast milk. *J Forensic Sci.* 2001; 46:1221-23.

Witter FR, Blake DA, Baumgardner R, Mellits ED, Niebyl JR. Folate, carotene, and smoking. *Am J Obstet Gynecol.* 1982;1:857.

Wonnacott S. The paradox of nicotinic acetylcholine receptor up regulation by nicotine. *Trends Pharmacol Sci.* 1990; 11:216-19.

Woodward A. Smoking and reduced duration of breast-feeding. *Med J Aust.* 1988; 148:477-78.

Woodward A, Douglas RM, Graham NM, Miles H. Acute respiratory illness in Adelaide children: breastfeeding modifies the effect of passive smoking. *J Epidemiol Community Health.* 1990; 44:224-30.

Woodward A, Grgurinovich N, Ryan P. Breast feeding and smoking hygiene: Major influences on cotinine in urine of smokers' infants. *J Epidemiol Community Health.* 1986; 40:309-15.

Woodward A, Miles H, Grgurinovich N. Cotinine in urine of smoker's infants. *Lancet.* 1984; 20:935.

Woolridge MW, Fisher C. Colic, "overfeeding", and symptoms of lactose malabsorption in the breastfed baby: a possible artifact of feed management? *Lancet.* 1988; 2:382-84.

Yildiz D. Nicotine, its metabolism and an overview of its biological effects. *Toxicon.* 2004; 43:619-32.

Yin SJ, Liao CS, Wu CW, Li TT, Chen LL, Lai CL, *et al.* Human stomach alcohol and aldehyde dehydrogenases: comparison of expression pattern and activities in alimentary tract. *Gastroenterology.* 1997; 112:766-75.

Young S, Sherrill DL, Arnott J, Diepeveen D, LeSouef PN, Landau LI. Parental factors affecting respiratory function during the first year of life. *Pediatr Pulmonol.* 2000; 29:331-40.

Zimmerberg B, Gray MS. The effects of cocaine on maternal behaviors in the rat. *Physiol Behav.* 1992; 52:379-84.

Zuardi AW, Crippa JA, Hallak JE, Moreira FA, Guimaraes FS. Cannabidiol, a cannabis sativa constituent, as an antipsychotic drug. *Braz J Med Biol Res.* 2006; 39:421-29.

Zuckerman B, Frank DA, Hingson R, Amaro H, Levenson SM, Kayne H, *et al.* Effects of maternal marijuana and cocaine use on fetal growth. *N Engl J Med.* 1989; 23:762-68.

Chapter 34

Study Design and Data Analysis for Assessing Drug Transfer into Milk

Kenneth F. Ilett and L. Peter Hackett

INTRODUCTION

Although drug transfer into milk has been a topic of considerable interest to various health professionals since the early 1970's, very limited attention has been given to the description and evaluation of study design. This is an important area, as good experimental design offers the prospect of generating robust data that can advance our ability to measure and interpret the safety of breastfeeding for the neonate whose mother needs to use drugs.

The seeds of study design and interpretation of infant dose/exposure were sown in the first edition of Peter Bennett's book entitled *Drugs and Human Lactation* and strengthened in the second edition (Bennett, 1988; Bennett, 1996). Bennett enunciated several key concepts:

(a) the quantification of drug concentration in maternal plasma and milk simultaneously, following either single or multiple drug doses.

(b) that the parameter milk/plasma drug concentration ratio (M/P) should be calculated from several paired samples of milk and plasma, or ideally from measurement of the areas under the milk and plasma concentration-time curves (AUC). Implicit in his discussion was the idea that if one could not readily measure drug concentration in milk (largely because of analytical sensitivity limitations), then it could be calculated as the product of M/P and drug concentration in the plasma.

(c) that an estimate of the dose received by the infant via milk ("Absolute Infant Dose" in mg/kg/day) could be calculated as the product of the average (C_{avg} in mg/L) or maximum (C_{max} in mg/L) drug concentration in milk over a dose interval and the average infant milk intake of 0.15 L/kg/day.

(d) that the absolute infant dose could be related to the mother's dose (in mg/kg/day) to yield a measure that has become known as the "Relative Infant Dose." This descriptor was expressed as a percentage of mother's dose for ease of use. An arbitrary limit of 10% for relative infant dose was suggested as being safe, but no convincing rationale for this choice was put forward.

(e) comparing the absolute infant dose to the pediatric dose was recognized as a useful yardstick of infant exposure for those drugs with a pediatric use.

(f) finally, measuring plasma concentration in the infant was recognized as an important means of assessing toxicity. For this measure, a limit of 25% of the lower end of the usual therapeutic range was suggested as being acceptable.

Unfortunately, optimal design for pharmacokinetic studies was in its infancy at the time of Bennett's first edition and for this reason, scant consideration was given to the optimal way to collect the milk and plasma concentration-time data. The first comprehensive review of methodology for lactation studies appeared in 2002 when Begg, Duffull, Hackett, and Ilett published on selected aspects of data collection and analysis for studies of drugs in milk and their interpretation (Begg *et al.*, 2002). This contribution built on Bennett's original work and integrated an understanding of contemporary pharmacokinetic sampling protocols (Anonymous, 2001; Anonymous, 2002), together with the improved understanding of the factors that influence the bidirectional transfer of drug from plasma to milk that had developed in the 1980's and 90's (Fleishaker *et al.*, 1987; Atkinson *et al.*, 1988a; Atkinson *et al.*, 1988b; Atkinson *et al.*, 1990; Begg *et al.*, 1991; Begg *et al.*, 1992; Begg *et al.*, 1993), and an invigorated discussion of how to interpret the "absolute and relative infant dose" data, and hence predict "safety" for the breastfed infant. Both prospective prediction of potential adverse effects in the breastfed infant and retrospective evaluation of adverse effect reports in infants were discussed.

In the sections that follow, we have summarized the various aspects of experimental design and data collection that can assist in obtaining robust estimates of infant dose and provide information on which parameters are important and which ones are unimportant and/or misleading in assessing infant safety. We have also tried to integrate our discussion with the draft "Guidance for industry. Clinical lactation studies - study design, data analysis, and recommendations for labeling" document that the US Food and Drug Administration (FDA) issued in February 2005 (PK in Pregnancy Working Group of the Pregnancy Labeling Task Force, 2005), as when finalized this initiative is likely to influence both academic- and industry-based research on drugs and lactation over coming years.

CATEGORIES FOR DRUG STUDIES IN LACTATION

Lactation studies for drugs can be considered in three main categories dealing with:

1. The extent to which drugs transfer from the maternal circulation into milk, and the drug dose that the infant receives (Category 1).
2. The level of exposure of the breastfed infant to drugs in mother's milk and the consequences, if any, of such exposure (Category 2).
3. The effects of drugs taken by the mother on milk production and/or composition (Category 3).

Category 1 studies mainly aim to estimate the infant's drug intake. This is most often quantified as the product of the concentration of drug in the milk (C_{milk} in mg/L) and the daily actual or average milk volume consumed by the infant (0.15 L/kg/day). These studies may also extend to evaluating the characteristics of the transfer of drug between plasma and milk by quantifying the drug concentration in plasma and hence estimating the milk/plasma ratio (M/P).

Category 2 studies aim to measure an infant's actual drug exposure. Both the bioavailability (F) of the drug orally ingested in milk, as well as the clearance of the drug by the infant's organs of elimination (liver, kidney, etc.) will influence the steady-state concentrations in the infant's plasma (C_{ss}). Importantly, infant studies should also include measurement of any short- or long-term pharmacodynamic or developmental effects of the drug.

Where a mother is already taking the drug of interest under the guidance of her physician, studies in the first and second categories are often undertaken together by studying mother-infant pairs. Such studies are most appropriately carried out when the mother has taken the drug for a length of time that ensures that her drug levels in both plasma and milk will be at a steady-state. This also means that the drug in the infant's plasma will have achieved a steady-state concentration and hence be interpretable.

These studies can also be undertaken following a single dose. Such designs suit the use of volunteer lactating mothers who may be prepared to participate in a drug study and to bottle-feed their nursing infant during the short period of the study. Drugs with an intermittent dosing schedule (e.g., antimigraine agents) (Wojnar-Horton *et al.*, 1996), and/or those with short half-lives are well suited to this style of investigation. As there is very limited, or no infant exposure, this type of study does not lend itself to evaluation of drug effects in the infant.

Category 3 studies aim to measure drug-related changes in the volume of milk produced and/or effects on the nutrient composition of milk. Drugs that decrease milk production can be largely anticipated on the basis of their pharmacological group classification or their effects on receptor function (e.g., decreased by estrogens, progestagens, or ergot alkaloids, and increased by drugs with dopamine D_2 receptor antagonist activity in the anterior pituitary, such as clonidine, domperidone, haloperidol, methyldopa, metoclopramide, quetiapine, and risperidone). We are not currently aware of any drugs that alter milk composition, although this is theoretically possible.

The FDA draft guidance document mentioned above also raised the possibility of a fourth study category in which the effects of lactation itself on the maternal pharmacokinetics (PK) and pharmacodynamics (PD) of the drug might be evaluated. Again, while this is theoretically possible, we are not aware of any examples. Given the small distribution volume of the "milk compartment" (relative to the total volume of distribution), and the related limited ability to clear a significant amounts of drug via the usual daily milk production, the excretion of drugs via milk is unlikely to influence maternal PK or PD.

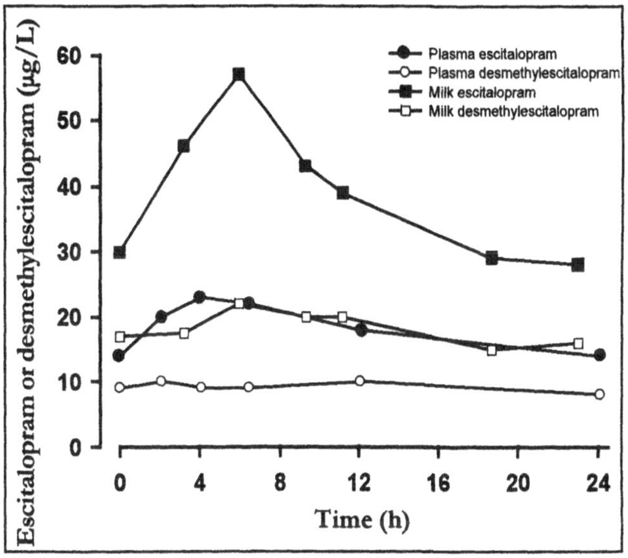

Figure 1. Steady-state milk and plasma concentration-time profiles for escitalopram and demethylescitalopram in a patient taking 20 mg escitalopram (299 µg/kg) daily.

STUDY DESIGN

Steady-State Experimental Designs

The majority of milk drug transfer studies are carried out using a steady-state (i.e., multi-dose) $AUC_{0-\tau}$ (where τ= dose interval) design. This arises because they are opportunistic in nature – i.e., the researcher identifies breastfeeding mothers (patients) who are already taking the drug of interest and who, in consultation with their physician, have already made the decision to continue breastfeeding.

The usual sample (milk and/or maternal blood) collection schedule starts with baseline samples immediately before the next dose of the drug taken, and continues at fixed or variable times for one or sometimes more dose interval(s). Sampling within each dose interval should be spaced so as to define the absorption phase, the peak concentration (C_{max}), and its time of occurrence after dose (T_{max}), as well as the elimination phase up to the end of the dose interval. Since the drug concentration in milk may vary from the start to the end of a feed (parallel change in fat content), it is important to collect a representative milk sample. One method of ensuring a uniform sample is to collect half the sample at the start of the feed and the other half at the end of the feed. An example of a study profile using this type of collection schedule is shown for a patient taking the antidepressant escitalopram in **Figure 1**. The relevant data for this example are summarized in **Table 1**.

For each of the drugs of interest, using the method outlined by Bennett for multiple-dose studies (Bennett, 1996), the absolute infant dose for this study is C_{avg} x

Table 1. Primary Pharmacokinetic Descriptors for Escitalopram and Its Metabolite Desmethylescitalopram in Milk and Plasma

Drug/Matrix	C_{max} (µg/L)	T_{max} (h)	$AUC_{0\text{-last}}$ (µg*h/L)	C_{avg} (µg/L)	Absolute infant dose (µg/kg/day) using C_{avg}	Relative infant dose (%)
Escitalopram						
Milk	57	5.92	886	38	5.7	1.9
Plasma	23	4.08	436	18	2.7	
Desmethylescitalopram						
Milk	22	5.92	416	18	2.7	0.9†
Plasma	10	2.08	222	9	1.4	

† expressed as escitalopram equivalents

Table 2. Primary Pharmacokinetic Descriptors for Sumatriptan in Milk and Plasma

Matrix	C_{max} (μg/L)	T_{max} (h)	Half-life (h)	$AUC_{0\text{-}last}$ (μg*h/L)	$AUC_{0\text{-}\infty}$ (μg*h/L)
Milk	61	3	2.2	284	350
Plasma	61	0.25	1.3	87	90

volume of milk ingested/day (0.15 L/kg), while relative infant dose is absolute infant dose (mg/kg/day) X 100 /maternal weight adjusted daily dose (20000 μg/67 kg = 299 μg/kg). The numerical values are summarized in **Table 2**. Alternatively, if C_{max} had been used in the above calculations, slightly higher infant doses would have resulted. In this case the differences are small because of the relatively flat concentration-time profile for both escitalopram and its metabolite. The M/P_{AUC} values are 2.0 for escitalopram and 1.9 for desmethylescitalopram. Where the times of the last data point differ slightly between milk and plasma, the respective C_{avg} values for milk and plasma can be used to derive a value for M/P_{AUC}.

The issue of quantifying metabolites in milk is important if they have significant pharmacological activity. In most cases we have calculated the contribution of the metabolite to the infant dose in "equivalents (on a molecular weight ratio basis)" of the parent drug. In this way, the contribution for parent and metabolite can be summed. However, this is often a conservative overestimate of the real dose, as metabolite activity is invariably less than that of the parent drug. A further problem is that the estimates of metabolite activity in relation to the parent drug are usually derived from animal or *in vitro* experiments and may not be exactly transferable to humans.

General guidance for the ideal distribution of sampling times can be found in FDA Guidance documents (Anonymous, 2001; Anonymous, 2002) and elsewhere (D'Argenio, 1981). Standard noncompartmental pharmacokinetic modeling can be used to estimate C_{max}, T_{max}, and $AUC_{0\text{-}\tau \text{ (milk and/or plasma)}}$ (Thomann, 1993), from which M/P, absolute infant dose, and relative infant dose can be derived. Over time, data from a group of several similar patients (usually n = 8-15) can be accrued to give mean parameters and their inter-patient variability. This is essentially what pharmacokineticists call a two-stage pharmacokinetic analysis. The individual patient data sets are termed "rich" because each contributes multiple samples allowing individual estimates of relevant parameters.

It is also possible to employ a population pharmacokinetic approach where a much larger group of patients (e.g., n=50-200) taking the drug are recruited, but each contributes only a small number of samples (e.g., 3-4) to the overall data set. Non-linear mixed effects pharmacokinetic modeling (Sheiner *et al.*, 1983) can then be used to estimate population values for the model parameters [e.g., half-life ($t_{1/2}$, clearance (CL), and volume of distribution (V)], and individual Bayesian estimates of directly applicable parameters such as C_{max}, T_{max} and $AUC_{0\text{-}\tau}$ in milk and/or plasma. As above, these data can then be used to derive M/P, absolute infant dose, and relative infant dose. The population approach is intuitively more attractive as it allows parameter variability to be analyzed in a more robust manner. However, its application is limited by the availability of large groups of patients taking the same drug. The only application of a "population style " data collection of which we are aware presently is from our own laboratory where the transfer of tramadol into colostrum/early milk in mothers who received the drug for pain management following cesarian section has been studied (Ilett *et al.*, submitted 6/2007).

Single-Dose Experimental Designs

Single-dose studies are best suited to volunteer studies where a cohort of breastfeeding women are recruited

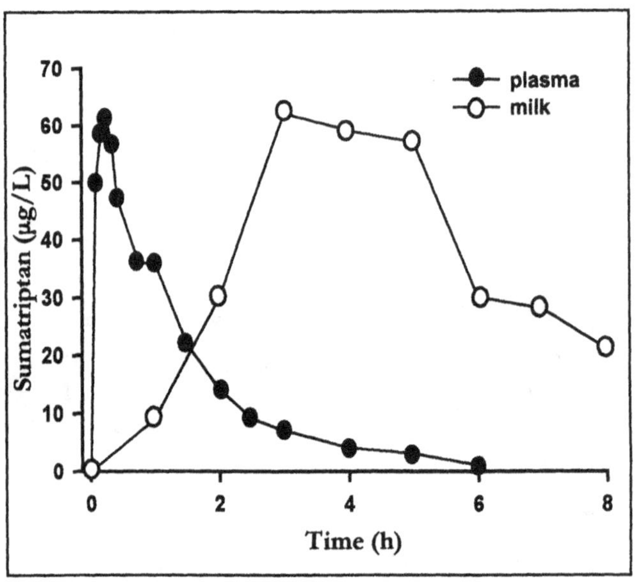

Figure 2. Concentration-time profile for sumatriptan in plasma and milk following a single subcutaneous dose of 6 mg (85.7 μg/kg) at zero time.

and all are administered one dose of the drug of interest under standardized conditions. Both two-stage and population pharmacokinetic methods of data analysis can be applied. As for steady-state studies, due attention must be paid to the distribution of sampling times and the same limitations of available numbers of patients apply. Ideally, in order to define the concentration-time profile adequately, milk sampling should continue for at least 2-3 x $t_{1/2}$ after absorption and distribution are complete. This will enable a robust estimation of the $t_{1/2}$, the elimination rate constant (k_{el}), and the extrapolated AUC from the last sampling time to infinity (where $AUC_{last-\infty} = C_{last}/k_{el}$). An example of a study profile using this type of collection schedule is shown for a volunteer (70 kg) taking the drug sumatriptan in **Figure 2**. The relevant data for this example are summarized in **Table 2**.

Using the method outlined by Bennett for single dose studies (Bennett, 1996), the absolute infant dose for this study is C_{max} x volume of milk ingested/day (0.03 L/kg, assuming five feeds/day) x maternal body weight (70 kg)/maternal single dose (6000 μg) = 2.1%. The M/P_{AUC} is 3.9 (350 μg*h/L/90μg*h/L). The delayed penetration of sumatriptan (later C_{max}) into the milk was not anticipated when the sampling schedule was designed. Hence, the sampling of milk did not really continue for long enough to ideally define the half-life ($t_{1/2}$) in milk. The estimated $t_{1/2}$ of 2.2 hours really should have been closer to that of 1.3 hours seen in plasma. As a consequence, the M/P is probably slightly overestimated.

As with steady-state studies as above, it should also be possible to use a population PK approach to sampling and analysis to give required parameters such as C_{max}, T_{max} and $AUC_{0-\infty}$ in milk and/or plasma.

Steady-State Versus Single Dose Experimental Designs

For assessment of M/P_{AUC}, the optimal measure for both milk and plasma is the AUC. Since the $AUC_{0-\tau}$ (where τ= dose interval) at steady-state is equal to $AUC_{0-\infty}$ following a single dose (Rowland *et al.*, 1995), both single-dose and multi-dose at steady-state experimental designs can ultimately yield estimates of M/P. Single dose studies use Cmax to calculate infant dose and thus may underestimate exposure where the drug acccumulates significantly when repeated doses are taken (i.e., steady-state). Steady state designs have the advantage that effects in the infants are also able to be measured.

Selecting Suitable Patients or Volunteers for Study

The selection of subjects for lactation studies is driven both by "ethics" and "study aims" considerations.

Patients are most often chosen for studies where the aim is to quantify infant exposure to therapeutic drugs ingested by the mother. A preliminary risk-benefit analysis (see Chapter 24) should have been done before a breastfeeding mother started on the medication, and thus recruitment for such studies is largely opportunistic and driven by a need to confirm the expected "safe/compatible" outcome. The timing of such studies depends on when the drug is needed in relation to the stage of lactation. They are usually conducted at maternal steady-state. Since the decision to breastfeed while the mother is taking the drug has already been made, the ethics considerations in these cases are mostly to do with the degree of invasiveness of the study prototcol and whether this may adversely affect the well-being of mother or her infant. If the drug is to be used in the first few days postnatally, then the extent of transfer into colostrum/transitional milk is a legitimate question. Methadone transfer into early milk is a good example of such a study (Jansson *et al.*, 2007). Similarly, if the drug to be used is an antidepressant, long-term treatment is likely and transfer into milk is best evaluated at the stage when mature milk is being produced. Since mature milk composition and production is relatively constant (Allen *et al.*, 1991) across the first year of life, the timing of these studies is not critical. However, if it is a question of confirming drug compatibility with breastfeeding, then timing should be in the first one to two months after birth. This is also a time when most mothers have developed a routine and are able to participate in a study without undue stress. Escitalopram transfer into mature milk is a good example of such a study (Rampono *et al.*, 2006).

Volunteer lactating mothers are most suited to assessing milk transfer following single doses of therapeutic drugs. Ethics considerations here relate mainly to ensuring that there is no chance of adverse effects in the volunteer and that infant exposure is limited or avoided. The timing of such studies in relation to lactation stage depends on the intended use of the drug. For example, colostrum/transitional milk would be used to assess infant exposure to analgesics that may be used in the immediate postnatal period. Volunteers producing mature milk are suitable for assessing milk transfer of drugs that may be needed at any time during established lactation. In our experience, volunteer studies are most suited to drug transfer studies when they are several months into lactation. At this time, their infants are often only partially breastfed, and bottle-feeding the infant over a 12-24 hour study period is practical and prevents infant exposure. The anti-migraine drug sumatriptan and the decongestant pseudoephedrine are relevant examples of single dose studies in volunteers (Wojnar-Horton *et al.*, 1996, Aljazaf *et al.*, 2003).

BREASTMILK SAMPLING AND RELATED ASPECTS

Samples may be collected by hand expression or by use of electric pumps. Both methods are effective. The electric pump is the best option where the study design specifies total available milk collection at discrete time intervals across the period of study. Both breasts would normally be emptied and a 2-phase pump, such as the Symphony® (Medela International, Baar, Switzerland), will give the best chance of a complete and reproducible series of samples.

Timing of Breastmilk Studies in Relation to Stage of Lactation

The composition of human milk varies considerably over the first year of breastfeeding (Neville *et al.*, 1991; Allen *et al.*, 1991). Colostrum, which is produced starting on day one to two after birth contains about 2% fat, 3% total protein, and 4% lactose (Hibberd *et al.*, 1982). By day five or so, mature milk, with about 3.6% fat, 1.8% total protein, and 5% lactose, is produced. Milk volume also increases from around 50 mL/day on day one to around 600 mL/day by day five (Neville *et al.*, 1988) and volumes of 700-800 mL/day are then maintained, according to infant demand, throughout the first six months of lactation or longer (Allen *et al.*, 1991). Both fat and protein content of milk may influence drug distribution into milk (Begg *et al.*, 1993) and time-dependent changes in their concentrations may therefore be important.

Although prescribed drug use in lactating women (4.3% prevalence) is lower than that in matched controls (7.5%) (Malm *et al.*, 2003), breastfeeding women still need to use a wide variety of both prescribed and non-prescribed medicines (Matheson *et al.*, 1990). Treatment for both acute disorders, such as hemorrhoids, cracked nipples, headache, upper respiratory infections, and genitourinary tract infections, as well as for chronic diseases, such as migraine, asthma, depression, diabetes, epilepsy, psoriasis, thyrotoxicosis, was documented in the first four months after birth (Matheson *et al.*, 1990).

For convenience, we will consider drug use in lactation in two main time periods. The first is days one to four after birth when drugs such as antiinfectives and analgesics are often needed. At this stage of lactation, the volume of milk (colostrum) consumed by the infant is small and this limits drug exposure, as does the duration of maternal drug use, which is usually short-term. On the other hand, the alveolar epithelial cell barrier still has open cell junctions at this time and in theory this could facilitate drug transfer into milk. Drugs whose transfer into colostrum has been studied include analgesics, such butorphanol (Pittman *et al.*, 1980), fentanyl (Steer *et al.*, 1992), indomethacin (Beaulac-Baillargeon *et al.*, 1993), morphine (Baka *et al.*, 2002), and methadone (Jansson *et al.*, 2007), the antifungal, tinidazole (Mannisto *et al.*, 1983), and the environmental pollutant, cotinine (Karmowski *et al.*, 1998). Nevertheless, there are relatively few studies of drug transfer into colostrum, and there is a need to accumulate further data.

The second and most important period of maternal drug use in lactation coincides with the time when mature milk is produced from about five days after birth and onwards, usually for several months. In this period, women may need to use a variety of medications from different pharmacological classes. The duration of use may vary from single or short-term use of drugs, such as analgesics, antiinfectives, and antifungals, through to chronic use of drugs, such as antipsychotics, antiepileptics, and antidepressants. Hence, the majority of drug studies are carried out at a time when mature milk is being produced.

Investigating Whether Milk Fat Content Influences Drug Transfer into Milk

Drugs with high lipid solubility may have their transfer into milk enhanced by co-transport in the lipid fraction of milk. The likelihood of co-transport in lipid can to some extent be predicted from a knowledge of the oil/water partition ratio (P) for the drug. This parameter (usually specified as the log P_{10} at pH 7.2) may be measured experimentally, as has been previously described (Ilett *et al.*, 1992). If experimental data are not available, appropriate software programs can be used to derive $\log P_{10}$ (at pH 7.2) from a knowledge of the physicochemical properties of the molecule (ACD I Lab Software version 8.14 for Solaris; ACD Labs, Toronto, Canada). The coefficient is estimated at pH 7.2 because this is the approximate pH of breastmilk (Rampono *et al.*, 2000). Fat content of milk can increase up to three-fold from the start (fore-milk) to the end of a feed (hind-milk) (Neville *et al.*, 1984). Hence, for such drugs, the sample collection may be modified to incorporate an assessment of cotransport in milk fat. The usual strategy is to collect a milk sample just before the infant starts feeding and a second 15 minutes later when the feed is completed or almost completed. For example, the increase (hind/fore) in drug concentration was 1.2-fold for escitalopram (Rampono *et al.*, 2006) and 2.3-fold for mirtazapine (Ilett *et al.*, 2003). It is not necessary to do these dual fore- and hind-milk samples at every sampling time, and one or two observations/patient (with an n=6-10) is usually adequate to assess any difference. The ideal sampling times for such investigations are those in the terminal elimination phase on the milk drug concentration-time profile and after the milk T_{max}. Fore- and hind-milk sampling should not be attempted early after dose, as the concentration-driven increase in drug in milk in the absorption phase can be much larger than any increase

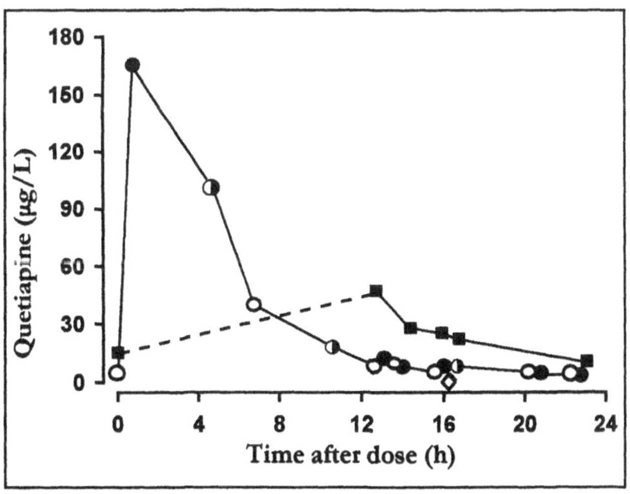

FIGURE 3. Steady-state milk and maternal plasma concentration-time profile for quetiapine in maternal plasma (■, dotted line to indicate limited data between 0 and 12.8 h), milk (fore ○, hind ●, mixed ◑) and infant plasma (◊). The evening dose (20:00 h) was taken at zero time. (Rampono *et al.*, 2007. Reprinted with permission from *The Annals of Pharmacotherapy*.)

attributable to cotransport in milk fat. An excellent example is shown in Figure 3 for quetiapine, where a large increase in hind/fore ratio would be predicted using samples taken during absorption, but in reality no change is seen in paired samples taken in the elimination phase.

To assist in interpretation of the drug concentration data, milk samples for fore/hind drug concentration assessment should also have their milk fat content measured to confirm the expected increase in fat content. Measuring the "creamatocrit" provides a quick and simple method for estimating fat content (Lucas *et al.*, 1978).

ASSESSING PARAMETERS RELATED TO INFANT DOSE

Estimating AUC and C_{avg} in Milk and Plasma

The AUC_{milk} and C_{avg} are critical parameters for estimating infant dose. Likewise AUC_{plasma} may be useful in estimating M/P. The timing of samples for AUC measurements is discussed in the section on Study Design. In this section, we wish to consider the measurement of AUC for lactation studies from a general perspective. In a drug concentration-time plot, the AUC can be estimated by dropping a series of vertical lines from each observed concentration (Y-axis) on the graph to the X-axis. This results in definition of a series of triangles and/or trapezoids across the time axis, and their areas can be calculated mathematically (Gibaldi *et al.*, 1982). The total AUC is calculated as the sum of the individual trapezoids. When the observations of drug concentration are made frequently and fairly evenly across the dose interval, as in a drug administration study at steady-state, the Y-axis plot is made on a linear scale and the linear trapezoidal rule is applied. In cases where sampling is less frequent as often occurs in the elimination phase of drug disposition, then it is more appropriate to use a $\log_{10}$ Y-axis plot and AUC is then estimated by applying the log trapezoidal rule. This prevents overestimation of the triangular section of each trapezoid that occurs because the elimination phase of drug disposition is an exponential function on a linear-linear plot.

Figure 4 shows a worked example of the calculation of AUC for the antiepileptic drug topiramate in milk and plasma of a patient who was studied across a dose interval (12 hours) at steady-state. Topiramate was measured by gas-liquid chromatography/mass

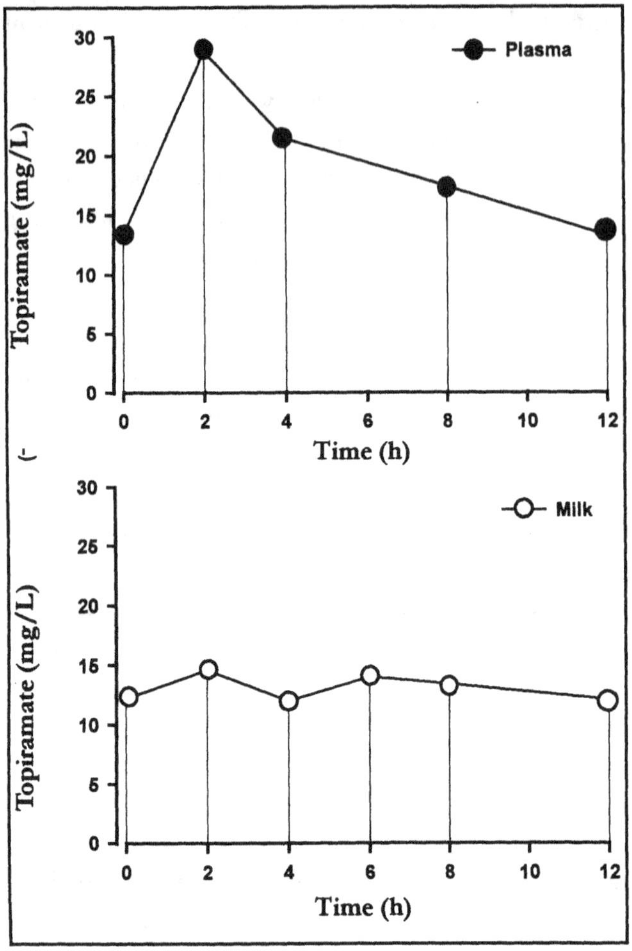

Figure 4. Topiramate in plasma (●) and milk (○) at steady-state. The figure shows how to calculate AUC from the concentration-time profile for a patient (56 kg) receiving the antiepileptic topiramate (200 mg at zero time at 8 am, followed by a further 300 mg at 8 pm) (Hale TW & Hackett LP, unpublished data). The daily weight-adjusted maternal dose for this patient is 500 mg/56 kg = 8.9 mg/kg.

spectrometry after on-column methylation, and concentrations in plasma and milk are shown in the figure. The area under each curve was estimated by the linear trapezoidal rule (series of trapezoids created by dropping vertical lines from each data point as shown). The areas under the plasma and milk concentration-time curves were 321 mg*h/L and 158 mg*h/L, respectively, and from these data an M/P_{AUC} of 158/321 = 0.5 can be calculated.

In addition, the C_{avg} in milk can be calculated as 158 mg*h/L/12 h = 13.2 mg/L for the 12 hour dose interval following the 200 mg maternal dose. Since the evening dose was 300 mg, the estimated C_{avg} (assuming no diurnal variation in drug disposition) is 13.2 mg/L *300/200 = 19.8 mg/L. C_{avg} across the whole day would then be (13.2 + 19.8)/2 = 16.5 mg/L). In turn, this daily C_{avg} can be used to calculate absolute (16.5 mg/L x 0.15 L/kg/day = 2.48 mg/kg/day) and relative (2.48 mg/kg/day *100/8.9 mg/kg/day = 28%) infant doses. The latter figure indicates that there was extensive transfer of topiramate into milk, as has been found by others (Ohman *et al.*, 2002).

As noted earlier, estimating AUC can also be useful when single dose drug studies are performed. **Figure 5** shows an example of milk AUC following a single dose of the decongestant pseudoephedrine. Drug concentration measurements should be made for at least 3 x the $t_{1/2}$ after absorption is complete, so as to allow an accurate measurement of the latter and of the elimination rate constant ($k_{el} = 0.693/\ t_{1/2}$). The AUC from zero time to the last data point ($AUC_{0\text{-}last}$) is added to that from the last measurable time point to infinity (estimated as C_{last}/k_{el}) to give the total $AUC_{0\text{-}\infty}$.

$AUC_{0\text{-}17.5h}$ estimated by the mixed log-linear trapezoidal rule (linear trapezoidal rule to 3.1 h and log-linear from 3.1 to 17.5 h) was 3259 mg/L*h (Thomann, 1993). The elimination $t_{1/2}$ from log-linear regression of the last four data pairs was 4.5 h, giving a k_{el} of 0.154 h^{-1} ($0.693/\ t_{1/2}$). The extrapolated $AUC_{17.5\text{-}\infty}$ (shaded blue and bounded by the dashed line and the X-axis) can then be estimated as C_{last} (42 µg/L) divided by k_{el}, or 272 µg*h/L. This gives a total $AUC_{0\text{-}\infty}$ of 3531 µg*h/L.

Assuming linear kinetics apply, the steady-state $AUC_{0\text{-}\tau}$, is the same as the single-dose $AUC_{0\text{-}\infty}$ (Rowland *et*

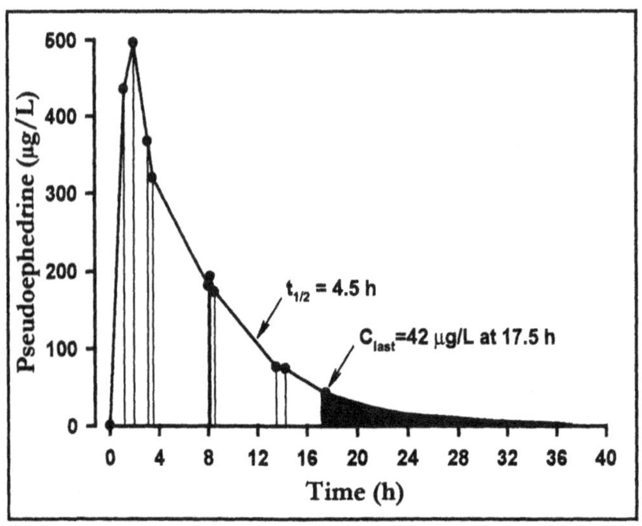

Figure 5. Illustrates the estimation of AUC for volunteer # 3 (Aljazaf *et al.*, 2003), who received a single 60 mg dose of pseudoephedrine at zero time with serial milk samples collected over the next 17.5 hours.

al., 1995). Hence, we can use $AUC_{0-\infty}=AUC_{0-\tau}$ to estimate the C_{avg} at steady-state. To illustrate the process, let us assume that the same 60 mg dose of pseudoephedrine was given four times daily (i.e., τ = 6 h) (maternal dose 4 * 60,000 μg/93 kg = 2580 μg/kg/day) until steady-state was achieved. Hence, the C_{avg} concentration at steady state will be $AUC_{0-\tau}$/6 or 3531 μg*h/L divided by 6 = 589 μg/L. Absolute infant dose at steady-state then becomes (589 μg/L*0.15 L/kg/day = 88 μg/kg/day) and relative infant dose is 3.4% (88 μg/kg/day *100/2580 μg/kg/day) of the weight-adjusted maternal dose.

The above calculation can be compared to the single-dose C_{max}- based method recommended by Bennett (Bennett, 1996). In his calculation, he assumes that the infant feeds once at C_{max}. The infant dose is then C_{max} (496 μg/L) * 0.03 L/kg (average milk volume ingested by infant in one of five daily feeds)* 93 kg (maternal body weight) *100/maternal single dose (60,000 μg) = 2.3% of the weight-adjusted maternal dose.

In some lactation studies, total milk collections are made using an electric pump at fixed or variable intervals following dose. AUC_{milk} may be obtained from a histobar plot of milk volume versus drug concentration versus time as the mid-point of each collection period. A typical dataset from one subject in a study conducted in our laboratory (Wojnar-Horton *et al.*, 1996) is shown in **Table 3**.

In this study, all milk available was collected by use of an electric breast pump at hourly intervals for eight hours following administration of the s.c. dose. The concentration of drug in each sample was measured by high performance liquid chromatography, and this was multiplied by the sample volume to calculate the amount of drug (ng) in each hourly sample. These are cumulated over time to give the total amount excreted in milk (RHS column **Table 3**). A histobar plot of the amount of sumatriptan in each milk sample versus the mid point of the collection period is shown in **Figure 6**.

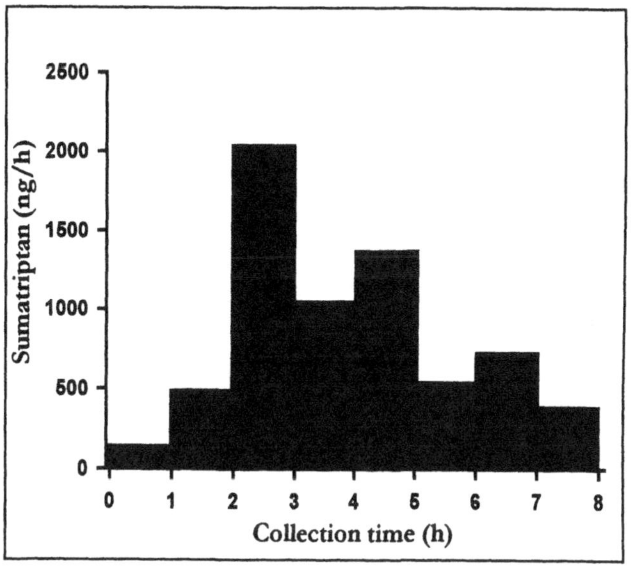

Figure 6. Histobar plot of the amount of sumatriptan in total milk collections made at hourly intervals. Figure drawn from raw data for patient HO in the study by Wojnar-Horton *et al.*, 1996.

The total cumulative excretion of 6722 ng over the eight hours of the study can be said to represent the amount of a breastfed infant's exposure if all milk produced was ingested. In absolute terms, over the eight hours of the study, this amount is some 0.1% of the maternal dose. However, the dose can also be considered on the more familiar percent of the weight-adjusted maternal dose. The C_{avg} would be 6722 ng/169 mL = 40 μg/L. Multiplying this by an average infant milk intake of 0.15 L/kg/day gives an absolute infant dose of 6 μg/kg/day or 2 μg/kg/8 hours (the period of the study). Mother's single dose for this eight hour period is 6000 μg/70 kg = 85.7 μg/kg. Hence, the relative infant

Table 3. Excretion of Sumatriptan in Milk Following a 6 mg s.c. Dose at Zero Time

Collection time (h)	Sumatriptan (μg/L)	Volume of milk (mL)	Sumatriptan excreted (ng/h)	Sumatriptan cumulative excretion (ng)
0	0.0	25[1]	0.0	0.0
1	9.1	15	136.5	136.5
2	30.3	16	484.8	621.3
3	61.5	33	2029.5	2650.8
4	58.5	18	1053.0	3703.8
5	56.9	24	1365.6	5069.4
6	29.9	18	538.2	5607.6
7	27.8	26	722.8	6330.4
8	20.6	19	391.4	6721.8

[1] Necessary for zero time sample but not included in total volume

dose on a single-dose basis is approximately 2 μg/kg/8h *100/85.7 μg/kg/8h = 2.3%.

In the above example, the individual rectangular areas of the histobars (amounts of sumatriptan/hour) have essentially been summed to give the total exposure amount from which a C_{avg} is calculated. The trapezoidal rule can also be applied to rectangular area datasets by plotting the drug concentration versus the time of collection. Interestingly, we have previously shown that there are only minor differences in AUC estimates obtained by the rectangular area and trapezoidal rule methods (Begg *et al.*, 2002).

The rectangular AUC approach could be applied to most lactation studies, but is particularly useful for assessing milk production. However, if it is used for estimating infant dose, consideration should be given to the possibility that the total volume collected over a dose interval might differ from that which an infant would normally ingest (i.e., the volume may not be physiological), and this could alter interpretation of the data.

Measuring M/P Ratio

There is an erroneous view among some medical and other health care providers that the magnitude of M/P is an indicator of infant dose and hence of drug safety in breastfeeding. M/P merely reflects the transfer ratio between the plasma and milk compartments, and the prime reason for measuring it is to gain information about the nature of the transfer process itself (e.g., active or passive transfer). It has no direct application in assessing infant dose or safety.

M/P can be measured from single paired observations of drug concentration (in milk and plasma) made at approximately the same time after dose. However, because the concentration-time profiles of drug in milk and plasma are not necessarily parallel, M/P is best measured as the ratio of AUC_{milk}/AUC_{plasma} (Begg *et al.*, 2002). The profile of milk and plasma concentration-time curves can differ, particularly in the early absorption phase following a dose. The physicochemical properties of the drug may allow rapid absorption into the blood, but transfer from blood across the breast alveolar epithelium into milk may be less rapid, resulting in T_{max} being later in milk than in plasma. In turn, such differences ultimately lead to a two- to three-fold variability in M/P calculated from single-point estimates for drugs, such as bupropion (Briggs *et al.*, 1993) and sumatriptan (Wojnar-Horton *et al.*, 1996). Not all drugs show marked differences in M/P as illustrated by the approximately parallel milk and plasma concentration profiles for citalopram (Rampono *et al.*, 2000) and escitalopram (Rampono *et al.*, 2006).

M/P can also be influenced by the milk creamatocrit (Hale *et al.*, 2002) and such variability can be reduced when M/P is estimated from AUC data. What follows from the above discussion is that AUC data will give the most robust estimate of M/P. However, where only single point measurements in milk and plasma are available, then the best estimate will be obtained from a mixed fore- and hind-milk sample and a paired plasma sample taken after the C_{max} in milk.

Nevertheless, where only plasma concentration measurements for drug (C_{plasma}) are available and M/P is known from experimental observation or has been calculated theoretically from physicochemical data (Atkinson *et al.*, 1990; Begg *et al.*, 1991; Begg *et al.*, 1992; Doogue *et al.*, 2004), the concentration in milk (C_{milk}) may be estimated as the product of M/P and C_{plasma}. Since this calculation could be imprecise because of variation in C_{plasma} across time, the average drug concentration in plasma across the dose interval would provide the most robust estimate of C_{plasma}. However, this method is useful for newly marketed drugs where there is no experience with their use in lactation. Inability to quantify drug concentration in milk could also predicate its use, but is a less likely scenario, given the quality of modern analytical methodologies.

ASSESSING DRUGS THAT ALTER MILK PRODUCTION

Some hormones and therapeutic drugs may alter milk production. Collecting all milk produced across a representative period (daily or more frequently) and measuring the volume produced/time is a common method for such studies. Initially, studies in this area used oxytocin to stimulate milk let-down (Neville *et al.*, 1988). However, modern electric breast pumps can simulate the actions of infant suckling closely and give reliable milk collections (Mitoulas *et al.*, 2002a; Mitoulas *et al.*, 2002b; Aljazaf *et al.*, 2003; Kent *et al.*, 2003; Mitoulas *et al.*, 2004).

Another method of estimating milk production involves weighing the infant before and after each feed to obtain the weight (and hence volume, assuming a weight/mL of 1) of milk consumed. Individual feed volumes are then summed over time (usually 24 hours). This method gives the infant demand volume, rather than the total production capability estimated, using the electric breast pump as described above.

Experimental designs for milk production studies may include the use of a parallel randomized control group or a randomized cross-over design where each mother serves as her own control. An example of the parallel control group can be seen with the increase in milk production caused by domperidone (da Silva *et al.*, 2001), while a cross-over design (pseudoephedrine vs placebo) was used to demonstrate a decrease in milk production after pseudoephedrine (Aljazaf *et al.*, 2003). In the domperidone study, the women with low milk supply pumped milk from both breasts at several intervals each day and volumes were summed to give daily production. In the pseudoephedrine study, milk production was measured by test weighing the baby (Baby Weigh™ Scale, Medela Inc.) before and after each feed, (Arthur *et al.*, 1987) over a period of 24 hours, commencing at the time of the pseudoephedrine or placebo dose. As with all clinical trials, the study design may be enhanced by administering the drug either single-blind or double-blind.

Finally, an investigation by Lai *et al.* raised yet another way of assessing milk production. They investigated the use of 10-15 minute pumping sessions for both breasts, at hourly intervals over a six hour period (Lai *et al.*, 2004). Milk production averaged 50-65 ml/hour at the initial zero time collection, decreased to 20-30 ml after the first hour, and thereafter remained at a steady rate of 15-20 mL/hour through to six hours. There were minor differences between the right and left breast production in the first two hours. The authors proposed that the plateau production seen between two to six hours might be used as a measure of basal production capacity for the individual. We have also used a modification of this method for assessing milk production in mothers with inadequate milk supply (Wan, 2004).

ANALYTICAL METHODOLOGY

At a minimum, it is necessary to quantify the drug in milk, but as explained above, it may also be important to measure drug in plasma of the mother and/or her breastfed infant. There are two previous reviews of analytical methods for drugs in milk (Rossi *et al.*, 1997; Begg *et al.*, 2002). The primary focus of analysis is on developing sample preparation methods that will produce a clean extract that is suitable for subsequent separation and quantitation by chromatographic or other methods. Hence, the sections that follow provide selected insights into preparative clean-up and quantitative analysis of drugs in milk.

Plasma

Quantifying drugs in plasma is a well established process, usually involving a preliminary clean-up/concentration stage where the drug is separated from other substances in the matrix. Protein precipitation, liquid-liquid extraction, and solid-phase extraction are commonly used for this process. The next step is separation of the drug from other components in the extract using techniques, such as gas-liquid chromatography, high performance liquid chromatography, or capillary electrophoresis. Finally, the drug is quantified using its physicochemical properties (e.g., UV or fluorescence absorption or mass spectrometry). Such methods are well described in standard texts (Siek *et al.*, 1999; Moffat *et al.*, 2004).

Milk

In addition to its protein and carbohydrate content, milk also contains a significant and variable amount of fat, and hence separating the drug of interest from the other components of the matrix may present a greater analytical challenge than for plasma. Nevertheless, the same range of analytical methods used for plasma are also suitable for milk.

The average amounts of protein and fat in mature milk are around 1.8% and 3.6%, respectively (Hibberd *et al.*, 1982). However, as outlined above, the fat content is highly variable, particularly from the start to the end of a feed and overall can range from 1-20%. By contrast, plasma contains 5-7% total protein and around 0.35-0.85% total lipids (Anonymous, 1970). Hence, sample clean-up and subsequent analysis of drugs in milk is made more difficult by the presence of a high and variable concentration of fat in the matrix.

The potential matrix problems with milk may be addressed by using the "method of addition." In this method, drug concentrations in milk are determined by taking four equal aliquots of each milk sample (with internal standard added), and spiking three of these with increasing concentrations of authentic drug (and/or metabolite) standard. The samples are then extracted and analyzed according to the usual assay method, a standard curve (peak height ratio drug: internal standard versus added drug concentration) is constructed, and drug concentrations are determined from the negative x-axis intercept of the plot. This method has been used widely in our laboratories (Ilett *et al.*, 1992; Rampono *et al.*, 2000; Kristensen *et al.*, 2002; Hackett *et al.*, 2006). However, while it overcomes a matrix problem, it is very labor intensive because each sample generates four assays.

Assay Validation

Validation criteria for drug assay in plasma and milk are clearly set out in previous documents/reviews (Anonymous, 1999). Measures such as linearity, range, accuracy, precision, recovery, detection and quantitation limits, and specificity and interferences should all be documented. In addition, stability of the drug and any metabolites that are to be assayed should be demonstrated for relevant periods of frozen storage, as well as during the short time between extraction and quantitation, while samples are at a controlled laboratory or autosampler temperature. Recovery of the internal standard through the assay procedure should also be demonstrated.

Separate validations are necessary for plasma and milk. Because of the high and variable fat content in milk, it is advisable to perform recovery, precision, and accuracy measures using milk samples with high and low fat content. Again, attention should be paid to both the analyte(s) of interest and to the internal standard, as any differential recovery could compromise the assay reliability.

ASSESSING THE BREASTFED INFANT

Assessment of the general health and well being of the breastfed infant is an important part of any formal lactation study. The breastfed infant has exposure to a drug that he/she does not need and is thus exposed to potential adverse effects, i.e., the infant is essentially an "innocent bystander" in the maternal therapeutic regimen (Begg, 2003).

The primary method of assessing adverse effects in exposed infants should be done within the normal post-natal clinical assessment of infant progress by infant clinic nurses, neonatologists, or pediatricians. Standard charts giving population ranges for weight, head circumference, and length (3rd to 97th percentiles) can be used to monitor the infant's general progress (Anonymous, 2006). Some investigators have also used standard pediatric health assessment instruments, such as the Denver Development Score (Frankenburg *et al.*, 1967; Frankenburg *et al.*, 1992), the Brazelton Score (Als *et al.*, 1977; Brazelton, 1978), or the Finnegan Neonatal Abstinence Score (Finnegan *et al.*, 1975; Finnegan, 1990) to quantify infant well being and progress. The Denver and Brazelton scoring instruments were not designed for assessment of the subtleties of a drug-related adverse event, and thus may be quite blunt probes in this context. The Finnegan score was designed specifically for assessment of opiate withdrawal in neonates, but has been used successfully in evaluation of the effects of drugs, such as selective serotonin reuptake inhibitor (SSRI) antidepressants (Rampono *et al.*, 2004, Levinson-Castiel *et al.*, 2006). Others have designed neonatal behavioral evaluation scoring systems that specifically target the adverse effects of SSRIs (Zeskind *et al.*, 2004). Despite limitations of individual systems, they nevertheless provide a structured assessment process that facilitates comparison of the exposed infant with an appropriate control population. Specially trained staff are required for the successful administration of these instruments. Less complex measures, such as reports of the infant's general progress as assessed by medical and nursing staff and the mother, should also be sought. No matter what assessment procedure is used, a pre-determined questionnaire or data collection checklist should be used for all infant assessments, so that the results can be assessed in a structured manner.

In any lactation study protocol, one should also take the opportunity to analyze drug/metabolite content in a sample of the infant's blood. The concentration of drug or its metabolite(s) in the infant's plasma is really the ultimate measure of the extent of exposure. It represents the balance between oral ingestion of drug and infant clearance. Blood samples should be taken (at steady-state) at a known time in relation to the mother's last drug dose. The exact timing within the mother's dose interval is probably not critical as most infants feed several times per day, and hence peak-trough variation is likely to be small. We generally aim to collect a minimum 0.5 mL volume of heparinised blood. However, the volume required for analysis will be influenced by the sensitivity of the individual analytical technique. It should be noted that the expectation of low levels of drug transfer to the infant usually means that a lower limit of quantitation will be needed for the infant than for maternal plasma samples. For some drugs (e.g., venlafaxine), metabolism in the maternal and/or infant circulations may make it more likely that the metabolite(s) (e.g., *O*-desmethylvenlafaxine) will be detected in the infant's plasma (Ilett *et al.*, 1998; Ilett *et al.*, 2002). The concentration of drug in the infant's plasma can be interpreted as a percentage of that in the mother's plasma concentration at around the same time after dose and/or by comparison to the usual therapeutic range if this is known. A limit of 25% of the lower end of the usual therapeutic range has been suggested as being acceptable infant exposure (Bennett, 1996).

Measurements of drug concentration in the infant's plasma have also been recommended as a routine means of monitoring infant exposure for drugs, such as lamotrigine (Pennell, 2003) and lithium (Moretti *et al.*, 2003), where relative infant dose is often significantly greater than 10% and concentration in infant plasma can be up to 50% of that in maternal plasma.

Assessment of Long-term Adverse Effects in Infants Exposed to Drugs During the Normal Course of Lactation

For some infants, exposure to maternal medications which need to be taken chronically will continue throughout lactation (usually three to 12 months). Therefore, it may be equally, if not more important, to follow-up these infants over the longer-term (e.g., up to seven years). Such studies require an epidemiological approach with repeated measurement of a range of physical and cognitive behavioral parameters in the exposed breastfed infants versus an age- and sex-matched cohort of infants whose mothers breastfed, but did not take drugs. Since many environmental factors may influence infant progress and cognitive development over the long-term, such studies necessarily require large numbers of exposed infants and controls. They are both logistically difficult and expensive to conduct. For many drug classes, long-term assessment of adverse effects may be impractical because the number of exposed infants is small. This could perhaps be overcome by coordinated multi-center studies. To our knowledge, the antidepressants are the main drug class where infants exposed to the drug via milk have been studied over longer time periods. For example, data for infant exposure to doxepin over five years (Buist *et al.*, 1995), fluoxetine over six years (Nulman *et al.*, 2002), or citalopram over one year (Heikkinen *et al.*, 2002) showed no differences in cognitive development.

Assessment of Acute Adverse Events in Breastfed Infants That are Suspected of Being Related to Maternal Drug Therapy

The reporting of adverse effects thought to be related to drug exposure via milk is an area that has been characterized by inadequate data reporting standards and misinterpretations. First, the misinterpretations have often been caused by the association of adverse events/effects with breastfeeding in the first one to two weeks after birth. While such events were real, their association with exposure via breastmilk was often incorrect. Many women need to take drugs during pregnancy, and we and others have documented that infant exposure to maternal drugs via the placenta is 1-2 orders of magnitude greater than that via milk (Rosen *et al.*, 1975, Rosen *et al.*, 1976, Laine *et al.*, 2003, Heikkinen *et al.*, 2003, Rampono *et al.*, 2004). Hence, when considering adverse events, one must carefully discriminate between placental and milk exposure to maternal medicines.

In addition, the connection between the suspected adverse event and the drug in mother's milk must be carefully examined in the broader context of all possible differential diagnoses. A review of all published "adverse events related to drug exposure via milk" published up to 2003 (Anderson *et al.*, 2003) found only 100 cases. Using a structured method of assessing adverse drug reactions (Naranjo *et al.*, 1981), 47% of the events were classified as "possible," 53% as "probable," and only 1% as "definite." Interestingly, over 78% of the infants in the case reports were under two months of age. Hence, for assessment of possible adverse effects in the breastfed infant, we recommend a careful differential diagnosis, use of the Naranjo scoring system to clarify association with the suspected drug, and finally measurement of the concentration of suspected drug/metabolite in the infant's plasma.

THE LACTATION STUDY TEAM

The composition of the team will of course vary with the drug being investigated as well as with local expertise available at the study site. However, from the above discussion, it should be apparent that the following areas of expertise are necessary in most studies:

- General or specialist clinical medicine
- Neonatal or pediatric medicine
- Analytical chemistry
- Study design, coordination, data analysis, and statistics
- Research nursing for sample collection and documentation on the study day(s)

In our view, all of these diverse areas need to be covered, although perhaps to differing extents for different drugs and study types. In our experience, study design is often left to pharmacologists or pharmacists with these skills, but an experienced biostatistician may be needed for some protocols. The choice of a medical person for the study is usually determined by the drug class and/or the mother's disease, while an experienced neonatologist or pediatrician is absolutely essential for infant assessment. Research nurses generally have excellent patient handling skills and are accustomed to strict adherence to formal study protocols and hence are a valuable part of the team. Last but not least, an experienced analytical chemist is absolutely essential for lactation studies.

CONCLUSION

The aim of this chapter has been to comprehensively review experimental designs used in the investigation of drugs in lactation. There is a clear need to generate data on drug effects on milk production, the transfer of drugs into milk, as well as their effects on the breastfed infant. This need is present for many older drugs already on the market and also for newly developed drug molecules. Good experimental design and clear study objectives are critical to obtaining meaningful data that can optimize how we use drugs during lactation and improve drug safety for the breastfed infant.

In considering the various study areas, we have tried to provide worked examples so that the new investigator can readily appreciate practical aspects of data collection and analysis. The majority of drug studies in lactation have been done by academics with a research or clinical interest in this topic, while the need for such studies has largely been driven by the lactating mother and/or her medical advisors as they try to grapple with the assessment of the risk and benefits of drug use during breastfeeding. However, for new drugs, such studies ideally should be an integral part of the normal drug development process undertaken by the pharmaceutical industry. It is encouraging to see that the US Food and Drug Administration is presently in the process of developing Guidelines for Industry in all aspects of the study of drugs and lactation.

References

Aljazaf K, Hale TW, Ilett KF, Hartmann PE, Mitoulas LR, Kristensen JH, *et al.* Pseudoephedrine - effects on milk production in women and estimation of infant exposure via breastmilk. *Br J Clin Pharmacol.* 2003; 56:18-24.

Allen JC, Keller RP, Archer PC, Neville MC. Studies in human lactation; milk composition and daily secretion rates of macronutrients in the first year of life. *Am J Clin Nutr.* 1991; 54:69-80.

Als H, Tronick E, Lester BM, Brazelton TB. The Brazelton Neonatal Behavioral Assessment Scale (BNBAS). *J Abnorm Child Psychol.* 1977; 5:215-31.

Anderson PO, Pochop SL, Manoguerra AS. Adverse drug reactions in breastfed infants: less than imagined. *Clin Pediatr (Phila).* 2003; 42:325-40.

Anonymous. *Scientific tables.* 7th Ed. Basle, Switzerland: Ciba-Geigy Limited; 1970.

Anonymous. *Guidance for industry. Validation of analytical procedures.* Rockville, MD, USA: U.S. Department of Health and Human Services, Food and Drug Administration, Center for Veterinary Medicine; 1999.

Anonymous. *Guidance for industry: Statistical approaches to establishing bioequivalence. Appendix D.* Rockville, MD, USA: U.S. Department of Health and Human Services, Food and Drug Administration, Center for Drug Evaluation and Research; 2001.

Anonymous. *Guidance for industry. Food-effect in bioavailability and fed bioequivalence studies.* Rockville, MD, USA: U.S. Department of Health and Human Services, Food and Drug Administration, Center for Drug Evaluation and Research; 2002.

Anonymous. *National Centre for Health Statistics, Clinical growth charts.* 2006.

Arthur PG, Hartmann PE, Smith M. Measurement of the milk intake of breast-fed infants. *J Pediatr Gastroenterol Nutr.* 1987; 6:758-63.

Atkinson HC, Begg EJ. Prediction of drug concentrations in human skim milk from plasma protein binding and acid-base characteristics. *Br J Clin Pharmacol.* 1988a; 25:495-503.

Atkinson HC, Begg EJ. Prediction of drug distribution into human milk from physicochemical characteristics. *Clin Pharmacokinet.* 1990; 18:151-67.

Atkinson HC, Begg EJ, Darlow BA. Drugs in human milk. Clinical pharmacokinetic considerations. *Clin Pharmacokinet.* 1988b; 14:217-40.

Baka NE, Bayoumeu F, Boutroy MJ, Laxenaire MC. Colostrum morphine concentrations during postcesarean intravenous patient-controlled analgesia. *Anesth Analg.* 2002; 94:184-87, table.

Beaulac-Baillargeon L, Allard G. Distribution of indomethacin in human milk and estimation of its milk to plasma ratio in vitro. *Br J Clin Pharmacol.* 1993; 36:413-16.

Begg EJ. *Instant clinical pharmacology.* 1st Ed. Oxford, UK: Blackwell Publishing Ltd; 2003.

Begg EJ, Atkinson HC. Partitioning of drugs into human milk. *Annals Acad Med Sing.* 1991; 20:51-55.

Begg EJ, Atkinson HC. Modelling of the passage of drugs into milk. *Pharmacol Ther.* 1993; 59:301-10.

Begg EJ, Atkinson HC, Duffull SB. Prospective evaluation of a model for the prediction of milk:plasma drug concentrations from physicochemical characteristics. *Br J Clin Pharmacol.* 1992; 33:501-5.

Begg EJ, Duffull SB, Hackett LP, Ilett KF. Studying drugs in human milk: time to unify the approach. *J Hum Lact.* 2002; 18:319-28.

Bennett PN. *Drugs and human lactation: A guide to the content and consequences of drugs, micronutrients, radiopharmaceuticals, and environmental and occupational chemicals in human milk.* 1st Ed. Amsterdam: Elsevier; 1988.

Bennett PN. Use of the monographs on drugs. In: Bennett PN (ed.). *Drugs and human lactation.* 2nd Ed. Amsterdam: Elsevier; 1996. p. 67-74.

Brazelton TB. The Brazelton Neonatal Behavior Assessment Scale: introduction. *Monogr Soc Res Child Dev.* 1978; 43:1-13.

Briggs GG, Samson JH, Ambrose PJ, Schroeder DH. Excretion of bupropion in breast milk. *Ann Pharmacother.* 1993; 27:431-33.

Buist A, Janson H. Effect of exposure to dothiepin and northiaden in breast milk on child development. *Brit J Psychiatry.* 1995; 167:370-73.

D'Argenio DZ. Optimal sampling times for pharmacokinetic experiments. *J Pharmacokinet Biopharm.* 1981; 9:739-56.

da Silva OP, Knoppert DC, Angelini MM, Forret PA. Effect of domperidone on milk production in mothers of premature newborns: a randomized, double-blind, placebo-controlled trial. *Can Med Assoc J.* 2001; 164:17-21.

Doogue MP, Gardiner SJ, Begg EJ. Prediction of milk/plasma concentration ratio of drugs. *Ann Pharmacother.* 2004; 38:174-76.

Finnegan LP. *Neonatal abstinence syndrome. Current therapy in neonatal perinatal medicine-2.* Toronto, Canada: BC Dekker Inc; 1990. p. 314-20.

Finnegan LP, Connaughton JF, Jr., Kron RE, Emich JP. Neonatal abstinence syndrome: assessment and management. *Addictive Dis.* 1975; 2:141-58.

Fleishaker JC, Desai N, McNamara PJ. Factors affecting the milk-to-plasma drug concentration ratio in lactating women - physical interactions with protein and fat. *J Pharm Sci.* 1987; 76:189-93.

Frankenburg WK, Dodds J, Archer P, Shapiro H, Bresnick B. The Denver II: A major revision and restandardization of the Denver Developmental Screening Test. *Pediatrics.* 1992; 89:91-97.

Frankenburg WK, Dodds JB. The Denver development screening test. *J Pediatr.* 1967; 71:181-91.

Gibaldi M, Perrier D. *Estimation of areas. Pharmacokinetics.* 2nd Ed. New York: Marcel Dekker Inc; 1982. p. 445-49.

Hackett LP, Ilett KF, Rampono J, Kristensen JH, Kohan R. Transfer of reboxetine into breastmilk, its plasma concentrations and lack of adverse effects in the breastfed infant. *Eur J Clin Pharmacol.* 2006; 62:633-38.

Hale TW, Ilett KF. *Drug therapy and breastfeeding. From theory to clinical practice.* 1st Ed. London: The Parthenon Publishing Group; 2002.

Heikkinen T, Ekblad U, Kero P, Ekblad S, Laine K. Citalopram in pregnancy and lactation. *Clin Pharmacol Ther.* 2002; 72:184-91.

Heikkinen T, Ekblad U, Palo P, Laine K. Pharmacokinetics of fluoxetine and norfluoxetine in pregnancy and lactation. *Clin Pharmacol Ther.* 2003; 73:330-37.

Hibberd CM, Brooke OG, Carter ND, Haug M, Harzer G. Variation in the composition of breast milk during the first 5 weeks of lactation: implications for the feeding of preterm infants. *Arch Dis Child.* 1982; 57:658-62.

Ilett KF, Hackett LP, Dusci LJ, Roberts MJ, Kristensen JH, Paech M, *et al.* Distribution and excretion of venlafaxine and *O*-desmethylvenlafaxine in human milk. *Br J Clin Pharmacol.* 1998; 45:459-62.

Ilett KF, Hackett LP, Kristensen JH, Rampono J. Distribution and excretion of the novel antidepressant mirtazapine in human milk. Sydney, Australia: 2003 Conference and Annual Meeting of the International Lactation Consultant Association; 2003.

Ilett KF, Kristensen JH, Hackett LP, Paech M, Kohan R, Rampono J. Distribution of venlafaxine and its *O*-desmethyl metabolite in human milk and their effects in breastfed infants. *Br J Clin Pharmacol.* 2002; 53:17-22.

Ilett KF, Lebedevs TH, Wojnar-Horton RE, Yapp P, Roberts MJ, Dusci LJ, *et al.* The excretion of dothiepin and its primary metabolites in breast milk. *Br J Clin Pharmacol.* 1992; 33:635-39.

Jansson LM, Choo RE, Harrow C, Velez M, Schroeder JR, Lowe R, *et al.* Concentrations of methadone in breast milk and plasma in the immediate perinatal period. *J Hum Lact.* 2007; 23:184-90.

Karmowski A, Sobiech KA, Dobek D, Terpilowski L, Palczynski B, Mis-Michalek M. The concentration of cotinine in urine, colostrum and amniotic fluids within the system mother-baby. *Ginekologia Polska.* 1998; 69:115-22.

Kent JC, Ramsay DT, Doherty D, Larsson M, Hartmann PE. Response of breasts to different stimulation patterns of an electric breast pump. *J Hum Lact.* 2003; 19:179-86.

Kristensen JH, Hackett LP, Kohan R, Paech MJ, Ilett KF. The amount of fluvoxamine in milk is unlikely to be a cause of adverse effects in breastfed infants. *J Hum Lact.* 2002; 18:139-43.

Lai CT, Hale TW, Kent JC, Simmer K, Hartmann PE. Hourly rate of milk synthesis in women. *Proceedings 12th ISRHML International Conference.* Cambridge, UK, September 10 2004.

Laine K, Heikkinen T, Ekblad U, Kero P. Effects of exposure to selective serotonin reuptake inhibitors during pregnancy on serotonergic symptoms in newborns and cord blood monoamine and prolactin concentrations. *Arch Gen Psychiatry.* 2003; 60:720-26.

Levinson-Castiel R, Merlob P, Linder N, Sirota L, Klinger G. Neonatal abstinence syndrome after in utero exposure to selective serotonin reuptake inhibitors in term infants. *Arch Pediatr Adolesc Med.* 2006; 160:173-76.

Lucas A, Gibbs JA, Lyster RL, Baum JD. Creamatocrit: simple clinical technique for estimating fat concentration and energy value of human milk. *Br Med J (Clin Res Edn).* 1978; 1:1018-20.

Malm H, Martikainen J, Klaukka T, Neuvonen PJ. Prescription drugs during pregnancy and lactation--a Finnish register-based study. *Eur J Clin Pharmacol.* 2003; 59:127-33.

Mannisto PT, Karhunen M, Koskela O, Suikkari AM, Mattila J, Haataja H. Concentrations of tinidazole in breast milk. *Acta Pharmacol Toxicol (Copenh).* 1983; 53:254-56.

Matheson I, Kristensen K, Lunde PK. Drug utilization in breast-feeding women. A survey in Oslo. *Eur J Clin Pharmacol.* 1990; 38:453-59.

Mitoulas LR, Lai CT, Gurrin LC, Larsson M, Hartmann PE. Effect of vacuum profile on breast milk expression using an electric breast pump. *J Hum Lact.* 2002a; 18:353-60.

Mitoulas LR, Lai CT, Gurrin LC, Larsson M, Hartmann PE. Efficacy of breast milk expression using an electric pump. *J Hum Lact.* 2002b; 18:340-48.

Mitoulas LR, Ramsay DT, Kent JC, Larsson M, Hartmann PE. Identification of factors affecting breast pump efficacy. *Adv Exp Med Biol.* 2004; 554:325-27.

Moffat AC, Osselton DM, Widdop B. *Clarke's analysis of drugs and poisons in pharmaceuticals, body fluids and postmortem material.* 3rd Ed. London: Pharmaceutical Press; 2004.

Moretti ME, Koren G, Verjee Z, Ito S. Monitoring lithium in breast milk: An individualized approach for breast-feeding mothers. *Ther Drug Monit.* 2003; 25:364-66.

Naranjo CA, Busto U, Sellers EM, Sandor P, Ruiz I, Roberts EA, *et al.* A method for estimating the probability of adverse drug reactions. *Clin Pharmacol Ther.* 1981; 30:239-45.

Neville MC, Allen JC, Archer PC, Casey CE, Seacat J, Keller RP, *et al.* Studies in human lactation: milk volume and nutrient composition during weaning and lactogenesis. *Am J Clin Nutr.* 1991; 54:81-92.

Neville MC, Keller R, Seacat J, Lutes V, Neifert M, Casey C, *et al.* Studies in human lactation: milk volumes in lactating women during the onset of lactation and full lactation. *Am J Clin Nutr.* 1988; 48:1375-86.

Neville MC, Keller RP, Seacat J, Casey CE, Allen JC, Archer P. Studies on human lactation. I. Within-feed and between-breast variation in selected components of human milk. *Am J Clin Nutr.* 1984; 40:635-46.

Nulman I, Rovet J, Stewart DE, Wolpin J, Pace-Asciak P, Shuhaiber S, *et al.* Child development following exposure to tricyclic antidepressants or fluoxetine throughout fetal life: a prospective, controlled study. *Am J Psychiatry.* 2002; 159:1889-95.

Ohman I, Vitols S, Luef G, Soderfeldt B, Tomson T. Topiramate kinetics during delivery, lactation, and in the neonate: Preliminary observations. *Epilepsia.* 2002; 43:1157-60.

Pennell PB. Antiepileptic drug pharmacokinetics during pregnancy and lactation. *Neurology.* 2003; 61:S35-S42.

Pittman KA, Smyth RD, Losada M, Zighelboim I, Maduska AL, Sunshine A. Human perinatal distribution of butorphanol. *Am J Obstet Gynecol.* 1980; 138:797-800.

PK in Pregnancy Working Group of the Pregnancy Labeling Task Force. Guidance for industry. Clinical lactation studies - study design, data analysis, and recommendations for labeling. Draft February 2005. Available from: http://www.fda.gov/cder/guidance/index.htm.

Rampono J, Hackett LP, Kristensen JH, Kohan R, Page-Sharp M, Ilett KF. Transfer of escitalopram and its metabolite demethylescitalopram into breastmilk. *Br J Clin Pharmacol.* 2006; 62:316-22.

Rampono J, Kristensen JH, Hackett LP, Paech M, Kohan R, Ilett KF. Citalopram and demethylcitalopram in human milk; distribution, excretion and effects in breast fed infants. *Br J Clin Pharmacol.* 2000; 50:263-68.

Rampono J, Kristensen JH, Ilett KF, Hackett LP, Kohan R. Quetiapine and breastfeeding. *Ann Pharmacother.* 2007; 41:711-4.

Rampono J, Proud S, Hackett LP, Kristensen JH, Ilett KF. A pilot study of newer antidepressant concentrations in cord and maternal serum and possible effects in the neonate. *Int J Neuropsychopharmacol.* 2004; 7:329-34.

Rosen TS, Pippenger CE. Disposition of methadone and its relationship to severity of withdrawal in the newborn. *Addictive Dis.* 1975; 2:169-78.

Rosen TS, Pippenger CE. Pharmacologic observations on the neonatal withdrawal syndrome. *J Pediatr.* 1976; 88:1044-48.

Rossi DT, Wright DS. Analytical considerations for trace determinations of drugs in breast milk. *J Pharmaceut Biomed Analysis.* 1997; 15:495-504.

Rowland M, Tozer TN. *Multiple-dose regimens. Clinical pharmacokinetics. Concepts and applications.* 3rd Ed. Baltimore: Williams and Wilkins; 1995. p. 66-105.

Sheiner LB, Beal SL. Evaluation of methods for estimating population pharmacokinetic parameters. III. Monoexponential model: routine clinical pharmacokinetic data. *J Pharmacokinet Biopharm.* 1983; 11:303-19.

Siek T, Cole K, Levine B, Stafford ET, Smith ML, Cody J. *Principles of forensic toxicology.* Washington DC, USA: American Association for Clinical Chemistry Inc; 1999.

Steer PL, Biddle CJ, Marley WS, Lantz RK, Sulik PL. Concentration of fentanyl in colostrum after an analgesic dose. *Can J Anaesth.* 1992; 39:231-35.

Thomann P. Non-compartmental analysis methods manual. In: Heinzel G, Woloszcak R, Thomann P (eds.). *TopFit 2.0 Pharmacokinetic and pharmacodynamic data analysis system for the PC.* Stuttgart: Gustav Fischer; 1993. p. 5-66.

Wan W-Z. *Domperidone; defining an effective dose schedule as a stimulant of milk production.* Postgraduate Diploma in

Pharmacology, School of Medicine and Pharmacology, University of Western Australia; 2004.

Wojnar-Horton RE, Hackett LP, Yapp P, Dusci LJ, Paech M, Ilett KF. Distribution and excretion of sumatriptan in human milk. *Br J Clin Pharmacol.* 1996; 41:217-21.

Zeskind PS, Stephens LE. Maternal selective serotonin reuptake inhibitor use during pregnancy and newborn neurobehavior. *Pediatrics.* 2004; 113:368-75.

Chapter 35

Herbal Therapeutics During Lactation

Sheila Humphrey

INTRODUCTION

This chapter gives an overview of herbal medicine and discusses safety and efficacy issues surrounding the use of herbal medicine during breastfeeding. It seeks to educate health care professionals about herbal medicine and provide sources of accurate information, including scientific evidence for use during lactation when this is available.

The health care provider today is expected to be able to provide sound anticipatory guidance about herbs using the principles of evidence-based care. The practice of suggesting or prescribing herbal remedies is growing in acceptance as the evidence base favoring this treatment option continues to develop. Yet, the breastfeeding mother with a health problem presents a conundrum for the practitioner as few drugs and no herbal products have been exhaustively researched for their safety during breastfeeding or for their efficacy for breastfeeding problems. Evidence for drug safety accumulates through case reports, limited trials with a handful of mothers, or through clinical experience and experimentation when other options for treatment are not acceptable. After years of data accumulation, lactation experts at least feel fairly confident in predicting drug risk during lactation. Interpretation of evidence is assisted by written resources that reflect consensus for many drugs. The situation is more complex for herbs, demanding some measure of expertise for both herbal medicine and lactation pharmacology. Yet, a search of the scientific literature on herbs and lactation shows a remarkable lack of studies, despite the fact that nursing mothers commonly use herbs (Westfall, 2003).

Long-term human use has accumulated a body of astute observations about plants, identifying uses as well as potential safety concerns. Plant use during lactation has generated its own body of empirical knowledge. Animal research has focused either on milk supply effects or toxic effects known from human use. Published adverse events are few despite the apparent ease in getting incomplete case reports into the medical literature, while a very large number of positive case reports are confined to the grey literature and oral traditions. Human lactation studies are few, though some research has been done with the most promising herbs. Further discussion can be found in the tables on toxins and potential toxins and in the discussion of galactogogue herbs.

Herbal medicine remains a mostly empirical discipline, especially regarding lactation. Although allopathic and thus amenable to rational use, the general nature of herbal remedies differs from drugs in many ways. Serious in-depth study of herbal medicine as a discipline is only now being re-introduced into medical schools in the West. Like the field of lactation, it is in the process of being recognized as a medical specialty in its own right. During this transition time, a more detailed analysis of information sources on herbs and breastfeeding is pertinent.

Most lactation reviews focus on infant safety issues. While the focus must be on the infant, effects on milk supply cannot be overlooked. Not all breastfeeding dyads are at equal risk, though this fact is not discussed in most herb safety reviews. Yet, the same relative risk factors that apply for drugs apply to herbs: premature infants are high risk, toddlers are very low risk. The amount of breastmilk and the weight of the child determine the pediatric dose. A mother nursing a two or three-year-old at bedtime or her health care provider may incorrectly apply safety concerns of herbs as if she were nursing a near-term infant with health problems. Concern needs to be focused not just on the ingested substance, but also on the inherent risks for the particular mother and baby dyad.

LESS THAN USEFUL HERB SAFETY REVIEWS

Expert review of herbs for safety during breastfeeding has generated differing findings, depending on the expertise of the reviewers with herbal medicine, lactation, or perhaps both. Some widely distributed texts aimed at professionals have contraindicated almost all herbs (Feltrow & Avila, 1999), a highly implausible conclusion. This stance favors a drug option, regardless of circumstance, also implausible. A blanket contraindication approach to herbs is like the PDR guidance for drugs, essentially meaningless and perhaps more rooted in legal considerations of the authors than clinical reality. Relying on such negative sources alone for clinical guidance has its drawbacks. If the mother feels her health care provider will "just say no," she will go elsewhere for help and may be reluctant to tell her doctor about herb use in the future. In situations where no safe alternative drug therapy is available, it could be argued that withholding knowledge of potentially useful herbal options would be unethical, even though they may not meet the highest evidence standards usually demanded of Western medicine. This is certainly the reality of galactogogue therapy in the U.S. at this time.

SYSTEMATIC SAFETY REVIEWS

Some published texts of herb safety that systematically reviewed lactation and so provide more guidance are listed below.

The German Commission E

An English language edition (Blumenthal *et al.*, 1998) was published in 1998, providing reliable risk and efficacy analyses and further assessed risk of approved herbs for use during lactation. This German government panel of both herb and medical experts found few contraindications for breastfeeding in approved herbs. Contradicted herbs were stimulant laxative herbal agents, except senna pod, kava kava, Indian snakeroot, and uva ursi. The Commission did not approve any herb as a galactogogue. The monographs do not contraindicate the essential oils, niauli (tea tree) oil and camphor, but note that these substances can induce respiratory problems when used near the face and nose of infants. In Blumenthal's edition, they were included in a summary table of contraindications. As a governmental agency, the Commission E did not make public any documents or references supporting their conclusions, limiting critique and discussion.

The Botanical Safety Handbook

An expert panel of the American Herbal Products Association (AHPA) (McGuffin *et al.*, 1997) reviewed herb safety to provide guidance on herbal product labeling for the American market. The panel of herb experts systematically reviewed issues for lactation separate from pregnancy. Compared to the German Commission E, the AHPA lists a larger number of herbs, those containing caffeine for example, that should be labeled with a specific lactation warning against self-use without supervision. In a few instances, their findings confuse pediatric versus lactation considerations. For example, garlic is contraindicated for lactation based on reports of ingestion of fresh garlic being dangerous and even fatal to young children. The Handbook also reviewed potentially problematic plant constituents and actions and is extensively referenced.

Medications and Mother's Milk (Hale, 2006)

Hale's handbooks contain the first systematic lactation risk analyses written from the perspective of a lactation pharmacology expert. The inclusion of referenced sources upon which these conclusions were made is invaluable, allowing further study and discussion. In the 2004 edition, a total of 23 herbs are reviewed. Five of these herbs received the lowest safety rating (L5): cannabis (illegal *and* anti-lactogogue), kombucha tea, kava kava, blue cohosh, and comfrey. Two more were rated L4: black cohosh and sage. Coffee and St. John's wort were graded L2. St. John's wort was upgraded in the 2004 edition to L2 on the strength of well-evidenced benefits for depression, reassuring measures of constituent serum levels and milk entry, and a lack of negative findings during lactation in published surveys. All the other herbs were rated L3, similar to the rating for most drugs. Most of the L5 rated herbs are known toxins or have serious toxicity associated with their use (**Table 4**). Other herbs chosen for review are top-selling herbs or herbs widely used by mothers to manage milk supply. Hale's reviews of black cohosh and fennel reflect a concern for their reported phytoestrogenic activity, speculating that if similar to synthetic estrogens, milk supply may be reduced. There are no studies to determine if this oft-repeated idea has value. The common occurrence of a wide range of active plant estrogens in traditional galactogogues (Farnsworth *et al.*, 1975) argues the opposite outcome may be more generally true. Black cohosh is now thought to lack estrogenic activity (Upton, 2002). Others do not consider the typical short-term use during lactation a reason to contraindicate black cohosh (Upton *et al.*, 2002; Humphrey, 2003).

The Nursing Mother's Herbal

Humphrey (Humphrey, 2003) classified 500 herbs according to their overall safety issues as well as those pertinent to lactation. Allergic or photosensitizing potential and the potential for altering milk supply were accounted for separately. A relative safety category was chosen based on the power of effects, the severity of overdose or other adverse effects, known contraindications for medical conditions, pregnancy, and the potential for drug interaction. Appropriate use of a quality product was assumed, but the advisability of self-use was the final determination of safety.

Herbal Medicines, A Guide for Health-Care Professionals

Newall *et al.* published extensively referenced monographs of British herbs (Newall *et al.*, 1996). The authors take an overly conservative view of herb use during lactation, stating in their introduction:

"A drug substance taken by a nursing mother presents a hazard if it is transferred to the breastmilk in pharmacologically or toxicologically significant amounts. Limited information is available regarding the safety of conventional medicines taken during breastfeeding. Much less information exists for herbal ingredients, and generally the use of herbal remedies is not recommended during lactation."

While quite correct in every sentence, the authors reflect a negative attitude toward drug use, which they then extend to herbs. Their drug statement is not accompanied by the necessary statement that almost all medications can be used during breastfeeding because the dose in milk is usually not sufficient to cause any effects in the infant. Why should general herb safety be assumed to differ from what we know about drug safety? Is it even a logical conclusion, given that the majority of herbs are 'weak drugs' and do not generally have strong effects or severe side effects? Such a general negative stance does not focus proper attention on those few herbs that should be avoided. Otherwise, the text is an excellent reference for general herb information.

Standard Herbal Reference Texts

It is usually necessary to look at multiple sources for herb information as no one text can provide all the information needed or cover all herbs. And, not all reference texts contain accurate information! These books provide detailed, reliable information on folk use, indications, dose ranges, actions, cautions, and adverse reactions: *The German Commission E* (Blumenthal *et al.*, 1998), *The Herbal PDR* (2nd or 3rd edition, but not the 1st edition) (Gruenwald *et al.*, 2000), Duke's *Handbooks on Medicinal Herbs* (1st and 2nd edition) (Duke, 1985; 2002), *Herbal Drugs* (Bissett, 1994), Weiss' *Herbal Medicine* (6th edition) (Weiss, 1985), *The WHO Monographs on Selected Herbs* (WHO, 2004) and Newall *et al.*'s *Herbal Medicines* (1997). Detailed herb monographs are also available from the European Scientific Cooperative on Phytomedicine (www.escop.com) and from the American Herbal Pharmacopoeia (e.g., Upton, 2002).

HERBALISM, HERBS, AND HERBAL PRODUCT

Herbal medicine is the employment of complex plant products for the purposes of preventing or healing disease. A herbal product contains a significant proportion of the original complex of plant chemicals for the plant in a range of amounts naturally found in the living plant species. With this definition, essential oils are sometimes included as herbal medicines, as many contain hundreds of plant chemicals. Worldwide, systems of understanding health and illness may appear to differ from Western Medicine's model. Disregarding homeopathic or energetic models that do not employ material doses, most of the world's cultures use herbal medicine in material doses. Thus, herbal medicine is allopathic and pharmacological principles can be used to explain mechanisms of action and physiological effects. Despite diversity in the practice of herbal medicine, some generalities are found (Mills & Bone, 1999). Weiss (1985) sums up what is important to understand about herbal medicine:

- Do not confuse rapid onset of effects with effective.
- Do not confuse strong effects with effective.
- Do not confuse gentle effects with ineffective.
- Do not mistake lack of immediate side effects with safe.
- The need for exact dose increases as the power of the agent increases.

The following points are useful when considering herbal safety during lactation.

Medicinal herbs generally have gentle effects. Medicinal plants with powerful effects are the source of many valuable Western medicines: morphine from opium poppy, atropine from belladonna, digitoxin from foxglove. Safe use of such powerful agents is only possible by controlling the dose of these constituents, bolstered by extensive knowledge of exactly how, when, and where they are metabolized in the body. Compared to these medicines, most medicinal herbs are 'weak' or gentle agents. But, some herbs are gentler than others. Rudolf Weiss, famed German physician and educator, points out that gentle does not always mean entirely safe.

The most important predictor for effects is dose. The more powerful the herbal agent, the more pharmacokinetic and pharmacodynamic information is needed to determine a safe dose. Most herbs are gentler than drugs and have a wide dose range where adverse effects are not expected. Herb constituents entering the maternal serum are likely to enter milk, a fact that in and of itself is insignificant, as we know for drugs. With most herbs, it is interesting, but not usually essential, to know the degree of milk entry in nanograms, or the half-life, etc. Like drugs, not all plant constituents are bioavailable, many do not reach the serum or are unable to enter milk easily. Only tiny amounts would be expected to be in the milk. Information confirming milk entry of constituents is limited to those herbs known to cause problems during lactation, with the exception of St. John's Wort (**Table 1**).

Just because a plant is natural does not make it safe. More powerful medicinal plants may be beneficial over a small dose range, yet show serious toxicity in overdose (**Table 2, Table 3**). There is general expert consensus on which herbs a nursing mother should avoid (**Table 3**). A few plants are too toxic to justify continued use in herbal medicine, causing irreversible organ damage (**Table 4**).

When the need for efficacy is high, proof of efficacy is required. As yet, few herbs have a high level of proof of efficacy for serious acute conditions, though a complementary role cannot be ignored.

While a large number of herbs have been identified as contraindicated during pregnancy, fewer plants have safety concerns during lactation. Contraceptive effects, uterotonicity, menstrual cycle "influences," and "hormonal effects" all indicate concern during pregnancy, but not necessarily for lactation. Indeed, such effects may indicate utility as a galactogogue (Bingel & Farnsworth, 1994; Farnsworth *et al.*, 1975a; 1975b; Patisaul *et al.*, 1999).

Mothers using prescription and other drugs may be at risk of drug-herb interactions, though this risk is not a lactation-related risk *per se*. Knowledge of interactions among drugs, herbs, and foods is a rapidly expanding field. Research trends indicate that it is simply wise to avoid consumption of large doses of any one food or herb while taking powerful pharmaceutical agents.

Maternal use of herbs contraindicated for liver or kidney dysfunction is of greatest concern with premature or high-risk infants.

Mothers with health problems must be especially careful to avoid inappropriate herbs for the sake of their own health.

REPORTS OF LACTATION RELATED ADVERSE EVENTS

Medical reports of adverse events involving lactation alone are rare, and in the cases of internal use, the two cases known describe unexpected events. These case reports should be viewed in the context of much more common and well-known adverse events caused by plants. For example, allergic responses in the infant to maternal food plant constituents are common. It is to be expected that hypersensitive infants may also react to allergenic medicinal plants that their mothers consume. It is also well-known that a young infant can become overly alert or fussy from maternal use of coffee, tea, chocolate or other CNS stimulant plants. Laxative herbs, such as senna, can cause diarrhea in the infant as well. Adverse event reports involving herb use that started in pregnancy are not considered here as it is not possible to determine to what degree lactation contributed to the outcome.

Garlic - external use on the breast (Roberge *et al.*, 1997). A woman presented to the emergency room with second degree burns on her breast where she had applied freshly crushed garlic to a rash that she had taken to be "thrush." The garlic poultice was covered and left there for several days, despite immediate and increasing pain. The baby continued to nurse without harm throughout her self-treatment. The application of freshly crushed garlic is well-known to cause severe skin reactions including burns when left in contact with skin for a number of hours. The authors speculated that lactating breast tissue may have a heightened sensitivity to external agents. This incident was well documented. In particular, the authors took pains to distinguish the inappropriate external use from the internal use of fresh garlic.

Roman chamomile *(Chamaemelum nobile)* - allergic dermatitis of the nipple (McGeorge, 1991). Two cases of allergic dermatitis of the nipple were reported with the use of Kamillosan® ointment. At that time in the UK, this product contained Roman chamomile essential oil, lanolin, peanut oil, paraben, and beeswax. One mother was using it for cracked nipples at ten weeks postpartum. The other mother was apparently using it to prevent sore nipples, having used the product without reaction with a previous child. Both developed severe exudative eczema on both nipples and areola. This well-documented report identified a specific allergic reaction to the essential oil. The other ingredients failed to elicit reaction in a skin patch test. Roman chamomile is a known allergenic plant and should not be used on nipples.

Dong quai *(Angelica sinensis)* – transient high blood pressure in infant (Nambiar *et al.*, 1999). A mother of Chinese-Malaysian origin presented to a U.S. emergency room at three weeks postpartum, suffering sudden onset of headache, weakness, lightheadedness, and vomiting. Although normotensive during a normal pregnancy, her blood pressure was consistently measured at 195/85. She quickly normalized after 12 hours. She reported eating a postpartum soup twice that was reported to contain dong quai, prepared for her by her mother who had recently arrived from Malaysia. The patient denied use of any other herbal remedies. The next day the infant (no symptoms reported) was evaluated by a pediatrician and found to have a blood pressure above the 90th percentile for age. Breastfeeding was temporarily discontinued for two days and his blood pressure "normalized" (repeat measures not given). The history describes customary use of a soup made with dong quai and chicken bone stock, widely used in many Asian cultures to speed recovery in the postpartum period. The episode is fairly well-documented. The authors were not able to verify the identity of the soup ingredients, although they did obtain "dong quai" from the same shop in Malaysia where the source material was purchased. This material was identified by an expert in Chinese medicine, but this is not a definitive botanical verification. While the authors state that they could not determine the dose consumed, they failed to state that hypotension is a known side effect of dong quai use, not hypertension. This appears to be an isolated report, not otherwise reported despite widespread similar usage.

Herbal tea mixture – infant toxicity (Rosti *et al.*, 1994) Two neonates (15 and 20 days old) were admitted to the hospital with multiple toxicity symptoms. The mothers reported ongoing feeding difficulties, then emesis and restlessness on the day before admission. The infants showed multiple signs of CNS involvement: hypotonia, lethargy, emesis, weak cry, and poor suckling. Septic and other lab studies were negative. One of the mothers complained of drowsiness and weakness. The mothers reported having consumed large volumes of "herbal tea mixtures" containing "extracts of licorice, fennel, anise, and galega officinalis" for unspecified reasons. Within 24 to 36 hours after withdrawing the tea (and temporarily discontinuing breastfeeding), all symptoms in mothers and babies resolved. The infants resumed breastfeeding and were healthy at one year follow-up. The amount of tea reportedly consumed was more than two liters per day, which may represent an overdose. The actual doses for any of the herbs were not documented, nor were their identities confirmed. The occurrence of unusual symptoms in two mother-baby pairs at the same time and place could indicate that a local herbal product contained misidentified plants. It is pertinent to note that there are documented cases of hemlock being misidentified as fennel (Bisset, 1994).

Table 1. Milk Entry of Medicinal Plant Constituents

Constituents	Plant source	Lactation Effects
(+)nor-pseudoephedrine	Khat (*Catha edulis*)	Present in human milk of khat users and in infant urine as well, but no information on infant effects. Suspected of causing frequent complaints of low milk supply in Yemen (Kristiansson *et al.*, 1987; Luqman & Danowski, 1976).
Rhein and other anthraquinones	Senna pod, senna leaf, cascara, rhubarb and other herbs containing anthranoids have not been studied for milk entry, but it is assumed on the basis of empirical evidence.	Rhein metabolite, rheinanthrone, is known to enter milk in animal studies. In one human study, laxative effects were rare in infants exposed through milk (Hale, 2006). German Commission E contraindicates use of senna leaf and other stimulant laxative herbs during lactation, but allows use of senna pod (Blumenthal *et al*,, 1998).
Dicoumarol	Product of fungal metabolism of coumarin – i.e., a contaminant of herbal products (Farnsworth, 1993). Safety concerns about coumarin, the drug preparation, have little bearing on herb use (Felter *et al.*, 2006). Herbs containing coumarin have no such effects per se (Booth *et al.*, 2004).	Has induced bleeding diasthesis in breastfed infants of mothers who consumed contaminated herbal elixers (Pansatiankul & Mekmanee, 1993).
Unsaturated Pyrrolizidine alkaloids (UPAs)	E.g., Russian comfrey, *Senecio* species (see Table 4 Toxic Herbs)	The German Commission E notes that animal studies demonstrated milk entry (Blumenthal *et al*,, 1998).
Isoflavones: daidzein, genistein, glycitein, formononetin, biochanin-A	E.g., Soy	Human milk total isoflavone content: 0.2 micromol/L after ingestion of soy beans containing 37 mg total isoflavones (Franke, 1998)
Vicine , convicine	Fava beans	Favism induced in 2 glucose-6-phosphate dehydrogenase-deficient infants after mothers had consumed fava beans. Milk entry of the oxidant glycones of vicine and convicine into milk is presumed (Kaplan *et al.*, 1998).
Hypericin, hyperforin	St. John's Wort	A single patient study could not detect hypericin in milk (< 0.2 ng/mL). Hyperforin detected in milk was 0.58 to 18.2 ng/mL and none was detectable in the infant's plasma. No known effect on infants. (Hale, 2004).

Plant constituents usually employed as pharmaceutical drugs, such as digoxin, morphine, caffeine, and ephedrine, are not included nor are food plant constituents, such as vitamins, minerals, beta-carotene, peanut allergens, or gliadin.

Goat's rue and licorice also have look-alike toxic relatives. The possibility that the toxic effects represented an overdose was not discussed by the authors. No data on infant gestational age, weight loss, degree of jaundice, maternal nipple trauma, or any other indicators of breastfeeding adequacy were included in the report. The widespread and apparently safe use of lactogogue teas in Europe was not mentioned by the authors. This report is worrisome yet remains an isolated and critically incomplete report.

HERBAL PRODUCT ISSUES

Crude natural substances naturally vary in quality and constituent quantity, manufacturing is a human enterprise, and market regulation is a function of governmental resources, therefore:

- Even herbs with well-evidenced efficacy do not always show therapeutic effect.
- Products may vary significantly from manufacturer to manufacturer.
- A small, but persistent risk of contamination exists even with good production values and government oversight (as is true with foods) (**Table 5**).

PREFERRED HERBAL PRODUCTS

Advanced Products are Generally Preferred over Crude Products, Based on their Safety Track Record.

Most cases of adverse events from herb use involve crude rather than more advanced forms of herbal medicine (Farnsworth, 1993). Crude herbal medicines

Table 2. Herbs with Dose-Related Toxicity

Potential toxin	Actions	Plants of concern
Alkylbenzenes: beta-asarone, safrole estragole	Weak potential carcinogen and mutagen.	Essential oils of sassafras, sweet flag, cinnamon, nutmeg, basil, tarragon.
Atropine	Powerful CNS effects – dose with narrow therapeutic window.	Belladonna, henbane, mandrake, jimson weed (Duke, 2002). Likely to lower milk supply.
Berberine, sanguinarine	Moderately powerful - cardiac depression in overdose. Poorly absorbed from GI tract.	Goldenseal, bloodroot, coptis, celandine.
Cardiac glycosides	Powerful cardiac effects – dose with narrow therapeutic window.	Lily of the valley, pleurisy root, spreading dogbane. Blue cohosh should not be used.
Iodine	Daily adult intake of up to 1100 mg is considered the tolerable limit. Iodine concentrates in milk and depresses infant thyroid function.	Brown algae (kelps, bladderwrack) can contain up to 8165+/- 373 μg/gram. Note: the red alga nori (*Porphyra*), used in sushi, contains only 16 μg/g (Teas *et al.*, 2004).
Lectins	Glycoproteins that can cause hemagglutination. Vary in toxicity: low in green beans to extreme in castor beans (ricin). Pokeweed lectins mitogenic in tiny doses (J Duke, personal communication, 1997).	High toxicity: mistletoe leaves, all parts of poke weed, castorbean seed, but not expressed oil. Raw legumes can cause GI disturbances.
Oxalates	Kidney irritation and stone formation.	Large doses of shepherd's purse, purslane, sorrel, dock, black haw, rhubarb.
Methyl salicylate	CNS excitement, convulsions, anti-coagulant interactions known after external use.	External use of wintergreen or sweet birch essential oils is hazardous.
Tannic acid – in tinctures of high tannin plants	Potential for GI disturbance, rarely kidney irritation or liver damage.	Tinctures of *Quercus* oak galls should not be used on sore nipples (author's opinion).
Thujone	Neurotoxic in high doses, e.g., sage essential oil, wormseed oil. Chronic ingestion has caused seizures, delerium.	Crude garden sage (*Salvia officinalis*) is not associated with toxicity. Thujone is not soluble in water. Other sages (*Salvia, Artemesia*) often contain thujone and many are of undetermined safety. Absinthe apparently contains little thujone.

German or Swiss Manufactured Products Standardized to Contain Defined Amounts of UPAs.

Comfrey -
True medicinal comfrey leaf (*Symphytum officinalis*) contains small amounts of toxic PAs, but 25% of surveyed North American products were found to contain highly toxic echimidine (Farnsworth, 1993). The Commission E contraindicates use of even well-characterized comfrey products during pregnancy or nursing (Blumenthal *et al.*, 1998). Safer alternative herbs are available.

Butterbur -
Petasites hybridus - Advanced products contain low to negligible levels of total UPAs, being processed to reduce PA content. Germany restricts internal use to <1 μg/day for four to six weeks/year and contraindicates use during pregnancy or nursing. However, prophylactic use for migraine may justify use. Clinical studies of adults, as well as children as young as six, have not shown toxicity in humans (Danesch & Rittinghausen, 2003; Pothmann & Danesch, 2005). Only products made in Germany or Switzerland should be considered for use (Brown, 2003).

Table 3. Herbs of Greatest Concern during Nursing

Herb	Lactation Concern
Aloes leaf cortex *Aloe* species	GI cathartic. Although the gel inside the leaf contains little of the laxative principle, drinking large volumes can cause diarrhea in adults. Conservatively, do not use aloe gel on nipples; it is somewhat bitter.
Bladderwrack *Fucus* species	Very high iodine content.
Kelp E.g., *Laminaria, Nereocystis* species	Very high iodine content.
Black walnut *Juglans nigra*	Juglones are carcinogenic. Avoid use on the nipple.
Blue cohosh *Caulophyllum thalictroides*	Cardiac glycosides.
Borage leaf *Borago officinalis*	Leaf contains unsaturated pyrrolizidine alkaloids (UPAs), known to be toxic.
Buckthorn fruit *Rhamnus cathartica*	GI cathartic.
Bugle weed leaf *Lycopus* species	Anti-thyroid effects, may decrease milk supply (Sourgens & Winterhoff, 1982).
Cinchona bark *Cinchona* species	GI cathartic.
Comfrey leaf or root *Symphytum* species	UPAs or high potential for product contamination with UPAs.
Coltsfoot leaf *Tussilago farfara*	Controversial by association with adverse event, but toxicity of pyrolizzidine alkaloids not demonstrated in follow-up studies.
Kava kava rhizome *Piper methysticum*	Controversial as kava is suspected, but not clearly evidenced, as a liver toxin. Kava is very well evidenced as an anxiolytic (Ernst, 2006).
Ma huang *Ephedra sinensis*	Ephedrine alkaloids are CNS stimulants and probably also anti-galactogogue (Aljazaf *et al.*, 2003).
Queen of the Meadow Joe Pye weed, gravel root *Eupatorium purpureum*	UPAs.
Queens' Delight *Stillingia sylvatica*	Fresh latex is emetic, cathartic, mucous membrane irritant. Properly dried latex is weaker, but still considered to have strong GI actions.
Senecio, ragwort *Senecio* species	UPAs.
Wormwood leaf *Artemesia absinthium*	Thujone (up to 0.6%) and has known toxic effects in humans.
Uva ursi leaf *Arctostaphylos uva-ursi*	Contraindicated by the German Commission E. Controversial due to hydroquinone content, but milk entry or effects through lactation not studied. Use should be avoided with a high risk infant.

refer to bulk plant materials that may be further prepared by the consumer as teas or decoctions for example, but also include dried plant material in capsules or tea bags. Advanced herbal products refer to prepared materials: tinctures or other liquid extractions or dried extracts in capsule or pill form. These may range from simple alcoholic extractions to very specific fractionations of a plant's constituents. See the WHO website for definitions of crude and advanced herbal medicines (WHO, 2000). Herbs sold in bulk have no label to guide the consumer. While many quality herbals can be obtained from such sources, it is mainly up to the consumer to judge their identity and quality.

Traditional use of Herbs and Herbal Combinations

The WHO defines traditional use of herbal medicines as having "long historic use," being "well established and widely acknowledged to be safe and effective, and may be accepted by national authorities" (WHO, 2000). Traditional use has recently been defined in Europe to mean documented use of an herb or of specific herbal combinations for over 30 years (www.ESCOP.com). Simple herbal preparations, those containing one plant, are advantageous to nursing mothers as the source of any allergic reaction can be quickly identified. Yet, most herbal medicine uses a combination of herbs.

Table 4. Toxic Herbs

Toxic plants and detoxified products		
Constituent	**Plant**	**Potential adverse effects**
Aristolochic acid – no safe dose range known.	*Aristolochia, Asarum* species and probably all other members of the Aristolochiaceae family. *Stephania tetranda* - plant does not contain aristolochic acid, but *Aristolochia fangchi* is often substituted for *Stephania* in Chinese products. Canada does not allow sale as a precaution.	Known renal toxin. Documented multiple occurrences of irreversible kidney damage, kidney failure, death. Constituent occurs in all Aristolochia species and probably all members of the Aristolochiaceae, but not found outside of this plant family (Yang *et al.*, 2002; DeSmet, 1999).
Toxic pyrrolizidine alkaloids - those with a 1,2 unsaturated necine structure and their N-oxides (UPAs). E.g., Echimidine, senkirkine, intermedine, lycopsamine, indicine, lithosenine, senecionine. Pyrrolizidine alkaloids with saturated rings are not considered toxic, though their intake should be limited and chronic use avoided.	Plants with historic medicinal use, but that should not be ingested: *Senecio* species *Symphytum asperum* (prickly comfrey) *Symphytum* X *uplandicum* - Russian comfrey *Symphytum caucasicum* *Symphytum tuberosum* *Lithospermum officinale* - stone seed *Myosotis scorpioides* (syn. *M. palustris*) - forget-me-not *Eupatorium cannabinum* - hemp agrimony *Anchusa officinalis* - common bugloss *Alkanna tinctoria* - alkanet *Petasites spurius* - spurius pestilence - wort *Petasites hybridus* - butterbur in crude form *Adenostyles alliariae* - grey alpendost *Emilia sonchifolia* *Heliotropium arborescens* (syn. *H. corymbosum*) *Cynoglossum officinale* -Hound's Tongue *Crotalaria* species *Borago officinalis* - borage - low levels in leaf; seed oil has also been found to contain UPAs in the range of 0.5- 5 μg/g. Use of unassayed seed oil could be hazardous and should be avoided during pregnancy and lactation (Robbers & Tyler, 1999; De Smet, 1991).	Irreversible & cummulative liver damage, death. Children are more vulnerable to effects, though recovery more likely. Use of *Petasites* with *Tussilago* in pregnancy and early lactation resulted in infant death (Farnsworth, 1993). UPAs documented to enter milk in rodents. Herbal product label should indicate the near absence of UPAs (less than 1 ppm). German regulation limits daily oral intake of total UPA content to 1 microgram per day. German regulation contraindicates even external use during pregnancy and nursing (Blumenthal *et al.*, 1998). AHPA recommends label statement, "Do not apply to broken or abraded skin. Do not use when nursing." Canada disallows use in food. Australia does not allow sale of comfrey other than in a low concentration homeopathic preparation (McGuffin *et al.*, 1997).
This is not an exhaustive list of UPA-containing plants. A more complete list can be found at www.inchem.org/documents/ehc/ehc/ehc080.htm.		

Table 5. Contamination of Herbal Products

Contaminants A quality control program should be continually monitoring their products in all categories.	**Examples of known contamination events**
Toxic plants or toxic constituents	*Digitalis*, *Atropa belladonna*, *Teucrium*, aristolochic acid, unsaturated forms of pyrrolizidine alkaloids
Micro-organisms	*Staph aureus*, *E.coli*, *Salmonella*
Microbial toxins	Bacterial endotoxins, aflatoxins
Pesticides	Chlorinated pesticides, organophosphates
Fumigation agents	Ethyl oxide, methyl bromide, phosphine
Radioactivity (contaminated soils)	Cs-134, Cs-137, Ru-103, I-131, Sr-90
Toxic metals (contaminated soils)	Lead, cadmium, mercury, arsenic
Synthetic pharmaceuticals (illegal additions)	Analgesics, anti-inflammatory agents (e.g., indomethacin), corticosteroids, HCTZ, diazepam
Animal substances	Thyroid hormones
Source: Reprinted with permission from DeSmet PAGM. Overview of herbal quality control. Drug Inf J. 1999; 33:717-24. Copyright 1999, Drug Information Association.	

Traditional combinations are used to lessen potential side effects or to increase beneficial effects, as observed through generations of use. Their use by nursing mothers may be acceptable if there are no identified lactation concerns known. There are no data to guide the lactation use of new plant preparations, such as grapefruit seed extract, or non-traditional combination products that may contain dozens of herbs or be mixed with vitamins, minerals, or other additions. There are no data to guide the lactation use of isolated plant constituents, amino acids, or the host of other non-botanical dietary supplement products of natural origin.

Formulations with Evidence of Safety or Efficacy in Clinical Trials

Herbal products of European origin for sale in the U.S. have known performance in clinical trials and are high quality as reflected in price. Reference texts that identify specific products include *Handbook of Clinically Tested Herbal Remedies* (Barrett, 2004) and *ABC's Clinical Guide to Herbal Remedies* (Blumenthal *et al.*, 2003). Brands with evidence of quality control measures, such as a "standardized" constituent content, may also be preferred when marketed by long-established firms. But refer to reliable sources for the established standardization content for a herb; an abnormally high amount is a sign of a spiked product, not a quality product. Standardization ranges should reflect the range of natural occurrence in the plant. High quality herbal material should contain this amount, so that a manufacturer need only blend batches of plant material to make a uniform product. Spiking of cheap, low quality herbal material with a specific isolated constituent can allow a label to be "truthful," but the herbal product should not be expected to work well. The amounts of other equally important plant constituents will be low. Be aware that some labels have a "standardization" statement that merely guarantees the weight of the herb or extract contained in each capsule. Price remains the most useful indicator of quality, but buyer beware.

Products with Accurate, Detailed Information on the Label

A good label should have a batch number, manufacturer contact number, proper botanical identification of contents, and complete dosage information. Expiration dates are reassuring, but not research-based. Labels should use either acceptable common names (per AHPA) or, preferably, include proper botanical names (*Genus species*). Incorrect spelling is a good reason to avoid a product as it reflects the manufacturer's lack of sophistication. Some herbal products originating in Asia continue to show serious heavy metal problems, likely from soil contamination. U.S. companies selling Asian herbs must have good quality control on an ongoing basis. In the U.S., packaged herbal products should provide "Supplement Facts" on the label. Any health claim statements should be acceptable to the FDA and be accompanied by a proper FDA disclaimer statement. American products without these required label statements reflect a lack of sophistication by the manufacturer and should be avoided.

GALACTOGOGUE HERBS

Herbs and drugs that are used with the intention to increase milk supply are called galactogogues (galactagogues, lactagogue, or lactagogues). Mechanisms of action may act through stimulation of milk synthesis or production. Increasing the ease and volume of milk flow will stimulate milk synthesis if this increases breast emptying significantly. Increasing milk flow gives immediate positive feedback to the mother. Although placebo response may play a particularly important role with galactogogues, folk selection of herbs used to increase milk appears pharmacologically sophisticated (Bingel & Farnsworth, 1994). Galactogogue herbs have been the subject of a number of brief reviews (e.g., Westfall, 2003; Ayers, 2000; Bruckner, 1989; Academy of Breastfeeding Medicine, 2006; Kopek 1999, Betzold, 2004; Tustanovskyj, 1996; Nice *et al.*, 2000). The most valuable and extensive review of ethnobotanical and scientific literature was published by Bingel and Farnsworth (1994). These well-respected plant pharmacologists reviewed the ethnobotanical, clinical, and experimental plant literature in a well-defined extensive literature search. They identified over 400 galactogogue plants in use world-wide. Their commentary discussed potential mechanisms of action with numerous examples where scientific study lent support for folk customs. Summaries of animal experiments, clinical trials, and 247 references were cited in this review. Potential mechanisms of action were discussed: Doctrine of Signatures (therapeutic suggestion), diuretic and sudorific effects, sedative effects, appetite stimulation and nutritional effects, as well as hormonal effects. A number of hormone-related effects known from the experimental study of medicinal plants were detailed. The authors described plants with oxytocic, estrogenic, insulinotropic, and thyroid-related activities that could promote lactation as well as those found to increase prolactin release. This article is required reading by anyone with a serious interest in understanding the potential of galactogogue herbs. The rapidly advancing field of plant medicinal chemistry continues to provide evidence for this list of the world's traditional galactogogue plants. Here are two recent examples: *Moringa oleifera* (malunggay) was recently found to have lactagogue activity in a controlled human trial of lactagogue drugs and herbs (Co *et al.*, 2002). Another plant on this list, *Acacia nilotica* ssp. *adansonii*, was found to increase milk, increase mammary gland proliferation, and stimulate prolactin release in a controlled study of rats (Lompo-Ouedroaogo *et al.*, 2004).

Yet, few herbs familiar to Westerners have a strong ethnobotanical record backed by experimental evidence in both animal studies and human trials. But the most noted galactogogues of Western herbal medicine do: fenugreek, goat's rue, and chasteberry. Non-Western herbs with scientific evidence include: shatavari, black seed, and torbangun. To date, other common Western galactogogues, such as blessed thistle, nettle, alfalfa, marshmallow, milk thistle, and the aromatic seeds of fennel, anise, dill, cumin, and caraway lack study. Russian studies have been done for many of these and other common herbs, but are not yet available in full English translation (Tustanovskyj, 1996). Given the popularity and apparent clinical efficacy of fenugreek and goat's rue, these herbs are discussed in the most detail.

Fenugreek *(Trigonella foenum-gracum)*

The seeds contain the saponin diosgenin (0.1-0.9%) and smaller amounts of other saponins: fenugrin B, sarsasapogenin, smiligenin, and yuccagenin (Habel *et al.*, 1996). Diosgenin has been found to induce mammary tissue growth in ovarectomized mice (Aradhana *et al.*, 1992). Other constituents are coumarin, betaines (trigonelline, gentianine, carpaine), flavones (vitexin, iso-orientin), and mucilagenous fiber (50%) (Habel *et al.*, 1996). The mucilage contributes short-chain fatty acids to the diet through bacterial metabolism in the large bowel as is known with other plant mucilages (Mills & Bone, 1999). The seeds contain sotolone, a harmless source of the maple syrup-like odor. When fenugreek is eaten in sufficient amounts, this odor can be detected in sweat, urine, breastmilk, and even in amniotic fluid. Lectins are present in the unprocessed seed and, along with the saponins, may be responsible for bloating and diarrhea sometimes associated with capsule use. The seed contains a unique amino acid, 4-hydroxy-isoleucine, an insulin-sensitizing constituent (Broca *et al.*, 1999; 2004). Both fenugreek and 4-hydroxyleucine, the major amino acid in fenugreek, have been studied for hypoglycemic (Broca *et al.*, 2000) and antilipidemic (Sharma *et al.*, 1990) effects in diabetic states. 4-Hydroxy-isoleucine improves hyperglycemic states, but has little effect at normal levels in animal models. Human studies show a decrease in high blood sugar in diabetics when very large doses of 15-100 g/day fenugreek seed are used (Sharma *et al.*, 1986). The seed also contains trigonelline and fenugreekine, which have weak, but attenuated hypoglycemic activity (Duke, 1985). Fenugreek was approved as an appetite stimulant in Germany (Blumenthal *et al.*, 1998).

Fenugreek is a well-known allergen in topical applications. Inhalation of the powder has induced asthmatic symptoms and sensitization in industrial workers. There are reports of reaction in asthmatic mothers (Hale, 2006). Powdered seed forms should be avoided in allergy-prone or asthmatic individuals and alternative herbal galactogogues sought. Fenugreek seed can stimulate uterotonic activity, so avoidance in pregnancy is often cautioned (McGuffin *et al*, 1997), though the German Commission E did not do so (Blumenthal *et al*, 1998). Dietary restriction for pregnancy throughout the Middle East and Asia is not known. Fenugreek was recently found to be non-genotoxic according to standard test procedures (Flammang *et al.*, 2004). There are occasional, informal reports on Lactnet of light-headedness and lowered blood pressure in mothers using fenugreek, which are resolved upon discontinuation.

Complex dose-dependent effects on thyroid hormones and liver and spleen enzymes are documented in animal studies (Tahiliani & Kar, 2003a; 2003b; Choudhary *et al.*, 2001; Thakran *et al.*, 2004). In a series of rat studies, garlic and/or fenugreek were found equally able to lower thyroid hormones T3 and T4 in induced hyperthyroidism (Tahiliani & Kar, 2003a; 2003b). Bingel and Farnsworth (1994) point out that anti-thyroid plants that increase TSH may also induce prolactin release, though this mechanism of action remains to be documented in lactation studies. The potential for fenugreek to alter thyroid function in humans has not been reported or studied. The self-use of fenugreek (9 g/day) did complicate the medical and lactation assessment of a mother on Synthroid and found to have low thyroid hormone levels at three months postpartum (Latterner, personal correspondence, 2005).

Fenugreek seed has been used as a lactagogue since antiquity. At least three Ayurvedic and Middle Eastern medical texts describe a specific lactation dose of 3-6 g/day (Bingel & Farnsworth, 1994; Kapoor, 1990). The fixed seed oil has been used in India to increase milk, a practice investigated in the 1950s by El Ridi who reported galactogogue effects in a controlled rat study (Bingel & Farnsworth, 1994). Fenugreek use in the West has become increasingly popular; it is undoubtedly the most suggested herbal remedy for low milk supply. Clinical reports over the last 20 years in the U.S. describe very few adverse effects for mothers and even fewer for infants. One survey of lactation consultants and La Leche League Leaders reported positive supply responses in about 75% of mothers (Renfree, 2004). Respected lactation practitioners have published detailed protocols for use (Newman & Pitman, 2000; Huggins, 1998) that are congruent with ethnobotanical information. Use is typically described as three capsules taken three times daily, often combined with an equal number of capsules of blessed thistle (e.g., Newman & Pitman, 2000). Blessed thistle may counter adverse GI effects of the uncooked seed. The Academy of Breastfeeding Medicine's galactogogue protocol (ABM, 2006) suggests a fenugreek dose of one to four capsules, three to four times/day for capsules weighing 580-610 mg each (yielding a daily dose range of 1.74 - 4.9 g). However, capsule size varies by product. Many practitioners introduce fenugreek slowly, increasing the dose over two to three days to prevent diarrhea in the mother and, more rarely, in the baby. Fenugreek tinctures are thought to give more consistent effects. The tincture may also be easier to take than multiple capsules. Combination teas and tinctures of fenugreek have a positive reputation (Humphrey, 2003). Although fenugreek is relatively well studied for other indications, such as diabetes, formal investigation as a lactagogue in women is limited to one small (n=10) U.S. study (Swafford & Berens, 2000). Exclusively pumping women served as their own controls, keeping record of milk volume for two weeks as baseline. After two weeks use of six capsules of powdered fenugreek/day, significantly increased pumped milk volumes were reported. Average milk volumes increased from 207 to 464 mL/day. Unfortunately, the study did not include a study of milk volumes after withdrawal of fenugreek (Swafford & Berens, 2000).

Fenugreek Versus Torbangun

A recent study (Damanik *et al.*, 2006) provides some additional evidence of fenugreek efficacy. Researchers investigated a local lactagogue soup called torbangun, using fenugreek and a vitamin product for comparison. Seventy-five women were assigned to three groups receiving one of three different treatments starting on the second day postpartum and continuing for one month. Sixty-seven women completed the study, with each study arm losing the same number of women. The study group (n=23) received a daily dose of soup made with 150 g/day of 'torbangun' leaf (*Plectranthus amboinicus*, syn. *Coleus amboinicus*) prepared and delivered daily by health workers. The fenugreek group (n=22) took 600 mg fenugreek capsules supplied from New Zealand, one capsule three times/day for a daily dose of 1.8 g/day. The other "reference" group (n=22) were given Moloco B12, a combination product containing 20 micrograms of vitamin B12 and 15 grams of a placental extract, not further described. The study measured total milk production by conducting before and after weighing with every feeding for 24 hours, using a scale accurate to ± 10 grams. Fenugreek showed a 20% increase in milk production from day 14 to 28, compared to a 10% increase for the vitamin supplement. The soup treatment group showed a 65% increase in milk volume over the same period. Milk volumes were sustained in the soup group after the soup was discontinued, unlike the fenugreek and vitamin groups. However, the only statistically significant different effect was a higher milk volume at two months for torbangun as compared to the vitamin supplement. No significant statistical difference in milk volume was noted at any time between the torbangun and fenugreek groups. This study employed a low dose of fenugreek, yet some positive effects are suggested, even for women without supply issues. This study does not answer the real question: can fenugreek help the woman with a pre-existing low supply?

Goat's Rue *(Galega officinalis)*

The aerial parts of the plant (the part used for lactation) contain a number of guanidine derivative alkaloids:

galegine (0.1-0.3%), vasicine (0.3%), vasicinone (0.3 or less), and two additional trimethylene alkaloids. The actions of the plant are strongly associated with these alkaloidal derivatives of guanidine. The coumarin medicagol is reported at very low levels (0.00024%). The plant also contains a variety of flavonoids, but apparently no isoflavones. Goat's rue contains the flavones: rutin, kaempherol, quercitin, and mauritianin, and the flavonoids: sativan and medicarpin. Other reported constituents are allantoin, a sesquiterpene, and the triterpene saponin, soyasapogenol B. The flavone galuteolin is reported from the seed, but not the leaf or flower (NAPRALERT, 2006).

The use of goat's rue goes back to at least the Middle Ages in Europe, where it was considered a cure for plague and other infections. The plant can induce sweating, an action often interpreted as anti-infective, as well as being a galactogogue in folk medicine. In folk medicine, it is still considered a relatively powerful treatment for diabetes. With fenugreek, it shares the reputation of building breast tissue, as well as increasing milk supply (Hoffman, 1992). Other folk uses of the plant include the treatment of gout and topical applications for sprains, dislocations, and to heal old sores. In vitro studies have found anti-platelet effects (Atanasov & Tchorbanov, 2002) and broad-spectrum anti-bacterial activity (Pundarikakshudu *et al.*, 2001).

Like a remarkable number of other galactogogue herbs (Bingel & Farnsworth, 1994), goat's rue shows promising anti-diabetic activity (Marles & Farnsworth, 1995). One positive human study, done in 1935, used 2 g/day to successfully treat adult diabetes (NAPRALERT, 2006). The guanidine derivative galegine (also spelled galagrin) is considered the main active hypoglycemic constituent. Research of galegine's effects led to the development of metformin, a synthetic biguanidine derivative. Descriptions of the development of metformin erroneously state that galegine is "too toxic to use" so synthetic derivatives had to be developed from it (Witters, 2001). What was actually discovered was that subcutaneous injection of alcoholic extracts of goat's rue or of galegine sulfate (77.5 mg/kg) into mice was indeed immediately lethal (Kohler, 1969). Yet even large oral doses in herbal preparation do not appear acutely toxic to mice, according to new animal studies. A study of mice fed as much as a 10% diet of goat's rue showed significant fat loss and reduced serum glucose compared to controls (Palit *et al.*, 1999). Genetically obese mice showed fat loss, reduced food intake, and lowered insulin levels. In normal rats, food intake was independent of fat loss and no insulin-lowering effect was seen. The researchers could not establish a statistically significant weight loss when animals were fed smaller doses in the range of 1-6 g/kg. In this study, no toxic effects were seen at any dose level, though the authors failed to determine the actual galegine content of their plant material. An acute toxicity study in rats (Rasekh *et al.*, 2004) showed no sign of toxicity or weight loss after oral administration of as much as 5 mL/kg of an alcoholic extract.

Still, goat's rue was not approved by the German Commission E due to insufficient evidence for efficacy in treating diabetes or other conditions. The Commission expressed concern for potential toxicity, noting that "Poisoning by goat's rue herb has been observed in grazing animals." The Commission was mainly concerned with its use for treating diabetes, stating, "It cannot be justified for diabetes mellitus because of the severity of the disease and the availability of effective therapeutic alternatives." Data supporting use for low milk supply were considered "not documented" (Blumenthal *et al.*, 1998). Goat's rue is still used in Europe as a traditional medicine for diabetes and as a galactogogue. It is increasingly popular in North America.

Lactagogue effects in livestock have been known in France. The 1918 *Dispensary of the United States* records:

"In 1873, Gillet-Damitte, in a communication to the French Academy, stated that this plant, when fed to cows, would increase the secretion of milk from 35 to 50 per cent; since which time Cerisoli, Goubeaux, Masson d'Aury, Millbank, and Carron de la Carriere have affirmed that goat's rue is a powerful galactogogue" (Low Dog & Micozzi, 2005).

In the U.S., goat's rue is classified by the FDA as a "plant of undetermined safety" and as a noxious weed of agriculture. Sheep willingly consume large amounts of goat's rue and are well known to suffer immediate toxic and even fatal effects from such uncontrolled grazing or when fed acute overdoses. However, when fed smaller controlled doses, they quickly build tolerance to even previously toxic doses (Low Dog & Micozzi, 2005).

In a modern controlled animal study, a dose of 2 g/kg/day dried goat's rue given to sheep for three months increased milk production 17% in the first month and 11% over the full three month lactation period (Gonzalez-Andres *et al.*, 2004).

Weiss (1985) describes this herb as an effective and safe lactagogue for women, citing a study by Heiss (1968). Two experiments were described in this study. In the first, 50 randomly selected, newly postpartum women were given Galegran (2 tablets/day), containing goat's rue as well as phosphorus, calcium, and iron salts, while another group of 50 were given placebo tablets. While a control group had a milk volume increase of 75% between day three and five, the study group milk volume increased 125%. In a separate experiment with 100 additional women, half were given Galegran, half placebo. In the goat's rue group, milk constituents increased in proportion to the increased volume. Lactogenic effects were strongly suggested, but not statistically significant. The authors reported that mothers felt Galegran improved milk ejection and breast emptying. No details are available on how milk volumes were attained or the amount of goat's rue in Galegran, apparently a historic compound. Other German language studies of goat's rue have been done (Heiss, 1968). One early study used Galegran in 336 women who were formally determined to have low milk supply on day four. A milk production increase of 30-60% was described, including one woman who had failed to produce milk with four previous children (Typi, 1961).

Goat's rue has a quite variable reported dose range for lactation (Humphrey, 2003), though a range of approximately 1-5 grams/day dried aerial parts is the most common range cited in textbooks. The German Teedrogen (Bissett, 1994) describes using one teaspoon (0.5-1 g)/150 mL in boiling water, taken as a tea, three to five times per day. This is a very similar description to the dose provided in the 1918 *Dispensary of the United States* for an aqueous extract to be given in doses of 0.5-1.0 g, three to five times per day (Remington *et al.*, 1918). A smaller dose of 1 g/150 mL taken as a tea two times per day is suggested for low supply by Hoffman (Hoffman, 1992). American lactation tinctures and solid extract products also suggest a low dose. One brand (Motherlove) contains 333 mg dried plant weight equivalent/gel capsule, with instruction to use one to two capsules four times per day, representing 2.66 g/day. For a woman weighing 100 lbs or 45 kg, the maximal dose suggested on the label would be 0.06 g/kg/day.

No adverse effects from lactation use are published in the scientific literature, excepting one poorly documented report by Rosti (Rosti *et al.*, 1994). Motherlove® company provides much of the goat's rue purchased for lactation in the U.S. and has received no negative reports after several years of sales (K Huggins, personal communication, 2006). Internet sources describe maternal side effects ranging from headache and nausea to dizziness and light-headedness (www.kellymom.com). It is not known if these effects are speculative or based on actual occurrences. The plant is known to induce sweating, and the unpleasant bitter taste of the alkaloid fraction can cause nausea and a loss of appetite. GI irritation may be possible. The herbs's potential to lower blood sugar to less than normal levels is unstudied in humans.

The mechanism of action for goat's rue is unknown and uninvestigated. It may be reasonable to speculate that it's guanidine constituent, galegine, has the same mechanism of action as it's biguanidine derivative, metformin. If so, then it would act to normalize high blood sugar without causing hypoglycemia. Indeed, sensitization of the insulin receptor may be a main mechanism of action as a galactogogue. It has been more recently observed that some women with PCOS have poor milk supply and, in some instances, mammary hypoplasia (Marasco *et al.*, 2000). With the growing use of metformin to treat PCOS, there are now reports of metformin also improving milk supply (L Marasco, personal communications, 2004-6). It is plausible to speculate that both goat's rue and metformin are galactogogues of particular value for women who show the many manifestations of PCOS, including obesity, Type II diabetes, and underdeveloped breasts.

Very positive reports about goat's rue continue to be circulated by clinicians and mothers despite the paucity of modern human study. The use of goat's rue by mothers continues to grow, probably because it works. There is little human lactation data to guide use. This is of particular concern in high risk situations, such as when mothers are pumping for sick premature infants. In these situations, drug alternatives are few. No drug is formally indicated for low milk supply in the U.S. Off-label, domperidone is not easily available in the U.S., and metoclopramide is considered to be a drug of concern while breastfeeding (AAP). Commonly used herbs such as fenugreek do not always work for every mother. What if a mother finds goat's rue enables her to increase her volume enough to preserve breastfeeding? Is the milk safe for these vulnerable infants? Without some evidence of safety, health care providers may understandably not want to feed her milk to her child. But would all-formula feeds really be safer for the infant? Indeed, the mother may not ask or may simply "forget" to tell the doctor about her herb use, fearing that she will be told to dump the milk. These are not theoretical situations, but current clinical dilemmas. Given the historic use, current positive reputation of this particular lactagogue, the existence of animal and human studies showing lactogenic activity, and the inevitable and understandable concerns for its safety, it is clear that goat's rue should be given the highest priority for investigation. New use surveys, case reports, and animal studies would all help. Some measure of actual alkaloidal content in expressed milk would be useful as well. Placebo controlled lactagogue trials are entirely possible with this herb as it is available in well-defined doses in sealed capsule form.

Blessed Thistle *(Cnicus benedictus)* *(syn. Carbinia benedicta, Carduus benedictus)*

Blessed thistle is more widely known as a digestive bitter, but traditional use as a lactagogue is described in Grieve (1982) as well as Bingel & Farnworth (1994). The aerial parts contain lignans, polyacetylenes, terpenoids, including the bitter sesquiterpene cnicin (considered the bitter principle) (Newall *et al.*, 1997), unspecified tannins (8%), volatile oils, lithospermic acid, and mucilage. In herbal medicine, a herb constituent is considered a bitter if it acts to stimulate secretion of saliva and gastic juices (Blumenthal *et al.*, 1998). It was approved by the German Commission E to treat loss of appetite and dyspepsia in doses of 4-6 g/day. No human studies have been done on this plant, though it has been found to have anti-biotic, anti-tumor, and anti-inflammatory effects. It is not considered toxic (Newall, 1997). In a 1975 literature survey of anti-fertility herbs, its traditional use to prevent pregnancy and the presence of lithospermic acid plus anti-gonadotropic effects in animal studies were noted. Farnsworth concluded it should be evaluated further for its contraceptive potential (Farnsworth 1975a; 1975b). Blessed thistle is commonly combined with fenugreek (Newman & Pitman, 2000; Huggins, 1999). It may improve GI tolerance by increasing digestive processes. Being a member of the daisy family, blessed thistle has some potential for allergic reaction, though no record of occurrence is known (Blumenthal *et al.*, 1998).

Marshmallow *(Althaea officinalis)*

The powdered root is usually prepared as a cold infusion of the powdered root and immediately taken (Bissett, 1994; Blumenthal *et al.*, 1998). It is considered a demulcent and nutritious due to its high mucilage content. Plant mucilages are partially digested to short chain fatty acids in the large bowel (Mills & Bone, 1999). Marshmallow has the highest betaine content in the USDA plant database (40,000 ppm) (Duke, 1992). The German Commission E approved use of 6 g/day for irritations of the mouth and throat and mild irritation of the gastric mucosa (Blumenthal *et al.*, 1998). There is little research and no lactation studies of this herb. The mucilage is likely to slow drug absorption if taken at same time as medications.

Barley, Oats, Brown Rice

These whole grains are excellent sources of minerals, choline, and the beneficial soluble fiber, beta-glucan. Oatmeal and barley have recently been found to improve blood glucose and insulin responses in both diabetic (Rendell *et al.*, 2005) and overweight women (Behall *et al.*, 2005). The soluble fiber, beta-glucan, is metabolized by intestinal bacteria to short-chain fatty acids. The choline content of the whole grains is much higher than "instant" cereals and refined grain products listed in the USDA table (USDA, 2003). Choline is metabolized to betaine, a methyl donor able to reduce homocysteine levels in the body and is thought to buffer negative effects of fluxuating osmotic states (Randall *et al.*, 1996). Betaine and choline levels were found to be increased in the lactating breast (Rudolph *et al.*, 2006). Choline requirements during lactation are increased (Zeisel *et al.*, 1995; 2006), but no dietary choline studies of lactating women could be found. Although choline deficiency in the diet is thought to be rare, women may differ in their requirement for choline (da Costa *et al.*, 2006). Traditional use of choline-rich grains to improve lactation performance is worldwide (Jacobson, 2004). For example, the recorded use of the specific combination of fennel and barley water dates back to

Dioscorides of Ancient Greece. Current use of this specific combination is described in herbals from the U.S. (Weed, 1985), Europe (Jacobson, 2004), and the Ukraine (Tustanovskyj, 1996).

Nettle *(Urtica dioica)*

Nettle effects may be mainly nutritional and anti-inflammatory – the plant has a high mineral and flavonoid content and also contains betaines and choline. It is likely to have nutritional, anti-inflammatory, anti-oxidant, and hormonal effects (Newall *et al.*, 1997). German Commission E had approved use of the aerial parts for rheumatism and as "irrigation therapy" against kidney stones (Blumenthal *et al.*, 1998). Traditional use is usually in combination with other galactogogue herbs. No lactation studies are known. Hemostatic and hypoglycemic effects are known as well as GI irritant effects with excessive use (Newall *et al.*, 1997). The plant accumulates metals, including heavy metals when present, so it is important to use only quality products (see Nature's Way report: FDA, 2002).

Alfalfa *(Medicago sativa)*

This most ancient of fodder crops contains significant amounts of the most powerful phytoestrogen, coumestrol, as well as a diverse number of isoflavone phytoestrogens (biochachin, daidzein, formononetin, and genistein). The betaine fraction contains stachydrine and homostachydrine. The plant also contains 2-3% saponins (Newall *et al.*, 1997). Coumestrol, stachydrine, and saponins have all been described as possible lactogenic plant constituents (Bingel & Farnsworth, 1994). The plant is considered a good source of the minerals calcium, potassium, phosphorus, and iron, as well as vitamins A, C, E, and K. It is likely to have nutritional, anti-inflammatory, anti-oxidant, and hormonal effects (Newall *et al.*, 1997). Traditionally, the aerial parts are used to improve lactation in women and dairy animals (Bingel & Farnsworth, 1994). There are no human lactation studies. Alfalfa sprouts produced gynomastia in a man eating large amounts of alfalfa sprouts daily (Duke, 1985). The saponin content may cause GI distress. In animals, alfalfa is mixed with other hay plants to lessen the risk of bloat. Alfalfa products that contain alfalfa seed may exacerbate lupus, an effect associated with the high canavanine of the seed. The leaf contains considerably less canavanine (Newall *et al.*, 1997).

Milk Thistle *(Silybum marianum)*

This plant is well-documented as a liver-protectant against many toxins and for supportive therapy in chronic liver disease. Well-defined concentrated extracts standardized to contain at least 70% silimarin content were approved for such use in Germany. Silimarin is a mixture of flavonoids, mainly silibinin, silydianin, and silichrystin. Crude preparations of the seed were also approved by the German Commission E for dyspeptic complaints. Neither form was contraindicated for lactation (Blumenthal *et al.*, 1998). Traditionally, the fresh, young aerial parts or the seeds have long been used to increase milk supply (Bingel & Farnsworth, 1994; Low Dog & Micozzi, 2005). There are no human lactation studies.

Fennel *(Foeniculum vulgare)*
Anise *(Pimpinella anisum)*
Caraway *(Carum carvi)*
Coriander *(Coriandrum sativum)*
Cumin *(Cuminum cyminum)*
Dill *(Anethum graveolens)*

All of these aromatic seeds are considered effective digestive aids (Weiss, 1985) as well as lactagogue, either as simples or in combinations. Fennel and anise contain significant amounts of anethole, a weak estrogenic compound (Farnsworth *et al.*, 1975). There are no human lactation studies, though one controlled animal study of cumin found no lactogenic effect (Agrawala *et al.*, 1968)

Shatavari *(Asparagus racemosa)*

The fleshy rhizomes of the plant contain the steroidal saponins - shatavarins and sarsapogenin, the alkaloid - asparagamine, a dihydrophenanthrene compound, and a large amount of mucilage (Sharma *et al.*, 1996). Shatavari is considered a major female tonic and a specific for low milk supply in Ayurveda (Sharma *et al.*, 1996; Puri, 2003; Kapoor, 1990). Lactation use is widespread throughout Asia. Shatavari is often combined with ashwaghanda (*Withania somnifera*), licorice, fenugreek, and garlic in small amounts. This traditional Ayurvedic combination (Puri, 2003) is marketed as Lactare® in Asia. A number of positive lactation studies with shatavari and Lactare® have been done with dairy animals as well as women (Goyal *et al.*, 2003). One small randomized controlled trial (Sharma *et al.*, 1996) did not find significant differences between a combination herb pill containing a small amount of shatavari versus a placebo pill preparation. This study used prolactin response as the primary outcome. Women with persistent low supply despite assistance were selected and randomly placed in study and placebo groups. The treatment group was given pills containing only 30 mg/day of shatavari, compared to the traditional lactogogue dose of 3-5 g/day (Sharma *et al.*, 1996) or 600 mg shatavari/day when combined with other lactagogue herbs (Puri, 2003).

Black Seed *(Nigella sativa)*

Black seed or black cumin is a traditional lactogogue in Middle Eastern and Ayurvedic medicine (Kapoor, 1990). Seeds contain essential oil, fixed oil, alkaloids, and a remarkable number of plant sterols. Both the essential and fixed oil fractions and alkaloid constituents have a fairly large body of evidence of efficacy for various diseases, reflecting its many uses. Findings generally indicate anti-inflammatory and anti-oxidant effects (Suboh *et al.*, 2004). A controlled study of lactating rats fed cumin or black seed showed lactogenic and mammotropic effects of the whole blackseed (Agrawala *et al.*, 1968). These effects were later identified with the oil fractions as the defatted seed was inactive (Agrawala *et al.*, 1971). No negative effects during lactation are documented.

Torbangun *(Plectranthus amboinicus) (syn. Coleus amboinicus)*

This plant, along with fenugreek, was recently investigated in breastfeeding women in Indonesia (see fenugreek for study details) (Damanik & Wahlqvist, 2006). Little information on this species' constituents could be found, though phenolics, monoterpenes, diterpenes, and sesquiterpenes are commonly found in other *Plectranthus* species. Forskolin, a labdane diterpenoid widely used in cell research, occurs in large amounts in the related species *Plectranthus barbaras*, as well as several other *Plectranthus* species. Not enough is known about the chemistry of torbangun to explain its traditional use as a lactogogue.

Chasteberry *(Vitex agnus-castus)*

This plant has been used since ancient times to assist breastfeeding. Dioscorides described use of the leaf extracted in wine "to make the milk come down" (McKenna, 2001). Minor but persistent use of the fruit continues by lactation specialists in Europe, Britain, and North America. Several positive clinical lactation studies were done in Germany in the late 1940s through 1954 (McKenna, 2001), using a simple alcoholic tincture of the berries. Animal studies of the time also showed lactogogue activity. More recent studies have shown dopaminergic and anti-prolactin effects. An in vivo rat study using an injected extract (Winterhoff *et al.*, 1991) and in vitro studies of special extracts (Sliutz *et al.*, 1993; Jarry *et al.*, 1994) showed anti-prolactin and dopaminergic effects, later attributed to specific diterpene fractions of these special extracts (Meier *et al.*, 2000). Men given higher doses of a defined extract also showed lowered prolactin, but when given smaller doses, their prolactin levels were increased (Merz *et al.*, 1996). The German Commission E approved use of aqueous-alcoholic extracts equivalent to 30-40 mg dried fruit for "menstrual cycle irregularities, premenstrual complaints, and mastodynia," recommending physician consultation for diagnosis (Blumenthal *et al.*, 1998). In Witchl's English translation (Bissett, 1994), the monograph notes, "In animal experiments, a negative influence on the nursing performance was observed." Although chasteberry is currently assumed to lower milk supply by lowering prolactin, this has not been established to occur in vivo in humans (Bissett, 1994), and no modern studies of lactating women have been done to confirm the effects. Current human and laboratory studies are of specific extracts developed to treat premenstrual syndrome and related hormone imbalances, which may have quite different actions than more traditional extracts. As one of the best-evidenced herbs for treatment of symptoms of premenstrual syndrome, chasteberry should be studied in lactating women (e.g., mothers of older nursing toddlers.)

PREFERRED HERBS FOR BREAST AND NIPPLE PROBLEMS

Engorgement - Cabbage

Cabbage is used to relieve the pain and tenderness of engorgement. Sulphur compounds and flavonoids are the likely constituents able to affect the apparent anti-inflammatory, anti-edematous effects. Sulphur compounds may increase skin penetration by plant constituents through the skin. Cabbage leaves have been found to work as well as cold packs for symptomatic relief (Rossier, 1998; Roberts, 1995). When mothers used cabbage and cold packs together, one on each breast, they reported a significant and equal degree of pain reduction for each treatment, but preferred the cabbage leaves (Roberts, 1995). Other studies found cabbage more pain-relieving than cold packs (Nikodem *et al.*, 1993). Cabbage leaf remains popular with a large body of case reports and anecdotes supporting its complementary use for engorgement. The proteolytic enzyme combination, bromelain/trypsin, has been found to relieve engorgement (Low Dog & Micozzi, 2005). No comparison of cabbage versus proteolytic enzymes has yet been done. There is speculative concern that cabbage has anti-galactogogue activity, so extended use could lead to loss of milk supply. Lactation failure as a consequence of extended, unrelieved engorgement resulting from lack of milk removal would be a more likely possibility. Allergy to cabbage family proteins (Dannaker & White, 1987) and hypersensitivity to isothyocyanates (released from the chopped plant) is known (Focke *et al.*, 1998). No documented evidence was found that sulfa allergy predicts cabbage allergy.

Thrush - Myrrh *(Commiphora molmol)*

Nipple thrush can be treated by anti-fungal pharmaceuticals when applied locally to the nipple and to the baby's mouth, though non-prescription formulations may contain substances not suitable for infant ingestion. Gentian violet, a synthetic chemical, and mupirocin are widely used clinically. In herbal medicine, myrrh has long been used for thrush, but has not yet been studied. The gum resin is anti-inflammatory, astringent, vulnerary, and anti-candidal (Newall *et al.*, 1997). Given the antiquity of documented use and extensive current use in herbal medicine, it is surprising how few human studies have been done. A recent study documents its utility as a local antiseptic (El Ashry *et al.*, 2003). German health authorities (Blumenthal *et al.*, 1998) approved myrrh for oral inflammations. A German pediatric herbal medicine textbook (Schilcher, 1997) suggests myrrh for thrush - a 1:1 tincture of myrrh diluted 1:2 or 1:3 with boiled water, applied with cotton swabs to the baby's mouth. For nipples, a 1:1 dilution has been suggested (Low Dog & Micozzi, 2005). Myrrh is a gum resin and must be extracted in 80-90% alcohol; dilution of the tincture before use avoids tissue irritation. Infant treatment in this manner appears safe (Low Dog & Micozzi, 2005). Myrrh is considered non-toxic, non-sensitizing, and non-allergenic (Newall *et al.*, 1997). Mothers must be very clear on how to use myrrh tincture appropriately due to the high alcohol content.

Tea tree oil (*Melaleuca alternifolia*) and black walnut (*Juglans nigra*) have potentially toxic effects (Newall *et al.*, 1997) and they should not be used on the nipple where a young infant may ingest them. Grapefruit seed extracts have no traditional use to back their use in nursing mothers. Contamination of most brands of grapefruit seed extract with synthetic toxic antiseptics has been found (Ganzera *et al.*, 2006). The extract is bitter to taste and potentially sensitizing. Use on nipples should be avoided.

Mastitis - Garlic, Echinacea *(Echinacea species)*

These herbs can be used to complement basic lactation management of mastitis. The immune-boosting and anti-infective properties of garlic are well documented (Koch & Lawson, 1996). The use of garlic to prevent and fight infections is ancient and global. Garlic contains wide-spectrum anti-biotic activity, including activity against *Staph* species and *Candida albicans* (Blumenthal *et al.*, 1998; Newall *et al.*, 1997). While some herbal literature has suggested garlic be contraindicated during lactation (McGuffin *et al*, 1997), no serious adverse effects are known to occur. While there are reports that direct feeding of freshly crushed garlic has resulted in infant death (McGuffin *et al*, 1997), no severe reactions are seen when babies are exposed to the much smaller doses through milk. Onions and garlic can cause GI upset or colic in some babies as it can in sensitive adults (Mohrbacher & Stock, 2003). One study has demonstrated that babies will nurse longer when milk has a garlic flavor (Menella & Beauchamp, 1993). Garlic should not be used in conjunction with blood-thinners or before surgery (McKenna, 2001).

Echinacea is thought to stimulate the immune system, thus strengthening the body's own defenses to fight off infections. The German government approved the use of *Echinacea pallida* root tincture and *E. purpurea* aerial parts as expressed juice for viral infections (Blumenthal *et al*, 1998). Echinacea products in North America vary in quality (Blumenthal *et al.*, 2003). Using herbs, such as echinacea and garlic, to complement antibiotic drugs is common, though research is needed to explore interaction or efficacy. Short-term antibiotic therapy to prevent neonatal sepsis at birth is standard practice. It has been suggested (Lactnet) that prophylactic dietary use of garlic and probiotics (Lactobacillus, yogurt) may prevent mastitis and thrush. Research is clearly indicated. Appropriate antibiotic treatment remains the primary intervention to treat bacterial mastitis in order to prevent abscess and other serious consequences. Reliance on herbal remedies alone to treat serious, acute conditions, such as mastitis or abscess, should be avoided, although some mothers may still choose this course. Clear communication of risks with the mother and ensuring proper lactation management and follow-up support is vital.

Pokeweed (*Phytolacca americana*) has been used, dangerously, to treat mastitis by American herbalists. The plant has significant potential for toxicity and should be avoided (Duke, 1985).

Nipple Trauma - Calendula

Any nipple preparation should be non-toxic, non-sensitizing, non-allergenic, and not bitter. Colostrum remains the preferred topical treatment and correction of the latch remains the primary intervention. Calendula (*Calendula officinalis*) flower petals may be used to complement basic lactation management of nipple trauma. The petals contain triterpenes, flavonoids, carotenoids, and essential oils and are considered anti-inflammatory, anti-microbial, and vulnerary. The plant is non-toxic, non-sensitizing, and non-allergenic (Newall *et al.*, 1997; Blumenthal *et al.*, 1998). Calendula was approved for external wound healing in Germany (Blumenthal *et al.*, 1998). The dried petals can be moistened and applied as a poultice or the tea used to make cool compresses. Commercial calendula cream preparations contain multiple ingredients that should be reviewed before use. German chamomile (*Matricaria recutita*) is also used for sore nipples, although a slight risk of allergic reaction may exist. It has been approved for external skin and mucous membrane inflammations and irritations by the German Commission E.

On the other hand, Roman chamomile (*Chamaemelum nobile*) is allergenic and associated with two cases of contact dermatitis of the nipple (McGeorge & Steele, 1991). Roman chamomile was not approved by the German Commission E due to a lack of evidence and incidents of anaphylaxis with use (Blumenthal *et al.*, 1998).

One study found an association with mastitis and nipple creams, especially those containing papaya (Low Dog & Micozzi, 2005). Using black tea bags for nipple trauma is controversial. One study found black tea bags used four times a day as effective as water compresses and superior to placebo (LaVergne, 1997). However, black tea is bitter and infants may develop aversion. Green tea is much milder and has superior antioxidant, anti-inflammatory effects as Low Dog discussed in her textbook (2005). Further study of green tea and other strongly anti-inflammatory, anti-bacterial herbs is clearly indicated.

ANTI-LACTAGOGUES

No studies exist to either support or refute the use of sage, parsley, or peppermint to reduce milk supply. Their use is evidenced by a long history of traditional use for weaning (Humphrey, 2003). Current clinical experience is mixed, even for sage, which has the strongest traditional reputation (Low Dog & Micozzi, 2005).

The possibility that certain herbs can indeed lower supply is bolstered by experimental study of jasmine flowers (*Jasminum officinale*), traditionally used in India for rapid weaning. In women suffering fetal demise, jasmine flowers were compared with bromocryptine (Shrivastav *et al.*, 1988). Women were randomly assigned to either receive bromocryptine 2.5 mg every eight hours for five days or a garland of fresh jasmine flowers taped to the breast and refreshed daily for five days. No control group was used. After five days, prolactin levels decreased significantly in both groups, though more so for the bromocryptine group. Hand expression produced similar volumes in each group and engorgement ratings were also similar. An earlier study (Abraham *et al.*, 1979) had demonstrated inhibited milk production and involution of breast tissue following jasmine flower contact by lactating mice. These studies deserve follow-up to determine jasmine's impact on lactation, given its popularity as an essential oil. A recent controlled study of jasmine demonstrated improved sleep, mood, and cognitive function in college students exposed to jasmine odor (Raudenbush *et al.*, 2003).

Large doses of fresh parsley is reputed to lower milk supply, intentionally and unintentionally. Unconfirmed reports of reduced milk supply are associated with tabouli salad made with large amounts of fresh parsley and "green drinks" made with parsley juice. Fresh parsley is remarkable for its relatively high apigenin content (225 mg/kg), according to the USDA database (USDA, 2006). Apigenin is phytoestrogenic and a very strong aromatase inhibitor, compared to other flavones or isoflavones (Rice *et al.*, 2006).

While peppermint leaf is not noted to lead to milk supply problems, peppermint essential oil is reported to reduce oversupply (Humphrey, 2003). There are historic descriptions of camphor and menthol applied externally to reduce engorgement with weaning (Ellingwood, 1919). Infants exposed to the strong odors of peppermint essential oil or menthol ointments may react with breathing difficulties. Cases of respiratory collapse are described with application to the face or nares of infants (Duke, 1985; Burkhard *et al.*, 1999).

Sage (*Salvia officinalis*) is commonly used as a food spice and due to the presence of thujone, content standards have been set. Internal use of 3-6 g/day of the crude powdered herb given in divided doses was approved by German authorities (Blumenthal *et al.*, 1998) for dyspepsia and excessive perspiration. The Commission did not contraindicate the use of the whole herb during pregnancy or lactation. Although it is a widely reputed weaning aide, Commission E did not specifically address this use. No studies have been done to determine its anti-lactogogue effects. Thujone, with cineol and camphor, are the principle components of the essential oil. Essential oil extracts of sage should never be used internally as they cause seizures. Avoidance with tincture forms may be warranted as well. The whole herb also contains tannins, caffeic acids, including rosmarinic acid, diterpene bitter principle, triterpenes, steroids, flavones, including apigenin and luteolin, and other flavonoids. In crude form, no adverse effects have been noted in humans using medicinal doses (Blumenthal *et al.*, 1998). It is important to use in divided doses. Overdose symptoms (sensation of heat, vertigo) are known with single doses over 15 grams (Duke, 1985). Doses used to slow milk production range from ¼ teaspoon to 1 tablespoon (0.75 g) per dose repeated up to six times per day (Humphrey, 2003). The higher dose range should probably be restricted to rapid weaning.

Colic Treatments

Colic places enormous stress on parents and has been identified as a trigger for postpartum depression. A number of recent infant colic studies have demonstrated safety and efficacy for a number of herbal combination preparations (Savino *et al.*, 2005; Alexandrovich *et al.*, 2003; Weizman *et al.*, 1993), though adverse events are also documented (Sas *et al.*, 2004; Minodier *et al.*, 2003) as expected with direct feeding of herbal preparations to young infants. Aromatic herbs, such as fennel, anise, dill, caraway, and catnip (*Nepeta cataria*) are traditionally also taken by the mother to treat her infant's colic. This option is described in the ethnobotanical and western herbalist literature (Gladstar, 2001; Humphrey, 2003), but has not yet been investigated. Yet, for the exclusively breastfed child, this route minimizes risks. For example, fennel contains a toxic essential oil constituent, estragole, which is metabolized on first pass through the liver (McGuffin *et al.*, 1997), thus avoiding infant exposure. The active volatile essential oils likely penetrate the milk compartment easily.

POSTPARTUM DEPRESSION

St. John's Wort (*Hypericum perforatum*) has been shown to be as efficacious and to have fewer side effects in trials of side-by-side comparison to prescription anti-depressants (Hale, 2006). A recent double blinded prospective trial comparing Paxil® for patients with acute moderate-to-severe depression found both more effective than a placebo, but St. John's wort had fewer side effects (Szegedi *et al.*, 2005). The anti-depressant effect derives from a growing list of identified active constituents: the napthadianthrones - hypericin and hyperforin, and more recently the more ubiquitous flavones - quercitin and rutin (Wurglics & Schubert-Zsilavecz, 2006).

Studies with breastfeeding women are few. A prospective cohort observational study was done with 33 breastfeeding women using St. John's wort for postpartum depression. The researchers followed mothers who had contacted a Canadian teratogen/toxicant counseling service (Motherwise), seeking safety information about St. John's wort (Lee *et al.*, 2003). The study found no significant negative effects for mothers. No significant differences with infant weight gain at one year or change in milk supply were seen in comparison to two control groups: a disease-matched group (n=101) and an age and parity-matched, non-disease matched group (n=33). However, maternal reports of infant "colic" (2) and "lethargy" (1) were significantly increased in the study group using St. John's wort. The three mothers sought medical evaluation, but no specific treatment was required for their infants. It is surprising that out of a total of 134 babies in the control groups, there were only two reports of colic. One would expect more. One report of lethargy among the entire study group is not much above what one would find surveying hundreds of mothers. A much bigger study is, of course, needed.

The German Commission E (Blumenthal *et al.*, 1998) did not contraindicate use during lactation and animal lactation studies do not show adverse effects (Low Dog & Micozzi, 2005). Given the accumulated evidence, St. John's wort appears to be a reasonable choice for treatment of postpartum depression. A detailed consideration of complementary and alternative therapies for postpartum depression is recommended reading (Low Dog & Micozzi, 2005). Any recommendation for use of St. John's wort for such a serious condition as postpartum depression necessitates the use of only the highest quality products, preferably those evaluated in European trials (Blumenthal *et al.*, 2003; Barrett, 2004).

HERBS AND INFLAMMATION

Herbal and dietary sources of flavonoids may protect the milk supply. The School of Hippocrates, 400 CE, is famous for writing, "Let food be your medicine and medicine be your food." Diet is indeed a basis for health and modern research is rapidly uncovering how the complex array of constituents in our food assists the body to work well. Beyond the constituents long identified as essential are the complexes of secondary products of plant metabolism that give color, fragrance, and flavor to our foods, which are now being studied for their many contributions to health maintenance. In particular, the flavonoid plant constituents are now intensely studied for their role in the reduction of inflammatory states. As engorgement and mastitis are inflammatory states, herbs with particularly strong anti-inflammatory actions may be beneficial, so a further discussion of flavonoids is warranted.

Some food plants and many herbs are very rich sources of flavonoids (USDA, 2006). This extremely common and diverse class of plant constituents function as plant pigments, taking their name from the Latin *flavus*, meaning yellow, though not all types are yellow or even have color. Flavonoids are polyphenolic compounds, having a single benzene ring joined to a benzo-gamma-pyrone structure, and are further classified into several groups: flavanones, flavanonols, flavonols, leucoanthocyanidins, catechins, chalcones, aurones, and isoflavones. Other closely related anti-inflammatory compounds include the red, blue or purple anthocyanidins that lend color to blueberries and cranberries for example. Flavonoids play an important role in reducing the negative consequences of fluid stasis in tissues (Mills & Bone, 1999). As mixed moities, they have been shown to strengthen fragile capillary membranes by improving the surrounding connective tissue tone. They work with and extend the beneficial effects of Vitamin C. They are thought to help prevent edema associated with inflammation and fluid stasis. Flavonoids inhibit some key enzymes involved in the inflammatory process, including xanthine oxidase (XO). Products of XO enzymatic activity, uric acid and superoxide radicals, produce inflammation in fluid stasis. Recent structure-activity work has identified which flavonoid structures inhibit XO, which are only anti-oxidant, and which do both (Cos *et al.*, 1998). Almost all tested flavones and to a smaller degree flavonols were XO inhibitors. XO has long been known to occur in high concentration within the lactating breast. It is now thought to play a vital structural role in the formation of milk fat globules during milk synthesis (McManaman *et al.*, 2004). A study of mice with defective XO found them unable to maintain milk production due to failure of micelle formation (Vorbach *et al.*, 2002). It is tempting to speculate that dietary flavonoids may directly assist milk production by maintaining XO in a structural state. Through inhibition of XO enzyme activity, flavonoids may also further reduce breast inflammation during periods of milk stasis. A correlation of low inflammatory states in the body with a high diversity flavonoid intake has recently been demonstrated in women (Thompson *et al.*, 2006). This study found differing oxidative biomarker levels with two diet regimes in women. The control diet contained five plant families versus a diet drawing on 18 plant families, which manipulated the range of flavonoids and carotenoids. The low diversity diet had larger amounts of certain types of flavonoids and reduced inflammation, but not as much as the diet with more diverse flavonoids, even though the amount of any one flavonoid was smaller. Increasing the intake and diversity of flavonoid-rich plants may assist those women prone to severe engorgement or inflammatory mastitis with subsequent low milk supply. No information regarding flavonoid or uric acid content of human milk could be found, other than measures of low milk entry for the chemically related isoflavones (Franke *et al.*, 1998).

CO-EVOLUTION OF PLANTS AND MAMMALS

Human lactation is perhaps the essential element in ancient infant survival and like other mammalian features co-evolved with plants. Our mammalian ancestors not only ate plants to survive, but survived the eating of plants. Plants have probably evolved a complex array of secondary compounds in order to deter herbivores, and animals evolved many adaptations in order to survive. In humans, exclusive breastfeeding for six months delays the need for direct plant consumption by the extremely immature human infant while providing frequent small doses of vitamins, minerals, and anti-inflammatory constituents derived mainly from the plants in the mother's diet, along with the essential macronutrients and immune factors critical for survival. Lactation would strongly favor infant survival when a mother naively consumed potentially toxic plants or was forced to depend on them in times of starvation. The consumption of colostrum may have been more hazardous under such conditions. The effects of plant toxin accumulation in the neonate could well have inspired the custom of colostrum avoidance.

Future research about herbs and breastfeeding will find the theory of coevolution of plants and humans a fruitful path of study. While not specifically addressing lactation in his book, Johns (1990) has developed a useful theoretical framework for such future research.

References

Abraham M, Devi NS, Sheela R. Inhibiting effect of jasmine flowers on lactation. *Indian J Med Res.* 1979; 69:88-92.

Agrawala P, Achar MVS, *et al.* Galactogogue action of Cuminum cyminum and Nigella sativa. *Indian J Med Res.* 1968; 56(6):841-44.

Agrawala P, Achar MVS, *et al.* Galactogogue action of Nigella sativa. *Indian J Med Res.* 1971; 25(8):535-37.

Alexandrovich I, Rakovitskaya O, Kolmo E, Sidorova T, Shushunov S. The effect of fennel (Foeniculum Vulgare) seed oil emulsion in infantile colic: a randomized, placebo-controlled study. *Altern Ther Health Med.* 2003; 9(4):58-61.

Academy of Breastfeeding Medicine. Protocol # 9: Galactogogues. Available from: www.bfmed.org. Accessed 12-11-06.

Aradhana, Rao AR, Kale RK. Diosgenin - a growth stimulator of mammary gland of ovariectomized mouse. *Indian J Exp Biol.* 1992; 5:367-70.

Atanasov AT, Tchorbanov B. Anti-platelet fraction from Galega officinalis L. inhibits platelet aggregation. *J Med Food.* 2002; 5(4):229-34.

Ayers JF. The use of alternative therapy in the support of breastfeeding. *J Hum Lact.* 2000; 1:52-56.

Barrett M (ed). *Handbook of clinically tested herbal remedies. Vol 2.* Binghampton, NY: Haworth Herbal Press; 2004.

Behall KM, Scholfield DJ, Hallfrisch J. Comparison of hormone and glucose responses of overweight women to barley and oats. *J Am Coll Nutr.* 2005; 24(3):182-88.

Betzold CM. Galactogogues. *J Midwifery Womens Health.* 2004; 49(2):151-54.

Bingel AS, Farnsworth NR. Higher plants as potential sources of galactogogues. In: Wagner H, Hikino H, Farnsworth NR (eds.). *Economic and medicinal plant research.* Vol 6. New York, NY: Academic Press; 1994. pp. 1-54.

Bisset NG (ed.). *Herbal drugs and phytopharmaceuticals: A handbook for practice on a scientific basis.* Boca Raton, LA: CRC Press; 1994.

Blumenthal M, Brinkermann J, Wollschlaeger B (eds.). *The ABC clinical guide to herbs.* Austin, TX: American Botanical Council; 2003.

Blumenthal M, Gruenwald J, Hall T, Riggins CW, Rister RS (eds). *German Commission E monographs: Therapeutic monographs on medicinal plants for human use.* Austin, TX: American Botanical Council; 1998.

Booth N, Nikolic D, van Breemen R, *et al.* Confusion regarding anticoagulant coumarins in dietary supplements. *Clin Pharmacol Therap.* 2004; 76(6):511-16.

Broca C, Breil V, Cruciani-Guglielmacci C, *et al.* Insulinotropic agent ID-1101 (4-hydroxyisoleucine) activates insulin signaling in rat. *Am J Physiol Endocrinol Metab.* 2004; 287(3): E463-71. Epub 2004 Apr 13.

Broca C, Gross R, Petit P, Sauvaire Y, *et al.* 4-Hydroxyisoleucine: experimental evidence of its insulinotropic and antidiabetic properties. *Am J Physiol.* 1999; 277(4 Pt 1):E617-23.

Brown D. Standardized butterbur extract for migraine treatment: a clinical overview. *Herbalgram.* 2003; 58:18-19.

Bruckner C. Use and value of common European lactation-promoting medicinal plants (galactogogues). *Padiatr Grensgeb.* 1989; 28(6):403-10.

Burkhard PR, Burkhardt K, Haenggeli CA, Landis T. Plant-induced seizures: reappearance of an old proble. *J Neurol.* 1999; 246(8):667-70.

Choudhary D, Chandra D, Choudhary S, Kale RK. Modulation of glyoxalase, glutathione S-transferase and antioxidant enzymes in the liver, spleen and erythrocytes of mice by dietary administration of fenugreek seeds. *Food Chem Toxicol.* 2001; 39(10):989-97.

Co MM, Hernandez EA, Co BG. A comparative study on the efficacy of the different galactogogues among mothers with lactational insufficiency. Abstract, AAP Section on Breastfeeding, NCE; November, 2002.

Cos P, Ying L, *et al.* Structure-activity relationship and classification of flavonoids as inhibitors of xanthine oxidase and superoxide scavengers. *J Nat Prod.* 1998; 61(1):71-76.

da Costa KA, Kozyreva OG, Song J, Galanko JA, Fischer LM, Zeisel SH. Common genetic polymorphisms affect the human requirement for the nutrient choline. *FASEB J.* 2006; 20(9):1336-44.

Damanik R, Wahlqvist ML, Wattanapenpaiboon N. Lactagogue effects of Torbangun, a Bataknese traditional cuisine. *Asia Pac J Clin Nutr.* 2006; 15(2):267-74.

Danesch U, Rittinghausen R. Safety of a patented special butterbur root extract for migraine prevention. *Headache.* 2003; 43(1):76-78.

Dannaker CJ, White IR. Cutaneous allergy to mustard in a salad maker. *Contact Dermatitis.* 1987; 16(4):212-14.

De Smet PAGM. Overview of herbal quality control. *Drug Information J.* 1999; 33:717-24.

De Smet PAGM. Safety of borage seed oil. *Can Pharm J.* 1991; 124:5.

Duke JA. *Handbook of medicinal herbs.* 2nd Ed. Boca Raton: CRC Press; 2002.

Duke JA. *Handbook of phytochemical constituents of GRAS herbs and other economic plants.* Boca Raton: CRC Press; 1992.

Duke JA. *Handbook of medicinal herbs.* 1st Ed. Boca Raton: CRC Press; 1985.

El Ashry ES, Rashed N, Salama OM, *et al.* Components, therapeutic value and uses of myrrh. *Pharmazie.* 2003; 58:163-68.

Ellingwood F. *American materia medica, therapeutics and pharmacognosy 1919.* Sandy, OR: Eclectic Medical Publications; 1983 facsimile edition.

Ernst E. Herbal remedies for anxiety – a systematic review of controlled clinical trials. *Phytomed.* 2006; 13:205-8.

Farnsworth NR. Relative safety of herbal medicines. *Herbalgram.* 1993; 29: 36A-H. Classic Reprint.

Farnsworth N, Bingel AS, Cordell GA, Crane FA, Fong HS. Potential value of plants as sources of new antifertility agents. Part I. *J Pharm Sciences.* 1975a; 64(5): 535-98.

Farnsworth N, Bingel AS, Cordell GA, Crane FA, Fong HS. Potential value of plants as sources of new antifertility agents. Part II. *J Pharm Sciences.* 1975b; 64(5):717-54.

Felter SP, Vassallo JD, Carlton BD, Daston GP. A safety assessment of coumarin taking into account species-specificity of toxicokinetics. *Food Chem Toxicol.* 2006; 44:462-75.

FDA. Nature's Way Products, Inc. recall nettle because of possible health risk. Springville, UT: Nature's Way Products; [originated 2002 June 28; cited 2006 Oct. 30]. Available from: www.fda.gov/oc/po/firmrecalls/nettle06_02.html.

Feltrow CW, Avila JR. *Professional's handbook of complementary & alternative medicines.* Springhouse, PA: Springhouse Corporation; 1999.

Flammang AM, Cifone MA, Erexson GL, Stankowski LF Jr. Genotoxicity testing of a fenugreek extract. *Food Chem Toxicol.* 2004; 42(11):1769-75.

Focke M, Hemmer W, Hayek B, *et al.* Identification of allergens in oilseed rape (Brassica napus) pollen. *Int Arch Allergy Immunol.* 1998; 117(2):105-12.

Franke AA, Custer LJ, Tanaka Y. Isoflavones in human breast milk and other biological fluids. *Am J Clin Nutr.* 1998; 68(6 Suppl):1466S-73S.

Ganzera M, Aberham A, Stuppner H. Development and validation of an HPLC/UV/MS method for simultaneous determination of 18 preservatives in grapefruit seed extract. *J Agric Food Chem.* 2006; 54(11):3768-72.

Gladstar R. *Rosemary Gladstar's family herbal.* North Adams, Massachusetts: Storey Books; 2001.

Gonzalez-Andres F, Redondo PA, Pescador R, Urbano B. Management of Galega officinalis L. and preliminary results on its potential for milk production improvement in sheep. *New Zealand Journal of Agricultural Research.* 2004; 47(2):233-45.

Goyal RK, Singh J, Lal H. Asparagus racemosus – an update. *Indian J Med Sci.* 2003; 57(9);408-14.

Gruenwald J, Brendler T, Jaenicke C (eds). *PDR for herbal medicines.* 2nd Ed. Montvale, NJ: Medical Economics Co; 2000.

Habel SK, *et al.* (eds). Fenugreek. In: *The Lawrence review of natural products.* St Louis: Wolters Klewer; 1996.

Hale TW. *Medications and mother's milk.* 12th Ed. Amarillo, TX: Pharmasoft Publishing; 2006.

Heiss H. Clinical and experimental contribution on the question of the lactogenic effect of Galega officinalis. *Wein Med Wochenschr.* 1968; 118(24):546-8. English translation: H Jacobson, pers comm.

Hoffman D. *The new holistic herbal.* 3rd Ed. Rockport, MA: Element Books; 1992.

Huggins K. *The nursing mother's companion.* 4th Ed. Boston: Harvard Common Press; 1999.

Huggins KE. Fenugreek: One remedy for low milk production. *Medela Rental Round-up.* 1998; 15(1):16-17.

Humphrey S. *The nursing mother's herbal.* Minneapolis, MN: Fairview Press; 2003.

Jacobson H. *Motherfoods.* 2004. Available from: www.mother-food.com.

Jarry H, Leonhardt S, Gorkow C, Wuttke W. In vitro prolactin but not LH and FSH release is inhibited by compounds in extracts of Agnus Castus: direct evidence for a dopaminergic principle by the dopamine receptor assay. *Exp Clin Endocrinol.* 1994; 102:448-54.

Johns T. *The origins of human diet and medicine: chemical ecology.* Tucson: University of Arizona Press; 1990.

Kaplan M, Vreman HJ, *et al.* Favism by proxy in nursing glucose-6-phosphate dehydrogenase-deficient neonates. *J Perinatol.* 1998; 18(6 Pt 1):477-79.

Kapoor LD. *CRC Handbook of ayurvedic medicinal plants.* Boca Raton: CRC; 1990.

Koch HP, Lawson LD (eds.). *Garlic: The science and therapeutic application of Allium sativum L. and related species.* 2nd Ed. Baltimore: Williams & Wilkins Publishing Co; 1996.

Kohler H. Researches on *Galega* species regarding their content of toxins by means of biological methods. I. Toxicity of goat's rue (*Galega officinalis* L.) for warmblooded animals. *Biol Zbl.* 1969; 88:165-77.

Kristiansson B, Abdul Ghani N, Eriksson M, Garle M, Qirbi A. Use of khat in lactating women: a pilot study on breast-milk secretion. *J Ethnopharmacol.* 1987; 21(1):85-90.

LaVergne NE. Does application of tea bags to sore nipples while breastfeeding provide effective relief? *J Obstet Gynecol Neonatal Nurs.* 1997; 26(1):53-58.

Lee A, Minhas R, Matsuda N, *et al.* The safety of St. John's wort (Hypericum perforatum) during breastfeeding. *J Clin Psychiatry.* 2003; 64:966-68.

Lompo-Ouedraogo Z, van der Heide D, *et al.* Effect of aqueous extract of Acacia nilotica spp adansonii on milk production and prolactin release in the rat. *J Endocrinol.* 2004;182(2): 257-66.

Low Dog T, Micozzi MS. *Women's health in complementary and integrative medicine: a clinical guide.* St. Louis, MO: Elsevier; 2005.

Luqman W, Danowski DS. The use of khat (Catha edulis) in Yemen. Social and medical observations. *Annals Internal Medicine.* 1976; 85:246-49. Available from: http://members.aol.com/yalnet/KHAT.html. Accessed Nov 1, 2006.

Marasko L, Marmet C, Shell E. Polycystic ovary syndrome: a connection to insufficient milk supply? *J Hum Lact.* 2000; 16(2):143-48.

Marles RJ, Farnsworth NR. Antidiabetic plants and their active constituents. *Phytomedicine.* 1995; 2(2): 137-89.

McGeorge BCL, Steele MC. Allergic contact dermatitis of the nipple from Roman chamomile ointment. *Contact Derm.* 1991; 24:139-40.

McGuffin M, Hobbs C, Upton R, Goldberg A, (eds). *Botanical safety handbook: Guidelines for the safe use and labelling for herbs in commerce.* Boca Raton, FL: CRC Press; 1997.

McKenna D (ed). *Botanical medicines: the desk reference for major herbal supplements.* Binghamton, NY: Haworth Press; 2001.

McManaman JL, Palmer CA, Anderson S, Schwertfeger K, Neville MC. Regulation of milk lipid formation and secretion in the mouse mammary gland. *Adv Exp Med Biol.* 2004; 554:263-79.

Meier B, Berger D, Hoberg E, Sticher O, Schaffner W. Pharmacological activities of Vitex agnus-castus extracts in vitro. *Phytomedicine.* 2000; 7(5):373-81.

Mennella JA, Beauchamp GK. The effects of repeated exposure to garlic-flavored milk on the nursling's behavior. *Pediatric Res.* 1993; 34: 805-8.

Merz PG, Gorkow C, Schrodter A, Rietbrock S, Sieder C, Loew D, *et al.* The effects of a special Agnus castus extract (BP1095E1) on prolactin secretion in healthy male subjects. *Exp Clin Endocrinol Diabetes.* 1996; 104(6):447-53.

Mills S, Bone K. *Principles and practice of phytotherapy.* Edinburgh: Churchill Livingstone; 1999.

Minodier P, Pommier P, Moulene E, Retornaz K, Prost N, Deharo L. Star anise poisoning in infants. *Arch Pediatr.* 2003; 10(7):619-21.

Mohrbacher N, Stock J. *The breastfeeding answer book.* 3rd Ed. Schaumburg IL: La Leche League International; 2003.

Nambiar S, Schwartz RH, Constantino A. Hypertension in mother and baby linked to ingestion of Chinese herbal medicine (letter). *West J Med.* 1999; 171(3):152.

NAPRALERT. Natural products alert *Galega officinale.* Chicago: University of Illinois at Chicago Program for Collaborative Research in the Pharmaceutical Sciences;. cited 2006 Nov 24. Available from: www.napralert.org.

Newall CA, Anderson LA, Phillipson JD. *Herbal medicines: A guide for health-care professionals.* London: The Pharmaceutical Press; 1996.

Newman J, Pitman T. *The ultimate breastfeeding book of answers.* Rocklin, CA: Prima Publishing; 2000.

Nice, FJ, Coghlan RJ, and Birmingham BT: Herbals and breastfeeding. *U.S. Pharmacist.* 2000; 25: 28, 31-32, 34, 41-42, 45-46. Available from: http://www.uspharmacist.com/oldformat.asp?url=newlook/files/comp/acf1e63.htm.

Nikodem VC, Danziger D, Gebka N, Gulmezoglu AM, Hofmeyr GJ. Do cabbage leaves prevent breast engorgement? A randomized controlled study. *Birth.* 1993; 20(2):61-64.

Palit P, Furman BL, Gray AI. Novel weight-reducing activity of *Galega officinalis* in mice. *J Pharm Pharmacol.* 1999;51(11):1313-19.

Pansatiankul BJ, Mekmanee R. Dicumarol (sic) content in alcoholic herb elixers: one of the factors at risk induced IVKD-I. *SE Asian J Trop Med Public Health.* 1993; 24 Suppl 1:201-3.

Patisaul HB, Whitten PL, Young LJ. Regulation of estrogen receptor beta mRNA in the brain: opposite effects of 17beta-estradiol and the phytoestrogen, coumestrol. *Brain Res Mol Brain Res.* 1999; 67(1):165-71.

Pothmann R, Danesch U. Migraine prevention in children and adolscents; results of an open study with a special butterbur root extract. *Headache.* 2005; 45(3):196-203.

Pundarikakshudu K, Patel JK,Bodar MS, Deans SG. Anti-bacterial activity of Galega officinalis L. (Goat's Rue). *J Ethnopharmacol.* 2001;77(1):111-12.

Puri HS. *Rasayana: Ayurvedic herbs for longevity and rejuvenation.* London: Taylor & Francis; 2003.

Randall K, Lever M, Peddie BA, Chambers ST. Natural and synthetic betaines counter the effects of high NaCl and urea concentrations. *Biochim Biophys Acta.* 1996;1291(3):189-94.

Rasekh H, Hoseinzadeh I, *et al.* Acute toxicity of Galega officinalis alcoholic extract in wistar rats. Poster abstract. M2nd International Congress on Traditional Medicine and Materia Medica. *Journal of Pharmaceutical Research.* 2004; Supplement 2:45-45.

Raudenbush B, Koon J, *et al.* Effects of odorant administration of objective and subjective measures of sleep quality, post-sleep mood and altertness, and cognitive performance. *North Am J Psychol.* 2003; 5(2):181-92.

Remington JP, Wood HC, *et al.* (eds.). The dispensary of the United States of America. 1918. Finland: Henriette Kress; [updated 2005 Oct 7; cited 2006 Nov 25]. Available from: www.henriettesherbal.com/eclectic/usdisp/galega.html.

Rendell M, Vanderhoof J, *et al.* Effect of a barley breakfast cereal on blood glucose and insulin response in normal and diabetic patients. *Plant Foods Hum Nutr.* 2005; 60(2):63-67.

Renfree C. Herbal galactagogue use for the breastfeeding mother. Scottsdale, Arizona: ILCA Conference; 2004.

Rice S, Mason HD, Whitehead SA. Phytoestrogens and their low dose combinations inhibit mRNA expression and activity of aromatase in human granulosa-luteal cells. *J Steroid Biochem Mol Biol.* 2006; 101(4-5):216-25. Epub 2006 Sep 11.

Robbers JE, Tyler VE. *Tyler's herbs of choice: the therapeutic use of phytomedicinals.*: Birmingham, NY: The Hawthorn Herbal Press; 1999.

Roberge RJ, Leckey R, Spence R, Krenzelok EJ. Garlic burns of the breast (letter). *Am J Emer Med.* 1997;15(5):548.

Roberts K. A comparison of chilled cabbage leaves and chilled gelpaks in reducing breast engorgement. *J Human Lact.* 1995; 11(1):17-20.

Rossier W. Cool cabbage compresses. *Breastfeed Rev.* 1988; 12:28-31.

Rosti L, Nardini A, Bettinelli ME, Rosti D. Toxic effects of a herbal tea mixture in two newborns(letter). *Acta Paediatrica.* 1994; 83(6):683.

Rudolph MC, McManaman J, Phang T, Russell T, Kominsky DJ, Serkova NJ, *et al.* Metabolic regulation in the lactating mammary gland: A lipid synthesizing machine. *Physiol Genomics.* 2006; Nov 14 [Epub ahead of print].

Sas D, Enrione MA, Schwartz RH. Pseudomonas aeruginosa septic shock secondary to "gripe water" ingestion. *Pediatr Infect Dis J.* 2004; 23(2):176-77.

Savino F, Cresi F, *et al.* A randomized double-blind placebo-controlled trial of a standardized extract of *Matricariae recutita, Foeniculum vulgare* and *Melissa officinalis* (ColiMil) in the treatment of breastfed colicky infants. *Phytother Res.* 2005; 19(4):335-40.

Schilcher H. *Phytotherapy in paediatrics: Handbook for physicians and pharmacists.* Stuttgart: Medpharm Scientific Publishers; 1997.

Sharma S, Ramji S, *et al.* Randomized controlled trial of Asparagus racemosa (shatavari) as a lactogogue in lactational inadequacy. *Indian Pediatr.* 1996; 33:675-77.

Sharma, PV. *Classical uses of medicinal plants.* Varanasi India: Chaukhambha Visvabharati Publishers;1996.

Shrivastav P, George K, Balasubramaniam N, Jasper MP, Thomas M, Kanagasabhapathy AS. Suppression of puerperal lactation using jasmine flowers (Jasminum sambac). *Aust NZ J Obstet Gynaecol.* 1988; 28(1):68-71.

Sliutz G, Speiser P, Schultz AM, *et al.* Agnus castus extracts inhibit prolactin secretion of rat pituitary cells. *Hormone Metab Res.* 1993; 25:253-55.

Suboh SM, Bilto YY, Aburjai TA. Protective effects of selected medicinal plants against protein degradation, lipid peroxidation and deformability loss of oxidatively stressed human erythrocytes. *Phytother Res.* 2004; 18(4):280-84.

Swafford S, Berens P. Effect of fenugreek on breast milk volume. Meeting Abstract. *ABM News and Views.* 2000; 6(3):2000.

Szegedi A, Kohnen R, Dienel A, Kieser M. Acute treatment of moderate to severe depression with hypericum extract WS5570 (St John's wort): randomized controlled double blind non-inferiority trial versus paroxetine. *BMJ.* 2005; 330:503.

Tahiliani P, Kar A. Mitigation of thyroxine-induced hyperglycaemia by two plant extracts. *Phytother Res.* 2003a; 17(3):294-96.

Tahiliani P, Kar A. The combined effects of Trigonella and Allium extracts in the regulation of hyperthyroidism in rats. *Phytomedicine.* 2003b; 10(8):665-68.

Teas J, Pino S, Critchley A, Braverman LE. Variability of iodine content in common commercially available edible seaweeds. *Thyroid.* 2004; 14(10):836-41.

Thakran S, Siddiqui MR, Baquer NZ. *Trigonella foenum graecum* seed powder protects against histopathological abnormalities in tissues of diabetic rats. *Mol Cell Biochem.* 2004; 266(1-2):151-59.

Thompson HJ, Heimendinger J, *et al.* Dietary botanical diversity affects the reduction of oxidative biomarkers in women due to high vegetable and fruit intake. *J Nutr.* 2006; 136(8):2207-12.

Tustanovskyj GB. Medicinal herbs effect on lactation. *Farmacevtychnyj J.* 1996: 5-6:106-9. English translation: V Nesterova, personal communication, Jan 2007.

Typi H. The effect of Galega officinalis on milk production. *Zentralblatt fuer Gynaekologie.* 1961;18(83). English translation: H Jacobson, personal communication, 2006.

Upton R (ed.) *Black cohosh rhizome standards of analysis, quality control, and therapeutics.* Santa Cruz: American Herbal Pharmacopoeia and Therapeutic Compendium; 2002.

USDA. USDA database for the flavonoid content of selected foods. Release 2 (2006). Beltsville MD:USDA; (updated 2006 Aug 31; cited 2006 Oct 14). Available from: www.ars.usda.gov/Services/docs.htm?docid=6231.

USDA. USDA database for the flavonoid content of selected foods – 2003. (Accessed 1-27-07). Available from: www.nal.usda.gov/fnic/foodcomp/Data Flav/flav.html.

USDA. USDA database for the choline content of common food 2004. (Accessed 1-27-07). Available from: www.nal.usda.gov/fnic/foodcomp/Data/Choline/Choline.html.

Vorbach C, Scriven A, Capecchi MR. The housekeeping gene xanthine oxidoreductase is necessary for milk fat droplet enveloping and secretion: gene sharing in the lactating mammary gland. *Genes Dev.* 2002; 16:3223-35.

Waller DP, Martin AM, Farnsworth NR, Awang DVC. Lack of androgenicity of siberian ginseng (letter). *JAMA.* 1992; 267:2329.

Weed, S. *Wise woman herbal for the childbearing year.* Woodstock, NY: Ash Tree; 1985.

Weiss R. *Weiss' herbal medicine* (classic ed). New York, NY: Thieme New York; 1985.

Weizman Z, Alkrinawi S, Goldfarb D, Bitran C. Efficacy of herbal tea preparation for infantile colic. *J Pediatr.* 1993; 122(4):650-52.

Westfall RE. Galactagogue herbs: a qualitative study and review. *Canadian Journal of Midwifery Research and Practice.* 2003; 2(2):22-27.

WHO. Traditional medicines: definitions. Geneva, Switzerland: World Health Organization. (Originated 2000; cited 2006 Oct 27). Available from: www.who.int/medicine/areas/traditional/definitions/en/index.html.

WHO. WHO monographs on selected medicinal plants. Vol 2. Geneva, Switzerland: World Health Organization. (Originated 2004). Available from: http://www.who.int/medicinedocs/library.fcgi?e=d-0edmweb--00-1-0--010---4----0--0-10l--1en-5000---50-about-0---01131-0011%2eb%29Wd2zx9ee80c740000000043f40c62-0utfZz-8-0-0&a=d&c=edmweb&cl=CL2.1.6&d=Js4927e.

Winterhoff H, Munster CG, Behr B. Reduced lactation in rats followed Vitex extract application - evidence for prolactin inhibiting activity. *Zeitschrift fur Phytotherapie.* 1991; 12:175-79.

Witters L. The blooming of the French lilac. *J Clin Invest.* 2001; 108(8):1105-7.

Wurglics M, Schubert-Zsilavecz M. Hypericum perforatum: a 'modern' herbal antidepressant: pharmacokinetics of active ingredients. *Clin Pharmacokinet.* 2006; 45(5): 449-68.

Yang SS, Chu P, Lin A, Lin SH. Aristolochic acid-induced Fanconi's syndrome and nephropathy presenting as hypokalemic paralysis. *Am J Kidney Dis.* 2002; 39(3):E14.

Zeisel SH, Mar MH, Zhou Z, da Costa KA. Pregnancy and lactation are associated with diminished concentrations of choline and its metabolites in rat liver. *J Nutr.* 1995; 125(12):3049-54.

Zeisel SH. Choline: critical role during fetal development and dietary requirements in adults. *Annu Rev Nutr.* 2006; 26:229-50.

INDEX

Symbol

ß-1,4 galactosyl transferase, 40
ß-glycosidic bond, 39
ß-lactalbumin, 40
α-hemolytic streptococci, 193
α-Lactalbumin, 81, 169
α-lactalbumin, 4, 69, 93, 95
α–Lactalbumin, 70
β-1,4 galactosyltransferase, 6

A

Absolute Infant Dose, 611, 614
Abstinence, 315
Acarbose, 568
Acetaminophen ± Codeine, 491
Acne, 346
Active transport as a mechanism for
drug transfer into milk, 470
Adhesins, 161, 169
Adipocyte-containing stroma, 388
Albendazole, 523
Albumin, 257
Alcohol, 407-410, 577
Alcohol on breastmilk composition, 578
Alcohol's effect on the
breastfed infant, 580
Alcohol's effect on the breastfeeding
process, 578
lactation performance, 578
milk ingestion by infant, 579
Alfalfa, 644
Alveolar epithelium, 466
Alveolar subunit of the breast, 465
Alveoli and Secretory
epithelial Cells, 37
cuboidal lactocyte, 37
Amenorrhea, 310, 343
Amisulpride, 547
Amitriptyline, 542
Amoxapine, 545
Amphetamine, dextroamphetamine, and
methamphetamine, 576
Amylase, 83
Anaerobes, 193
Analgesia, 359, 501
Anesthesia, 359, 501
Anesthetic techniques, 502
Angiotensin converting
enzyme inhibitors, 559
Angiotensin II receptor blockers, 559
Anise, 644
Anthelmintics, 523
Anthrax, 203
Antibiotics, 513
Antibodies, 167
Anticholinergics, 566
Anticoagulants, 561
Antigen Presenting Cells,
the APCs., 162
Antihypertensives, 557
Antimalarials, 526
Antimycobacterials, 531
Antiprotozoals, 523
Antipsychotics, 545
Anxiety spectrum disorders, 535
Apocrine glands, 5
Apoptosis, 20, 26
Arachnoid mater, 501
Aripiprazole, 547
Aspirin, 493
Assay validation, 622
Assessing the function of the
breast during lactation, 101
Atypical antipsychotics, 547
Autocrine Control, 99
Azotemia, 216

B

Baby-Friendly Hospital Initiative, 364
Bacteroides thetaiotamicron, 160
Barrier methods, 315
Bedsharing, 274
Beneficial effects of maternal drug
therapy in the breastfed
infant, 474
Benefits of the Cellular Components to
Infants, 44
Bile stimulated lipase, 83
Bilirubin Encephalopathy, 263
Bioenergetics, 319
Bipolar mood disorder, 535
Birth spacing, 305, 306
Black Seed, 645
Blessed Thistle, 640, 643
Body fat, 388
Body mass index, 387
Botanical Safety Handbook, 630
Bradycardia, 557
Breast abscess, 194
Breast changes, 394
Breast Engorgement, 362
Breastfeeding, autoimmune, and other
inflammatory diseases, 178
Breastfeeding, infant mortality, and
episodes of illness, 171
Breastfeeding and allergy, 176
Breastfeeding and diarrhea, 173
Breastfeeding and long term protection
against infections, 175
Breastfeeding and proposed protection
against other infections, 175
Breastfeeding and protection against
neonatal infections, 172
Breastfeeding and protection against
urinary tract infections, 174
Breastfeeding and respiratory
tract infections, 174
Breastfeeding and tumors, 179
Breastfeeding the late
preterm infant, 236
Breastfeeding the NICU graduate, 237
Breastmilk jaundice, 255
Breast size, 101
Brucellosis, 202
Bupivacaine/Lidocaine, 509
Buprenorphine, 495
Bupropion, 545
Butorphanol, 496
Butterbur, 635

C

Cabbage, 645
Calcium, 375, 382
Calcium channel blockers, 559
Calculation of infant dose and
its interpretation, 472
absolute infant dose, 472
relative infant dose, 472
risk-benefit analysis, 473
Calendula, 647
Calorie restriction, 372
Candida breast infections, 363
Candidosis, 205
Caraway, 644
Carbohydrate components, 169
Carnitine, 77
Casein micelles, 43
Caseins, 4, 78
Casecidin, 79
Celecoxib, 493
Cells in Breastmilk, 41
Cells of the mammary gland, 36
Cesarean delivery, 357
Cesarean section, 389, 392
Chasteberry, 645
Chemical receptor proteins, 403
Chemical Senses, 403
Chickenpox, 197
Chlorine, 382
Chloroquine, 527
Chlorpromazine, 546
Cholecalciferol, 429
Chromium, 382
Chyle, 27
Citalopram, 536
Clarithromycin, 531
Clinical and subclinical mastitis, 180
Clofazimine, 531
Clomipramine, 543
Clostridia,, 160
Clozapine, 547
Club drugs, 599
CMV, 195
Co-sleeping, 274
Coagulase negative staphylococci, 193
Cocaine Case studies, 583
Cocaine pharmacokinetics and
effect on breastfed infants, 582
Colic, 648
Colonization resistance, 160
Colostrum corpuscles, 9
Combined Spinal-Epidural (CSE), 506
Common analgesics, 491
Complementary foods, 415, 420
Computerized Breast
Measurement (CBM), 89
Contraceptive Use, 314
Cooper's dissections, 21
Copper, 382
Coriander, 644
Corticosteroids, 571
betamethasone, 571
budesonide, fluticasone and
mometasone, 571
hydrocortisone, 571
hydrocortisone, 571
methylprednisolone, 572
mometasone, 571
prednisolone, 572
prednisone, 572
triamcinolone, 571
Cracked nipples, 194
Crotamiton, 526
Cumin, 644
Cyanosis, 557
Cystic atrophy, 26
Cytokeratins, 39
Cytokines, growth factors, and other
signals from mother to
infant, 170
Cytomegalovirus, 198
Cytomegalovirus, 231
Cytomegalovirus (CMV), 182

D

DC-SIGN, 72
Defensins and cathelicidin, 170
Define and Achieve
Growth Standards, 220
Delayed Lactogenesis II and Lactation
Failure, 106
Delay in Commencement of Breast
Emptying, 106
Depression, 535
Desipramine, 543
Development during pregnancy –
mammogenesis and
lactogenesis I, 89
Development of the breast, 19
blood supply, 26
ethnicity, 23
ethnic morphology, 23
fetal development, 20
gross anatomy of the lactating
breast, 24
gross anatomy of the mature
non-lactating breast, 21
innervation, 27
lymphatic drainage, 27
axillary nodes, 27
neonatal and pre-pubertal
development, 21
post-lactation involution, 26
postmenopausal involution, 26
pregnancy, 23
human placental lactogen, 23
lactogenesis II, 23
mammogenesis, 23
puberty, 21
Development of the
Immune System, 219
Dietary Reference Intakes, 373, 435
Dietary volatiles, 406
Digestive development, 218
Dill, 644
Diphenhydramine, 565
Diphtheroids, 193
Diuretics, 559
Domperidone, 482, 484
Dong quai, 633
Donor human milk for preterm
infants, 232
donor Milk Banking, 232
donor Milk Recipients, 232
Donor human milk for preterm infants:
benefits, 234
Donor human milk for preterm infants:
concerns, 234
infection concerns, 235
nutritional concerns, 234

Dothiepin, 543
Doula, 356
Doxepin, 543
Doxycycline, 526
Doxylamine, 565
Drug transfer into milk, 611
Ductal epithelial cells, 36
Duloxetine, 541

E

E. coli, 160, 161
Early induced preterm delivery, 389
Early parenteral nutrition, 223
Early pregnancy loss, 321
Echinacea, 646
Ecstasy (MDMA), 599
Ectodermal ridges, 20
Effects of breastfeeding on inflammatory diseases and tumors in the infant, 176
Effects of Gut Lumenal Starvation, 224
Endocrine drugs, 567
Endometriosis, 328
Energy content of human milk, 85
Energy intake and infant growth, 85
Energy requirements, 371
Engorgement, 194, 362, 645
Enhancing and long-term effects on the infant's immune system by breastfeeding, 175
Enterobacter, 161
Enteromammary system, 220, 226
Enterovirus, 198
Environmental issues, 220
Eosinophilic granulocytes, 166
Epidural, 505
Epidural Anesthesia, 356
Epithelial-Derived Populations, 42
Epstein-Barr Virus, 197
Ergocalciferol, 429
Erythropoietin, 220
Escitalopram, 536
Estimated intrauterine nutrient accretion rate, 221
Estrogen, 479
Estrogenic methods, 315
Exercise, 372
Exercise induced menstrual irregularities, 319
Exocrine glands, 168, 180
Exocytosis, 40, 70
Experimental animal studies, 577
Expressed milk, 195
Extrauterine life, 393

F

Factors affecting gastric emptying, 218
Factors associated with lactation problems and failure, 103
Family planning, 305, 306
Fat, 378
Fat Content of Human Milk, 50
Feedback Inhibitor of Lactation, 99
Fennel, 644
Fentanyl, 494
Fenugreek, 639
Ferguson Reflex, 148
Fertility, 305, 319
Fertility suppression, 308
First immunization, 226
Flash heating, 201
Flavor memories, 406
Flavor perception, 403
Flavor profiles, 403
Flavor Programming, 404
Fluoxetine, 538
Fluvoxamine, 539
Folate, 381
Follicle-stimulating hormone, 308, 319
Fungal infections, 205

G

Galactagogues, 483
Galactography, 22
Gamma hydroxybutyrate (GHB), 599
Garlic, 633, 646
Gastrointestinal development, 226
Gastrointestinal tract, 217
Gestational cocaine use and its effects on the infant postnatally, 581
Gestational diabetes mellitus, 389
Gestational diabetes mellitus (GDM), 389
Glucocorticoid Receptor, 97
Glucocorticoids, 96
Goat's Rue, 640
Golgi-apparatus, 6
Gonadotropin-releasing hormone, 305
Gonadotropin releasing hormone, 319
Gonadotropin suppression, 331
Gram negative rods, 193
Gross Anatomy of the
 lactating Breast, 19
 clinical Implications, 28
 breast surgery, 28
 periareolar incisions, 28
 milk removal, 29
 pathology galactoceles, 29
 histology of the breast
  adipose cells, 31
 basal lamina, 31
 morphogenesis, 31
 lactocyte alveolus, 30
 milk ducts, 31
 myoepithelial cells OTR, 31
 paraventricular nuclei, 30
 supraoptic nuclei, 30
Group B ß-hemolytic streptococcus, 202
Growth charts, 419
Growth factors, 83
Growth patterns, 418

H

Haloperidol, 547
Hansen's disease, 196
Hepatitis A, 199
Hepatitis B, 199
Hepatitis C, 200
Hepatitis E, 200
Hepatitis G, 200
Herbal Galactagogues, 486
Herbal medicine, 629, 631
Herbal tea, 633
Heroin, 584
Heroin and the breastfed infant, 584
Herpes simplex virus, 198
Hirsutism, 343
Histology and Cytology of the Mammary Gland, 39

Histology and cytology of mammary gland and breastmilk, 35
HIV, 195, 200, 216, 231
HIV-1, 181
HIV-2, 182
Hoechst dye, 38
Host defense, 225
HTLV-1, 195, 200
HTLV 1, 231
Human Growth Hormone, 97
Human Milk Composition - Fat, 49, 51
triacylglycerols, 51
NEFA, 52
VLCPUFA, 51
fat content of human milk, 50
milk fat globule (MFG), 50
milk fat globule membrane (MFGM), 50
variation in total fat content of human milk, 50
Human milk for preterm infants, 229
fortification concerns, 230
hindmilk "Fortification", 229
multinutrient fortification, 229
new directions in fortification, 231
volume, 229
Human T cell leukemia virus (HTLV), 182
Hydrocodone, 496
Hyperammonemia, 216
Hyperandrogenism, 343
Hyperbilirubinemia, 255
Hyperinsulinemia, 343
Hyperprolactinemia, 322
Hypotension, 557
Hypothalamic amenorrhea, 322
Hypovitaminosis D, 443

— *I* —

Imipramine, 544
Immunoglobulins, 81
Impaired tubal motility and obstruction, 327
Indomethacin, 493
Indomethacin therapy, 224
Infant's own host defense compared to that of the adult, 161
Infant Dose; controlling factors and interpretation, 471
absolute infant dose, 472
calculation of infant dose and its interpretation, 472
drug disposition in mother and infant, 471
Inflammation, 649
Inflammatory response, 6
NF-κB, 6
RANKL, 6
Tumour Necrosis Factor, 6
xanthine oxidoreductase, 6
inhibition of the milk ejection reflex, 149
Inhibit milk production, 480
Initiation of breastfeeding, 395
Initiation of milk synthesis, 101
Insulin, 99, 567
Insulin resistance, 343
Intrathecal, 502
In utero growth curves, 221
Involution, 93
Involuting Mammary Gland, 41
Iodine, 382
Iron, 375, 381
Iron deficiency, 415, 420
Isoniazid, 531
IUD, 315
Ivermectin, 524

— *J* —

Jaundice, 255

— *K* —

Kernicterus, 261
Ketamine, 503
Ketamine, 599
Ketorolac, 494
Klebsiella, 160, 161

— *L* —

Labor Support, 356
Lactadherin, 170
Lactational amenorrhea, 421
Lactational amenorrhea method, 307
Lactational infertility, 307
Lactation consultants, 365
Lactation cycle, 35, 89
apoptosis, 35, 36
Lactiferous sinus, 25, 29
Lactobacillus rhamnosus, 161
Lactoferrin, 80, 93, 169
Lactogenesis I, 90, 101, 466
Lactogenesis II, 91, 92, 94, 97, 98, 102, 103, 105, 395
Lactogenesis III, 395
Lactose structure, 70
UDP-galactose, 69
La Leche League, 365
LAM, 314
LCPUFA, 77
Leptin, 320
Leucocytes in human milk, 170
Leukocyte population, 42
Levofloxacin, 531
Lithium, 547
Lobule development, 36
Local anesthetic, 502
Long term benefits of human milk for preterm infants
immunomodulation, 227
neurodevelopmental outcome, 226
other potential benefits, 227
Low gestational weight gain, 391
LSD, 586, 599
Lysozyme, 5, 79

— *M* —

M. avium subsp paratuberculosis, 196
Macrosomic infants, 392
Magnesium, 382, 509
Malathion, 526
Male factor infertility, 329
Mammalia, 3
Mammalian Flavor Learning, 404
Mammary Gland: Past, Present and Future, 3
Mammary Gland Growth and Development, 35
Mammary parenchyma, 9, 20
Mammary stemcells, 38
Mammary stem cellsfrom breastmilk, 44
Mammogenesis, 89

Managing breastfeeding in the
NICU, 238
Maprotiline, 544
Marijuana, 587
effect on lactation and the
breastfeeding infant, 589
Marijuana and brain development, 590
effects of marijuana on the
fetus and infant, 589
motor development, 589
Marshmallow, 643
Mastitis, 180, 194, 646
Maternal adioposity, 390
Maternal anemia, 362
Maternal diabetes, 104
Maternal obesity, 104, 387
M cells, 168
Measles, 196
Measuring M/P ratio, 620
Mebendazole, 523
Medications and Mother's Milk, 630
Meet the unique nutritional needs of
prematurity, 221
Mefloquine, 527
Meglitinides, 569
Melioidosis, 202
Meningitis, 160
Menses, 308
Meperidine, 503
Mescaline, 598
Metabolic acidosis, 216
Metabolism of heroin, 584
Metformin, 346
Methadone, 494
Methamphetamine, 599
Metoclopramide, 482, 483
Metronidazole, 524
Mianserin, 544
Microbes present in human milk, 180
Microbial flora, 160
Micronutrients, 418
Midazolam, 508
Milk/Plasma (M/P) ratio, 471
Milk/Plasma drug concentration
ratio, 611
Milk and plasma concentration-time
curves, 611
Milk composition, 373, 378
Milk Ejection, 143
Milk Fat Globule Membrane
proteins, 82
oxidoreductase, 82
Milk production, 479
Milk Synthesis and Secretion, 92
Minimal Enteral Nutrition (MEN)
(AKA "trophic feeds" or "GI
priming"), 224
Minimizing infant exposure to
drugs in milk, 474
Minocycline, 531
Mirror neuron system, 8
Mirtazapine, 541
Mode of Delivery, 103
Monoamine oxidase inhibitors, 545
Morphine, 495, 504
Mother-infant interactions, 291
Mumps, 196
Myoepithelial Cells, 37
Myrrh, 646

N

N-desmethylsertraline, 539
Nalbuphine, 496
Naltrexone, 496
Naproxen, 493
Narcotic analgesia, 356
Natural family planning methods, 315
Necrotizing
enterocolitis, 160, 216, 224, 225
Neonatal hypoglycemia, 393
Neonatal septicemia, 160
Nettle, 644
Neuraxial Analgesia, 502, 504
Nicotine, 590
factors influencing nicotine
concentrations in
breastmilk, 591
neuronal nicotinic receptor up
regulation, 596
nicotine and cotinine in
breastfeeding infants, 591
nicotine patch and smokeless
tobacco, 592
passive smoke, nicotine, and
cotinine, 592
polydrug use, 597
postnatal obesity, hypertension,
and diabetes mellitus, 596
risk for pulmonary
emphysema, 596
Nicotine's effect on mammary glands,
breastmilk yield, 593
lack of motivation to
breastfeed, 594
Mammary gland abscesses, 593
role of prolactin, 593
Nicotine's effect on the breastfeeding
infant, 594
poor bodyweight, colic, & infant
development, 594
Nipple dissymmetry, 194
Nipple trauma, 647
Non-protein Nitrogen, 75
Nonsteroidal anti-inflammatory drugs
(NSAIDs), 493
Norfluoxetine, 538
Normogonadotropic ovulatory
dysfunction, 324
Nortriptyline, 544
Nosocomial, 220
Nosocomial pathogens, 226
NRI antidepressants, 541
Nucleotides and nucleosides, 76
Nursing Mother's Herbal, 631
Nutritional "Best Practices" for the
preterminfant, 223
Nutritional goals for preterm
infants, 220
Nutritional recommendations for lactat-
ing women, 371

O

Obesity, 343, 387, 419
Obsessive compulsive disorder, 535
Ofloxacin, 531
Olanzapine, 548
Oligo-amenorrhea, 322, 343
Oligosaccharides, 5
Oocytes, 320
Opiate, 502
Opiates/Opioids, 503
Opioid, 502

Opioids and Antagonists, 494
Optimize Long-Term Outcomes, 223
Oral antidiabetic agents, 568
Osmosis learning, 8
Osteoporosis, 425
Other Organs/Systems
Development, 219
Overview of the lactation cycle, 103
Ovulation, 311
Ovulation, 308
Ovulation Induction, 319, 333
Oxycodone, 496
Oxytocin, 98, 141
Oxytocin Nasal Spray, 148
Oxytocin Receptor, 145
Oxytocin Release, 146

P

p-Aminosalicylic Acid, 531
Pain Management, 355
Panic disorder, 535
Parasitic Infections, 204
Parathyroid hormone, 431
Parecoxib, 493
Parenchymal branching, 20
Parenchymal mass, 395
Parity, 103
Paroxetine, 539
Parturition, 399
Passage of drugs across the alveolar epithelium, 467
Passive diffusion as a pathway for drug transfer into milk, 467
bioavailability of drugs in mother and infant, 469
drug concentration and
protein binding in plasma, 468
lipid solubility of the drug and co-transport into milk, 468
milk pH and drug pKa, 468
molecular weight of the drug, 467
Pasteurization, 195
Patient-controlled analgesia, 502
Patient-Controlled Epidural Analgesia (PCEA), 508
PCOS, 348
Pectoral fascia, 28
Pediculicides, 526
Peritonitis, 225
Permethrin, 526
Peyer's patches, 168
Phagocytosis, 162
Pharmacodynamics, 613
Pharmacokinetics, 613
Phencyclidine (PCP), 597
effect on prolactin and oxytocin, 598
pharmacokinetics, 597
Phosphorus, 382
Phosphorylation, 69
Physiologic jaundice, 259
Pia mater, 502
Pili, 169
Piperaquine, 527
Pituitary luteinising hormone, 308, 319
Placenta, 166
Placental Lactogen, 98
Polycystic ovary syndrome, 333, 343
Polydrug abuse of cocaine and alcohol, 582
Polydrug use, 585
Postpartum amenorrhea, 319
Postpartum contraception, 310
Postpartum depression, 648
Postpartum hemorrhage, 389
Post traumatic stress disorder, 535
Potassium, 382
Praziquantal, 524
Preeclampsia, 389
Premature ovarian failure, 322
Premature rupture of membranes, 389
Preterm developmental physiology, 217
Pretoria pasteurization, 201
Prevent Feeding-Related Morbidities, 223
Primary hypothyroidism, 326
Problem nutrients, 421
Progesterone, 98, 479
Progestin-only methods, 315
Proguanil, 529
Prolactin, 94, 480
Prolactin Receptor, 95
Promethazine, 565
Propionibacteria, 193
Propofol, 503
Protein, 78, 373, 378
Protriptyline, 545
Psilocybin, 599
Puerperium, 355
Pulsatile gonadotropin releasing hormone, 335
Pyrantel, 524
Pyrethrins, 526
Pyrimethamine, 529
Pyrizinimide, 531

Q

Q-fever, 204
Quetiapine, 548
Quinine, 529

R

Reboxetine, 541
Recommended nutrient intakes, 416
Regional anesthesia, 502
Relative Infant Dose, 611, 614
Remifentanil, 504
Reproduction, 305, 319
Reproductive health, 305
Retronasal olfaction, 403
Rifampicin, 531
Risperidone, 548
Rofecoxib, 493
Rohypnol, 599
Roman chamomile, 633
RT-PCR, 39
Rubella, 197

S

S. aureus, 161
Salmonellosis, 203
Scabicides, 526
Scabies, 205
Scheduled breastfeeding, 12
Schizophrenia, 535
Sebaceous glands, 5
Secondary amenorrhea, 322
Sedatives/Hypnotics, 503
Selenium, 382
Sensory-specific satiety, 410

Sepsis, 216
Sertraline, 539
Sexually transmitted diseases, 327
Shatavari, 644
Short term benefits of human milk for preterm infants, 225
Shoulder dystocia, 392
SIDS, 273
Single-dose experimental designs, 614
Skin-to-skin, 308, 355
SNRI's, 536
Social phobia, 535
Sodium, 382
Sore nipples, 363
Sources of vitamin D, 429
Special nutrition, 226
Spina/Intrathecal, 505
SSRI's, 536
Staphylococcus aureus, 161, 193, 194, 202, 364
Starvation jaundice, 255
STAT3, 93
STAT5, 93
Steady-state experimental designs, 613
Stimulate milk production, 482
St John's Wort, 542
Stress in Labor and Delivery, 105
Strongyloidiasis, 204
Sulfadoxine, 529
Sulfonylureas, 568
Sulpiride, 485
Synthesis and Exocytosis of Major Breastmilk Components, 39
Synthesis and Secretion of Human Milk Proteins, 85
Syphilis, 204

— *T* —

Taste receptors, 404
Terminal Ductal Lobular Units (TDLU), 21
T helper cells, 164
Theory of evolution, 273
Thiabendazole, 524
Thiazolidinediones, 346, 569
Thiopental, 503
Thoracoacromial artery, 26
Thrush, 646
Thyroid and anti-thyroid drugs, 569
  Carbimazole and methimazole, 569
  Levothyroxine and liothyronine, 569
  Propylthiouracil, 571
Tinidazole, 526
Toll-like receptors (TLRs), 162
Torbangun, 640, 645
Tramadol, 495
Transfer of alcohol into breastmilk, 577
Transfusion-Transmitted Virus, 200
Transitional/ mature milk, 466
Transnatal chemosensory continuity, 403
Trazodone, 542
Triacylglycerols, 51
Tricyclic antidepressants, 542
Tuberculosis, 195, 231
Tuboperitoneal Factors, 327
Tumor Necrosis Factor, 164
Two-stage pharmacokinetic analysis, 614

— *U* —

Urea, 77
Urinary tract infections, 389
Use of Human Milk, 225
Use of pasteurized donor human milk in the NICU, 236
  commercial Development of Donor Human Milk Products, 236
  logistics, 236

— *V* —

Varicella-Zoster virus, 197
Vas menstrualis, 9
Vegans, 375
Virgin Mammary Gland, 39
Vitamin B12, 380
Vitamin B12 deficiency, 421
Vitamin B6, 381
Vitamin C, 380
Vitamin D-fortified foods, 441
Vitamin D deficiency, 421, 437, 440
Vitamin D requirements, 434
Vitamin D supplementation, 449
Vitamin E, 380
Vitamin K, 380
Vitamin losses, 381
Vitamins, 376, 379

— *W* —

Water-soluble vitamins, 380
Weight loss during breastfeeding, 372
West Nile Virus, 201
Wound infection, 389

— *Z* —

Zinc, 382
Ziprasidone, 548
Zoster, 197

www.ingramcontent.com/pod-product-compliance
Lightning Source LLC
Chambersburg PA
CBHW081717040526
44405CB00026B/485
* 9 7 8 0 8 2 6 1 6 0 0 9 6 *